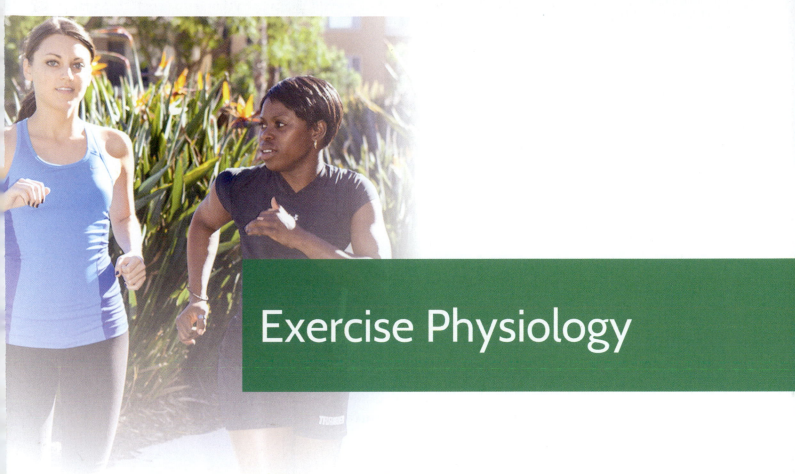

# Exercise Physiology

### John P. Porcari, PhD, RCEP, MAACVPR, FACSM
Program Director
Clinical Exercise Physiology
University of Wisconsin La Crosse
Executive Director
La Crosse Exercise and Health Program
La Crosse, Wisconsin

### Cedric X. Bryant, PhD, FACSM
Chief Science Officer
American Council on Exercise
San Diego, California

### Fabio Comana, MA, MS
Faculty Instructor
San Diego State University, School of Exercise & Nutritional Sciences
National Academy of Sports Medicine
San Diego, California

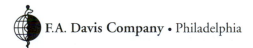 F.A. Davis Company • Philadelphia

F. A. Davis Company
1915 Arch Street
Philadelphia, PA 19103
www.fadavis.com

Printed in the United States of America

Last digit indicates print number: 10 9 8 7 6 5 4 3 2 1

*Publisher:* Quincy McDonald
*Director of Content Development:* George W. Lang
*Developmental Editor:* Nancy J. Peterson
*Art and Design Manager:* Carolyn O'Brien

As new scientific information becomes available through basic and clinical research, recommended treatments and drug therapies undergo changes. The author(s) and publisher have done everything possible to make this book accurate, up to date, and in accord with accepted standards at the time of publication. The author(s), editors, and publisher are not responsible for errors or omissions or for consequences from application of the book, and make no warranty, expressed or implied, in regard to the contents of the book. Any practice described in this book should be applied by the reader in accordance with professional standards of care used in regard to the unique circumstances that may apply in each situation. The reader is advised always to check product information (package inserts) for changes and new information regarding dose and contraindications before administering any drug. Caution is especially urged when using new or infrequently ordered drugs.

**Library of Congress Cataloging-in-Publication Data**

Porcari, John P., 1955- , author.
  Exercise physiology / John P. Porcari, Cedric X. Bryant, Fabio Comana.
    p. ; cm.
  Includes bibliographical references and index.
  ISBN 978-0-8036-2555-6 (alk. paper)
  I. Bryant, Cedric X., 1960- , author. II. Comana, Fabio, author. III. Title.
  [DNLM: 1. Exercise—physiology. 2. Physical Fitness—physiology. QT 256]

  QP301
  612'.044—dc23

                    2014038201

I dedicate this book to my parents, Virginia and Michael (deceased) Porcari. There is a book by Robert Fulghum entitled *All I Really Need to Know I Learned in Kindergarten: Uncommon Thoughts on Common Things.* I would say that everything I needed to learn about life I learned at 110 Wheeler Avenue in Orange, Massachusetts...my home. My parents raised four children and treated us all with selflessness and unequivocal love. For that, my brother, my two sisters, and I will be forever grateful. –J.P.

To my late parents, Joe and Buelah, who are without question the two people most responsible for any success I have experienced personally or professionally. I thank them for instilling in me a love of learning and a commitment to "doing the right things the right way." I share any and all accomplishments with them. –C.X.B.

To my parents...the beacons in my life. Words will never convey my gratitude for all you have given to me. Thank you for your relentless and unwavering support. –F.C.

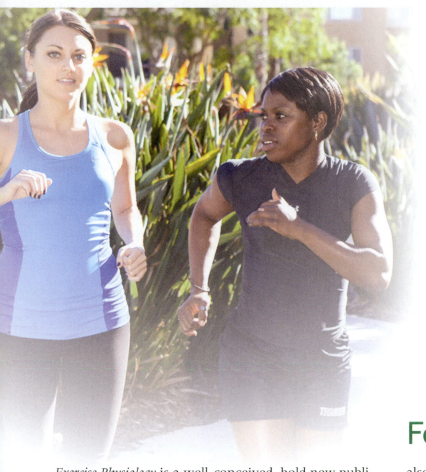

# Foreword

*Exercise Physiology* is a well-conceived, bold new publication that wonderfully bridges the gap between the theory and practice of all areas in exercise physiology. This book is sensibly targeted to students who are seeking careers in exercise physiology, exercise science, physical education, physical therapy, occupational therapy, sports nutrition, athletic performance, and sports medicine. *Exercise Physiology* also clearly provides a relevant, evidence-based source for professionals in the fitness industry, including group fitness instructors, personal trainers, strength and conditioning specialists, athletic coaches, and health coaches. This resource is optimally targeted for students who have completed basic college course work in general biology, chemistry, and anatomy and physiology.

One of the overriding achievements that the editors of and contributors to this textbook successfully accomplish is providing educational material that is applicable, meaningful, and understandable. Each chapter proceeds in a logical and readable format, beginning with specific learning outcomes that are followed by a real-world vignette, which immediately captures and engages the interest of the reader. The original vignettes are descriptive narratives that reveal meaningful issues based on the chapter topic. They introduce a tone for the chapter with resonating questions that are resolved at the end of the chapter. The authors thoughtfully showcase a breadth and depth of individuals by age, sex, and ethnicity with the vignettes. They also transcend different careers, so the diverse readership of the text will actually be able to identify with the situations. The book content is richly supported with numerous graphics, tables, illustrations, photographs, and ancillary materials.

One of the highlights of *Exercise Physiology* is the use of enlightening practical examples of complex physiological and/or metabolic principles. In each chapter, various sport, clinical, health, and fitness examples are included that supplement and expand on the content. These examples are written to stimulate students to analyze and better understand scientific principles of exercise physiology.

Compelling features throughout the text include Research Highlights. The Highlights are succinctly written briefs that convey the core findings of eye-opening research, insight into thought-provoking research questions, answers to controversial concepts, and/or interview responses from preeminent researchers. These self-contained objective statements describe a larger investigation with informative and useful study findings.

The authors positively engage the readers with the use of In Your Own Words features within chapters, which are interactive questions to the reader. These experiential learning events help the student integrate the concepts of the chapter with a student-centered learning approach. Also, the Critical Thinking Questions at the end of chapters motivate the student to synthesize some all-inclusive learning outcomes, thus increasing the student's curiosity for, and engagement with, the chapter material.

Another special feature of *Exercise Physiology* is the Doing the Math section in certain chapters. The authors provide the reader with the tools to do the necessary physiological calculations and then provide real-world associations to functional concepts. By teaching the reader how to execute the calculations, a better understanding of the framework of the question is developed.

Perhaps the most significant difference between this 30-chapter textbook and others currently on the market is Part IV: Physiology of Training. This part includes the following seven chapters: Principles of Exercise Training, Stability and Mobility Training, Cardiorespiratory Training, Resistance Training, Flexibility Training, Skill-Related Training, and Mind–Body Exercise and Fitness. These subjects are so timely and relevant in providing the reader with the skills, knowledge, and "hands-on" tools to apply the theory in a real-world situation. The Physiology of Training chapters represent a unique blending of exercise physiology with exercise and practical application.

*Exercise Physiology* is going to have a dominant and long-lasting influence in the field of exercise physiology. This text is a welcome new addition to some vintage resources that have not addressed the needs of present-day students and professionals. The authors methodically incorporate contemporary principles of exercise physiology, scrupulously researched material, compelling figures and graphics, and mind-opening pedagogical strategies into an easy-to-understand textbook. All of this combined will truly capture the interest of the exercise physiology student and hopefully inspire her or him to read and learn with a passion to understand.

Len Kravitz, PhD
Coordinator of Exercise Science
Department of Health, Exercise
and Sports Sciences
University of New Mexico
Albuquerque, New Mexico

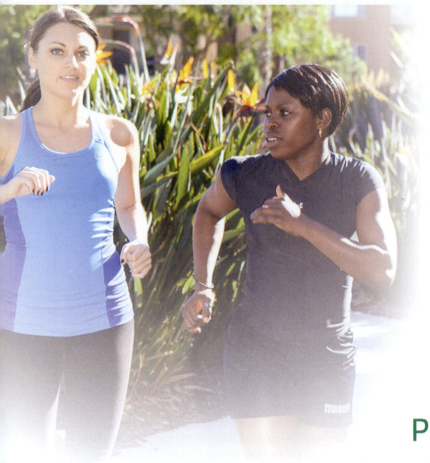

# Preface

Over the past several years, curricula in exercise science programs have been moving toward a more applied direction, integrating science with practice. Much of this movement has been triggered by growth in the job market in the fitness industry and students' desire to acquire the necessary knowledge, skills, and abilities to compete for those jobs. Current textbooks and training materials tend toward a theoretical and scientific approach, often leaving students confused about the relevancy of this education to their future careers. Therefore, the burden has fallen on educators to connect knowledge with application.

The partnership of F.A. Davis with the American Council on Exercise (ACE) has provided the opportunity to create a textbook package that is application based and geared toward today's students and future exercise science professionals. This text marries a robust group of features with technologically driven ancillaries to provide students and educators with a complete teaching and learning package endorsed by one of the most credible organizations in the health and fitness industry.

Founded in 1985, ACE is a nonprofit organization that is committed to America's health and well-being. Over the past 30 years, ACE has become an established resource for both fitness professionals and consumers, providing comprehensive, unbiased, scientific research impacting the fitness industry and proving to be a trusted authority on fitness.

Today, ACE educates, certifies, and represents more than 55,000 fitness professionals, health coaches, and other allied health professionals. ACE advocates for a new intersection of fitness and health care, bringing the highly qualified professionals that ACE represents into the healthcare continuum so they can contribute to the national solution to physical inactivity and obesity. ACE is the largest certifier in its space; all four of its primary certification programs are accredited by the National Commission for Certifying Agencies (NCCA), the gold standard in the U.S. for assessing professional competence. ACE also plays an important public-service role, conducting research and making available science-based information and resources on safe and effective physical activity and sustainable behavior change.

ACE's leadership on this endeavor has resulted in a relevant, timely, and comprehensive primary course textbook on exercise physiology. This text meets the needs of exercise science students who take an exercise physiology course as part of their coursework toward a degree in exercise science, athletic training, coaching, exercise physiology, fitness, health and human performance, physical education, nutrition, physical therapy, or sports medicine. It will also benefit individuals who already are members of the fitness industry, including personal trainers, medical or clinical exercise specialists, group fitness instructors, and health coaches, who are preparing for examinations or simply strengthening their knowledge base.

As an edited text, *Exercise Physiology* utilizes experts from diverse areas within the field to author chapters on their specialty topics. Combined with a rigorous review and development process, the text has benefited from the guidance and expertise of many of the brightest and most active minds in the field.

## GUIDING PRINCIPLES

Several philosophical principles guide the tone and content of this textbook:

- Application—The main distinguishing feature of this textbook is its applied approach: a hands-on, application-based manual that is practical and relevant. This approach is evident through in-text examples, special features, and the art program.
- Focus on Diverse Populations—This textbook focuses on exercise physiology principles that are applied to a wide variety of populations, not just athletes.
- Affective Domain—This textbook includes the emotional/affective aspect of exercise physiology practice, such as interpersonal communication and exercise as an experience, in translating the science into practical knowledge.
- Forward Looking—This textbook looks forward, focusing on current trends and research, without extensive historical coverage.

## ORGANIZATION

*Exercise Physiology* is organized for an intuitive, logical flow of content in the following manner:

- **Part I: Introduction to Exercise Physiology** gives students an appreciation of the field of exercise physiology as a discipline and an understanding of how it fits into the "real world." It clarifies the differences and interrelationships among physical activity, fitness, and health.
- **Part II: Fueling Physical Activity** explains the relationship between energy and physical activity and exercise, beginning with the macronutrients and micronutrients in the diet and their specific roles within the body, and continuing with the energy pathways that make it possible to perform physical work.
- **Part III: Physiological Systems** describes the many physiological systems that must work in a coordinated fashion to allow the body to maintain sustained physical exertion: the respiratory system, cardiovascular system, muscular and nervous system, endocrine system, and thermoregulatory system, including both acute and chronic (adaptive) responses of these systems to exercise.

- **Part IV: Physiology of Training** focuses on the practical application and incorporation of many of the principles presented in earlier chapters. General principles of exercise training are followed by chapters covering specific topics such as stability and mobility, cardiorespiratory training, resistance training, flexibility training, skill-related training, and mind–body exercise.
- **Part V: Nutritional Strategies** outlines the latest information relative to nutrition, hydration, and ergogenic aids for exercise and sports.
- **Part VI: Obesity and Weight Management** covers an area of major concern for many of the clients with whom health and fitness professionals work on a daily basis.
- **Part VII: Fitness Across the Life Span** addresses information relative to exercising during all decades of life—from the growth and maturation process in young exercisers to specific programming guidelines for older adults.
- **Part VIII: Special Considerations** explains common medical conditions and environmental challenges that are likely to be encountered by health and fitness professionals as they work with clients. This part also provides the latest guidelines for programming exercise for special populations. Exercise-related injuries are described, followed by guidelines for safely progressing individuals during the recovery process.

## UNIQUE FEATURES

Educators and students alike find special features to be useful in helping the learner comprehend and retain new information, as well as envision how it will apply to practice. *Exercise Physiology* offers several unique pedagogical features:

- **Vignettes** open each chapter and pose a thought-provoking question or concept to grab the reader's interest and showcase the relevance of content. Vignettes progress through the chapter and are resolved in a Vignette Conclusion at the end. Importantly, they are extremely diverse in terms of individuals (i.e., age, ethnicity, and sex), types of professionals/careers (i.e., athletic trainers, physical therapists, and exercise physiologists), and settings (i.e., gym, field, or laboratory), so students from all fields will see themselves in the "story."
- **In Your Own Words** entries provide students with opportunities to focus on and practice essential affective skills that will help to make them successful professionals. For example, students are presented with a situation and then asked to articulate, in their own words, how they would respond. This feature encourages professional behavior in students and future professionals.

- **Research Highlight** features emphasize evidence-based practice by presenting key research and how it applies to practice today.
- **From Theory to Practice** features showcase real-world examples of how an exercise physiology principle affects fitness and sports performance, and how it can be manipulated by health and fitness professionals to improve performance.
- **Doing the Math** examples give an applications perspective to math calculations, giving the students the context for how the numbers are used in practice and why they matter.
- **Sex Differences** features highlight significant differences in male and female responses to activity and other exercise physiology concepts.
- **Critical Thinking Questions** wrap up each chapter to give students problem-solving experience. Answer prompts are provided in the Instructor Resources.
- **Additional Resources** lists supplemental content available to readers to support understanding of chapter content.
- **Practice What You Know** features are the laboratory component of the text, presenting step-by-step experiential exercises to expand the student's knowledge base and practical experience.

## EDITORIAL AND ART GOALS

The editors of *Exercise Physiology* have worked with the contributors to ensure an open, accessible tone and consistent writing level that will engage students—it is not overly theoretical. Students and educators can also be assured of a sound evidence base supporting all content, evidenced by current references for all statistics, exercise guidelines, and other sensitive information. Rigorous development and review processes were followed to ensure the most timely, clearly organized and written, and fully accurate and relevant content.

A completely new, full-color art program including photographs and illustrations has been created to bring the words to life and clarify what can be complex topics for students.

## STUDENT AND EDUCATOR RESOURCES

Go beyond the book to Davis*Plus* for additional resources that support and reinforce content. Learners can see concepts from the book come to life via 18 animated videos that describe physiological processes within the context of body movement and exercise. Online quizzes for each chapter help learners assess their understanding of chapter concepts. To keep learners up to date on the latest news and career trends related to exercise physiology, podcasts featuring ACE experts will be posted quarterly. Finally, learners will be able to access links to nutrition calculators to aid their study and practice.

For educators, Davis*Plus* features a test bank with optional ExamView Pro software, which makes it easy to customize tests. PowerPoint presentations for each chapter support lectures, and an instructor's guide and an image bank help in planning and pacing courses. To access these valuable online student and instructor resources, go to Davis*Plus* at: http://davisplus.fadavis.com.

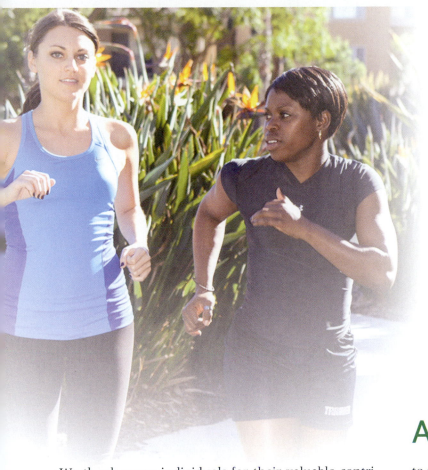

# Acknowledgments

We thank many individuals for their valuable contributions to this textbook. A book of this magnitude cannot be produced without the collective efforts of a talented group of professionals.

We are privileged to have had so many knowledgeable and dedicated chapter contributors. We are indebted to them for sharing their expertise and creativity in helping us realize our vision of developing a science-based, yet application-oriented textbook. We extend our sincere thanks to our development editor, Nancy J. Peterson, who played a critical role behind the scenes in helping keep us focused and on schedule in a very professional manner. Our supporters at F.A. Davis Company's Health Professions/Medicine division included Quincy McDonald, Publisher, George Lang, Director of Content Development, and Liz Schaeffer, Developmental Editor/Electronic Products Coordinator.

A very special thanks is extended to Daniel J. Green and Sabrena Merrill, MS, for their assistance with various aspects of the writing, reviewing, and editing tasks related to this massive project.

The illustrations and photographs in an exercise physiology textbook are critical for many reasons, the most important of which is to help students understand key—and sometimes complicated—concepts. It takes a keen understanding of the content and a creative mind to translate those concepts into ideas for artwork to be rendered by professional illustrators. Jeff Janot, PhD, ACSM-CES, and Lance Dalleck, PhD, ACSM-RCEP, deserve special mention and recognition for their invaluable assistance in helping to develop the art program for this textbook. In addition to contributing chapters to the textbook, they spent countless hours reviewing content and contributors' art ideas, generating their own ideas, creating graphs from research data, and pulling everything together into a cohesive art program. We are immensely grateful for their contribution.

Special thanks also go to the individuals who assisted with the photo shoot for this textbook. Our photographer, Jason Torres of J. Torres Photography, was patient and enthusiastic as he applied his artistic eye to the job. Jessica Yeager and Jessie Bradley helped with coordination and served as models. Pete McCall, MA, and Mark Kelly, PhD, served as subject-matter experts. Other models included Sarah Chambers, Zach Clayton, Michael Davis, Makeba Edwards, Robin Floyd, Chris Gagliardi, Nancy Garcia, Alex Link, Tyler Pagano, Belinda Thompson, and Stacy Wong.

Over the course of an individual's career, many people contribute to the development of one's theories, knowledge, and expertise. We have continued to learn from our former professors and past and current students and colleagues who have helped shape and challenge our thoughts and perspectives.

Finally, words cannot express our gratitude and appreciation to our friends and family for their support and understanding in affording us the necessary time to devote to this project.

John P. Porcari, PhD
Cedric X. Bryant, PhD
Fabio Comana, MS, MA

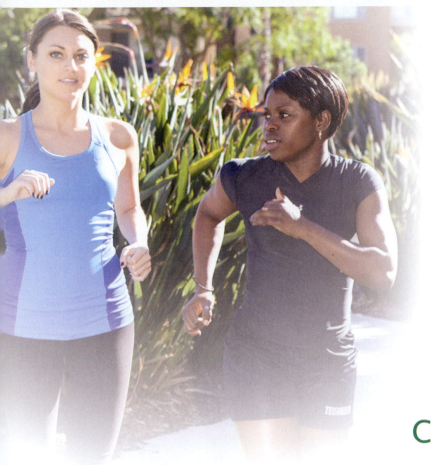

# Contributors

**Don Bahneman, MS**
Well Equipped, LLC
Boca Raton, Florida

**Lawrence Biscontini, MA**
Mindful Movement Specialist
Fajardo, Puerto Rico

**Anthony Carey, MA**
CEO, Function First
San Diego, California

**Scott W. Cheatham, DPT, PhD(c), ATC**
Assistant Professor
Director, Pre-physical Therapy Program
Division of Kinesiology and Recreation
California State University Dominguez Hills
Carson, California
President/CEO
National Institute of Restorative Exercise, Inc.

**Lance C. Dalleck, PhD, ACSM-RCEP**
Assistant Professor of Exercise and Sport Science
Recreation, Exercise & Sport Science Department
Western State Colorado University
Gunnison, Colorado

**J. Jay Dawes, PhD**
Assistant Professor
University of Colorado-Colorado Springs
Colorado Springs, Colorado

**Natalie Digate Muth, MD, MPH, RD**
Senior Advisor for Healthcare Solutions, American
    Council on Exercise
San Diego, California
Pediatrician and Obesity Medicine Specialist
Vista, California

**Scott Drum, PhD**
Assistant Professor
Exercise Physiology
Undergraduate Sport Science Coordinator
School of Health and Human Performance
Northern Michigan University
Marquette, Michigan

**Avery D. Faigenbaum, EdD**
Professor
Department of Health and Exercise Science
The College of New Jersey
Ewing, New Jersey

**Jeffrey M. Janot, PhD**
University of Wisconsin-Eau Claire
Associate Professor of Kinesiology
Eau Claire, Wisconsin

**Len Kravitz, PhD**
Coordinator of Exercise Science
Department of Health, Exercise and Sports Sciences
University of New Mexico
Albuquerque, New Mexico

**Pete McCall, MS**
Science Officer
Institute of Motion
San Diego, California

**Sabrena Merrill, MS**
Exercise Scientist/Curriculum Development Specialist
Seattle, Washington

**Christopher R. Mohr, PhD, RD**
Co-owner, Mohr Results, Inc.
Louisville, Kentucky

**Brad A. Roy, PhD**
Executive Director
The Summit Medical Fitness Center
Kalispell Regional Medical Center
Kalispell, Montana

**Cody Sipe, PhD**
Associate Professor, Director of Clinical Research
Physical Therapy
Harding University
Co-founder, Vice-President
Functional Aging Institute
Searcy, Arkansas

**Gary P. Van Guilder, PhD**
Assistant Professor of Exercise Science
Department of Health and Nutritional Sciences
South Dakota State University
Brookings, South Dakota

**Kara A. Witzke, PhD**
Program Lead, Exercise and Sport Science
Oregon State University, Cascades Campus
Bend, Oregon

**Glenn A. Wright, PhD**
Program Director
Graduate Program in Human Performance
University of Wisconsin-La Crosse
La Crosse, Wisconsin

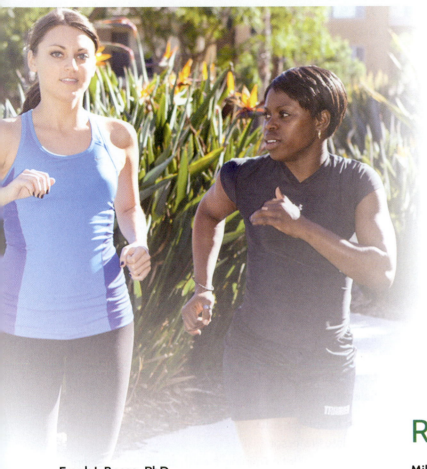

# Reviewers

**Frank J. Bosso, PhD**
Professor
Human Performance and Exercise Science
Youngstown State University
Youngstown, Ohio

**William Marvin Collman, BS, MA**
Assistant Professor of Physical Education and Biology
Health and Life Sciences
William Penn University
Oskaloosa, Iowa

**Douglas Crowell, MS**
Program Director–Applied Exercise Science
Department of Exercise and Sport Science
Azusa Pacific University
Azusa, California

**Charles R. Darracott, EdD**
Associate Professor
Kinesiology and Health Science
Augusta State University
Augusta, Georgia

**Mike Diede, PhD**
Program Director
Exercise Science
Brigham Young University
Provo, Utah

**Gina S. Evans, PhD**
Assistant Professor
School of Kinesiology
Marshall University
Huntington, West Virginia

**Elizabeth Frechette, MS**
Lecturer
Kinesiology
University of Massachusetts
Amherst, Massachusetts

**Matthew J. Garver, PhD**
Assistant Professor
Kinesiology and Nutrition
Abilene Christian University
Abilene, Texas

**Trevor L. Gillum, PhD**
Assistant Professor
Kinesiology
California Baptist University
Riverside, California

**Helen A. Hartman**
Sr. Lecturer of Kinesiology Science
Penn State Berks
Reading, Pennsylvania

**Tamara D. Hew, DPM, PhD**
Assistant Professor
Exercise Science
Oakland University
Rochester, Michigan

**David Hydock, PhD**
Assistant Professor
School of Sport and Exercise Science
University of Northern Colorado
Greeley, Colorado

**Dean E. Jacks, PhD**
Assistant Professor
Kinesiology and Integrative Physiology
Hanover College
Hanover, Indiana

**George William Lyerly, Jr., PhD**
Assistant Professor
Exercise and Sport Science
Coastal Carolina University
Conway, South Carolina

**Craig Mattern, PhD**
Associate Professor
Kinesiology, Sports Studies, and Physical Education
The College at Brockport, State University of New York
Brockport, New York

**Jacalyn McComb, PhD**
Professor in Exercise Physiology
Health, Exercise, and Sport Sciences
Texas Tech University
Lubbock, Texas

**Fred L. Miller III, PhD**
Assistant Professor, Kinesiology
Anderson University
Anderson, Indiana

**Ronald Otterstetter, PhD**
Assistant Professor
Sport Science and Wellness Education
The University of Akron
Akron, Ohio

**Jennie Phillips, PhD**
Instructor
Kinesiology
University of Maryland
College Park, Maryland

**Jeffrey P. Rudy, PhD**
Director of Athletic Training Education
Nutrition and Health Sciences
University of Nebraska
Lincoln, Nebraska

**Shannon Simmons**
Doctor of Health Science
Assistant Professor
Human Performance
Corban University
Salem, Oregon

**David K. Spierer, EdD**
Associate Professor
Division of Athletic Training, Health and Exercise Science
Long Island University, Brooklyn
Brooklyn, New York

**Robert Stow, PhD**
Director, Athletic Training Education Program/Assistant Professor
Kinesiology
University of Wisconsin–Eau Claire
Eau Claire, Wisconsin

**Toni Torres-McGehee, PhD**
Assistant Professor
Physical Education & Athletic Training
University of South Carolina
Columbia, South Carolina

**Wayland Tseh, PhD**
Associate Professor
School of Health and Applied Human Sciences
University of North Carolina Wilmington
Wilmington, North Carolina

**Molly Winke, PhD**
Assistant Professor
Kinesiology and Integrative Physiology
Hanover College
Hanover, Indiana

**Amanda J. Wooldridge, MS**
Adjunct Professor
Fitness and Health Management
University of the Sciences in Philadelphia
Plymouth Meeting, Pennsylvania

# Contents in Brief

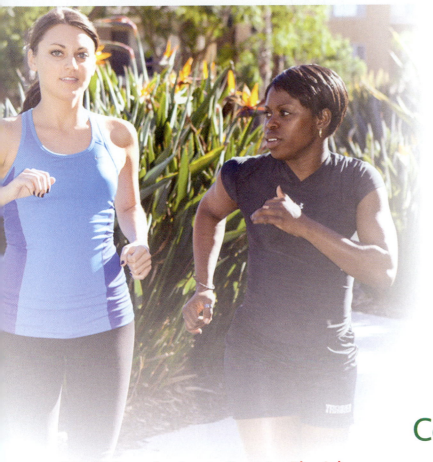

# Contents

## Chapter 9: Structure and Function of Muscle and the Nervous System   230

Glenn A. Wright, PhD

## Chapter 10: Acute and Chronic Neuromuscular Responses to Exercise   254

Glenn A. Wright, PhD

## Chapter 11: Endocrine System and Hormonal Responses to Exercise   276

Glenn Wright, PhD
Sabrena Merrill, MS

## Chapter 29: Altitude, Pollution, and Underwater Diving: Effects on Exercise Capacity   802

John Porcari, PhD

Scott Drum, PhD

## Chapter 30: Common Musculoskeletal Injuries   830

Dr. Scott Cheatham, PT, DPTATC

## Appendix A: American Council on Exercise Fitness Certifications   858

## Glossary   860

## Subject Index   882

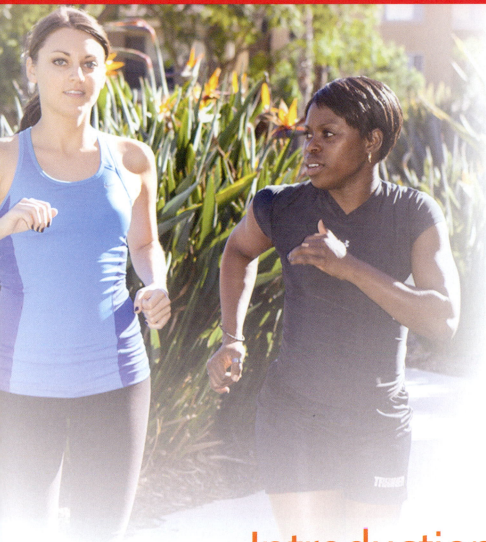

# PART I

# Introduction to Exercise Physiology

This part of this textbook is designed to give you an appreciation of the field of exercise physiology as a discipline. Chapter 1 provides a brief historical perspective of the field of exercise physiology so you will understand the relevance of the profession within the context of health professions. It is also intended to give you a foundational understanding of how the field of exercise physiology fits into the "real world" and how it can impact consumers. Chapter 2 defines the differences and interrelationships among physical activity, fitness, and health. The focus is on how physical activity and exercise impact the risk for development of chronic diseases, as well as quality of life and longevity.

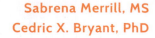

Sabrena Merrill, MS
Cedric X. Bryant, PhD

CHAPTER 1

# Welcome to the Field of Exercise Physiology

## CHAPTER OUTLINE

## LEARNING OUTCOMES

1. Define *exercise physiology*.
2. Identify the various areas of professional opportunity for exercise physiologists.
3. Briefly describe the history of exercise physiology, including the influence of ancient Greece, early pioneers who studied exercise-related topics, and advancements in science-related technology.
4. Define *physical education*.
5. Briefly describe the origins of physical education as a school curriculum.
6. Explain the general evolution of physical education programs in the United States.
7. Describe the modern fitness movement, including current and future emphases of research in exercise science.

## ANCILLARY LINK

Visit Davis*Plus* at http://davisplus.fadavis.com for study and practice resources, including online quizzes, animations that help explain physiological processes, podcasts concerning news and career trends in exercise physiology, and practice references.

## VIGNETTE

■ Upon graduating from high school, Charlotte decided that she wanted to go to college to study human physiology, as she had always had an interest in learning about science and biology. Initially, Charlotte was undecided on a major for her studies, so she enrolled in a collection of entry-level biology, anatomy, and physiology courses during her freshman year. The more Charlotte learned about the human body's incredible potential for adaptation as a response to physical exertion, the more she realized she was interested in studying exercise physiology. Now all she had to decide was how she could apply her education to a profession that she would enjoy and that included helping people improve health through exercise.

What are Charlotte's professional options in exercise physiology?

Exercise physiology has its roots in the fundamental disciplines of anatomy and physiology, which explore the structure and function of the human body. Studying the specific challenges to the body's interrelated systems as experienced through the stress of an acute bout of exercise and as a result of chronic physical training are the core tenets of exercise physiology.

This chapter presents a brief historical review of the field of exercise physiology, as well as the importance of exercise physiology in the development of the academic disciplines of exercise science, physical education, sports, and other health professions. The principles of exercise physiology, as they apply to the general population and to society as a whole, are also covered.

## WHAT IS EXERCISE PHYSIOLOGY?

Exercise presents a form of stress to the bodily systems that brings about distinct changes in physiology. Essentially, any type of physical activity disrupts the body's internal **homeostasis**, or internal state of physiological balance. Consequently, the cellular changes that occur as a response to exercise are designed to limit internal stress so that homeostasis can return or be maintained. If exercise is performed consistently over a period (e.g., weeks or months), chronic physiological adaptations occur to prepare the exerciser for the ongoing demands of the activity. **Exercise physiology** is the field of study devoted to examining the body's response to any type of physical activity. Exercise physiologists study how physical activity influences the body's cardiovascular, endocrine, and musculoskeletal systems.

Fundamentally, there are two key areas of specialization in exercise physiology: fitness and rehabilitation. Exercise physiology professionals who work in fitness may help athletes to improve performance or train private clients to enhance overall conditioning and lose weight (Fig. 1-1). Rehabilitation services in the field of exercise physiology are performed by professionals who specialize in helping people who are recovering from injuries or living with chronic medical conditions (Fig. 1-2). In these cases, the use of exercise is part of a comprehensive treatment plan to improve overall health and address specific problems associated with the condition.

Although these two areas of specialization exist, it is not uncommon for professionals working in exercise physiology to be involved with both fitness and rehabilitation as the proportion of the aging population increases, and the need for health improvement and increased performance obtained through exercise are sometimes goals established by one individual.

For more information on careers in exercise physiology, visit the links to the professional organizations listed in Table 1-1.

### FROM THEORY TO PRACTICE

The following positions are a sampling of career options available for individuals working in the field of exercise physiology:

**Careers in Exercise Physiology**

**Sports Programs**
- Director of state and national teams
- Sports management director
- Strength and conditioning coach
- Athletic trainer

College and University Programs
- Professor
- Researcher
- Administrator
- Wellness coordinator

Community/Private Practice
- Manager of health and wellness programs
- Manager of fitness and athletic programs
- Director of corporate fitness/wellness programs
- Health and fitness club instructor
- Health/fitness director in correctional services
- Sport psychologist
- Biomechanist
- Health-risk manager
- Physical education teacher

- Personal health/fitness coach
- Personal fitness trainer
- Group fitness instructor

Clinical Practice
- Medical physician
- Dietitian/sports nutritionist
- Cardiopulmonary rehabilitation specialist
- Physical therapist
- Occupational therapist
- Evaluation and supervision of special populations, including individuals with the following conditions:
  - Diabetes
  - Obesity
  - Rheumatoid arthritis
  - Dyslipidemia
  - Hypertension
  - Low functional capacity
  - Pregnancy

Government and Military Services
- Fitness director/manager in military, including the air force and army
- Other positions within military services

## VIGNETTE continued

■ Charlotte graduated college with a Bachelor of Science degree in Exercise Science. Her education provided her with basic knowledge of human physiology and how the body responds to the challenges of exercise. Now she wants to apply this knowledge in the real world to help people become healthier. One area that sparked Charlotte's interests was corporate wellness. During her undergraduate program, she interned as a fitness instructor at a large insurance corporation. During her internship, Charlotte helped employees with their fitness assessments and exercise programs. She also gave several brown bag lunch seminars on the benefits of eating healthy and being physically active.

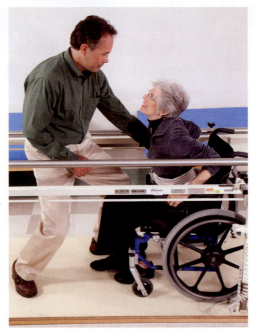

**Figure 1-2.** Some exercise physiology professionals pursue careers in rehabilitation services to help people recover from injuries or live more fully with their chronic medical conditions. *(From Johansson C, Chinworth SA. Mobility in Context: Principles of Patient Care Skills. Philadelphia: F.A. Davis; 2012:399, with permission.)*

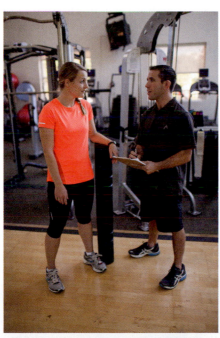

**Figure 1-1.** Some exercise physiology professionals work in fitness to help athletes improve performance or they train private clients to enhance overall conditioning.

### Table 1-1. Professional Organizations in the Field of Exercise Physiology

| ORGANIZATION | WEBSITE |
| --- | --- |
| American Association of Cardiovascular and Pulmonary Rehabilitation | http://aacvpr.org |
| American Alliance for Health, Physical Education, Recreation, and Dance | http://aahperd.org |
| American College of Sports Medicine | http://acsm.org |
| American Council on Exercise | http://acefitness.org |
| American Kinesiology Association | http://american-kinesiology.org |
| American Society of Exercise Physiologists | http://asep.org |
| National Strength and Conditioning Association | http://nsca-lift.org |

## BRIEF HISTORY OF EXERCISE PHYSIOLOGY

Bodily responses to exercise in various environmental conditions (e.g., heat, cold, and altitude) and the effects of exercise, or physical activity, on health, disease, and wellness have been studied extensively by exercise physiologists since the early 19th century. Although rigorous scientific research in exercise physiology began in the late 1800s, the benefits of regular exercise were extolled by leaders in medicine long before then. The famous Greek physician Hippocrates (ca. 460–370 BC)—who is often called the Father of Preventive Medicine—has been quoted as saying, "If we give every individual

## RESEARCH HIGHLIGHT

### Research as a Career Option

The field of exercise physiology has been, and continues to be, advanced by scientists who conduct both basic and applied research studies. Basic researchers typically conduct studies with a focus on cellular and molecular processes, such as how organ systems respond to various factors (e.g., the stress of different types of exercise). Applied researchers usually conduct studies with a focus on more practical issues that can be applied in current practice, such as ways to increase athletic performance or improve health and reduce disease.

Both types of research require the scientist to obtain a terminal degree, such as a PhD, which involves at least 4 to 5 years beyond the undergraduate level. Most researchers are employed in universities and clinical settings.

the right amount of nourishment and exercise, not too little and not too much, we would have found the safest way to health" (Fig. 1-3).

Five hundred years after Hippocrates, another influential and well-known physician, Claudius Galenus, or Galen, practiced the ideals of the Hippocratic school of medicine that touted logical science based on experimentation and observation. Galen wrote extensively about various aspects of health including personal hygiene, human anatomy and physiology, nutrition, growth and development, benefits of exercise, consequences of being inactive, and treatment of disease. On exercise, Galen wrote, "The criterion of vigorousness is changes of respiration; those movements which do not alter respiration are not called exercise."[1] Thus, even more than two millennia ago, those who studied the human body understood the benefits of being active, as well as the health risks associated with being sedentary.

The development of exercise physiology as a science includes important contributions from European and American researchers that have led the way for future studies on how the body responds to the challenges of exercise. Although an in-depth discussion of the complete history of exercise physiology and physical education is beyond the scope of this chapter, the following sections present a selection of important leaders and events that shaped how exercise is studied today.

## Ancient Greece

The first gymnasium was built in ancient Greece and it coincided with the first Olympic Games, which is traced back to 776 BC. The Greeks were the first to invent public athletic contests, with the games staged on the plains of Olympia (Fig. 1-4). These competitions were significant to the overall culture of ancient Greece as they were dedicated to the Olympian gods. Thus, the gymnasium environment supplied the means of training

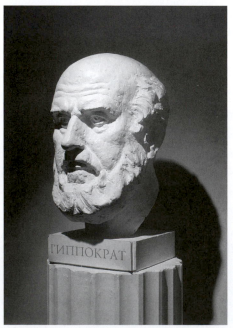

**Figure 1-3.** The famous Greek physician Hippocrates (ca. 460–370 BC) is often called the Father of Preventive Medicine.

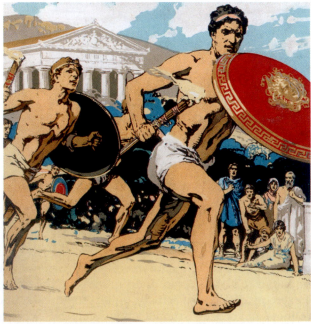

**Figure 1-4.** Artist depiction of the relay race in ancient Olympic games. *(© Getty Images)*

and competition that formed an important part of the social and spiritual life of the ancient Greeks. The public interest in the training of Greek athletes was so great that special buildings were provided by the state as gymnasiums for such use. When an athlete won a competition in one of the grand Olympic festivals, the victory was considered an honor for the entire state. The ancient Olympic Games continued for almost 12 centuries until they were banned by Emperor Theodosius in 393 AD.

## In Your Own Words

Have you decided which career path to take in exercise physiology? If not, answering the following questions might help make the decision clearer for you:

- Do you participate in exercise as it relates to health, fitness, or athletics?
- Are you interested in any of the specialty areas or fields of study previously mentioned in the Careers in Exercise Physiology section, such as medicine, teaching, research, or leading exercise classes?
- Have you enjoyed classes in high school or college such as physical fitness, health and wellness, or nutrition?
- Do you enjoy helping and working with people?
- Do you get excited about the possibility of working in sports medicine or exercise science environments?

Over time, the ancient Greek gymnasium developed into a place for more than just the training of athletes. The Greeks acknowledged a robust association among athletics, education, and health, which led to the gymnasium becoming a place for the education of children (both physical and intellectual) and medicine. Several hundred years after the introduction of the first Greek gymnasium, Hippocrates improved on the gymnastic exercises used at the time. Following Hippocrates, Galen wrote prolifically about the importance of proper and frequent use of gymnastics in the promotion of health and well-being. The observations and writings of these two important physicians set the stage for the interest in and eventually the study of modern exercise physiology.

### Foundations of Modern Medical Science

Galen's influence was so significant that his ideas on the structure and function of the body remained unchallenged for almost 14 centuries. In 1543, the foundations of what would become modern anatomy and physiology were introduced by Belgian physician Andreas Vesalius (1514–1564) with the publication of *De Humani Corporis Fabrica* (*On the Fabric of the Human Body*). Figure 1-5 illustrates a sample drawing from this text. *De Humani Corporis Fabrica* contained the most detailed human anatomical drawings that had

ever been created, along with theories that conflicted with Galen's concepts. Vesalius's literary works paved the way for the subsequent advancement of modern science.

In the mid-1600s, the invention of the microscope opened the gate for researchers to begin observing anatomical structures on a cellular level, which furthered the understanding of human physiology. During the 1700s to the late 1800s, important discoveries made by numerous European scientists in the areas of respiration, nutrition, digestion, and metabolism served as examples for emerging experimental anatomists and physiologists in the United States. Throughout the 1700s and into the late 1800s, the United States founded its first medical schools and produced graduates with medical degrees who either taught in medical schools and conducted research or became associated with departments of physical education and hygiene (health).

### Pioneers in Exercise Science

Edward Hitchcock (1793–1864) and his son Edward Hitchcock Jr. (1828–1911) were both physicians and professors at Amherst College in Massachusetts. Together, they wrote the physical education textbook *Elementary Anatomy and Physiology: For Colleges, Academies, and Other Schools.*[2] Of particular importance was the assertion by Edward Hitchcock Jr. that the study of **anthropometry**, or the proportions of the human body, was crucial to demonstrate that engaging in daily, vigorous exercise produced beneficial results, especially for muscular development.

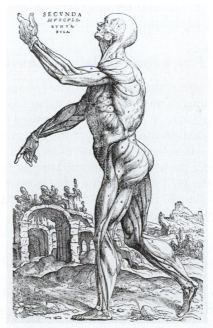

**Figure 1-5.** Anatomical drawing by Andreas Vesalius from *De Humani Corporis Fabrica* (*On the Fabric of the Human Body*). This illustration depicts the superficial musculature of the human body. (© Getty Images)

Through his studies on several cohorts of exercising college-aged men between the years 1861 and 1900, Hitchcock Jr. was able to compare bodily stature and strength measurements for physical education students at the beginning of their enrollment and at graduation. These data were presented in the first American textbook on anthropometry, *Anthropometry and Physical Examination*, published in 1896 by Jay W. Seaver, MD (1855–1915).

Also during the 1860s, the U.S. military was performing anthropometric, spirometric (the measuring of breath), and muscular strength assessments on Civil War soldiers. These protocols led the way for future studies on body dimensions and muscular strength as seen in both the military and the field of exercise physiology today.

Early in the 20th century, the U.S. medical community began to promote endeavors based on collaborations among scientific laboratories (both national and international), which created an environment where free scientific exchange, discussion, and debate were encouraged. The beginnings of exercise physiology began to take hold as researchers in this era started to focus on the energy demands of exercising muscle as a means to clarify the processes of cellular metabolism.

In 1922, Archibald Vivian (A. V.) Hill, a professor of physiology at the prestigious University College in London, won the Nobel Prize for his findings on energy metabolism. Other notable Nobel laureates, such as Albert Szent-Györgyi, Otto Meyerhof, August Krogh, and Hans Krebs, were also studying cellular metabolism and respiration at that time. Through international meetings and organizations such as the International Union of Physiological Sciences, the sharing of the discoveries made by leaders in biochemistry and physiology made it possible for advances in anatomy and physiology to continue around the world.

## Exercise Physiology at Harvard University

From 1927–1946, the Harvard Fatigue Laboratory (HFL) attracted many of the great exercise scientists of the 20th century. In 1926, A. V. Hill visited Harvard University, which spurred on the creation of the HFL 1 year later. Lawrence J. Henderson, MD (1878–1942), a renowned biochemistry professor at Harvard Medical School, established the HFL. To direct the laboratory, Henderson appointed David Bruce (D. B.) Dill (1891–1986), a biochemist from Stanford University.

During his tenure at the HFL, Dill coordinated the research efforts of scientists from 15 different countries and oversaw the publication of hundreds of research papers in the areas of exercise physiology, which included blood chemistry analysis methods, exercise and aging, and acute responses and chronic adaptations to exercise under environmental stresses (e.g., exposure to altitude, heat, and cold). These studies laid the groundwork for research conducted in the exercise physiology laboratories of today and helped to shape the methodologies necessary for military research throughout the modern world. The influence of the HFL was so significant that a majority of today's prominent exercise physiologists can attribute their training to the leaders who conducted research at the HFL.

## European Contributions to Exercise Science

In the early 1900s at the University of Copenhagen in Denmark, a physiological chemistry scientist named August Krogh (1874–1949) conducted many classic experiments on gas exchange in the lungs, the utilization of carbohydrate and fat during exercise, blood redistribution during physical activity, and cardiorespiratory dynamics in exercise. Through collaboration with the HFL, research on these topics continued at the University of Copenhagen for several decades by important Danish scientists, including Erik Hohwü-Christensen, Erling Asmussen, and Marius Nielsen.

Research conducted in Sweden has also significantly influenced the field of modern exercise physiology. The world-renowned exercise physiologist Per-Olof Åstrand, MD (b. 1922) studied at The College of Physical Education at the Karolinska Institute Medical School in Stockholm. Åstrand's research on the physical working capacity of children and adults of both sexes—together with the collaboration of his wife, Irma Rhyming—established him as an international leader in the emerging science of experimental exercise physiology.

Also at the Karolinska Institute, two Swedish scientists, Jonas Bergström and Erik Hultman, pioneered the technique of using needle muscle biopsy in the 1960s to study various conditions of exercise and nutritional status on working muscle (Fig. 1-6). Along with Bengt Saltin, a fellow Swedish scientist at the College of Physical Education, and two researchers from the United States (Philip Gollnick at Washington State University and David Costill at Ball State University), Bergström and Hultman contributed to a turning point in exercise physiology by creating a way to analyze muscle tissue biochemistry through their work in needle muscle biopsy.

Researchers from Norway and Finland who were trained in the 1940s made contributions to exercise physiology that are frequently cited today. In 1947, Norwegian scientist Per Scholander (1905–1980) developed a method to analyze carbon dioxide and oxygen in expired air that inspired the gas analyzer technologies used in exercise physiology laboratories today. Finnish researcher Martti Karvonen, MD (1918–2009), developed an often-used method for predicting optimal exercise training heart rate, known as the Karvonen formula. In addition, Karvonen conducted important research in the areas of exercise performance and exercise in health and longevity.

## Advances in Technology

Technological advances beginning in the late 1950s propelled the field of exercise physiology forward as they

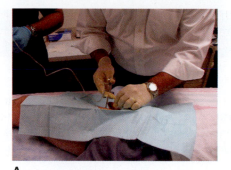

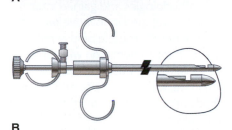

A

B

**Figure 1-6.** Muscle biopsy technique used to measure metabolic conditions in a sample of skeletal muscle. A. An incision is made in the skin, and the biopsy needle (B) is inserted into the muscle. The needle is removed after the small muscle sample is gathered and then can be analyzed under a microscope. *(Reprinted from Kraemer WJ, Fleck SJ, Deschenes MR. Exercise Physiology: Integrating Theory and Applications. Baltimore, MD: Wolters Kluwer/Lippincott Williams & Wilkins; 2012:76, by permission.)*

allowed researchers to perform difficult analyses more efficiently and they permitted the more in-depth study of cellular responses to exercise. The methods developed in the U.S. space program to measure and analyze respiratory gases and to monitor heart rate and body temperature were used by exercise physiologists in the 1960s.

Figure 1-7 shows different methods used to collect and analyze expired gases to determine energy expenditure or aerobic fitness, or both. Figure 1-7A shows a gas collection method called the *Douglas bag technique*. In this photo, the subject is breathing into a collection bag, which will be analyzed later to determine the overall amount of air expired, oxygen concentration, and carbon dioxide production. Figure 1-7B is a modern gas analyzer that can display expired air data in real-time during an exercise test. Figure 1-7C is a portable version of the technology in Figure 1-7B that can be used to measure expired air in field settings such as on a track, field of play, or skating rink.

Concurrently in the 1960s, research was being introduced by prominent U.S. biochemists that resulted in a more biochemical approach to studying exercise. John Holloszy at Washington University in St. Louis, Charles Tipton at the University of Iowa, and Phil Gollnick at Washington State University were using biochemical methods to study rat muscle metabolism and to explore factors related to muscle fatigue. These researchers led the field in the studies that examined human muscle fiber characteristics during exercise and muscle fiber adaptations as a result of chronic exercise training.

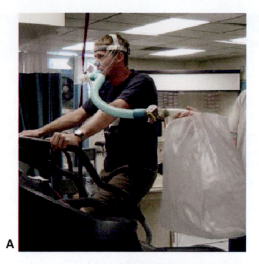

A

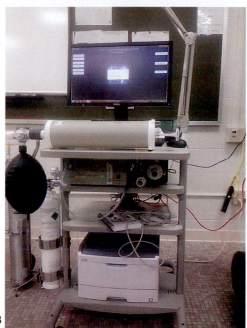

B

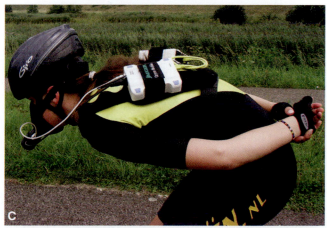

C

**Figure 1-7.** Methods of measuring expired gas technology. A, The Douglas bag method evolved to not only measure energy expenditure, but also to determine aerobic fitness or endurance potential. B, More modern technology can measure these variables in real time in a laboratory setting using a metabolic analyzer or field setting using a portable metabolic analyzer (C). *(A: courtesy of Lance Dalleck; B: courtesy of Jeffrey Janot; C: Courtesy of CareFusion)*

## RESEARCH HIGHLIGHT

### Women in Exercise Physiology

The restrictions imposed on female scientists throughout most of history explain the dearth of scientific contributions made by women up until the middle of the 20th century. Opposition to include female colleagues in the sciences was strong, and the few women who did break through experienced significant hurdles. Nonetheless, several female exercise physiologists have conducted significant research and added important discoveries to the growing field of exercise physiology.

In the area of human muscle fiber research, two women advanced the methodologies and gained international acclaim on publishing their findings. In the 1970s, Birgitta Essén from Sweden developed innovative procedures for analyzing microbiochemical characteristics of muscle tissue obtained from the needle muscle biopsy procedure. In the same decade, another woman from Sweden, Karen Piehl, presented important evidence on which muscle fiber types the body relies on during different categories of physical activity (i.e., anaerobic vs. aerobic exercise).

Two women in the 1970s and 1980s contributed cornerstone research in the area of exercise and environmental stress. Scandinavian researcher Bodil Nielsen published data on the body's responses to environmental heat stress and dehydration. Concurrently, U.S. exercise physiologist Barbara Drinkwater at the University of California at Santa Barbara (UCSB) was conducting research on similar topics in UCSB's Environmental Physiology Laboratory. Drinkwater is also well-known for her contributions to the physiological problems associated with the female athlete triad, focusing on changes in bone density. She went on to be the first female President of American College of Sports Medicine (ACSM) in 1988.

More and more women continue to enter the field of exercise physiology as evidenced by their key positions as deans, chairs of departments of exercise science and kinesiology, principal investigators on research studies, and directors of exercise physiology laboratories. Relative to the history of the field of exercise physiology, female researchers' influences on and contributions to the study of how the body responds to the challenges of exercise have just begun.

## PHYSICAL EDUCATION

Modern physical education programs refer to courses taken within primary and secondary school curricula that encourage psychomotor learning in a play or movement-exploration setting. Similar to exercise physiology, physical education has its roots in ancient cultures and sports. The Persians, Assyrians, Greeks, and Romans of ancient times all had fitness training regimens associated with the requirement that their young men served in the military. Playing competitive games was a method for males to develop the fitness and skills necessary to be a warrior. As such, young women were typically excluded from sports because those activities were associated with military training. Thus, the history of physical education for centuries was about the athletics and performance skills related to war and less about the health aspects of physical activity.

### In Your Own Words

Physical education teachers are professionals who work in the field of exercise physiology who have the opportunity to directly influence many lives. Talk with a friend or fellow student about your experiences with physical education in your childhood. How did they shape your current attitudes about physical activity and exercise? Did your physical education teacher significantly impact your physical fitness development?

## The First Physical Education Curriculum

The introduction of physical education into public school curricula can be traced back to Sweden in the 1800s. Per Henrik Ling (1776–1839) became the first director of Stockholm's Royal Central Institute of Gymnastics in 1813. Ling soon developed and introduced to Sweden his own program of gymnastics, which included: (1) educational gymnastics, (2) military gymnastics, and (3) medical gymnastics. Ling believed that exercise was important for the health of each individual. His strong belief in using science based on anatomy and physiology to better understand fitness required that physical educators who graduated from the Royal Central Institute of Gymnastics were well schooled in basic biological sciences. Ling's gymnastics program became part of Sweden's school curriculum in 1820.

Another important figure in physical education was Archibald MacLaren, who promoted the importance of fitness and regular exercise throughout Great Britain in the late 1800s. MacLaren believed that weariness and stress could be cured with exercise, and that individualized training and progression within training were important programming principles. MacLaren's system of physical training was adopted by the British Army and implemented into the public school curriculum in the late 19th century. Because of the importance that the Europeans placed on the societal benefits of physical education, it was woven into the public school systems.

## Physical Education in America

There was less interest in physical fitness in the United States during the 1800s than in European countries. However, after the Civil War, physical education was introduced into many public school and college curricula. A medical professor at Harvard University, John Collins (J. C.) Warren (1778–1856), was a major proponent of physical activity and made significant contributions to the advancement of physical education in America. Although Warren was best known for his contributions to understanding the use of anesthesia during surgery, he was also deeply involved in attempts to promote the importance of exercise on health with his publications *Physical Education and the Preservation of Health*[3] and *The Preservation of Health*.[4]

Catharine Beecher (1800–1878) was another important leader in early physical education (Fig. 1-8). Through self-study, Beecher learned the subjects not offered in schools for young women, and by 1824 she had opened a private school for young women in Hartford, Connecticut, known as the Hartford Female Seminary. Among her many accomplishments were the fitness programs she created with the needs of women in mind, including a system of calisthenics performed to music. Beecher also advocated for the health, exercise, and dress reform of women and children.

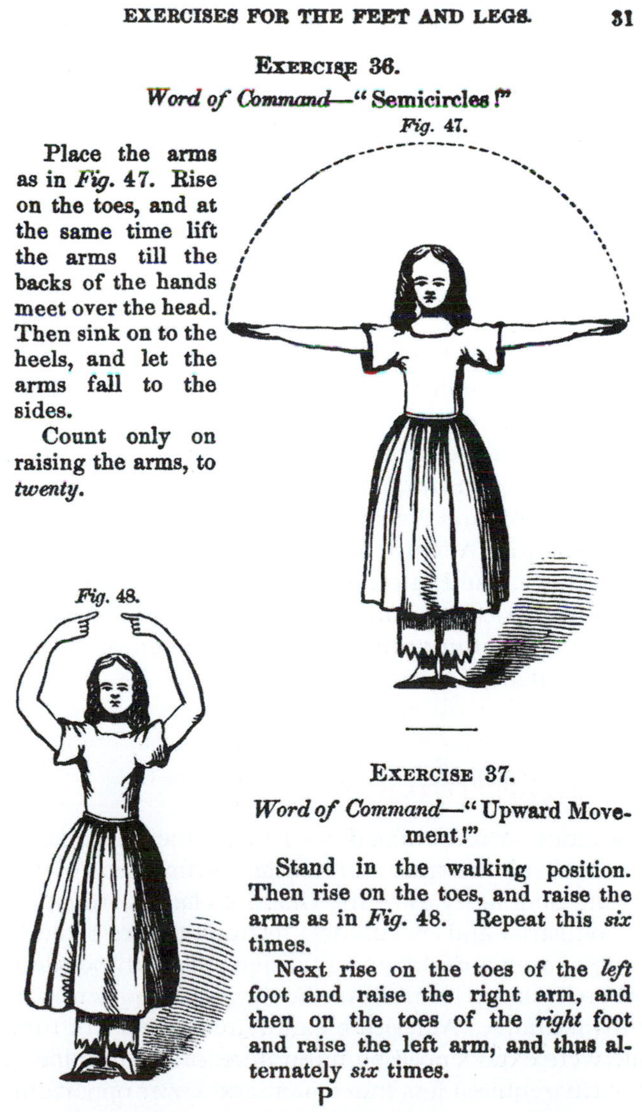

The post-Civil War period in the United States also brought about an increased interest in competitive sports. The revival of the modern Olympic Games and the formation of the International Olympic Committee (IOC) in 1894 occurred during this period in history. Consequently, the beginnings of physical education in the United States coincided with the country's growing support of sports. Thus, a large part of the evolution of physical education in the United States revolved around a focus on sports and games. However, many physical educators at the time believed that the value of incorporating exercise curricula into public schools was that it would improve each individual's health-related fitness. Still a topic of debate today is the role of physical education programs and whether their focus should be on health-related fitness or on athletic, skill-related performance.

As the approach of World War I loomed, draft examinations revealed an enormous number of deferrals because of various health problems. Thus, following the war, a "new" physical education was proposed based on biological, psychological, sociological, and educational foundations. Legislation was passed to improve physical education programs within the public schools, but because of lack of funding and the poor economy during the Great Depression, the emphasis on improving physical education waned.

Several decades later, when the United States entered World War II with the bombing of Pearl Harbor in 1941, draft examinations revealed once again that many of the draftees were not fit for combat. In fact, almost half of all draftees were rejected or given noncombat positions because of poor health or fitness. This alarming data led to the recognition that improving fitness in America's youth was an important objective, which played a significant role in shifting the focus from sport and recreation activity in physical education programs to an emphasis on physical fitness activities.

The U.S. Army instituted a fitness training regimen to improve the combat readiness and effectiveness of soldiers entering the armed forces through the draft. The World War II fitness test was developed in 1942 to determine the functional fitness of draftees who were soon to be sent into combat. This test included the following exercises: pull-ups, squat jumps, push-ups, sit-ups, and a 300-yard run.

**EXERCISES FOR THE FEET AND LEGS.** **31**

**EXERCISE 36.**

*Word of Command—"Semicircles !"*

*Fig. 47.*

Place the arms as in *Fig. 47*. Rise on the toes, and at the same time lift the arms till the backs of the hands meet over the head. Then sink on to the heels, and let the arms fall to the sides.

Count only on raising the arms, to *twenty*.

*Fig. 48.*

**EXERCISE 37.**

*Word of Command—"Upward Movement !"*

Stand in the walking position. Then rise on the toes, and raise the arms as in *Fig. 48*. Repeat this *six* times.

Next rise on the toes of the *left* foot and raise the right arm, and then on the toes of the *right* foot and raise the left arm, and thus alternately *six* times.

P

**Figure 1-8.** Through her writings and the schools she founded, Catharine Beecher advocated that women be taught health and exercise principles. *(From Beecher C. Physiology and Calisthenics. For schools and families. New York: Harper & Brothers, Publishers; 1856.)*

## In Your Own Words

Discuss this question with a peer: Which approach do you think is more valuable for youth programs: sport-related activities or health/fitness-focused activities? Why?

In the middle of the 20th century, two important leaders in the promotion of physical activity as a means to improve health in the United States emerged. First, in 1941, Professor Thomas K. Cureton created an exercise physiology laboratory at the University of Illinois. For the following 30 years, Cureton would teach many of today's leaders in physical fitness, lead research studies that resulted in improvement in individual exercise recommendations, and develop fitness tests for cardiorespiratory endurance, muscular strength, and flexibility. Second, in 1968, physician and researcher Kenneth Cooper published *Aerobics*, a book that explained a physiological rationale for using exercise to promote a healthy lifestyle.[5] Cooper's pioneering vision helped to change the social norm around exercise, making its preventive health benefits accessible to athletes and the general public alike (Fig. 1-9). Consequently, popular acceptance of regular exercise as an important aspect of optimal health began to take hold in the late 1960s.

## Current Trends in Physical Education

Today, physical education is institutionalized in most schools in the United States (Fig. 1-10). In the most recent School Health Policies and Practices Study conducted by the U.S. Centers for Disease Control and Prevention (CDC), it was reported that 63% of elementary schools, 83.9% of middle schools, and 95.2% of high schools require physical education.[6] However, a recent trend in many schools is that physical education classes and recess have been squeezed out because of increasing educational demands and tough financial times. The same CDC study found that only 3.8% of elementary schools, 7.9% of middle schools, and 2.1% of high schools provide the nationally recommended daily physical education or its equivalent for the entire school year for students in all grades in the school.[6]

During difficult economic times, states and school districts often examine ways to decrease spending

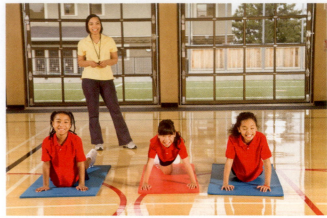

**Figure 1-10.** A background in exercise physiology can help physical educators design and implement appropriate curricula to improve health-related fitness and promote physical activity in school-aged children.

and balance the budget. As a result, physical education often is targeted for reduction or elimination. In addition, intense pressure to improve academic performance and increase test scores has led school administrators to reduce the amount of time that students are physically active during the school day. This approach is counterproductive, however, considering the research that suggests that physical activity and physical education positively impact student attendance, participation, and enthusiasm for academic subjects and motivation to learn, as well as reduce behavior and discipline problems.[7] In addition, numerous studies show significant positive relationships between physical fitness and academic achievement, including improved performance on standardized tests.[8–10]

To combat the trend of reduced physical education in schools, organizations such as the National Association for Sport and Physical Education, an association of the American Alliance for Health, Physical Education, Recreation, and Dance, are working to promote high-quality physical education programs, supported by the school and community, to further the education and development of the whole child.[11]

## MODERN FITNESS MOVEMENT

The industrial revolution of the 1950s in the United States was one of the most influential occurrences in the health and lifestyles of the U.S. population. Advances in industrial and mechanical technologies resulted in the replacement of labor-intensive jobs with positions wherein sitting for most of the day was the norm. The urbanization of America meant that the rigors of rural life were experienced by fewer people, and that life in the city required less movement and fewer opportunities for physical activity.

The costs of a more industrialized and urbanized society are evidenced by the health trends of a developed

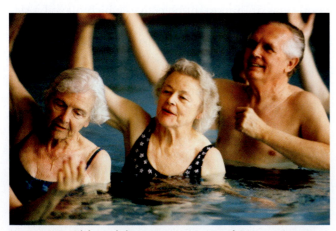

**Figure 1-9.** Older adults engaging in aerobic exercise as popularized and recommended by Dr. Kenneth Cooper of the Cooper Clinic.

nation. Instead of death and illness from infectious causes (such as influenza, polio, and rubella, as was common at the beginning of the 20th century), most of modern society's mortality and morbidity stem from hypokinetic diseases related to physical inactivity such as **cardiovascular disease (CVD)**, obesity, and type 2 diabetes. This realization led to efforts by the medical and physical education communities to inform the general public about the health risks of being physically inactive.

In the 1950s, several organizations got involved in the promotion of fitness as an important component of overall health. The American Heart Association, the American Medical Association, the American Association for Physical Education, Recreation, and Dance, and the President's Council on Youth Fitness were all important in providing education and resources for Americans interested in improving health through increased physical activity. Furthermore, these organizations added merit and legitimacy to the burgeoning fitness movement. Another notable organization formed in the mid-1950s, the American College of Sports Medicine, promotes and integrates scientific research and practical applications of sports medicine and exercise science in the areas of physical performance, fitness, and health.

The American Council on Exercise (ACE) is a non-profit organization committed to America's health and well-being. ACE is an established resource for both exercise professionals and consumers, providing comprehensive scientific research impacting the fitness industry. ACE offers fitness certification, education, and training to more than 50,000 certified professionals.

## Current and Future Emphases in Exercise Science

As the average life expectancy continues to increase through advances in medical technologies, the years that many people live with some sort of disability because of poor health have also increased. The alarming increase in the prevalence of lifestyle-related conditions, such as obesity, CVD, and type 2 diabetes, has necessarily shifted the focus from health practices that treat symptoms to health-care recommendations for the prevention of chronic disease. Fluctuating economies and skyrocketing increases in the cost of health care has put mounting pressure on individuals and communities to take part in programs that promote overall health improvement. An integral part of a healthy lifestyle that proactively reduces the risk for many chronic diseases (e.g., CVD, some forms of cancer, type 2 diabetes, and **stroke**) is regular exercise.

## Healthy People 2020

Beginning in 1979 with the Surgeon General's Report, *Healthy People: The Surgeon General's Report on Health Promotion and Disease Prevention*, Healthy People initiatives have provided science-based, 10-year national objectives for improving the health of all Americans. For three decades, Healthy People has allowed the government to establish benchmarks and monitor progress over time to: (1) encourage collaborations across sectors, (2) guide individuals toward making informed health decisions, and (3) measure the impact of prevention activities.[12]

In December 2010, the Healthy People 2020 initiative was presented. The vision for Healthy People 2020 is to create a society in which all people live long, healthy lives. The following overarching goals have been established to achieve this end[12]:

- Attain high-quality, longer lives free of preventable disease, disability, injury, and premature death.
- Achieve health equity, eliminate disparities, and improve the health of all groups.
- Create social and physical environments that promote good health for all.
- Promote quality of life, healthy development, and healthy behaviors across all life stages.

Each of the overarching goals of Healthy People 2020 can be achieved, in part, by implementing some type of physical activity for improved health. Thus, a large portion of future exercise research in the United States will most likely be related to discovering methods to increase each individual's access to and participation in regular physical activity. This includes conducting more research on often understudied population groups such as women and children.

As defined in the 2008 release of *Physical Activity Guidelines for Americans*, regular physical activity includes participation in moderate and vigorous physical activities and muscle-strengthening activities. Also described in the 2008 guidelines was the alarming percentage of Americans who do not get enough physical activity. For example, it was reported that more than 80% of adults do not meet the guidelines for both aerobic and muscle-strengthening activities. Similarly, more than 80% of adolescents do not do enough aerobic physical activity to meet the guidelines for youth.[13]

The objectives related specifically to physical activity for Healthy People 2020 reflect the significant contributions of exercise science in supporting the health benefits of regular physical activity among youth and adults. Healthy People 2020 also points to a multidisciplinary approach to promoting physical activity. This approach brings about traditional partnerships, such as that of education and health care, with nontraditional partnerships representing, for example, transportation, urban planning, recreation, and environmental health. The Physical Activity objectives for 2020[12] highlight how physical activity levels are positively affected by structural environments, such as the availability of sidewalks, bike lanes, trails, and parks, and legislative policies that improve access to facilities that support physical activity.

Healthy People 2020 also established objectives related to policies that target younger children through:
- increasing physical activity in child-care settings.
- decreasing television viewing and computer usage.
- supporting recess and physical education in public and private elementary schools.

Healthy People 2020, together with other emerging general public and community efforts to incorporate more physical activity into daily life, reflects the increased acceptance and understanding of the important role that regular exercise plays in overall health. This continued focus on discovering the many health benefits of physical activity helps to drive future research in the still evolving field of exercise physiology.

## V I G N E T T E  *conclusion*

■ Charlotte's first job after graduating college was at the same corporate wellness center where she completed her internship. She started as an entry-level floor instructor and gained more experience applying the principles of exercise physiology to

design safe and effective exercise programs for the employees of the corporation. Charlotte also pursued continuing education in nutrition and wellness concepts, and became certified as a health coach. After several years of working at the same corporate facility, Charlotte was promoted to employee fitness director in charge of managing the entire facility, developing health and wellness programs for facility members, and promoting healthy nutrition and regular physical activity among all the corporation's employees for the purposes of improving worker productivity and reducing chronic illness. Charlotte enjoys helping hundreds of employees improve their health and wellness as she continues to apply in her work the foundations of exercise physiology together with core concepts rooted in nutritional science, behavior change, and stress management.

## CRITICAL THINKING QUESTIONS

1. Exercise physiology and health care are often interrelated. What are the driving forces responsible for the bridge between the two practices in today's health-care environment?

2. What circumstances in ancient Greece led to the cultural acceptance of exercise physiology and physical education?

3. How did the industrial revolution in the United States affect the lifestyles and overall health of its general population?

4. A lack of physical activity has led to a wide variety of the so-called hypokinetic diseases in our country. What steps can community planners make to engineer their communities to foster increased levels of physical activity in their residents?

## ADDITIONAL RESOURCES

Beecher CE. *Physiology and Calisthenics*. New York: Harper & Brothers; 1858.

Berryman JW. *Out of Many, One: A History of the American College of Sports Medicine*. Champaign, IL: Human Kinetics; 1995.

Berryman JW. Exercise is medicine: a historical perspective. *Curr Sports Med Rep*. 2010; 9(4):195-201. doi: 10.1249/JSR.0b013e3181e7d86d.

Hill AV. *Muscular Movement in Man: The Factors Governing Speed and Recovery From Fatigue*. London: McGraw-Hill; 1927.

Messengale JD, Swanson RA, eds. *History of Exercise and Sport Science*. Champaign, IL: Human Kinetics; 1996.

## References

1. Green RM. *A Translation of Galen's Hygiene*. Springfield, IL: Charles C. Thomas Publisher; 1951.
2. Hitchcock E, Hitchcock EJ. *Elementary Anatomy and Physiology: For Colleges, Academies, and Other Schools*. New York: Ivison, Phinney & Co; 1860.
3. Warren JC. *Physical Education and the Preservation of Health*. Boston: W.D. Ticknor & Company; 1845.
4. Warren JC. *The Preservation of Health*. Boston: W.D. Ticknor & Company; 1854.
5. Cooper KH. *Aerobics*. New York: Evans; 1968.
6. U.S. Centers for Disease Control and Prevention. SHPPS: School Health Policies and Practices Study. 2006. http://cdc.gov/HealthyYouth/shpps/. Accessed October 2012.
7. Strong W, Maline R, Blimkie C, et al. Evidence-based physical activity for school-age youth. *J Pediatr*. 2005;146:732–737.
8. California Department of Education. *A Study of the Relationship Between Physical Fitness and Academic Achievement in California Using 2004 Test Results*. Sacramento, CA; 2005.
9. Texas Education Agency. *Physically Fit Students More Likely to Do Well in School, Less Likely to Be Discipline Problems*. Austin, TX: Texas Education Agency; 2009.
10. U.S. Centers for Disease Control and Prevention. *The Association Between School-Based Physical Activity, Including Physical Education, and Academic Performance*. Atlanta, GA: U.S. Department of Health and Human Services; 2010.
11. National Association for Sport and Physical Education & American Heart Association. *Physical Education Is Critical to Educating the Whole Child*. Reston, VA; 2011.
12. U.S. Department of Health and Human Services. *Healthy People 2020: Topics and Objectives*. 2010. http://healthypeople.gov/2020/
13. U.S. Department of Health and Human Services, Office of Disease Prevention and Health Promotion. *2008 Physical Activity Guidelines for Americans*. 2008. http://health.gov/PAGuidelines/pdf/paguide.pdf.

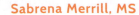

Sabrena Merrill, MS

## CHAPTER 2

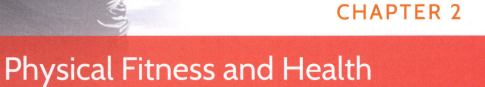

# Physical Fitness and Health

## CHAPTER OUTLINE

## LEARNING OUTCOMES

1. Define *physical activity*, *exercise*, and *physical fitness*.
2. Describe the major categories of physical fitness that contribute to total daily energy expenditure.
3. Differentiate among the components of health-related physical fitness and skill-related physical fitness.
4. Describe the impact of participation in regular physical activity on public health.
5. Explain the dose–response relationship of physical activity and health status.
6. List general physical activity guidelines for improving health.
7. Describe the general physiological mechanisms by which physical activity positively impacts health.
8. Explain the effect of increasing rates of obesity on public health.
9. Describe the relationship between physical activity and longevity.
10. Explain how older adults can use physical activity as a means for reducing the risk for chronic disease and improving quality of life.

## ANCILLARY LINK

Visit Davis*Plus* at http://davisplus.fadavis.com for study and practice resources, including online quizzes, animations that help explain physiological processes, podcasts concerning news and career trends in exercise physiology, and practice references.

## VIGNETTE

■ Vince is a 50-year-old news journalist who travels at least 3 weeks a month and works long, unpredictable hours. He has gained approximately 50 pounds since he was in his 30s and often complains of stiff, aching joints and chronic low-back pain. Because of his joint ailments, Vince visited his physician to explore therapies for the treatment of pain. The physician advised Vince to take over-the-counter pain relievers to ease his joint pain, and more importantly, to address the root of the problem—excess body weight. The physician notified Vince that his weight placed him in the obese category and that his blood pressure was elevated. She recommended a weight-management program that included increased daily physical activity.

How can incorporating more habitual physical activity into Vince's daily life help him manage his weight?

Participation in regular physical activity provides numerous health and physical performance benefits. Ample incontrovertible evidence has been reported that physical inactivity is a major modifiable risk factor for a wide variety of chronic diseases and that it leads to premature mortality.[1–3] Despite these data, the high prevalence of physical inactivity in many individuals causes concern about the burden of avoidable chronic diseases on public health-care systems.[4]

Professionals working in the health and fitness fields are presented with a challenging task as they take on the roles of resource provider, motivator, and coach in the effort to get more people physically active. This chapter reviews the current evidence linking physical activity to health status and presents practical definitions for commonly used terminology in exercise science and public health research. Further, information on the impact of physical activity on chronic disease and longevity is presented, together with guidelines that health/fitness professionals can use to recommend appropriate levels of physical activity to their clients.

## DEFINING PHYSICAL ACTIVITY, EXERCISE, AND PHYSICAL FITNESS

In any field of study, it is important to define the items under investigation so that a standardized terminology can be used to promote greater understanding of the concepts being measured. In the area of exercise physiology, the terms *physical activity* and *exercise* are sometimes stated as synonyms, but they actually have different definitions. In addition, the term *physical fitness* is often misunderstood as it relates to an individual's overall health.

Physical activity, exercise, and physical fitness were first defined in the mid-1980s by epidemiologists at the Centers for Disease Control and Prevention (CDC) in a Public Health Report entitled *Physical Activity, Exercise, and Physical Fitness: Definitions and Distinctions for Health-related Research*.[5] The definitions of the terms contained in this report have served as a framework for comparing studies that relate physical activity, exercise, and physical fitness to health (Table 2-1).

### Physical Activity

**Physical activity** is defined as any bodily movement produced by skeletal muscles that results in energy expenditure (Fig. 2-1).[5] Energy expenditure is measured as a value of heat production. A **kilocalorie (kcal)**, the amount of heat required to raise the temperature of 1 kg of water 1°C, is commonly used as a comparison value to measure human energy expenditure. Technically, a **kilojoule (kJ)** is a more accurate representation of energy measurement (1 kcal is equivalent to 4.184 kJ), but the kilocalorie has been used so extensively to describe energy expenditure, that it is an accepted form of quantification for the energy requirements of physical activity. A kilocalorie is also called a **calorie**, which is the term most commonly used when describing energy factors related to physical activity and nutrition. More detailed information on capturing and calculating an individual's energy expenditure can be found in Chapter 5.

Because individual factors influence the amount of energy expended by a person during physical activity, there is always a range of caloric expenditure associated with any given activity. For example, the amount of a person's muscle mass that is producing bodily movement and the intensity, duration, and frequency of

## Table 2-1. Comparison of Health and Fitness Terms

| PHYSICAL ACTIVITY | EXERCISE | PHYSICAL FITNESS |
|---|---|---|
| • Any bodily movement that contributes to daily energy expenditure<br>• Positively associated with physical fitness | • Planned, structured, and repetitive bodily movement that contributes to daily energy expenditure<br>• Very positively associated with physical fitness<br>• A subcategory of physical activity | • A set of attributes that a person has or achieves<br>• Health-related components:<br>  √ Cardiorespiratory endurance<br>  √ Muscular endurance<br>  √ Muscular strength<br>  √ Flexibility<br>  √ Body composition<br>• Skill-related components:<br>  √ Agility<br>  √ Balance<br>  √ Coordination<br>  √ Speed<br>  √ Power<br>  √ Reaction time |

Data from Caspersen CJ, Powell KE, Christenson GM. Physical activity, exercise, and physical fitness: Definitions and distinctions for health-related research. *Public Health Rep.* 1985;100:126–131.

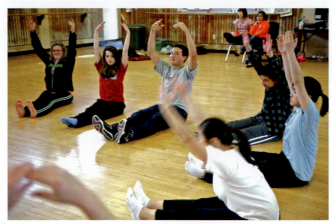

**Figure 2-1.** Physical activity is defined as any bodily movement produced by skeletal muscles that results in energy expenditure. *(Photo courtesy of Arthur Hsieh)*

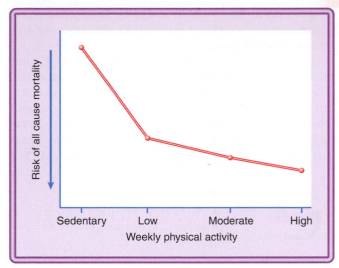

**Figure 2-2.** Relationship between weekly physical activity and risk for all-cause mortality.

muscular contraction all contribute to the total calories used during physical activity. As such, energy expenditure (expressed as calories per unit of time) is a continuous variable, ranging from low to high.

Identifying physical activity during daily life is made simpler when different activities are categorized according to segments of a typical day. The following formula expresses a simple way to categorize the total energy expenditure due to physical activity:

$$Kcal_{sleep} + kcal_{occupation} + kcal_{leisure} = kcal_{total\ daily\ physical\ activity}$$

*Note: The caloric expenditures in these categories of physical activity are above* **basal metabolic rate (BMR)** *and the thermic effect of food. BMR is defined as the number of calories expended in a neutrally temperate environment while in the postabsorptive state. Sleep outside of a clinical/ laboratory setting (such as sleep the average person gets each night) is not true BMR; thus, it counts as part of a person's activity calories.*

Leisure-time physical activity includes subcategories such as sports, exercise conditioning, household tasks, and other activities that may or may not contribute significantly to a person's energy expenditure throughout the day. Accordingly, how a person spends his or her leisure time has the potential to influence health. For example, classic research on physical activity and mortality has suggested that greater levels of physical activity (e.g., >2,000 kcal/week) result in a lower risk for "all-cause mortality" (i.e., from any cause) compared with reduced levels of physical activity[6,7] (Fig. 2-2).

## Exercise

Although exercise has some commonalities with physical activity, exercise and physical activity are not the same. **Exercise** is defined as physical activity that is planned, structured, repetitive, and performed with the intention of improving or maintaining one or more components of physical fitness (see Table 2-1). Thus, exercise is a subcategory of physical activity. Most conditioning routines and sports activities are performed to improve or maintain components of physical fitness and are considered exercise (Fig. 2-3). Also, work tasks and household activities may be considered exercise if they are performed in a less efficient manner and structured to expend more energy to increase health benefits.[5] For example, a factory worker might move inventory by purposely lifting boxes manually instead of using a machine lift, with the intention of developing greater upper body strength. A person performing yard work might choose to use a push mower instead

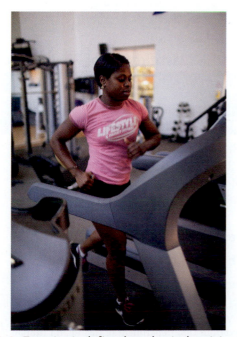

**Figure 2-3.** Exercise is defined as physical activity that is planned, structured, repetitive, and performed with the intention of improving or maintaining one or more components of physical fitness.

of a riding mower to trim the lawn to create a more significant calorie "burn" to assist in his or her weight-management efforts.

Intensity, or level of physical exertion, is a commonly measured variable in exercise science research. There are numerous methods for assessing exercise intensity, including percentage of **maximal oxygen consumption ($\dot{V}O_{2max}$), oxygen consumption reserve ($\dot{V}O_2R$), heart rate reserve, maximal heart rate ($HR_{max}$),** and **metabolic equivalents (METs).**

Each method has its advantages and limitations. Professionals in exercise physiology must choose the most appropriate protocol to use for determining exercise intensity depending on the individual and the situation. Chapter 15 covers these methods in more detail. It is important to clearly quantify physical activity in terms of intensity, because a wide range of possible exertion levels are associated with physical activity. Table 2-2 presents classifications of various levels of physical activity intensity.

## FROM THEORY TO PRACTICE

METs have been established as a convenient and practical way to determine the intensity of various physical activities. The amount of oxygen consumed by a person performing physical activity is directly proportional to the energy expended. The MET method assumes that the body uses approximately 3.5 mL of oxygen per kilogram of body weight (2.2 lb) per minute (3.5 mL/kg/min) at rest. Thus, resting metabolic rate is comparable with 1 MET. That is, 1.0 MET = 3.5 mL/kg/min. Using the MET system allows physical activities to be classified by intensity according to their oxygen requirements in relation to the body at rest. For example, an activity that is rated at 3.0 METs, such as walking at 2.5 miles per hour (mph; 4 km/h), requires three times the resting metabolic rate, or 10.5 mL/kg/min. Table 2-3 lists some physical activities and their MET values.

The MET system is a practical way to describe intensity and is a relatively simple method to use for recommending physical activity. The American College of Sports Medicine (ACSM) and CDC have defined light physical activity as requiring less than 3 METs, moderate activity between 3 and 6 METs, and vigorous activity more than 6 METs.[8] MET values are so common that many cardiorespiratory endurance exercise machines display them on their consoles as a measure of workout intensity. As such, it is important for professionals working in the fitness field to understand the concept of METs and be able to explain them to their clients.

The main drawback of using the MET system is that MET values are only approximations of energy expenditure. That is, there are potential errors in using 1.0 MET as a constant resting value because metabolic efficiency varies between individuals. Also, the MET system does not account for individual variations in age, sex, muscle mass, and disease states (e.g., cardiac disease, pulmonary disease, and neuromuscular diseases), nor does it factor in environmental conditions. Nonetheless, MET values can be useful guidelines for training in a general sense.

## Table 2-2. Classification of Physical Activity Intensity

| INTENSITY | RELATIVE INTENSITY | | ABSOLUTE INTENSITY RANGES (METS) ACROSS FITNESS LEVELS | | | |
| | $\dot{V}O_2R$ (%) HRR (%) | MAXIMAL HR (%) | 12 MET $\dot{V}O_{2MAX}$ | 10 MET $\dot{V}O_{2MAX}$ | 8 MET $\dot{V}O_{2MAX}$ | 6 MET $\dot{V}O_{2MAX}$ |
|---|---|---|---|---|---|---|
| Very light | <20 | <50 | <3.2 | <2.8 | <2.4 | <2.0 |
| Light | 20–39 | 50–63 | 3.2–5.3 | 2.8–4.5 | 2.4–3.7 | 2.0–3.0 |
| Moderate | 40–59 | 64–76 | 5.4–7.5 | 4.6–6.3 | 3.8–5.1 | 3.1–4.0 |
| Hard (vigorous) | 60–84 | 77–93 | 7.6–10.2 | 6.4–8.6 | 5.2–6.9 | 4.1–5.2 |
| Very hard | ≥85 | ≥94 | ≥10.3 | ≥8.7 | ≥7.0 | ≥5.3 |
| Maximal | 100 | 100 | 12 | 10 | 8 | 6 |

HR, heart rate; HRR, heart rate reserve; MET, metabolic equivalent unit (1 MET = 3.5 mL/kg/min); $\dot{V}O_{2max}$, maximal oxygen consumption; $\dot{V}O_2R$, oxygen uptake reserve.

Adapted from U.S. Department of Health and Human Services. *Physical Activity and Health: A Report of the Surgeon General.* Atlanta, GA: Centers for Disease Control and Prevention; 1996; American College of Sports Medicine. The recommended quantity and quality of exercise for developing and maintaining cardiorespiratory and muscular fitness, and flexibility in healthy adults. *Med Sci Sports Exerc.* 1998;30:975–991; and Howley ET. Type of activity: Resistance, aerobic and leisure versus occupational physical therapy. *Med Sci Sports Exerc.* 2001;33:S364–S369.

## Table 2-3. Metabolic Equivalent Values of Common Physical Activities Classified as Light, Moderate, or Vigorous Intensity

| LIGHT (<3 METs) | MODERATE (3–6 METs) | VIGOROUS (>METs) |
|---|---|---|
| **Walking** | **Walking** | **Walking, jogging, and running** |
| Walking slowly around home, store, or office = 2.0* | Walking 3.0 mph = 3.0* <br> Walking at very brisk pace (4 mph) = 5.0* | Walking at very, very brisk pace (4.5 mph) = 6.3* <br> Walking/hiking at moderate pace and grade with no or light pack (<10 lb) = 7.0 <br> Hiking at steep grades and pack 10–42 lb = 7.5–9.0 <br> Jogging at 5 mph = 8.0* <br> Jogging at 6 mph = 10.0* <br> Running at 7 mph = 11.5* |
| **Household and occupation** <br> Sitting while using computer, work at desk, using light hand tools = 1.5 <br> Standing while performing light work, such as making bed, washing dishes, ironing, preparing food, or store clerk = 2.0–2.5 | **Household and occupation** <br> Cleaning, heavy—washing windows, car, clean garage = 3.0 <br> Sweeping floors or carpet, vacuuming, mopping = 3.0–3.5 <br> Carpentry—general = 3.6 <br> Carrying and stacking wood = 5.5 <br> Mowing lawn/walk power mower = 5.5 | **Household and occupation** <br> Shoveling sand, coal, etc. = 7.0 <br> Carrying heavy loads, such as bricks = 7.5 <br> Heavy farming, such as bailing hay = 8.0 <br> Shoveling, digging ditches = 8.5 |
| **Leisure time and sports** <br> Arts and crafts, playing cards = 1.5 <br> Billiards = 2.5 <br> Boating—power = 2.5 <br> Croquet = 2.5 <br> Darts = 2.5 <br> Fishing—sitting = 2.5 <br> Playing most musical instruments = 2.0–2.5 | **Leisure time and sports** <br> Badminton—recreational = 4.5 <br> Basketball—shooting around = 4.5 <br> Bicycling on flat surface—light effort (10–12 mph) = 6.0 <br> Dancing—ballroom slow = 3.0; ballroom fast = 4.5 <br> Fishing from riverbank and walking = 4.0 <br> Golf—walking, pulling clubs = 4.3 <br> Sailing boat, wind surfing = 3.0 <br> Swimming leisurely = 6.0† <br> Table tennis = 5.0 <br> Tennis doubles = 5.0 <br> Volleyball—noncompetitive = 3.0–4.0 | **Leisure time and sports** <br> Basketball game = 8.0 <br> Bicycling on flat surface—moderate effort (12–14 mph) = 8; fast (14–16 mph) = 10 <br> Skiing cross-country—slow (2.5 mph) = 7.0; fast (5.0–7.9 mph) = 9.0 <br> Soccer—casual = 7.0; competitive = 10.0 <br> Swimming—moderate/hard = 8–11† <br> Tennis singles = 8.0 <br> Volleyball—competitive at gym or beach = 8.0 |

Note. A more complete list of physical activities (and their associated MET values) can be found in the updated version of the "Compendium of Physical Activities" by Ainsworth and colleagues.[65]
*On flat, hard surface.
†MET values can vary substantially from person to person during swimming as result of different strokes and skill levels.
MET, metabolic equivalent; mph, miles per hour.
Reprinted from American College of Sports Medicine. *ACSM's Guidelines for Exercise Testing and Prescription* (9th ed.). Philadelphia: Lippincott Williams & Wilkins; 2014, by permission.

## In Your Own Words

How would you describe the difference between physical activity and exercise to a sedentary person who has come to you for advice on becoming more physically active?

## Physical Fitness

Physical activity and exercise essentially refer to the performance of movement, whereas **physical fitness** is defined as a set of measurable attributes that a person has achieved.[5] A person who is physically fit has achieved a physiological state of well-being that allows him or her to successfully meet the demands of daily living or that provides the basis for sport performance. The most frequently cited components of physical fitness are divided into two groups: health-related attributes and performance-related skills.

The five health-related components of physical fitness are: (1) **cardiorespiratory endurance**, (2) **muscular endurance**, (3) **muscular strength**, (4) **flexibility**, and (5) **body composition** (Fig. 2-4). These attributes are important to public health, as individuals with favorable measures of these components tend to enjoy an increased quality of life.

The skill-related components of physical fitness include: (1) **agility**, (2) **coordination**, (3) **balance**, (4) **power**, (5) **reaction time**, and (6) **speed** (Fig. 2-5).

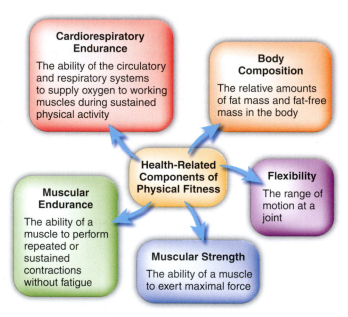

**Figure 2-4.** The health-related components of fitness.

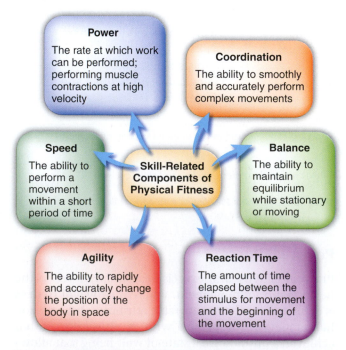

**Figure 2-5.** The skill-related components of fitness.

Individuals who perform exercises to enhance these components typically have already achieved a certain level of conditioning, as these skills are required for the performance of most sport activities. That is, skill-related physical fitness components are commonly pursued by athletes who want to maintain or improve their abilities in their chosen sport. As such, the health-related components of physical fitness are more important to public health than are the components related to athletic ability. Thus, research on physical fitness and health primarily focuses on the health-related components.

## VIGNETTE continued

■ Since his physician's recommendation last month to become more physically active, Vince has committed to incorporating more physical activity during his frequent travel. This includes walking laps around airport terminals while he waits to board his airplane (9 days per month, total). When he stays in hotels, Vince takes the stairs instead of using elevators, and he always handles his luggage himself. Essentially, Vince is incorporating more physical activity into his lifestyle, and he has noticed that he has more energy throughout the day when he is active. On the days that Vince is not active, he feels lethargic and emotionally depressed. Spurred into action from these negative feelings, Vince decides that he wants to incorporate more physical activity into his schedule each day, instead of only when he travels.

## IMPACT OF PHYSICAL ACTIVITY ON PUBLIC HEALTH

In the mid-1990s, three prominent organizations published landmark reports on the association between physical activity and health. The U.S. Surgeon General,[2] the National Institutes of Health,[9] and the ACSM in conjunction with the CDC[10] all issued recommendations that clarified the role of physical activity in improving health parameters. These reports were milestones because they presented for the first time information on the health benefits associated with regular physical activity that did not meet the criteria for improving fitness levels. These guidelines suggested that improved health, lowered susceptibility to chronic disease, and decreased mortality could be obtained by performing physical activity that was below the threshold for improving physical fitness (e.g., <20 minutes per session and <50% of aerobic capacity). Notably, it was documented that some activity is better than none, and more activity, up to a point, is better than less, which suggests a dose–response relationship between physical activity and health. Table 2-4 lists evidence-based benefits of participation in regular physical activity, exercise, or both.

### Table 2-4. General Benefits of Regular Physical Activity, Exercise, or Both

| HEALTH PARAMETER | IMPACT OF PHYSICAL ACTIVITY AND/OR EXERCISE |
|---|---|
| Cardiovascular function | Increased |
| Cardiorespiratory function | Increased |
| Coronary artery disease risk factors | Decreased |
| Morbidity | Decreased |
| Mortality | Decreased |
| Anxiety and depression | Decreased |
| Feelings of well-being | Increased |
| Performance of work, recreational, and sport activities | Increased |
| Risk for falls and injuries (older adults) | Decreased |
| Physical function and independent living (older adults) | Increased |

Data from American College of Sports Medicine. *ACSM's Guidelines for Exercise Testing and Prescription* (9th ed.). Philadelphia: Lippincott Williams & Wilkins; 2014, by permission.

## Dose–Response Relationship Between Physical Activity and Health

Evidence supports the wide-held practice of recommending regular physical activity as an effective method in the **primary prevention** (i.e., intervention to prevent the initial occurrence) and **secondary prevention** (i.e., intervention after the onset) of chronic health conditions, including cardiovascular disease (CVD), diabetes mellitus, cancer (colon and breast), obesity, hypertension, bone and joint diseases (osteoporosis and osteoarthritis), and depression.[7,11–16] Both laboratory-based studies and large-scale, population-based observational studies have clearly documented a dose–response relationship between physical activity and the risk for CVD and premature mortality in men and women, and in ethnically diverse participants.[8]

There appears to be a curvilinear relationship between physical activity and health, such that those individuals who are sedentary or get minimal physical activity benefit the most from relatively modest increases in physical activity and physical fitness in terms of improvements in health status.[10,16,17] However, individuals who already meet the recommended minimum levels of weekly physical activity (i.e., 30 minutes of moderate-intensity physical activity most days of the week) are likely to derive some additional health and fitness benefits from becoming more physically active.[10]

There is also evidence showing a dose–response relationship (Fig. 2-6) between physical activity and numerous health outcomes, such as high-density lipoprotein cholesterol and cardiorespiratory fitness (i.e., $VO_{2max}$). Furthermore, individuals who are inactive show an increased risk for all-cause mortality, overweight, obesity, type 2 diabetes, colon cancer, poor quality of life, and difficulty with independent living (in older adults).[6]

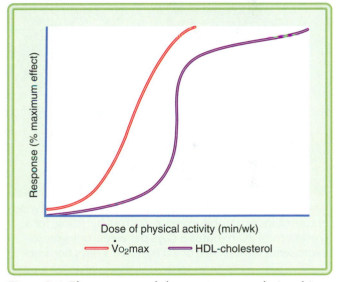

**Figure 2-6.** The conceptual dose–response relationship between weekly physical activity and improvements in both high-density lipoprotein cholesterol and cardiorespiratory fitness (i.e., maximal oxygen consumption [$VO_{2max}$]).

## General Physical Activity Guidelines

More than a decade ago, in an attempt to increase public awareness about the importance and health-related benefits of moderate physical activity, the CDC and the ACSM issued the recommendation that "every U.S. adult should accumulate 30 minutes or more of moderate physical activity on most, preferably all, days of the week."[10] Unfortunately, it has been reported that less than half (49.1%) of U.S. adults meet the CDC-ACSM recommendations.[18] In 2007, the ACSM and American Heart Association issued updated recommendations for physical activity and health in an effort to reduce confusion about the 1995 guidelines and to improve the rate of physical activity among

Americans.[8] The most significant recommendations from the 2007 update include:

- All healthy adults aged 18 to 65 need moderate-intensity **aerobic exercise** (e.g., walking, bicycling, and rowing) for a minimum of 30 minutes 5 days per week, or vigorous exercise for a minimum of 20 minutes 3 days per week (Fig. 2-7).
- Moderate and vigorous exercise intensities can be combined to meet this recommendation.
- An accumulation of 30 minutes of moderate-intensity aerobic exercise can be accomplished by performing bouts lasting 10 minutes or longer throughout the day.
- All adults should engage in muscular strength and endurance activities at least 2 days per week.
- Exceeding the minimum amount of recommended weekly physical activity may result in further improvements in fitness, risk reduction

for chronic diseases and disabilities, and the prevention of unhealthy weight gain.

One year after the CDC-ACSM physical activity update, the U.S. Department of Health and Human Services published the *2008 Physical Activity Guidelines for Americans*.[14] This report presented practical information to guide Americans in choosing appropriate physical activity and incorporating it into a healthy lifestyle. The significance of the *2008 Guidelines* report is that it is accessible to and appropriate reading for the general public. The authors aimed to keep the content straightforward and clear, while remaining consistent with complex scientific information. Four levels of physical activity were classified (inactive, low, medium, and high). The classification of physical activity is useful because these categories show how the total amount of weekly physical activity is related to health benefits (Table 2-5). Low amounts of activity provide some benefits, medium amounts provide substantial benefits, and high amounts provide even greater benefits.

The dose–response relationship clarifies how varying amounts of weekly physical activity contribute to health status. Notably, the minimum recommended level of weekly physical activity (i.e., 150 min/week) provides health benefits, but it does not prove effective in managing or preventing weight gain or obesity. Nonetheless, the health benefits of physical activity are generally independent of body weight. This means that individuals who need to lose weight can still receive major health benefits from regular physical activity, no matter how their weight changes over time.

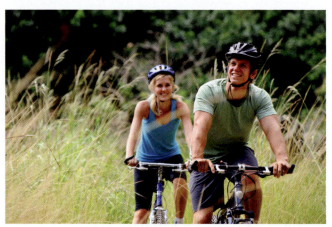

**Figure 2-7.** Healthy adults aged 18 to 65 years need moderate-intensity aerobic exercise, such as bicycling, for a minimum of 30 minutes 5 days per week, or vigorous exercise for a minimum of 20 minutes 3 days per week.

## In Your Own Words

Describe to a friend who is new to exercise how to divide up his or her weekly physical activity so that the minimum recommended level (i.e., 150 min/week) is achieved.

## Table 2-5. Classification of Total Weekly Amounts of Aerobic Exercise

| PHYSICAL ACTIVITY LEVEL | MODERATE-INTENSITY ACTIVITY PER WEEK | GENERAL HEALTH BENEFITS | LIFESTYLE APPLICATION |
|---|---|---|---|
| Inactive | No activity beyond baseline* | None | Being inactive is unhealthy. |
| Low | Activity beyond baseline but fewer than 150 min/week | Some | Low levels of activity are clearly preferable to an inactive lifestyle. |
| Medium | 150–300 min/week | Substantial | Activity at the high end of this range has additional and more extensive health benefits than activity at the low end. |
| High | >300 min/week | Additional | There is no identifiable upper limit of activity above which there are no additional health benefits. |

*Baseline activity refers to the light-intensity activities of daily life, such as standing, walking slowly, and lifting lightweight objects.
From the U.S. Department of Health and Human Services, Office of Disease Prevention and Health Promotion. *2008 Physical Activity Guidelines for Americans*. 2008. www.health.gov/PAGuidelines/pdf/paguide.pdf.

## RESEARCH HIGHLIGHT

### The Hazards of Occupational Sitting

Traditionally, the term *sedentary* has been defined as the absence of physical activity.[19] However, sedentary behavior has begun to evolve to mean prolonged sitting. Many adults in Western and developed countries are in occupations that require times of prolonged sitting. In the United States and Australia, about two thirds of adults are employed, with 83% of those working adults putting in a minimum of 35 hours per week.[20,21] Evidence also suggests that these working adults spend up to half of the workday sitting down (Fig. 2-8).[22,23] Further, time-use surveys have shown that full-time U.S. employees spend an average of just over 2 hours per day watching television or playing computer games, or both.[24] Thus, for full-time employees in jobs that require no physical activity, occupational sitting is likely to be the largest component of overall daily time.

As discussed previously, the association between physical inactivity and health status has been established, such that low levels of or the absence of physical activity can increase the risk for chronic disease (e.g., CVD, diabetes mellitus, and cancer). The high incidence of prolonged occupational sitting among full-time workers has prompted investigations into the association of prolonged sitting and health status, even in individuals who exercise regularly. Healy and colleagues[25] found that prolonged periods of sedentary time, even in people who also regularly performed moderate- to vigorous-intensity exercise, were associated with indicators of declining cardiometabolic function and increased systemic inflammation, such as larger waist circumferences, lower levels of high-density lipoprotein, or "good" cholesterol, and higher levels of C-reactive protein (an important marker of inflammation) and triglycerides (blood fats). The researchers also found that, even in people who sat for prolonged periods, the more breaks workers took during this time, the smaller their waists and the lower their levels of C-reactive protein.[25]

These findings have important implications for full-time employees who spend most of their workday sitting. Namely, long periods of uninterrupted sitting throughout the day increase the risk for chronic health problems, such as obesity and CVD. This increased risk even holds true for individuals who are physically active outside of the workplace.

One approach to thwart the increased risks associated with prolonged sitting is to provide workers with a desk station set up around a treadmill, called a treadmill desk (Fig. 2-9). This setup allows office workers to slowly walk on a treadmill while completing their normal work-related tasks. Preliminary research in this area has suggested that the treadmill desk offers a way to reduce sedentariness in the workplace and has the potential to reduce employee obesity and health-care costs.[26] For example, it was found that medical transcriptionists expended 100 calories per hour more when they transcribed while walking than when they transcribed while sitting. However, the same study showed that the speed of transcription was 16% slower while walking than while sitting.[26]

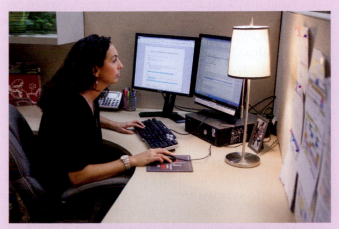

**Figure 2-8.** Many adults in Western and developed countries are in occupations that require periods of prolonged sitting, often using poor posture, with a forward head position and rounded shoulders.

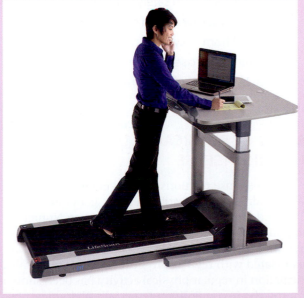

**Figure 2-9.** Desk stations set up around a treadmill, or treadmill desks, can reduce the risks associated with prolonged sitting. Photo courtesy of LifeSpan Fitness.

*Continued*

## RESEARCH HIGHLIGHT—cont'd

so employee productivity while using the treadmill desk is a factor for consideration. Furthermore, the cost of incorporating the treadmill desk (ranging from several hundred to several thousands of dollars each) at all employee workstations could become prohibitive for many companies.

Less costly and more practical strategies for decreasing health risks include advising employees to break up their prolonged periods of sitting with some type of physical activity. In the office-based workplace, for example, individuals could be encouraged to:

- Stand up to take phone calls.
- Walk to see a colleague rather than phoning or e-mailing.
- Have standing meetings or regular breaks during meetings wherein people are allowed to stand.
- Go to a restroom on a different level, using the stairs to get there.
- Walk to distant trash receptacles and printers rather than using these items close to his or her desk.
- Take the stairs instead of the elevator whenever possible.

Healy GN, Matthews CE, Dunstan DW, Winkler EAH, Owen N. Sedentary time and cardio-metabolic biomarkers in U.S. adults: NHANES 2003–06. *Eur Heart J.* 2011;32:590–597.

Thompson WG, Levine JA. Productivity of transcriptionists using a treadmill desk. *Work.* 2011;40:473–477.

## VIGNETTE *continued*

■ After successfully increasing his daily physical activity by walking and taking the stairs more often, Vince has not noticed much of a weight change. In addition, his joints are still painful and his lower back still gives him trouble. Vince realizes that he would be better off following a schedule of planned exercise to help him in his weight-loss efforts, in addition to being more physically active throughout his day. To this end, Vince hires a personal fitness trainer to assist him in safely and effectively exercising to lose weight. In doing so, Vince has progressed from daily physical activity to a program of structured exercise, including aerobic and resistance training, a minimum of 3 days per week.

## IMPACT OF PHYSICAL ACTIVITY ON CHRONIC DISEASE

The dose–response relationship between physical activity and health status described earlier generally relates to CVD and premature death from all causes. Numerous biological mechanisms may be responsible for the reduction in the risk for chronic disease and all-cause mortality associated with regular physical activity. Specifically, participation in regular physical activity has been shown to improve body composition (especially abdominal obesity),[15] enhance lipoprotein profiles,[15] improve glucose homeostasis and insulin sensitivity,[3,11,15] reduce blood pressure,[27] reduce systematic inflammation,[28–31] decrease blood coagulation,[9] and enhance endothelial function.[32–34]

Another important area of overall health, psychological well-being, is also positively impacted by routine physical activity. People who engage in regular physical activity experience reduced stress, anxiety, and depression.[15,35] In addition to playing a factor in the prevention and management of CVD, improved psychological well-being also has implications in the prevention and management of other chronic diseases such as diabetes mellitus, osteoporosis, hypertension, obesity, cancer, and depression.[15]

One of the most pernicious conditions that impacts the development of chronic disease is obesity. As such, the prevention and treatment of obesity are public health concerns that, if successful, could reduce the risk for development of many chronic diseases that result in reduced quality of life and disability. Because of the prevalence of inactive lifestyles and increased caloric consumption in modern society, as well as genetic factors that may lead to the excess accumulation of body fat, the incidence of overweight and obesity continues to grow at an alarming rate. Obesity is defined as a **body mass index** ≥30 kg/m², whereas overweight is classified as a body mass index between 25 and 29.9 kg/m². Together, overweight and obesity affect more than approximately two-thirds of the adult population in the United States, which is a trend that has been increasing for more than a century, with a substantial increase noted in the past several decades.[36,37]

Obesity is associated with many other adverse health conditions including CVD, type 2 diabetes, and **metabolic syndrome** (i.e., a cluster of factors associated with increased risk for coronary heart disease and diabetes—abdominal obesity, dyslipidemia, and elevated levels of triglycerides, blood pressure, and fasting blood glucose).[38] Chapter 27 addresses these cardiometabolic-related conditions in more detail. In addition, chronic obesity may lead to functional impairment[39] and reduced quality of life,[40] as well as to greater mortality.[41] Fortunately, when treatment is successful at producing small amounts of weight loss (even as little as 10 pounds), obese individuals experience many health benefits, including prevention of disease (especially type 2 diabetes)[42] and reduced mortality rate.[43] These factors, in combination with the estimated direct and indirect costs of obesity-related conditions that exceed $117 billion in the United States annually, make treating obesity a national health-care concern.[44]

The basis for managing body weight is founded on energy balance, which is influenced by energy intake (i.e., caloric consumption) and energy expenditure. Physical activity and structured exercise programs play an important role in weight management because they contribute to long-term weight loss by facilitating energy expenditure. Overweight and obese individuals can exhibit weight loss when they expend more daily calories on average than they consume.

Although any energy expenditure provided by increased physical activity and/or structured exercise can lead to weight loss for obese individuals, the effect is even more pronounced after the initial 6 months of adopting an intervention program.[38] Regular physical activity appears to be important in the long term for sustaining significant weight loss and preventing weight regain.[45] Furthermore, a review of the literature suggests that diet plus exercise, rather than diet only or exercise only, produces significantly greater weight loss at 12 months, 18 months, and 36 months after the adoption of a weight-loss intervention.[46] Thus, the influence of managing caloric intake through healthy eating behaviors is an important factor in long-term weight-loss success that must not be overlooked.

## In Your Own Words

After regularly exercising for 1 month, an obese colleague has lost only 4 pounds. He is discouraged by this slow rate of weight loss. How would you explain his progress to him in a way that would encourage him to continue with his exercise program?

## PHYSICAL ACTIVITY AND LONGEVITY

Assuming that physical activity improves health status, researchers have studied the association between physical activity and longevity. Classic research data on health and longevity among London bus conductors and postmen in the 1950s revealed that men in physically active jobs had less coronary heart disease during middle age compared with men in physically inactive occupations (Fig. 2-10). For example, the drivers of London's double-decker buses were more likely to die suddenly of heart complications than the conductors, who spent most of their time walking the aisles of the buses and climbing up and down the stairs to collect fares. It was also found that government clerks, who spent most of their time sitting at a desk, suffered more

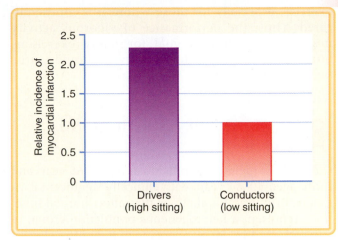

**Figure 2-10.** According to the data in this figure, men who sat more hours per week (conductors vs. drivers) while at work had a 125% greater incidence of experiencing a myocardial infarction compared with those who were more active during the work day. *(Data from Morris JN, Heady JA, Raffle PA, Roberts CG, Parks JW. Coronary heart disease and physical activity of work. Lancet 1953;265:1053–1057.)*

often from fatal heart attacks than did postmen, who spent most of their days walking.[47] These findings sparked the beginning of the field of **physical activity epidemiology**, or the formal study of epidemiological investigation into the associations of physical activity with many health outcomes.[48]

Indeed, evidence does support the current recommendations that emphasize moderate-intensity physical activity, such as brisk walking, as having a positive impact on increasing the duration of life. Further, the evidence is even stronger for an association between vigorous activity and longevity.[49] For example, the estimation of remaining life expectancy among 50-year-old men in the Framingham Heart Study showed an approximate 4-year longer life expectancy for men reporting high levels of physical activity and a slightly less than 2-year longer life expectancy for men reporting medium levels of physical activity compared with a sedentary group.[1,50]

These data indicate that participation in moderate-intensity physical activities showed a trend toward lower mortality rates, whereas greater energy expended in vigorous activities clearly predicted lower mortality rates. In contrast, participation in light-intensity physical activities, regardless of energy expenditure, does not reduce mortality rates. These findings are in line with the physical activity and health dose–response relationship described earlier in the chapter such that more activity is associated with greater health benefits. Another advantage of performing vigorous exercise is its efficiency in increasing energy expenditure. That is, one half hour of vigorous exercise expends as much energy as does moderate activity carried out for two to three times as long.

Although vigorous activity provides the most benefits in terms of longevity, it is not feasible to expect all individuals to be capable of performing high-intensity exercise, especially for those whom it is contraindicated. Thus, the performance of vigorous activity might be an ultimate goal for many exercisers, but the benefits of moderate activity should not be overlooked.

## CHRONIC DISEASE AND THE AGING POPULATION

Older adults (defined as individuals aged ≥65 years and those aged 50–64 years with clinically significant conditions or physical limitations that affect normal function) represent a heterogeneous population group, in which the individuals vary greatly in their physiological capabilities.[48] Among older adults, chronic diseases and their associated health limitations are a major problem that can reduce seniors' health-related quality of life. These conditions can cause years of pain, disability, and loss of function and independence. At least 80% of older Americans live with at least one chronic condition, and 50% have at least two.[52] The percentage of older adults who report very good or excellent health decreases with age. Based on research collected from the 2001 National Health Interview Survey, the CDC reports that 43% of men and women aged ≥65 years reported very good or excellent health, compared with 34% of those aged 75 to 84 years and only 28% of those aged ≥85 years.[53]

Because life expectancy in the United States has increased dramatically in the 20th century, from about 47 years in 1900 to about 75 years for males and 80 years for females in 2003, older adults are living for an extended period with chronic ailments that tend to appear in the fourth decade of life.[54] Conditions such as CVD, cancer, diabetes, arthritis, and cognitive impairment are challenges that many seniors must manage as they advance in age.

Regardless of age and health limitations, older adults can expect to experience significant physiological and psychological benefits from regular physical activity including decreased risk for clinical depression and anxiety, and a reduced risk for cognitive decline and dementia. (Fig. 2-11).[11] Table 2-6 lists some of the benefits experienced by previously sedentary older adults after they participated in regular cardiorespiratory and resistance training programs.

Although the benefits of physical-activity participation by older adults are well-known, only about 21% of individuals aged ≥65 years engage in regular physical activity. As people get older, even fewer individuals engage in physical activity (i.e., <10% of those older than 85 years regularly participate in some form of physical activity).[55] This presents a public health-care challenge as a greater proportion of the population advances into old age and many older adults succumb unnecessarily to preventable chronic diseases that could be improved or eliminated through regular participation in physical activity.

---

## RESEARCH HIGHLIGHT

### Exercise and Longevity: It's Never Too Late to Start

Research on the association between physical activity and mortality rates has suggested that the introduction of regular exercise even later in life can positively influence longevity. In an investigation of mortality rates in sedentary versus physically active middle-aged men, researchers found that changes in physical activity between the ages of 50 and 60 were associated with mortality.[51] Swedish researchers categorized 2,205 male study subjects (first surveying them from 1970 to 1973 when the men were 50 years old) into 4 groups based on their levels of physical activity—sedentary, low, medium, or high. Follow-up surveys were performed on the subjects at the ages of 60, 70, 77, and 82 years.

Byberg and colleagues[51] discovered that after a 10-year period of increased physical activity, the mortality rate for the previously inactive men was reduced to the same levels of mortality as seen in physically active men. The study team found that more physical activity translated to lower mortality rates; for those in the low-, medium-, and high-level groups, the absolute mortality rates were 27.1, 23.6, and 18.4 per 1,000 person-years, respectively. The researchers reported, however, that the improvement in mortality rate was observed 10 years after the change in habitual activity. That is, for the first 5 years of follow-up, men who had increased their physical activity still experienced higher mortality, as compared with those who had continuously been highly active throughout the years. This suggests that a sustained period of regular physical activity of at least 5 years would be necessary for low-level exercisers to receive the same longevity benefits as high-level exercisers.

The authors of the study also reported that the improved longevity associated with increased physical activity in midlife (compared with continued inactivity) was similar to that seen after smoking cessation (compared with continued smoking).[51] Thus, efforts for promotion of physical activity, even among middle-aged individuals, are important.

Byberg L, Melhus H, Gedeborg R, et al. (2009). Total mortality after changes in leisure time physical activity in 50-year-old men: 35-year follow-up of population based cohort. *Br Med J.* 2009;338:b688.

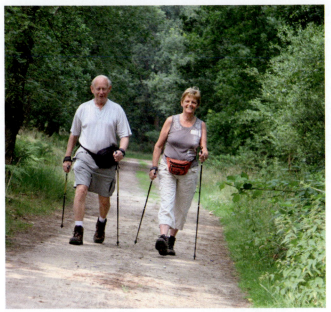

**Figure 2-11.** Older adults can expect to experience significant physiological and psychological benefits from regular physical activity.

## Quality of Life

Factors such as physical, social, cognitive, and emotional functioning can influence the overall quality of an individual's life.[56] Regular physical activity has a positive impact in many of these domains (Table 2-7). The benefits of physical activity are especially important for older adults, because they are more likely to develop chronic diseases and are more likely to have conditions that can affect their physical function.[57] For example, one study of older men demonstrated that leisure-time physical activity was more important for protecting against heart disease in men older than 65 years than in younger men.[58]

One of the most significant factors of quality of life for older adults is the ability to live independently. Evidence suggests that the mobility and functioning of frail and very old adults can be improved by regular physical activity.[57] For midlife and older adults of all ages and abilities, adopting regular physical activity as part of a healthy lifestyle may extend years of active independent life, reduce or prevent chronic disease and

## Table 2-6. Select Benefits of Regular Exercise in Previously Sedentary Older Adults

| TYPE OF TRAINING | EFFECT |
| --- | --- |
| Cardiorespiratory Endurance Training<br>• ≥60% $\dot{V}O_{2max}$ pre-exercise training<br>• ≥3 days/week<br>• ≥16 weeks | |
| Aerobic exercise capacity | Significantly increases in healthy middle-aged and older adults |
| Cardiovascular function | Enhanced in healthy middle-aged and older adults |
| Body composition | Total body fat is reduced in overweight, healthy middle-aged and older adults |
| Metabolic function | Enhanced in healthy middle-aged and older adults |
| Resistance Training<br>Variety of methods including:<br>  • Isometric<br>  • Isokinetic<br>  • 1-RM and 3-RM protocols | |
| Muscle strength | Substantially increases in older adults |
| Muscle power (torque of muscular power × velocity) | Substantially increases in older adults |
| Muscle endurance | Improved after moderate- and high-intensity protocols, but not after low-intensity protocols |
| Body composition | Improved after moderate- and high-intensity protocols |
| Bone health | Improved bone mineral density* |

*Bone mineral density is a measure of the amount of minerals (mainly calcium) contained in a certain volume of bone.
1 RM, one-repetition maximum; 3 RM, three-repetition maximum.
Adapted from American College of Sports Medicine. Position stand: Exercise and physical activity for older adults. *Med Sci Sports Exerc.* 1998;30:992–1008.

**Table 2-7. Health Domains Positively Influenced by Regular Physical Activity in Older Adults**

| | |
|---|---|
| Physiological well-being | Lower overall mortality<br>Lower risk for coronary heart disease<br>Lower risk for colon cancer<br>Lower risk for diabetes<br>Lower risk for development of high blood pressure; decreased blood pressure in individuals who have hypertension<br>Lower risk for obesity<br>Lower risk for certain cancers |
| Physical well-being | Improved dyspnea<br>Decreased fatigue<br>Decreased pain<br>Improved symptom perception<br>Improved appetite<br>Improved sleep patterns<br>Improved quality of life<br>Improved performance of activities of daily living<br>Lower risk for falls and injury |
| Psychological well-being | Improved self-concept<br>Increased self-esteem<br>Improved mood<br>Reduced anxiety<br>Lower risk for development of depression |
| Social function (in group programs) | Increased social interaction<br>Increased social support<br>Decreased social isolation |

From the Centers for Disease Control and Prevention. *Physical Activity and Older Americans: Benefits and Strategies*. Agency for Healthcare Research and Quality and the Centers for Disease Control and Prevention. 2002. http://www.ahrq.gov/ppip/activity.html; and Shephard RJ. *Aging, Physical Activity and Health*. Champaign, IL: Human Kinetics; 1997.

disability, and improve overall quality of life.[2,44,59–61] Clearly, few factors contribute as much to successful aging as having a physically active lifestyle.

## In Your Own Words

How would you explain to one of your grandparents the importance of regular exercise as it affects quality of life?

## Musculoskeletal Fitness in Older Adults

As noted earlier in this chapter, much of the research on physical activity and health has been focused on the benefits of engaging in cardiorespiratory exercise. However, the importance of musculoskeletal fitness (i.e., muscle strength, muscle power, muscle endurance, and flexibility), especially in older adults, cannot be overlooked. Figure 2-12 highlights the differences in all-cause mortality rate across different levels of muscular fitness.[62] The ability to perform **activities of daily living** does not require a large aerobic output, but depends on one or more of the musculoskeletal fitness components. For example, older adults who experience declines in musculoskeletal function may find it difficult to get out of a chair or climb stairs. This could lead to a cycle of decline wherein reduced musculoskeletal

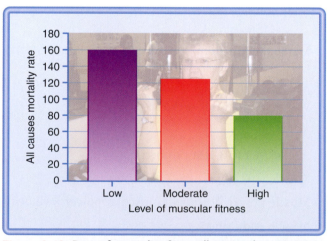

**Figure 2-12.** Rate of mortality from all causes (per 10,000 person-years) by levels of muscular fitness. According to this data, individuals who are at the lowest end of the muscular fitness range have a much greater risk of death (160 individuals per 10,000 people in a population per year) than individuals who are moderately or highly fit. *(Data from Ruiz JR, Sui X, Lobelo F, Morrow JR Jr, Jackson AW, Sjostrom M, Blair SN. Association between muscular strength and mortality in men: prospective cohort study. BMJ 2008;337:a439. doi:10.1136/bmj.a439.)*

fitness results in inactivity and further dependence. Thus, improving and maintaining musculoskeletal fitness later in life has a significant impact on delaying or eliminating the onset of disability, dependence, and chronic disease (e.g., diabetes mellitus, stroke, arthritis, coronary artery disease, and pulmonary disorders).[15,63,64] Chapter 26 provides additional content about this population.

## VIGNETTE conclusion

■ Three months after beginning his structured exercise program, in addition to making healthier nutrition choices on the advice from his fitness trainer, Vince has lost 20 pounds and feels great. His joints are no longer aching, and he claims to have a more positive outlook most of the time. Vince still has slight discomfort in his lower back (especially when he travels long distances), but he reports that as his trunk musculature becomes stronger and better able to stabilize his spine as a result of his core training, he continues to notice a decrease in the level of pain.

At a recent doctor's visit, Vince is pleased that his physician has categorized him in the overweight rather than the obese category, and that his blood pressure has normalized. He has only 10 more pounds to lose to reach his ideal body weight. The physician encourages him to continue his new healthy lifestyle, which includes exercise and healthy eating habits.

At the beginning of Vince's transformation, he performed minimal amounts of physical activity and reported feeling more energy and a positive mood on the days he was active. If Vince would have stopped his progression of activity and remained at very low daily activity levels, he would have continued to notice small improvements in his overall health status and quality of life. However, because Vince chose to progress his activity to incorporate a structured exercise program, he experienced even more health benefits and lost weight in the process. This represents the dose–response relationship between physical activity and health such that some activity is better than none, and more activity, up to a point, is better than less.

## CRITICAL THINKING QUESTIONS

1. Explain how a person who is lacking in any one of the health-related components of physical fitness might be affected in his or her daily activities.

2. How does regular physical activity benefit obese individuals, even if it does not result in weight loss?

3. Considering the evidence that vigorous-intensity exercise provides a more efficient path to increased fitness, explain why recommending moderate-intensity exercise for overweight/obese individuals is appropriate.

4. How can encouraging obese individuals to become more physically active ultimately slow the progression of chronic disease that is prevalent in many developed nations?

5. How does a disproportionately large aging population impact public health-care costs?

## ADDITIONAL RESOURCES

**Books and Articles**

American College of Sports Medicine. *ACSM's Guidelines for Exercise Testing and Prescription* (9th ed.). Philadelphia: Lippincott Williams & Wilkins; 2014.

American College of Sports Medicine. Position stand: Appropriate physical activity intervention strategies for weight loss and prevention of weight regain for adults. *Med Sci Sports Exerc.* 2009;41:459–471.

American College of Sports Medicine. Position stand: Exercise and physical activity for older adults. *Med Sci Sports Exerc.* 1998;30:992–1008.

American College of Sports Medicine. Position stand: Physical activity, physical fitness, and hypertension. *Med Sci Sports Exerc.* 1993;25:i–x.

Warburton ER, Whitney-Nichol C, Bredin SD. Health benefits of physical activity: The evidence. *Can Med Assoc J.* 2006;174:801–809.

Warburton ER, Whitney-Nichol C, Bredin SD. Prescribing exercise as preventive therapy. *Can Med Assoc J.* 2006;174:961–974.

**Websites**

American Council on Exercise: www.acefitness.org
American College of Sports Medicine: www.acsm.org
American Heart Association: www.heart.org
The Obesity Society: www.obesity.org
International Council on Active Aging: www.icaa.cc

## References

1. Jonker JT, De Laet C, Franco OH, Peeters A, Mackenbach J, Nusselder WJ. Physical activity and life expectancy with and without diabetes: Life table analysis of the Framingham Heart Study. *Diabetes Care.* 2006; 29:38–43.
2. U.S. Department of Health and Human Services. *Physical activity and health: A report of the Surgeon General.* Atlanta, GA: Centers for Disease Control and Prevention; 1996.
3. Warburton ER, Whitney-Nichol C, Bredin SD. Health benefits of physical activity: The evidence. *Can Med Assoc J.* 2006;174:801–809.
4. Katzmarzyk PT, Gledhill N, Shephard RJ. The economic burden of physical inactivity in Canada. *Can Med Assoc J.* 2000;163:1435–1440.
5. Caspersen CJ, Powell KE, Christenson GM. Physical activity, exercise, and physical fitness: Definitions and distinctions for health-related research. *Public Health Rep.* 1985;100:126–131.
6. Kesaniemi YK, Danforth Jr E, Jensen MD, Kopelman PG, Lefebvre P, Reeder BA. Dose-response issues concerning physical activity and health: An evidence-based symposium. *Med Sci Sports Exerc.* 2001;33:S351–S358.
7. Lee IM, Skerrett PJ. Physical activity and all-cause mortality: What is the dose-response relation? *Med Sci Sports Exerc.* 2001;33:S459–S471.
8. Haskell WL, Lee IM, Pate RR, et al. Physical activity and public health: Updated recommendation from the American College of Sports Medicine and the American Heart Association. *Med Sci Sports Exerc.* 2007;39:1423–1434.
9. National Institutes of Health. Physical activity and cardiovascular health. NIH Consensus Development Panel on Physical Activity and Cardiovascular Health. *J Am Med Assoc.* 1996;276:241–246.
10. Pate RR, Pratt M, Blair SN, et al. Physical activity and public health: A recommendation from the Centers for Disease Control and the American College of Sports Medicine. *J Am Med Assoc.* 1995;273:402–407.
11. American College of Sports Medicine. Position stand: Exercise and physical activity for older adults. *Med Sci Sports Exerc.* 1998;30:992–1008.
12. Shephard RJ. Absolute versus relative intensity of physical activity in a dose-response context. *Med Sci Sports Exerc.* 2001;33:S400–S418.
13. Taylor RS, Brown A, Ebrahim S, et al. Exercise-based rehabilitation for patients with coronary heart disease: Systematic review and meta-analysis of randomized controlled trials. *Am J Med.* 2004;116:682–692.
14. U.S. Department of Health and Human Services. Office of Disease Prevention and Health Promotion. *2008 Physical Activity Guidelines for Americans.* 2008. www.health.gov/PAGuidelines/pdf/paguide.pdf.
15. Warburton DE, Gledhill N, Quinney A. The effects of changes in musculoskeletal fitness on health. *Canadian Journal of Applied Physiology* 2001;26:161–216.
16. Williams PT. Physical fitness and activity as separate heart disease risk factors: A meta-analysis. *Med Sci Sports Exerc.* 2001;33:754–761.
17. American College of Sports Medicine. *ACSM's Guidelines for Exercise Testing and Prescription* (9th ed.). Philadelphia: Lippincott Williams & Wilkins; 2014.
18. Centers for Disease Control and Prevention. Trends in leisure time physical inactivity by sex, age, and race/ethnicity: United States—1994–2004. *Morb Mrtl Wkly Rep.* 2005;54:1208–1212.
19. Hamilton MT, Hamilton DG, Zderic TW. Role of low energy expenditure and sitting in obesity, metabolic syndrome, type 2 diabetes, and cardiovascular disease. *Diabetes.* 2007;56:2655–2667.
20. Australian Bureau of Statistics. Labour Force, Australia. Canberra, ACT: Australian Bureau of Statistics; 2009.
21. Van Uffelen JGZ, Wong J, Chau JY, et al. Occupational sitting and health risks: A systematic review. *Am J Prev Med.* 2010;39:379–388.
22. Brown WJ, Miller YD, Miller R. Sitting time and work patterns as indicators of overweight and obesity in Australian adults. *Int J Obes Relat Metab Disord.* 2003; 27:1340–1346.
23. Jans MP, Proper KI, Hildebrandt VH. Sedentary behavior in Dutch workers: Differences between occupations and business sectors. *Am J Prev Med.* 2007;33: 450–454.
24. Bureau of Labor Statistics. News. U.S. Department of Labor, June 24, 2009. http://www.bls.gov/news.release/archives/atus_06242009.pdf
25. Healy GN, Matthews CE, Dunstan DW, Winkler EAH, Owen N. Sedentary time and cardio-metabolic biomarkers in U.S. adults: NHANES 2003–06. *Eur Heart J.* 2011;32:590–597.
26. Thompson WG, Levine JA. Productivity of transcriptionists using a treadmill desk. *Work.* 2011;40:473–477.
27. Paffenbarger RS, Wing AL, Hyde RT, et al. Physical activity and hypertension: An epidemiological view. *Ann Med.* 1991;23:319–327.
28. Adamopoulos S, Parissis J, Kroupis C, et al. Physical training reduces peripheral markers of inflammation in patients with chronic heart failure. *Eur Heart J.* 2001;22:791–797.
29. Church TS, Barlow CE, Earnest CP, Kampert JB, Priest EL, Blair SN. Associations between cardiorespiratory fitness and C-reactive protein in men. *Arterioscler Thromb Vasc Biol.* 2002;22:1869–1876.
30. Mora S, Lee IM, Buring JE, Ridker PM. Association of physical activity and body mass index with novel and traditional cardiovascular biomarkers in women. *J Am Med Assoc.* 2006;295:1412–1419.
31. Panagiotakos DB, Pitsavos C, Chrysohoou C, Kavouras S, Stefanadis C. The associations between leisure-time physical activity and inflammatory and coagulation markers related to cardiovascular disease: The ATTICA study. *Prev Med.* 2004;40:432–437.
32. Gokce N, Vita JA, Bader DS, et al. Effect of exercise on upper and lower extremity endothelial function in patients with coronary artery disease. *Am J Cardiol.* 2002;90:124–127.
33. Kobayashi N, Tsuruya Y, Iwasawa T, et al. Exercise training in patients with chronic heart failure improves endothelial function predominantly in the trained extremities. *Circ J.* 2003;67:505–510.
34. McGavock J, Mandic S, Lewanczuk R, et al. Cardiovascular adaptations to exercise training in postmenopausal women with type 2 diabetes mellitus. *Cardiovasc Diabetol.* 2004;3:3.
35. Dunn AL, Trivedi MH, O'Neal HA. Physical activity dose–response effects on outcomes of depression and anxiety. *Med Sci Sports Exerc.* 2001;33:S587–S597.
36. Helmchen LA, Henderson RM. Changes in the distribution of body mass index of white US men, 1890–2000. *Ann Hum Biol.* 2004;31:174–181.
37. Ogden CL, Carroll MD, Curtin LR, McDowell MA, Tabak CJ, Flegal KM. Prevalence of overweight and obesity in the United States, 1999–2004. *J Am Med Assoc.* 2006;295:1549–1555.
38. National Heart, Lung and Blood Institute (NHLBI). *Obesity Education Initiative Expert Panel. Clinical Guidelines on the Identification, Evaluation, and Treatment of*

*Overweight and Obesity in Adults: The Evidence Report* [NIH publication No. 98-4083]. Bethesda, MD: National Institutes of Health; 1998.

39. Jensen GL. Obesity and functional decline: Epidemiology and geriatric consequences. *Clin Geriatr Med.* 2005; 21:677–687.

40. Fontaine KR, Barofsky I. Obesity and health-related quality of life. *Obes Rev.* 2001;2:173–182.

41. Fontaine KR, Redden DT, Wang C, et al. Years of life lost due to obesity. *J Am Med Assoc.* 2003;289:187–193.

42. Knowler WC, Barrett-Connor E, Fowler SE, et al. Reduction in the incidence of type 2 diabetes with lifestyle intervention or metformin. *N Engl J Med.* 2002;346:393–403.

43. Bray GA. The missing link—lose weight, live longer. *N Engl. J Med.* 2007;357:818–820.

44. Stewart AL. Community-based physical activity programs for adults age 50 and older. *J Aging Phys Act.* 2001;9(Suppl.):71–91.

45. American College of Sports Medicine. Position stand: Appropriate physical activity intervention strategies for weight loss and prevention of weight regain for adults. *Med Sci Sports Exerc.* 2009;41:459–471.

46. Avenell A, Broom J, Brown TJ, et al. Systematic review of the long-term effects and economic consequences of treatments for obesity and implications for health improvement. *Health Technol Assess.* 2004;21:1–465.

47. Morris JN, Crawford MD. Coronary heart disease and physical activity of work. *Br Med J.* 1958;2:1485–1496.

48. Shiroma EJ, Lee I. Physical activity and cardiovascular health: Lessons learned from epidemiological studies across age, gender, and race/ethnicity. *Circulation.* 2010;122:743–752.

49. Lee IM, Paffenbarger RS. Associations of light, moderate, and vigorous intensity physical activity with longevity: The Harvard Alumni Health Study. *Am J Epidemiol.* 2000;151:293–299.

50. Franco OH, De Laet C, Peeters A, Jonker J, Mackenbach J, Nusselder W. Effects of physical activity on life expectancy with cardiovascular disease. *Arch Intern Med.* 2005;165:2355–2360.

51. Byberg L, Melhus H, Gedeborg R, et al. Total mortality after changes in leisure time physical activity in 50-year-old men: 35-year follow-up of population based cohort. *Br Med J.* 2009;338:b688.

52. Centers for Disease Control and Prevention. Public health and aging: Trends in aging—United States and worldwide. *Morbid Mrtl Wkly Rep.* 2003;52:101–106.

53. Centers for Disease Control and Prevention and The Merck Company Foundation. *The State of Aging and Health in America 2007.* Whitehouse Station, NJ: The Merck Company Foundation; 2007. www.cdc.gov/aging/pdf/saha_2007.pdf.

54. Arias E. United States life tables, 2006. *Natl Vital Stat Rep.* 2010;58:21.

55. Federal Interagency Forum on Aging-related Statistics. *Older Americans 2004: Key Indicator of Well-being.* Washington, DC: U.S. Government Printing Office; 2004.

56. Rejeski WJ, Brawley LR, Shumaker SA. Relationships between physical activity and health-related quality of life. *Exerc Sport Sci Rev.* 1996;24:71–108.

57. Centers for Disease Control and Prevention. *Physical Activity and Older Americans: Benefits and Strategies.* Rockville, MD: Agency for Healthcare Research and Quality and the Centers for Disease Control and Prevention; 2002. www.ahrq.gov/ppip/activity.htm

58. Talbot LA, Morrell CH, Metter EJ, Fleg JL. Comparison of cardiorespiratory fitness versus leisure time physical activity as predictors of coronary events in men aged ≤65 years and >65 years. *Am J Cardiol.* 2002;89:1187–1192.

59. Atienza AA. Home-based physical activity programs for middle-aged and older adults: Summary of empirical research. *J Aging Phys Act.* 2001;9(Suppl.):38–58.

60. Eakin E. Promoting physical activity among middle-aged and older adults in health care settings. *J Aging Phys Act.* 2001;9(Suppl.):29–37.

61. Linnan LA, Marcus B. Worksite-based physical activity programs and older adults: Current status and priorities for the future. *J Aging Phys Act.* 2001;9(Suppl.): 59–70.

62. Ruiz JR, Sui X, Lobelo F, et al. Association between muscular strength and mortality in men: Prospective cohort study. *BMJ* 2008;337:a439. doi:10.1136/bmj.a439

63. Katzmarzyk PT, Craig CL. Musculoskeletal fitness and risk of mortality. *Med Sci Sports Exerc.* 2002; 34:740–744.

64. Warburton DE, Gledhill N, Quinney A. Musculoskeletal fitness and health. *Can J Appl Physiol.* 2001;26: 217–237.

65. Ainsworth BE, Haskell WL, Whitt MC, et al. Compendium of physical activities: an update of activity codes and MET intensities. *Med Sci Sports Exerc.* 2000;32:S498–S504.

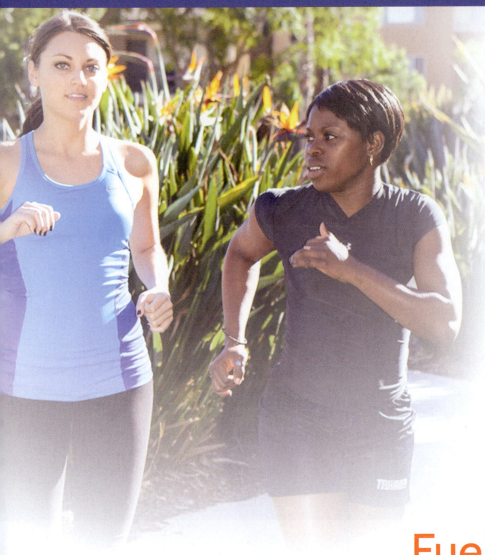

# PART II
## Fueling Physical Activity

This section of the textbook presents information relevant to providing energy for physical activity and exercise. Chapter 3 focuses specifically on the macronutrients and micronutrients in the diet, and their specific roles within the body. Chapter 4 then details the specific energy pathways that provide the energy to perform physical work. A major focus is on the interplay between the anaerobic and aerobic pathways, and how they seamlessly interact to supply energy when the body is at rest all the way up to maximal exertion. Chapter 5 introduces the concept of energy balance (i.e., the balance between caloric intake vs. caloric expenditure) and how that impacts weight management.

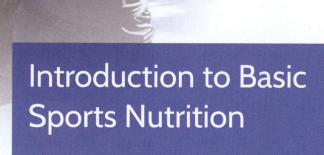

Christopher Mohr, PhD
Fabio Comana, MA, MS

CHAPTER 3

# Introduction to Basic Sports Nutrition

## CHAPTER OUTLINE

## LEARNING OUTCOMES

1. Define *macronutrients* and *micronutrients*.
2. Describe the structure, function, and storage locations for carbohydrates.
3. Describe the structure, function, and storage locations for fats.
4. Describe the structure, function, and storage locations for proteins.
5. Differentiate structure, functions, and roles among the three macronutrients.
6. Explain the concept and importance of glycemic index and glycemic load.
7. Identify key health benefits and concerns of fiber and fructose.
8. Explain protein quality scoring systems.
9. Identify the key functions of vitamins and minerals within the body.

## ANCILLARY LINK

Visit Davis*Plus* at http://davisplus.fadavis.com for study and practice resources, including online quizzes, animations that help explain physiological processes, podcasts concerning news and career trends in exercise physiology, and practice references.

## VIGNETTE

■ Catherine is confused about what she should be eating. She constantly reads in magazines that carbohydrates should be avoided and how they are often blamed for "fattening America." She has also talked with friends who have suggested that she start eating low-carbohydrate alternatives to help her reduce her weight and transform her body from "flab-to-fab." Although she would like to lose weight, she has also heard that reducing or eliminating carbohydrates from her diet can be harmful. Consequently, she is frustrated over this conflicting information and does not clearly understand the roles that food plays within the body. Catherine visits with Becky, a sports nutritionist who, in addition to working with local college sports teams, specializes in helping clients achieve and maintain weight loss.

What advice could Becky give Catherine to help her make a healthy decision about how to get started on her weight-loss journey?

The term nutrition refers to the overall process of ingestion, digestion, absorption, and metabolism of food. All of these processes allow nutrients from food to be assimilated and used by the tissues of the body. The guidelines for healthy nutrition apply to both physically active and sedentary individuals alike, although some recommendations do differ between these two populations (e.g., timing of nutrient intake and amount of carbohydrates needed). Considering the fact that the needs of athletes and physically active individuals are primarily driven by the demand for additional calories, any increase in caloric intake will typically translate into an increase in both macronutrients (carbohydrates, fats, and proteins) and micronutrients, assuming the additional calories come from nutritious foods. The nutritional and hydration needs of active individuals and athletes are discussed in Chapter 20.

This chapter explores the basic, underlying principles of good nutrition and nutrients, including how this information can be applied in practice. You will learn the difference between macronutrients and micronutrients, and the needs that the body has for each. The structure, function, and storage of the three macronutrient categories are described, as well as fundamental information on hydration, vitamins, and minerals.

## NUTRIENTS

The foods we eat provide nutrients. A **nutrient** can be classified as essential or nonessential; it is a basic component of food that contributes to cell growth, plays a role in cell repair, and is necessary for cell maintenance.[1] **Essential nutrients** must be obtained from the diet—they cannot be manufactured within the body and, therefore, must be obtained directly from food sources. In contrast, **nonessential nutrients** are nutrients that can be manufactured by the body as needed. Nutrients work synergistically to maintain physiological function.

Foods are considered nutrient-dense when they provide high quantities of essential and nonessential nutrients relative to the calories they provide. In contrast, foods are considered calorically dense when they provide a high quantity of calories relative to the nutrients they provide.

There are six general categories of nutrients, each of which serves different functions within the body. They are traditionally subdivided into **macronutrients** (carbohydrates, proteins, and fats) and **micronutrients** (water, minerals, and vitamins). The word *macro* implies larger quantities, whereas the word *micro* implies smaller quantities. For example, a 140-pound (63.6 kg) female may need 51 g protein each day, but only 75 mg vitamin C daily. Ironically, although water has traditionally been classified as a micronutrient, it is actually needed in far greater quantities by the body than any macronutrient to survive (e.g., the Institute of Medicine daily water recommendation

for sedentary females is 91 oz. [2.7 L]).[2] Furthermore, although adults can survive for approximately 30 days without food, they could survive only about 10 days without water.[3]

Although both macronutrients and micronutrients are essential for health, the primary focus of this chapter is on the macronutrients: carbohydrates, fats, and proteins, including their general structure, function, and storage within the body. Vitamins and minerals are briefly introduced in this chapter, and water is discussed in detail in Chapter 12.

## Macronutrients

Macronutrients not only provide nutrients, but also calories, which are needed to fuel all physiological functions within the body. A key function of carbohydrates is to provide energy for the body, specifically for the brain and muscles. Fats, although providing the largest source of energy, are a necessary structural component of every cell. Fats help protect internal organs against injury and provide many essential nutrients (fat-soluble vitamins and essential fatty acids [EFAs]). Proteins help build and repair tissues, and provide essential amino acids.

## Micronutrients

Micronutrients, which include water, vitamins, and minerals, do not provide energy, but they are needed to regulate various body processes. Water comprises approximately 60% of total body weight. It provides a medium for transportation, structural integrity to cells, and is crucial for numerous chemical reactions within the body.[4] Vitamins and minerals contribute to our health and function in many ways, including supporting normal growth and development, metabolism of macronutrients to energy, healthy bone and red blood cell development, and good immune function.[5,6]

## CARBOHYDRATES

**Carbohydrates** are made up of three basic elements: carbon, hydrogen, and oxygen, hence the name "carbo" (implying carbon) and "hydrate" (implying water or hydrogen and oxygen). Carbohydrates serve various functions within the body. One key function includes providing energy as glucose to the brain, central nervous system, and red blood cells, and as a fuel to working muscles for exercise and activity. Carbohydrates located in tissue are stored as glycogen, the storage form of glucose, and found primarily within muscle and liver tissue.

**Glycogen** provides fuel for sustained periods of exercise or activity in muscle tissue, whereas liver glycogen helps maintain normal blood levels for physiological function. A defining characteristic of liver glycogen is that it can be released as glucose into blood circulation. By comparison, muscle glucose cannot be released into circulation because the glucose molecules released from muscle glycogen undergo a small structural change (phosphorylation, or the addition of phosphate to the glucose units); this essentially traps glucose molecules inside the cell. Therefore, the body relies on liver glycogen to maintain blood sugar and to help deliver additional glucose to the working muscles.

Because there are no essential carbohydrates, the body can always make glucose from other carbohydrates consumed in our diet or from noncarbohydrate sources during extreme situations, such as with fasting or very low-carbohydrate diets. This process of creating glucose from noncarbohydrates sources occurs within the liver and is termed **gluconeogenesis**. Carbohydrates are also considered a "fat primer," which means that the complete metabolism of fats requires the presence of carbohydrates. This concept is discussed in detail in Chapter 4.

## Structure

Although a scientific classification system based on chemical structures exists, carbohydrates are broadly classified as either simple or complex. These are more commonly referred to as sugars (simple) and starches (complex). The scientific nomenclature of carbohydrates is derived from their chemical structure and size. Carbohydrates are divided into three general groups of sugar units called *saccharides:* **monosaccharides**, or single sugar units; **oligosaccharides**, with 2 to 10 sugar units (including **disaccharides**, or 2 sugar units, which represent the most common form of oligosaccharides); and **polysaccharides**, which contain more than 10 sugar units. With the exception of glycogen and lactose (milk sugar), all carbohydrate forms originate from plant sources.

## Simple Carbohydrates

Simple carbohydrates, also known as sugars, represent the monosaccharides (single sugar units) and disaccharides (two sugar units). Monosaccharides represent the only form of carbohydrate that the body can absorb; thus, all forms of carbohydrates eaten must be digested to this single sugar unit form before they can be absorbed into the body.

The three nutritionally important monosaccharides are (Fig. 3-1):
- Glucose
- Fructose (sometimes called *fruit sugar*)
- **Galactose** (found primarily in milk and other dairy products)

All three monosaccharides share the same molecular structure of $C_6H_{12}O_6$ and the same caloric density (4 kcal/g), but the structural arrangement of atoms within each molecule differs, giving each unique characteristics that make them significantly different. For example, glucose is absorbed more rapidly from the intestinal tract via a more active process, triggering an insulin response on entering the blood. Glucose is the preferred fuel used by the body and the most prevalent carbohydrate form found in the body, present as either blood glucose or as a sequence of glucose chains forming glycogen, the storage form of glucose in the body.[7]

Fructose is absorbed more slowly through the intestinal wall via a passive process. It does not trigger an insulin release on entry into the blood and is usually transported to the liver for conversion to glucose (if needed) or to fats (when carbohydrates are consumed in excess).

Galactose is absorbed by a similar process as glucose and is used in a limited capacity by the body to help build glycolipids and glycoproteins, cellular components that help develop our immune function (e.g., antibodies). Galactose is either derived from dietary sources (e.g., milk and sugar beets) or manufactured within the body. Mannose and ribose are other biological monosaccharides, but they hold no real nutritional or caloric value to the body.

Disaccharides are composed of two monosaccharides bonded together. The three nutritionally important disaccharides are (Fig. 3-2):
- Sucrose, which is a combination of one glucose and one fructose molecule

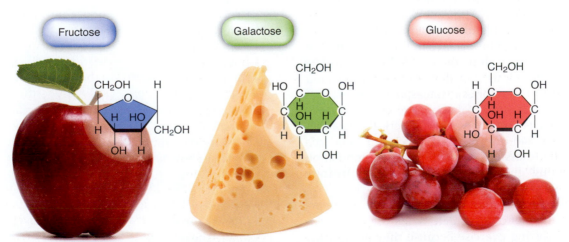

**Figure 3-1.** The three nutritionally important monosaccharides are glucose, fructose, and galactose.

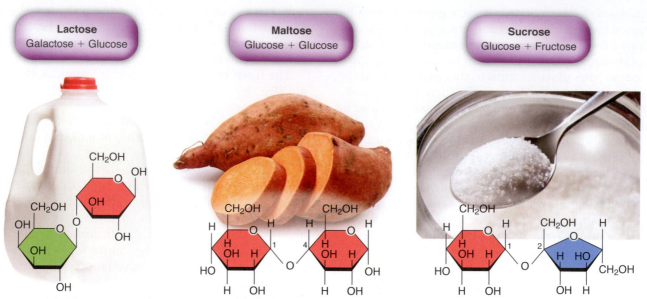

**Figure 3-2.** The three nutritionally important disaccharides are sucrose, lactose, and maltose.

- Lactose, which is a combination of one glucose and one galactose molecule
- Maltose, which is a combination of two glucose molecules

Each of these nutritionally important simple carbohydrates (monosaccharides and disaccharides) generally converts to glucose so the body can use it as fuel, store it as glycogen, or convert it to fat when consumed in excess. There are many forms of simple carbohydrates in our diets, such as honey, table sugar, fruits, and the sugar found in soft drinks and candy.

Most of the added sugars in our diets come from soft drinks and candy; the average American currently consumes a whopping 22 to 28 teaspoons of added sugar each day (equal to 350–440 empty calories), which is the equivalent of drinking 2 to 3 cans of soda daily.[8] To add another example of how much sugar is consumed in our diets, sugars make up approximately 50% of the carbohydrates we consume daily and almost 25% of all the total calories we consume daily. Current U.S. Department of Agriculture (USDA) dietary guidelines recommend that sugars constitute no more than 10% of our total caloric intake.[9] The American Heart Association guidelines recommend a maximum of 9 teaspoons daily, whereas Center for Science in the Public Interest recommends women limit their added sugars to 100 calories (6½ teaspoons) per day, and men limit their added sugars to 150 calories (9½ teaspoons) per day.[8,10] Considering the amount of sugar we currently consume and the fact that the average American consumes approximately 540 cans of 12 oz. (355 mL) soda each year, it is safe to assume that the general population is not meeting guidelines for simple carbohydrate intake.[11]

However, simple carbohydrates also play an important role in the diet of an athlete when used at appropriate times during exercise because they are quickly assimilated into the body to become available as a fuel for working muscles. Still, it is important to remember that they constitute only a small portion of the overall caloric intake of an athlete's diet. Carbohydrate recommendations during exercise are discussed in greater detail in Chapter 20.

In addition, although sugar content must be included on a food label, it is often "hidden" under different names. Do not be fooled, because these are all essentially simple carbohydrates. Common names of sugars found on food labels are listed in Box 3-1.

## Box 3-1. Common Names of Sugars Found on Food Labels

- Brown sugar
- Sucrose
- Sugar
- Confectioner's sugar
- High-fructose corn syrup (HFCS)
- Maltodextrin
- Turbinado sugar
- Glucose
- Lactose
- Date sugar
- Fruit sugar
- Dextrose
- Honey
- Corn syrup
- Molasses
- Caramel
- Brown rice syrup
- Molasses powder
- Maple syrup
- Dextrin
- Fructose
- Chicory syrup
- Maple sugar

## Complex Carbohydrates

Starches and dietary fiber constitute the complex carbohydrates. These structures generally contain longer chains of glucose molecules. Although oligosaccharides include some simple sugars, their structures contain up to 10 units, so they are known as complex carbohydrates. Examples include raffinose and stachyose, carbohydrates found in beans and some vegetables that are partially digestible and are known to cause some gastrointestinal (GI) distress (e.g., gas). Beano is a commercially available product that contains an enzyme called *alpha-galactosidase* that is capable of breaking down these oligosaccharides to reduce gas in the digestive tract. This improves digestion by reducing bloating and discomfort caused by gas formation from these carbohydrates during digestion.

Various more obscure oligosaccharides also exist and represent a small percentage of the carbohydrates we consume. For example, fructo-oligosaccharides, found in various vegetables, consist of short chains of fructose molecules. Galacto-oligosaccharides, found in various natural sources and breast milk, consist of short chains of galactose molecules. However, both of these compounds are only partially digested by humans.

Most carbohydrates in nature, in our diets, and in our bodies exist in longer chains ranging from more than 10 to many thousand units. These are called *polysaccharides,* and it is important to note that glucose units constitute these longer chains. These polysaccharides—starch, fiber, and glycogen—are found in three basic forms (Fig. 3-3):

- **Amylose:** Contains a straight chain format of glucose units that undergo digestion and absorption more slowly by the digestive enzymes because they can only break the molecule apart from its two open ends.
- **Amylopectins/Glycogen:** Contain a branched-chain format of glucose units that undergo digestion and absorption more rapidly because the digestive enzymes can break the molecule apart from its multiple open ends. Amylopectin is found

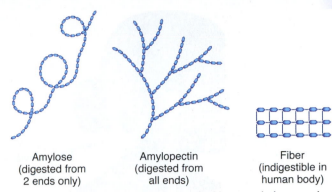

Amylose
(digested from
2 ends only)

Amylopectin
(digested from
all ends)

Fiber
(indigestible in
human body)

**Figure 3-3.** Polysaccharides (starch, fiber, and glycogen) are found in the following three basic forms: amylose, amylopectin, and fiber.

in plants, whereas glycogen is found in animals. Interestingly, the branched structure of these carbohydrates allows for the formation of stable starch gels that better retain water, thus proving ideal for making sauces and gravies.

- **Fiber:** Contains a blocklike chain format of glucose units in which the bonds holding each monosaccharide together ($\beta$-1, 4 bonds) are resistant to human digestive enzymatic activity; thus, these structures are not well digested or absorbed, but they play an important role in maintaining digestive health.

The general classifications of carbohydrates are outlined in Table 3-1. As described earlier, all carbohydrates, regardless of their original form, undergo digestion to monosaccharide forms before absorption. This basic sequence is illustrated in Figure 3-4. Some individuals are "lactose intolerant" and may suffer from a variety of GI distresses such as diarrhea when they consume dairy products. These individuals lack the enzyme lactase that is needed to digest the disaccharide lactose, so they cannot break this disaccharide down into its monosaccharide units (glucose and galactose). Therefore, it remains in the

## Table 3-1. General Classifications of Carbohydrates

| DESCRIPTION | NO. OF SUGAR UNITS | SOURCES |
|---|---|---|
| Simple sugar (monosaccharides) | Smallest carbohydrate unit<br>1 sugar unit<br>Absorbable form | Glucose<br>Fructose<br>Galactose |
| Simple sugar (disaccharides) | 2 sugar units | Sucrose (sugar) = 1 glucose + 1 fructose<br>Lactose (milk) = 1 glucose + 1 galactose<br>Maltose = 2 glucose |
| Complex carbohydrates (oligosaccharides) | 3–10 sugar units<br>Not well digested | Raffinose<br>Stachyose |
| Complex carbohydrates (polysaccharides) | Starch<br>>10 sugar units | Amylose<br>Amylopectin |
| Complex carbohydrates (fiber) | Indigestible starch | Soluble fiber (e.g., pectin)<br>Insoluble fiber (e.g., cellulose) |

*Note*: Carbohydrates are ordered by sweetest to least sweet.

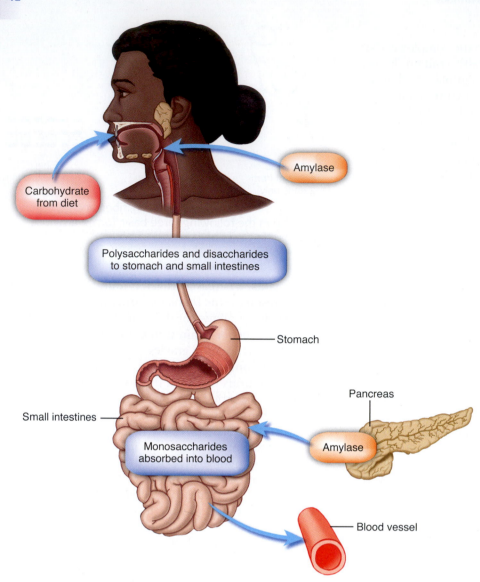

**Figure 3-4.** Overall process of carbohydrate digestion. Dietary carbohydrate is digested early by the enzyme amylase released from salivary glands in the mouth. This digestion forms polysaccharides and disaccharides. These sugars are further digested into monosaccharides through the stomach and small intestine with the use of pancreatic amylase and other enzymes in the gastrointestinal tract. The monosaccharides are absorbed through the lining of the small intestine and transported to the blood.

intestinal tract, where intestinal bacteria feed on it, causing some GI distress and discomfort. For these individuals, the solution is either to consume a "predigested" milk (i.e., lactose is broken down to glucose and galactose before consumption by adding the enzyme to the milk) or to take a pill that contains lactase before consuming dairy products. Table 3-1 shows that, as carbohydrates break down into monosaccharide forms, they generally become sweeter in taste. Thus, lactose-free milk has a slightly sweeter taste than regular milk.

## In Your Own Words

You are given the opportunity to present a brief educational session on healthy eating to a small group of 12-year-old children. Your focus is to help them make better dietary choices when selecting carbohydrate sources and help them understand differences between simple and complex carbohydrates. How would you explain these topics in an understandable way to these children? Remember to include food examples to help illustrate your point.

## VIGNETTE continued

■ Becky educates Catherine on the different kinds of carbohydrates and about the many important roles that carbohydrates play in the human body. Given her recent commitment to living a healthier, more active lifestyle with Becky's guidance, Catherine is particularly struck by the fact that carbohydrates are the body's preferred source of energy during physical activity. She agrees to limit, but not exclude, carbohydrates from her diet given this knowledge and is pleased that she has decided to ignore the quick-fix advice of her friends. She is more interested in adopting a healthier approach geared toward long-term weight-maintenance success and would like to now learn more about fats and proteins.

## Key Functions of Specific Carbohydrates

Glucose and blood sugar continue to receive significant attention through research, given their health and performance implications, but fiber and fructose have also become subjects of research, considering how they can positively and negatively impact an individual's health. Although glucose and the concept of glycemic index and glycemic load (GL) are discussed later in this chapter, this section focuses on the health risks and benefits of fiber and fructose.

## Fiber and Health

The whole-grain kernel is composed of several parts that include the husk, or brush (outermost shell), the bran (contains fiber), the endosperm (contains starch), and the innermost germ (contains minerals and vitamins), as illustrated in Figure 3-5. During the processing of whole grains, the husk, bran, and part of the germ are removed, leaving not much more than the endosperm, which has little nutrient value. In contrast, 100% whole-wheat grains contain an intact kernel loaded with health-promoting bran, fiber, vitamins, minerals (particularly the B vitamins, vitamin E, magnesium, and zinc), and various antioxidants. The general rule of thumb is to choose carbohydrates when the first ingredient on the label has the word *whole* in it and states 100% (e.g., 100% whole wheat or whole oats). In addition, many natural foods are also good sources of dietary fiber; these include:

- Cereals and other grains (All Bran, Kashi, whole-grain nuggets, Raisin Bran, whole-wheat spaghetti, and oatmeal)
- Fruits and vegetables (raspberries, blueberries, blackberries, pear with skin, broccoli, all potatoes with skin, corn, green beans, apples with skin, and bananas)

- Beans and nuts (pinto beans, black beans, kidney beans, lentils, almonds, pistachios, and walnuts)

Fiber can be classified as **soluble** and **insoluble**. Generally, fiber is known to provide several beneficial functions within the body, such as decreasing food intake by providing a feeling of fullness in the stomach, helping to maintain stable blood sugar (glucose) levels, improving intestinal health, preventing constipation, and decreasing fat and cholesterol absorption.[12]

Figure 3-6 provides a general comparison between soluble and insoluble fiber. It is important to remember that both types of fiber provide health benefits. Insoluble fibers help control the appetite by slowing gastric emptying and promoting a greater sensation of fullness (satiety). They attract water, which adds bulk to matter in our intestinal tract, resulting in greater movement of material through our intestinal tract and more frequent bowel movements. Furthermore, the presence of insoluble fiber can also slough away dead cells that line the intestinal tract or reduce the potential for food to become lodged within the folds of the tract, which can lead to colorectal cancer.

Soluble fibers bind to bile, a fat emulsifier manufactured in the liver from cholesterol and other substances. Bile is stored, released from, and reabsorbed back into the gallbladder. In doing so, soluble fibers not only potentially impede lipid absorption by interfering with bile function, but can also reduce bile reabsorption after fat digestion is complete, thus eliminating cholesterol from the body.

Fiber is therefore crucial for optimal health. Total fiber intake among adults in the United States is well below the recommended amounts. Table 3-2 provides the average and recommended daily intakes of fiber (grams) for adults.[12] Although fiber provides no calories, it may reduce the risk for heart disease, obesity,

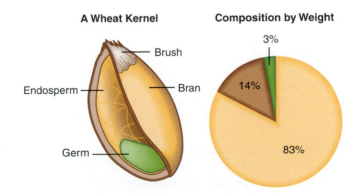

**A Wheat Kernel** — Brush, Endosperm, Bran, Germ

**Composition by Weight** — 3%, 14%, 83%

**Figure 3-5.** The basic parts of the whole-grain kernel are germ, endosperm, and bran. The pie chart shows the percent composition of each of these parts, with the endosperm making up the majority of the kernel. The table indicates the nutritional value of macronutrients within each part of the kernel. The bran constitutes the greatest value for fiber, the endosperm for carbohydrate, and the germ for protein and fat plus other micronutrients.

| | Carb/g | Protein/g | Fat/g | Fiber/g | Iron (% daily req.) | Others |
|---|---|---|---|---|---|---|
| Bran | 63 | 16 | 3 | 43 | 59 | Vitamin Bs |
| Endosperm | 79 | 7 | 0 | 4 | 7 | |
| Germ | 52 | 23 | 10 | 14 | 35 | Vitamin Bs Omega-3/6 lipids |

Nutritional value (per 100 g)

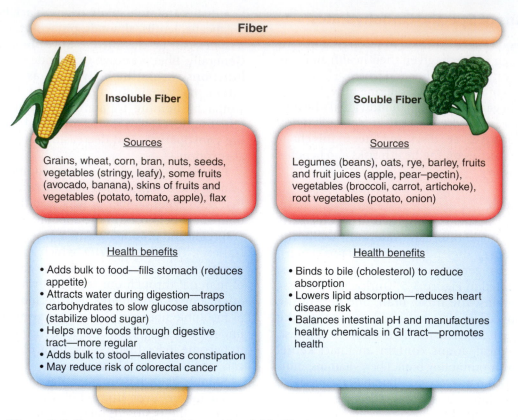

**Figure 3-6.** Comparison of soluble and insoluble fiber.

## Table 3-2. Average and Recommended Daily Intakes of Fiber (Grams) for Adults

| SEX/AGE | AVERAGE INTAKE | RECOMMENDED INTAKE |
|---------|----------------|--------------------|
| Men | | |
| 19–50 years | 13.7 g/day | 38 g/day |
| >50 years | 11.4 g/day | 30 g/day |
| Women | | |
| 19–50 years | 13.2 g/day | 25 g/day |
| >50 years | 11.2 g/day | 18 g/day |

Data from Food and Nutrition Board. *Dietary Reference Intakes: Proposed Definition of Dietary Fiber.* Washington, DC: Institute of Medicine of the National Academy of Sciences; 2001.

certain cancers, and even diabetes. It is also important to help slow food digestion, which can be beneficial by controlling appetite and caloric intake; however, it can also be detrimental to the body at times, such as during performance. Although slowing the passage of food and the digestive process may provide sustained energy over longer periods, it may also impede delivery of a quick burst of energy that might sometimes be needed. Therefore, it may have a negative effect on an individual when consumed too close to or during exercise. Thus, an effective strategy is needed to optimize nutrition and performance, which is discussed in detail in Chapter 20.

## FROM THEORY TO PRACTICE

Now that you understand the benefits of fiber in your diet and the recommended quantities to consume, estimate how much fiber you are actually consuming on a daily basis.

- Take a typical day and try to write down everything you eat during that 24-hour period, including portion sizes, to the best of your ability. Focus on your intake of fruits, vegetables, grains, and beans—the better sources of fiber.
- Using food labels that list the amount of fiber, record the total number of grams of fiber consumed.
- Because fruits and vegetables do not contain labels, use the following guideline to help calculate your intake: One serving of fresh fruit or vegetables contains an average of 3 g fiber. Examples of one serving include one medium-sized piece of fruit (size of a tennis ball), a 5-inch banana, a level handful of berries or grapes, 1/2 cup of fresh, chopped fruit or vegetables, 1 cup of leafy or starchy vegetables, and 1/2 cup of vegetable or fruit juice (with pulp).
- Compare your estimated intake with the recommendations presented in Table 3-2. If you are below the recommended guidelines, devise basic strategies to increase your fiber intake.

## Fructose and Health

Although fructose can be used by cells, the body generally favors glucose as a fuel. Consequently, fructose travels to the liver, where it undergoes metabolic processing for conversion to glucose. A growing body of evidence is beginning to show strong correlations among fructose consumption, obesity, health, and liver disease.[13,14] In the liver, fructose may not convert to glucose, but may actually convert to fats (triglycerides [TGs]) that are stored within liver tissue. This results in the development of a fatty liver (as seen with cirrhosis from excessive alcohol consumption) or increased levels of blood TGs that increase the risk for obesity and heart disease. Furthermore, evidence shows that fructose may also increase levels of uric acid in the body (which increases the potential for gout) and reduce circulating levels of leptin, an essential hormone that helps control satiety and appetite.[15,16] Researchers are beginning to devote more attention to the effects of excessive fructose consumption on health. Table 3-3 provides a breakdown of the amounts of fructose in various fruits and sweeteners.

**High-fructose corn syrup (HFCS)** is a sweetener derived from corn that has also gained the attention of researchers and the public, most of it being negative. HFCS is a group of corn starches (glucose chains) that have undergone enzymatic processing to increase their sweetness to resemble sugar, which consequently increases the fructose content. This compound is then mixed with pure corn syrup (100% glucose) to create various alternative, and less expensive, commercial sweeteners than sugar. Commercially manufactured types of HFCS are listed in Box 3-2.

Sodas and sweet beverages contribute significant calories to the U.S. diet and contribute to obesity. In fact, 20% of children drink at least three sweetened beverages each day, constituting almost one third of their total daily calories (Fig. 3-7).[11] Many of these beverages are sweetened with HFCS, so the question arises whether there is a correlation between obesity and HFCS, or whether obesity rates would remain unchanged if HFCS was replaced with regular sugar. In other words, would our obesity rates be any different if sucrose cost the same? Many experts agree that it is

## RESEARCH HIGHLIGHT

### Fructose Consumption as a Risk Factor for Nonalcoholic Fatty Liver Disease

As increases in **nonalcoholic fatty liver disease (NAFLD)** appear to parallel increases in obesity, diabetes, and dietary fructose consumption in industrialized nations (primarily because of increased consumption of sugar and high-fructose corn syrup from soft drinks), the study examined 73 patients, comparing individuals with NAFLD without liver cirrhosis against a control group.

The research demonstrated that patients with NAFLD consumed two to three times more fructose than the control group (365 kcal from fructose vs. 170 kcal), leading researchers to conclude that a key pathogenic mechanism behind the development of NAFLD may be associated with excessive dietary fructose consumption.

Ouyang X, Cirillo P, Sautin Y, et al. Fructose consumption as a risk factor for non-alcoholic fatty liver disease. *J Hepatol.* 2008;48:993–999.

## Table 3-3. Fructose Levels in Various Foods

| FRUIT OR SWEETENER | FRUCTOSE (g/100 g) | SUCROSE (g/100 g) | TOTAL FRUCTOSE (g/100 g) | TOTAL SUGARS (g/100 g) | % FRUCTOSE |
|---|---|---|---|---|---|
| Apples | 7.6 | 3.3 | 9.3 | 13.3 | 70.0 |
| Grapes | 7.6 | 0.0 | 7.6 | 18.1 | 42.0 |
| Strawberries | 2.5 | 1.0 | 3.0 | 5.8 | 51.8 |
| Mango | 2.9 | 9.9 | 7.9 | 14.8 | 53.4 |
| Papaya | 2.7 | 1.8 | 3.6 | 5.9 | 61.0 |
| Sucrose | 0.0 | 97.0 | 48.5 | 97.0 | 50.0 |
| Honey | 42.4 | 1.5 | 43.2 | 81.9 | 52.7 |
| High-fructose corn syrup–55 | 42.4 | 0.0 | 42.4 | 77.0 | 55.1 |

## Box 3-2. Commercially Manufactured Types of High-Fructose Corn Syrup

- HFCS-90 (90% fructose, 10% glucose) is used primarily to produce HFCS-55 and HFCS-42. It is sweeter than regular sugar (sucrose).
- HFCS-55 (55% fructose, 45% glucose) is the most common form often used to sweeten drinks (e.g., soft drinks, sports drinks). It is comparable in sweetness and fructose-glucose ratio to sucrose, and thus is often used as a cheap alternative to sugar.
- HFCS-42 (42% fructose, 58% glucose) is used in a variety of other foods (e.g., baked goods).

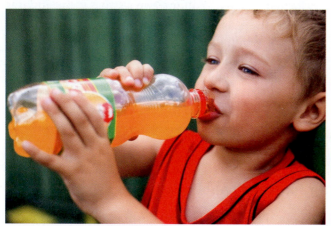

**Figure 3-7.** Soft-drink consumption in children and adults has been one factor linked to obesity trends in the United States. In many cases, consumption of calories from soft drinks (e.g., soda, juices) represents a significant portion of daily caloric intake.

the excessive consumption of sweetened beverages and not the caloric sweetener that is to blame.[11] However, research has also examined the potential health consequences of consuming sucrose instead of HFCS. As mentioned previously, studies link fructose to increased risks for obesity and heart and metabolic diseases (e.g., diabetes), because it stimulates liver production of TGs. Because HFCS contains higher levels of fructose than sucrose, do they increase these risks for disease? Furthermore, carbonyl compounds, a substance derived from carbohydrates, are found in higher concentrations in individuals with diabetes and tend to cause diabetic complications (e.g., foot ulcers and eye/nerve damage). Because these compounds are found in concentrations that are 10 times higher in HFCS than in sugar, researchers are expressing additional concerns about the use of HFCS.[17]

## Storage in the Body

Once carbohydrates enter the body, they are either used for immediate energy or transported to the cells for storage as glycogen in chains ranging from 100 to 30,000 glucose molecules. Once the body's immediate energy needs are met, excesses are converted to glycogen until this capacity is maximized. Any additional carbohydrates are then converted to fats. This biochemical process is discussed in Chapter 4. Glycogen formation or glycogenesis takes place inside cells under the influence of the enzyme glycogen synthetase, which is most active immediately following meals and exercise. Carbohydrates are generally stored in three primary regions of the body (Fig. 3-8)[1,6]:

- As glucose in the blood (5–15 g)
- Within the liver (90–110 g)
- Within muscle tissue (250–600 g)

The total amount stored within the body equals approximately 2,000 Kcal, increasing toward and beyond 3,000 Kcal in trained athletes, given their capacity for increased carbohydrate storage. For the average adult, this provides adequate fuel for about 20 miles of running (at a 100 kcal/mile average for many adults). With the appropriate training and eating strategies, liver and muscle can temporarily double their stored glycogen levels. The application of carbohydrate feeding strategies to improve performance is discussed in Chapter 20.[1]

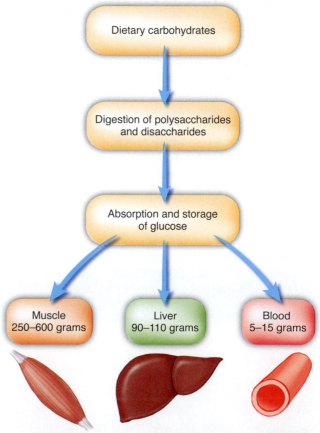

**Figure 3-8.** Carbohydrate storage within the body begins with intake and digestion of polysaccharides and disaccharides, and eventual absorption of the monosaccharide glucose. A small amount of glucose remains in the blood, but most is stored as glycogen within skeletal muscle and liver. Glycogen is broken down by the muscle for energy and by the liver to maintain blood glucose.

## Blood Glucose

Glucose serves various roles in the blood that include delivery of fuel and helping to maintain blood osmolality (concentration). Our brain, central nervous system, and red blood cells all depend on glucose as their primary fuel. In fact, red blood cells lack mitochondria (organelles in which aerobic respiration occurs) and only generate fuel anaerobically. The brain accounts for 2% of our body weight, but uses 25% of our blood glucose.

Blood glucose levels are maintained by the liver. Carbohydrates located in muscle tissue are essentially trapped within the cells and cannot be released into circulation directly. It is the phosphorylation of glucose in muscle cells (adding a phosphate group to the molecule) that prevents it from being released into circulation. Carbohydrates in liver cells, however, can be released into circulation. These topics are explored in detail in Chapter 4.

## Glycemic Index

The **glycemic index** is a ranking system used to score carbohydrates (foods and beverages) according to their ability to increase blood glucose levels. Essentially, this system assigns a numeric value between 0 and 100 to all carbohydrate sources based on how quickly they are digested and absorbed into the body, and how they impact blood sugar. Although older standards still exist, the most current ranking system is based on how quickly 50 g of available carbohydrate increases blood sugar, when measured against the rate of glucose, which is considered the standard and assigned a value of 100. The scoring system categorizes carbohydrates as high-, moderate-, or low-glycemic foods (Fig. 3-9):

- **High:** score ≥ 70
- **Medium:** score 56–69
- **Low:** score ≤ 55

With the exception of specific times (e.g., fueling during or immediately following exercise), consuming high-glycemic sources is generally not recommended. These foods are ingested rapidly by the body, causing larger blood sugar spikes (**hyperglycemia**), followed by rapid drops (**hypoglycemia**, or "crashes") caused by large doses of insulin being released into the blood. These wide fluctuations in blood sugar can cause extreme changes in hunger and energy levels, but more importantly, can lead to a progressive desensitization of insulin receptors located on the cell wall (insulin resistance), increasing the potential for development of type 2 diabetes.

Foods with lower glycemic scores, by contrast, are digested more slowly and do not cause the extreme fluctuations in blood sugar. These foods also are believed to help control appetite, delay hunger cues, and help reduce the risk for insulin resistance. Figure 3-10 shows the blood sugar response to consuming a low- versus high-glycemic carbohydrate source.

From a health and cognitive standpoint (e.g., mental performance), we should always strive to avoid large fluctuations in blood sugar, which can negatively impact health and influence mood and mental performance. Extensive glycemic index ranking lists are available online or in books, and Table 3-4 also provides the glycemic index scores for various carbohydrate sources.

Notably, this glycemic index scoring system is not perfect. The rate at which a carbohydrate food impacts

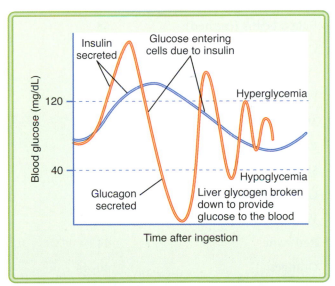

**Figure 3-10.** Blood glucose and hormone (insulin and glucagon) responses to low- versus high-glycemic carbohydrates. The blue line represents the blood glucose response following ingestion of low glycemic index carbohydrates. Note the slow rise, lower peak, and gradual return of blood glucose to within normal ranges following the secretion of insulin. The orange line represents blood glucose responses to high glycemic index food. Note that blood glucose concentration increases quickly, peaks at a higher level compared with low glycemic index carbohydrates, and quickly drops following a greater release of insulin. This rapid drop triggers the production of glucagon, a hormone that stimulates the breakdown of glycogen to glucose in the liver, to stabilize blood glucose. Thus, a greater fluctuation of blood glucose following high-glycemic carbohydrates is less desirable from a health standpoint.

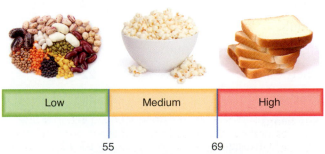

**Figure 3-9.** Cutoff values used to determine low, medium, and high glycemic index foods. Also shown are sample foods for each index level.

**Table 3-4.** Glycemic Index Scores for Various Carbohydrate Sources

| FOOD | GLYCEMIC INDEX SCORE | FOOD | GLYCEMIC INDEX SCORE |
|---|---|---|---|
| Glucose | 100–103 | Vanilla wafers | 77 |
| Hard candy | 95–100 | Potato/Corn chips | 60–77 |
| Rice (instant) | 91 | Rice cakes | 77 |
| Carrot juice | 90 | Watermelon | 72–76 |
| Honey | 87 | Bran cereal | 75 |
| Most candy | 80–95 | French fries | 75 |
| Cakes and most desserts | 70–85 | Banana (ripe) | 74 |
| Corn flakes | 85 | Beer | 73 |
| Potatoes (baked/instant) | 84 | Bagel (plain) | 72 |
| Pretzels | 82 | Saltines | 72 |
| White bread | 81 | Rice (regular/white) | 70 |
| Carrots | 65–80 | Corn tortilla | 70 |
| Wheat Thin crackers | 68 | Rye bread (regular) | 64 |
| Rice (brown) | 68 | Orange juice | 60 |
| Raisins | 68 | Popcorn | 60 |
| Baked beans (canned) | 68 | Soft drinks | 59 |
| Grape-Nuts cereal | 68 | Pita bread | 58 |
| Oatmeal (instant) | 66 | Potatoes (boiled with skin) | 57 |
| Pineapple | 66 | Mango | 56 |
| Melons | 65 | Sweet corn | 55–60 |
| Pasta (white) | 65 | Pasta (protein enriched) | 55 |
| Sucrose | 65 | Sweet potatoes | 55 |
| Grapefruit juice | 49 | Apples | 30–38 |
| Whole-wheat pasta | 45 | Yogurt (with fruit) | 38 |
| Red wine | 44 | Pinto beans | 38 |
| Oranges | 40–44 | Tomatoes | 38 |
| Bananas (unripe) | 43 | Pears | 36 |
| Soy milk | 43 | Other berries | 32 |
| Grapes | 43 | Milk (skim) | 32 |
| Kidney beans (canned) | 42 | Lentils | 25–30 |
| Apple juice | 41 | Grapefruit/Plums | 25 |
| Blueberries | 40 | Cherries | 22 |
| Peanut butter | 40 | Fructose | 20 |
| Chocolate | 40 | Soy beans | 18 |
| Peaches | 30–40 | Meats/Fish/Eggs | 10–12 |

Data from http://Glycemic-Index.org.

blood sugar levels is affected by numerous factors, such as:

- Carbohydrate form (simple vs. complex)—Generally, smaller molecules exhibit higher glycemic index scores because they require less digestion.
- Monosaccharide form—Glucose and galactose are absorbed faster (active process) than fructose (passive process). Only glucose increases blood sugar and elicits an insulin response, and thus has the highest glycemic index scores, whereas fructose has the lowest glycemic index scores.
- Starch form—Amylose versus amylopectin: amylopectin is digested faster given its multiple open ends, thus increasing glycemic index scores.
- Food form—Liquid versus solid: food is essentially liquefied to chyme before it leaves the stomach, so solid foods will remain in the stomach longer, thus decreasing the glycemic index score.
- Presence of fiber—Fiber slows gastric emptying and digestion, thus lowering the glycemic index score.
- Degree of processing and cooking—Cooking and reheating starches develops greater resistance to digestion, thus lowering glycemic index scores. In contrast, cooking fibrous starches may break apart or break down fiber, increasing the glycemic index score.
- Presence of other macronutrients (e.g., protein and fats)—These collectively slow digestion, thus decreasing the glycemic index score.
- Human variability in digestion and absorption.

Consequently, these differences have resulted in glycemic score variations ranging from 20 to 40 points for the same foods. Furthermore, the glycemic index score largely ignores the cephalic insulin response, or the stimulation of the pancreas to secrete insulin in anticipation of food. This is greatly influenced by environmental triggers (e.g., sight of food) and hunger levels. Because this scientific discovery occurred after the creation of the glycemic index scoring system, it may play a large role in influencing blood sugar responses to eating carbohydrates.

## Glycemic Load

An additional limitation to the glycemic index scoring system is that the total amount of carbohydrates consumed is not considered, which can also affect the impact of a food on blood sugar. For example, consuming 1 g of a high-glycemic carbohydrate will not impact blood sugar levels when we have between 5 and 15 g glucose in our blood, but can the same be said for a moderate glycemic index carbohydrate when we consume 30 g? Consequently, some nutritional experts favor the use of a **glycemic load (GL)** rather than the glycemic index score. GL is basically a weighted average that characterizes the glycemic effect, specific to the carbohydrate and amount consumed, and calculated using the following formula:

$$GL = (\text{glycemic index score} \times \text{grams of carbohydrate}) \div 100$$

Example 1: Carrot juice (glycemic index score = 90) and you consume 6 g:
- $90 \times 6 \text{ g} = 540 \div 100 = \text{GL score of } 5.4$

Example 2: Popcorn (glycemic index score = 60) and you consume 20 g:
- $60 \times 20 \text{ g} = 1,200 \div 100 = 12$

Much like the glycemic index ranking system, GLs can be ranked as low, medium, and high (Fig. 3-11):
- High: score ≥ 20
- Medium: score between 10 and 19.9
- Low: score < 10

---

### FROM THEORY TO PRACTICE

Although menu planning for others generally falls within the scope of practice of a dietitian, many of us plan our own menus. Using your knowledge of the glycemic index scoring system and the factors that influence these scores, draft a list of carbohydrate sources you would consume under the two following scenarios:
1. Breakfast and lunch menu that would stabilize blood sugar levels and prevent any "crash" when participating in high-level business meetings and decisions
2. Snack and feeding menu to fuel your body before and during a 2-hour endurance training session

---

### DOING THE MATH:
Calculate the GL for the following foods using the glycemic index scores presented in Table 3-4.
1. 5 g pretzels
2. 10 g grapes
3. 15 g cherries

Which of the three has the highest GL score?

**ANSWERS:**
1. Glycemic index score for pretzels = $82 \times 5 \text{ g} = 410 \div 100 = 4.1$
2. Glycemic index score for grapes = $43 \times 10 \text{ g} = 430 \div 100 = 4.3$
3. Glycemic index score for cherries = $22 \times 15 \text{ g} = 330 \div 100 = 3.3$

## RESEARCH HIGHLIGHT

### Low Glycemic Index Diets Are Easier and Healthier to Follow

Researchers at the New Balance Foundation Obesity Prevention Center at Boston Children's Hospital recruited 21 male and female subjects, aged 18 to 40 years. After losing 10% to 15% of their body weight, participants followed each of the following three diets for 4 weeks (in random order):
- Low-fat diet (60% carbohydrates, 20% fat, and 20% protein), emphasizing whole grains, fruits, and vegetables
- Low-glycemic diet (40% carbohydrates, 40% fat, and 20% protein), emphasizing minimally processed grains, vegetables, healthy fats, and fruits
- Low-carbohydrate diet, modeled after the Atkins diet with 10% carbohydrates, 60% fat, and 30% protein

Total energy expenditure for each subject was measured, as well as other markers such as insulin, cortisol, and C-reactive protein levels, an inflammatory marker in the blood that correlates with several diseases including heart disease.

Of the three diets, although the low-carbohydrate diet stimulated the greatest improvements in metabolism, it also increased levels of cortisol that often lead to increased inflammation (C-reactive protein levels) and insulin resistance, which may increase the risk for heart disease. The low-glycemic diet also improved metabolism but did not elicit many of the same negative effects of the low-carbohydrate diet.

By comparison, the low-fat diet did not yield the same benefits and increased insulin resistance. The researchers concluded that, given how low glycemic index diets are easier to follow than both low-carbohydrate and low-fat diets, and because they do not eliminate whole food groups, these diets may be easier and healthier to follow.

Ebbeling CB, Swain JF, Feldman HA, et al. Effects of dietary composition on energy expenditure during weight loss maintenance. *J Am Med Assoc.* 2012;307:2627–2634.

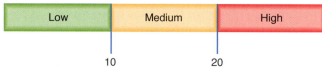

**Figure 3-11.** Cutoff values used to determine the relative glycemic load for carbohydrates.

## FATS

Fats can be classified as **hydrocarbons**, because they contain carbon and hydrogen elements in their backbone. It is the arrangement and number of carbons that determines the type of fat.

### Structure

The most common type of fat in the body is a fatty acid that contains a methyl group ($CH_3$) at one end of its chain and a carboxylic acid (COOH) at the other end of its chain.[3–11] The two basic classifications of fats are based on the number of hydrogen ions present within the hydrocarbon chain (Fig. 3-12):
- **Saturated fats (SFAs)** contain only single bonds within the carbon backbone, and thus are capable of bonding with a maximal number of hydrogen ions, hence the term *saturated*.
- **Unsaturated fats (UFAs)** contain double bonds, and thus are incapable of maximizing the opportunities to bond with hydrogen ions, hence the term *unsaturated*.

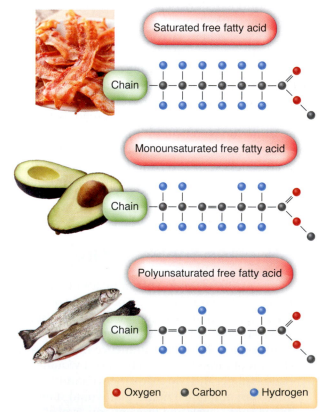

**Figure 3-12.** Structural differences between saturated and unsaturated fats. Note that saturated fats do not contain any double bonds between carbon molecules, whereas monounsaturated fats contain one double bond and polyunsaturated fats contain more than one. Also pictured are common sources of these fats.

UFAs are further subdivided into **monounsaturated fats (MUFAs)** and **polyunsaturated fats (PUFAs)**. These terms denote the number of carbon double bonds (unsaturated carbon atoms) within the carbon chain.

- A MUFA has only one double carbon bond within the backbone, whereas a PUFA has more than one double carbon bond within the carbon chain.
- Omega-3 and omega-6 fatty acids are examples of PUFAs and are named accordingly because of the unique position of the first double carbon bond within the carbon chain.

Because we are unable to manufacture some of these fatty acids in the body, they must be obtained through our diet, and thus are classified as **essential fatty acids (EFAs)**. Docosahexaenoic acid (DHA) and eicosapentaenoic acid (EPA), more commonly referred to as omega-3 fatty acids, are examples of EFAs that provide numerous health benefits but must be obtained from food sources such as cold-water fish (e.g., salmon, sardines, mackerel, herring, and tuna), krill (shrimplike crustaceans approximately 1/2 to 2 inches long), and in seaweed to a lesser extent. Nonessential fatty acids are those we can manufacture within our body and constitute the majority of fats we consume in our diet.

Fatty acids are joined together to a parent backbone called glycerol to form a molecule called a **triglyceride (TG)**. Figure 3-13 shows the general structure of a TG (one glycerol joined to three fatty acids), depicting the methyl and carboxylic acid ends of each hydrocarbon chain. TGs represent the most abundant fat found in the human body, accounting for approximately 95% to 98% of all fats in the body.[18] They also are known as simple fats and comprise the saturated, unsaturated, trans fats, and omega-3 fats mentioned previously. Compound and derived fats constitute the remaining fats in our body (2%–5%) and include compounds such as cholesterol, high-density lipoproteins (HDLs), and low-density lipoproteins (LDLs), each performing specific physiological functions.[18]

Although TGs consist of one glycerol molecule bound to three free fatty acids, these fatty acids may vary in length between 4 and 28 carbons. It is the length of the hydrocarbon backbone (i.e., number of carbon atoms) that designates the classification of the fatty acid. Furthermore, the length of the hydrocarbon chain also changes some physical properties of the fatty acid:

- Short chain fatty acids (SCFA) contain four to six carbon atoms within their backbone and are generally more liquid at room temperature.
- Medium chain fatty acids (MCFA) contain 8 to 14 carbon atoms within their backbone and can be liquid or solid at room temperature.
- Long chain fatty acids (LCFA) contain greater than 14 carbon atoms within their backbone and are generally more solid at room temperature.

Although fatty acids are generally classified by degree of saturation (e.g., MUFA, PUFA, SFAs), it is the trans fats and omega-3 fats that have garnered the most attention in recent years. First, it is helpful to clarify some facts and dispel some misconceptions about saturated and unsaturated fats. Box 3-3 highlights *true* statements about saturated and unsaturated fats.

## Box 3-3. True Statements About Saturated and Unsaturated Fats

- Saturated fats are generally more stable and tend to be more solid at room temperature; thus, they are preferred for storage (shelf-life) and cooking.
- Unsaturated fats are less stable and tend to be more liquid (oils) at room temperature; thus, they are less desirable when manufacturing many baked products.
- Saturated fats are generally believed to increase the risks for many health issues and diseases including heart disease in comparison with unsaturated fats, although some research on some MCFAs (e.g., lauric and myristic acids in coconut oil) demonstrates some health benefits.[19]
- Animal sources of fats contain cholesterol, a known fat that increases the risk for heart disease when consumed in excess. MUFAs such as olive and canola oil are associated with improved heart health.
- PUFAs are not unhealthy, as EFAs such as omega-3 and omega-6 fatty acids are PUFAs.
- Saturated fats are not exclusively derived from animal sources. In fact, coconut oil and palm kernel oil, both plant fats, contain higher levels of saturated fats than animal sources. Their high degree of stability and low cost provide some explanation why these two fats are frequently found in baked products (various cereals, cookies, etc.).

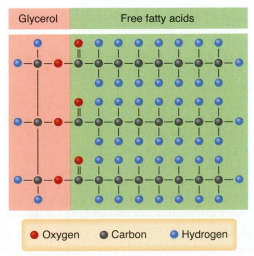

Glycerol | Free fatty acids

● Oxygen   ● Carbon   ● Hydrogen

**Figure 3-13.** General structure of a triglyceride. The backbone of the triglyceride is the water-soluble alcohol molecule, glycerol. Attached to each carbon is a free fatty acid chain.

## Trans (Hydrogenated) Fats

Hydrogenation dates back to the late 1800s, but it was not until the early 1900s that companies began marketing the first hydrogenated shortening known as Crisco, composed largely of partially hydrogenated cottonseed oil. Although this shortening enjoyed its popularity, studies in the mid-1900s began to examine causal relationships between the consumption of trans fats and the incidence of diseases such as heart disease. The major negative health impact associated with consuming trans fats is the increased risk for coronary heart disease because of its effect on elevating levels of "bad" LDL cholesterol and lowering levels of "good" HDL cholesterol in the bloodstream.[20]

Although animal fats were believed to contain greater quantities of saturated fats, which improved their stability and consistency (i.e., being more solid), they also contained higher levels of cholesterol. Thus, scientists experimented with vegetable oils that contain lower levels of saturation in the hopes of engineering a vegetable fat devoid of cholesterol, yet possessing the same physical properties of an animal fat (i.e., solid and stable). This process, called *hydrogenation*, essentially transforms an unsaturated fat to a saturated fat by breaking the unsaturated carbon atoms (double bonds), and then infusing hydrogen atoms that bond with these carbon atoms in the hydrocarbon backbone. Although the end product physically resembles and functions like a saturated fat, the molecule's chemical configuration differs from naturally occurring fats.

The terms *trans*-form and *cis*-form reflect the chemical configuration of hydrogen ions located around the carbon double bond. Whereas the *cis*-form represents the alignment of a fat in its natural form, the *trans*-form was created from the hydrogenation process. As illustrated in Figure 3-14, the *cis*-form contains kinks within the hydrocarbon chain, whereas the trans-fat form appears more as a straight chain.[6] This physical difference allows these trans fats to be more tightly packed into cell membranes, increasing an individual's risk for coronary heart disease, cancer, and other diseases. This fact has spurred greater awareness to the harmful effects of these fats, to the point at which, in 2010, the USDA dietary guidelines recommended avoiding trans fats completely.[9] Box 3-4 lists fats and oils that are good for you (A-list) and those to avoid.

## Omega-3 Fatty Acids

Much has been written about the health benefits associated with consuming additional quantities of omega-3 fatty acids. Omega-3 and omega-6 fatty acids are both essential to our health, but it is a balance between the two that is most important. Eicosanoids are signaling molecules made from EFAs that exert complex control over many physiological functions within the body, in particular with regard to inflammation or immunity. Eicosanoids are derived from omega-3 or omega-6 EFAs, with the omega-6 eicosanoids being generally proinflammatory, whereas the omega-3 eicosanoids are generally anti-inflammatory. As mentioned previously, the omega-3 fats EPA (20-carbon compound) and DHA (22-carbon compound) are found primarily in cold water fish. Alpha-Linolenic acid, an 18-carbon compound, is often labeled as or associated with omega-3 fatty acids and is found in various plant sources such as flaxseed, canola oil, chia seeds, and walnuts. Although it can be converted to EPA or DHA in the body, it does so at low conversion rates between 8% and 20% into EPA, and between 0.5% and 9% into DHA.[21–24]

DHA and EPA are biologically active substances that are responsible for many beneficial processes such as blood vessel and airway dilation, reduced blood clotting (blood thinning), improved blood lipid profiles, reduced coronary vessel inflammation and levels of inflammatory agents in circulation (e.g., cytokines), improved cell-wall permeability, and a gradual slowing of cellular aging.[25–27]

## Omega-6 Fatty Acids

The omega-6 fatty acids (linoleic acid, gamma-linoleic acid, and arachidonic acid), found in higher quantities

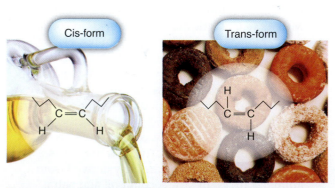

**Figure 3-14.** Structural difference between the *cis*-form versus *trans*-form fats. Olive oil is a food source high in oleic acid (in the *cis*-form) and good for heart health. Fried foods such as doughnuts are high in the *trans*-form of oleic acid (elaidic acid) and possibly linked to the promotion of heart disease. *(Doughnuts are from Comstock Images, © Getty Images.)*

### Box 3-4. Fats and Oils: A-List and Avoid List

**A-list "Good" fats:**
- PUFAs—fish oils, flaxseed (oil), canola oil, chia seeds, almonds
- MUFAs—olive oil, canola oil
- Saturated fats—coconut oil

**Avoid list:**
- Trans fats
- PUFAs—excessive amounts of corn oil, safflower oil, sunflower oil, sesame oil, peanut oil, and palm kernel oil
- Saturated fats—high-fat meats such as USDA prime beef cuts (e.g., ribs), regular ground beef, sausage, salami, and bologna; whole milk; and regular cheese

in corn, peanuts, safflower, sunflower, and other grains, produce unhealthy eicosanoids that promote inflammation and many of the opposite effects of EPA and DHA. Excessive blood vessel and airway dilation, cell-wall permeability, and blood thinning can all be potentially harmful; thus, good health requires a healthy balance between omega-3 and omega-6 fatty acids. Some researchers suggest that 1:1 to 4:1 omega-6/omega-3 is a healthy ratio.[28,29]

Whereas our Paleolithic ancestors maintained a healthy balance by eating diets rich in fish and with less grain, traditional western diets are low in fish oils and include greater consumption of corn, peanut, safflower oil, and sunflower oil that has increased omega-6/omega-3 ratios to 10:1 to 20:1. This disproportionate ratio has significantly increased risks for heart disease, cancer, and other diseases (e.g., colitis and irritable bowel syndrome), and should be considered when making healthy eating choices. Essentially, we need to increase consumption of omega-3 fatty acids, while simultaneously reducing consumption of omega-6 fatty acids. In fact, the current dietary guidelines suggest a minimum of two servings of fish per week to increase our intake of omega-3 fatty acids.[9] Furthermore, we should aim to increase consumption of healthy oils with better omega-3/omega-6 ratios. For example, flaxseed and canola oil contain a 4:1 and 1:2 omega-3/omega-6 ratio, respectively, whereas peanut oil has no omega-3 fats and corn oil has a 1:59 omega-3/omega-6 ratio. Table 3-5 outlines the composition of SFAs, MUFAs, omega-3, and omega-6 fatty acids in various foods, which can serve as a guide to making healthier choices.

**Table 3-5.** Saturated, Monounsaturated, Omega-3, and Omega-6 Fatty Acids: Composition in Various Foods

| DIETARY FAT | SATURATED FATTY ACID | MONOUNSATURATED FATTY ACID | LINOLEIC ACID (OMEGA-6): PUFA | ALPHA-LINOLENIC ACID (OMEGA-3): PUFA |
|---|---|---|---|---|
| Almond | 5% | 78% | 60% | 20% |
| Avocado | 20% | 70% | 10% | 0% |
| Canola (Rapeseed) | 6% | 62% | 22% | 10% |
| Chia seed | 0% | 0% | 40% | 30% |
| Coconut | 92% | 6% | 2% | 0% |
| Corn | 15% | 25% | 59% | 1% |
| Cottonseed | 25% | 21% | 50% | 0% |
| Flaxseed | 9% | 19% | 14% | 58% |
| Grape seed | 12% | 17% | 71% | 0% |
| Hemp | 8% | 12% | 60% | 20% |
| Margarine | 17% | 49% | 32% | 2% |
| Olive | 15% | 76% | 8% | 1% |
| Palm kernel | 85% | 13% | 2% | 0% |
| Peanut | 18% | 49% | 33% | 0% |
| Pumpkin | 9% | 34% | 42%–57% | 0%–15% |
| Rice bran | 17% | 48% | 35% | 1% |
| Safflower | 11% | 13% | 75% | 1% |
| Sesame | 13% | 42% | 45% | 0% |
| Soybean | 15% | 26% | 52% | 7% |
| Sunflower | 12% | 23% | 65% | 0% |
| Vegetable shortening | 28% | 44% | 26% | 2% |
| Walnut | 11% | 28% | 51% | 5% |
| Wheat Germ | 18% | 25% | 50% | 5% |

*Continued*

**Table 3-5.** Saturated, Monounsaturated, Omega-3, and Omega-6 Fatty Acids: Composition in Various Foods—cont'd

| DIETARY FAT | SATURATED FATTY ACID | MONOUNSATURATED FATTY ACID | LINOLEIC ACID (OMEGA-6): PUFA | ALPHA-LINOLENIC ACID (OMEGA-3): PUFA |
|---|---|---|---|---|
| Beef fat | 52% | 44% | 3% | 1% |
| Butter | 66% | 30% | 2% | 1% |
| Lard | 41% | 47% | 11% | 1% |

PUFA, polyunsaturated fats.
Data from Pennington JA. *Bowes & Church's Food Values of Portions Commonly Used.* 17th ed. Philadelphia, PA: Lippincott Williams & Wilkins; 1998; and Fat content and fatty acid composition of seed oils. http://curezone.com. Accessed November 20, 2012.

As research continues to shed more light on the risks and benefits of consuming various quantities and types of fats and oils, it is reasonable to assume that some confusion will exist with respect to what constitutes healthy oils. The list in Box 3-4 provides several key A-list and avoid-list items that may help steer individuals toward making better choices.

## In Your Own Words

You are given the opportunity to present a 5-minute educational session on "choosing healthy fats" to first-year college students who have chosen to attend a series of "Healthy Eating at College" seminars. Your focus is to help them make better dietary choices and understand key differences between the various types of fats discussed in this chapter. How would you present the information in lay terms to increase their awareness and encourage them to make healthier choices? Don't forget to include food examples to help illustrate your points.

## Key Functions

Although fats are most commonly known as a vast reserve of energy for the body, they serve numerous vital functions that are critical to physiological function and survival. These functions include:
- Manufacture of key hormones (e.g., cortisol, testosterone)
- Formation of cell membranes
- Vital structural component in brain and nerve cells (e.g., myelin sheath in neurons)
- Transport of substances within the body (e.g., cholesterol, fat-soluble vitamins)
- Insulation against the cold
- Padding against potential trauma
- Source of EFAs needed by the body

## Storage

The digestion of fats occurs predominantly in the small intestine, although some digestion starts in the stomach. In the small intestine, bile emulsifies fats into smaller droplets so that digestive enzymes (pancreatic lipases) can break TGs into fatty acids and glycerol. The fatty acids then diffuse across the intestinal wall, where small and medium chain fatty acids pass into the blood. Long chain fatty acids are too big to pass into the blood, and thus are repackaged with other larger compounds into molecules called *chylomicrons*, composed of fats and proteins. They pass to the lymphatic system before slowly entering circulation at the thoracic duct (above the heart) via the left subclavian vein. This is a slow process that limits the availability of larger fatty acids as a fuel after eating (it may take several hours before entering the blood circulation). In the liver and while in circulation, chylomicrons can be broken apart by lipoprotein lipase, an enzyme located on the cell membrane (e.g., fat or muscle cells) that facilitates the passage of fatty acids and glycerol into the cells for storage or for energy. The metabolism of fatty acids is discussed in Chapter 4.

The majority of TGs and fatty acids are stored in adipose cells (fat cells) or within muscle and liver cells, although small portions of each are also present in the circulation. As depicted in Figure 3-15, the average adult stores between 7,500 and 12,000 g (approximately 265–420 oz.) of fat in adipose tissue (subcutaneous [under the skin] and visceral [around the organs]), about 150 to 300 g (approximately 5–10 oz.) in muscle tissue, and about 5 g in the blood.[1,18]

## VIGNETTE continued

■ Catherine had always assumed that all animal fats were "bad" because they increased risks for heart disease. After learning about the various classifications of fats and their function within the human body, she now understands the importance of making healthier choices when it comes to fats and oils. Becky takes this opportunity to teach Catherine about the various types of fat commonly found in foods, including which ones to limit as much as possible–trans fats, SFAs, and oils high in omega-6 fatty acids.

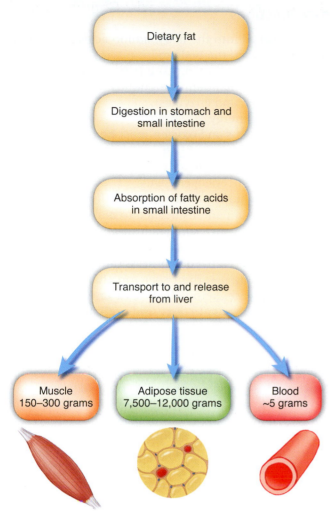

Figure 3-15. Fat storage within the body commences with the digestion of fat in the stomach and small intestine. These fatty acids are then absorbed in the small intestine and eventually transported to the liver for release to peripheral tissues such as muscle and adipose. A small amount of fatty acids remain in and circulate through the blood.

## PROTEINS

It is well established that proteins constitute a major portion of muscle tissue, and that muscle tissue represents a significant portion of overall body weight, comprising approximately 36% to 40% of a woman's total body weight and 40% to 45% of a man's total body weight.[1] This may partly explain why some people believe that eating dietary protein correlates directly to large muscles. This misguided belief is particularly true among strength athletes, who regularly consume an abundance of dietary protein, protein supplements, and amino acids. The truth is that eating protein does not build muscle. It is the stimulus of exercise, primarily resistance training, that ultimately builds muscles. Dietary proteins, however, are the crucial ingredient needed for building or rebuilding muscles during the recovery process.

## Structure

Amino acids differ from fats and carbohydrates in that their backbone contains nitrogen in addition to carbon, hydrogen, and oxygen. As illustrated in Figure 3-16, the elements that constitute the amino acid backbone contain an amino group at one end, a carboxyl group at the other end, a central or alpha carbon, and a side chain that differentiates the 20 nutritionally important amino acids from each other.[18] Amino acids are called the "building blocks" of proteins because every single protein is made up of various amino acids, uniquely linked together by a peptide bond (Fig. 3-17), that build into peptide chains (longer chains of amino acids). It is the unique arrangement of amino acids within the peptide chain that differentiates proteins (e.g., steak and tofu will have different amino acid combinations and structures).

Amino acids are categorized as essential and nonessential. An **essential amino acid** is one that cannot be synthesized by the body; therefore, it must be obtained from foods we consume. A **nonessential amino acid** implies that it can be produced by the body and is thus not

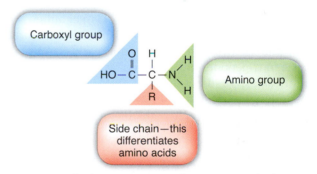

Figure 3-16. The basic amino acid structure with the three important parts labeled: carboxyl group, amino group, and side chain. The alpha carbon is in the middle of the structure with the three parts branched off from it.

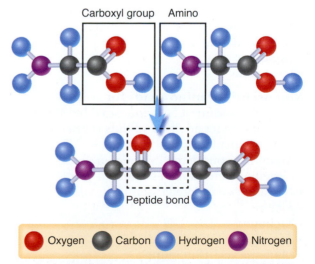

Figure 3-17. The formation of a peptide bond when combining the carboxyl group of one amino acid with the amino group of another amino acid. Following formation of this bond, water is released.

required to come from our diet (Box 3-5). Eight essential amino acids are needed by adults, each with its own Recommended Dietary Allowance (RDA); additional amino acids are needed in children.

If insufficient essential amino acids are consumed, the body will attempt to conserve what it can. It may slow production of new proteins (e.g., muscles, organs, hair, and nails) until the proteins in the body begin to break down faster than they can be resynthesized. The results of this can be seen during starvation, or when an individual follows a very low carbohydrate or extremely low calorie diet.

## Digestion of Dietary Protein

Protein digestions begins in the stomach through the action of gastric acid that breaks the structures apart, allowing the enzymatic action of pepsin, a protein digestive enzyme, to break the primary structures into smaller chains that pass into the small intestine.[6,18] Pancreatic enzymes complete the digestive process, creating amino acids, amino pairs (dipeptides), and groups of three amino acids (tripeptides) that can then be absorbed through the intestinal wall. Although amino acids compete for absorption, a unique group of larger amino acids called *branched-chain amino acids* (BCAAs) are absorbed faster than many of the smaller amino acids, and dipeptides and tripeptides are absorbed faster than the single amino acids. In the intestinal wall, however, these dipeptides and tripeptides are further digested to amino acids, which can then enter the blood.

## Box 3-5. Amino Acids

**Essential Amino Acids for Adults**
- Isoleucine (BCAA)
- Leucine (BCAA)
- Valine (BCAA)
- Lysine
- Methionine
- Phenylalanine
- Threonine
- Tryptophan

**Nonessential Amino Acids for Adults**
- Histamine—cannot be synthesized by children and some older adults, and thus is essential in these populations
- Arginine—considered essential in youth
- Cysteine—considered essential in youth
- Tyrosine—considered essential in youth
- Alanine
- Arginine
- Asparagine/Aspartic acid
- Glutamic acid/Glutamine
- Glycine
- Proline
- Serine

## Key Functions

Once absorbed into the body, amino acids are used in different areas of the body to:
- synthesize/maintain tissue (e.g., muscle).
- synthesize/maintain compounds (e.g., muscle, hormones, and enzymes).
- generate energy.
- transport fats and oxygen (e.g., hemoglobin, albumin).
- become a substrate for the manufacture of glucose (gluconeogenesis).
- maintain blood pH, acting as a buffer.
- provide components needed to make nonprotein compounds (e.g., some neurotransmitters).

Any excess amino acids travel to the liver, where the amino group is removed (a process called *deamination*), leaving a residual carbon skeleton that can be converted to glucose, ketone bodies, or fatty acids. These metabolic processes are discussed in Chapter 4.

## Recommendations on Protein Intake

Much confusion persists regarding optimal protein recommendations. Currently, the RDA for adults is set at 0.8 g/kg body weight per day or 0.364 g/lb body weight per day for a sedentary population. Currently, women in the United States consume approximately 0.95 g/kg body weight (up to 20% more than the RDA), whereas men consume 1.15 g/kg body weight (44% more than the RDA).[30] However, it is well established that athletes have higher requirements because of the additional need for protein to synthesize muscle tissue and contribute to the energy pathways.

Because so many factors play a role in determining protein requirements, it is nearly impossible to make specific recommendations for active individuals. Protein needs are not only determined by activity level, but by length of time training (untrained vs. trained), sex, age, timing of intake, carbohydrate intake, total energy intake, quality of protein, and more. In 2009, however, in response to a growing need for some direction, a joint position statement by the American Dietetic Association (now known as the Academy of Nutrition and Dietetics), Joint Dietitians of Canada, and American College of Sports Medicine provided recommendations for endurance- and resistance-trained athletes[31]:
- Endurance athletes, defined as engaging in sport-specific training or participating in more than 10 hours of vigorous weekly exercise: 1.2 to 1.4 g/kg body weight
- Resistance-trained athletes: 1.4 to 1.8 g/kg body weight

Other organizations and institutions have also made their own recommendations based on their own research, and although their suggestions may vary in minor ways, they are all quite similar. Protein needs and dietary strategies for more active individuals are described in Chapter 20.

**DOING THE MATH:**
Using an example of a 175-lb male, calculate his RDA and how this amount would change if he were either an endurance-trained athlete or a resistance-trained individual. Remember to convert pounds to kilograms (2.2 lb = 1 kg).

**ANSWERS:**
- 175 lb ÷ 2.2 = 79.5 kg
- RDA = 0.8 g/kg body weight = 0.8 × 79.5 kg = 63.6 g
- Endurance-trained athlete = 1.2 to 1.4 g/kg body weight = 95.4 to 111.3 g
- Resistance-trained athlete = 1.4 to 1.8 g/kg body weight = 111.3 to 143.1 g

Using your own body weight (convert to kilograms), calculate your daily protein requirement following the RDA guidelines. Next, calculate how this amount would change if you were either an endurance athlete or a resistance-trained individual.

## Storage

Unlike fats and carbohydrates that can be stored as such in the cells, once proteins enter the body, they are used to complete any of the functions presented earlier, with any excesses converted to fat. However, at any point, the body may rely on proteins as a substrate from which we can manufacture glucose as needed. This implies breaking down any usable forms of protein, i.e., any dietary protein or the 99% of protein within our body that exists as living tissue (e.g., muscle tissue). The remaining 1% (approximately 6–7 oz. or 170–200 g) exists as free amino acid pools located in cells (e.g., liver cells) and is used primarily for repair and maintenance of cells and tissue.

## Protein Quality

Not all proteins are created the same. Animal sources of protein are generally considered to be of better quality because they contain greater quantities of essential amino acids in ratios that better correlate to the individual RDAs for each essential amino acid, and they are absorbed more efficiently. Proteins that offer a complete amino acid profile are sometimes referred to as **complete proteins**, whereas those that do not provide all the essential amino acids are referred to as **incomplete proteins** (Fig. 3-18).

Various scoring systems exist to rank the quality of a protein. Numerical scoring systems similar to glycemic index rank protein quality against a reference food, which was originally developed around the whole egg, considered the most complete protein food. **Biological value (BV)** is one such ranking system that measures the proportion of an absorbed food protein that becomes incorporated into protein tissue within the body.[6] Essentially, it summarizes the efficacy of how we break down proteins for use in protein synthesis in the body, but it fails to account for efficacy of protein digestion and absorption.

More recently, **Protein Digestibility Corrected Amino Acid Score (PDCAAS)** has been adopted as a more accurate scoring system based on a food's amino acid profile and its digestibility.[6] This scoring system ranks protein sources between zero and one, with higher numbers reflecting better sources of protein. Table 3-6 provides examples of PDCAAS and BV scores, and the digestibility efficiency of various protein sources.

An understanding of protein quality allows vegans and various types of vegetarians to plan effectively to ensure they consume the appropriate quality and quantity of protein. A **limiting amino acid (LAA)** in a protein source reflects that the essential amino acid is present in insufficient quantities to support protein-adequate protein synthesis (i.e., the food contains an LAA not aligned with the RDS requirements for essential amino acids). Although vegetarians are more

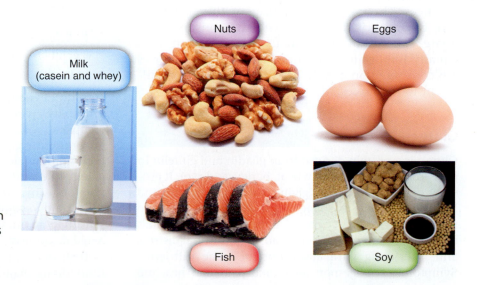

**Figure 3-18.** Sources of quality protein in the diet. With the exception of nuts and other vegetable proteins, all of the proteins shown are sources of complete proteins.

### Table 3-6. Protein Quality Scores

| PROTEIN | PROTEIN DIGESTIBILITY CORRECTED AMINO ACID SCORE | BIOLOGICAL VALUE | PROTEIN DIGESTIBILITY (%) |
|---|---|---|---|
| Whey protein | 1.00 | 100 | 99 |
| Whole egg | 1.00 | 88–100 | 98 |
| Casein | 1.00 | 80 | 99 |
| Beef protein | 0.92 | 80 | 98 |
| Soy protein concentrate | 0.91 | 74 | 95 |
| Wheat gluten | ~ <0.60 | 54 | 91 |

limited in their protein choices, if they consume adequate levels of calories from a variety of foods, they should meet their protein needs. However, given their choices and preferences, and given the LAA present in foods, they should consider incorporating complementary proteins in their diet. The practice of complementing proteins is one in which two or more proteins are combined in one meal or over the course of a day to compensate for essential amino acid deficiencies present within each protein. For example, rice and beans are each limited in different amino acids; however, when combined, all the essential amino acid requirements are provided. If someone was to live solely on rice as their protein source, they would not obtain sufficient quantities of lysine, and would therefore limit their ability to synthesize proteins. Table 3-7 provides a listing of the LAA found within many common protein food sources.

Until recently it was generally believed that, because the body does not readily store amino acids, it was essential for vegetarians to combine complementary proteins at each meal. Debate continues over this issue, but it appears the general consensus is that this practice is not strictly necessary. However, it may still have some advantages and appears to be a sensible way for vegans to approach their dietary practices. The take-home message with vegetarianism, however, is that it is possible to consume adequate sources of high-quality proteins, but it is equally important to ensure that adequate calories are consumed on a daily basis from a variety of different food sources.

## Gluten

Gluten is a protein derived from gliadin and glutelin in grass-related grains (e.g., wheat, barley, and rye). It provides elasticity to dough, giving it a chewy texture and helping maintain its shape, yet it allows the dough to stretch and rise (as occurs in baking). Some individuals experience gluten sensitivity, causing intestinal distress and interfering with absorption of some nutrients. Symptoms of indigestion, abdominal pain, diarrhea, and

### Table 3-7. Limiting Amino Acids in Common Protein Sources

| SOURCE | LIMITING AMINO ACID |
|---|---|
| Whole eggs | Not applicable |
| Milk | Methionine |
| Egg whites | Tryptophan |
| Beef | Methionine |
| Fish | Tryptophan |
| Oats | Lysine |
| Rye | Tryptophan |
| Rice | Lysine |
| Corn | Tryptophan |
| Wheat | Lysine |
| Soybean | Methionine, tryptophan |
| Legumes | Methionine |
| Nuts/seeds | Lysine |
| Potato | Methionine |
| Cereals | Lysine, threonine |
| Grains | Threonine |
| Vegetables | Methionine, lysine, tryptophan |

chronic fatigue (low energy) are characteristic of gluten sensitivity. Avoiding gluten-rich foods can reduce these complications, especially when intestinal diseases are present (e.g., celiac disease), and can improve mineral/vitamin deficiencies and fatigue. Consuming gluten-free foods (e.g., rice, corn, flax, most oats, millet, potatoes, soy, and buckwheat), whole-grain foods, fruits, and vegetables enables individuals with gluten sensitivity to attain the needed fiber and nutrients, yet avoid discomfort.

Historically, gluten-free diets were prescribed for individuals diagnosed with celiac disease, affecting about 1% of the U.S. population, although almost 5% of the population has some form of gluten sensitivity that is generally undiagnosed. Although regarded as a therapeutic diet for a GI disease, gluten-free eating has become increasingly popular to resolve many unexplained ailments or for weight management, and now represents approximately $2.6 billion in gluten-free products in 2010.[32]

## In Your Own Words

Using the knowledge acquired in this section, what concerns would you have and what recommendations would you make to a vegan who also suffers from gluten sensitivity and competes as an endurance athlete? Be sure to consider protein needs, quality, digestibility, and efficiency, as well as limiting amino acids and complementing proteins.

## VITAMINS AND MINERALS

Vitamins and minerals contribute to virtually all structural, functional, and regulatory reactions within the body. Although all vitamins and minerals have their own unique properties, they typically work synergistically with enzymes, hormones, and other compounds to ensure appropriate physiological functions. Key physiological functions include:

- Bone formation and health: Calcium and phosphorous are two major minerals found in bone. Although most bone growth stops by age 20 to 24 years, the skeleton continues to undergo constant remodeling (replacement of existing bone cells). In fact, it is estimated that the entire skeleton is replaced every 10 years via the action of osteoblasts (bone-forming cells) and osteoclasts (bone-reabsorbing cells).
- Cardiorespiratory function and blood formation: Iron is a vital component of hemoglobin that is found in red blood cells that need vitamins $B_6$, $B_{12}$, and folate (folic acid) for their development. Iron, folate, and vitamin $B_{12}$ allow red blood cells to mature, whereas vitamin C enhances iron absorption.
- Production of energy: The body's energy pathways depend on vitamin B complex and vitamin C that perform various functions in metabolizing macronutrients as fuel.
- Antioxidant roles: Although oxygen is essential for life, it can also damage cells by reacting with compounds to form free radicals or unstable compounds. To combat and remove these unstable compounds, the body manufactures antioxidants that are composed of various vitamins and minerals including vitamin A, vitamin C, and selenium.

Vitamins are essential organic molecules that cannot be synthesized within the body. Like essential amino acids and EFAs, they must be obtained from food. There are two categories of vitamins: fat-soluble and water-soluble vitamins (Box 3-6).

Vitamin and mineral deficiencies reduce the body's physiological function and can impair health. However, overconsuming vitamins and minerals is also not healthy. Fat-soluble vitamins can all be stored in the body, increasing the likelihood of toxicity if megadoses are consumed. Water-soluble vitamins can be excreted in urine, but they can still place undue stress on the body when consumed in excess. Both extremes (i.e., deficiency or excess) can be avoided by eating a wide variety of whole foods. Although it is also possible to satisfy the RDA for each vitamin and mineral through dietary supplements (e.g., pills and powders), whole foods provide a more optimal way to obtain nutrients.

## Box 3-6. Water- and Fat-Soluble Vitamins

**Essential Amino Acids for Adults**
- Fat-soluble vitamins:
- Vitamin A
- Vitamin D
- Vitamin E
- Vitamin K
- Water-soluble vitamins:
- Vitamin $B_1$ (thiamin)
- Vitamin $B_2$ (riboflavin)
- Vitamin $B_3$ (niacin)
- Vitamin $B_6$ (pyridoxine)
- Cobalamin
- Pantothenic acid
- Biotin
- Folic acid

## VIGNETTE conclusion

It is now 4 months after Catherine's initial visit with Becky. She has lost 15 pounds, but more importantly, she has successfully adopted a program of healthy eating and physical activity. Early on in their relationship, Becky realized how much Catherine thrives on truly understanding the science behind nutrition and the functions of the foods she eats, so she has consistently seized educational opportunities during their sessions together. Although Catherine has had brief lapses like any other weight-loss client, she has been able to adhere to her program and is excited to keep learning and maintain her new way of life.

## CRITICAL THINKING QUESTIONS

1. Armed with your understanding of the structure and function of the macronutrients, prepare key talking points to share with a peer to increase his or her knowledge and understanding of the benefits to low-glycemic food sources and the impact on overall health and functionality.

2. Although research is still evolving, a diet with favorable omega-6/omega-3 fatty acid ratios appears to be beneficial. Compile a rationale argument for selecting olive oil, canola oil, and coconut oil as healthy oils to include in one's diet.

3. What strategies would you suggest to a resistance-trained vegan to meet his or her daily requirements for protein quantity, yet achieving the necessary protein quality to sustain tissue maintenance and growth?

## ADDITIONAL RESOURCES

American Council on Exercise. ACE Fitness Nutrition Manual. San Diego, CA: American Council on Exercise; 2013.
Center for Nutrition Policy and Promotion. *Dietary Guidelines for Americans*. Washington, DC: United States Department of Agriculture, 2010.

Harvard Health Letter (a monthly newsletter). Boston, MA: Harvard Health Publication, Harvard Medical School.
Nutrition Action Newsletter (a monthly newsletter). Washington, DC: Center of Science in the Public Interest.

## REFERENCES

1. Jeukendrup A, Gleeson M. *Sport Nutrition: An Introduction to Energy Production and Performance*. Champaign, IL: Human Kinetics; 2004.
2. Food and Nutrition Board. *Dietary Reference Intakes: Water, Potassium, Sodium, Chloride, and Sulfate*. Washington, DC: Institute of Medicine of the National Academy of Sciences; 2004.
3. American Council on Exercise. *ACE's Essentials of Exercise Science for Fitness Professionals*. San Diego, CA: American Council on Exercise; 2010.
4. Mahan LK, Escott-Stump S. *Krause's Food Nutrition and Diet Therapy*. 10th ed. Philadelphia, PA: W.B. Saunders Company; 2000.
5. Wardlaw GM. *Contemporary Nutrition: Issues and Insights*. 5th ed. Boston, MA: McGraw-Hill; 2003.
6. Berardi J, Andrews R. *The Essentials of Sports and Exercise Nutrition*. 2nd ed. Toronto, ON, Canada: Precision Nutrition, Inc.; 2012.
7. Fink HH, Mikesky AE, Burgoon LA. *Practical Applications in Sports Nutrition*. 3rd ed. Burlington, MA: Jones & Bartlett Learning; 2012.
8. Jacobsen ME, ed. *Sugar Belly: How Much Is Too Much?* Washington, DC: Center of Science in the Public Interest; 2102.
9. Center for Nutrition Policy and Promotion. *Dietary Guidelines for Americans*. Washington, DC: U.S. Department of Agriculture; 2010.
10. Johnson RK, Appel LJ, Brands M, et al. Dietary sugars intake and cardiovascular health: a scientific statement from the American Heart Association. *Circulation*. 2009;120:1011–1020.
11. Trust for America's Health (TFAH) and Robert Wood Johnson Foundation (RWJF). *F as in Fat: How Obesity Threatens America's Future*. Washington, DC: TFAH; 2011.
12. Food and Nutrition Board. *Dietary Reference Intakes: Proposed Definition of Dietary Fiber*. Washington, DC: Institute of Medicine of the National Academy of Sciences; 2001.
13. Harvard Health Letter. *Abundance of Fructose Not Good for the Liver, Heart*. Boston, MA: Harvard Health Publication, Harvard Medical School; 2011.
14. Targher G, Day CP, Bonora E. Risk of cardiovascular disease in patients with non-alcoholic fatty liver disease. *N Engl J Med*. 2010;363:1341–1350.
15. Choi HK, Curhan G. Soft drinks, fructose consumption, and the risk of gout in men: prospective cohort study. *Br Med J*. 2008;336:309–312.
16. Shapiro A, Mu W, Roncal C, Cheng K, Johnson RJ, Scarpace PJ. Fructose-induced leptin resistance exacerbates weight gain in response to subsequent high-fat feeding. *Am J Physiol Regul Integr Comp Physiol*. 2008; 295:R1370–R1375.
17. Lo CY, Li S, Tan D, Wang Y. (2007). Food bioactives and nutraceuticals: Production, chemistry, analysis and health effects: Health Effects. Presented at 234th National Meeting, American Chemical Society, Boston, MA; Aug. 23, 2007.
18. Wardlaw GM, Hampl JS, DiSilvestro RA. *Perspectives in Nutrition*. 6th ed. Boston, MA: McGraw-Hill; 2004.
19. Clegg ME. Medium-chain triglycerides are advantageous in promoting weight loss although not beneficial to exercise performance. *Int J Food Sci Nutr*. 2010;61:653–689.
20. Kris-Etherton PM. Trans-fats and coronary disease. *Crit Rev Food Sci Nutr*. 2010;50:29–30.
21. Talahalli RR, Vallikannan B, Sambaiah K, Lokesh BR. Lower efficacy in the utilization of dietary ALA as compared to preformed EPA + DHA on long chain n-3 PUFA levels in rats. *Lipids*. 2010;45:799–808.
22. Gerster H. Can adults adequately convert alpha-linolenic acid to eicosapentaenoic acid and docosahexaenoic acid? *Int J Vitam Nutr Res*. 1998;68:159–173.
23. Brenna JT. Efficiency of conversion of alpha-linolenic acid to long chain n-3 fatty acids in man. *Curr Opin Clin Nutr Metab Care*. 2002;5:127–132.
24. Burdge GC, Calder PC. Conversion of alpha-linolenic acid to longer-chain polyunsaturated fatty acids in human adults. *Reprod Nutr Dev*. 2005;45:581–597.
25. Karr JE, Alexander JE, Winningham RG. Omega-3 polyunsaturated fatty acids and cognition throughout the lifespan: A review. *Nutr Neurosci*. 2011;14:216–225.
26. Kiefer D. That fish you ate might protect against colorectal cancer. *Integr Med Alert*. 2012;15:97–100.
27. Harris KA, Hill AM, Kris-Etherton PM. Health benefits of marine-derived omega-3 fatty acids. *ACSM Health Fitness J*. 2010;14:22–28.
28. Simopoulos AP. The importance of the ratio of omega-6/omega-3 essential fatty acids. *Biomed. Pharmacother*. 2002;56:365–379.

29. Okuyama H. High omega-6 to omega-3 ratios of dietary fatty acids rather than serum cholesterol as a major risk factor for coronary heart disease. *Eur J Lipid Sci Technol.* 2001;103:418–422.

30. Jacqueline D, Wright JD, Wang CY. *Trends in Intake of Energy and Macronutrients in Adults from 1999–2000 through 2007–2008.* National Center for Health Statistics, Hyattsville, MD; 2010:49.

31. American Dietetic Association (ADA), Dietitians of Canada (DC), American College of Sports Medicine (ACSM). Nutrition and Athletic Performance. *Med Sci Sports Exerc.* 2009;41:709–731.

32. National Foundation for Celiac Awareness website. http://celiaccentral.org. Accessed November 21, 2012.

## *Practice What You Know:* Using Glycemic Index and Glycemic Load to Evaluate a Meal

Recall the most recent meal you have eaten. On a piece of notebook paper, list the food items and estimate their portion sizes. Next, find the glycemic index of the food items using Table 3-4: Glycemic Index Scores for Various Carbohydrate Sources or a reputable website (e.g., http://glycemicindex.com). Then calculate the GL of each food item: GL = (glycemic index score × grams of carbohydrate) ÷ 100.

- What is the average glycemic index score for your meal?

  _____

  _____

  _____

  _____

  √ Use Figure 3-9 to score this meal as high, medium, or low.

  _____

  _____

  _____

  _____

- What is the average GL score for your meal?

  _____

  _____

  _____

  _____

  √ Use Figure 3-11 to score this meal as high, medium, or low.

  _____

  _____

  _____

  _____

- What might account for the differences observed between the two scores?

  _____

  _____

  _____

  _____

- Are there changes you could make to this meal to make it healthier in terms of the body's insulin response?

  _____

  _____

  _____

  _____

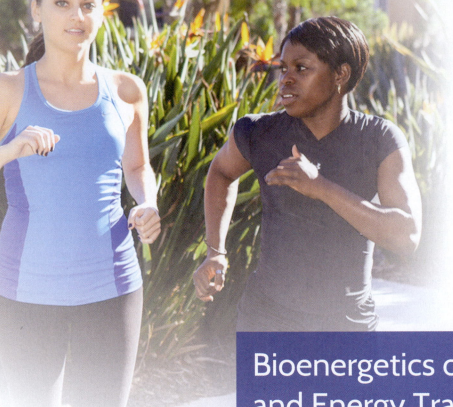

Lance C. Dalleck, PhD

# CHAPTER 4

# Bioenergetics of Exercise and Energy Transfer

## CHAPTER OUTLINE

## CHAPTER OUTLINE—cont'd

## LEARNING OUTCOMES

1. Explain the key bioenergetic concepts that are fundamental to energy metabolism.
2. Describe the general energy pathways and their fundamental differences.
3. Explain the mechanics of each energy pathway.
4. Describe adenosine triphosphate (ATP) generation for each energy pathway.
5. Identify the molecules used as substrate during exercise at different intensities.
6. Describe the function of specific enzymes in cellular biochemical reactions.
7. Identify the rate-limiting enzyme for each energy pathway.
8. Identify the ATP total produced from carbohydrate and lipid metabolism.
9. Explain the factors that contribute to fatigue with each energy pathway.
10. Describe the integrated function of the energy systems.
11. Explain key sex differences regarding the energy pathways.
12. Identify the effects of aging on the energy pathways.

## ANCILLARY LINK

Visit Davis*Plus* at http://davisplus.fadavis.com for study and practice resources, including online quizzes, animations that help explain physiological processes, podcasts concerning news and career trends in exercise physiology, and practice references.

## VIGNETTE

■ Felicia Rodriguez is a doctoral student in exercise science and is teaching an undergraduate-level course as part of her studies. While preparing to teach her students about bioenergetics, she remembers the confusion that she and her classmates experienced when first learning about the various energy pathways and which nutrients serve as the primary fuel during different forms of physical activity. Once Felicia was able to understand the difference between activities fueled mainly by carbohydrate sources (i.e., high-intensity, short-duration activities that primarily call upon the anaerobic energy systems) versus those fueled by an increased proportion of free-fatty acids (i.e., low- to moderate-intensity, long-duration activities that mainly rely on the aerobic energy pathway), she fared much better in her studying efforts.

What real-world examples can Felicia use to illustrate this complex topic to her students?

The onset of intense exercise can elicit an adenosine triphosphate (ATP) energy demand that is 500 to 1,000 times higher than that required at rest.[1] This sudden increase in energy demand necessitates a concurrent increase in energy supply that must equal the demand for energy for exercise to continue. To accomplish this feat, various physiological systems undergo rapid changes to ensure delivery of the necessary substrate (fuel, oxygen) to the working cells that then generate the needed energy.

At the cellular level, a complex series of chemical reactions involving fuels and gases occur that ultimately generate energy to perform work. The field of science that examines how our body accomplishes this amazing feat is called **bioenergetics** and can be defined as the study of energy transfer in living organisms.[2] Bioenergetics certainly raises questions regarding the science and application of energy production as it pertains to fuel utilization and exercise intensity, performance, fatigue, the accumulation of lactate, and even differences between individuals. This chapter explores the answers to these questions and explains other important topics related to cellular metabolism and its application into practice.

## BIOENERGETICS SURVIVAL GUIDE

The study of bioenergetics is among the most challenging of all the topics in the field of exercise physiology. Thus, it may be helpful to review a few key concepts and nomenclature that will facilitate comprehension of the subject matter.

Five key elements of bioenergetics are:
1. Coupled reactions
2. Enzymes
3. Oxidation-reduction reactions
4. Substrates and products
5. Shuttles and transporters

Numerous reactions that occur in exercise metabolism are coupled together. More specifically, one reaction releases energy (technically termed *free energy*) that is required to drive another reaction. In **coupled reactions**, a reaction that releases free energy is termed **exergonic**, whereas a reaction that requires energy is coined **endergonic**. Sometimes the word *exothermic* is used interchangeably with exergonic because they both define the release of heat or energy during a reaction. An exothermic reaction is one wherein energy is released from a system usually in the form of heat. Examples of exothermic reactions that release heat are the combustion of fuels, such as wood, coal, or oil, or mixing chemicals (e.g., acids and alkalis) that liberate heat. Exergonic literally means "outside work," which means releasing energy in the form of work. Examples of exergonic reactions are those that release energy to complete work, representing many reactions occurring within the body, namely, catabolism, respiration, and the breakdown of sugars to energy through cellular metabolism. In a similar fashion, the terms endothermic and endergonic can be used interchangeably.

An **enzyme** is a biological catalyst that enhances the rate of chemical reactions (i.e., speeds up the rate of a reaction). Enzymes do not cause reactions to occur; rather, it is the enzymatic activity that controls the rate of reactions. Enzyme activity can be upregulated (increased via activators) and downregulated (decreased via inhibitors) by various molecules. These features permit enzymes to play an integral role in regulating exercise metabolism.

Removal of an electron from a molecule or atom is termed **oxidation**. Conversely, the addition of an electron to a molecule or atom is referred to as **reduction**. Oxidation and reduction reactions always occur together and, therefore, are referred to as **oxidation-reduction reactions**. Among the numerous chemical reactions that occur in the energy pathways, one oxidation-reduction reaction involves the transfer of hydrogen atoms ($H^+$) that hold an electron. This hydrogen atom transfer is essential to energy production and is explained in greater detail later in this chapter. Two common molecules in the energy pathways that transfer hydrogen atoms via oxidation-reduction reactions are flavin adenine dinucleotide (FAD) and nicotinamide adenine dinucleotide (NAD).

**Substrates** are the molecules acted on by enzymes in chemical reactions that result in the manufacture of various end products. In the field of bioenergetics, common substrates for the three energy systems include phosphocreatine, carbohydrates (in the form of glucose and glycogen), lipids (in the form of free fatty acids [FFAs]), and proteins (in the form of amino acids). The fate of each of these substrates is also explained in detail throughout this chapter. **Products** refer to molecules manufactured from the substrates that are involved in enzymatically catalyzed reactions. Interestingly, many reactions in energy metabolism are reversible, which means that the substrates and products are interchangeable (i.e., substrate is acted on to form a product, but in reverse, the product is altered to resynthesize substrate).

Another important concept within bioenergetics is the movement of molecules within the cell (e.g., sarcoplasm), across membranes (e.g., mitochondrial wall), and between the plasma and cellular environments (e.g., moving from blood into the cell). Although some molecules can diffuse easily across membranes, others require specialized **shuttles**, or **transporters**, to move from one environment to another. For example, the carnitine shuttle moves FFAs entering the muscle cell to the mitochondria, and the glucose transporter type 4 (GLUT-4) transporter protein helps move glucose molecules across membranes.

## THERMODYNAMICS

Bioenergetics is part of the larger field of study of the science of energy transfer called **thermodynamics**.

A basic appreciation of the laws of thermodynamics provides a foundation for better understanding of bioenergetics. Bioenergetics is essentially governed by two laws of thermodynamics that always hold true in the physical world. The first law relates to conservation of energy, and the second to directionality of reactions.

## First Law of Thermodynamics: Conservation of Energy

The first law of thermodynamics states that *energy can be neither created nor destroyed, but* can be transferred from one form to another and ultimately degrades to heat.[3] This is what transpires when we consume food. The chemical energy harnessed from the foods we eat is liberated to support cellular work, such as muscle contraction. Any unused energy, as well as the energy used to perform that work, is ultimately converted to heat that is either preserved or removed from the body as needed. Although there certainly is an exchange of energy, there is no net change in the total energy content during the process.

## Second Law of Thermodynamics: Directionality of Reactions

Although the first law of thermodynamics implies no net change in energy, it does not provide insight into why various biochemical reactions involved in energy transfer proceed in a given direction. For example, why do certain chemical reactions proceed in one direction during specific conditions, but then reverse direction when other cellular conditions prevail? It is the second law of thermodynamics that governs directionality of biochemical reactions. Although more complicated to understand, this law states that *the entropy of a system never decreases, because it progresses spontaneously toward a thermodynamic equilibrium.* First, consider the definition of the term *entropy*: a measure of the disorder that exists in a system. More simply stated, entropy is the measure of energy in a system that is unavailable to do work. To help illustrate this concept, consider the action of curling a dumbbell (Fig. 4-1): a portion of the energy released from the breakdown of energy molecules cannot be harnessed to perform actual work (i.e., muscle contraction), but any free energy released from the bonds can be used to perform work (i.e., muscle contraction). Another example is burning gasoline in a vehicle. Only a portion of that combusted fuel is used to perform work (i.e., turn the drive shaft to rotate the wheels).

Although entropy permits chemical reactions to occur, it may not directly benefit cellular performance because only the release of free energy in the reaction is used to drive cellular function.[4] Within biological systems, such as the human body, energy transfer always proceeds in the direction of increased entropy and the release of free energy, moving toward thermodynamic equilibrium where differences

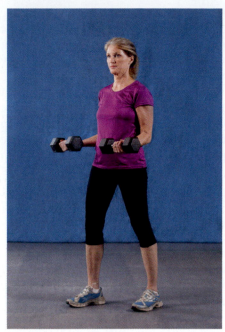

**Figure 4-1.** The action of curling a dumbbell illustrates the second law of thermodynamics.

(e.g., temperature, pressure, chemical potential between two points) decrease.[3]

It is important to recognize that only basic concepts of these laws have been presented in this section; more detailed information concerning the laws of thermodynamics can be obtained from the resources and references listed at the end of the chapter.

## ENERGY: THE CAPACITY TO DO WORK

All living organisms share the ability to produce, store, and transfer energy. Energy originates as light from the sun that is then converted into the energy forms of carbohydrates, proteins, and fats in plants and animals. Humans consume these energy sources, and through digestion (a catabolic or breakdown reaction) and absorption, we assimilate them into our bodies. In the body, they are either used immediately to produce energy to fuel biological work or are stored for later use. The form of energy used by the body is called **adenosine triphosphate (ATP)** and is considered the body's energy currency. When used, it liberates calories, which is defined as a unit of energy.

### Calorie

Energy is described as the capacity to do work, but it is often conceptually difficult to understand this definition and how work is quantified. In the same way that mass can be measured in kilograms or pounds, the amount of work performed can be quantified through **calories**, abbreviated Kcal, or by kilojoules (1 Kcal or food calorie is equivalent = 4.184 kJ). The concept of measuring calories via calorimetry is presented in Chapter 5. By definition, a calorie (Kcal) is defined as the quantity of heat required to raise the temperature of 1 Kg (1,000 mL, 1 L, or 33.8 ounces) of water by 1°C from 14.5°C (58°F) to 15.5°C (60°F).

For individuals who are not familiar with the metric system, let's quantify this definition in more understandable terms and provide a practical example. First, the metric system is based off of water where 1 Kg water equals 1 L water (33.8 ounces). A temperature range of 14.5°C to 15.5°C is equivalent to 58°F to 60°F. As a practical example, imagine a chemistry experiment where you have 1 L water in a container placed above a heat source (e.g., flame). Imagine, too, that this container does not absorb any heat but transfers all heat from the source directly to the water. Place a thermometer in the water at 58°F and turn on your heat source. If you could capture the heat (from the source) that would be needed to raise the temperature of that water to 60°F, this would represent 1 calorie. Given our hypothetical container, this would take less than a minute to accomplish.

## Adenosine Triphosphate

ATP consists of three components: adenine, a nucleobase (nitrogen-containing biological compound); ribose, a sugar; and three phosphate molecules, with the two outermost phosphates representing high-energy bonds that store the potential energy within the ATP molecule (Fig. 4-2).

ATP is formed by combining the molecules adenosine diphosphate (ADP) and inorganic phosphate (Pi) through a reaction catalyzed by the enzyme ATP synthase. Synthesis of ATP requires energy derived from the catabolism of other molecules (e.g., muscle glycogen), part of which becomes stored in the chemical bond linking ADP and Pi, creating a high-energy bond. During activity or exercise, this bond is broken and free energy becomes available to facilitate biological processes, including muscle contraction, molecular transport across cell membranes, and cell growth and development. The enzyme ATPase promotes the splitting of ATP, releasing 7.3 kcal of energy from the outermost high-energy phosphate bond.[5] Breakdown of the ATP molecule to ADP and Pi is commonly referred to as hydrolysis because of involvement of a water molecule in this reaction (Fig. 4-3).

In recovery or during lower-intensity bouts of exercise (following more vigorous bouts that rapidly used ATP), the depleted ATP stores can be replenished by the reverse process of joining ADP and Pi in a reaction driven by the presence of energy.

Given that ATP is essential for repeated muscle contraction, it would seem logical that large stores of ATP exist within skeletal muscle. However, this is not the case; the body stores only small amounts of ATP within cells, containing a total of approximately 3 ounces or 90 g in an entire adult body.[6] We therefore rely on the rapid regeneration of ATP when any work is performed. In fact, if ATP could not be rapidly regenerated, the stores of ATP would quickly be depleted during high-intensity exercise scenarios.[7] It is important to recognize that it is the demand for ATP from skeletal muscle contraction that stresses cellular homeostasis; that is, it is this disruption of ATP stores that stimulates increased metabolism and sets in motion all of the biochemical reactions needed to maintain muscle ATP,

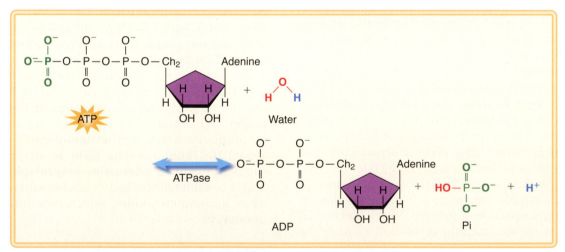

Figure 4-2. Chemical structure of adenosine triphosphate (ATP) and products of ATP hydrolysis.

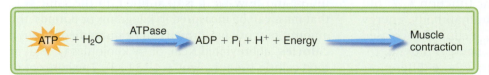

Figure 4-3. Adenosine triphosphate hydrolysis. Substrates and products of the chemical reaction.

which subsequently stimulates the energy pathways to meet that ATP demand.[1]

## ENERGY PATHWAYS

As illustrated in Figure 4-4, the body contains two basic energy systems: the aerobic pathway (oxidative or mitochondrial), which functions with the presence of oxygen, and the anaerobic pathways, which function without oxygen. The anaerobic pathway is further subdivided into two systems: the more immediate phosphagen system and the glycolytic system, sometimes referred to as the fast-glycolytic or lactate system. Each of these systems can generate ATP.

There are fundamental differences between the aerobic and anaerobic pathways:

- The aerobic pathway is capable of generating large amounts of ATP, whereas the anaerobic pathways generate smaller, limited quantities of ATP.
- The aerobic pathway generates ATP slowly, whereas the anaerobic pathways have the capacity to generate ATP more rapidly, as illustrated in Figure 4-5. This characteristic provides insight into the activity of different energy pathways during various exercise conditions.
- Aerobic respiration occurs within the mitochondria of the cell, whereas anaerobic respiration takes place within the cell sarcoplasm.

Generally speaking, the aerobic and anaerobic pathways can be differentiated by their relative contributions to maximal efforts of differing durations, as illustrated in Figure 4-6. In practical terms, Table 4-1 illustrates how the different pathways contribute energy to fuel events of different intensities and durations.

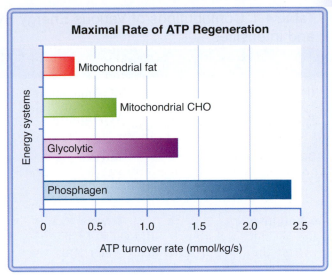

Figure 4-5. Maximal rate of adenosine triphosphate (ATP) regeneration for each energy system. Maximal rate of ATP regeneration can be quantified by ATP turnover rate in the units of millimoles per kilogram per second (mmol/kg/sec).

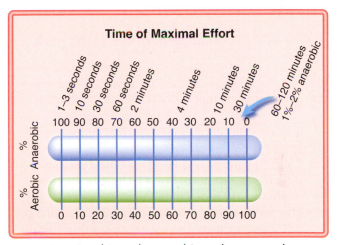

Figure 4-6. Aerobic and anaerobic pathways can be differentiated by their relative contributions to maximal efforts of differing durations.

## Phosphagen System

The most rapid means for generating ATP is through the **phosphagen system**.[8] This pathway comprises two components: molecules of ATP and a larger quantity of **phosphocreatine** or **creatine phosphate**: (CrP). The sequence of how this system generates ATP might be best understood if it is presented as a sequence that is illustrated in Figure 4-7.

- The demand for ATP increases because of the onset of activity, especially high-intensity exercise.
- The hydrolysis of ATP catalyzed by the action of ATPase increases levels of ADP.
- Increased levels of ADP activate (upregulate) the enzyme creatine kinase, which is responsible for facilitating the hydrolysis of CrP to creatine (Cr) and phosphate (P), in the process liberating some free energy. Conversely, this creatine kinase

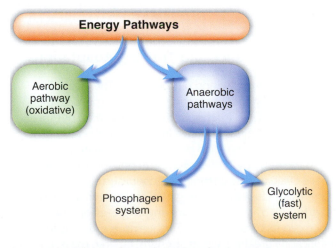

Figure 4-4. The body contains two basic energy systems: the aerobic pathway (oxidative or mitochondrial), which functions with the presence of oxygen, and the anaerobic pathways, which function without oxygen.

**Table 4-1.** Contributions of Various Energy Systems During Events of Differing Durations and Intensities

| DURATION OF EVENT | EVENT INTENSITY | PRIMARY ENERGY SYSTEM |
|---|---|---|
| 0–5 seconds | Maximal effort | Phosphagen (predominantly) |
| 6–30 seconds | Very intense | Phosphagen (becoming depleted around 10 sec) Fast glycolytic (assuming primary role) |
| 30–120 seconds | Intense | Fast glycolytic (predominantly) |
| 2–3 minutes | Moderate | Fast glycolytic (becoming depleted) Aerobic (assuming primary role) |
| >3 minutes | Lower | Oxidative (almost exclusively) |

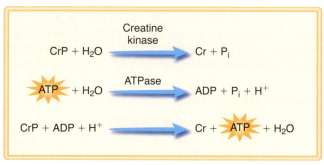

**Figure 4-7.** Coupled reaction. The creatine kinase reaction and adenosine triphosphate rephosphorylation.

activity is inhibited when normal concentrations of ATP are present.

- This free energy is used to manufacture (phosphorylate) a molecule of ATP by adding phosphate to ADP molecules.[9]
- This process continues as long as the demand for ATP exists or until the concentrations of CrP diminish to the point at which it can no longer

provide free energy to phosphorylate ATP from ADP and phosphate, as shown in Figure 4-8.

The design of this system permits an almost instantaneous capacity to match ATP demand with a swift supply,[10] and the maximal rate of ATP production from the phosphagen system is twice as rapid as in glycolysis. Unfortunately, the skeletal muscle concentration of CrP is limited, and within a duration of approximately 10 seconds at near-maximal efforts, the resting CrP stores become rapidly depleted.[11]

Examples of activities that rely heavily on the phosphagen system for ATP provision include sprinting 100 m, pole vaulting, chopping wood, jumping rope, and any other high-intensity exercise repeated over multiple bouts for a short duration (Fig. 4-9).[12] Recovery from CrP degradation becomes critical in these instances if high-intensity exercise performance is to continue. After severe, high-intensity exercise in which the phosphagen system is completely depleted, research has reported it may take 5 to 15 minutes for CrP levels to become completely restored.[1,13–15] It has also

## RESEARCH HIGHLIGHT

### Effects of Creatine Supplementation on Performance and Training Adaptations

Creatine still remains a highly popular and well-researched supplement in exercise and performance. The rationale behind creatine supplementation is the premise that if the body's stores of phosphocreatine can be augmented, the regeneration of ATP by this mechanism would be enhanced, thus allowing high-intensity effort to be carried out for a longer period. This literature review examined more than 500 research studies that have investigated the effects of creatine supplementation on muscle physiology or exercise capacity, or both, in varied populations. Creatine supplementation has been reported to increase total creatine content in the body by 10% to 30% and phosphocreatine stores by 10% to 40%. Of the approximate 300 studies that have evaluated its potential ergogenic effects, about 70% report statistically significant improvements in performance. This includes improving maximal power/strength by 5% to 15%, improving work capacity during sets of maximal effort by 5% to 15%, improving single-effort sprint performance by 1% to 5%, and improving repetitive performance events by 5% to 15%. Furthermore, creatine supplementation during training has been reported to promote significantly greater gains in strength, fat-free mass, and performance (primarily high-intensity exercise) compared with placebo-controlled trials.

Kreider RB. Effects of creatine supplementation on performance and training adaptations. *Mol. Cell. Biochem.* 2003;244:89–94.

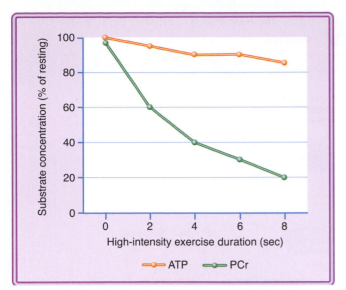

Figure 4-8. The decline in concentrations of phosphocreatine (PCr) associated with short-duration, high-intensity exercise.

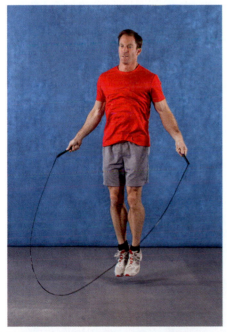

Figure 4-9. Jumping rope is an example of an activity that relies heavily on the phosphagen system for adenosine triphosphate provision—a high-intensity exercise repeated over multiple bouts for a short duration.

been shown that an active recovery appears to facilitate more rapid CrP regeneration compared with a passive recovery,[16] and higher cardiorespiratory fitness levels also influence recovery because of improved delivery of oxygen to assist with recovery.[17] In addition, phosphocreatine levels are restored more rapidly in slow-twitch muscle fibers than in fast-twitch muscle fibers.

Given the fact that the overall capacity for the phosphagen system at maximal rates is limited to a duration of approximately 10 seconds, an alternative pathway capable of regenerating ATP in an expedited

fashion must exist for exercise to continue at relatively high intensities.

## Glycolysis

By definition, **glycolysis** represents the metabolic pathway that catalyzes (breaks down) glucose ($C_6H_{12}O_6$) or muscle glycogen into two pyruvate (three-carbon) or two lactate structures.[18] Although pyruvate is technically the end product of glycolysis, it is then converted to lactate in the absence of sufficient oxygen or is shuttled into the mitochondria for aerobic respiration. It is important to note, however, that the fate of pyruvate does not follow an all-or-nothing principle; it can lead to either or both simultaneously, depending on the availability of oxygen.

Glycolysis is a sequence of 10 reactions that involve intermediate compounds that result in the manufacture of 2 pyruvate structures. Glycolysis uses energy to complete specific steps and also releases free energy at specific steps that are used to phosphorylate ATP molecules. In addition, throughout this process, hydrogen atoms are transferred to a specific electron carrier, nicotinamide adenine dinucleotide (NAD) + hydrogen (H), or NADH. These steps and the electron carrier transferring hydrogen atoms away from the glycolysis pathway are illustrated in Figure 4-10. These intermediate compounds of glycolysis also provide entry and exit points for other substances into glycolysis. For example, the intermediate dihydroxyacetone phosphate manufactured in step 5 is a source of entry or production for glycerol (from triglycerides: glycerol + three fatty acids). A common approach to studying glycolysis is to break this pathway into two phases. Phase 1 can be thought of as the energy investment phase, and phase 2 represents the energy generation phase.

### Phase 1

Phase 1 of glycolysis requires an initial investment of either one or two ATP molecules to proceed. To help explain this concept, let's use a simple example: Think of someone bowling; without a backswing, the ball will not have much momentum. However, by incorporating a backswing, which costs energy to execute, the ball will roll with greater momentum. In a similar fashion, to enable glycolysis to complete all 10 steps, it helps if we give the reaction a "backswing" to start. As indicated, phase 1 requires an initial investment of either one or two ATP molecules.

This analogy offers a simplified explanation of why we use energy to initiate glycolysis, but it does not explain the difference between the need for one or two ATP molecules. The difference is explained by whether the original carbohydrate source is glucose or glycogen. Essentially, glucose must be transported into the muscle cell from the blood via a specific protein carrier, and this costs more energy. Therefore, we must contribute two ATP molecules: one during step 1 and the second during step 3 (see Fig. 4-10). Glycogen, in contrast, is already stored within the cell, and it does not require transportation nor does it incur any cost to initiate its

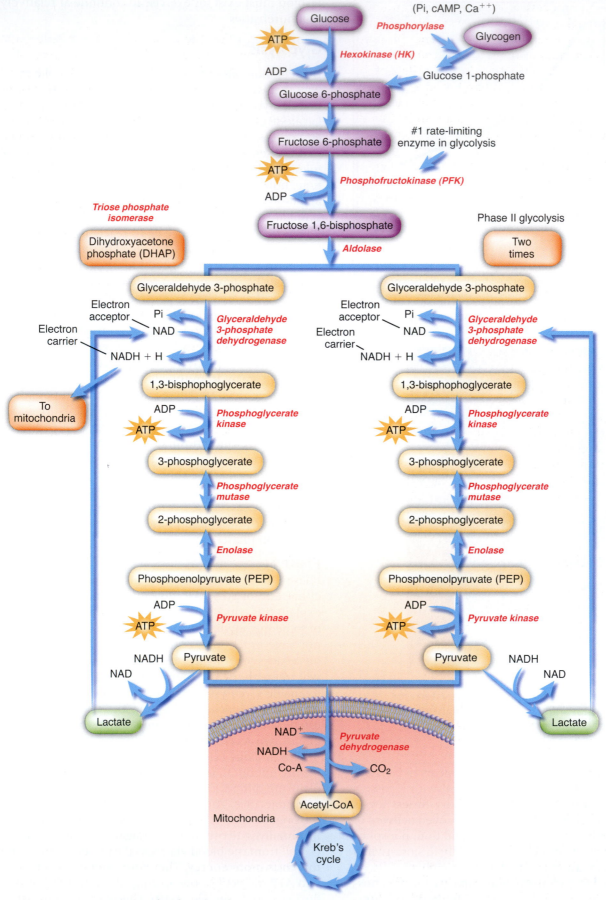

**Figure 4-10.** Reactions involved in glycolysis.

breakdown. The process of breaking glycogen down into individual glucose units requires only one ATP molecule to be invested during step 3. The third glycolytic step is the conversion to the intermediate fructose, 1,6-diphosphate (see Box 4-1). Regardless of the source of the carbohydrate, glucose or glycogen, this step will require the use of one ATP. In summary, as a starting substrate, glycogen requires an initial investment of one ATP molecule, whereas glucose requires an initial investment of two ATP molecules.

The final step of phase 1 involves the cleavage of fructose-1,6-disphosphate (a six-carbon molecule) into two 3-carbon molecules. Each of these molecules subsequently enters into the energy generation phase of glycolysis.

## Phase 2

The second phase of glycolysis involves the remaining reactions from which four ATP molecules (steps 7 and 10) and two pyruvate (step 10) molecules are produced. As illustrated in Figure 4-10, during glycolysis, the six-carbon structure divides into two 3-carbon structures that ultimately are converted to two pyruvate molecules. During the remaining reactions, there are two steps in which enough free energy is liberated in the formation of the intermediate products to drive the formation of ATP molecules from an ADP and Pi (phosphorylation).

This generates four ATPs (two for each side), whereas phase 1 requires an initial investment of one or two ATP molecules, pending the initial substrate. Thus, when examining the net ATP production of glycolysis:

- Net yield = two ATP when the initial substrate is glucose.

- Net yield = three ATP when the initial substrate is glycogen.

In addition, two molecules of $NAD^+$ are reduced to NADH during phase 2 of glycolysis from the glyceraldehyde-3-phosphate dehydrogenase reaction (Box 4-2). These will ultimately move to the electron transport chain (ETC; discussed later) to produce ATP.

Under steady-state exercise intensity conditions, the electrons and protons from NADH are passed into the mitochondria, where they are used to generate ATP (Fig. 4-11). Steady-state exercise can be briefly defined

## Box 4-2. Nicotinamide Adenine Dinucleotide

**Nicotinamide adenine dinucleotide ($NAD^+$)**, synthesized from dietary niacin (vitamin $B_3$), is a critical cofactor (nonprotein chemical compound) involved in reduction-oxidation reactions in cells (involving the transfer of electrons). The enzymes involved in these reactions require a high-energy electron carrier that can transfer hydrogen and electrons, and $NAD^+$ is one such carrier that exists in glycolysis. The addition of two electrons and their associated hydrogen atoms converts $NAD^+$ into NADH. Conversely, a reaction in which the substrate gains electrons from NADH will convert this carrier back to $NAD^+$. A second carrier, FAD, another cofactor involved in metabolism, functions predominantly during aerobic respiration and is discussed later.

## Box 4-1. Phosphofructokinase

The rate of glycolysis (also known as glycolytic flux) is principally controlled by the activity of one of the many enzymes involved in the 10 steps of glycolysis. This enzyme is **phosphofructokinase (PFK)**, which is the enzyme involved in step 3 that converts fructose 6-phosphate to fructose 1,6-diphosphate. It is considered the main rate-limiting step in glycolysis, and its action requires the utilization of one ATP molecule (see Fig. 4-10).[76]

Activity levels of PFK are increased by elevated levels of ADP and Pi, all molecules likely to increase under exercising conditions where we witness an increased demand for ATP.[77] The activity of this enzyme is swiftly upregulated at the onset of intense exercise.[78] Conversely, PFK is inhibited by higher elevations of ATP (rest or recovery) and also by a decrease in pH levels. In other words, if blood acidity increases (lower pH), as occurs with the accumulation of protons in the muscle cell, the rate of the glycolytic flux is reduced, potentially offering one explanation for why exercise capacity decreases when lactate levels in the tissue increase.

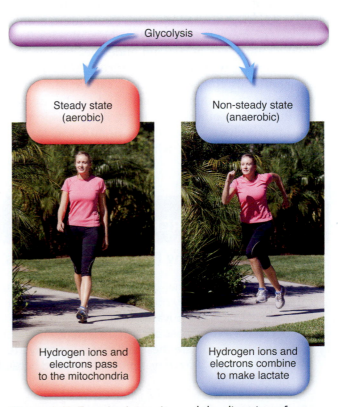

**Figure 4-11.** Exercise intensity and the direction of hydrogen ions.

as exercise intensities that remain relatively constant where the energy needs are met aerobically. Under non–steady-state exercise intensity conditions, NADH can pass its protons and electrons back to pyruvate to form lactate.

As mentioned previously, it is important to remember that the fate of pyruvate is not an all-or-nothing concept, implying that both outcomes can occur simultaneously (i.e., conversion to lactate and shuttling into the mitochondria). The quantity of pyruvate that enters the mitochondria is contingent on the capacity of the aerobic pathway (e.g., availability of oxygen, size, and number of mitochondria), whereas any excess pyruvate is converted to lactate. Although lactate production is frequently associated with fatigue, we will learn in the next section that lactate production is paramount to continued functioning of glycolysis.

In summary, the process of glycolysis, which takes place within the sarcoplasm in muscle cells, produced two pyruvate molecules, two NADH, and either two or three ATP molecules. As mentioned earlier, pyruvate suffers two fates: conversion to lactate within the sarcoplasm or transfer to the mitochondria, where it will continue through aerobic respiration.

## Lactate Production

Our understanding of the role of lactate has changed from one where it was perceived as a dead-end metabolic waste product of glycolysis and a major cause of skeletal muscle fatigue to a compound that now plays an important role in the energy pathways.[19] The human body is constantly producing lactate, as cells such as red blood cells lack mitochondria and, therefore, can only generate energy through the anaerobic pathways (i.e., glycolysis). However, at rest and under steady-state exercise conditions, we maintain a balance between lactate production and removal, as lactate can be converted back to pyruvate within some cells and can be used as substrate (fuel) by others (e.g., heart, liver, muscles).[2]

During glycolysis, blood glucose or muscle glycogen is converted to pyruvate, which will either enter the mitochondria to continue aerobic respiration or be converted to lactate, depending on the intensity of exercise and availability of oxygen (Fig. 4-12). Keep in mind that both can occur simultaneously. Almost all pyruvate enters the mitochondria at rest or during low-intensity exercise, but at higher intensities when the capacity for mitochondrial respiration is exceeded, more pyruvate is converted to lactate. At higher exercise intensities, there is an increased reliance on the rate at which glucose transfers to pyruvate through glycolysis to make ATP. Researchers believe that, at higher rates of glycolysis, pyruvate is produced faster than it can enter into the mitochondria for mitochondrial respiration.[20] Thus, the excess pyruvate that cannot enter the mitochondria is converted to lactate, which can then be used as fuel elsewhere in the body (e.g., heart, liver, nonexercising muscles).

## Proton Buffering

Lactate is formed from pyruvate (reduction process) via a reaction catalyzed by the enzyme lactate dehydrogenase.[21] As a result of this reaction, the cells regenerate $NAD^+$ and consume (remove) a $H^+$ proton in the process—both contribute to the continued rapid rate of ATP production. In the following section, we explain these concepts in more detail.

During our discussion of the second phase of glycolysis, we highlighted that a key step involved the glyceraldehyde-3-phosphate dehydrogenase reaction, in which two molecules of $NAD^+$ are reduced to NADH. This step precedes the phosphoglycerate kinase and pyruvate kinase reactions from which four ATP molecules are produced. During steady-state–type exercise, the electrons and protons from NADH are passed into the mitochondria, but at higher exercise intensities this does not occur. Consequently, NADH begins to accumulate in the cytosol, whereas $NAD^+$ becomes limited. If $NAD^+$ is not regenerated in the lactate dehydrogenase reaction, the glycolytic flux becomes compromised and ATP regeneration is reduced.

The consumption of protons is beneficial in that it combats the development of metabolic acidosis, a condition

## RESEARCH HIGHLIGHT

### Emerging Research in Glycolysis

Traditionally, glycolysis has been presented as a series of 10 bidirectional steps. However, some research has indicated that glycolysis may not actually occur in reverse in vivo (i.e., in skeletal muscle) because of the irreversible reactions of PFK and pyruvate kinase, key enzymes involved in glycolysis.[1] These researchers concluded that any gluconeogenesis that does occur from lactate, other amino acids, or glycerol must take place in the liver and not in skeletal muscle, where these substrates are converted back to glucose as needed. However, more research demonstrating this discovery is probably needed because this could have significant implications in the field of bioenergetics.

Baker JS, McCormick MC, Robergs RA. Interaction among skeletal muscle metabolic energy systems during intense exercise. *J. Nutr. Metab.* 2010;2010:1–13.

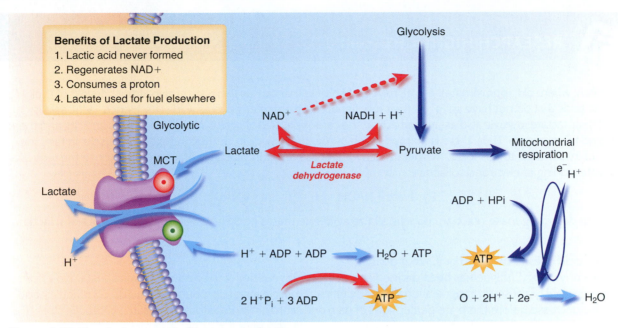

**Figure 4-12.** Metabolic control of lactate production.

marked by the accumulation of hydrogen ions (protons) in the cell or blood that reduce the pH level. In fact, it is this proton accumulation that plays a more significant role in muscle fatigue than lactate. This is because of the inhibitory effect of lower pH levels on the activity of PFK and ATPase, enzymes necessary for the production and utilization of ATP. Proton accumulation is also believed to negatively impact muscle contraction by interfering with calcium release from the sarcoplasmic reticulum, thereby interfering with its ability to bind to troponin and allow for muscle contraction. These concepts are presented in detail in Chapter 9. Furthermore, an accumulation of protons is also believed to increase pain receptor sensitivity within muscles. This may explain why individuals experience a muscle "burn" at higher exercise intensities. Therefore, lactate production should not necessarily be viewed as a fatigue-inducing event.

## RESEARCH HIGHLIGHT

### Lactate and Metabolic Acidosis: An Interview with Robert A. Robergs, PhD

EDITOR'S NOTE: *Dr. Robergs is the Head of Human Movement Studies at Charles Sturt University in Australia. He is an accomplished author with more than 110 published peer-reviewed articles and is an internationally recognized expert on lactate and metabolic acidosis.*

#### Q: Can you tell us briefly about the history of lactic acid?
Lactic acid has a long history. For centuries it had been known that if milk is left to go bad, then something was formed in the milk that caused a sour taste. In 1780, Carl Scheele, a Swedish chemist, was able to document that this "something" was lactic acid. By the 1830s, lactic acid had also been found in muscle from stressed animals, fresh milk, and blood. In the 1920s, the Nobel Prize-winning research of Hill and Meyerhof established that intense muscle contractions caused increased lactic acid production, and that lactic acid was produced from pyruvic acid, which was the final product of the glycolytic pathway. Hill's and Meyerhof's work occurred 20 years before L. J. Henderson proposed computations of acid-base chemistry. Such acid-base chemistry principles revealed the pH dependence of acids, and that given the pH of biological solutions was close to neutral (pH 7), cellular conditions were far from the severe acidity needed (pH ~3.8) for the existence of metabolic acids produced from cellular metabolism.

#### Q: Why is there no such thing as lactic acidosis in the body?
I have tried to remain solidly grounded in science when explaining the biochemistry of metabolic acidosis; however, there remains a strong bias for some physiologists to continue to "blame" lactic acid for this condition. The scientific reality is that numerous chemical reactions in the body involve hydrogen ions ($H^+$), with some consuming $H^+$ and others releasing $H^+$. An acid metabolite is able to release $H^+$ to solution. For the carboxylic acids of cellular

*Continued*

## RESEARCH HIGHLIGHT—cont'd

metabolism, where pH approximates 7.0, all have a pH profile that causes them to remain almost devoid of their $H^+$. Metabolic acids that do not have an $H^+$ on their functional group are referred to as acid salts. Hence, lactic acid is referred to as lactate; pyruvic acid as pyruvate. Thus, no carboxylic acid of glycolysis is produced as an acid, and therefore has no $H^+$ to release. Thus, there is no production of metabolic acids in contracting skeletal muscle. In fact, the reaction of importance to this topic, the lactate dehydrogenase reaction, actually consumes a proton in the reduction of pyruvate (adding of electrons) to lactate.

$$Pyruvate + NADH + H^+ \leftrightarrow lactate + NAD^+$$

The lactate dehydrogenase reaction alone is all the evidence that is needed to refute the construct of a lactic acidosis!

### Q: If lactic acid doesn't cause fatigue, what does?

In exercise physiology, fatigue has been defined as a decrease in muscle force or power despite sustained effort. There is evidence of muscular fatigue even before significant muscle lactate production. Muscle contractility and power also decrease before there are perceptions of pain or discomfort, and before significant metabolic stress (i.e., large increases in protons). Such early-onset fatigue has to be largely neural in origin, and may reside in the neural pathways descending from the motor cortex to the spinal cord that determine motor unit recruitment. Unfortunately, most of the research of muscular "fatigue" has focused on the physiology and muscle metabolic biochemistry that occurs when a subject terminates exercise. The end of exercise is not the start of "fatigue," and one can criticize past research of a clear bias in researching "fatigue" at exercise termination when there has been evidence for a long time that actual muscular fatigue starts far earlier in the exercise bout! This latter point is important for muscle lactate production. The biochemical evidence reveals that during intense exercise, muscle must produce lactate to regenerate cytosolic $NAD^+$ and in doing so sustain a high rate of ATP turnover from glycolysis. In other words, muscle needs to produce lactate to sustain repeated intense muscle contractions.

### Q: What is the practical application of this new way of thinking for exercise professionals?

Science and education are meant to be about factual evidence, or in more simple terms, the truth. When science deviates from the truth, it is no longer science. The key issue that needs to change is the incorrect interpretation that muscle lactate production causes acidosis, and that muscle lactate production impairs muscle contractile function. The acidosis interpretation is just blatantly incorrect. The impaired contractile function issue requires added research, as we still do not know enough of the independent contribution of lactate to muscular fatigue. Lactate may not be a detrimental molecule to muscle contractile function. Rather, muscle must produce lactate to sustain intense exercise. Lactate is not the "bad" molecule that we have been led to believe.[22]

## Lactate Removal and Disposal

As described previously, small amounts of lactate production occur at rest, which indicates the presence of a lactate removal process that prevents lactate accumulation. Lactate produced in skeletal muscle can be shuttled out of the cell through a transporter protein called a monocarboxylate transporter (MCT), which removes both lactate and proton molecules from the muscle cell (see Fig. 4-12).[23]

The primary means of lactate disposal include uptake by the heart, liver, kidneys, and within less active skeletal muscle as a metabolic fuel.[24] In particular, during exercise, lactate produced in the skeletal muscle is shuttled out of the muscle cell and transported by the blood to the liver.[25] Within the liver, lactate contributes to glucose production (a process known as gluconeogenesis). This manufactured glucose can then be subsequently released back into the bloodstream and transported back to the exercising skeletal muscle and used as fuel. This lactate-to-glucose cycle between skeletal muscle and the liver is known as the **Cori cycle** and represents an effective means to manage accumulation of blood lactate (see explanatory animation of the Cori cycle on the Davis*Plus* site at http://davis*plus*.fadavis.com).

The Cori cycle represents a mechanism that occurs within the liver by which the body regenerates lactate back to pyruvate. The pyruvate can then either regenerate glucose by moving backward through glycolysis or move into the aerobic pathway. Recalling how the process of converting glucose to pyruvate generated two to three ATP molecules, it stands to reason that converting two pyruvate molecules back to glucose will cost energy. How, then, does the body fuel this metabolic process? It is believed that within the Cori cycle, some pyruvate passes to the mitochondria and enters the aerobic pathways, generating energy to fuel the conversion of lactate to pyruvate and back to glucose (Fig. 4-13).

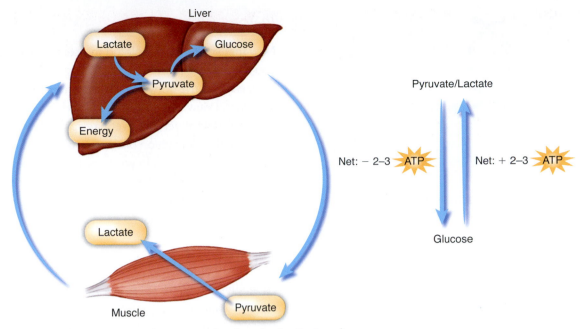

**Figure 4-13.** Lactate-to-glucose production via the Cori cycle.

Once the protons, transported to the bloodstream via MCT proteins, spill over into the blood, the process of proton disposal involves binding with a buffer within the blood. Although various buffers exist in the blood, each with a unique function, sodium bicarbonate ($NaHCO_3$), commonly referred to as baking soda, acts as our principal proton buffer. Figure 4-14 presents a general overview of how the buffer works to prevent proton accumulation and metabolic acidosis. Sodium or potassium in the blood binds with lactate to form a compound that can enter the cell for use as a fuel or for entry into the Cori cycle. The remaining bicarbonate binds with hydrogen to form carbonic acid ($H_2CO_3$), a weak acid that can disassociate into water and carbon dioxide. Although we have no real need to remove this

metabolic water from the body, the carbon dioxide can be expelled via the lungs. An understanding of how this buffer works has led researchers and athletes to experiment with the consumption of sodium bicarbonate. The goal is to increase the quantity of this buffer in our blood to tolerate greater levels of lactate and protons, thereby enabling one to maintain higher intensities of exercise for longer periods.

## Lactate Threshold and Onset of Blood Lactate Accumulation

As mentioned previously, although there are always small amounts of lactate in our blood at all times, it is the progressive increases that occur during exercise that interest researchers and coaches. As exercise intensity

## RESEARCH HIGHLIGHT

### Sodium Bicarbonate Supplementation and Performance

Research has shown that muscle buffering capacity can be augmented by nutritional strategies. Alkalizing agents (e.g., sodium bicarbonate) have been studied extensively for their potential to enhance performance by reducing the extent to which the metabolic acidosis contributes to fatigue during high-intensity exercise performance. The mechanism by which sodium bicarbonate ingestion improves performance is by promoting removal of protons. Removing protons prevents a decline in pH within the muscle that contributes to fatigue. Results of the meta-analysis indicate that ingestion of sodium bicarbonate can enhance endurance performance in events where a rapid buildup of lactate impacts performance (e.g., 400-m dash). The main drawback to using sodium bicarbonate is that some individuals experience gastrointestinal distress with its ingestion. Accordingly, it has been recommended that exercise professionals purposefully experiment with the sodium bicarbonate loading protocols for clients to maximize the alkalizing effects and minimize the risk for potential symptoms. The recommended dosage and timeframe for sodium bicarbonate ingestion (normally delivered via capsule or flavored beverage) is 0.2 to 0.4 g/Kg body weight (0.1–0.18 g/lb) taken with 1 L (33.8 oz) of fluids at 60 to 120 minutes before exercise.

Peart DJ, Siegler JC, Vince RV. Practical recommendations for coaches and athletes: a meta-analysis of sodium bicarbonate use for athletic performance. *J. Strength Cond. Res.* 2012;26:1975–1983.

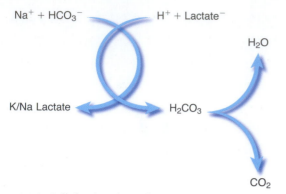

**Figure 4-14.** Cellular-level mechanisms responsible for the buffering of protons.

## In Your Own Words

Now that you have completed this section, we hope you have a new-found understanding of the role of lactate within the body. Considering how many individuals still view lactate as a dead-end, metabolic waste product, it generally requires professionals to share a little information of the role of lactate, hydrogen ions, and acidosis. In your words, what are the key scientific points and takeaways that you can use to help educate individuals who still share this outdated way of thinking about lactate?

progresses, there is a gradual switch from fats as a primary fuel to carbohydrates as a primary fuel because of the increased efficiency of using carbohydrates to produce energy. Furthermore, this also represents a shift from using our more aerobic, type I muscle fibers with a greater capacity for aerobic work toward increased recruitment of our larger, more anaerobic type II fibers that rely more on anaerobic pathways.[26] This represents a slight but manageable increase in lactate levels, reflecting a small imbalance between lactate production (spillover into the blood) and uptake (removal from the blood).[27]

This first accumulation of blood lactate above resting concentrations is defined as the **lactate threshold (LT)**. Technically, this point represents an intensity where carbohydrates now become the body's primary fuel source and corresponds to a respiratory exchange ratio score of approximately 0.85 to 0.87, which is explained in Chapter 5. This marker also represents the point at which the body begins to lose its aerobic efficiency (i.e., the ability to burn fats as a primary fuel) and starts relying on the anaerobic systems to assist in producing energy (see Chapter 15).[28]

Further increases in exercise intensity continue to raise blood lactate levels, suggesting a greater mismatch between lactate production and disposal that ultimately leads to a disproportionate increase in blood lactate. This is known as the **onset of blood lactate accumulation (OBLA)**, which is the point at which the ability to sustain high-intensity exercise cannot be sustained much longer.[29] Physiologically, this marker indicates an inability by the body to dispose or manage the rate at which lactate (produced in muscle cells) is entering the blood. Essentially, at this point, the body's ability to dispose of blood lactate becomes overwhelmed. OBLA represents the intensity that athletes and coaches refer to as LT, or the highest sustainable intensity of exercise (i.e., immediately below OBLA). From a performance standpoint, implementing any strategies to boost OBLA or expand the body's lactate buffer to tolerate greater quantities of lactate spillover into the blood and improve performance is of paramount importance. Chapter 15 will discuss the practical applications of these metabolic indicators to programing.

## Role of the Energy Systems in Exercise Fatigue

Fatigue refers to the inability to continue exercise at a given intensity (Fig. 4-15).[28] In all sports and exercise training, the onset of fatigue will vary depending on numerous factors, including fitness level and training status, exercise intensity, and environmental conditions (e.g., heat, humidity, and altitude).[30] This section provides a brief overview of the role these anaerobic energy systems play in exercise fatigue (i.e., short-term, more intense exercise).[3]

During vigorous exercise bouts such as sprinting, short-burst interval training, and high-intensity resistance exercise, continued muscle contraction is dependent on the formation of ATP to meet the high demand for energy. Under these exercise conditions, CrP, which resynthesizes ATP, and glucose breakdown (glycolysis) are primarily responsible for maintaining ATP levels. During intense muscle contraction, CrP becomes rapidly depleted, providing an inadequate supply of ATP.[30] The skeletal muscle concentration of CrP is limited, and within a duration of approximately 10 seconds, the resting CrP stores are rapidly depleted.[31]

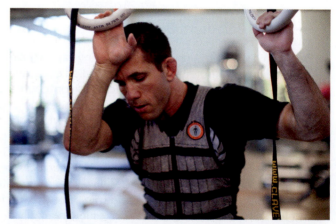

**Figure 4-15.** The onset of fatigue, or the inability to continue exercise at a given intensity, depends on fitness level and training status, exercise intensity, and environmental conditions.

To offset a potential ATP deficiency, glycolytic flux (glycolysis) increases, producing additional ATP. However, the increased output of glycolysis results in the accumulation of by-products, including lactate and protons ($H^+$), both of which will lead to fatigue. It is the proton accumulation discussed earlier in this chapter that contributes to a decreased cellular pH (acidosis), which impairs muscle contraction through a number of mechanisms, including inhibition of the rate-limiting enzymes ATPase and PFK.

The protons produced from increased glycolytic flux also often interfere with calcium ions reacting with proteins at the myofilament site in muscle where contraction is occurring, further inhibiting the muscle's ability to contract. Furthermore, enzymes involved in the cellular regulation of sodium and potassium during muscle contraction also become impaired by increased proton accumulation.[3]

Both within the blood and intramuscular cellular environment there exists a natural buffering capacity system to help combat increased acidosis (i.e., proton accumulation). Given the link between metabolic acidosis and fatigue, there has long been considerable interest in training strategies that can augment this natural buffering capacity. The cellular environment possesses a buffering capacity system to help combat increased acidosis (i.e., proton accumulation); however, in untrained individuals, this system is easily overwhelmed during high-intensity exercise conditions. Correct exercise training confers an increased muscle buffering capacity, which ultimately contributes to an increased ability to tolerate high-intensity exercise conditions, delay fatigue, and improve recovery. High cellular concentrations of protons manufactured during intense exercise provide a needed stimulus for improving muscle buffering capacity. For example, it has been demonstrated that high-intensity interval-type training (6- to 12-interval bouts of 2 minutes each at a workload of 90%–100% $\dot{V}O_2max$ with 1-minute rest intervals) is a successful strategy for eliciting favorable buffering capacity adaptations.[32]

## VIGNETTE continued

■ After presenting a series of lectures on the rather complex science required to understand the bioenergetics of exercise, Felicia simplifies things by going back to the basics, telling her students that the process of digestion breaks the macronutrients into their simplest components (i.e., glucose, fatty acids, and amino acids), which are absorbed into the blood and transported to metabolically active cells, such as nerve or muscle cells. These substances either immediately enter a metabolic pathway to produce ATP or are stored for later use.

To clarify how the human body uses the three energy systems–phosphagen, anaerobic glycolysis, and aerobic–Felicia discusses physical activities with which her students are familiar.

- 100-m run: This activity derives approximately 50% of the fuel needed from the phosphagen system and 50% from the anaerobic glycolysis system, with an insignificant contribution from the aerobic system. This is because a rapid production of ATP is required to fuel this high-intensity, short-duration activity.
- 10,000-m run: In contrast, this low-intensity, long-duration activity derives 97% of the fuel needed from the aerobic system and only 3% from the anaerobic glycolysis system.
- Soccer game: A soccer game is a perfect example of how most activities and sports require a combination of fuel sources, as 10% of the energy required comes from the phosphagen system, 70% from anaerobic glycolysis, and 20% from the aerobic system. A soccer game requires a tremendous amount of stamina, but also short bursts of energy for high-intensity sprints.

## AEROBIC RESPIRATION: MITOCHONDRIAL RESPIRATION

The third pathway by which ATP is produced is through mitochondrial (aerobic) respiration. In terms of overall quantity, the production of ATP molecules in this pathway is greatest, but the rate of ATP production is considerably slower than from either the phosphagen system or glycolysis. Another benefit of this system is that all three macronutrients serve as substrate (fuel) for energy production. Figure 4-16 illustrates the continued process of carbohydrate metabolism into the mitochondria after pyruvate formation, and Figure 4-17 shows the entire aerobic pathway and the interplay of all three macronutrients.

As mentioned previously, carbohydrates in the form of glucose or glycogen pass through glycolysis to form pyruvate molecules. Pyruvate is either converted to lactate or to acetyl-coenzyme A (CoA) (irreversible) that enters mitochondrial respiration. Triglycerides are composed of FFAs and glycerol, and enter the bioenergetics pathways via:

- beta-oxidation, a process of cleaving longer fatty acids into two-carbon structures to form acetyl-CoA.
- glycolysis, the pathway followed by glycerol, a three-carbon structure that resembles pyruvate.

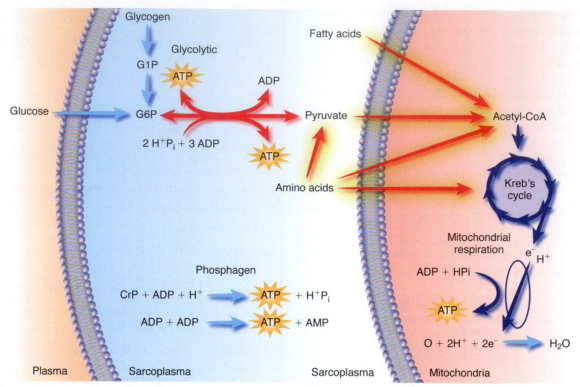

**Figure 4-16.** Overview of the three energy systems capable of resynthesizing adenosine triphosphate: the phosphagen system, glycolytic system, and mitochondrial respiration.

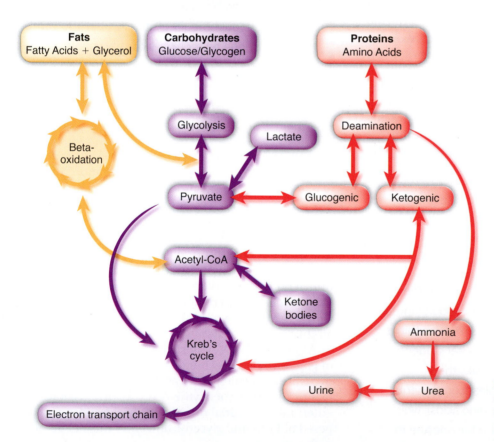

**Figure 4-17.** Overview of how each macronutrient (fats, carbohydrates, and proteins) is involved in mitochondrial respiration.

Proteins contain nitrogen atoms in addition to carbon, hydrogen, and oxygen; thus, they must first undergo deamination, the process of removing the nitrogen group from the amino acid. The remaining amino acid skeleton will either enter the aerobic pathway as acetyl-CoA or other intermediate products of the Krebs cycle (discussed in upcoming sections), or be converted to pyruvate. Those entering the aerobic pathway are called **keto-genic** amino acids and are essentially used to produce energy, whereas those amino acids being converted to pyruvate (**glucogenic**) are used to manufacture glucose. An additional component illustrated in Figure 4-17 is the manufacture of ketone bodies, derived from incomplete metabolism of fatty acids. These structures remain popular and controversial with weight loss and carbohydrate-restricted diets, and are discussed later in this chapter.

## Pyruvate Entry Into the Mitochondria

The end product of glycolysis is the production of two pyruvate molecules that move through the sarcoplasm to enter the mitochondria where they undergo further oxidation (Fig. 4-18). Although carbohydrates that are used anaerobically only pass through glycolysis, two additional steps remain to complete carbohydrate metabolism aerobically: the Krebs cycle and **Electron Transport Chain (ETC)**.

Movement into the Krebs cycle and ETC occur in the presence of sufficient oxygen and when the rate of pyruvate production from glycolysis does not exceed the capacity for the mitochondria to receive pyruvate. Under the influence of the enzyme pyruvate dehydrogenase, pyruvate (a three-carbon structure) moves into the mitochondria and in the process, it is converted to acetyl-CoA (a two-carbon structure), whereas simultaneously producing a molecule of NADH + H+ and releasing a molecule of carbon dioxide ($CO_2$). Perhaps the most critical point to note with this step is that this reaction is **NOT** bidirectional. This means that, once pyruvate is converted to acetyl-CoA, this process cannot be reversed. The implication is that, if acetyl-CoA is formed from fats or some proteins, they cannot then be used to form glucose. Only substrates entering the bioenergetics pathway as pyruvate or as an intermediate product of glycolysis (e.g., glycerol) can form glucose. As we will learn in the subsequent sections, the FFA portion of fats and some proteins enter the energy pathways as acetyl-CoA and, therefore, cannot be converted to carbohydrates. Acetyl-CoA represents the common substrate to which all three macronutrients are converted before entering the aerobic pathway.

## Krebs Cycle

The **Krebs cycle** is named after the German-born British biochemist and physician Hans Krebs, whose research furthered our understanding of this cycle and how it functions within mitochondrial respiration. The Krebs cycle completes the oxidation of pyruvate formed from glycolysis and involves a series of enzymatically catalyzed reactions illustrated in Figure 4-18. This cycle begins by combining acetyl-CoA, a two-carbon structure, with oxaloacetate, a four-carbon structure, to form citrate, a six-carbon structure.

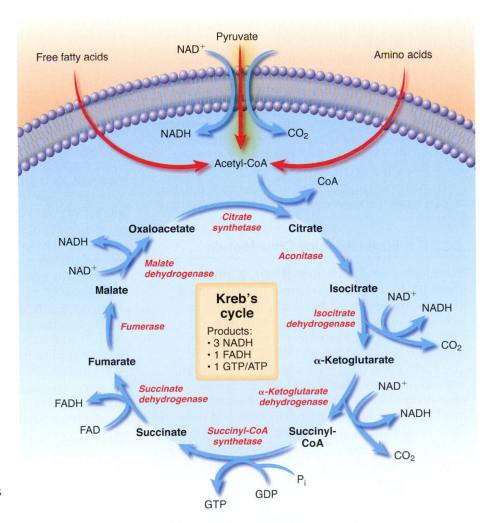

**Figure 4-18.** Pyruvate entry into the mitochondria and the reactions involved in the Krebs cycle.

Acetyl-CoA molecules entering the Krebs cycle subsequently pass through a full turn of this cycle, yielding molecules of ATP (step 8: "substrate phosphorylation"), $CO_2$ (steps 5 and 7), $FADH_2$ (step 9), and $NADH + H^+$ (steps 5, 7, and 11). The main function of the Krebs cycle is to remove hydrogen and harness the energy held within these molecules from other compounds that are part of the cycle. $NAD^+$ and $FAD^+$ molecules are reduced to $NADH + H^+$ and $FADH_2$ to remove hydrogen. The $NADH + H^+$ and $FADH_2$ molecules produced during glycolysis, during the conversion of pyruvate to acetyl-CoA, and from the Krebs cycle all move to the ETC where significant quantities of ATP are generated (Box 4-3).

The final step of the Krebs cycle involves the formation of oxaloacetate (four-carbon structure), a substrate that binds with acetyl-CoA to form citrate to initiate the Krebs cycle. Without adequate oxaloacetate, the ability for acetyl-CoA to enter the Krebs cycle becomes limited, which may result in an accumulation of these molecules.

Enzymes also play a role in controlling the rate at which the Krebs cycle turns. Isocitrate dehydrogenase (step 5) is the main rate-limiting enzyme of the Krebs cycle, and its activity is upregulated (increased) by the presence of increased quantities of ADP and Pi (i.e., during activity). In addition, increased concentrations of $NAD^+$ will also upregulate isocitrate-dehydrogenase activity. Viewed from a different perspective, isocitrate dehydrogenase activity is inhibited by increased concentrations of ATP and NADH.[33]

Remember, one glucose molecule split into two pyruvate molecules, and both subsequently form acetyl-CoA molecules that enter the Krebs cycle. Although Figure 4-18 illustrates one turn of the Krebs cycle from one acetyl-CoA (manufactured from one pyruvate), we need to recognize that one glucose molecule actually generates two turns of the Krebs cycle (one from each acetyl-CoA).

Thus, when tallying the total number of intermediate products formed from one glucose molecule, everything generated during glycolysis and after the formation of pyruvate must be doubled.

- *Glycolysis:*
  - Two NADH formed during glycolysis
  - Two to three ATP formed during glycolysis
  - Two NADH formed during the conversion of pyruvate to acetyl-CoA
- *Krebs Cycle:*
  - Six NADH formed during the Krebs cycle
  - Two FADH formed during the Krebs cycle
  - Two ATP formed during the Krebs cycle

## Electron Transport Chain

The $FADH_2$ and $NADH + H^+$ molecules produced from glycolysis and the Krebs cycle will donate protons and electrons (from hydrogen) to the electron transport chain (ETC) (Fig. 4-19). The electrons are passed along a series of electron-carrier **cytochromes**, iron-containing electron carriers, bound to the inner mitochondrial membrane that are primarily responsible for participating in the stepwise transfer of electrons (hydrogen ions) passed from $NADH + H^+$ and $FADH_2$. Each cytochrome alternately accepts and releases an electron at a slightly lower energy level in the order designated: cytochrome $b$, cytochrome $c_1$, cytochrome $c$, cytochrome $a$, and cytochrome $a_3$. Ultimately, at the end of the chain, electrons are passed along to molecular oxygen, and it is only here that oxygen consumption in aerobic respiration takes place, forming water, an end product of respiration.

Concurrent to this process, the protons released from $NADH + H^+$ and $FADH_2$ are pumped from the inner membrane to the outer mitochondrial membrane and in the process create a gradient. At the end of the chain, these protons diffuse back into the inner membrane, providing energy required to phosphorylate ATP. More simply stated, at specific steps throughout the ETC, sufficient free energy is released to phosphorylate ATP molecules from ADP and Pi. The oxidation of compounds in the ETC, coupled with the phosphorylation of ATP, is referred to as oxidative phosphorylation.[34]

The two primary electron carriers entering the ETC yield different quantities of ATP, as illustrated in Figure 4-19. NAD releases its protons and electrons at the beginning of the chain, whereas flavin adenine dinucleotide (FAD) does not release its protons and electrons until further along the chain, at the second cytochrome. This difference results in the generation of less potential energy that is used to phosphorylate ATP molecules. Consequently, each NADH molecule available for passage through the ETC generates three ATP molecules, whereas each FADH molecule generates two ATP molecules. Because oxygen is the final acceptor of electrons in the chain, any reduction in the availability of oxygen will retard the entire oxidative phosphorylation process.

## Box 4-3. Flavin Adenine Dinucleotide

Flavin adenine dinucleotide (FAD), synthesized from dietary riboflavin (vitamin $B_2$), is a critical cofactor (nonprotein chemical compound) involved in reduction-oxidation reactions in cells (involving the transfer of electrons). The enzyme succinate dehydrogenase involved in step 9 of the Krebs cycle (Fig. 4-18: conversion of succinate to fumarate) requires a high-energy electron carrier to transfer hydrogen and electrons to the ETC. The addition of two electrons and their associated hydrogen atoms converts FAD into $FADH_2$. Conversely, a reaction in which the substrate gains electrons from $FADH_2$ will convert this carrier back to FAD.

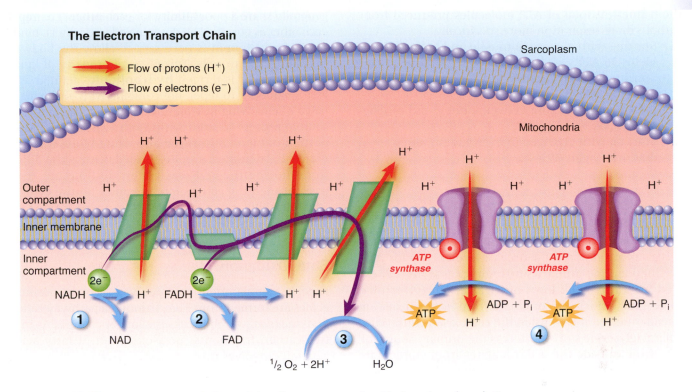

**Figure 4-19.** Electron transport chain and the phenomenon of oxidative phosphorylation.

## Overall Adenosine Triphosphate Total From Carbohydrates

Although we have already established that the anaerobic yield of energy from glycolysis is two or three ATP molecules, we need to tally the total from mitochondrial (aerobic) respiration. Before doing so, we still need to address an exception that occurs within specific cells that impacts the total number of ATP molecules produced (Table 4-2). Mitochondria located in muscle and brain cells are uniquely different from those located in liver, kidney, and cardiac cells. In these cells, the two NADH + H+ carriers manufactured during glycolysis are unable to pass through the mitochondrial membrane, and therefore must pass their electrons (and hydrogen) to FAD (forming $FADH_2$), which can pass through the mitochondrial membrane and enter the ETC. Consequently, these two carriers will lose some of their energy-generating potential and, rather than producing three ATP molecules each, they will only be capable of yielding two ATP molecules each. In liver, kidney, and cardiac cells, however, the two NADH + H+ carriers manufactured during glycolysis are able to pass through the mitochondrial membrane, and thus will join the ETC and yield three ATP molecules each.

Understanding the differences in ATP yield from glucose and glycogen, and between muscle and brain cells versus liver, kidney, and cardiac cells, we can determine

## Table 4-2. Adenosine Triphosphate Total From Carbohydrates

| SOURCE | NO. OF ATP |
|---|---|
| Directly from glycolysis | 2–3 ATP |
| 2 NADH + H+ produced during glycolysis | 4–6 ATP |
| 2 NADH + H+ produced during the conversion of 2 pyruvate molecules to acetyl-CoA molecules | 6 ATP |
| 6 NADH + H+ produced during the Krebs cycle (two turns, each producing three molecules) | 18 ATP |
| 2 $FADH_2$ produced during the Krebs cycle (two turns, each producing two molecules) | 4 ATP |
| Substrate phosphorylation, manufactured directly in the Krebs cycle (two turns, each producing one molecule) | 2 ATP |
| **Total:** | **36–39 ATP** |

the numerical total of ATP molecules produced from carbohydrate respiration more specifically.

- Starting with glucose in muscle and brain cells yields 36 ATP.
- Starting with glycogen in muscle and brain cells yields 37 ATP.
- Starting with glucose in liver, kidney, and cardiac cells yields 38 ATP.
- Starting with glycogen in liver, kidney, and cardiac cells yields 39 ATP.

## LIPID OXIDATION

In addition to carbohydrates, the oxidation of lipids also serves as an important source of free energy for ATP production. The primary source of lipids is FFAs liberated from the breakdown of triglycerides (glycerol + three fatty acids) that originate from either inside or outside the cell. FFAs inside the cell exist as intramuscular triglyceride stores, whereas the primary source of FFA from outside the cell originates from stored adipose tissue and FFAs found within the blood. In Chapter 3, the structure of FFAs was discussed, where we learned that FFAs vary in length from 4 to 28 carbons, but it is palmitate, a 16-carbon fatty acid, that is the primary FFA oxidized in skeletal muscle.

Activation of the sympathetic nervous system (SNS) provides a signal to begin the breakdown of stored triglycerides in muscle or adipose tissue. SNS activation occurs in response to stress imposed on the body, and larger stressors (e.g., moderate-to-more vigorous exercise) trigger the release of the hormone epinephrine, a major SNS hormone. This hormone activates hormone-sensitive lipase, the enzyme responsible for the breakdown of stored triglycerides.

FFAs manufactured in adipose tissue move into circulation, and most are bound to the protein carrier **albumin**.[35] Considering how water and lipids (oils, fats)

generally share a poor affinity for each other (i.e., repel each other as observed by dropping oil into water), binding FFA to albumin is necessary to allow the body to transport FFAs to cells. This physical property of lipids repelling water is termed **hydrophobic**, defined as a lipid's tendency to repel, not combine with, or be incapable of dissolving in water. Albumin is a large, water-soluble protein located within our plasma (the fluid portion of blood minus red and white blood cells) in which particulates are suspended. Once the FFAs from outside the cell reach their destination, they pass through the cell membrane and into the cytosol (the intracellular fluid or cytoplasmic matrix located inside cells) by specific transporters.

### Beta-Oxidation

Here, in a similar manner to pyruvate, acetyl-CoA molecules are formed from FFAs through a pathway called *beta-oxidation*, which breaks the longer chain FFAs into two-carbon fragments. Beta-oxidation of fatty acids generally involves three stages:

- Activation of the FFAs in the cytosol
- Transport of activated FFAs into mitochondria via a transport carrier (carnitine shuttle)
- Beta-oxidation proper in the mitochondrial matrix

Activation of FFAs occurs by the addition of CoA, and is facilitated by the enzyme acyl-CoA synthetase, forming a fatty acyl-CoA molecule. This activation process requires two ATP molecules and need only occur once, regardless of the length of the FFA carbon chain. The transport of the fatty acyl-CoA molecule across the impermeable inner mitochondrial membrane is facilitated by the carnitine shuttle (Fig. 4-20). Upon entry into the mitochondria, the fatty acyl-CoA molecule passes through the beta-oxidation sequence of four enzymatically catalyzed reactions, as illustrated in Figure 4-21. Each beta-oxidation sequence removes a two-carbon segment that results in the manufacture

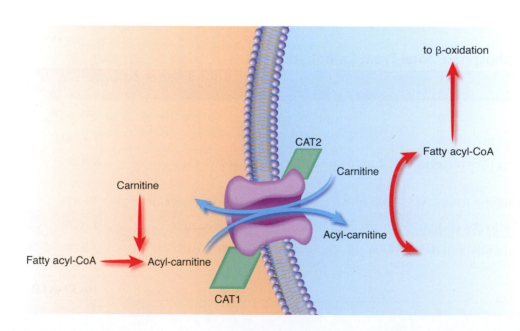

**Figure 4-20.** The carnitine shuttle whereby fatty acyl-CoA is shuttled into the mitochondria for entry into beta-oxidation.

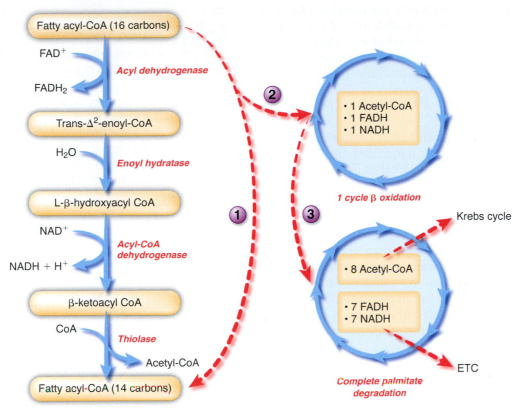

**Figure 4-21.** Sequence of beta-oxidation in the mitochondria. Upon entry into the mitochondria, fatty acyl-CoA molecules pass through the beta-oxidation sequence of four enzymatically catalyzed reactions (1). Each cycle of beta-oxidation produces one acetyl-CoA, one FADH, and one NADH (2). The complete degradation of palmitate (the most common free fatty acid oxidized in skeletal muscle) results in eight acetyl-CoA, seven FADH, and seven NADH (3).

of one acetyl-CoA, whereas simultaneously removing electrons (and hydrogen), reducing $NAD^+$ and $FAD^+$ to $NADH + H^+$ and $FADH_2$ as illustrated. As discussed previously, these carriers will make their way to the ETC.

Using palmitate, a 16-carbon FFA, as our example, the complete degradation of this FFA will yield:

- Eight acetyl-CoA ($8 \times 2$-carbon fragments)
- Seven $NADH + H^+$ (as the beta-oxidation sequence must occur seven times to yield eight 2-carbon fragments)
- Seven $FADH_2$ (as the beta-oxidation sequence must occur seven times to yield eight 2-carbon fragments)

FFAs may vary in size, but all entering the Krebs cycle must pass through beta-oxidation and be systematically cleaved into these two-carbon fragments to produce acetyl-CoA.

## Odd-Numbered Free Fatty Acid Chains

Some odd-numbered FFA chains do exist in nature (e.g., some plants, some marine organisms). FFA with odd-numbered carbon atoms follow the same oxidation sequence as the even-numbered FFA chains but produce an additional final product in addition to acetyl-CoA, namely, propionyl-CoA. The compound passes through a series of reactions that ultimately forms succinyl-CoA, which then enters the Krebs cycle, but rather than enter this cycle by joining to oxaloacetate (as we witness with acetyl-CoA),

succinyl-CoA joins the pathway as a principal in its own right.

## Glycerol

Glycerol forms the backbone of the triglyceride molecule and is also oxidized through the bioenergetic pathways. As mentioned previously, glycerol is a three-carbon structure that resembles a three-carbon intermediate product formed during glycolysis. Thus, when metabolizing triglycerides, the FFAs move through beta-oxidation, whereas the glycerol portion enters the glycolytic pathway, where it ultimately forms one pyruvate molecule. Because glycerol will manufacture only one pyruvate molecule, which, in turn, will produce one acetyl-CoA, the net yield from the glycerol molecule is approximately 19 ATP molecules.

## Overall Adenosine Triphosphate Total From Lipids

Because FFAs vary in length, the net ATP yield will vary from structure to structure, but if we use our previously mentioned example of palmitate, the predominant fat used during exercise, we can tally a total presented in Table 4-3. The complete oxidation of palmitate through beta-oxidation yields eight acetyl-CoA, seven $NADH + H^+$, and seven $FADH_2$ molecules.

Each acetyl-CoA enters the Krebs cycle and produces three NADH + H⁺, one FADH₂ molecule, and one ATP molecule via substrate phosphorylation. Considering that each NADH + H⁺ yields three ATP molecules, and each FADH₂ yields two ATP molecules, the net ATP production from the electron carriers produced during beta-oxidation is 35 ATP (7 × 3 NADH + H⁺ plus 7 × 2 ATP from FADH₂).

If we now combine fatty acids into a triglyceride (e.g., three palmitate + one glycerol), it increases the ATP total significantly, producing a grand total of approximately 406 ATP (129 × 3 − 3 palmitate + 19 ATP − glycerol). This example and Table 4-3 illustrate how much more energy lipids can yield in comparison with glucose, but they do so more slowly and less efficiently (i.e., yield less ATP per molecule of oxygen) than glucose; thus, lipids are best used when oxygen is readily available and the demand for energy is low (i.e., lower-to-moderate levels of exercise). (See explanatory animation of Fat Utilization on the Davis*Plus* site at http://davisplus.fadavis.com). The concept of fuel efficiency will be discussed in Chapter 15.

## PROTEIN OXIDATION

Proteins represent an additional substrate that can be catabolized and eventually provide the free energy required to manufacture ATP during exercise conditions.[36,37] Proteins must be broken down to amino acids, after which the nitrogen amino group is removed (deamination), leaving a carbon skeleton that can enter the energy pathways at different points (glycolysis, beta-oxidation, or the Krebs cycle). A major point of entry for amino acid skeletons into the energy pathways, specifically the Krebs cycle, is as acetyl-CoA. In the same way that pyruvate is converted to acetyl-CoA, the three-carbon amino acid skeletons are also broken down into a two-carbon structure to form acetyl-CoA.

Previously, we mentioned how amino acids that feed into glycolysis can be used to manufacture glucose

### Table 4-3. Adenosine Triphosphate Total From Palmitate (16-carbon structure)

| SOURCE | NO. OF ATP |
|---|---|
| • Fatty acid activation | −2 ATP |
| • Beta-oxidation: 7 cycles producing 7 NADH + H⁺ | 21 ATP |
| • Beta-oxidation: 7 cycles producing 7 FADH2 | 14 ATP |
| • 8 turns of Krebs cycle: (eight Acetyl-CoA) = 24 NADH + H⁺ | 72 ATP |
| • 8 turns of Krebs cycle: (eight Acetyl-CoA) = 8 FADH2 | 16 ATP |
| • 8 turns of Krebs cycle: Substrate phosphorylation | 8 ATP |
| **Total:** | **129 ATP** |

**DOING THE MATH:**
Conceptually, using a 14-carbon FFA that passes through beta-oxidation, how many sequences of beta-oxidation are needed? How many acetyl-CoA are produced? How many NADH + H⁺ and FADH₂ molecules would be produced through the Krebs cycle? And what would you calculate as the total ATP yield if this were a triglyceride with three 14-carbon FFAs?
**ANSWER:**
- A 14-carbon structure requires 6 turns of beta-oxidation producing 6 NADH + H⁺ and 6 FADH₂
- 7 acetyl-CoA
- 7 turns of the Krebs cycle: 21 NADH + H⁺ and 7 FADH₂ and 7 ATP molecules via substrate phosphorylation
- Net ATP yield from one 14-carbon FFA = 112 ATP
  - FFA activation = −2 ATP
  - Beta-oxidation = 30 ATP
  - 7 turns of Kerbs cycle = 84 ATP
- Triglyceride (3 × 14-carbon FFA + 1 glycerol): = 355 ATP (112 ATP × 3 + 19 ATP)

via gluconeogenesis and are thus defined as **glucogenic**. In contrast, other amino acids are converted to acetyl-CoA or Krebs cycle intermediate products, and can only be used to produce energy. These amino acids are termed **ketogenic**.

Amino acid oxidation during short-duration, low-intensity exercise is negligible, whereas contributions during short-duration, high-intensity or sustained exercise in which glycogen depletion becomes a concern may be more significant. Because of the short-term nature of high-intensity exercise, the overall ATP production from amino acid breakdown remains relatively small, but prolonged exercise with glycogen depletion will elicit a greater stimulus for protein catabolism and increased amino acid oxidation. The maximal contribution of amino acid oxidation to total ATP production during exercise is between 5% and 10%.[2]

Notably, amino acid oxidation involves the production of ammonia ($NH_3$) molecules that occurs during the process of removing the amino group from the amino acids during deamination.[38,39] (Please refer to Chapter 3 for a more detailed explanation of amino acid structure.) Ammonia is toxic to cells and must therefore be removed. Accordingly, the ammonia is incorporated into other amino acids (a process called **transamination**) that can then either remain in skeletal muscle or be transported from skeletal muscle to the liver. This transportation process to the liver involves the formation of alanine, which is the most important amino acid synthesized to reach the liver.[2] On reaching the liver, the amino group is again removed, again producing ammonia. However, in the liver, this ammonia is processed to form urea that is eventually excreted in urine. The remaining alanine amino acid skeleton resembles pyruvate and can be converted to glucose through gluconeogenesis. The newly formed glucose molecule can subsequently be released back into circulation and taken up as fuel by exercising muscle cells. The process of alanine conversion to glucose in the liver is known as the **glucose-alanine cycle** (Fig. 4-22). Researchers have reported that the glucose formed from the glucose-alanine cycle may provide up to 5% of the total substrate used to manufacture ATP during prolonged exhaustive exercise.[40]

This pathway can indirectly supply glucose to exercising muscles from stores located elsewhere in the body. For example, during running, where muscle glycogen stores in the quadriceps may become depleted, it would be simple and logical to think that nonexercising muscles (e.g., deltoids) could contribute glucose to the quadriceps so that they do not become depleted. Unfortunately, any free glucose (i.e., not bound into a glycogen chain) in muscle tissue is found in a phosphorylated form as glucose-6 phosphate, which cannot leave the cell. Essentially, the glucose molecule is trapped within the cell and cannot escape. However, by partially degrading (breaking down) the glucose molecule through glycolysis to a three-carbon structure that resembles an amino acid, it can then be joined with an amino group to form alanine that can then be transported to the liver to enter the glucose-alanine pathway. Liver cells are unique in that they, unlike muscle cells, are able to release glucose into circulation.

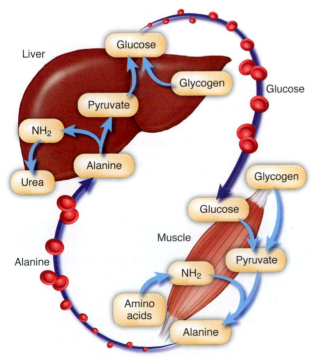

**Figure 4-22.** Glucose-alanine cycle that occurs in the liver.

## KETONE BODIES AND KETOGENESIS

Incompletely metabolized fats and proteins that cannot enter the Krebs cycle because of insufficient presence of oxaloacetate (due to low carbohydrate levels) are converted to ketone bodies, which have become a source of great interest to researchers and dieters. Although the body has some limited capacity to excrete ketone bodies in urine, controversy exists over the safety of accumulating ketones within our body. Manufactured ketones are typically found in various forms such as acetone, acetoacetone, and β-hydroxybutyrate. Although the first two are potentially harmful in larger quantities, the latter is a viable fuel that can be used by our brain when necessary (i.e., during periods of starvation when glucose stores are depleted).

Individuals who advocate low-carbohydrate (ketogenic) diets point to the fact that we, as did our ancestors, are able to function under conditions of carbohydrate depletion, because brain cells are capable of using β-hydroxybutyrate as a fuel. This may help explain how our Paleolithic ancestors survived the brutal cold winters without much more than fats and proteins from animal carcasses hunted during the fall months. However, support for low-carbohydrate diets fails to address how muscles continue to function at higher intensities without carbohydrates, given the fact that they do not favor the use of ketone bodies as a fuel. The only viable option in this scenario is to attack living muscle tissue from which we manufacture carbohydrates (gluconeogenesis). Although our ancestors managed to survive a few bitter months in hibernation without activity, contemporary humans have no need to hibernate; thus, muscle activity (i.e., exercise) while following low-carbohydrate diets poses legitimate causes for concern (Box 4-4).

## In Your Own Words

A friend is contemplating following a low-carbohydrate diet to lose weight, because she read that carbohydrates are what make people fat. Coupled with her diet, she plans to start a cardio program to achieve her goal. Given your understanding of the energy pathways and the need for carbohydrates, explain why carbohydrates are necessary in her diet to allow her to metabolize fats efficiently.

## THE METABOLIC MILL

Collectively, all three fuels serve integrated roles in contributing to the production of energy (see explanatory animation of the Metabolic Mill on the DavisPlus site at http://davisplus.fadavis.com). Note the following points:
- Pyruvate is transported into the mitochondria for conversion to acetyl-CoA (a nonreversible reaction) or converted to lactate in the sarcoplasm.

## Box 4-4. Overall Diet Comparisons

A 2012 ranking by *U.S. News & World Report* involving a panel of 22 nationally recognized experts in diet, nutrition, obesity, food psychology, diabetes, and heart disease were asked to weigh in on health benefits, weight-loss efficacy, and ease of following 25 common diets on the market. Of the 25 diets examined, the Paleo diet was rated last because experts took issue with the diet on every measure. It is important to mention that the ranking assumed a modernized offshoot of the true Paleo diet (modern diets emphasize low carbohydrates, approximately 23% of total calories, whereas a true Paleo diet is closer to 40% from carbohydrates). Proponents of the low-carbohydrate Paleo diet debated the panel outcome indicating that four of five recent studies that experimentally tested contemporary versions of this diet found them to be superior to most diets in regard to weight loss, cardiovascular disease risk factors, and risk factors for type 2 diabetes. However, the panel included these studies in their ranking and indicated the studies did not carry much weight as all five were small, of short duration, or both.

Best diets overall. *U.S. News & World Report.* 2012. http://health.usnews.com/best-diet/best-overall-diets. Accessed January 4, 2013.

- Triglycerides separate into FFAs before entering the mitochondria, where they undergo beta-oxidation for conversion to acetyl-CoA. Because FFA will enter the metabolic pathway at this point, they cannot be converted to glucose.
- Glycerol, a three-carbon structure, is capable of entering the glycolytic pathway where it can then be converted to either glucose (combining with another three-carbon structure) or pyruvate.
- Glucogenic amino acids are those that enter the pathway before the formation of pyruvate, and thus can be converted to glucose.
- Ketogenic amino acids enter the pathway as acetyl-CoA or as a Krebs cycle intermediate product; thus, they can only be used to produce energy.

The fate of excess macronutrients is evident in Figure 4-17 and displayed in Table 4-4. Although it is clear why excess carbohydrates are accused of making us fat, dietary protein that exceeds the quantity needed for tissue maintenance, growth, and repair can also be converted to fats. This dates back to our ancestral days, when the body needed to store energy to survive the frequent times when food was scarce.

## ROLE OF THE ENERGY PATHWAY IN EXERCISE FATIGUE

As mentioned previously, in all sports and exercise training, the onset of fatigue will vary depending on numerous factors, including fitness level and training status, exercise intensity, and environmental conditions (e.g., heat, humidity, and altitude).[30] This section provides a brief overview of a submaximal conditioning scenario leading to fatigue.[3]

During prolonged exercises such as cycling, cross-country skiing, and distance running, muscle contraction is also dependent on the ability of the metabolic pathways to continuously generate ATP. Mitochondrial respiration is the primary supplier of ATP, derived from fat, carbohydrates, and proteins made available for mitochondrial respiration. However, the two most important substrates, with regard to fatigue, are blood glucose and muscle glycogen. Fats as triglycerides are readily available for ATP production, but their breakdown is much slower than the rates of glucose and glycogen, thus creating a reliance on carbohydrates. Decreased levels of blood glucose and low levels of muscle glycogen have been primarily associated with the onset of fatigue during sustained exercise events.[30] In terms of optimizing exercise performance, a limiting factor to glycolysis, and maintenance of a maximal rate of ATP production, is the availability of muscle glycogen. Research has reported muscle glycogen stores become depleted after approximately 2 hours of exercise, under high-intensity exercise or maximal usage.[41] The point of glycogen depletion in muscles, commonly referred to as "bonking" or "hitting the wall" is a serious consideration for all endurance athletes.

## Table 4-4. Summary of the Fate of Excess Macronutrients

| MACRONUTRIENT | GLUCONEOGENIC POTENTIAL | POTENTIAL TO MANUFACTURE AMINO ACIDS | POTENTIAL TO MANUFACTURE FATS |
|---|---|---|---|
| Fats | Glycerol portion of fats | Rare instances (nonessential amino acids) | N/A |
| Carbohydrates | N/A | Nonessential amino acids | Yes (excess) |
| Proteins | Glucogenic amino acids | N/A | Ketogenic amino acids |

N/A, not applicable.

# INTEGRATED FUNCTION OF ENERGY SYSTEMS

To this juncture, our discussion of the energy systems has focused entirely on how each pathway functions individually. Although this singular approach is logical with an initial study of the topic, readers should not misinterpret the information to mean that each system functions independently to meet the ATP demand within the body. In reality, there is considerable overlap in the contributions from each energy system to various activities of daily living and athletic events.[42] Also, for any given activity or event, there is at least some contribution from each of the three energy systems. Overall, the relative contribution of each energy system will be dictated by the required energy demands.

The sequential overlapping of energy systems for two distinctively different exercise scenarios is shown in Figure 4-23. In Figure 4-23A, the contributions from each system from the beginning of an exercise bout to steady-state exercise are illustrated. Steady-state exercise refers to metabolic conditions where ATP demand is supplied exclusively with ATP generated from mitochondrial respiration. This is often referred to as achieving your "second wind" during exercise and generally takes between 45 and 90 seconds, or up to 4 minutes, to achieve. The time required to achieve steady state depends primarily on the intensity of exercise (higher intensities require more time to achieve steady state), but is influenced by other variables such as training status (i.e., more fit individuals will attain steady state faster). However, in the initial transition from rest to exercise, there is a brief time delay before steady state can be achieved. Under these circumstances, ATP contributions are made from both CrP hydrolysis and glycolysis.

In Figure 4-23B, the contributions from each energy system are shown during an incremental maximal exercise test. Throughout the range of low-intensity exercise (i.e., between 20% and 60% of maximal oxygen uptake or $\dot{V}O_2$max), ATP demand is supplied primarily from mitochondrial respiration. In particular, lipid catabolism makes a substantial contribution to ATP synthesis during this intensity range. However, as the intensity of exercise approaches approximately 60% $\dot{V}O_2$max, a decline in lipid catabolism is evident.[43] Given the increased rate of ATP demand required at higher exercise intensity, and the fact that the maximal rate of ATP generation from lipids is considerably slower compared with other substrates, a decreased reliance on lipid catabolism occurs. Gradually, the body begins to favor mitochondrial respiration from carbohydrates, a more efficient fuel that yields more ATP per molecule of oxygen and generates ATP more rapidly. As intensities continue to increase, glycolysis, resulting in lactate formation, begins to augment mitochondrial respiration. The contribution from glycolysis steadily increases

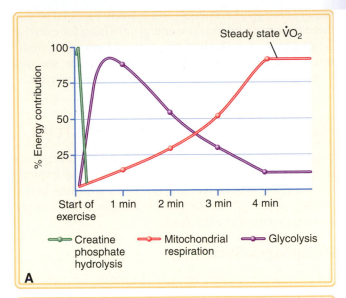

**A**

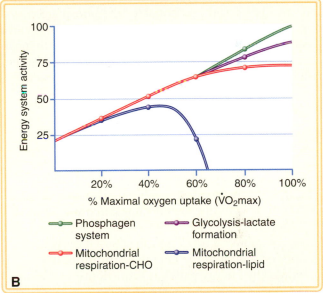

**B**

**Figure 4-23.** The blending and overlap of all three energy systems during two different exercise conditions: (A) moderate-intensity exercise from the onset to steady state, and (B) maximal-intensity exercise from the onset to volitional fatigue.

until maximal exercise intensity is achieved. At near-maximal exercise, the phosphagen system joins glycolysis (anaerobic outcome: lactate) and mitochondrial respiration in the task of ATP production. Given the tremendous amount of ATP required to sustain high-intensity exercise, the increased activity of both the phosphagen system and glycolysis (anaerobic) is needed given their capacity to maximally generate ATP. Despite the heightened activity of glycolysis and the phosphagen system at higher intensities of exercise, mitochondrial respiration continues to remain elevated and is subsequently making a significant contribution to overall ATP generation.

In summary, normal functioning of our energy pathways supports daily life. Regardless of our profession, whether training as an athlete or functioning as a stay-at-home parent, our activities of daily living require energy. This energy is collectively supplied by our three energy pathways. The energy provision for exercise is not simply the product of a series of energy systems *turning on* and *turning off*, but conversely the smooth blending and overlapping of all three energy systems.

## SEX DIFFERENCES IN ENERGY SYSTEMS

In this final section, we examine differences in the energy systems between men and women, and explore the effect of exercise training on the functioning of the energy systems. We also look at changes in the energy pathways across the life span.

### Phosphagen System

CrP stores are greater in type II muscle fibers.[49] The greater proportion of type II muscle fibers in men therefore means a greater potential for the phosphagen system. Accompanying increased CrP levels is greater creatine kinase activity. Both can be interpreted to mean that the ATP contribution from the phosphagen system will support greater anaerobic performance in men.[50]

### FROM THEORY TO PRACTICE

Think of three track events and performance times of better athletes: the 100-m sprint, lasting approximately 10 seconds; the 400 m or 1/4 mile, lasting approximately 50 to 55 seconds; and the 5,000-m (5K or 3.1-mile) run in about 13 to 15 minutes. Based on your understanding of the energy continuum, how would the energy pathways contribute to fueling each event from start to finish?

### Glycolysis

The key enzymes involved in glycolysis, including phosphorylase and PFK, have also been found to be in higher concentrations in male individuals.[51–53] This allows more and faster rates of glycolysis to produce greater quantities of ATP. Furthermore, lactate dehydrogenase activity has also been found to be greater in men. Collectively, these three key enzymatic differences contribute to an overall greater potential to generate ATP via glycolysis in male compared with female individuals.

### Mitochondrial Respiration

No differences have been reported between the sexes in the key enzymes involved in mitochondrial respiration (Krebs cycle and ETC) and beta-oxidation.[54] Why, then, are female individuals better suited to endurance performance? This fact is essentially attributed to a greater distribution of type I fibers and lower concentration of type II fibers.[55] With a lowered capacity for anaerobic ATP production, fatigue attributed to these pathways is reduced, thus delaying the onset of fatigue in females.

### EFFECT OF AGING ON ENERGY PATHWAYS

Our understanding of the effects of aging on the functioning of the various energy systems is somewhat limited. A common challenge when studying the effects of aging on any physiological parameter is partitioning out the decrease in function, which can be attributed to less than ideal levels of physical activity.[56] Simply put, it is often difficult for researchers to separate out the change in physiological function that occurs from age alone versus the effects of aging combined with physical inactivity.

### SEX DIFFERENCES

There are notable physiological differences between males and females in regard to muscle performance. Generally, males produce greater absolute muscle strength and power outputs relative to their female counterparts.[44] Conversely, females exhibit greater resistance to skeletal muscle fatigue and demonstrate a superior capacity for recovery from exercise.[45,46] Most of these contrasting properties can be explained by differences in muscle fiber types, and the corresponding energy system profile, that exist between the sexes.

In Chapter 9, you will learn that skeletal muscle can essentially be divided into two different fiber types: type I fibers (also commonly referred to as slow-twitch) and type II fibers (also commonly referred to as fast-twitch, and can be further subdivided to type IIa and type IIx). The biochemical and enzymatic profiles of each fiber type differ considerably.[33] Type I muscle fibers are more suited to aerobic respiration, and to the breakdown of lipids and carbohydrates for ATP synthesis through mitochondrial respiration. In contrast, type II fibers are better suited to generating ATP via the phosphagen system and glycolysis.[47]

Research has shown a greater distribution of type I muscle fibers and lower distribution of type IIx muscle fibers in female compared with male individuals.[48] Given these differences, it may seem intuitive that male athletes have a greater potential for sprint- and strength-related performance, whereas female athletes are better geared for endurance performance.

Nevertheless, research has quantified a number of key changes to the energy systems that occur with age (Fig. 4-24). Underpinning many of these changes is the fact that overall aging contributes to an overall decline in skeletal muscle fibers.[57] In particular, research has reported consistently that the number of type II muscle fibers declines more rapidly than type I fibers as an individual ages.[58,59]

Inherent to the loss of specific muscle fibers is the concomitant loss in the biochemical infrastructure required for ATP production. Given that type II muscle fibers specialize in manufacturing ATP via the phosphagen system and glycolysis, it is naturally to be expected that older

adults experience a gradual decline in the areas of muscle strength and power output. GLUT-4 transporter protein content is also decreased in older adult skeletal muscle,[60] reducing the capacity to bring glucose into the cell to fuel glycolysis during exercise and to facilitate glucose uptake after exercise for muscle glycogen synthesis. Both compromise the capacity for carbohydrate catabolism and the overall functioning of the glycolytic system for ATP production. In addition to an overall age-related decline in type I muscle fibers, within the remaining fibers there is also a decrease in mitochondrial volume and enzymatic activity.[61] These reductions reduce our capacity to generate ATP through mitochondrial respiration. From a whole-body perspective, the diminished potential of the mitochondrial respiration energy system contributes to the gradual decline in cardiorespiratory fitness (i.e., $\dot{V}O_2$max). (Also see Chapter 26.)

## Capacity of the Energy Pathways and Effects of Training

Each of the three energy systems undergoes favorable adaptations with exercise training (Table 4-5). Two of the most common types of exercise training include short-term, higher-intensity sprint or interval-type training and prolonged, submaximal endurance-type training. A discussion of the modifications within each energy system in response to these types of training follows.

### Short-Term, High-Intensity Training

The considerable ATP demands during higher-intensity exercise are highly dependent on the phosphagen system and glycolysis.[62] Chronic high-intensity training increases the capacity of these two systems to rapidly generate ATP in several ways[63]:

- Resting concentrations of CrP stores are significantly increased in skeletal muscle following short-term, high-intensity training.
- Creatine kinase, the rate-limiting enzyme of the phosphagen system, is also upregulated with training.[64]

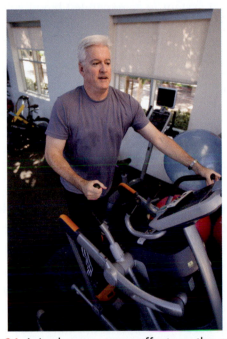

**Figure 4-24.** Aging has numerous effects on the energy pathways, including decreased glycolytic capacity and reduced mitochondrial volume and enzymatic activity. Collectively, the physiological changes associated with aging will result in older individuals having lower cardiorespiratory fitness levels compared with their younger counterparts.

## Table 4-5. Adaptations to Energy Systems from High-Intensity Training and Submaximal Endurance Training

| SYSTEM | HIGH-INTENSITY TRAINING ADAPTATIONS | SUBMAXIMAL ENDURANCE TRAINING ADAPTATIONS |
|---|---|---|
| Phosphagen | ↑ CrP concentration<br>↑ CK activity | No significant changes |
| Glycolysis | ↑ Glycogen stores<br>↑ Phosphorylase activity<br>↑ Phosphofructokinase activity<br>↑ Lactate dehydrogenase activity | ↑ Glycogen stores<br>↑ Phosphorylase activity<br>↑ Phosphofructokinase activity<br>↑ Lactate threshold |
| Mitochondrial respiration | No significant changes | ↑ Volume of mitochondria<br>↑ Activity of Krebs cycle enzymes<br>↑ Activity of beta-oxidation enzymes |

CK, creatine kinase; CrP, creatine phosphate.

Collectively, an increase in the primary substrate for the phosphagen system, coupled with the principal enzyme catalyzing the reaction, contributes to an increased capacity for rapidly manufacturing ATP (rapid production of ATP).

Short-term, high-intensity training also simulates improvements in glycolysis by:

- increasing glucose delivery to working muscles.[65]
- increasing resting concentrations of muscle glycogen.[3]
- elevating the two primary rate-limiting enzymes of glycolysis: phosphorylase and PFK.
- enhancing the body's capacity for tolerating proton accumulation and clearance.
- increasing activity of the enzyme lactate dehydrogenase, the enzyme that permits rapid conversion of pyruvate to lactate when pyruvate production exceeds the capacity for mitochondrial uptake. You may recall that the reduction of pyruvate to lactate under these circumstances is critical for regenerating $NAD^+$ to enable glycolysis to continue.

High-intensity interval training (also known as HIIT) has gained considerable interest lately as evidenced by the myriad of available HIIT programs. Part of their popularity lies with the efficiency with which they can improve cardiovascular fitness and various other physiological parameters. HIIT generally involves alternating bouts of higher-intensity exercise (20 seconds to 5 minutes) sessions with either true rest or light- to low-intensity recovery workloads throughout an exercise routine and has traditionally been used to train athletes who require high levels of both aerobic and **anaerobic fitness** (e.g., track, team sport athletes). The influx of this form of training with the mainstream and even special populations groups is raising concerns regarding overall safety and appropriateness.

The current physical activity recommendation for U.S. adults of 150 minutes per week of moderate-intensity exercise is designed to provide numerous health benefits, but the unfortunate reality is that the majority of the population falls short of this recommendation, citing *lack of time* as the primary barrier. Emerging research suggests HIIT may be a time-efficient strategy for improving the health of all populations if properly supervised. (Please refer to Chapter 15 for more detailed information concerning HIIT training.)

### Prolonged, Submaximal Endurance Training

The extended ATP demands during prolonged submaximal exercise are primarily reliant on mitochondrial respiration. Chronic endurance training increases the capacity of this system to generate ATP in numerous areas.[66,67] The hallmark adaptation is increased mitochondria mass and numbers (known as mitochondrial density).[68,69] The benefit of increased mitochondria volume includes augmented enzymatic activity within beta-oxidation and the Krebs cycle.

Endurance training also elicits increases in glucose and FFA delivery[67,70,71] and resting concentrations of muscle glycogen.[3] Collectively, these adaptations lead to a greater capacity for carbohydrate and lipid metabolism, and have important practical implications to performance.[72,73] The increased muscle glycogen content means glycolysis can continue at optimal rates for longer durations. Moreover, the greater capacity for pyruvate uptake and oxidation through mitochondrial respiration results in increased ATP production and the potential to sustain higher intensities of steady-state exercise.[74] The latter point is also supported by the fact that metabolic thresholds (i.e., LTs and CrP thresholds) are improved following endurance training (Fig. 4-25).[75]

However, the physiological adaptations to endurance training are not limited to events within the cell. For example, multiple adaptations within the cardiovascular system (e.g., expanded blood volume, left ventricular chamber size, capillary density) and pulmonary system (e.g., more conditioned respiratory muscles, larger air volumes) are all necessary to complement the cellular adaptions to improve overall metabolic efficiency.

## VIGNETTE conclusion

■ Felicia Rodriguez learned an important lesson as a student that she was able to leverage as a teacher—namely, that real-world examples are needed to bring some of the more intricate scientific concepts to life for students. This teaching technique will help her students turn theoretical concepts into practical tips that help them better understand the importance of not only *what* happens in the human body, but *why* it happens. This will serve Felicia's students well, whether they become personal trainers trying to explain the specificity principle to clients or professors teaching the next generation of students.

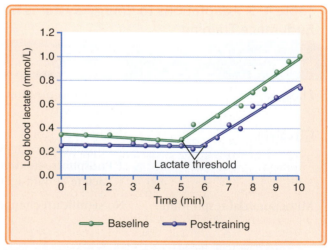

**Figure 4-25.** Increase in the lactate threshold after endurance training.

# CRITICAL THINKING QUESTIONS

1. You are an undergraduate student and have approached your exercise physiology course professor from the previous semester about taking an independent project with her. She has a study that might be suitable; however, she first wants to ensure your background exercise biochemistry knowledge and skills are sufficient. She asks you to calculate the ATP tally from (a) a molecule of glycogen from glycolysis only, and (b) a molecule of palmitate that is completely oxidized. What steps are involved with these calculations?

2. After reading a fitness magazine, a friend is contemplating following a low-carbohydrate diet and participating in HIIT-type workouts to lose weight. Using your knowledge of the energy pathways, provide scientific explanations why this combination is not recommended.

3. We often hear how carbohydrates make us fat, but can a high-protein diet also make us fat?

4. You are asked to share your expertise with a friend who is trying to improve his overall fitness to compete in a recreational basketball league. His is uncertain whether he should participate in slower, longer distance-type endurance training, follow a program of higher-intensity, shorter bouts of sprinting, or do both. Using your knowledge of bioenergetics and how each pathways works, think of the game of basketball and discuss your ideas on what an appropriate training program would involve for him to be successful.

## ADDITIONAL RESOURCES

American College of Sports Medicine. *ACSM's Guidelines for Exercise Testing and Prescription*. 9th ed. Baltimore, MD: Lippincott Williams & Wilkins; 2014.

Brooks GA, Fahey TD, Baldwin KM. *Exercise Physiology: Human Bioenergetics and Its Applications*. 4th ed. New York: McGraw-Hill Companies; 2005.

American Council on Exercise. *ACE's Essentials of Exercise Science for Fitness Professionals*. San Diego, CA: American Council on Exercise; 2010.

Power SK, Howley ET. *Exercise Physiology: Theory and Application to Fitness and Performance*. 7th ed. New York: McGraw-Hill Companies; 2009.

Robergs RA, Roberts S. *Exercise Physiology: Exercise, Performance, and Clinical Applications*. St Louis, MO: Mosby; 1997.

## REFERENCES

1. Baker JS, McCormick MC, Robergs RA. Interaction among skeletal muscle metabolic energy systems during intense exercise. *J. Nutr. Metab.* 2010;2010:905612.

2. Brooks GA, Fahey TD, Baldwin KM. *Exercise Physiology: Human Bioenergetics and Its Applications*. 4th ed. New York: McGraw-Hill Companies; 2005.

3. Robergs RA, Roberts S. *Exercise Physiology: Exercise, Performance, and Clinical Applications*. St Louis, MO: Mosby; 1997.

4. Houston M. *Biochemistry Primer for Exercise Science*. Champaign, IL: Human Kinetics; 2006.

5. Bangsbo J, Krustrup P, Gonzalez-Alonso J, Saltin B. ATP production and efficiency of human skeletal muscle during intense exercise: effect of previous exercise. *Am. J. Physiol. Endocrinol. Metab.* 2001;280:E956–E964.

6. Baechle TR, Earle RW, eds. *Essentials of Strength Training and Conditioning*. 2nd ed. Champaign, IL: Human Kinetics; 2008.

7. Gastin PB. Energy system interaction and relative contribution during maximal exercise. *Sports Med.* 2001;31:725–741.

8. Bogdanis GC, Nevill ME, Lakomy HK, Boobis LH. Power output and muscle metabolism during and following recovery from10 and 20 s of maximal sprint exercise in humans. *Acta Physiol. Scand.* 1998;163:261–272.

9. Spriet LL. Anaerobic metabolism in human skeletal muscle during short-term, intense activity. *Can. J. Physiol. Pharmacol.* 1992;70:157–165.

10. Greenhaff PL, Nevill ME, Soderlund K, et al. The metabolic responses of human type I and II muscle fibres during maximal treadmill sprinting. *J. Physiol.* 1994;478:149–155.

11. Walter G, Vandenborne K, McCully KK, Leigh JS. Non-invasive measurement of phosphocreatine recovery kinetics in single human muscles. *Am. J. Physiol.* 1997;272:C525–C534.

12. Glaister M. Multiple sprint work: physiological responses, mechanisms of fatigue and the influence of aerobic fitness. *Sports Med.* 2005;35:757–777.

13. Bessman SP, Carpenter CL. The creatine-creatine phosphate energy shuttle. *Annu. Rev. Biochem.* 1985;54:831–862.

14. McMahon S, Jenkins D. Factors affecting the rate of phosphocreatine resynthesis following intense exercise. *Sports Med.* 2002;32:761–784.

15. Sahlin K, Harris RC, Hultman E. Resynthesis of creatine phosphate in human muscle after exercise in relation to intramuscular pH and availability of oxygen. *Scand. J. Clin. Lab. Invest.* 1979;39:551–558.

16. Siegler JC, Bell-Wilson J, Mermier C, Faria E, Robergs RA. Active and passive recovery and acid-base kinetics following multiple bouts of intense exercise to exhaustion. *Int. J. Sport Nutr. Exerc. Metab.* 2006;16:92–107.

17. Tomlin DL, Wenger HA. The relationship between aerobic fitness and recovery from high intensity intermittent exercise. *Sports Med.* 2001;31:1–11.

18. Pilegaard H, Domino K, Noland T, et al. Effect of high intensity exercise training on lactate/H+ transport capacity in human skeletal muscle. *Am. J. Physiol.* 1999;276:E255–E261.

19. Robergs RA. Exercise-induced metabolic acidosis: where do the protons come from? *Sportscience*. 2001;5:1–20.

20. Wasserman K, Beaver WL, Whipp BJ. Mechanisms and patterns of blood lactate increase during exercise in man. *Med. Sci. Sports Exerc.* 1986;18:344–352.

21. Kaplan NO, Everse J. Regulatory characteristics of lactate dehydrogenase. *Adv. Enz. Regul.* 1972;10:323–336.

22. Roberts RA, Ghiasvand F, Parker D. Biochemistry of exercise-induced metabolic acidosis. *Am. J. Physiol. Regul. Integr. Comp. Physiol.* 2004;287:R502–R516.

23. Juel C, Halestrap AP. Lactate transport in skeletal muscle—role and regulation of the monocarboxylate transporter. *J. Physiol.* 1999;517:633–642.

24. Brooks GA. Anaerobic threshold: review of the concept and directions for future research. *Med. Sci. Sports Exerc.* 1985;17:22–34.

25. Brooks GA. Intra- and extra-cellular lactate shuttles. *Med. Sci. Sports Exerc.* 2000;32:790–799.

26. Anderson GS, Rhodes EC. A review of blood lactate and ventilatory methods of detecting transition threshold. *Sports Med.* 1989;8:43–55.

27. Chwalbinska-Moneta J, Roberts RA, Costill DL, Fink WJ. Threshold for muscle lactate accumulation during progressive exercise. *J. Appl. Physiol.* 1989;66:2710–2716.

28. Sjodin B, Jacbos I. Onset of blood lactate accumulation and marathon running performance. *Int. J. Sports Med.* 1981;16:49–56.

29. Katz A, Sahlin, K. Regulation of lactic acid production during exercise. *J Appl Physiol.* 1988;65:509–518.

30. Fitts R. Cellular mechanisms of fatigue. *Physiol. Rev.* 1994;74:49–94.

31. Ament W, Verkerke GJ. Exercise and fatigue. *Sports Med.* 2009;39:389–422.

32. Bishop D, Girard O, Mendez-Villanueva A. Repeated-sprint ability part II: recommendations for training. *Sports Med.* 2011;41:741–756.

33. Balaban RS. Regulation of oxidative phosphorylation in the mammalian cell. *Am. J. Physiol.* 1990;258:C377–C389.

34. Senior AE. ATP synthesis by oxidative phosphorylation. *Physiol. Rev.* 1988;68:177–231.

35. Nielsen S, Guo Z, Albu JB, et al. Energy expenditure, sex, and endogenous fuel availability in humans. *J. Clin. Invest.* 2003;111:981–988.

36. Gibala M. Protein metabolism and endurance exercise. *Sports Med.* 2007;37:337–340.

37. MacLean DA, Spriet LL, Hultman E, Graham TE. Plasma and muscle amino acid and ammonia responses during prolonged exercise in humans. *J. Appl. Physiol.* 1991;70:2095–2103.

38. Kemp GJ, Roussel M, Bendahan D, Le Fur Y, Cozzone PJ. Interrelations of ATP synthesis and proton handling in ischaemically exercising human forearm muscle studied by 31P magnetic resonance spectroscopy. *J. Physiol.* 2001;535:901–928.

39. Medbø JI, Burgers S. Effect of training on the anaerobic capacity. *Med. Sci. Sports Exerc.* 1990;22:501–507.

40. Brooks GA. Amino acid and protein metabolism during exercise and recovery. *Med. Sci. Sports Exerc.* 1987;19:S150–S156.

41. Coyle EF. Substrate utilization during exercise in active people. *Am. J. Clin. Nutr.* 1995;61:968S–979S.

42. Serresse O, Lortie G, Bouchard C, Boulay MR. Estimation of the contribution of the various energy systems during maximal work of short duration. *Int. J. Sports Med.* 1988;9:456–460.

43. Romijn JA, Coyle EF, Sidossis LS, et al. Regulation of endogenous fat and carbohydrate metabolism in relation to exercise intensity. *Am. J. Physiol.* 1993;265:E380–E391.

44. Billaut F, Bishop D. Muscle fatigue in males and females during multiple-sprint exercise. *Sports Med.* 2009;39:257–278.

45. Hunter SK, Enoka RM. Sex differences in the fatigability of arm muscles depends on absolute force during isometric contractions. *J. Appl. Physiol.* 2001;91:2686–2694.

46. Miller AEJ, MacDougall JD, Tarnopolsky MA, Sale DG. Gender differences in strength and muscle fibre characteristics. *Eur. J. Appl. Physiol.* 1993;66:254–262.

47. Karlsson J. Lactate and phosphagen concentrations in working muscle of man. *Acta Physiol. Scand. Suppl.* 1971;358:1–72.

48. Hicks AL, Kent-Braun J, Ditor DS. Sex differences in human skeletal muscle fatigue. *Exerc. Sports Sci. Rev.* 2001;29:109–112.

49. Bangsbo J. Quantification of anaerobic energy production during intense exercise. *Med. Sci. Sports Exerc.* 1998;30:47–52.

50. Komi PV, Karlsson J. Skeletal muscle fiber types, enzyme activities, and physical performance in young males and females. *Acta Physiol. Scand.* 1978;103:212–218.

51. Borges O, Essen-Gustavsson B. Enzyme activities in type I and II muscle fibres of human skeletal muscle in relation to age and torque development. *Acta Physiol. Scand.* 1989;136:29–36.

52. Green HJ, Fraser IG, Ranney DA. Male and female differences in enzyme activities of energy metabolism in vastus lateralis muscle. *J. Neurol. Sci.* 1984;65:323–331.

53. Jaworowski A, Porter MM, Holmback AM, Downham D, Lexell J. Enzyme activities in the tibialis anterior muscle of young moderately active men and women: relationship with body composition, muscle cross-sectional area and fibre type composition. *Acta Physiol. Scand.* 2002;176:215–225.

54. Carter SL, Rennie CD, Hamilton SJ, Tarnopolsky MA. Changes in skeletal muscle in males and females following endurance training. *Can. J. Physiol. Pharmacol.* 2001;79:386–392.

55. Fulco CS, Rock PB, Muza SR, et al. Slower fatigue and faster recovery of the adductor pollicis muscle in women matched for strength with men. *Acta Physiol. Scand.* 1999;167:233–239.

56. Pastoris O, Boschi F, Verri M, et al. The effects of aging on enzyme activities and metabolite concentrations in skeletal muscle from sedentary male and female subjects. *Exp. Gerontol.* 2000;35:95–104.

57. Coggan AR, Abduljalil AM, Swanson SC, et al. Muscle metabolism during exercise in young and older untrained and endurance-trained men. *J. Appl. Physiol.* 1993;75:2125–2133.

58. Kirkendall DT, Garrett WE Jr. The effects of aging and training on skeletal muscle. *Am. J. Sports Med.* 1998;26:598–602.

59. Williams GN, Higgins MJ, Lewek MD. Aging skeletal muscle: physiologic changes and the effects of training. *Phys. Ther.* 2002;82:62–68.

60. Gaster M, Staehr P, Beck-Nielsen H, Schroder HD, Handberg A. GLUT4 is reduced in slow twitch muscle fibers of type 2 diabetic patients: is insulin resistance in type 2 diabetes a slow, type fiber disease? *Diabetes.* 2001;50:1324–1329.

61. Lanza IR, Short DK, Short KR, et al. Endurance exercise as a countermeasure for aging. *Diabetes.* 2008;57:2933–2942.

62. Nevill ME, Boobis LH, Brooks S, Williams C. Effect of training on muscle metabolism during treadmill sprinting. *J. Appl. Physiol.* 1989;67:2376–2382.

63. Costill DL, Coyle EF, Fink WF, Lesmes GR, Witzmann FA. Adaptations in skeletal muscle following strength training. *J. Appl. Physiol.* 1979;46:96–99.

64. Jacobs I, Esbjornsson M, Sylven C, Holm I, Jansson E. Sprint training effects on muscle myoglobin, enzymes, fiber types, and blood lactate. *Med. Sci. Sports Exerc.* 1987;19:368–374.

65. Kraniou GN, Cameron-Smith D, Hargreaves M. Effect of short-term training on GLUT-4 mRNA and protein expression in human skeletal muscle. *Exp. Physiol.* 2004;89:559–563.

66. Gollnick PD. Metabolic regulation in skeletal muscle: influence of endurance training as exerted by mitochondrial protein content. *Acta Physiol. Scand.* 1986;128:53–66.

67. Thomas C, Bishop DJ, Lambert K, Mercier J, Brooks GA. Effects of acute and chronic exercise on sarcolemmal MCT1 and MCT4 contents in human skeletal muscles: current status. *Am. J. Physiol. Regul. Integr. Comp. Physiol.* 2012;302:R1–R14.

68. Holloszy JO. Muscle metabolism during exercise. *Arch. Phys. Med. Rehabil.* 1982;63:231–234.

69. Holloszy JO, Coyle EF. Adaptations of skeletal muscle to endurance exercise and their metabolic consequences. *J. Appl. Physiol.* 1984;56:831–838.

70. Dubouchaud H, Butterfield GE, Wolfel EE, Bergman BC, Brooks GA. Endurance training, expression, and physiology of LDH, MCT1, and MCT4 in human skeletal muscle. *Am. J. Physiol. Endocrinol. Metab.* 2000;278:E571–E579.

71. Fushiki T, Wells JA, Tapscott EB, Dohm GL. Changes in glucose transporters in muscle in response to exercise. *Am. J. Physiol.* 1989;256:E580–E587.

72. Gollnick PD. Metabolism of substrates: energy substrate metabolism during exercise and as modified by training. *Fed Proc.* 1985;44:353–357.

73. Hurley BF, Nemeth PM, Martin WH 3rd, Hagberg JM, Dalsky GP, Holloszy JO. Muscle triglyceride utilization during exercise: effect of training. *J. Appl. Physiol.* 1986;60:562–567.

74. Dudley GA, Tullson PC, Terjung RL. Influence of mitochondrial content on the sensitivity of respiratory control. *J. Biol. Chem.* 1987;262:1909–1914.

75. Apple FS, Tesch PA. CK and LD isozymes in human muscle fibers in trained athletes. *J. Appl. Physiol.* 1989;66:2717–2720.

76. Ren JM, Hultman E. Regulation of glycogenolysis in human skeletal muscle. *J. Appl. Physiol.* 1989;67:2243–2248.

77. Taylor AW, Bachman L. The effect of endurance training on muscle fiber types and enzymatic activities. *Can. J. Appl. Physiol.* 1999;24:41–53.

78. Casey A, Constantin-Teodosiu D, Howell S, Hultman E, Greenhaff PL. Metabolic response of type I and II muscle fibers during repeated bouts of maximal exercise in humans. *Am. J. Physiol.* 1996;271:E38–E43.

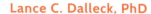

Lance C. Dalleck, PhD

## CHAPTER 5

# Energy Expenditure

## CHAPTER OUTLINE

## LEARNING OUTCOMES

1. Define the general dose-response relationship and the link between physical activity and all-cause mortality.

2. Describe the relationship between energy expenditure and risk for chronic disease.

3. Identify the different categories of calorimetry, and describe the advantages, disadvantages, and validity of each method.

4. Demonstrate how to calculate oxygen consumption, carbon dioxide production, respiratory exchange ratio (RER), and energy expenditure from gas exchange data via the Haldane transformation.

5. Define *oxygen deficit* and *excess post-exercise oxygen consumption* (EPOC), including the primary factors that contribute to the magnitude of each parameter.

## ANCILLARY LINK

Visit Davis*Plus* at http://davisplus.fadavis.com for study and practice resources, including online quizzes, animations that help explain physiological processes, podcasts concerning news and career trends in exercise physiology, and practice references.

## *VIGNETTE*

■ Norman is a 52-year-old man who was recently told by his doctor that he needs to start exercising to avoid the many complications that often accompany obesity. He is 5'10" (178 cm), weighs 260 lb (118.2 kg), and has been mostly sedentary his entire adult life. He is hesitant about working with a personal trainer at this point, but asks the advice of one of the trainers at his local health club. The trainer tells him that the safest way to get started is with recumbent cycling, because it is a non-weight-bearing activity that is perfectly suited for beginning exercisers. Norman commits to using the recumbent cycle three times each week for 20 minutes per session and successfully maintains that amount of exercise for 2 months before again seeking out Najat, the trainer who helped him get started. He tells Najat that he has lost 10 lb and feels ready for a more structured approach to improving his fitness.

How can Najat individualize and progress Norman's training regimen while maintaining high levels of both safety and effectiveness?

The study of energy expenditure and the means of quantifying energy expenditure has a long and rich history dating back to the early years within the field of exercise physiology. But what is energy expenditure? **Energy expenditure** is the collective energy cost for maintaining constant conditions within the human body, plus the amount of energy required to support daily physical activities.[1] **Physical activities** refer to any bodily movement produced by the contraction of larger skeletal muscles that increases energy expenditure (e.g., walking, gardening). This differs from exercise, which generally involves planned or structured movement that is repetitive in nature. As you have learned, both physical activity and exercise reduce the risk for premature morbidity and mortality, and may also improve mental and emotional health.[2]

Given the mounting scientific evidence implicating physical inactivity as a major modifiable risk factor for numerous chronic diseases and premature mortality (i.e., dying earlier in life from disease-related complications), the measurement of energy expenditure using various calorimetric techniques has become an increasingly important topic area within exercise physiology and public health.[1] The science of exercise prescription also uses energy expenditure to quantify both exercise intensity and overall exercise program volume.[3] Moreover, the measurement of energy expenditure can be used to assess metabolic needs, fuel use, and the relative energy costs of performing different activities. This chapter explores these fundamental and important topics.

## ENERGY EXPENDITURE AND EPIDEMIOLOGY/PUBLIC HEALTH

Scientific research has established a general dose–response relationship between physical activity and multiple health outcomes, including cardiorespiratory fitness, obesity, dyslipidemia, type 2 diabetes, colon cancer, and the relative risk for development of cardiovascular disease and mortality from all causes.[3,4] The **dose–response relationship** refers to the relationship between two variables, where any change in one parameter is associated with a concurrent change in the other parameter. **Relative risk** compares the degree of risk for development of a disease (e.g., cardiovascular disease) in one group compared with the same risk within another group, where the two groups generally differ by one or multiple variables (e.g., weekly levels of physical activity). The relative risk is expressed as a ratio that equates incidence or prevalence between two groups.

Based on these dose–response relationships, it has been noted that the health benefits of an exercise program are associated with total weekly energy expenditure.[4,5] Figure 5-1 illustrates the general relationship between total weekly energy expenditure and risk for all-cause mortality.

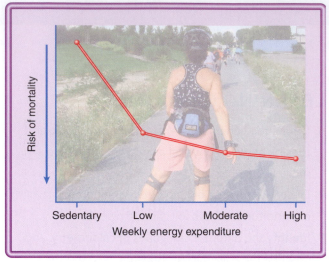

**Figure 5-1.** Relation between risk for mortality from all causes and weekly energy expenditure. (Photo courtesy of Crystal Taylor.)

Based largely on these findings, a number of organizations recommend an initial target for energy expenditure of 1,000 kilocalories (kcal)/week through physical activity for previously sedentary individuals (Box 5-1).[3] Exercise professionals, or others who design exercise programs, are then encouraged to gradually progress individuals toward an energy expenditure goal of 2,000 kcal/week to achieve or sustain weight loss.[4] The ultimate target goal is 3,000 kcal/week for weight and health maintenance. This upper target energy expenditure goal is based on evidence from the Harvard Alumni Study (Fig. 5-2) showing a graded inverse dose–response relationship between relative risk for all-cause mortality and levels of weekly physical activity.[6]

### Box 5-1. How Many Calories Improve Health?

Many research studies demonstrate how exercise programs that boost energy expenditure lead to significant improvements in cardiorespiratory fitness and other important risk factors for cardiovascular disease, including dyslipidemia, body composition, and insulin sensitivity.[32–35] As mentioned earlier, following the concept of a dose-related response, specific caloric expenditure targets have been proposed to improve health. Some targets even make recommendations based on an individual's body weight, because caloric expenditure during exercise can vary greatly based on body size. These estimates range from 14 to 23 kcal/kg/week. For example, a 165-lb (75 kg) person should target between 1,050 and 1,725 kcal/week (14 kcal/kg × 75 kg; 23 kcal/kg × 75 kg), whereas a 220-lb (100-kg) person should target between 1,400 and 2,300 kcal/week.

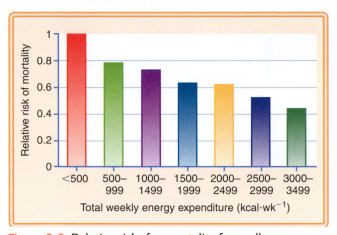

**Figure 5-2.** Relative risks for mortality from all causes across levels of weekly physical activity in the Harvard Alumni Study. *(Data from Paffenbarger Jr RS, Hyde RT, Wing AL, Hsieh CC. Physical activity, all-cause mortality, and longevity of college alumni. N Engl J Med. 1986;314:605–613.)*

## VIGNETTE continued

■ Najat begins by determining how many calories Norman has been burning each week and adjusts the duration of his workouts to reach an initial goal of 1,000 calories per week. She realizes, however, that Norman's program will need to achieve 2,000 calories per week to promote continued weight loss, a goal consistent with his doctor's overall recommendation.

After about 4 more months of exercising on the recumbent cycle, in addition to performing two full-body resistance training circuits each week, Norman is ready to add some variety to his workouts and start increasing his energy expenditure. Najat recommends that Norman now walk two or three nights each week after dinner to complement his current training program and add another weight-bearing activity, which is important for Norman's overall health. Najat estimates that these activities collectively will now exceed 2,000 kcal/week, the target to effectively allow Norman to lose weight.

## QUANTIFICATION OF ENERGY EXPENDITURE

It is fundamental to first have an appreciation and an understanding of how the science of calorimetry enables us to calculate energy expenditure. The first law of thermodynamics states that energy is neither created nor destroyed, but rather changes form (see Chapter 4). In the human body, a basic application of this principle is the transfer of energy from molecules

(e.g., adenosine triphosphate [ATP] or creatine phosphate) or stored reserves (e.g., carbohydrates and fats) to chemical energy to fuel cellular action, with the energy ultimately degrading to heat. Also mentioned in Chapter 4 is the fact that not all energy released from these molecules is made available to support cellular work (e.g., skeletal muscle contraction); in fact, the body is approximately 30% efficient in transferring energy from food molecules to mechanical work. The remainder of energy liberated from the breakdown of food molecules is released to the surrounding environment in the form of heat. Ultimately, the overall heat production will be proportional to the rate of reactions; consequently, the amount of heat generated is a reflection of the metabolic rate or energy expenditure. One technique to measure energy expenditure is to measure the heat released via actual or estimated techniques, which will be described later in this chapter.

**Metabolism** refers to the sum of all chemical reactions that occur in the human body that are required to support body function and survival.[7] The quantity of heat released from these chemical reactions can be measured and energy expenditure subsequently calculated. This is known as **calorimetry**, which is the measurement of metabolism determined from the quantity of heat released from the human body. Notably, the process of metabolism also requires oxygen; thus, the measurement of oxygen utilized can provide an estimate of energy expenditure. Three general categories of calorimetry exist:

1. **Direct calorimetry** refers to the direct measurement of heat dissipated from an individual.
2. **Indirect calorimetry (IC)** involves measurement of expired gases (oxygen consumption and carbon dioxide production). Because oxygen is needed to burn fuels, this method relies on the measurement of the amount of oxygen used to quantify calories.
3. **Noncalorimetric techniques** involve various scientific methods that predict the rate of heat production and energy expenditure via physiological measurements or observations, or both.

It is important to note that the advantages, disadvantages, and validity of each technique vary considerably.

## Direct Calorimetry

Direct calorimetry is the gold standard measurement for estimating calories and it involves estimating the energy value of food. Bomb calorimeters are designed to measure the amount of heat liberated when combusting (burning) food to assess the number of calories held within that food. To help understand this technique, think back to the definition of 1 calorie—the amount of energy needed to raise the temperature of 1 kg (33.8 oz) of water by 1°C from 14.5°C (58°F) to 15.5°C (60°F). Therefore, if we design a container surrounded by a known volume of water held at 14.5°C and then combust a food and measure how much heat is transferred into the water, then the caloric value of that food can be quantified. As illustrated in Figure 5-3, bomb calorimeters were designed to ignite a food surrounded by water, which then passed its heat into the adjacent water.

As a result of this research, scientists have quantified the calories derived from carbohydrates, fats, proteins, alcohol, and other carbon-based structures that hold energy (e.g., artificial sweeteners). Wilbur Atwater and his colleagues pioneered much of this research in the 19th century and gave us the Atwater Factor scores we now use today to calculate the available energy in foods.[7] Although they measured gross yields (i.e., total energy released), they also recognized that, as humans, we do not absorb food with 100% efficiency; thus, they needed to factor this into their figures (what they called a *coefficient of digestibility*). Table 5-1 outlines the net energy available from various food sources.

Obviously, this same technique is not applicable to humans, so the bomb calorimeter was modified to an insulated chamber in which a human could perform various activities while measuring heat production. As shown in Figure 5-4, pipes containing known volumes of water passed through these chambers and as the person released heat, it was transferred into the pipes. Although effective, the space required to house such a

**DOING THE MATH:**

Calculate the total caloric value of a meal containing the following nutrients:
- 30 g of carbohydrates
- 12 g of protein
- 5 g of fat

**ANSWER:**

248 kcal
$30 \times 4 = 120$
$12 \times 9 = 108$
$5 \times 4 = 20$
$120 + 108 + 20 = 248$

chamber or direct calorimeter presents a considerable barrier. Furthermore, the instrumentation and cost involved in building such a device can easily exceed $1 million; clearly this factor alone makes this technique prohibitive for many exercise physiology laboratories.

## Indirect Calorimetry

Indirect calorimetry (IC) is the method best suited to exercise physiology (Fig. 5-5). At rest and during exercise you constantly breathe air in and out. From a basic perspective, the difference between inspired and expired oxygen for a given time frame reflects the volume of oxygen consumed ($\dot{V}O_2$). The concentration of oxygen in expired air ($F_{EO_2}$) contains less oxygen

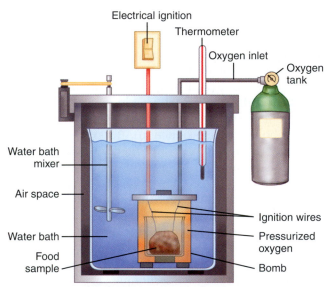

**Figure 5-3.** Bomb calorimeter. This device is capable of directly quantifying the heat released when macronutrients (i.e., carbohydrate, protein, fats) are combusted.

## Table 5-1. Net Energy Available From Various Food Sources

| CARBOHYDRATES | FATS | PROTEIN | ALCOHOL |
|---|---|---|---|
| 4 kcal/g | 9 kcal/g | 4 kcal/g | 7 kcal/g |

*Example:* A meal that contains 10 g of carbohydrates, 4 g of protein, and 2 g of fat would hold 74 kcal.
- 10 g × 4 kcal/g = 40 kcal
- 4 g × 4 kcal/g = 16 kcal
- 2 g × 9 kcal/g = 18 kcal

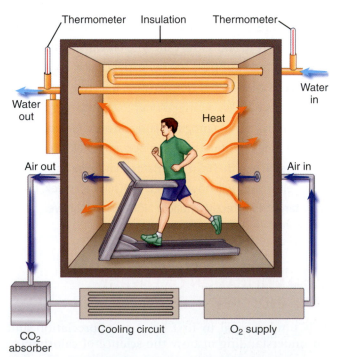

**Figure 5-4.** Example of direct calorimetry. A live-in metabolic chamber, which is a variation of the bomb calorimeter, is shown. The insulated chamber permits direct measurement of heat production during both activities of daily living and exercise.

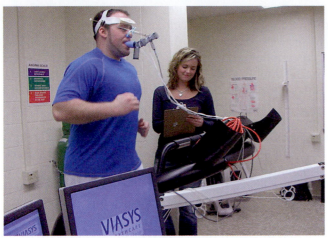

**Figure 5-5.** An individual performing a maximal exercise protocol on a treadmill. Gas exchange data are being collected and analyzed throughout the test by a metabolic cart; this is the most common type of indirect calorimetry performed in exercise physiology laboratories. *(Photo courtesy of Lance Dalleck)*

compared with that of inspired air ($FIO_2$); therefore, $\dot{V}O_2$ can be calculated using the following equation:

$$\dot{V}O_2 = (\dot{V}i \times FIO_2) - (\dot{V}e \times FEO_2)$$

where $\dot{V}i$ is the volume of air inspired (inhaled) and $\dot{V}e$ is the volume of air expired (exhaled).

**EXAMPLE:** During Norman's $\dot{V}O_2$ test, at one point his data reveal the following:

- $\dot{V}i$ = 80 L/min
- $FIO_2$ = 20.93%
- $\dot{V}e$ = 78.6 L
- $FEO_2$ = 18.6%

$$\dot{V}O_2 = (\dot{V}i \times FIO_2) - (\dot{V}e \times FEO_2)$$
$$\dot{V}O_2 = (80 \text{ L/min} \times 0.2093) - (78.6 \times 0.186)$$
$$\dot{V}O_2 = (16.744 \text{ L/min}) - (14.620 \text{ L/min}) = 2.12 \text{ L/min}$$

Conversely, the difference between inspired and expired carbon dioxide for a specific time frame equates to the volume of carbon dioxide ($\dot{V}CO_2$) production. Here, though, the concentration of carbon dioxide in expired air ($FECO_2$) contains more carbon dioxide relative to inspired air ($FICO_2$). $\dot{V}CO_2$ can be calculated using the following equation:

$$\dot{V}CO_2 = (\dot{V}e \times FECO_2) - (\dot{V}i \times FICO_2)$$

where $\dot{V}e$ is the volume of air expired (exhaled) and $\dot{V}i$ is the volume of air inspired (inhaled).

**EXAMPLE:** During Norman's $\dot{V}O_2$ test, at one point his data reveal the following:

- $\dot{V}i$ = 80 L/min
- $FICO_2$ = 0.03%
- $\dot{V}e$ = 78.6 L
- $FECO_2$ = 2.6%

$$\dot{V}CO_2 = (\dot{V}e \times FECO_2) - (\dot{V}i \times FICO_2)$$
$$\dot{V}CO_2 = (78.6 \text{ L} \times 0.026) - (80 \times 0.0003)$$

$$\dot{V}CO_2 = (2.044 \text{ L/min}) - (0.024 \text{ L/min}) = 2.02 \text{ L/min}$$

## Haldane Transformation

Ambient or environmental air consists of oxygen, carbon dioxide, and a combination of nitrogen and inert gases in the following concentrations:

- $O_2$ = 20.93%, expressed as $FIO_2$.
- $CO_2$ = 0.03%, expressed as $FICO_2$.
- $N_2$ and other inert gases = 79.04%, expressed as $FiN_2$.

Ambient air comprises all three gases and is expressed as $FIO_2 + FICO_2 + FiN_2$. Conversely, expired air is also composed of all three gases and expressed as $FEO_2 + FECO_2 + FEN_2$. Thus, although $FIO_2$ and $FICO_2$ are already known, the measurement of four variables is required to quantify $\dot{V}O_2$ and $\dot{V}CO_2$:

1. Volume of inspired air or inspired ventilation ($\dot{V}i$)
2. Volume of expired air or expired ventilation ($\dot{V}e$)
3. $FEO_2$
4. $FECO_2$

Most exercise physiology laboratories do not measure both inspired and expired ventilation because of the expense required to purchase two ventilation measurement systems. Therefore, the majority of commercially manufactured metabolic systems use a single ventilation measurement system that quantifies expired ventilation and then mathematically calculates the volume of inspired air via the **Haldane transformation**. This is a sequence of mathematical steps used to determine inspired volume when this value is not actually measured. This process ultimately permits exercise scientists to quantify oxygen consumption, carbon dioxide production, and energy expenditure across various conditions of exercise.

The mathematical calculation for measuring $\dot{V}O_2$ is $(\dot{V}i \times FIO_2) - (\dot{V}e \times FEO_2)$ or $\dot{V}iFIO_2 - \dot{V}eFEO_2$ and requires:

- $FIO_2$, which is known (20.93%)
- $\dot{V}e$ measured by the metabolic system
- $FEO_2$ measured by the metabolic system
- $\dot{V}i$ calculated via the Haldane transformation

**NOTE:** Because $N_2$ is inert and is not used by the body, the $\dot{V}i$ of $N_2$ or $\dot{V}iN_2$ = the $\dot{V}e$ of $N_2$ or $\dot{V}eN_2$.

Because $N_2$ is inert and is not used within the body, the Haldane transformation uses $N_2$ to determine $\dot{V}i$:

- *Step 1:* $\dot{V}i$ of $N_2$ = $\dot{V}e$ of $N_2$ or $[\dot{V}i \times FiN_2]$ = $[\dot{V}e \times FEN_2]$.
- *Step 2:* Rearrange that equation: $\dot{V}i$ = $[\dot{V}e \times FEN_2] \div FiN_2$.
- *Step 3:* $FEN_2$ is calculated from measuring expired gases where the collective totals of all three equal 100% or $FEO_2 + FECO_2 + FEN_2$ = 100%.
  - Rearrange the formula from 100% = $FEO_2 + FECO_2 + FEN_2$ to $FEN_2$ = 100% − $FEO_2 + FECO_2$ or $FEN_2$ = $(1 - [FEO_2] + [FECO_2])$ because we are working with percentages.
- *Step 4:* Rewrite the equation in step 2:
  - $\dot{V}i$ = $\dot{V}e \times [1 - (FEO_2) + (FECO_2)] \div FiN_2$.

• *Step 5:* Once you have calculated $\dot{V}i$, you can calculate $\dot{V}O_2$.

$$\dot{V}O_2 = [\dot{V}i \times F_{IO_2}] - [\dot{V}e \times F_{EO_2}]$$

• Solve for $\dot{V}CO_2$ in the similar manner: $\dot{V}CO_2 = [\dot{V}e \times F_{ECO_2}] - [\dot{V}i \times F_{ICO_2}]$.

## Doubly Labeled Water Method

Another form of IC is the doubly labeled water method. Although not ideally suited for assessment of energy expended during activity, it is regarded as a very accurate method for estimating total energy expenditure.[8] In this technique, baseline samples of blood, saliva, and urine are collected, after which non-radioactive isotopes ($^2H_2O$ and $H_2^{18}O$) are ingested by an individual. The isotopes become circulated uniformly throughout the body and subsequently are secreted gradually in the urine over the next 1 to 3 weeks. Regular urine samples are collected throughout the testing periods to quantify the elimination rate of each isotope; these measurements are then used to estimate the $\dot{V}CO_2$ production. The elimination rates of each isotope are proportional to

metabolic $\dot{V}CO_2$ production, which is influenced by the activity level of an individual. Ultimately, it is the estimated $\dot{V}CO_2$ production that is used to calculate oxygen consumption and total energy expenditure.

The doubly labeled method provides an accurate estimation of total energy expenditure, with a standard error between 6% and 8%. This error rate can be reduced with more frequent collection of urine samples.[9] Additional advantages to this method include its non-invasiveness and the capability to assess total energy expenditure under true free-living conditions. The primary drawback to the doubly labeled water method is cost; both the isotopes and the equipment required for analysis are expensive. Another limitation is that frequency, intensity, time, and type of physical activity or exercise cannot be quantified with this method.

## Noncalorimetric Techniques

An extensive list of different noncalorimetric techniques used to quantify energy expenditure exists. Noncalorimetric techniques can be further classified into objective and subjective methods. These methods all rely on the capacity to estimate energy expenditure based on a significant relationship existing between a given variable and energy expenditure in exercise. It is paramount that a noncalorimetric technique be validated against a standardized method to be considered robust. With objective methods, the instrument (e.g., accelerometers) is used to estimate energy expenditure and the results are compared against standardized methods. With subjective methods, energy expenditure is estimated based on an individual's interpretation and perception of their physical activities. The primary noncalorimetric techniques, objective and subjective, used in research, clinical, and field settings are examined in the following subsections.

## Objective Methods

The most common types of objective instruments for quantifying energy expenditure are pedometers, accelerometers, and heart rate monitors (Fig. 5-6). A major advantage with these instruments is that all are relatively lightweight and unobtrusive. Expense, however, can be a concern with some of the devices; certain accelerometers and heart rate monitors cost several hundred dollars. The inability to quantify specific types of activities is also a limitation with objective methods.

### Pedometers

Pedometers are simple, inexpensive devices that count the number of steps taken by an individual by detecting the motion of the person's hips (i.e., pendulum monitoring leg swing at the hip). But because individuals vary in size, so too will they vary in step length. Therefore, an initial step calibration is required to allow the device to total the number of steps taken, which translates into distance covered (distance = number of steps × step length). From the steps completed or distance covered, estimates of caloric expenditure can be determined.

---

**DOING THE MATH:**

If a person performs a treadmill test in which gas analysis is collected and it reveals the following information, what would be the $\dot{V}O_2$?

• $F_{IO_2}$ = 20.93%
• $F_{ICO_2}$ = 0.03%
• $FiN_2$ = 79.04%
• $\dot{V}e$ = 95 L/min (measured from flowmeter of the analyzer)
• $F_{EO_2}$ = 18.50% (measured from the analyzer)
• $F_{ECO_2}$ = 2.05% (measured from the analyzer)

1. Calculate $FeN_2$:

$FeN_2 = (1 - [F_{EO_2} + F_{ECO_2}])$
$FeN_2 = (1 - [18.50\% + 2.05\%])$
$FeN_2 = $ _____ .

2. Calculate $\dot{V}i$:

$\dot{V}i = (\dot{V}e \times FeN_2) \div FiN_2$
$\dot{V}i = (95.0 \text{ L} \times$ ____$) \div 0.7904$
$\dot{V}i = $ _____ L/min

3. Calculate $\dot{V}O_2$:

$\dot{V}O_2 = (\dot{V}i \times F_{IO_2}) - (\dot{V}e \times F_{EO_2})$
$\dot{V}O_2 = [$ ___ $\times .2093] - [95 \text{ L} \times .1850]$
$\dot{V}O_2 = $ _____ L/min

**ANSWERS:**
1. $FeN_2 = 0.7945$
2. $\dot{V}i = 95.5$ L/min
3. $\dot{V}O_2 = 2.41$ L/min

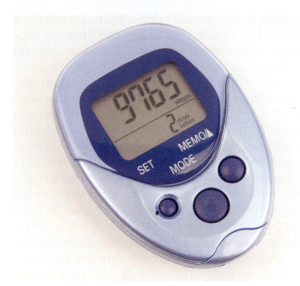

**Figure 5-6.** A pedometer is an objective device for quantifying energy expenditure that is available on the commercial market.

These devices range from very inexpensive or free items found in cereal packages or as giveaways at many events, to more advanced devices that can now estimate speed and distance. The cheaper pedometers often erroneously record movement that is not actual walking (i.e., motion artifact), but simply movement at the hips (e.g., bending down, movement in chairs). This falsely elevates the number of steps completed and calories expended.

Given standard step lengths for most adults, it is estimated that a total of 10,000 steps is equivalent to approximately 5 miles (8.0 km). The average adult should walk 1,000 steps in approximately 10 minutes and the target of 10,000 is recommended as a baseline to improve overall health, although this point is still debated among experts.[10] Unfortunately, most Americans fall far short of this target, but agencies continue to press the public to strive for that target. In a study conducted on 200 men and women, the men averaged 7,192 steps/day, whereas the women averaged 5,210 steps/day.[10]

## Accelerometers

An accelerometer is an instrument generally worn on either the trunk or limbs that determines the duration, frequency, and intensity of physical activity; this measurement is obtained by quantifying the acceleration and deceleration of the body. There are single-plane accelerometers and triaxial-plane (three planes) accelerometers. Single-plane accelerometers measure movement in the vertical plane, whereas triaxial-plane accelerometers measure movement in the horizontal, mediolateral (side-to-side), and vertical planes. The gathered values are recorded and then downloaded to a computer for analysis and interpretation. The primary advantages of accelerometers are that they are small, lightweight, and for the most part not cumbersome. Moreover, physical activity data can be recorded over prolonged periods, ranging from several days to even weeks.

From an economic perspective, the use of accelerometers can be hindered by the cost of the instrument, as well as the expense of the software and hardware required to analyze recorded data. Accelerometers also have some specific limitations in certain situations; for instance, single-plane accelerometers do not permit measurement of activities such as bicycling or weight lifting. Furthermore, both single and triaxial accelerometers are unable to detect increases in upper body movement (e.g., upper body resistance training), increased energy expenditure resulting from carrying a load (e.g., backpack), or alterations in energy expenditure ensuing from changes in surface type (e.g., walking uphill or walking in snow). In addition, the equations used to estimate energy expenditure from the movement recorded by accelerometers are based on data collected in the laboratory; accordingly, these equations may not always provide a valid estimate of energy expenditure for those activities performed in free-living

## RESEARCH HIGHLIGHT

### Amish Walk More Steps and are Less Obese

The Old Order Amish continue to live a labor-intensive lifestyle of farming and refrain from using many of the amenities of modern-day society (e.g., automobiles, electronic appliances). Researchers set out to quantify the physical activity levels of this population and also to examine different measures of adiposity.[11] Ninety-eight Amish adults (aged 18–75 years) were studied and were asked to wear an electronic pedometer for 7 days, while maintaining log sheets to record daily steps and physical activities. On average, the number of steps walked each day was 18,425 for men versus 14,196 for women. Although the Amish also engaged in various levels of moderate and vigorous activity, 0% of the men and only 9% of the women were classified as obese (BMI $\geq$ 30 kg/m²). By comparison, the prevalence of obesity in Americans is far greater, and as mentioned earlier, the average number of steps taken per day is far lower than the Amish population.

Bassett DR Jr, Schneider PL, Huntington GE. Physical activity in an Old Order Amish community. *Med Sci Sports Exerc.* 2004;36:79–85.

situations or on different populations. Nevertheless, accelerometers yield much important objective information regarding physical activity. Specifically, it has been recognized that accelerometers might provide the most objective and detailed data for research purposes.[12]

## Heart Rate Monitors

Heart rate monitors are perhaps the most popular electronic devices worn during exercise. They were originally designed to measure heart rate. Since the mid-2000s, however, research has advanced their functionality to the point where they can now quantify energy expenditure of a single exercise bout or over the span of an entire day.

Heart rate monitors vary considerably in overall capability. Whereas some monitors simply measure and display heart rate in real time, others have the potential to track heart rate data over prolonged periods, set target heart rate ranges with alerts, track improvements in overall fitness (e.g., lowered heart rate at rest or during specific submaximal workloads), or even estimate caloric expenditure using algorithms from heart rate responses. Although the notion of all this functionality is an exciting prospect for exercise professionals and clients alike, the reality is that the majority of these instruments have not yet been scientifically validated against gold standard methods for assessing energy expenditure, such as the doubly labeled water technique or IC.

Most monitors require a strap to be worn snugly around the chest (below the breast) that contains sensor pads that make direct contact with the skin. The strap also contains a transmitter that detects electrical activity of the heart in the same manner as an electrocardiogram (ECG), picking up electrical activity produced by the heart. The transmitter then relays this information to a display unit, usually in the form of a wristwatch, wrist strap, mobile application on your phone, or even to earphones, where each beat is converted to a sound. Many commercial brands are available and include Polar, Sunnto, and Garmin, but several issues exist with chest straps:

- They require the chest strap to make continuous good contact with the skin to pick up heart rate activity. This usually necessitates a need to dampen the strap electrodes with water or apply a saline gel.
- Straps can sometimes be uncomfortable for some individuals, although newer alternatives can alleviate this problem. These include the newer, more expensive soft straps (as opposed to the cheaper, molded plastic straps) and straps built into jogging bras and tank tops.
- Other electronic devices (e.g., radios, microwaves) or even synthetic fabrics (building static charges) can sometimes impede the strap's ability to pick up or transmit a signal.

Given some of these inconveniences, strapless monitors are becoming more popular and can now measure heartbeat without using a chest strap. Most strapless heart rate monitors are worn on the wrist (as a watch)

and function through one or two sensors. By placing a finger on a sensor, the unit reads and displays your heart rate. Other options include ring designs and arm sensors (upper arm) that use a strap around the arm.

Heart rate monitors are often used to estimate energy expenditure because of the significant linear relationship that exists between heart rate and oxygen uptake ($\dot{V}O_2$). Accordingly, these devices contain the means to predict the energy expenditure associated with various durations, intensities, and frequencies of exercise. It is important, however, for students and exercise professionals to recognize that the validity of these energy expenditure.estimates may be confounded by several factors.

- First, considerable interindividual variance for the relationship between heart rate and energy expenditure exists. For example, the increase in caloric expenditure for a given increase in heart rate will differ across individuals.
- Increases in heart rate can be elicited by various non–physical activity–related factors such as emotions, hydration status, and environment (e.g., temperature, humidity, and altitude all can increase heart rate independent of physical activity).

Nonetheless, researchers have found heart rate monitors to be reasonably accurate; it has been reported that there is a strong correlation between energy expenditure for activities of daily living when measured with indirect calorimetry compared with energy expenditure predicted from heart rate monitoring.[13]

## New Technologies for Estimating Energy Expenditure

Weight loss continues to drive the purchasing decisions of many individuals. In response, scientists continue their research in the hopes of developing new technology that can be implemented into portable, but affordable devices to help track caloric expenditure. Recently, a number of popular, commercially available portable devices with energy expenditure functionality, GPS capability, and more have emerged as solutions for tracking activity and caloric expenditure (e.g., Fitbit, Garmin Vivofit, Jawbone Up Wristband, and Nike FuelBand). Many track daily activity, comparing levels against established goals; map progress that can be downloaded or shared; and offer various engaging features to build motivation and adherence through their software or information-sharing applications. As fun, engaging, and interactive as they may be, the unfortunate reality is that they have not truly been validated in the scientific literature. This fact means that exercise professionals should assume that the reported energy expenditure of these devices may be erroneous. Consequently, the energy expenditure value reported from these instruments to the client may potentially be overestimated or underestimated. Exercise professionals and clients therefore are faced with the prospect of questioning whether the energy expenditure being reported is sufficient to achieve health and fitness goals.

## RESEARCH HIGHLIGHT

### New Technologies for Estimating Energy Expenditure—Are They Valid?

Accurate estimation of energy expenditure remains elusive for many who do not have access to expensive laboratory equipment. As technology continues to improve, manufacturers are constantly striving to validate the accuracy of using more affordable, commercially available pieces of equipment to measure energy expenditure. In one study, researchers examined the accuracy of the Polar S410 for estimating gross energy expenditure during exercise when using both predicted and measured maximal oxygen uptake ($\dot{V}O_{2max}$) and maximal heart rate (MHR) versus IC.[14] Ten males and 10 females had their initial $\dot{V}O_{2max}$ and MHR predicted by the S410, then performed a maximal treadmill test with gas analysis to determine their actual values. In the study design, the participants performed three submaximal exercise tests at ratings of perceived exertion (RPE) levels of 3, 5, and 7 on a treadmill, cycle, and rowing ergometer for a total of nine submaximal bouts. For all tests, the participants wore two S410 heart rate monitors: one collecting data based off their predicted (PRED) values and one measuring actual $\dot{V}O_2$ and HR values (ACT), while simultaneously measuring energy expenditure via gas analysis (IC). The results demonstrated no differences in energy expenditure values among all three collection methods (PRED, ACT, IC) for any intensity or exercise mode. In female subjects, the PRED significantly overestimated by 12%, whereas the ACT improved estimation of energy expenditure. It was concluded that the Polar S410 provided a good estimate of energy expenditure during running, rowing, and cycling.

Crouter SE, Albright C, Bassett DR Jr. Accuracy of the Polar S410 heart rate monitor to estimate energy cost of exercise. *Med Sci Sports Exerc.* 2004;36:1433–1439.

## Subjective Methods

The most common types of subjective methods for quantifying physical activity energy expenditure include questionnaires and diaries. Both of these strategies are relatively easy to administer and inexpensive, attributes that make them ideal for collecting data from large populations. Diaries are used by individuals to log their physical activity patterns over a given time frame. It is common to have people record their activity for 3 days (2 weekdays and 1 weekend day) of data collection to minimize the error involved with recording physical activity. Questionnaires can vary in intricacy; some instruments rely on a single question, whereas others are more extensive in detail and length. The more comprehensive questionnaires aim to identify the types of physical activity engaged in throughout the day and to specify the frequency, duration, and intensity of each activity performed.

Summarized data from diaries and questionnaires can then be analyzed further by linking a **metabolic equivalents (METs)** value to each physical activity performed over the collection period. METs are frequently used by fitness professionals to describe exercise intensity.[15] A single MET equates to the amount of energy expenditure during 1 minute of seated rest; in terms of oxygen consumption, 1 MET = 3.5 mL/kg/min. Figure 5-7 shows resting metabolic rate (i.e., 1 MET) being measured via IC.

The Compendium of Physical Activities[16] is a resource frequently used by fitness professionals to help develop exercise programs for clients. When using the Compendium of Physical Activities for this purpose, however, several things need to be kept in mind.

- The MET values in the compendium assume equivalency in skill; for instance, it is presumed that the

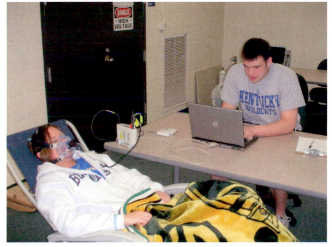

**Figure 5-7.** Resting metabolic rate (i.e., 1 MET) being measured via indirect calorimetry. *(Photo courtesy of Lance Dalleck)*

MET value of activities such as walking, gardening, and playing tennis are similar across the entire population. Clearly, it should be acknowledged that this scenario is not possible; consequently, there is error introduced by making this assumption.

- The MET cost of performing various physical activities is presumed to be equivalent for individuals of differing body masses; again, this assumption clearly does not hold true in the real-world population. Accordingly, you need to realize there is error introduced with this assumption.

Still, the ability to quantify energy expenditure based on data gathered via diaries and questionnaires provides valuable information for scientists, exercise physiologists, and clinicians alike.

## PREDICTION OF EXERCISE ENERGY EXPENDITURE WITH METABOLIC EQUATIONS

The capability to accurately estimate energy expenditure during exercise is a fundamental aspect of exercise physiology, with fitness professionals frequently relying on metabolic equations to prescribe exercise intensity and to determine the energy expenditure of different exercise modalities.[17] Such knowledge also permits students and fitness professionals to devise protocols that are more conducive to attaining valid results for the purpose of the exercise test. Previous studies using various exercise modalities including arm and cycle ergometers, elliptical machines, stair steppers, and treadmills have published prediction equations to estimate the oxygen consumption during exercise.[18,19]

From data collected in the laboratory, multiple regression analysis has been used to develop prediction equations based on the relationship between mechanical workloads and the corresponding metabolic cost. These equations have periodically been researched to evaluate their accuracy and usefulness to develop more accurate and valid estimates of oxygen consumption. Metabolic equations for the prediction of energy expenditure during common exercise modalities are presented in Table 5-2, as well as the standard error of the estimate (SEE) for each equation. The SEE is a measure of accuracy of the prediction equation; smaller SEE values can be interpreted to mean that the predicted energy expenditure value is more likely to reflect the actual energy expenditure value for the modality of exercise.

## OXYGEN CONSUMPTION

Volume of oxygen consumed, or $\dot{V}O_2$, is a measure of the overall total body oxygen consumption or use. It reflects the collective ability of the cardiovascular system

**Table 5-2.** Metabolic Equations for the Prediction of Energy Expenditure During Common Exercise Modalities (in Terms of Relative $\dot{V}O_2$, mL/kg/min)

| EXERCISE MODALITY | PREDICTION EQUATION FORMULA | SEE | RANGE OF ACCURACY |
|---|---|---|---|
| Arm ergometer* | $\dot{V}O_2 = 3.5 + (3 \times work\ rate)/mass$ | 1.3 | 150–750 kg/m/min (equates to 25–125 watts) |
| Cycle ergometer* | $\dot{V}O_2 = 3.5 + 3.5 + (1.8 \times work\ rate)/mass$ | 1.4–2.8 | 300–1,200 kg/m/min (equates to 50–200 watts) |
| Elliptical cross-trainer† | $\dot{V}O_2 = 3.5 + 0.15(cadence) + 1.22(resistance) - 0.11(mass)$ | 2.8 | Resistance of level 2–12; cadence of 90–135 strides/min for women and 90–150 strides/min for men |
| Recumbent stepper‡ | $\dot{V}O_2 = 3.5 + 0.016(W \times steps/min) + 0.092(steps/min) + - 0.053(mass)$ | 2.3 | Step/min of 60–100; W of level 1–7 |
| Stair stepping | $\dot{V}O_2 = 3.5 + 0.2\ (steps/min) + 1.33(1.8 \times step\ height \times steps/min)$ | 1.7 | Stepping rates between 12 and 30 steps/min |
| Treadmill running§ | $\dot{V}O_2 = 3.5 + 0.2(speed) + 0.9(speed)(grade)$ | 5.0 | Speeds >134 m/min (equates to >5.0 miles/hr) |
| Treadmill walking§ | $\dot{V}O_2 = 3.5 + 0.1(speed) + 1.8(speed)(grade)$ | 1.3–5.9 | Speeds between 50 and 100 m/min (equates to 1.9–3.7 miles/hr) |

Mass is given in kilograms. Convert from meters per minute to miles per hour by multiplying by 26.8.

*Arm ergometer and cycle ergometer work rate are given in kg/m/min.

‡Elliptical cross-trainer cadence in strides/min. Elliptical cross-trainer resistance in terms of level, which ranges from 1 to 20.

†Recumbent stepper W refers to stepper resistance level, which ranges from 1 to 10.

§Treadmill grade is expressed in decimal form (e.g., 5% = 0.05). Treadmill running and walking speed are given in m/min.

SEE, standard error of the estimate (in terms of mL/kg/min); $\dot{V}O_2$, oxygen consumption, mL/kg/min.

Adapted from American College of Sports Medicine. *ACSM's Guidelines for Exercise Testing* (p. 158). 9th ed. Baltimore, MD: Lippincott Williams & Wilkins; 2014; Dalleck LC, Kravitz L. Development of a metabolic equation for elliptical crosstrainer exercise. *Percept Mot Skills*. 2007;104:725–732; and Dalleck LC, Borresen EC, Parker AL, et al. Development of a metabolic equation for the NuStep recumbent stepper in older adults. *Percept Mot Skills*. 2011;112:183–192.

## VIGNETTE continued

■ Norman is now 8 months into his exercise program, including 6 months of working with Najat. Both Norman and his physician have been thrilled with the results, as Norman's weight has declined from 260 to 218 lb, and several key health markers have been positively affected (e.g., cholesterol levels and blood pressure). During this time, Norman also started working with Ella, a registered dietitian whom Najat had recommended. Although Najat is fairly well versed in nutrition, she knew it was outside her scope of practice to develop a detailed meal plan, which Norman had requested when he struggled with finding nutrient-dense foods that he enjoyed. In addition to imparting information on smart food choices, Ella taught Norman how to divide his caloric intake into segments throughout the day so that the timing of his meals and his workouts complemented each other for an optimal, individualized eating plan. His sessions with Ella were helpful, and Norman is committed to continue making progress. Therefore, Najat recommends that he try other exercise modalities to avoid boredom, and increase the duration of each of his cardiovascular workouts so that he can continue building toward the ultimate goal of burning at least 2,600 calories/week.

to deliver oxygenated blood to the exercising skeletal muscles, and also the capacity to extract oxygen from capillaries for utilization in mitochondrial respiration. $\dot{V}O_{2max}$ represents the maximal rate of oxygen consumption during exercise testing to volitional fatigue. The higher the $\dot{V}O_{2max}$ score, the greater the amount of oxygen utilization and capacity for physical work. Consequently, $\dot{V}O_{2max}$ (cardiorespiratory endurance or aerobic fitness) has long been considered a good indicator of health and performance. Oxygen consumption can be represented in both absolute and relative terms.

## Absolute $\dot{V}O_2$

Absolute $\dot{V}O_2$ represents the total amount of oxygen consumed by the entire body regardless of body size or weight. It is expressed in units of liters (L) or milliliters (mL). The rate of oxygen consumption (i.e., time) is expressed in minutes. Hence, the standard measurement unit for absolute $\dot{V}O_2$ is L/min or mL/min. However, it is misleading to compare scores of different individuals

using these units due to differences in body size, hemoglobin, and lean body mass content. Larger individuals, especially males, will always have higher absolute scores regardless of their fitness level. Consequently, this system of measurement is limited when attempting to make comparisons between individuals or when comparing scores with some standard reference.

The notion that oxygen is needed to burn fuel, which allows us to quantify calories and energy expenditure, was discussed previously. Therefore, if the absolute amount of oxygen consumed is measured, the number of calories expended can be determined. A standard estimate that every liter of oxygen consumed by the body yields approximately 5 kcal is generally used, although that statement is not 100% accurate. For purposes of estimating energy expenditure in exercise physiology, this estimate has become widely accepted. For example, if a person running on a treadmill is estimated to have an absolute $\dot{V}O_2$ of 2.5 L/min, this translates to 12.5 kcal/min, and if this person maintained that pace for 20 minutes, he or she would expend a total of 250 kcal. These values were calculated as follows:

- 1 L oxygen/min = 5 kcal
- 2.5 L/min = 5 kcal/L × 2.5 = 12.5 kcal/min
- 12.5 kcal/min × 20 minutes = 250 kcal

Operating software on today's cardiovascular training equipment work along this premise, estimating the user's absolute $\dot{V}O_2$ from the amount of work performed (speed, grade, watts) and then estimating calories expended.

## Relative $\dot{V}O_2$

Relative $\dot{V}O_2$ presents an alternative method to represent oxygen consumption. For comparative purposes, absolute $\dot{V}O_2$ is limited; however, if an individual's score is expressed relative to some standard that is consistent across individuals, then the validity of comparing scores improves. Absolute $\dot{V}O_2$ does not distinguish among different body sizes, as mentioned earlier; therefore, standardizing against a unit of weight removes the discrepancy of a size differential among people.

The conversion from absolute to relative requires consideration of body weight. Hence the individual's score is divided by his or her body weight to reflect a relative score. In doing this calculation, it is important to note that the units of measurement change. Use the following sequence to understand the change in units.

1. L/min (absolute $\dot{V}O_2$) is usually first converted to mL/min (absolute $\dot{V}O_2$) by multiplying by 1,000 because there are 1,000 mL in 1 L.
   - The purpose of this step is simply for convenience, to keep the final value greater than 1 once the score is divided by the person's body weight.
2. This value is then divided by body weight in kilograms to yield mL/kg/min (relative $\dot{V}O_2$).

Relative $\dot{V}O_2$ (mL/kg/min) represents milliliters of $\dot{V}O_2$ per kilogram of body weight per minute. For example, if Gary has a $\dot{V}O_{2max}$ score of 3.5 L/min and weighs 176 lb (80 kg), his relative $\dot{V}O_2$ can be calculated following the steps outlined earlier:

$$3.5 \text{ L/min} \times 1{,}000 = 3{,}500 \text{ mL/min}$$
$$3{,}500 \text{ mL} \div 80 \text{ kg} = 43.8 \text{ mL/kg/min}$$

Figure 5-8 presents a sequence to follow in converting absolute $\dot{V}O_2$ to relative $\dot{V}O_2$ for comparative purposes, and also for converting relative $\dot{V}O_2$ back to absolute $\dot{V}O_2$ to estimate energy expenditure.

## RESPIRATORY EXCHANGE RATIO

Chapter 4 explained that the body uses a combination of fuels to meet its energy needs. Red blood cells, for example, can only utilize glucose as a fuel; alternatively, skeletal muscle can use a mixture of fats/carbohydrates/proteins depending on exercise conditions. The amount of oxygen used during metabolism depends on the type of fuel being used. Because different fuels produce differing amounts of carbon dioxide relative to the amount of oxygen consumed, this can be represented as a ratio. This ratio is commonly referred to as the **respiratory exchange ratio (RER)** and is calculated from the volumes of both gases measured at the lungs. This reflects external respiration, or what is happening at the mouth where gases are exchanged with the environment. The **respiratory quotient (RQ)** is considered a measure of the same ratio, but it is considered a reflection of true cellular respiration (i.e., fuel use for metabolism at the cellular level). However, given our accessibility to external respiration (i.e., gas analyzers) versus true cellular respiration, it is acceptable to assume RER equates to RQ, but certain limitations to this assumption do exist that will be introduced later. Regardless, knowledge of RER or RQ values permits insight into the relative contributions of fat and carbohydrate to metabolism and also allows for calculation of energy expenditure. Table 5-3 presents the caloric equivalents for the range of RQ values.

RER is calculated using the following formula: RER $= \dot{V}CO_2 \div \dot{V}O_2$. If the same examples from earlier in this chapter are used, where $\dot{V}O_2$ was calculated at 2.12 L/min and $\dot{V}CO_2$ was calculated at 2.02 L/min, both values can be entered into the RER equation to

**DOING THE MATH:**

Compare relative $\dot{V}O_{2max}$ scores between Peter and Mary.
- Mary weighs 110 lb (50 kg) and is measured with an absolute $\dot{V}O_{2max}$ of 2.0 L/min.
- Peter weighs 220 lb (100 kg) and is measured with an absolute $\dot{V}O_{2max}$ of 3.0 L/min.

Is it fair to deduce that Peter is more fit than Mary because he has a higher absolute $\dot{V}O_{2max}$?

**Mary:**
- 2.0 L/min $\times$ 1,000 = _____ mL/min (1,000 mL in 1 L).
- If 50 kg body weight consumes ____ mL/min, then 1 kg consumes ____ mL/min.
- Her relative $\dot{V}O_2$ score becomes ___ mL/kg/min.

**ANSWERS:**

$$2.0 \text{ L/min} = 2{,}000 \text{ mL/min}$$
$$2{,}000 \text{ mL/min} \div 50 \text{ kg} = 40 \text{ mL/kg/min}$$

**Peter:**
- 3.0 L/min $\times$ 1,000 = _____ mL/min (1,000 mL in 1 liter).
- If 100 kg body weight consumes ____ mL/min, 1 kg consumes ___ mL/min.
- His relative $\dot{V}O_2$ score becomes ___ mL/kg/min.

**ANSWERS:**

$$3.0 \text{ L/min} = 3{,}000 \text{ mL/min}$$
$$3{,}000 \text{ mL/min} \div 100 \text{ kg} = 30 \text{ mL/kg/min}$$

Calculate the number of calories expended by Peter if he is running on a treadmill for 20 minutes at a $\dot{V}O_2$ of 2.4 L/min.
- 2.4 L/min $\times$ 5 kcal/L = ___kcal/min
- 20 minutes of exercise = total of ____ kcal

**ANSWERS:**

$$2.4 \text{ L/min} \times 5 \text{ kcal} = 12 \text{ kcal/min}$$
$$12 \text{ kcal} \times 20 \text{ min} = 240 \text{ kcal}$$

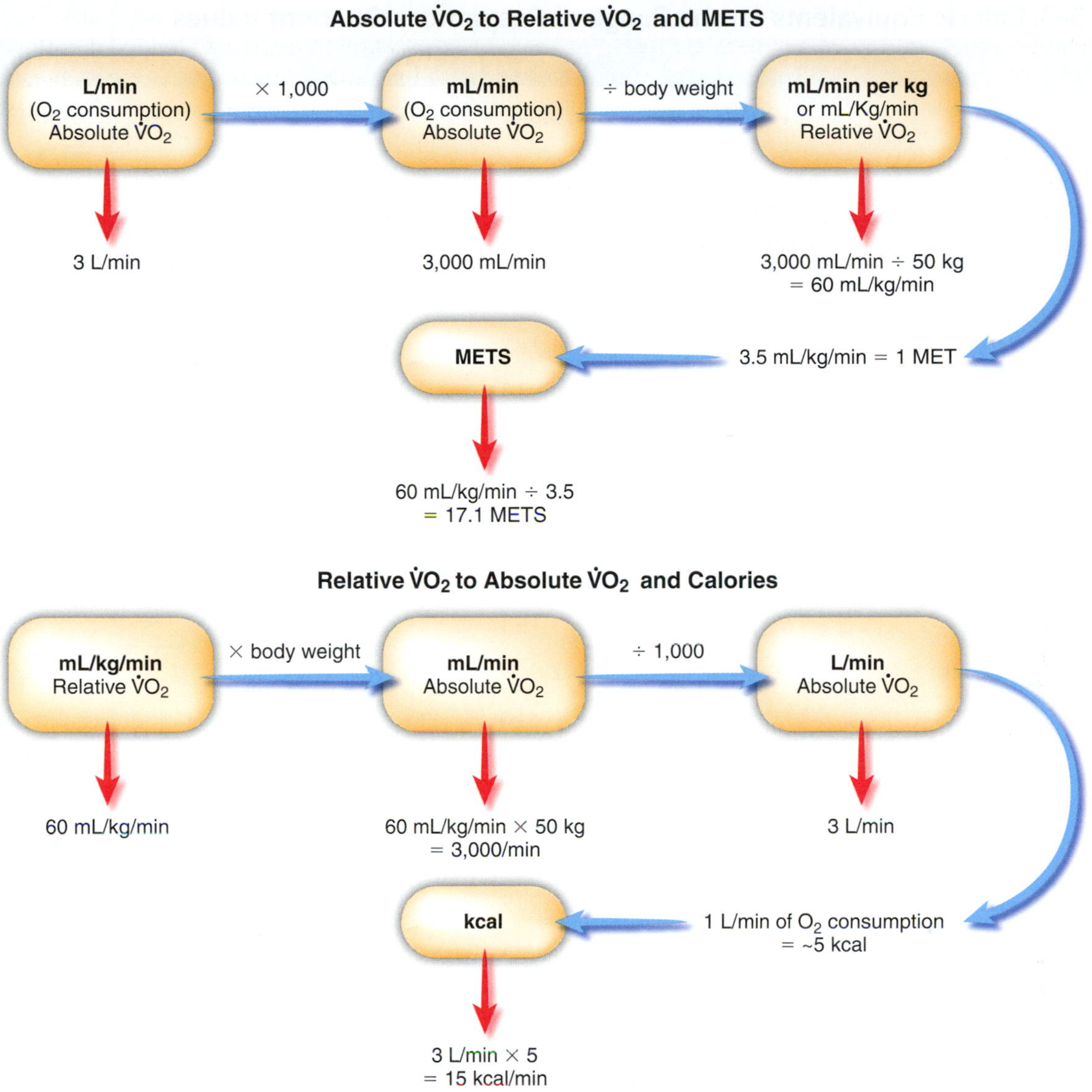

## Absolute $\dot{V}O_2$ to Relative $\dot{V}O_2$ and METS

L/min
($O_2$ consumption)
Absolute $\dot{V}O_2$

$\times$ 1,000

mL/min
($O_2$ consumption)
Absolute $\dot{V}O_2$

$\div$ body weight

mL/min per kg
or mL/Kg/min
Relative $\dot{V}O_2$

3 L/min

3,000 mL/min

3,000 mL/min $\div$ 50 kg
= 60 mL/kg/min

METS

3.5 mL/kg/min = 1 MET

60 mL/kg/min $\div$ 3.5
= 17.1 METS

## Relative $\dot{V}O_2$ to Absolute $\dot{V}O_2$ and Calories

mL/kg/min
Relative $\dot{V}O_2$

$\times$ body weight

mL/min
Absolute $\dot{V}O_2$

$\div$ 1,000

L/min
Absolute $\dot{V}O_2$

60 mL/kg/min

60 mL/kg/min $\times$ 50 kg
= 3,000/min

3 L/min

kcal

1 L/min of $O_2$ consumption
= ~5 kcal

3 L/min $\times$ 5
= 15 kcal/min

**Figure 5-8.** Steps for converting an absolute oxygen consumption value to its corresponding metabolic equivalent (METs) (top) and relative oxygen consumption to its equivalent in caloric expenditure (bottom).

determine the score. In this scenario, RER = 0.95 (2.02 ÷ 2.12). Using Table 5-3 as a reference, this ratio indicates a fuel utilization ratio of 84% carbohydrates and 16% fats.

As discussed earlier, RER ratios for fats and carbohydrates range between 0.70 and 1.00. However, it may be useful to first understand how these numbers were derived. When the balanced chemical reaction for aerobic respiration of glucose is examined, each glucose molecule requires 6 molecules of oxygen to be metabolized and, in turn, produces 6 molecules of carbon dioxide (Box 5-2). When calculating an RER score, this translates into 6 ÷ 6 ($\dot{V}CO_2$ ÷ $\dot{V}O_2$) and an RER score of 1.00. Table 5-3 demonstrates that an RER score of 1.00 indicates that 100% of the fuel utilization is derived from glucose.

In contrast, when the balanced chemical reaction for aerobic respiration of a fatty acid (palmitic acid, a 16-carbon fatty acid most commonly catabolized by skeletal muscle during exercise) is examined, each molecule requires 23 molecules of oxygen to be metabolized and, in turn, produces 16 molecules of carbon dioxide. When calculating an RER score, this translates into 16 ÷ 23 ($\dot{V}CO_2$ ÷ $\dot{V}O_2$) and an RER score of 0.70. Table 5-3 demonstrates that an RER score of 0.70 indicates that 100% of the fuel utilization is derived from fats.

At rest, the average person has a resting RER between 0.78 and 0.84, but this score can be influenced by dietary composition and training status to a lesser degree. The body generally burns what it eats; thus, higher carbohydrate diets generally increase resting RER scores, whereas higher fat diets, albeit unhealthy, decrease resting RER scores. Proteins contribute 2% to 5% of one's total daily energy expenditure, and thus have a small effect on resting RER scores. Protein metabolism yields RER scores of approximately 0.82, but varies slightly among the different amino acids. More conditioned individuals with greater capacities to use fats exhibit lower RER scores.

## Table 5-3. Caloric Equivalents for the Range of Respiratory Quotient Values

| RQ | KCAL/L $O_2$ | %KCAL CHO | KCAL/L $O_2$ CHO | % KCAL FAT | KCAL/L $O_2$ FAT |
|---|---|---|---|---|---|
| 1.00 | 5.047 | 100.00 | 5.047 | 0.00 | 0.000 |
| 0.99 | 5.035 | 96.80 | 4.874 | 3.18 | 0.160 |
| 0.98 | 5.022 | 93.60 | 4.701 | 6.37 | 0.230 |
| 0.97 | 5.010 | 90.40 | 4.529 | 9.58 | 0.480 |
| 0.96 | 4.998 | 87.20 | 4.358 | 12.80 | 0.640 |
| 0.95 | 4.985 | 84.00 | 4.187 | 16.00 | 0.798 |
| 0.94 | 4.973 | 80.70 | 4.013 | 19.30 | 0.960 |
| 0.93 | 4.961 | 77.40 | 3.840 | 22.60 | 1.121 |
| 0.92 | 4.948 | 74.10 | 3.666 | 25.90 | 1.281 |
| 0.91 | 4.936 | 70.80 | 3.495 | 29.20 | 1.441 |
| 0.90 | 4.924 | 67.50 | 3.324 | 32.50 | 1.600 |
| 0.89 | 4.911 | 64.20 | 3.153 | 35.80 | 1.758 |
| 0.88 | 4.899 | 60.80 | 2.979 | 39.20 | 1.920 |
| 0.87 | 4.887 | 57.50 | 2.810 | 42.50 | 2.077 |
| 0.86 | 4.875 | 54.10 | 2.637 | 45.90 | 2.238 |
| 0.85 | 4.862 | 50.70 | 2.465 | 49.30 | 2.397 |
| 0.84 | 4.850 | 47.20 | 2.289 | 52.80 | 2.561 |
| 0.83 | 4.838 | 43.80 | 2.119 | 56.20 | 2.719 |
| 0.82 | 4.825 | 40.30 | 1.944 | 59.70 | 2.880 |
| 0.81 | 4.813 | 36.90 | 1.776 | 63.10 | 3.037 |
| 0.80 | 4.801 | 33.40 | 1.603 | 66.60 | 3.197 |
| 0.79 | 4.788 | 29.90 | 1.432 | 70.10 | 3.356 |
| 0.78 | 4.776 | 26.30 | 1.256 | 73.70 | 3.520 |
| 0.77 | 4.764 | 22.30 | 1.062 | 77.20 | 3.678 |
| 0.76 | 4.751 | 19.20 | 0.912 | 80.80 | 3.839 |
| 0.75 | 4.739 | 15.60 | 0.739 | 84.40 | 4.000 |
| 0.74 | 4.727 | 12.00 | 0.567 | 88.00 | 4.160 |
| 0.73 | 4.714 | 8.40 | 0.396 | 91.60 | 4.318 |
| 0.72 | 4.702 | 4.76 | 0.224 | 95.20 | 4.476 |
| 0.71 | 4.690 | 1.10 | 0.052 | 98.90 | 4.638 |
| 0.707 | 4.686 | 0.00 | 0.000 | 100.00 | 4.686 |

RQ, respiratory quotient.
Adapted from Robergs RA, Roberts SO. *Exercise Physiology: Exercise, Performance and Clinical Applications*. St. Louis, MO: Mosby; 1997.

As mentioned earlier, the assumption of equality between RQ and RER is not appropriate under all conditions. During the following scenarios, RER will not reflect RQ:

- **Hyperventilation**: Generally, hyperventilation refers to a situation where an individual is

breathing in excess of what is required by the body. Frequently, this can occur during periods of anxiety or stress. A common scenario where hyperventilation may take place in the exercise physiology laboratory is when an individual has the equipment (i.e., head gear, mouthpiece, and

## Box 5-2. Oxygen Consumption, Carbon Dioxide Production, and Energy Released From the Breakdown of Glucose and Palmitate Molecules

### Glucose

$$C_6H_{12}O_6 + 6O_2 \leftrightarrow 6CO_2 + 6\ H_2O + energy$$
$$CO_2/O_2 = 6/6 = 1.0$$

### Palmitate

$$C_{16}H_{32}O_2 + 23O_2 \leftrightarrow 16CO_2 + 16H_2O + energy$$
$$CO_2/O_2 = 16/23 = 0.69$$

nose clip) required for exercise testing attached. Hyperventilation results in disproportionate exhalation that can subsequently increase the $\dot{V}CO_2$ exhaled from the lungs; if this occurs without a concurrent increase in $\dot{V}O_2$, the end result is an inflated RER value not representative of cellular metabolism.

- **Metabolic acidosis**: The $\dot{V}CO_2$ production within the cell cannot exceed $\dot{V}O_2$; the maximal ratio of $\dot{V}CO_2$ to $\dot{V}O_2$ is 1.0, which occurs when carbohydrate catabolism is exclusively providing the energy required for exercise. The metabolic responses to high-intensity exercise conditions are numerous; of primary interest to our current discussion on RER is the increased production of protons resulting from increased glycolytic flux. Increased proton production unchecked can lead to severe acidosis, of which the end result is decreased enzyme function and eventually an impaired ability to maintain optimal high-intensity exercise performance. Undoubtedly, this scenario is not altogether avoidable; however, the body does combat and delay acidosis initially by buffering the protons. An implication of this event is increased $\dot{V}CO_2$ production; it is important to note that this production of $\dot{V}CO_2$ is independent of cellular $\dot{V}CO_2$ production. Accordingly, $\dot{V}CO_2$ production will be disproportionate to $\dot{V}O_2$, and it is inevitable for RER values to exceed 1.0 under the metabolic conditions associated with high-intensity exercise.
- Non–steady-state exercise conditions: Steady-state exercise refers to metabolic conditions where ATP demand is supplied exclusively with ATP regenerated from mitochondrial respiration. In the transition from rest to exercise or the transition from a low-intensity exercise workload to a moderate-intensity workload, there is a time delay before steady-state can be achieved; under these circumstances, ATP contributions

are made from both creatine phosphate hydrolysis and glycolysis. The RER values can be higher during this non–steady-state changeover period, with the $\dot{V}CO_2$ and $\dot{V}O_2$ values not completely indicative of cellular metabolism. Therefore, any projections on the contributions of carbohydrate and fat to energy expenditure during the non–steady-state time frame would be flawed.

It is paramount that exercise science professionals recognize the earlier situations where making the assumption that RER equates to RQ does not hold true. Failure to adhere to these exceptions can result in critical errors when interpreting exercise responses or may lead to an erroneous conclusion while performing research.

## FROM THEORY TO PRACTICE

Given the information you have just learned on RER and fuel utilization, and considering how many individuals desire to burn more fats, then why don't individuals simply exercise at lower intensities*?

Let's examine this scenario using an example. If Jackie performs 30 minutes of lower-intensity exercise where her RER score is measured at 0.89 and her $\dot{V}O_2$ is measured at 1.4 L/min, calculate her total caloric expenditure, her percent contribution from fats, and the total number of fat calories expended.
**ANSWERS:**
- 1.4 L/min × 5 kcal/L = 7 kcal/min × 30 minutes = 210 kcal
- RER of 0.89 = approximately 36% contribution from fats
- 36% of 210 kcal = 76 kcal from fats

If Jackie performs 30 minutes of higher-intensity exercise where her RER score is measured at 0.94 and her $\dot{V}O_2$ is measured at 3.2 L/min, calculate her total caloric expenditure, her percent contribution from fats, and the total number of fat calories expended.
**ANSWERS:**
- 3.2 L/min × 5 kcal/L = 16 kcal/min × 30 minutes = 480 kcal
- RER of 0.94 = approximately 19% contribution from fats
- 19% of 480 kcal = 91 kcal from fats

*Back to the question — why don't individuals simply exercise at lower intensities to burn more fat?* The "fat burning zone" at low intensities of exercise does NOT exist. The best approach is to think of energy expenditure as "a calorie is a calorie is a calorie," rather than partitioning into carbohydrate and fat calories. To burn maximum calories in support of ongoing fat/weight loss, progress to a moderate-to-vigorous intensity/higher-volume exercise program and include interval training.

## OXYGEN KINETICS

Oxygen uptake into muscle cells increases rapidly during the first few minutes of exercise, reaching a plateau that generally takes between 45 seconds and 4 minutes to achieve after the onset of activity. This plateau is described as steady-state and is defined as the balance between the energy required by working muscles and the rate of aerobic ATP production. It is achieved when all the ATP required for muscle action is supplied from aerobic respiration. However, the time frame to reach steady-state varies considerably, depending on the magnitude of the increment in exercise intensity, conditioning level of the individual, and the modality of exercise. For example, the transition from rest to steady-state will be attained rather quickly when the exercise workload is low; conversely, it may take upward of 4 to 5 minutes to achieve steady-state at greater intensities. When transitioning from rest to the same given exercise workload, a more conditioned individual will achieve steady-state more rapidly than their lesser fit counterpart. Modalities involving upper and lower extremities (e.g., running versus cycling) or modalities with which the individual has less biomechanical efficiency may extend the time needed to reach steady-state.

### Oxygen Deficit

**Oxygen deficit** refers to the difference between oxygen uptake and the oxygen demand of exercise during exercise conditions that are non–steady-state. Until steady-state is achieved, the additional energy demands of the muscles are met by the anaerobic pathways. In other words, exercise is permitted to continue under non–steady-state conditions because of contributions from both creatine phosphate hydrolysis and glycolysis. This creates an energy deficiency, or oxygen deficit.

Most associate this deficit with very high-intensity exercise (e.g., sprints) where the energy demand from the working muscles exceeds the maximal capacity of aerobic respiration. However, it is important to appreciate that at any point of time when a change in activity or exercise intensity occurs (e.g., sitting to walking; standing to light jogging), the body may need to rely on the anaerobic systems to contribute ATP until the aerobic system achieves steady-state. In other words, there is a gradual transition in energy provision from anaerobic pathways to aerobic respiration during this deficit phase. The energy supplied for exercise is not simply the product of a series of energy systems "turning on" and "turning off," but rather the smooth blending and overlap of all three energy systems working synergistically, as described and illustrated in Chapter 4.

### Excess Post-exercise Oxygen Consumption

On termination of exercise, oxygen consumption ($\dot{V}O_2$) will gradually return toward baseline levels in an exponential manner, first demonstrating an initial rapid component followed by a slow, longer component (Fig. 5-9). The overall $\dot{V}O_2$ that is consumed above resting values during this phase is referred to as the **excess post-exercise oxygen consumption (EPOC)**. It was originally proposed in 1923[20] that the elevated $\dot{V}O_2$ post-exercise was an **oxygen debt**. This interpretation was based on the understanding that this additional oxygen consumption was repayment to replenish creatine phosphate and the oxidation of lactate produced from glycolysis during the oxygen deficit. More recently, it has been acknowledged that additional factors beyond those recognized by Hill contribute to this elevated post-exercise metabolism.[21] Elevated post-exercise metabolism is a product of widespread homeostatic perturbation of which the settlement of the oxygen deficit is only a fractional contribution. Accordingly, in 1984, the term *EPOC* was coined[21] to better represent the multiple factors that contribute to elevated post-exercise metabolism. (See explanatory animation of oxygen deficit and EPOC on the Davis*Plus* site at http://davisplus.fadavis.com.)

EPOC comprises two phases: the rapid and slow phases. The duration of the rapid phase generally lasts approximately 2 to 3 minutes but may extend out toward 30 to 60 minutes and primarily involves:
- restoration of the phosphagen system.
- removal and reconversion (oxidation) of lactate.
- reloading hemoglobin/myoglobin with oxygen.

At rest, hemoglobin molecules are almost completely saturated with oxygen when leaving the lungs, and given our low demand for oxygen, a significant proportion still contains oxygen when leaving the muscle cells. During exercise, more oxygen is delivered to the muscle cells, implying that less hemoglobin contains oxygen when leaving the muscle cells. During recovery, some inspired oxygen is not used for cellular respiration, but to replace the oxygen stores on hemoglobin. The same can be said for myoglobin, the oxygen-carrying protein molecule located inside muscle cells that transport oxygen from the cell wall to the mitochondria.

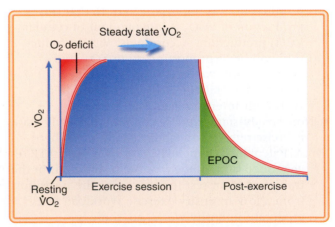

**Figure 5-9.** Oxygen deficit and excess post-exercise oxygen consumption (EPOC).

The slow phase lasts longer, depending on the magnitude of tissue stimulation (repair and adaptation) and the amount of recovery needed, and includes:

- continued thermoregulation.
- increased heart rate and ventilatory demand for anabolic processes.
- increased metabolism because of tissue repair and synthesis, and glycogen synthesis.
- residual effects of circulating sympathetic hormones (e.g., catecholamines).
- removal of accumulated carbon dioxide remaining within body tissues.

Exercise intensity and exercise duration contribute most notably to the magnitude of EPOC. Overall, it has been concluded that exercise intensity has a greater role in EPOC variability compared with exercise duration.[22–25] In other words, the higher the intensity of exercise, the greater the magnitude of the EPOC, which translates into a greater number of calories expended. Some studies have also examined the effect of repeated bouts of supramaximal intensity exercise (i.e., >100% $\dot{V}O_{2max}$) on EPOC and concluded that intermittent supramaximal exercise bouts elicit a greater EPOC responses when compared with moderate-intensity continuous exercise bouts.[26,27] One thing to be mindful of when making comparisons with interval-type research is the fact that many measured EPOC after the completion of the workout and not during the rest intervals. Consequently, it is possible that the magnitude of EPOC in these later studies has been underestimated. Only a few studies have compared EPOC between different modalities of exercise while controlling for the exercise duration and intensity.[28,29] No significant differences in EPOC were reported for either investigation.

Preliminary research findings with regard to EPOC heightened interest in its possible role in weight loss.

## CUSTOMIZING ENERGY EXPENDITURE GOALS

How can you customize an individually appropriate exercise program that does not underestimate or overestimate a client's energy expenditure requirements? Rather than design an exercise program that adheres to an absolute energy expenditure recommendation (1,000 kcal/week), aim rather for: (1) what is manageable at first, regardless of how many calories it expends; and (2) perhaps opt to follow an energy expenditure prescription that accounts for differences in body mass (e.g., 14 kcal/kg/week).

Based on the dose–response relationship between exercise volume and health benefits, it has been suggested that the major focus of exercise program design should

### RESEARCH HIGHLIGHT

#### Does Excess Post-exercise Oxygen Consumption Play a Significant Role in Weight Loss?

Early research led us to believe that EPOC played a large role in weight loss and contributed greatly to the overall caloric expenditure of exercise. LaForgia and colleagues[30] reviewed much of the research done on the topic of EPOC from the 1990s and early 2000s, and concluded that the earlier optimism concerning a critical role for EPOC in weight loss largely was unsubstantiated. Those studies that elicited substantial EPOC (e.g., >100 kcal) generally consisted of regimens that were high in intensity or long in duration, or both. In most circumstances, these types of programs would not be well tolerated by nonathletic populations. The authors concluded that EPOC generates approximately 7% of the total energy expenditure of exercise.

Knab and colleagues[31] studied 10 male participants who completed 2 separate 24-hour visits to a metabolic chamber (1 exercise day and 1 rest day). The exercise day consisted of 45 minutes of cycling at an intensity of 73% $\dot{V}O_{2max}$ (generally regarded as higher intensity with heart rates >85% of maximal effort). The exercise bouts expended 519 kcal and EPOC remained elevated above resting levels for 14 hours post-exercise, resulting in an impressive total of 190 kcal (13.5 kcal/hr average). However, it is important for students and exercise professionals to carefully note that the intensity of exercise performed by participants in this study was **vigorous**. For example, an exercise intensity of 70% to 75% $\dot{V}O_{2max}$ generally corresponds to the lactate threshold level of an endurance-trained individual. Accordingly, it should be evident that those individuals who are exercising to lose weight are probably unlikely to be capable of regularly performing the types of exercise workouts that research has found to be required for stimulating a meaningful EPOC.

In conclusion, although EPOC may be limited in its contribution to weight loss, there may be a role for it in terms of energy balance (i.e., weight maintenance). It has been suggested that the cumulative effect of the EPOC over a 1-year period may be the energy expenditure equivalent of 3 lb of adipose tissue.

LaForgia J, Withers RT, Gore CJ. Effects of exercise intensity and duration on the excess post-exercise oxygen consumption. *J Sports Sci.* 2006;12:1247–1264.
Knab AM, Shanely A, Corbin KD, Jin F, Sha W, Neiman DC. A 45-minute vigorous exercise bout increases metabolic rate for 14 hours. *Med Sci Sports Exerc.* 2011;43:1643–1648.

be the total weekly energy expenditure. Historically, this strategy has followed an absolute energy expenditure approach insensitive to differences between individuals, in particular, body mass. This approach increases the likelihood of overestimating or underestimating an individual's energy expenditure goals. Overestimation of the exercise energy expenditure requirements for an individual will almost certainly create an unrealistic goal; consequently, this increases the chances of overtraining, injury, discouragement, and decreased program adherence. Conversely, underestimation of the exercise energy expenditure requirements might lead to decreased health and fitness benefits, which can also contribute to lower program adherence. These issues are circumvented by establishing weekly goals with a relative energy expenditure prescription.[32–35]

As an exercise professional, the knowledge and skills you acquired from this chapter regarding recent research on the topic of energy expenditure and metabolic calculations permits you to better design exercise programs—programs that will maximize health and fitness benefits.

## VIGNETTE conclusion

■ Norman's case provides a good example of how to progress a client from completely sedentary to committed exerciser in a way that is safe, effective, and perhaps most importantly, individualized. Instead of using the generic recommendation of progressing from 1,000 to 2,000 and eventually to 3,000 kcal/week, Najat chose to first provide an appropriate program with progressions and then calculate specific energy expenditure for Norman, which was estimated to exceed 2,000 kcal/week. By doing so, Najat provided excellent service and made Norman feel like his exercise program was designed specifically for him, which can be a tremendous motivator.

## CRITICAL THINKING QUESTIONS

1. You are a personal trainer employed by a health club. A client comes to you after just completing a maximal exercise test on the treadmill at the local university. The professor who helped conduct the test calculated the target training intensity for the individual at 35 mL/kg/min (or 10 METs) and a goal of 350 calories per session. The client finds running at 6 miles/hr (mph) on the treadmill (0% grade) for 25 minutes an appropriate challenge. Your task is to use the metabolic calculation equation for treadmill running to identify whether this workload is consistent with the target intensity and whether the client is achieving the goal of 350 kcal per session. Assume he weighs 186 lb (84.5 kg).

2. You are employed as a clinical exercise physiologist at an outpatient cardiac rehabilitation program. Aidan (45 years and 80 kg) enters your program and you design an exercise program that achieves an exercise volume required to stabilize the process of atherosclerosis—expenditure goal of 1,500 kcal/week. You have been provided with target exercise intensity ($\dot{V}O_2$ = 18.9 mL/kg/min) by a technician who performed the baseline

exercise test, and you must now calculate the number of minutes per week of exercise needed to achieve the weekly energy expenditure goal of 1,500 kcal. What steps are involved with this calculation?

3. Your "old-school" exercise physiology professor, Dr. Jackson, has requested that you calculate $\dot{V}O_2$, $\dot{V}CO_2$, RER, and energy expenditure by hand, assuming that the individual spent 40 minutes exercising at these gas exchange values. You are provided with the following information:

| IME | $\dot{V}E$ (L/MIN) | $FEO_2$ | $FECO_2$ |
|---|---|---|---|
| — | 27.14 | 14.96% | 4.8% |
| | | (0.1496) | (0.048) |

4. If Mark performs 60 minutes of moderate-intensity exercise with an RER score of 0.91 and a $\dot{V}O_2$ measured at 2.4 L/min, would he burn more total calories and more fat calories than Pete, who performs 40 minutes of high-intensity exercise with an RER score of 0.97 and a $\dot{V}O_2$ measured at 3.6 L/min?

## ADDITIONAL RESOURCES

Compendium of Physical Activities Website: This site is accessible at: https://sites.google.com/site/compendiumofphysicalactivities. The purpose of this site is to provide the updated 2011 Compendium of Physical Activities* and additional resources. The 2011 update identifies and updates MET codes that have published evidence to support the values. In addition, new codes have been added to reflect the growing body of knowledge and popular activities.

*Ainsworth BE, Haskell WL, Herrmann SD, et al. *The Compendium of Physical Activities Tracking Guide*. Healthy Lifestyles Research Center, College of Nursing & Health Innovation, Arizona State University, 2011.
**Research Articles**
Ainsworth BE, Haskell WL, Herrmann SD, et al. 2011 compendium of physical activities: A second update of codes and MET values. *Med Sci Sports Exerc*. 2011;42:1575–1581.

Kohl HW III. Physical activity and cardiovascular disease: Evidence for a dose-response. *Med Sci Sports Exerc.* 2001; 33(6 Suppl):S472-S483.
Lee IM, Skerrett PJ. Physical activity and all-cause mortality: What is the dose-response relation? *Med Sci Sports Exerc.* 2001; 33(6 Suppl):S459–S471.

Oja P. Dose response between total volume of physical activity and health and fitness. *Med Sci Sports Exerc.* 2001;33 (6 Suppl):S428–S437.
Slentz CA, Houmard JA, Kraus WE. Exercise, abdominal obesity, skeletal muscle, and metabolic risk: Evidence for a dose response. *Obesity.* 2009;17(Suppl. 3):S27–S33.

## REFERENCES

1. American College of Sports Medicine. *ACSM's Resource Manual for Guidelines for Exercise Testing and Prescription.* 6th ed. Philadelphia, PA: Lippincott Williams & Wilkins; 2010.

2. Pleis JR, Ward BW, Lucas JW. Summary health statistics for U.S. adults: National Health Interview Survey, 2009. National Center for Health Statistics. *Vital Health Stat.* 2010;249(10). http://www.cdc.gov/nchs/data/series/sr_10/sr10_249.pdf

3. American College of Sports Medicine. *ACSM's Guidelines for Exercise Testing and Prescription.* 9th ed. Baltimore, MD: Lippincott Williams & Wilkins; 2014.

4. U.S. Department of Health and Human Services. *Surgeon General's Report: Physical Activity and Health.* Washington, DC: U.S. Department of Health and Human Services; 1996.

5. American College of Sports Medicine. *ACSM's Guidelines for Exercise Testing and Prescription.* 7th ed. Philadelphia, PA: Lippincott Williams & Wilkins; 2006.

6. Paffenbarger RS Jr, Hyde RT, Wing AL, Hsieh CC. Physical activity, all-cause mortality, and longevity of college alumni. *N Engl J Med.* 1986;314:605–613.

7. Robergs RA, Roberts SO. *Exercise Physiology: Exercise, Performance and Clinical Applications.* St. Louis, MO: Mosby; 1997.

8. Lagerros YT, Lagious P. Assessment of physical activity and energy expenditure in epidemiological research of chronic diseases. *Eur J Epidemiol.* 2007;22:353–362.

9. Levine JA. Measurement of energy expenditure. *Public Health Nutr.* 2005;8:1123–1132.

10. Tudor-Locke C, Bassett DR Jr. How many steps/day are enough? Preliminary pedometer indices for public health. *Sports Med.* 2004;34:281–291.

11. Bassett DR Jr, Schneider PL, Huntington GE. Physical activity in an Old Order Amish community. *Med Sci Sports Exerc.* 2004;36:79–85.

12. Welk GJ, Blair SN, Wood K, et al. A comparative evaluation of three accelerometry-based physical activity monitors. *Med Sci Sports Exerc.* 2000;32(9 Suppl):S489–S497.

13. Strath SJ, Swartz AM, Bassett DR Jr, et al. Evaluation of heart rate as a method for assessing moderate intensity physical activity. *Med Sci Sports Exerc.* 2000;32(9 Suppl): S465–S470.

14. Crouter SE, Albright C, Bassett Jr. DR. Accuracy of the Polar S410 heart rate monitor to estimate energy cost of exercise. *Med Sci Sports Exerc.* 2004;36:1433–1439.

15. Ainsworth BE, Haskell WL, Whitt MC, et al. Compendium of physical activities: An update of activity codes and MET intensities. *Med Sci Sports Exerc.* 2000;32 (9 Suppl):S498–S516.

16. Ainsworth BE, Haskell WL, Herrmann SD, et al. 2011 Compendium of physical activities: a second update of codes and MET values. *Med Sci Sports Exerc.* 2011;43: 1575–1581.

17. Swain DP. Energy cost calculations for exercise prescriptions. *Sports Med.* 2000;30:17–22.

18. Dalleck LC, Kravitz L. Development of a metabolic equation for elliptical crosstrainer exercise. *Percept Mot Skills.* 2007;104:725–732.

19. Dalleck LC, Borresen EC, Parker AL, et al. Development of a metabolic equation for the NuStep recumbent stepper in older adults. *Percept Mot Skills.* 2011; 112:183–192.

20. Hill AV, Lupton H. Muscular exercise, lactic acid, and the supply and utilisation of oxygen. *Q J Med.* 1923; 16:135–171.

21. Gaesser GA, Brooks GA. Metabolic basis of excess post-exercise oxygen consumption: A review. *Med Sci Sports Exerc.* 1984;16:29–43.

22. Gore CJ, Withers RT. Effect of exercise intensity and duration on postexercise metabolism. *J Appl Physiol.* 1990;68:2362–2368.

23. Quinn TJ, Vroman NB, Kertzer R. Post-exercise oxygen consumption in trained females: Effect of exercise duration. *Med Sci Sports Exerc.* 1994;26:908–913.

24. Phelian JF, Reinke E, Harris MA, Melby CL. Post-exercise energy expenditure and substrate oxidation in young women resulting from exercise bouts of different intensity. *J Am Coll Nutr.* 1997;16:140–146.

25. Smith J, McNaughton L. The effects of intensity of exercise on excess post-exercise oxygen consumption and energy expenditure in moderately trained men and women. *Eur J Appl Physiol.* 1993;67:420–425.

26. Laforgia J, Withers RT, Shipp NJ, Gore CJ. Comparison of exercise expenditure elevations after submaximal and supramaximal running. *J Appl Physiol.* 1997;82: 661–666.

27. Nummela A, Rusko H. Time course of anaerobic and aerobic energy expenditure during short-term exhaustive running in athletes. *Int J Sports Med.* 1995;16:522–527.

28. Sedlock DA. Post-exercise energy expenditure after cycle ergometer and treadmill exercise. *J Appl Sport Sci Res.* 1992;6:19–23.

29. Sedlock DA. Postexercise energy expenditure following upper body exercise. *Res Q Exerc Sport.* 1991;62:213–216.

30. LaForgia J, Withers RT, Gore CJ. Effects of exercise intensity and duration on the excess post-exercise oxygen consumption. *J Sports Sci.* 2006;24:1247–1264.

31. Knab AM, Shanely A, Corbin KD, Jin F, Sha W, Neiman DC. A 45-minute vigorous exercise bout increases metabolic rate for 14 hours. *Med Sci Sports Exerc.* 2011;43:1643–1648.

32. Duscha BD, Slentz CA, Johnson JL, et al. Effects of exercise training amount and intensity on peak oxygen consumption in middle-age men and women at risk for cardiovascular disease. *Chest.* 2005;128:2788–2793.

33. Houmard JA, Tanner CJ, Slentz CA, Duscha BD, McCartney JS, Kraus WE. Effect of the volume and intensity of exercise training on insulin sensitivity. *J Appl Physiol.* 2004;96:101–106.

34. Kraus WE, Houmard JA, Duscha BD, et al. Effects of the amount and intensity of exercise on plasma lipoproteins. *N Engl J Med.* 2002;347:1483–1492.

35. Slentz CA, Duscha BD, Johnson JL, et al. Effects of the amount of exercise on body weight, body composition, and measures of central obesity: STRRIDE—a randomized controlled study. *Arch Intern Med.* 2004;164:31–39.

## *Practice What You Know:* Ebbeling Single-Stage Treadmill Test

The single-stage treadmill test developed by Ebbeling and colleagues is an appropriate option for low-risk, apparently healthy, nonathletic adults aged 20 to 59 years. This test estimates $\dot{V}O_{2max}$ using a single-stage, 4-minute submaximal treadmill walking protocol.

### EQUIPMENT:

- Commercial treadmill
- Stopwatch
- RPE scale
- HR monitor (optional)

### PRETEST PROCEDURE:

- Measure pre-exercise HR, sitting and standing, and record the values on a testing form or data sheet.
- Estimate the submaximal target exercise HR using Gellish et al.'s formula for estimating MHR [$(206.9 - [0.67 \times age]) \times 50\%$ and $(206.9 - [0.67 \times age]) \times 70\%$] (see Chapter 15 for more information on this formula). These values represent the warm-up range. Record these values on the testing form.
- Discuss RPE and remind the subject that he or she will be asked for perceived exertion levels throughout the test.
- Describe the purpose of the treadmill test. This test consists of a 4-minute warm-up stage and a single 4-minute testing stage that should elicit steady-state heart rate (HR).
- Allow the subject to walk on the treadmill to warm up and get used to the apparatus (≤1.7 mph). He or she should avoid holding the handrails. If the subject is too unstable without holding on to the rails, consider using another testing modality. The results will not be accurate if the subject must hold on to the handrails the entire time.

### TEST ADMINISTRATION:

#### Warm-up stage:

1. The goal of the 4-minute warm-up phase is to determine a comfortable speed between 2.0 and 4.5 mph at a 0% grade that elicits a heart rate response within 50% to 70% of age-predicted MHR.
2. For more deconditioned or elderly subjects, target a warm-up intensity between 50% and 60% of MHR.
3. For apparently healthy individuals, target a warm-up intensity between 60% and 70% MHR.
4. If the HR response is not within that range at the end of the first minute, adjust the speed accordingly.

#### Test:

1. The goal of the exercise phase is to complete a submaximal 4-minute treadmill walk at the same speed determined during the warm-up phase, but at a 5% grade (Figure 1).

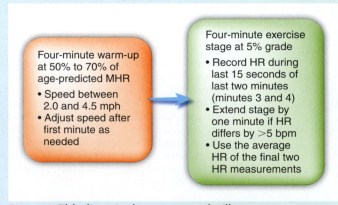

**Figure 1.** Ebbeling single-stage treadmill test. bpm, beats per minute; HR, heart rate; MHR, maximum heart rate.

2. After the warm-up phase and an appropriate treadmill speed has been determined, elevate the treadmill to a 5% grade and continue into the workout stage without any stoppages.
3. Record HR in the last 15 seconds of the last 2 minutes of this workload to establish steady-state HR.
4. If the HR varies by more than 5 beats/min (bpm) between the last 2 minutes, extend the workload by an additional minute and record the steady-state HR from the new final 2 minutes.
5. Use the average of the two last heart rates as the final HR score.
6. Record all values on a testing form.
7. Continue to observe the subject as he or she cools down, because negative symptoms can arise immediately post-exercise.
8. After performing the following calculation, use Table 1 to rank the subject's maximum oxygen uptake.

## Table 1. Percentile Values for Maximal Oxygen Uptake (mL/kg/min)

| | | | Age, yr | | |
|---|---|---|---|---|---|
| PERCENTILE* | 20–29 | 30–39 | 40–49 | 50–59 | 60–69 |
| **Men** | | | | | |
| 90 | 54.0 | 52.5 | 51.1 | 46.8 | 43.2 |
| 80 | 51.1 | 48.9 | 46.8 | 43.3 | 39.5 |
| 70 | 48.2 | 46.8 | 44.2 | 41.0 | 36.7 |
| 60 | 45.7 | 44.4 | 42.4 | 38.3 | 35.0 |
| 50 | 43.9 | 42.4 | 40.4 | 36.7 | 33.1 |
| 40 | 42.2 | 41.0 | 38.4 | 35.2 | 31.4 |
| 30 | 40.3 | 38.5 | 36.7 | 33.2 | 29.4 |
| 20 | 39.5 | 36.7 | 34.6 | 31.1 | 27.4 |
| 10 | 35.2 | 33.8 | 31.8 | 28.4 | 24.1 |
| **Women** | | | | | |
| 90 | 47.5 | 44.7 | 42.4 | 38.1 | 34.6 |
| 80 | 44.0 | 41.0 | 38.9 | 35.2 | 32.3 |
| 70 | 41.1 | 38.8 | 36.7 | 32.9 | 30.2 |
| 60 | 39.5 | 36.7 | 35.1 | 31.4 | 29.1 |
| 50 | 37.4 | 35.2 | 33.3 | 30.2 | 27.5 |
| 40 | 35.5 | 33.8 | 31.6 | 28.7 | 26.6 |
| 30 | 33.8 | 32.3 | 29.7 | 27.3 | 24.9 |
| 20 | 31.6 | 29.9 | 28.0 | 25.5 | 23.7 |
| 10 | 29.4 | 27.4 | 25.6 | 23.7 | 21.7 |

*Note.* $\dot{V}O_{2max}$ below the 20th percentile is associated with an increased risk for death from all causes.[3] Study population for the data set was predominately white and college educated. A modified Balke treadmill test was used with $\dot{V}O_{2max}$ estimated from the last grade/speed achieved. The following may be used as descriptors for the percentile rankings: well above average (90), above average (70), average (50), below average (30), and well below average (10).

*To realize the health benefits of aerobic conditioning, personal training clients should aim to achieve greater than 30th percentile.

Data from American College of Sports Medicine (2014). ACSM's Guidelines for Exercise Testing and Prescription (9th ed.). Baltimore: Wolters Kluwer/Lippincott Williams & Wilkins; Blair, S.N. et al. (1995). Changes in physical fitness and all-cause mortality: A prospective study of healthy and unhealthy men. Journal of the American Medical Association, 273, 14, 1093-1098.

*Practice What You Know:* Ebbeling Single-Stage Treadmill Test–cont'd

$\dot{V}O_{2max}$ **(mL/kg/min) Equation**

$\dot{V}O_{2max} = 15.1 + (21.8 \times mph) - (0.327 \times HR) - (0.263 \times mph \times age) + (0.00504 \times HR \times age) + (5.98 \times sex^*)$

*Females = 0, males = 1, to account for sex differences (lean mass and oxygen-carrying capacity).

Example: A 30-year-old male walked at 4.0 mph (5% grade) with a steady-state HR of 155 bpm.

$\dot{V}O_{2max} = 15.1 + (21.8 \times 4) - (0.327 \times 155) - (0.263 \times 4 \times 30) + (0.00504 \times 155 \times 30) + (5.98 \times 1) = 15.1 + 87.2 - 50.685 - 31.56 + 23.436 + 5.98 = 49.47$ mL/kg/min

## YMCA BIKE TEST

The YMCA bike test measures steady-state HR response to incremental (and predetermined) 3-minute workloads that progressively elicit higher heart rate responses. The steady-state HR responses are then plotted on a graph against workloads performed. Because exercise HR correlates to a $\dot{V}O_2$ score, the HR response line is extended to determine maximal effort (i.e., MHR) and estimate the individual's $\dot{V}O_{2max}$.

## EQUIPMENT:

- Cycle ergometer
- Stopwatch
- HR monitor with chest strap
- Metronome (optional)
- Sphygmomanometer
- RPE chart

## PRETEST PROCEDURES:

- Estimate the submaximal target exercise HR using Gellish et al.'s formula for estimating MHR [(206.9 − [0.67 × age]) × 85%] (see Chapter 15 for more information on this formula). Record this value on a testing form (this is one of the test end points). If an HR strap and monitor are unavailable, calculate a 15-second count for this value.
- Measure and record the subject's weight in pounds and convert that value to kilograms by dividing the weight by 2.2.
- Measure and record seated, resting BP.
- Discuss RPE and remind the subject that he or she will be asked for perceived exertion levels throughout the test.
- Adjust seat height and record the seat position for future tests to ensure consistency between tests:
  - Position the pedal at the bottom of a revolution so that the crank arm is orientated vertically. Have the subject place the heel of the foot on the pedal. The knee should be almost straight (5–10 degrees of flexion) in this position, with the ankle held in neutral (i.e., the toe should not be pointed in either direction). Test results may be inaccurately low if the seat is set too low.
  - The seat and pedal position should be comfortable for the subject.
- If a cadence meter is available on the bike, instruct the subject to ride at 50 revolutions/min (rpm). If the cadence meter is unavailable, use a metronome set to 100 bpm to coincide with each pedal stroke.
- Allow for a 2- to 3-minute warm-up period with tension on the cycle to allow the subject to practice and familiarize himself or herself with the cadence.
- Let the subject know that the test will be stopped once he or she has achieved a submaximal workload of 75% to 85% MHR. The subject can stop the test at any time and for any reason, but especially if he or she experiences chest pain, shortness of breath, dizziness, or nausea.

## TEST PROTOCOL AND ADMINISTRATION:

- Each stage is 3 minutes long. The first workload is set at 150 kilogram-meters per minute (kgm/min) or 0.5 kg (Figure 2).

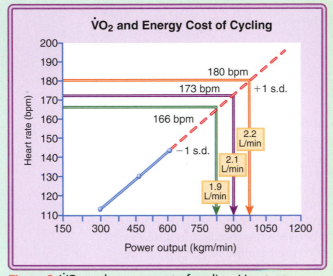

**Figure 2.** $\dot{V}O_2$ and energy cost of cycling. Heart rate responses to three submaximal work rates for a 50-year-old, sedentary man weighing 79 kg (174 lb). $\dot{V}O_{2max}$ was estimated by extrapolating the heart rate (HR) response to the age-predicted maximum HR of 173 beats/min (bpm; based on 208 – [0.7 × age]). The work rate that would have been achieved at that HR was determined by dropping a line from that HR value to the x-axis. $\dot{V}O_{2max}$ is estimated to be 2.1 L/min. The other two lines estimate what the $\dot{V}O_{2max}$ would have been if the subject's true maximum HR was ± standard deviation from the 173 bpm value.

- Continually coach the subject to maintain the 50-rpm cadence.
- Measure and record HR and RPE at the end of each minute; measure and record BP at the start of the third minute. Before progressing to the next stage, the HR at the end of the third minute must be within 5 bpm of the HR at the end of the second minute. If the subject has failed to achieve steady-state HR between these two timeframes, have him or her perform another minute at the same workload. During the last 15 seconds of stage 1, measure the subject's HR. This HR will determine which workload follows in stage 2. For example, if the subject's steady-state HR is 94 bpm at the end of stage 1, he or she will proceed to 450 kgm/min or 1.5 kg during stage 2; if the subject's steady-state HR is 88 bpm, he or she will proceed to 600 kgm/min or 2.0 kg during stage 2. Once a column is selected for stage 2, the next two workloads must remain consistent with each specific column (e.g., if stage 2 is performed at 600 kgm/min, then follow that same column to 750 and 900 kgm/min for the next two stages).
- Continue to record HR, RPE, and BP for each stage.
- The tension settings may loosen during the test. It is important for the tester to pay attention to both the settings and the cadence throughout the test to ensure consistent workloads. In addition, discourage the subject from talking during the test, as the effort to talk raises the heart rate, elevating the true HR response to the workload performed. The use and practice of signals should be encouraged.
- To ensure an accurate test, at least two stages must be completed to plot the appropriate HR response. These HR measurements must be between 110 and 155 bpm (and 85% of the age-predicted heart rate). Also, the exercise HR in the second and third minutes of stage 2 must be within 5 bpm of each other. This means that a

## *Practice What You Know:* Ebbeling Single-Stage Treadmill Test–cont'd

steady-state HR has been achieved for the particular stage/workload. If the HRs are more than 6 bpm apart between the second and third minutes, the subject will continue for 1 more minute at the same workload in an effort to achieve steady-state HR.

- **NOTE:** Approximately 10% of subjects will not achieve the steady-state HR, so the test should be discontinued, because it will not be valid (American College of Sports Medicine, 2008).

### POST-TEST PROCEDURE:

- The subject should cool down at a work rate equivalent to, or lower than, the first stage.
- As the subject cools down on the cycle, continue to observe him or her, because negative symptoms can arise immediately post-exercise.
- Plot HR against workload to estimate $\dot{V}O_{2max}$:
  - Determine the subject's MHR and draw a line across the graph at this value.
  - Plot two steady state heart rates between 110 and 155 bpm against the respective workload performed.
  - Draw a line through the HR coordinates and extend the line to MHR. If more than two points are used, draw a line of best fit between the coordinates if necessary.
  - Drop a line perpendicular from this point to the baseline to determine the estimated $\dot{V}O_{2max}$ indicated along the *x*-axis (Figure 3).

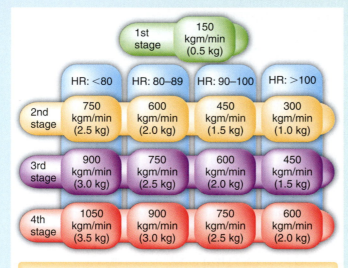

**Figure 3.** YMCA bike test protocol.
HR, heart rate. NOTE: Resistance settings shown here are appropriate for an ergometer with a flywheel of 6 m per revolution. Work rate is often expressed in watts; 1 watt = 6 kgm/min. *(Reprinted with permission from American College of Sports Medicine. ACSM's Guidelines for Exercise Testing and Prescription. 9th ed. Philadelphia, PA: Wolters Kluwer/Lippincott Williams & Wilkins; 2014.)*

$\dot{V}O_{2max}$ **Conversion**

Oxygen uptake is dependent on the size of the individual being tested. To compare $\dot{V}O_{2max}$ among individuals of different weights, oxygen uptake (in milliliters) must be divided by body weight (in kilograms). To calculate this conversion, perform the following steps:

- Convert L/min to mL/min by multiplying by 1,000.
- Convert body weight in pounds to kilograms by dividing by 2.2.
- Divide mL/kg.

  Oxygen uptake is always measured per minute, so the units become mL/kg/min.

Monark Exercise and Bodyguard both make suitable cycle ergometers. These cycles are more expensive than standard stationary cycles and are often used only for the purpose of fitness testing. Because they lack many of the features of modern electronic cycles, they are typically not used on the fitness floor. Consequently, testing with these protocols using traditional health club bikes is difficult, because the workloads or levels are predetermined and may not match the intensities required for the test protocol.

## *Practice What You Know:* Rockport Fitness Walking Test (1 Mile)

The purpose of the Rockport fitness walking test is to estimate $\dot{V}O_{2max}$ from a subject's steady-state HR response. This test involves the completion of a 1-mile (1.6-km) walking course as fast as possible. The $\dot{V}O_{2max}$ is calculated using the subject's steady-state HR, or immediate post-exercise HR, and his or her 1-mile walk time. This test is suitable for most individuals, is easy to administer, and is inexpensive to conduct. However, considering that walking may not elicit much of a cardiorespiratory challenge to conditioned individuals, this test will generally underpredict $\dot{V}O_{2max}$ in fit individuals, and is therefore not appropriate for that population group. A running track is the preferred testing surface. Most running tracks in the United States are a quarter-mile in distance, which means that walking four times around on the innermost lane will equal 1 mile. This test is also suitable for testing large groups of people, and subjects can periodically reassess their own fitness levels by self-administering this test. This method of testing would also be preferred for a subject who intends to walk/run outdoors as his or her mode of fitness training. When the weather is inclement and/or a track is not available, a treadmill test can be administered.

### EQUIPMENT:

- Quarter-mile track or suitable alternative (e.g., treadmill)
- Stopwatch
- RPE chart
- HR monitor with chest strap (optional)

### PRETEST PROCEDURE:

- After explaining the purpose of the 1-mile Rockport fitness walking test, define the 1-mile course.
- The goal of the test is to walk as fast as possible for 1 mile. Running is not permitted for this test. Pacing is strongly recommended throughout the test.
- Discuss RPE and remind the subject that he or she will be asked for perceived exertion levels throughout the test.

## *Practice What You Know:* Rockport Fitness Walking Test (1 Mile)–cont'd

### TEST PROTOCOL AND ADMINISTRATION:

- Record the subject's weight (in kg) and age.
- On the trainer's "go," the stopwatch is started and the subject begins.
- The subject's 1-mile (1.6-km) time, RPE, and HR during the first 15 seconds of recovery are recorded on the testing form. If a HR monitor is not used, a manual pulse count should be taken during the first 15 seconds of recovery and then multiplied by 4 to determine an accurate immediately post-exercise HR.
- Encourage a 3- to 5-minute cooldown, followed by stretching of the lower extremities.

### EVALUATION OF PERFORMANCE:

- The subject's information is plugged into one of the following formulas (American College of Sports Medicine, 2008):
  - Females: $\dot{V}O_2$ (mL/kg/min) = 132.853 – (0.1692 × weight in kg) – (0.3877 × age) – (3.265 × walk time expressed in minutes to the nearest 100th) – (0.1565 × HR)
  - Males: $\dot{V}O_2$ (mL/kg/min) = 139.168 – (0.1692 × weight in kg) – (0.3877 × age) – (3.265 × walk time expressed in minutes to the nearest 100th) – (0.1565 × HR)
- Record the values on the testing form. It is also important to include weather, surface conditions, or any other variables that may have an impact on overall time.
- Continue to observe the subject, because negative symptoms can arise immediately post-exercise.
- Evaluate the subject's score using Table 1 or Table 2 to classify performance based on the time to complete the one-mile walk.
- Example: Jessica, a 26-year-old subject weighing 125 lb (56.8 kg), completes the 1-mile walk in 16:40 with an steady-state HR of 132 bpm.
  - $\dot{V}O_{2max}$ = 132.853 – (0.1692 × body weight) – (0.388 × age) – (3.265 × time) – (0.1565 × HR) = 132.853 – (0.1692 × 56.8) – (0.388 × 26) – (3.265 × 16.67) – (0.1565 × 132) = 132.853 – 9.61 – 10.09 – 54.43 – 20.66 = 38.06 mL/kg/min

### Table 2. Normative Values for the Rockport Walking Test, Time (minutes:seconds)

| RATING | MALES (AGE 30–69 YR) | FEMALES (AGE 30–69 YR) |
|---|---|---|
| Excellent | 10:12 | 11:40 |
| Good | 10:13 to 11:42 | 11:41 to 13:08 |
| High average | 11:43 to 13:13 | 13:09 to 14:36 |
| Low average | 13:14 to 14:44 | 14:37 to 16:04 |
| Fair | 14:45 to 16:23 | 16:05 to 17:31 |
| Poor | 16:24 | 17:32 |
| PERCENTILE | MALES (AGE 18–30 YR) | FEMALES (AGE 18–30 YR) |
| 90 | 11:08 | 11:45 |
| 75 | 11:42 | 12:49 |
| 50 | 12:38 | 13:15 |
| 25 | 13:38 | 14:12 |
| 10 | 14:37 | 15:03 |

Adapted with permission from Morrow JR, et al. *Measurement and Evaluation in Human Performance.* 3rd ed. Champaign, IL: Human Kinetics; 2005.

# REFERENCES

American College of Sports Medicine. *ACSM's Health-Related Physical Fitness Assessment Manual.* 3rd ed. Philadelphia, PA: Lippincott Williams & Wilkins; 2008.

Ebbeling CB, Ward A, Puleo EM, Widrick J, Rippe JM. Development of a single-stage sub-maximal treadmill walking test. *Med Sci Sports Exerc.* 1991;23:966–973.

Foster C, Jackson AS, Pollock ML, et al. Generalized equations for predicting functional capacity from treadmill performance. *Am Heart J.* 1984;107:1229–1234.

Gellish RL, Goslin BR, Olson RE, McDonald A, Russi GD, Moudgil VK. Longitudinal modeling of the relationship between age and maximal heart rate. *Med Sci Sports Exerc.* 2007;39:822–829.

Pollock ML, Foster C, Schmidt D, Hellman C, Linnerud AC, Ward A. Comparative analysis of physiologic responses to three different maximal graded exercise test protocols in healthy women. *Am Heart J.* 1982;103:363–373.

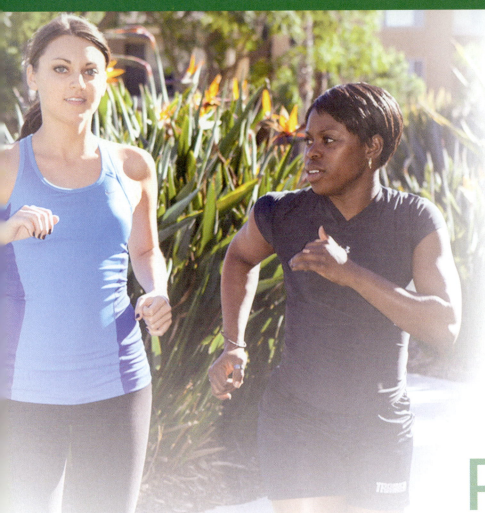

# PART III
# Physiological Systems

This part of the text describes the many physiological systems that must work in a co-ordinated fashion for the body to maintain sustained physical exertion. Chapter 6 details the respiratory system. The anatomy, mechanics, and control of respiration are described, including the diffusion and transport of oxygen and carbon dioxide. Then Chapter 7 focuses on the cardiovascular system, presenting the anatomy of the heart and the structure of the blood vessels, including the associated hemodynamics of circulation. Chapter 8 brings this material together and presents information on the acute and chronic responses to exercise. The changes that take place during incremental, steady state, and maximal exercise are presented, as well as the cardiovascular and respiratory adaptations to training.

Chapter 9 presents the structure and function of the nervous and muscular (collectively neuromuscular) systems and how they interact to provide bodily movement. Detail on the structure of muscle tissue and the contractile process is presented, with a specific focus on muscle fiber types and fiber recruitment patterns. The focus of the chapter on the nervous system is on how neural organization impacts the coordination of motor patterns and proprioception. Chapter 10 synthesizes all of the information presented in Chapter 9, highlighting the acute neuromuscular training responses and adaptations to exercise. There is a strong emphasis on the mechanism of muscle growth and muscle fiber adaptations to training.

An overview of the endocrine system and the hormonal responses to exercise is presented in Chapter 11, with an emphasis on the specific hormones that are influenced by exercise. The final chapter in this part, Chapter 12, focuses on thermoregulation, with an emphasis on how the body regulates core temperature in response to exercising in hot and cold environments. Because exercising in these types of climates can provide safety challenges to individuals, a major focus of this chapter is on providing practical suggestions for avoiding temperature-related problems.

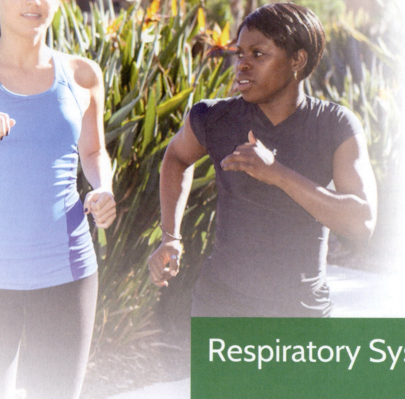

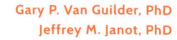

Gary P. Van Guilder, PhD
Jeffrey M. Janot, PhD

CHAPTER 6

# Respiratory System

## CHAPTER OUTLINE

# CHAPTER OUTLINE–cont'd

# LEARNING OUTCOMES

1. Outline the major anatomical structures of the respiratory system.
2. Explain the functional differences between respiration and ventilation.
3. Define *minute* and *alveolar ventilation,* and explain how to calculate these values.
4. Compare and contrast the functional components of the conducting and respiratory zones in the lungs.
5. Identify the respiratory control center in the brain.
6. Describe the major factors in the control of respiration.
7. Describe the factors that affect gas diffusion.
8. Explain how oxygen and carbon dioxide are exchanged at the lung and tissues.
9. Calculate the partial pressure of gases in the atmospheric air and alveoli.
10. Describe how gases are transported in the blood.
11. Explain the factors that affect hemoglobin-oxygen saturation during exercise.

# ANCILLARY LINK

Visit Davis*Plus* at http://davisplus.fadavis.com for study and practice resources, including online quizzes, animations that help explain physiological processes, podcasts concerning news and career trends in exercise physiology, and practice references.

## VIGNETTE

While leading a group of 10 exercisers through the warm-up portion of a beginner's boot camp class in a park near his downtown training studio, Joey notices that one of his newest clients seems to be having trouble catching her breath. Amanda is a physically fit college student, so seasoned trainer Joey is initially surprised to see her struggling during the body weight squats and dynamic lunges included in the warm-up. However, it is a particularly hot, humid summer day. He quickly approaches to ask Amanda how she is feeling. Amanda quietly says, "I'm okay," and continues exercising. Joey decides to keep a close eye on Amanda as her exercise intensity increases.

As soon as higher-intensity activities, such as jumping rope and box jumps, are introduced, it becomes clear that Amanda is struggling with shortness of breath, or dyspnea. Her respiratory rate (RR) is fast, and she looks uncomfortable. Joey comes to Amanda's side and can see that her breathing is labored, and her shortness of breath appears to be getting severe.

What could be causing Amanda's dyspnea?

tissue, gas is exchanged between the atmosphere and blood, which is referred to as **external respiration**, or pulmonary respiration. **Internal respiration** occurs between the blood and all of the other cells of the body. Pulmonary ventilation causes $O_2$ concentration and pressure ($O_2$ tension) in the lungs to exceed that of the blood. Consequently, $O_2$ will move from the lungs to the blood. Likewise, because $CO_2$ tension in the blood is greater than the lungs, it moves from the blood to the lungs, where it can be exhaled and removed from the body. The remarkable anatomical features of the respiratory system are designed to maximize efficient gas exchange.

Figure 6-1 provides an overview of the basic anatomy of the respiratory system. The primary anatomical structure of the human respiratory system is the lungs, a remarkable organ with a tremendous capacity for gas exchange. Indeed, it is estimated that the length of all the airway tubes in the lungs is a staggering 1,500 miles. To put this in geographical context, if each airway in the lungs were laid end to end, the total length would cover a distance equivalent to the distance from Boston, Massachusetts, to Omaha, Nebraska. Moreover, 600 miles of pulmonary capillaries supply the lungs with blood. Together, the vast number of airways, coupled with a massive blood supply, provides the lungs with the ability to exchange gas to supply the trillions of cells that make up the body. This section describes the main anatomical considerations of the respiratory system, including the thoracic cavity, lungs, and airways of the conducting zone and the respiratory zone.

The **respiratory system**, which consists of the airways, lungs, and respiratory muscles, works to continuously exchange gases between the external environment (atmosphere) and the body. Because it plays a major role in regulating oxygen and carbon dioxide levels in blood, maintains blood acid–base balance, and cleans and humidifies air, it is essential for the exercise physiology student to gain an understanding of the respiratory system. Accordingly, the objective of this chapter is to provide an overview of the essential structures and functions of the respiratory system as it relates to gas exchange and transport in the body. You will learn the basic structure, organization, and function of this system as it pertains to exercise physiology.

## ANATOMY OF THE RESPIRATORY SYSTEM

Breathing refers to the physical process by which gases are transported in and out of the lungs. During the breathing cycle, fresh, oxygen-rich air contained in the atmosphere is first brought into the lungs through **inhalation**, which is also called **inspiration**. Then, oxygen-depleted air that is rich in $CO_2$ is removed from the lungs by **exhalation**, or **expiration**. In the lung

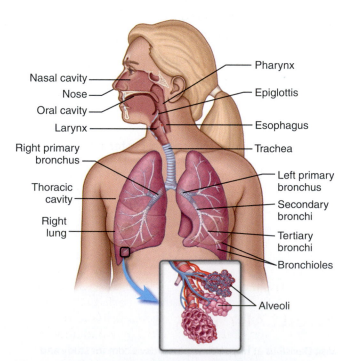

**Figure 6-1.** General organization of the respiratory system. Note that the system begins at the nose, where air is filtered and humidified, and concludes at the level of the alveoli, where gas exchange occurs.

## Thoracic Cavity

The *thoracic cavity*, also called the chest cavity, is a space located above the diaphragm that houses the lungs and the heart. This cavity is protected by the thoracic cage, which consists of several bones, including the ribs, spine, and sternum, and muscles that are involved in respiration. The volume of the thoracic cavity changes during the breathing cycle. During inspiration, the cavity gets larger, whereas during expiration it gets smaller. It is the main job of the respiratory muscles to control the size of the thoracic cavity to assist with inspiration and expiration.

The main muscles of the thoracic cavity are the 2 sets of internal and external intercostals, which connect the 12 rib pairs, and the sternocleidomastoid and scalene muscles, which connect the head and neck to the sternum and the first 2 pairs of ribs. Other muscles that play an important role in respiration, but are not considered muscles of the thoracic cavity, include the abdominal muscles (the rectus abdominis, internal and external obliques, and the transverse abdominis). A more detailed description of the role of these muscles during breathing is provided later in this chapter.

## Lungs

There are two lungs in the body, a right and a left lung, each located within the thoracic cavity. The lungs are separated by the heart, and enclosed and supported by the rib cage and respiratory muscles. Each lung is a cone-shaped organ composed primarily of a light, spongy tissue that contains hundreds of millions of microscopic air-filled sacs called **alveoli**. The weight of one lung is relatively small, averaging approximately 1 kg (2.2 lb) in a 70-kg (154 lb) adult. The right lung is subdivided into three lobes, (upper, middle, and lower) and is larger than the left lung, which contains only two lobes (upper and lower). The left lung is marginally smaller than the right lung because the heart protrudes into the left side of the thoracic cavity. Thus, the right lung is not as obstructed by the heart and represents approximately 55% of total lung volume. Connected to the base of the lungs is the diaphragm, a fatigue-resistant skeletal muscle that directs inspiration.

## Pleura and Pleural Cavity

Within the thoracic cavity, the lungs are completely enclosed by a very thin set of moist membranes called **pleura**. The inside layer of the pleura, referred to as the **parietal pleura**, lines the thoracic walls and the diaphragm. The **visceral pleura** is fused to the outer surface of each lung. Between these two membranous layers is a small space known as the **pleural cavity**. Within the pleural cavity is a tiny amount (10 mL) of viscous pleural fluid that works to lubricate and moisten the opposing parietal and visceral pleural membranes so that they can slide across one another with minimal friction during ventilation. The pleural fluid also helps to ensure that the lungs are connected tightly to the thoracic wall.

## Conducting Zone

The **conducting zone** of the respiratory system contains the air passages that transport air from the external environment to the areas of the respiratory system where gas exchange occurs. It accounts for a small portion of the total lung volume, typically about 10%. The structures of the conducting zone include the nose, nasal cavity, mouth, pharynx, larynx, trachea, bronchial tree, and terminal bronchioles. The primary function of the conducting zone, besides providing passageways for air, is to condition and clean the air that enters the body. Breathing through the nose instead of the mouth provides a greater opportunity for air conditioning. As air is inhaled through the nose, it swirls and slows. This swirling action facilitates air conditioning before it enters the conducting zone. Conditioning and cleaning the air is an essential step needed to prevent damage to the respiratory tract and lung surfaces caused by inhaled foreign bodies and pathogens. Air conditioning has three main components: warming, humidification, and filtration.

During air warming, the temperature of the air entering the body is rapidly warmed to body temperature (37°C). Indeed, by the time atmospheric air reaches the trachea, it has been warmed to body temperature. Air warming is important because it helps to prevent declines in core body temperature that may occur from breathing in very cold air. More so, warming the air before it reaches the respiratory zone helps protect the alveoli from cold damage.

Concomitant with air warming is air **humidification**. Water vapor is added to the incoming air, which is saturated to 100% humidity. Air humidification keeps the cell lining of the passageways moist and prevents it from drying out.

**Filtration** and cleaning occur as air is warmed and humidified. The air passages are extremely efficient at filtering and removing foreign particles that are contained in the atmospheric air. Thus, air filtration plays a vital role in defense against infections that may originate from breathing in environmental particles, such as dust, environmental pollutants, toxic chemicals, bacteria and other microorganisms, and airborne allergens (weed, grass, and tree pollens).

Filtration first occurs as air enters the nose and nasal cavity, which contains coarse hairs that help trap large particles. More importantly, however, is the fact that the air passages of the respiratory tract are lined with a unique cell layer called the *ciliated respiratory epithelium*. These cells secrete a sticky, moist, thick layer of mucus that traps many foreign airborne particles. In conjunction with mucous secretion is the sweeping motion of cilia. Cilia are microscopic, hairlike structures that project from the epithelial cells that continuously propel secreted mucus upward toward the oral cavity so that any foreign particles can be eliminated from the body by swallowing or coughing. The ciliated epithelium also secretes lysozyme, an enzyme that destroys inhaled bacteria.

Air first enters the conducting zone through the nose and **nasal cavity**. Most air enters the body through the nose; however, at higher breathing rates, especially during exercise, it increases through the **oral cavity** (mouth). Within the nasal cavity are three bony passages, called **nasal meatus**. Each meatus contains a narrow, constricted groove that increases airflow turbulence during inhalation. Increased air turbulence ensures that air remains in the nasal cavity for longer periods to warm, humidify, and filter.

After air passes through the nasal and oral cavity, it reaches the **pharynx**, or throat. The pharynx is subdivided into the nasopharynx, oropharynx, and laryngopharynx. The pharynx is the gateway for both inhaled and exhaled air and consumed food. For air to enter the **trachea**, the main conducting tube to the lungs, it must pass through the **larynx**. The larynx is a cartilaginous structure that is also called the *voice box*. It prevents food and other materials from entering the lungs. The conduction of air through the larynx into the trachea is directed by the opening and closing of the **epiglottis**. The epiglottis keeps the larynx closed when a person swallows. This helps to direct the flow

of food and liquids toward the esophagus, the main tube of the digestive system. Likewise, when a person inhales, the epiglottis moves in such a way to allow air to enter the trachea.

## Trachea

The trachea, also called the *windpipe*, is the passageway for air to the lungs (see Fig. 6-1). It is a semiflexible tube supported by 15 to 20 rings of cartilage. It is approximately 2.5 cm in diameter and 12 cm in length. The cartilage rings of the trachea are necessary to keep the airway open at all times. The rings also provide movement flexibility. During coughing, for instance, the tracheal diameter gets smaller through the contraction of the trachealis muscle. This helps to move air and objects up and out of the windpipe more rapidly. The lining of the trachea is also richly supplied by ciliated epithelium and mucus. The distal end of the trachea branches into the right and left primary bronchi, which initiate the **bronchial tree**.

## Bronchial Tree

Figure 6-2 displays the branching of the bronchial tree and the primary components of the conducting and respiratory zones. The bronchial tree is a progressively dividing network of airway passages that originates

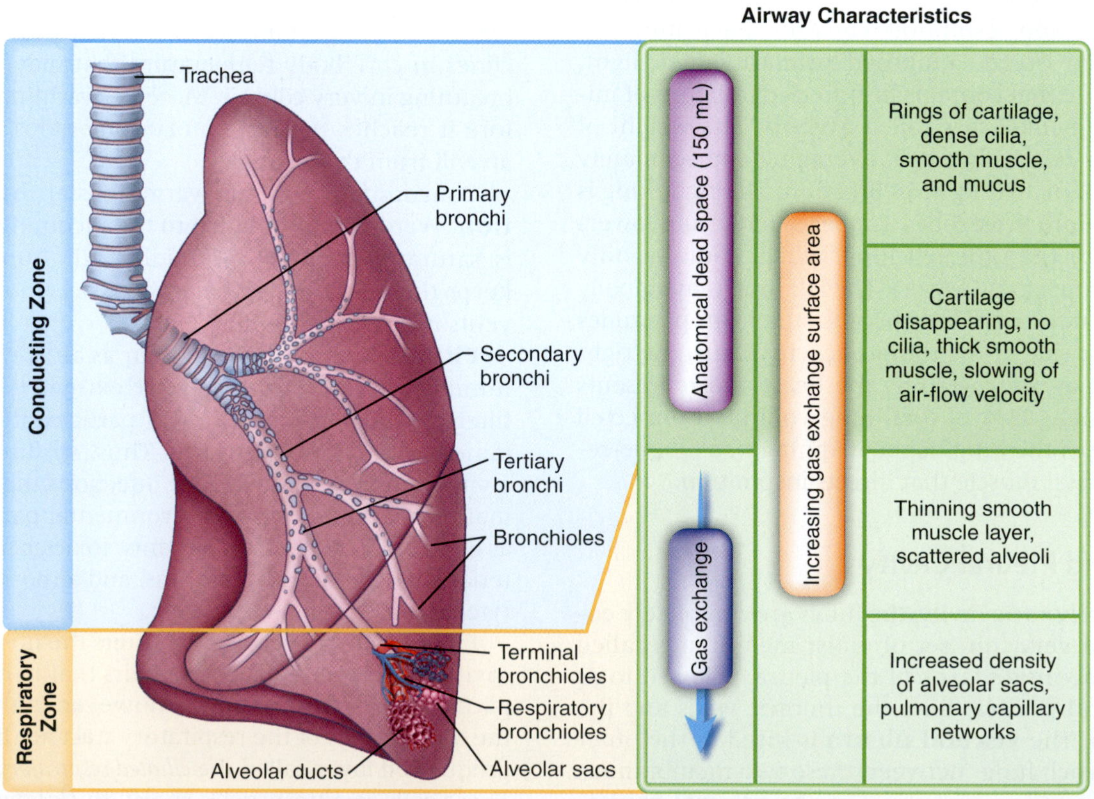

**Airway Characteristics**

**Figure 6-2.** The bronchial tree and the primary components of the conducting zone and respiratory zone. Remember, even though the conducting zone appears to make up a larger portion of the lung volume in this figure, it is the respiratory zone that makes up 90% of the total lung volume. Thus, the lung is the perfect tissue for gas exchange because of the large surface area in the respiratory zone.

from the first branching of the trachea (generation 1) into the right and left primary bronchi. In total, the bronchial tree contains approximately 23 generations of airways. The first 16 generations serve as airways for the conducting zone. The final seven generations are considered airways of the respiratory zone. The right primary bronchus aerates the right lung, whereas the left bronchus aerates the left lung. The right and left primary bronchi branch to form two sets of narrower **secondary bronchi**, which further divide into a series of **tertiary bronchi** that aerate a particular part of the lung. Typically, the right lung contains 10 tertiary bronchi, whereas the left, being slightly smaller, contains approximately 8 tertiary bronchi. From the tertiary bronchi, the bronchial tree continues to branch extensively into narrower tubes of smaller bronchi, up to about generation 10. Eventually, the bronchi lose all cartilage and reach a diameter of less than 1 mm, at which point they become **bronchioles**. The bronchioles continue to diverge before they end with the **terminal bronchioles** deep in the lungs. The terminal bronchioles mark the end of the conducting zone; they transport air into the respiratory zone for gas exchange.

The structure of the airways gradually changes as the generation number increases throughout the bronchial tree. The first change is that the airways become smaller and narrower. In addition, upon each successive airway branching, rings of cartilage become less numerous, the amount of mucous-producing cells declines, and cilia declines. Eventually, cartilage is replaced by a thicker layer of smooth muscle. The smooth muscle layer controls the internal diameter of the bronchioles and, therefore, controls the rate of airflow through the bronchial tree.

When the smooth muscle relaxes, it causes the bronchioles to dilate, which is referred to as **bronchodilation**. When the smooth muscle contracts, it causes the bronchioles to constrict, referred to as **bronchoconstriction**.

To facilitate the increased demand for oxygen at the start of exercise, the airways in the conducting and respiratory zone dilate to bring in more air from the atmosphere. Bronchodilation makes it substantially easier to deliver air into the lungs because it decreases airway resistance.

## Respiratory Zone

The **respiratory zone** marks the beginning of gas exchange in the lung. It accounts for 90% of total lung air volume. The structures of this zone include the respiratory bronchioles, alveolar ducts, and alveoli. Further branching of the terminal bronchioles at generation 16 creates **respiratory bronchioles**. These airways continue to divide through generation 19 into numerous smaller respiratory bronchioles that, to a limited degree, participate in gas exchange because they contain scattered alveoli. The smallest respiratory bronchioles end with tiny airway tubules called **alveolar ducts**. Each lung contains approximately 2 million alveolar ducts. The alveolar ducts divide and end with clusters of **alveolar sacs**, the terminal respiratory unit of the bronchial tree.

An alveolar sac contains several tiny pouches of air-filled semispherical compartments called *alveoli*. An alveolus is 0.25 mm in diameter. It is the primary site where gas is exchanged between the lungs and the blood. There are approximately 300 to 500 million alveoli in the human lung, which are blanketed with blood supplied by the pulmonary capillaries. Indeed, coupled with the massive airway branching and vast blood supply, the hundreds of millions of alveoli provide the lungs with a surface area for gas exchange of 75 m², or the equivalent of a racquetball court. Some medical conditions, such as exercise-induced asthma (EIA), involve constriction of the bronchioles (see Box 6-1).

## Box 6-1. Exercise-Induced Asthma

Dyspnea, or shortness of breath, is a symptom that many people experience while engaging in activities. The increased RR can be uncomfortable, but typically does not pose a significant concern. However, episodes of severe shortness of breath that occur with asthma can last for minutes to hours. In these situations, breathing becomes labored, difficult, and may be inadequate to meet the body's energy requirements. Breathlessness of this severity can be life-threatening and may require rapid emergency medical treatment.

Asthma that develops during exercise, referred to as **exercise-induced asthma (EIA),** can substantially limit performance. Individuals with EIA may notice the onset of asthma symptoms after a few minutes of activity, such as shortness of breath and unusual fatigue that persists and may worsen throughout the exercise bout.

EIA can transpire during any activity that increases ventilation. EIA is triggered by the rapid transport of cold, dry air or warm, humid air into the lungs before it is adequately conditioned. As a result, the variability in temperature and humidity of the inspired air aggravates the lining of the airways, causing asthma symptoms. If an individual's asthma is triggered by other causes, such as high pollen counts or air pollution, he or she may experience a worsening of EIA in specific places or during certain times of the year.

Individuals who have EIA experience limitations in exercise performance. The decrease in exercise performance with EIA depends largely on the severity of asthma and if there are other triggers involved besides exercise. Sustained exercise or activities that are performed in cold weather may trigger an asthma attack. These may include long-distance running,

*Continued*

## Box 6-1. Exercise-Induced Asthma—cont'd

hockey, cross-country skiing, or mountaineering. However, if rest periods are incorporated into the activity and it is performed in a comfortable climate, then the likelihood of an attack is reduced.

EIA can be effectively treated through lifestyle modification and medical management. Individuals need to consult with their physicians, acquire medical clearance to exercise, and develop an asthma action plan. Asthma action plans have been developed by a variety of organizations including the National Institutes of Health in collaboration with the Department of Health and Human Services. Please refer to the National Institutes of Health and the Centers for Disease Control and Prevention websites (see Additional Resources at the end of this chapter) for published asthma action plans that are available for people with asthma and their health-care team. Overall, an appropriate action

plan should include detailed instructions of the tasks that need to be completed before exercise to prevent an asthma attack, a list of specific asthma triggers, guidelines to follow in the event of an attack, and when to contact a health-care provider and/or seek emergency medical treatment.

Currently, there is no cure for asthma. If uncontrolled, asthma can be a life-threatening condition. However, the disease can be properly managed through medical treatment using bronchodilators to open up constricted bronchioles and inhaled corticosteroids to manage airway inflammation that can cause narrowing of the bronchioles (see Fig. 6-3). In addition, lifestyle modification can also be an effective way to avoid acute attacks of EIA. Most individuals with EIA can continue to enjoy the benefits of regular exercise without significant limitations.

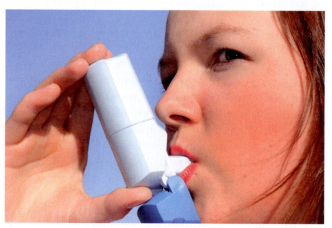

**Figure 6-3.** Using an inhaler before exercise can help individuals with asthma control symptoms and improve exercise performance.

## Respiratory Membrane

The alveoli are the fundamental site for gas exchange in the lung. Figure 6-4 shows the surface of the alveoli. Notice that alveoli are predominately lined by a single layer of epithelial cells called the *type 1 alveolar cells*. Type 1 cells form part of the **respiratory membrane**, a very thin wall separating the alveolar surface and the blood. It contains the cell membrane of a type 1 cell, a pulmonary capillary endothelial cell, and their fused basement membranes. Thus, the space for gas exchange is only two cell layers thick (alveolar type 1 cell and capillary endothelial cell).

An alveolus and its network of pulmonary capillaries are known as an alveolar-capillary unit. This unique anatomical organization between the alveolus and the capillary is specialized to promote efficient diffusion of oxygen and carbon dioxide. In a typical alveolar-capillary

unit, the distance covered by gases to diffuse across the fused membranes is less than 0.5 μm. $O_2$ diffuses from the alveolus across the respiratory membrane into the pulmonary capillary where it can be loaded onto the red blood cell for delivery to all cells of the body. In contrast, $CO_2$ diffuses from the pulmonary capillary in the opposite direction across the respiratory membrane and into the alveolus so that it can be expelled from the body (see Fig. 6-4). The diffusion of gases is explained later in this chapter.

The intimate relationship between the respiratory system and the cardiovascular system is exemplified at the alveolar-capillary unit. Each alveolus is almost completely enveloped by an extensive network of pulmonary capillaries. About 90% of the surface of an alveolus is covered with blood vessels, creating a blanket of blood that is as close to the air-filled alveoli as possible. The extreme proximity of the blood to the alveolar gas exchange surface ensures the rapid diffusion of gases across the respiratory membrane. Rapid diffusion of gases is also facilitated by the fact that the internal diameter of a pulmonary capillary is only about 8 μm, a space barely wide enough to fit a single red blood cell (Fig. 6-5).

The surface of the alveoli is also lined, to a lesser degree, by type 2 alveolar cells. The primary role of these cells is to produce and secrete a substance called **surfactant**. A fluid composed of lipids and proteins that lines the inside of the alveoli, surfactant helps to keep the airways open, improves lung compliance, and decreases the work of breathing. A third cell, the alveolar macrophage, protects the alveoli from foreign bodies and bacteria.

## Alveolar Interdependence

Each alveolus is mechanically tethered to one another to establish a degree of structural support called **alveolar interdependence**. Alveolar interdependence helps to

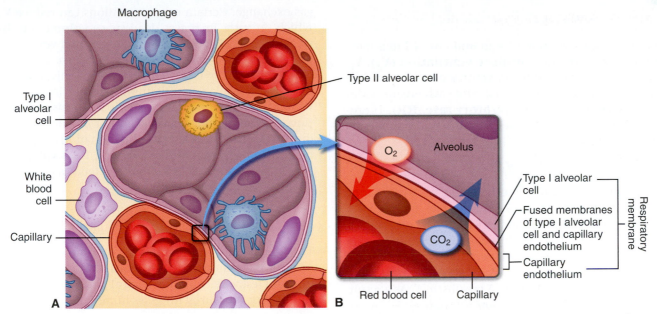

**Figure 6-4.** General organization of an alveolar-capillary unit. (A) An alveolus is lined by type I alveolar cells and the surfactant-secreting type II cells. (B) The respiratory membrane is composed of an alveolar type I cell, a pulmonary capillary endothelial cell, and their fused basement membranes. Oxygen diffuses from the alveolus into the pulmonary capillary, whereas carbon dioxide diffuses into the alveolus.

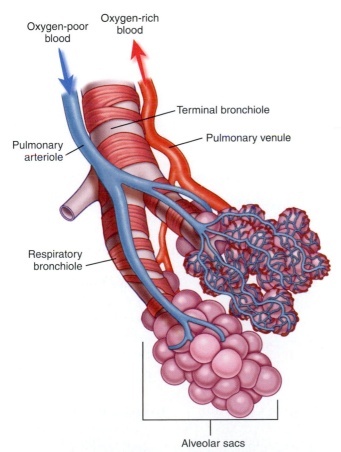

**Figure 6-5.** An alveolar sac and its network of pulmonary blood vessels. Notice that each alveolus is blanketed with pulmonary capillaries to facilitate rapid exchange of oxygen and carbon dioxide. Oxygen-poor blood from the right side of the heart travels to alveoli, whereas oxygen-rich blood travels to the left side of the heart.

stabilize the alveoli and prevent their collapse. If an alveolus were to begin to collapse spontaneously, the tension experienced by the tethered adjacent alveoli would act to pull open the collapsing alveolus. The tethered alveoli tend to hold the collapsing alveolus open. Alveolar interdependence is important during the respiratory cycle because it helps to establish uniformity in ventilation across the lung tissue to maximize gas exchange.

## In Your Own Words

A friend who has recently been diagnosed with EIA wants to begin a moderate-intensity exercise program. Share some exercise safety tips that your friend can use before this exercise program to minimize the risk for EIA.

## VIGNETTE continued

■ Joey suspects that Amanda is experiencing EIA. In addition to shortness of breath, Amanda has begun wheezing and coughing, and she is complaining of chest tightness. Joey also recalls that she exhibited some difficulty talking during the warm-up, another telltale sign of an asthma attack. He can tell that she is breathing with her abdominal, chest, and back muscles. She looks sweaty and is beginning to act panicky. Joey needs to act quickly before her symptoms become even more severe.

## MINUTE VENTILATION

The air that is transported into and out of lungs each minute is referred to as **minute ventilation ($\dot{V}_E$)**. $\dot{V}_E$, also referred to as pulmonary ventilation, is the product of the volume of air exchanged with each breath (**tidal volume [$V_T$]**) and the **respiratory rate (RR)**. Therefore, $\dot{V}_E$ is expressed mathematically by the following equation:

$$\dot{V}_E = V_T \times RR$$

As you can imagine, $\dot{V}_E$ can change relatively easily. For instance, breathing more deeply (i.e., increased $V_T$) and more often (i.e., increased RR) during exercise increases $\dot{V}_E$. Conversely, a reduced rate of breathing during sleep, or a decline in $V_T$, will decrease $\dot{V}_E$. In a healthy, average-sized man at rest, $V_T$ is about 500 mL, and breathing frequency is about 15 breaths/min. As a result, $\dot{V}_E$ is equivalent to about 7,500 mL/min (7.5 L/min). However, $\dot{V}_E$ increases abruptly during exercise and can reach upward of 150 L/min during maximal exercise. With respiratory disease or respiratory failure, $\dot{V}_E$ may decline to dangerously low levels (<6 L/min), at which point the respiratory system is unable to supply adequate oxygen to the tissues and effectively remove carbon dioxide.

An important concept to understand is that not all of the fresh air that enters the lungs during ventilation reaches the alveoli. Some of this air is trapped in the conducting airways, particularly the trachea and large bronchi, and is unavailable for gas exchange. The air that is trapped in the conducting airways is referred to as the **anatomical dead space** and is called **dead space ventilation ($V_D$)**. The volume of anatomical dead space that remains in the conducting airways is about 150 mL. Even though 500 mL of fresh air has entered the lungs with each breath, only about 350 mL of that volume reaches the alveoli. The remaining 150 mL is stale anatomical dead space air that mixes with the fresh air. If we consider the anatomical dead space air, we obtain a more accurate estimation of ventilation at the gas exchange surface, referred to as **alveolar ventilation ($\dot{V}_A$)**. $\dot{V}_A$ is the volume of inspired *fresh* air that reaches the alveoli for gas exchange in 1 minute. To calculate $\dot{V}_A$, first subtract the anatomical dead space from $V_T$. Thus, $\dot{V}_A$ is calculated by the following equation:

$$\dot{V}_A = (V_T - \text{anatomical dead space volume}) \times RR$$

For example, given a $V_T$ of 500 mL, dead space volume of 150 mL, and a breathing frequency of 15 breaths/min, the $\dot{V}_A$ would equal 5,250 mL/min.

$$\dot{V}_A = (500 \text{ mL} - 150 \text{ mL}) \times 15 \text{ breaths/min}$$
$$\dot{V}_A = 350 \text{ mL} \times 15 \text{ breaths/min}$$
$$\dot{V}_A = 5,250 \text{ mL/min}$$

Thus, although 7,500 mL of air entered the lungs in 1 minute, only 5,250 mL reached the respiratory zone and alveoli. Consequently, the dead space volume essentially decreases the volume of air that participates in gas exchange. Certain other conditions can reduce $V_A$, which, in turn, increases dead space volume. For instance, if a blockage occurs in a lung blood vessel (i.e., pulmonary embolism), then gas exchange in that region of the lung will be impaired because of a mismatch between perfusion and ventilation.[1] This will increase the volume of air that does not participate in gas exchange (increased anatomic dead space). For additional learning, review the explanatory animation of Alveolar Ventilation and Changes with Increasing Tidal Volume on the Davis*Plus* site at http://davisplus.fadavis.com.

## LUNG VOLUMES AND CAPACITIES

The function of the respiratory system can be assessed using a technique called **spirometry**, a pulmonary function test widely used in clinical practice. In general, spirometry measures lungs volumes throughout the

### DOING THE MATH:

Your client, a 35-year-old woman, comes to your facility for a pulmonary assessment at rest and during exercise. As part of the assessment, you gather information on variables specific to ventilatory performance. The data are as follows:

| VARIABLE | RESTING CONDITION | EXERCISE CONDITION |
|---|---|---|
| RR | 14 breaths/min | 30 breath/min |
| $V_T$ | 0.4 L/breath | 1.2 L/breath |

Calculate the client's $\dot{V}_E$ and alveolar ventilation at rest and during exercise.

**Calculate $\dot{V}_E$ at rest and during exercise.**

**Resting Condition**
$\dot{V}_E = V_T \times RR$
$\dot{V}_E = 0.4 \text{ L/breath} \times$ 14 breaths/min
$\dot{V}_E = 5.6 \text{ L/min}$

**Exercise Condition**
$\dot{V}_E = V_T \times RR$
$\dot{V}_E = 1.2 \text{ L/breath} \times$ 30 breaths/min
$\dot{V}_E = 36 \text{ L/min}$

**Calculate $V_A$ at rest and during exercise.**

**Resting Condition**
$\dot{V}_A = (V_T - V_D) \times RR$
$\dot{V}_A = (400 \text{ mL/}$ breath − 150 mL) × 14 breaths/min
$\dot{V}_A = 0.25 \text{ L/breath} \times$ 14 breaths/min
$\dot{V}_A = 3.5 \text{ L/min}$

**Exercise Condition**
$\dot{V}_A = (V_T - V_D) \times RR$
$\dot{V}_A = (1,200 \text{ mL/}$ breath − 150 mL) × 30 breaths/min
$\dot{V}_A = 1.05 \text{ L/breath} \times$ 30 breaths/min
$\dot{V}_A = 31.5 \text{ L/min}$

various stages of the respiratory cycle and can assess airflow. Spirometry is useful to health professionals and exercise physiologists because it provides important data that may indicate depressed lung function or pulmonary disease. For example, the maximum amount of air expired in the first second of expiration, that is, the **forced expiratory volume (FEV$_1$)**, can help to diagnose asthma or bronchitis.

To assess lung volumes, a person breathes through a mouthpiece into a device called a *spirometer*, which measures the volume of air ventilated during inspiration and expiration (Fig. 6-6). Figure 6-7 shows a typical spirogram and its associated lung volumes and capacities

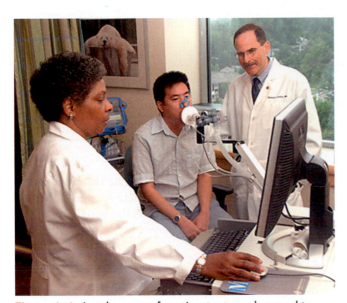

**Figure 6-6.** A pulmonary function test can be used to evaluate lung function and identify the presence and severity of diseases such as asthma and emphysema.

during quiet breathing, and Table 6-1 defines key terms related to lung volume and capacity.

## Lung Volumes

Four lung volumes can be assessed using spirometry:

- **Tidal Volume (V$_T$)**—V$_T$ is the volume of air exchanged with each breath. More specifically, it is the volume of air inspired and expired during unforced quiet breathing. V$_T$ averages about 500 mL per inspiration or expiration.
- **Inspiratory reserve volume (IRV)**—At the end of a quiet inspiration, the amount of air that a person can maximally inhale is referred to as the IRV. It represents the reserve volume for inhaled air. A typical IRV is 3,000 mL (six times the value of V$_T$) but varies substantially between males and females. The IRV for females is about 25% less than their age-matched male counterparts.
- **Expiratory reserve volume (ERV)**—The opposite of IRV is the ERV. To measure ERV, a person is instructed to maximally exhale as much air as possible immediately after a normal quiet expiration. It represents the additional volume of air that can be forcefully exhaled from the lungs. A normal ERV is about 1,100 mL for males and 900 mL for females.
- **Residual volume (RV)**—The RV is the volume of air remaining in the lungs after a forced maximal expiration. No matter how hard a person exhales, there will still be a small volume of air left over inside the lungs. It may not seem obvious to you why the lungs would need a certain volume of air to remain in the lungs. If you could exhale all the air out of your lungs, then the airways and alveoli would collapse. A collapsed airway is

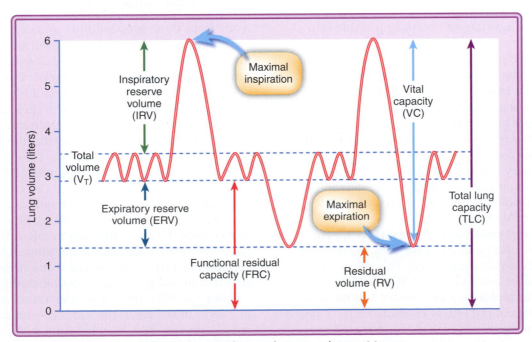

**Figure 6-7.** General spirogram showing lung volumes and capacities.

## Table 6-1. Key Terminology Related to Lung Volumes and Capacities

| TERM | DEFINITION |
| --- | --- |
| **Lung Volumes** | |
| Tidal volume ($V_T$) | The volume of air inspired or expired during quiet breathing |
| Inspiratory reserve volume (IRV) | The maximum volume of air that can be inspired following a normal inspiration |
| Expiratory reserve volume (ERV) | The maximum volume of air that can be expired following a normal expiration |
| Residual volume (RV) | The volume of air that remains in the lungs following a maximal expiration |
| **Lung Capacities** | |
| Vital capacity (VC) | The maximum volume of air that can be expired following a maximal inspiration |
| Inspiratory capacity (IC) | The maximum volume of air that can be inspired following a normal expiration |
| Functional residual capacity (FRC) | The volume of air remaining in the lungs after a normal expiration |
| Total lung capacity (TLC) | The total volume of air in the lungs after a maximal inspiration |

extremely difficult to open because of the tremendous inflation pressures. A modest RV keeps the airways open and minimizes the amount of pressure needed to inflate the lungs.

## Lung Capacities

Four lung capacities can be estimated from various combinations of the aforementioned lung volumes:

- **Vital capacity (VC)**—Mathematically, the VC is the sum of IRV, $V_T$, and ERV. Physiologically, VC is the maximum amount of air that can be expired following a maximal inspiration. Thus, a person must exhale as large a breath as possible into a spirometer to get an accurate assessment of VC. Because VC is a general indicator of lung size, it is logical to suggest that larger and taller individuals will have a higher VC. This is the case. Generally, men have a greater VC than women because of their larger body stature. VC declines with aging, which may reflect structural changes in the lung tissue that reduce compliance.
- **Inspiratory capacity (IC)**—The maximum amount of air that can be inspired following a normal expiration is referred to as the IC. It is the sum of $V_T$ and IRV.
- **Functional residual capacity (FRC)**—The sum of the ERV and RV is the FRC. Although it cannot be directly measured with spirometry, it indicates the amount of air left in the lungs after a quiet normal resting expiration. It is important to understand the FRC is estimated after a *quiet* tidal expiration, whereas RV is estimated after *maximal* expiration.

- **Total lung capacity (TLC)**—The total volume of air the lungs can accommodate is approximately 5 to 6 L. This is the TLC. TLC is the sum of all four lung volumes and is displayed by the following equation:

$$TLC = IRV + TV + ERV + RV$$

To put it another way, it is the total volume of air in the lungs after a maximal inspiration, plus the RV.

## Forced Expiratory Volume in 1 Second/ Forced Vital Capacity Ratio

Aside from these lung volumes and capacities, it may be important for a health-care professional to assess maximal airflow rate. The maximal volume of air that can be expired over a specified time is a good indicator of respiratory function and is particularly useful for diagnosing obstructive lung diseases that increase airway resistance (e.g., asthma, chronic obstructive pulmonary disease). For example, as explained at the beginning of this section, the volume of air that is forced out of the lungs in the first second of expiration ($FEV_1$) is a good indicator of airway resistance and can be used to diagnose lung disease. The $FEV_1$ is expressed as a proportion of the forced vital capacity (FVC; $FEV_1$/FVC ratio). To reiterate, the VC is the volume of air that a person can exhale after a maximal inspiration. A **forced vital capacity (FVC)** simply means that a person forces all air out of the lungs as fast as possible during expiration.

Normally, $FEV_1$/FVC is greater than 0.80, meaning that 80% of the air in the lungs is exhaled in the first second of expiration. This indicates that airflow out of the lung is not hindered; that is, airway resistance is low.

However, with airway obstruction, such as that caused by asthma (a disease that substantially increases airway resistance), it would be expected that the $FEV_1/FVC$ ratio is reduced. Indeed, in patients with asthma, it is typical for the $FEV_1$ to approach 40% of FVC.[2]

## CONTROL OF RESPIRATION

Most people tend to take breathing for granted until something goes wrong with it. Certainly, for much of the time throughout a day, you don't need to think about inhaling or exhaling; it just happens automatically, and the body regulates how fast and how deep a person needs to breathe. Under these circumstances, the control of respiration is largely involuntary. On the contrary, people with pulmonary disease and people who exercise, especially at high altitudes, become very aware of their breathing patterns. Likewise, there are times when we can directly control the rate and depth of breathing, for example, during a swim meet, while singing, or when a person goes deep-water diving. In this manner, the control of respiration is voluntary. Breathing is also influenced by changes in body posture and movement, by the time of day, by various states of emotional stress, and by eating and speaking.

The control of respiration is extremely complex. Despite this fact, the brain, in coordination with sensory information received from peripheral and central areas, precisely controls the rate and depth of breathing to achieve one primary goal: to provide the tissues with adequate oxygen to meet their metabolic needs. Consequently, changes in oxygen and carbon dioxide can have profound effects on respiratory control mechanisms. In general, RR and the depth of breathing, that is, the *rhythmicity* of breathing, is controlled by specialized areas in the brainstem known as the **respiratory control center**. The control of respiration during resting conditions is the focus of this chapter.

### Respiratory Control Center

Figure 6-8 illustrates the anatomical location of the respiratory control center in the brainstem. The **medulla oblongata** contains most of the respiratory control center. Within the medulla are two specialized groups of neurons that control the natural rhythmicity of breathing: the dorsal respiratory group (DRG) and the ventral respiratory group (VRG). Although still under intense investigation, it is thought that the DRG and VRG are reciprocal in their efforts to establish a sustained rhythmic pattern of inspiration and expiration. The DRG is thought to contain respiratory neurons that control mainly inspiration. Neurons travel via the phrenic nerve to stimulate the diaphragm and via the intercostal nerves to stimulate the external intercostal muscles during inspiration. In contrast, the VRG is thought to contain mainly neurons that control active expiration (remember, normal expiration is a passive process) and large inspirations.

**VIGNETTE continued**

■ Joey guides Amanda to gradually reduce her exercise intensity so that she is able to easily administer rescue medication via her prescribed inhaler. At first, Amanda says she can "push through" the episode, but Joey knows this goes against protocol for managing an EIA incident. Once Amanda's symptoms subside, Joey instructs Amanda to sit in the shade and drink some fluids to cool off. He reminds her to breathe deeply, in through the nose and out through the mouth. After class, Joey discusses the incident with Amanda. He learns that it had been quite a while since she had an attack, and therefore did not think it was important to discuss her condition with Joey. They agree to meet before her next scheduled exercise session to complete a full health history questionnaire.

In addition to the exercise being performed, in Amanda's case, an additional asthma trigger was likely environmental—possibly toxins present in the downtown park where they are exercising or the result of the hot, humid summer afternoon. Now that Joey knows about Amanda's asthma, in the future he should recommend that she avoid exercising at those times of day when allergens are at their peak—typically during morning and evening rush hour traffic—or during the hot afternoon hours.

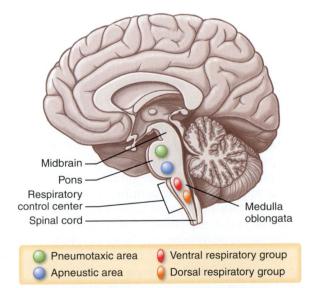

Midbrain
Pons
Respiratory control center
Spinal cord
Medulla oblongata

| ● Pneumotaxic area | ● Ventral respiratory group |
| ● Apneustic area | ● Dorsal respiratory group |

**Figure 6-8.** General location of the respiratory control centers in the medulla and pons. This area integrates and organizes all feedback from the central and peripheral nervous systems, and sends out signals to make adjustments in ventilation to meet metabolic demands.

Therefore, the VRG sends motor impulses to stimulate the abdominal muscles and the internal intercostals during active expiration and vigorous inhalations, but is largely inactive during normal quiet breathing.

Two additional regions of the brainstem, albeit to a lesser degree, are involved in respiratory control. These areas are located in the **pons** and work to fine tune the depth of breathing. These areas are referred to as the apneustic area and the pneumotaxic area. The apneustic area, derived from the word apnea, meaning cessation of breathing, appears to terminate inspiration. In this manner, the apneustic area may limit the depth and length of the inspiratory cycle by inhibiting the DRG so that expiration can proceed. The pneumotaxic area appears to inhibit both the inspiratory activity of the DRG and the apneustic area. Together, the apneustic and pneumotaxic areas modulate the pattern of inspiration and expiration to coordinate efficient breathing.

## Humoral Control

The respiratory control center adjusts ventilation in response to changes in the chemical composition of the peripheral and central internal environments. Alterations in the arterial partial pressure of carbon dioxide ($Pa_{CO_2}$), arterial partial pressure of oxygen ($Pa_{O_2}$), and changes in blood pH exert the most important influences on ventilation. For instance, increased partial pressure of carbon dioxide ($P_{CO_2}$), decreased partial pressure of oxygen ($P_{O_2}$), and decreased pH all cause increased ventilation. Conversely, an increase in ventilation tends to offset these changes and will, in turn, reduce $P_{CO_2}$, increase $P_{O_2}$, and elevate pH.

Ventilation is increased because specialized bodies of neuronal cells, termed **chemoreceptors**, sense mild changes in blood gases and $H^+$ concentrations. When a chemoreceptor senses a change in its local environment, it relays output messages to the respiratory control center, where adjustments are made in the rate and depth of breathing. This process returns the blood gas parameters back to normal. In this manner, the internal environment and the respiratory control center are partnered in negative-feedback loops that maintain normal concentrations of blood gases. The response of these receptors is very rapid, and their sensitivity is such that they are able to detect very small changes in blood gas variables on a breath-by-breath basis. Two main types of chemoreceptors modulate activity of the respiratory control center: peripheral chemoreceptors and central chemoreceptors. Collectively, the primary goals of the peripheral and central chemoreceptors are to fine-tune ventilation by supplying the control center with continuous breath-by-breath information on blood gas variables and pH levels.

## Peripheral Chemoreceptors

The primary **peripheral chemoreceptors** that help regulate the respiratory control center are located in the aortic arch and in the common carotid artery of the cardiovascular system. The receptors localized in the aorta are called **aortic bodies**, and those located in the carotid artery are called **carotid bodies**. Each of these chemoreceptors detects decreases in $Pa_{O_2}$, increases in $Pa_{CO_2}$, and decreases in blood pH (increased $H^+$ concentrations). Although less understood, there is some evidence to suggest that other peripheral receptors (chemoreceptors and mechanoreceptors) exist in the lungs, muscles, joints, and heart that help to increase ventilation during exercise.[3–7]

### VIGNETTE continued

■ Joey does some research later and learns that EIA can be effectively treated through lifestyle modification and medical management. With medical clearance to exercise and an asthma action plan in place, he will ensure that Amanda completes the appropriate tasks before exercise to prevent an asthma attack, identifies her specific asthma triggers, and knows what to do in the event of an attack, including when to contact her health-care provider or seek emergency medical treatment, or both. Importantly, her medications will always be on hand while she is exercising.

## Central Chemoreceptors

The **central chemoreceptors** are located in the medulla (Fig. 6-9). Although not in direct contact with the arterial blood, they are exposed to the cerebrospinal fluid and sense increases in $P_{CO_2}$ and $H^+$ concentrations. The central chemoreceptors do not respond to changes in $P_{O_2}$. Carbon dioxide rapidly diffuses from the blood across the blood–brain barrier. Increased cerebrospinal fluid, $P_{CO_2}$, or $H^+$ stimulates the central chemoreceptors to transmit signals to the respiratory control center, whereby the rate and depth of ventilation is increased. In turn, a rise in ventilation results in removal of carbon dioxide.

## Effect of Increased Arterial Partial Pressure of $CO_2$

As previously mentioned, $CO_2$ is a normal waste product of aerobic cellular metabolism and must be continuously removed from the body. One of the most efficient ways to remove this gas is to exhale it into the ambient air after it has been transported to the lungs. Therefore, it would make physiological sense for the respiratory system to increase ventilation when $CO_2$ concentrations rise. Indeed, an increased level of $CO_2$ in the arterial blood and cerebrospinal fluid is arguably the most powerful stimulus to increase ventilation. Figure 6-10 displays the changes in $V_E$ as a function of increased $P_{CO_2}$. Within physiological levels of carbon dioxide, ventilation increases linearly

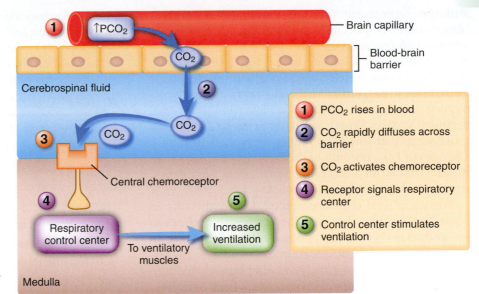

**Figure 6-9.** Control of ventilation through the central chemoreceptors. This is a visual description of how the brain directly influences the control of ventilation.

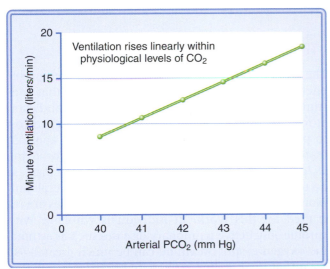

**Figure 6-10.** The influence of increasing arterial $P_{CO_2}$ on minute ventilation is demonstrated. The concentration of $CO_2$ in the blood is a potent stimulator of ventilation, and the relationship between $P_{CO_2}$ and minute ventilation is linear.

with an increase in $P_{CO_2}$. $Pa_{CO_2}$ is tightly regulated, and under normal circumstances, it is held remarkably constant (40–45 mm Hg), even during intense exercise. In general, an increase in $P_{CO_2}$ of 1 mm Hg leads to a 2- to 2.5-L/min increase in ventilation. When $Pa_{O_2}$ is reduced, the ventilatory response to increased $P_{CO_2}$ is amplified.

With respect to the peripheral chemoreceptors, the carotid bodies, probably because of their unique anatomical location (carotid arteries are the major blood supply vessel for the brain), appear to be more effective at sensing increased $Pa_{CO_2}$ than the aortic bodies. Similarly, the central chemoreceptors, located uniquely in the medulla at the interface with the cerebrospinal fluid, are in position to detect rapid increases in $P_{CO_2}$. Neural signals are then immediately sent from the central receptors to the respiratory control center

to increase ventilation. Notably, a decrease in $Pa_{CO_2}$ will have the opposite effect on the chemoreceptors. For example, hyperventilation will cause a decline in alveolar, arterial, and cerebrospinal fluid $P_{CO_2}$, which will decrease chemoreceptor activity (Box 6-2). As a result, the drive to ventilate is reduced.

### Effect of Decreased Arterial $PO_2$

Interestingly, reduced $Pa_{O_2}$ has little effect on the control of ventilation, especially in healthy people at sea-level

### Box 6-2. A Performance Benefit of Hyperventilation?

Have you ever observed a swimmer breathing rapidly before swimming underwater or maybe tried it yourself? If so, you experienced or witnessed a strategy that these individuals use with the thought that it will improve their performance. Voluntary hyperventilation, a deliberate increase in $\dot{V}_E$ beyond metabolic needs, can increase the duration a swimmer or diver can hold their breath. It is well-known that the most potent stimulus to breathe is an increase in carbon dioxide concentration in the blood. During hyperventilation, the concentration of carbon dioxide in the blood declines substantially, lowering the drive to breath; thus, you can hold your breath longer. However, the belief that hyperventilation will significantly increase blood oxygen content is incorrect and potentially dangerous. Blood oxygen levels may decrease significantly during the activity well before the concentration of carbon dioxide increases enough to stimulate breathing. Consequently, swimmers or active divers who hyperventilate may lose consciousness before they reach the surface. As the adage goes, "Don't try this at home!"

atmospheric pressure. Typically, ventilation is not stimulated until $Pa_{O_2}$ declines to less than 60 mm Hg, as when ascending to higher altitudes with lower atmospheric pressures. The increased $\dot{V}_E$ that occurs in response to decreased $Pa_{O_2}$ is called the **hypoxic ventilatory response** (hypoxic means "low blood oxygen") and can be observed in Figure 6-11.[8] As $Pa_{O_2}$ declines, $\dot{V}_E$ rises slowly at higher pressures, and then more steeply at lower pressures (hypoxic threshold). Changes in $P_{CO_2}$ potentiate the hypoxic ventilatory response; that is, for a given increase in $P_{CO_2}$, ventilation rises more abruptly at a similar $Pa_{O_2}$.

The peripheral chemoreceptors, mainly the carotid bodies rather than the aortic bodies, sense declines in $P_{O_2}$ and relay this information to the respiratory control center to increase ventilation. In turn, increased ventilation will lead to more oxygen being transported into the lungs in an attempt to increase $Pa_{O_2}$ back to normal values. As mentioned earlier, the central chemoreceptors are not involved in monitoring $Pa_{O_2}$.

### Effect of Decreased Arterial pH

A reduction of blood pH (acidosis) in response to increased $H^+$ levels is another mechanism that increases ventilation. Recall the influence of increased $Pa_{CO_2}$ on $H^+$ concentrations in the tissues. As $P_{CO_2}$ increases in arterial blood, carbonic acid rapidly dissociates to bicarbonate and $H^+$. Under normal circumstances, ventilation rises linearly with changes in $H^+$ concentrations. As the blood becomes more acidic (pH <7.40), the peripheral chemoreceptors send impulses to the brain to increase ventilation. $CO_2$ is then exhaled from the body and $Pa_{CO_2}$ decreases, leading to a reduction in $H^+$ concentrations (i.e., an increase in blood pH back to normal). The central

chemoreceptors also respond to changes in the pH level of the cerebrospinal fluid. However, their influence takes a bit longer to ensue because it is relatively difficult for $H^+$ to cross the blood–brain barrier. Figure 6-12 illustrates the chemoreceptor control of ventilation.

## In Your Own Words

Your grandfather loves to backpack in the high altitudes of the Rocky Mountains. However, in the first few days of ascending to altitude, he feels noticeably fatigued, short of breath, and somewhat nauseated. He mentions to you that these signs and symptoms tend to limit his enjoyment and, in some cases, have led him to end his backpacking trips early. How would you describe to your grandfather the changes that occur to the respiratory system that might explain his high-altitude symptoms?

## THE WORK OF BREATHING

The work of breathing is associated with a measurable energy cost, as the body calls upon muscles that consume oxygen in the act of moving the lungs and chest at rest and especially during exercise. The oxygen cost to perform the work of breathing at rest is approximately 5% of total oxygen consumption, or 6 mL $O_2$/min. During exercise, the oxygen cost may increase up to 30% of total oxygen consumption as overall pulmonary ventilation increases and more muscles are recruited for this work. In individuals who live with chronic obstructive pulmonary diseases such as asthma, the oxygen cost of breathing can be much greater—so great that their ability to exercise or perform activities of daily living is severely limited. In this section, the basic mechanics of inspiration and expiration are reviewed, followed by a discussion of the accessory muscles of ventilation that are used during exercise.

### Mechanics of Inspiration and Expiration at Rest

Ventilation can be split into two separate events: inspiration and expiration. At rest, the process of inspiration is much more active compared with the more passive function of expiration. During exercise, it is a much different story for expiration.

### Inspiration

Inspiration, or flow of air into the lungs, is primarily controlled by the contraction of the diaphragm during quiet breathing. This muscle is thin and dome-shaped, and sits just above the abdominal contents where it anchors to the lower rib cage. The phrenic nerve, originating from nerves in the cervical spine region (third to fifth vertebrae), innervates the diaphragm to stimulate the muscle to contract. Any damage to the spinal cord

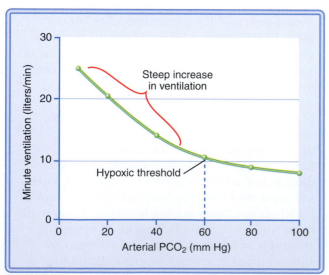

**Figure 6-11.** The influence of decreasing $P_{O_2}$ on minute ventilation. Compared with $P_{CO_2}$, $P_{O_2}$ has a nonlinear relationship with minute ventilation. Following the line from right to left, once the $P_{O_2}$ reaches a certain level (60 mm Hg), minute ventilation increases sharply. The point at which you observe a large increase in ventilation is termed the *hypoxic threshold*.

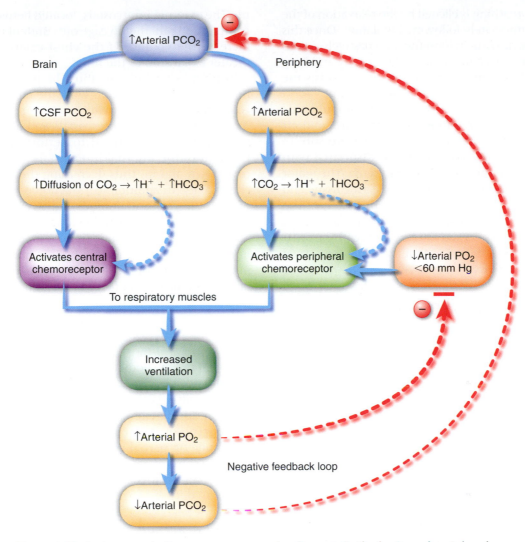

**Figure 6-12.** An increase in $P_{CO_2}$ causes a cascade of events in the brain and peripheral vasculature that both lead to the eventual stimulation of the muscles of ventilation to contract and increase the rate of ventilation.

above this region (or to the nerve itself) can cause paralysis of the diaphragm, in which case the individual can no longer breathe on his or her own.

The contraction of the diaphragm causes a slight increase in the volume (vertical and horizontal displacement) of the chest cavity, which allows the lungs to expand. This expansion causes a decrease in intrapulmonic pressure below that of atmospheric pressure, and air will flow inward from an area of higher pressure to lower pressure. The relatively small reduction of intrapulmonic pressure needed to inflate the lungs is due to the excellent compliance of the alveoli and low airway resistance in a normal lung. When compliance is low and/or airway resistance (as in asthma) is high, the difference between intrapulmonic and atmospheric pressure must be greater. Figure 6-13 shows the differences between atmospheric and intrapulmonic pressures at sea level for both inspiration and expiration.

## Expiration

The passive nature of expiration, or airflow out of the lungs, does not call for muscular contraction. Expiration

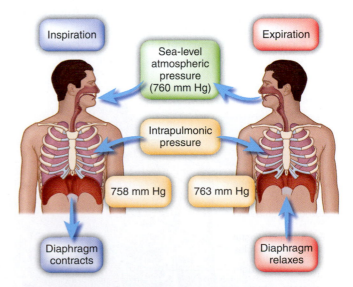

**Figure 6-13.** The mechanics of quiet breathing at rest. Note on the left, the diaphragm contracts down, increasing the volume of the lungs and decreasing intrapulmonic pressure. On expiration, the diaphragm relaxes, the lungs recoil, and pressure is increased in the lung.

during quiet breathing is elicited by the relaxation of the diaphragm immediately following inhalation. Once this occurs, the elastic tissue within the lung passively recoils in conjunction with a decrease in chest cavity and lung volumes. Surface tension within the alveoli assists the elastic recoil function in decreasing lung volume.

This movement causes an increase in intrapulmonic pressure above that of atmospheric pressure, and air will flow outward from an area of higher pressure to lower pressure. A pulmonary disease associated with the destruction of lung tissue is emphysema. The major problem with this disease is the loss of elastic tissue and the ability to expel air normally. Overinflation of the lung occurs simultaneously because of increased lung compliance, which overtaxes accessory breathing muscles involved with expiration that are usually reserved for use during activity.

## Muscles of Ventilation During Exercise

As discussed earlier, during quiet inspiration, the most important muscle at rest is the diaphragm. However, as exercise intensity increases, assistance from other muscles is necessary for proper ventilation. Collectively, these muscles are labeled the **accessory muscles of ventilation** and are specifically recruited during exercise. They rely greatly on aerobic metabolism for energy because they have to contract during each breath; thus, endurance exercise training will have the greatest impact at improving the work capacity of these muscles. Figure 6-14 illustrates the accessory muscles that are used to support inspiration and expiration as ventilation increases because of activity.

During inspiration, the lungs are required to fill with more air for greater gas exchange and can only do so with greater chest wall movement. The diaphragm is still engaged in this process as it is during rest through contraction and pulling down on the lungs. Additional muscles used during inspiration include the scalenes and sternocleidomastoid, both located superior to the clavicle, that contract and pull the rib cage and sternum

up. The external intercostals, located between the ribs, contract and pull the rib cage out. Both of these actions increase the volume of the chest cavity to allow for greater expansion of the lungs.

During expiration, air must be pushed out of the lungs more forcefully than what the natural elastic recoil of the lungs can provide for the removal of carbon dioxide. The internal intercostals and abdominal wall musculature are recruited to perform this task. The function of the internal intercostals is to pull the rib cage down and in, thus decreasing the volume of the chest cavity. In addition, contraction of the abdominal wall by the rectus abdominis, transversus abdominis, and external and internal oblique muscles pushes the abdominal contents and diaphragm up toward the lungs, increasing the intrapulmonic pressure to expel more air. The abdominal muscles are extremely important for the process of forced expiration.

## GAS DIFFUSION

The ability of the body to diffuse gases in and out of the alveoli and the tissues (muscle, in particular) quickly and efficiently is an essential physiological process at rest and during exercise performance. In this section, the concepts of partial pressure of gases and the impacts of altitude on partial pressures are explained. In addition, the sites for gas diffusion are described, as well as how certain factors affect the ability of the lungs and tissues to diffuse oxygen and carbon dioxide.

## Partial Pressure of Gases

The three main gases that require our attention in this section are oxygen, carbon dioxide, and nitrogen. In a gas mixture, each gas exerts an individual pressure unique from the others relative to the total pressure, which is referred to as the **partial pressure** of that gas. Also in this mixture, the overall or total pressure is equal to the sum of the partial pressures uniquely exerted by

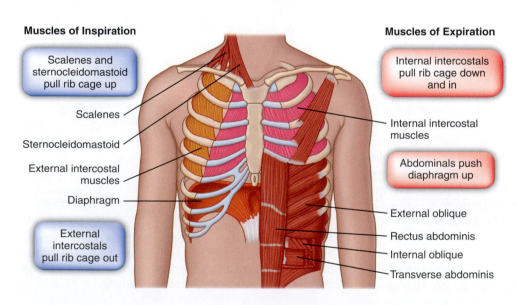

**Muscles of Inspiration**

Scalenes and sternocleidomastoid pull rib cage up

Scalenes

Sternocleidomastoid

External intercostal muscles

Diaphragm

External intercostals pull rib cage out

**Muscles of Expiration**

Internal intercostals pull rib cage down and in

Internal intercostal muscles

Abdominals push diaphragm up

External oblique

Rectus abdominis

Internal oblique

Transverse abdominis

**Figure 6-14.** Accessory muscles of ventilation.

each individual gas (**Dalton's law**). Thus, if the total pressure of a gas mixture is 500 mm Hg, then each individual partial pressure when added together will equal 500 mm Hg: $P_{Total} = P_1 + P_2 + P_3$, where P represents partial pressure of each gas or total pressure.

The partial pressure of a gas is determined by its specific percent or fractional content in the gas mixture. Thus, to calculate $PO_2$ in the atmosphere, we need to first discern how much oxygen there is in the atmosphere. The air in the atmosphere is made up of 20.93% (or 0.2093) oxygen, 0.03% (or 0.0003) carbon dioxide, and 79.04% (or 0.7904) nitrogen no matter what altitude you are at, be it sea level or high altitude. Calculating the partial pressure of a gas is as simple as multiplying the barometric or atmospheric pressure (i.e., the force exerted against a surface by the weight of air above that surface) by the fractional content of that gas (see later Doing the Math section to review the calculation of partial pressure in atmospheric air at sea level and at higher altitude).

The partial pressures for the gases, in particular, oxygen, are much lower at altitude compared with sea level. At higher altitude, the misconception is that there is less oxygen (content) in the air compared with lower altitudes. The difference between sea-level and higher altitude conditions is that atmospheric pressure is lower at higher altitude, not the content of oxygen. This pressure difference ultimately affects the partial pressure of gases. The pressure difference is due, in part, to the effects of gravity, which forces gas molecules closer together in air nearer to Earth's surface. As altitude increases and the effects of gravity on the air are lessened, gas molecules spread out, lowering the partial pressure of each gas. Individuals or athletes who are active at higher altitudes often report more difficulty in breathing, or that their breathing is more labored and subsequently their exercise performance is poorer. This feeling is due to a greater ventilatory drive needed to help maintain alveolar oxygen pressure gradients in the lung when atmospheric partial pressure is decreased.

## Factors That Affect Gas Diffusion

In general, gases diffuse along their individual pressure gradient from areas of high concentration to low concentration. In addition, three more factors are linked to the rate of gas diffusion in the lungs and tissues, and the interaction among these factors is best described through **Fick's law for diffusion**. This law establishes the directly proportional relationship between the rate of gas diffusion and gas solubility, pressure gradient, and surface area. The relationship between gas diffusion and diffusion space is inversely proportional according to this law. Figure 6-15 illustrates the factors that affect gas diffusion.

## Gas Solubility

Carbon dioxide has a 20-fold higher solubility coefficient in blood (factor 1 in Fig. 6-15) compared with

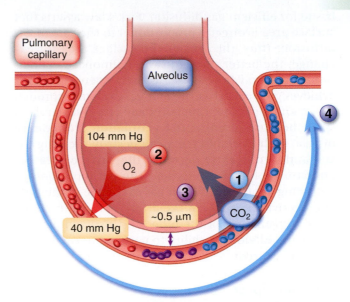

**Figure 6-15.** The four factors that influence the rate of diffusion: (1) gas solubility, (2) pressure gradient, (3) diffusion space, and (4) surface area for exchange. Gas solubility, pressure gradient, and surface area are positively related to an increase in the rate of gas diffusion. Diffusion space is inversely related to the rate of gas diffusion.

oxygen. Just based on this factor, better solubility permits a much greater rate of exchange for carbon dioxide. Thus, gas solubility is directly proportional to the ability to diffuse gas. In addition, this greater solubility affords for a much smaller pressure gradient for carbon dioxide diffusion, whereas oxygen diffusion requires a much greater pressure gradient to drive oxygen from alveolus to red blood cell.

### Pressure Gradient

For gases to move from alveoli to blood or blood to tissue, an appropriate pressure gradient or difference between the partial pressures across the gas exchange interface must be present (factor 2 in Fig. 6-15). In the case of oxygen, gas molecules will move down their gradient from high pressure in the alveoli to low pressure in the pulmonary capillary. This diffusion will continue to occur until the partial pressures across the alveoli and capillary equilibrate, and a gradient no longer exists. According to Fick's law, a greater pressure gradient translates into a greater diffusion rate for a gas. The pressure gradient for oxygen must be considerably higher than that of carbon dioxide to overcome poor solubility in the fluid medium and to maintain the same rate of exchange for both gases.

### Surface Area for Exchange

Surface area refers to the total area of contact where gas exchange will occur, either between alveoli and capillary (factor 4 in Fig. 6-15) or tissue and capillary. As described earlier, the total surface area for gas exchange is very large ($\sim$65–70 m²); this, combined with a small diffusion space, makes the lung an ideal tissue for efficient gas diffusion. Fick's law asserts that surface area is directly proportional to the rate of gas diffusion; thus, the greater the surface area for exchange, the better the diffusion. Pulmonary ventilation and blood flow increase with exercise, which achieves greater surface area for gas exchange through the opening of more capillaries and less alveolar dead space because of enhanced ventilation. Pulmonary disease such as emphysema can destroy the lung tissue and significantly decrease the surface area between alveoli and capillaries. The pathophysiology will bring about insufficient gas exchange in the lung and decrease the $PO_2$ in the arterial blood. In effect, poor oxygenation of the blood in this example will affect an individual's ability to perform normal activities and exercise.

### Diffusion Space

Diffusion space (factor 3 in Fig. 6-15) is the physical distance that gas must travel across the alveolar–capillary interface (between red blood cell and inside of the alveoli) and the tissue–capillary interface (between red blood cell and tissue). This distance is determined by the individual thickness of the alveolar membrane (or tissue membrane) and capillary wall, plasma, and the interstitial space between capillary and alveoli (or tissue). This space is filled with fluid that, along with plasma in the capillary, can affect the exchange of gases (i.e., oxygen) that have poor solubility in liquid.

Diffusion space is inversely related to the rate of gas diffusion; thereby the greater the distance a gas must travel for exchange, the poorer the diffusion rate. Certain issues linked to pulmonary disease can increase the diffusion space through increasing the interstitial fluid (e.g., edema) or thickness of the alveolar membrane (e.g., pulmonary fibrosis), which can greatly affect the oxygenation of the blood. The thickness of the alveolar–capillary interface is normally very small, with estimations of less than 0.5 μm thick. This structural characteristic greatly aids in the quick diffusion of gases to and from the alveoli. In contrast with the alveolar–capillary interface, the distance between capillary and muscle cell is considerably greater at rest. However, during exercise, this problem is solved by increasing muscle blood flow through the opening of more capillaries in the muscle, thus improving the surface area for gas exchange and decreasing diffusion differences. These two factors improve the diffusion rate of gases to and from the tissues during exercise.

## VIGNETTE continued

■ Although medication is very effective in managing EIA, Amanda and Joey can implement other measures to limit her asthma symptoms during and after future workouts. One of the most effective strategies is to properly warm up before exercise and adequately cool down after exercise. A proper warm-up may help the airways adjust to the stress imposed by changes in temperature and humidity of the inspired air. Joey recommends that Amanda warm up for 10 to 15 minutes *before* beginning her exercise routine. This strategy can decrease the severity of asthma symptoms experienced during exercise and may improve the effectiveness of Amanda's pre-exercise inhaled bronchodilators (it may take up to 10 minutes for bronchodilators to achieve maximal effects).

## RESEARCH HIGHLIGHT

### Exercise-Induced Hypoxemia: Causes and Concerns

It is generally accepted that the respiratory system does not limit performance of prolonged submaximal exercise in healthy people. Indeed, the concentration of oxygen in the arterial blood is held stable throughout various intensities of dynamic exercise in untrained and trained men. However, in the early 1980s and 1990s, a series of studies conducted by Powers and colleagues and Dempsey and coworkers strongly indicated that, at near-maximum exercise intensities (>90% $\dot{V}O_{2max}$), the respiratory system appears to limit performance in elite endurance-trained cyclists and runners.[4-6] It was reported that approximately 50% of highly trained endurance male athletes experience significant reductions in oxygen saturation, a phenomenon called *exercise-induced hypoxemia* (EIH; hypoxemia means "low blood oxygen"). Recent data indicate that this problem may be more frequent in women[9] and in people of various ages, including elderly men,[10] but large descriptive data on its widespread prevalence are currently limited.

Currently, the precise mechanisms that contribute to EIH in elite athletes are not completely understood, but intense investigations have recently provided important insight into this issue. It was originally thought that the velocity of red blood cells moving through the alveolar–capillary networks was too fast for red blood cells to adequately load

## Sites for Gas Diffusion

The two main sites for gas diffusion in the body are at the alveoli and at the tissues. For discussion purposes, this section focuses on the tissues and cells that involve skeletal muscle. Figure 6-16 illustrates the changes in $P_{O_2}$ and $P_{CO_2}$ throughout the cardiovascular and pulmonary system at rest.

## Diffusion at the Alveoli: External Respiration

Gas exchange at the alveoli is termed **external respiration**. The difference between atmospheric and alveolar air (at sea level and altitude) for $P_{O_2}$ and $P_{CO_2}$ can be seen in the sample calculations in the following Doing the Math section. As air is drawn into the lungs, it is warmed to normal body temperature (~37°C) and fully humidified. When air is 100% humidified, water vapor occupies space in the air, forcing gas molecules to spread out, which decreases the total gas pressure by 47 mm Hg at a temperature of 37°C. Thus, when any calculation of partial pressure of gas is made in the lung, the atmospheric pressure must be adjusted for water vapor partial pressure.

Figure 6-16 shows that the $P_{O_2}$ and $P_{CO_2}$ in alveolar air are approximately 104 and 40 mm Hg, respectively. The gas partial pressures in blood entering the lung are 40 mm Hg for oxygen and 45 mm Hg for carbon dioxide. Thus, a significant pressure gradient is set to facilitate appropriate gas exchange from alveoli (higher pressure) to capillary (lower pressure) for oxygen and capillary (higher pressure) to alveoli (lower pressure) for carbon dioxide. Remember, the pressure gradient for carbon dioxide does not need to be as great as oxygen's because of a superior solubility coefficient.

As blood passes through the pulmonary capillaries, the time it takes for gas partial pressures in blood to fully equilibrate with the alveoli is in the order of 0.25 second at rest. This time decreases as the rate of blood flow through the lung increases (e.g., during exercise). Once the exchange occurs at the alveoli, the blood leaving the lung has a partial pressure of 100 mm Hg for oxygen and 40 mm Hg for carbon dioxide. These partial pressures are maintained until the arterial blood is circulated into the tissues.

## Diffusion at the Tissues: Internal Respiration

Gas exchange at the level of the tissues is termed *internal respiration*. Figure 6-16 shows that the oxygen and carbon dioxide partial pressures in blood entering the muscle are 100 and 40 mm Hg, and within the muscle tissues 40 and 45 mm Hg, respectively. Thus, another considerable pressure gradient exists to facilitate appropriate gas exchange from capillary (higher pressure) to tissue (lower pressure) for oxygen and from tissue (higher pressure) to capillary (lower pressure) for carbon dioxide.

As blood passes through the muscle capillaries, the time it takes for gas exchange to occur is similar to that in the lungs (0.25 second at rest). After the exchange occurs, the blood leaving the muscle has a partial pressure of 40 mm Hg for oxygen and 45 mm Hg for carbon dioxide. These partial pressures are maintained until the blood is circulated back to the lungs.

During maximal exercise, the $P_{O_2}$ can be as low as 3 mm Hg, and the $P_{CO_2}$ can be as high as 90 mm Hg in the muscle. This widening of the pressure gradient for oxygen ensures an appropriate diffusion rate into the muscle and to the mitochondria, where it is needed for regenerating ATP through oxidative energy pathways. The increased pressure gradient for carbon dioxide facilitates a greater release from metabolic pathways within muscle to the blood where it can be blown off at the lung. The important processes of loading, transporting, and unloading these two gases are described in the next section.

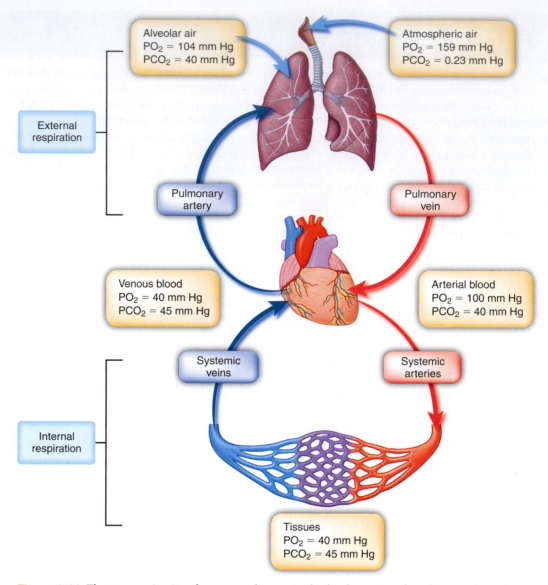

**Figure 6-16.** The two main sites for gas exchange in the body: external and internal respiration. Also, note the differences in the partial pressure of gases among alveolar air, arterial blood, muscle tissue, and venous blood at rest.

## DOING THE MATH:

Calculate the partial pressure of nitrogen, oxygen, and carbon dioxide in the atmospheric air at sea level ($P_B = 760$) and at higher altitude conditions (Pike's Peak at $P_B$ ~460), and calculate oxygen and carbon dioxide partial pressures in the alveoli under these same conditions. Remember to correct barometric pressure using the water vapor pressure when calculating partial pressure of gases within the lung (use 47 mm Hg at 37°C body temperature). Use 14.6% and 5.6% for oxygen and carbon dioxide percent content, respectively.

**Calculate partial pressure of gases at sea level: atmospheric air (assume 0% humidity)**

*Oxygen: 760 mm Hg × 0.2093 = 159.1 mm Hg
*Carbon dioxide: 760 mm Hg × 0.0003 = 0.23 mm Hg
*Nitrogen: 760 mm Hg × 0.7904 = 600.7 mm Hg

**Calculate partial pressure of gases at altitude: atmospheric air (assume 0% humidity)**

*Oxygen: 460 mm Hg × 0.2093 = 96.3 mm Hg
*Carbon dioxide: 460 mm Hg × 0.0003 = 0.14 mm Hg
*Nitrogen: 460 mm Hg × 0.7904 = 363.6 mm Hg

**DOING THE MATH:–cont'd**

*The numbers indicate that as altitude increases, total atmospheric pressure decreases along with partial pressures of gases, and content of gases remains the same.

**Calculate partial pressure of gases at sea level: alveolar air (assume 100% humidity)**

*Oxygen: 760 mm Hg – 47 mm Hg = 713 mm Hg × 0.146 = 104.1 mm Hg
*Carbon dioxide: 760 mm Hg – 47 mm Hg = 713 mm Hg × 0.056 = 40 mm Hg

**Calculate partial pressure of gases at altitude: alveolar air (assume 100% humidity)**

*Oxygen: 460 mm Hg – 47 mm Hg = 413 mm Hg × 0.146 = 60.3 mm Hg
*Carbon dioxide: 460 mm Hg – 47 mm Hg = 413 mm Hg × 0.056 = 23.1 mm Hg

*These numbers indicate that as altitude increases, the partial pressures of gases decrease within the alveoli, which lead to a change in pressure gradient that ultimately affects gas exchange.

## TRANSPORT OF OXYGEN AND CARBON DIOXIDE

The means of transport and delivery of oxygen and carbon dioxide through the cardiovascular and pulmonary circulatory systems vary based on several factors, such as the individual solubility of the gases in solution, the partial pressure of the gases in the blood, and the presence of hemoglobin in the blood.

### Oxygen Transport in the Blood

The two means of oxygen transport in the blood are: (1) dissolved in the plasma and (2) bound to hemoglobin. As you will discover in this section, the overall amount of oxygen transported through each method is very different.

### Dissolved Oxygen in the Blood

Dissolved oxygen in plasma accounts for approximately 1.5% of total oxygen in the blood. This is due to the very low solubility coefficient of oxygen in plasma, especially when compared with the coefficient for carbon dioxide. The dissolvability of oxygen (or any gas) is proportional to the individual $PO_2$ (Henry's law). At a partial pressure of 100 mm Hg, a value that is observed in arterial blood, the total volume of oxygen dissolved per liter of blood is equal to 3 mL oxygen. Consider that the total blood volume in the cardiovascular system is normally around 5 L and the human heart recirculates this total volume every minute. Doing the math, the total amount of dissolved oxygen in the blood is equal to 15 mL (3 mL $O_2$/L blood × 5 L blood). At rest, the body uses approximately 250 mL oxygen per minute for metabolic processes, and the cardiovascular system delivers only 15 mL dissolved oxygen per minute. Clearly, there is a mismatch between demand and supply in this example. Therefore, the blood requires a more effective method for transporting sufficient amounts of oxygen to active tissues at rest and during exercise.

### Hemoglobin and Oxygen Carrying Capacity of Blood

**Hemoglobin** is an oxygen binding protein on the red blood cell. Roughly 98.5% of oxygen in the blood is bound to and transported by hemoglobin, and the presence of this protein increases the total blood oxygen capacity 70 times. It helps to understand the basic characteristics of hemoglobin. It is made up of an iron-containing compound called *heme*, which is directly involved in the oxygen binding process, and a protein structure called *globin*. There are approximately 250 million hemoglobin molecules on each red blood cell, and there are 20 to 30 trillion red blood cells in the blood. That is a lot of hemoglobin! Hemoglobin can bind one molecule of oxygen at each heme group for a total of four oxygen molecules per hemoglobin. The specific terms used to describe hemoglobin when oxygen is reversibly bound to it is **oxyhemoglobin**, and when oxygen is not bound to hemoglobin, it is called **deoxyhemoglobin**. In the following equation, oxyhemoglobin is formed from left to right, and deoxyhemoglobin is formed from right to left:

$$O_2 + Hb \leftrightarrow HbO_2$$

The content of oxygen in arterial blood ($CaO_2$) and the content of oxygen in mixed venous blood ($CvO_2$) are affected by the amount of oxygen bound to 1 g hemoglobin, the total concentration of hemoglobin in the blood, and the relative amount of hemoglobin that is saturated with oxygen. For example, the following equation can be used to determine $CaO_2$:

$$CaO_2 = 1.34 \text{ mL } O_2/g \text{ Hb} \times \text{grams Hb/L blood} \times \%O_2 \text{ saturation}$$

$CvO_2$ is also calculated using the same equation. When fully saturated, every gram of hemoglobin in the blood has an oxygen binding capacity of 1.34 mL oxygen. Hemoglobin concentrations normally vary between 140 and 180 g Hb/L blood for adult males and 120 and 160 g Hb/L blood for adult females. In addition, hemoglobin concentrations can be influenced by activity level (i.e., endurance athletes will have a higher concentration), disease state (e.g., anemia), ethnicity, hormones, and even where you reside (e.g., high altitude vs. sea level). Blood oxygen content is also affected by the saturation of hemoglobin with oxygen. Represented as a percentage, the **oxygen saturation** is the ratio between oxyhemoglobin and the oxygen carrying capacity of blood (arterial or mixed venous). Nearly 98% of all hemoglobin molecules are saturated with oxygen under sea-level or low-altitude conditions. This number will change based on factors such as the presence or severity of chronic pulmonary disease, blood pH, and $PO_2$ changes (e.g., altitude). These concepts are applied in some of the following calculations.

## Fick Equation

The Fick equation illustrates the factors and the relationship between those factors that determine whole body **oxygen consumption**, or $\dot{V}O_2$. The Fick equation is as follows:

$$\dot{V}O_2 = \dot{Q} \times (a - v)O_2 \text{ diff}$$

### DOING THE MATH:

Your female client has a resting arterial and mixed venous blood oxygen saturation of 97% and 75%, respectively; a mixed venous blood oxygen saturation of 30% during exercise; and a hemoglobin concentration of 140 g Hb/L blood. Calculate your client's $Cao_2$ and $Cvo_2$ at rest and $Cvo_2$ during exercise.

**Resting $Cao_2$**

  *$Cao_2 = 1.34$ mL $O_2$/g Hb × g Hb/L blood × %$O_2$ saturation
  *$Cao_2 = 1.34$ mL $O_2$/g Hb × 140 g Hb/L blood × 0.97
  *$Cao_2 = 182$ mL $O_2$/L blood

**Resting $Cvo_2$**

  *$Cvo_2 = 1.34$ mL $O_2$/g Hb × g Hb/L blood × %$O_2$ saturation
  *$Cvo_2 = 1.34$ mL $O_2$/g Hb × 140 g Hb/L blood × 0.75
  *$Cvo_2 = 141$ mL $O_2$/L blood

**Exercise $Cvo_2$**

  *$Cvo_2 = 1.34$ mL $O_2$/g Hb × g Hb/L blood × %$O_2$ saturation
  *$Cvo_2 = 1.34$ mL $O_2$/g Hb × 140 g Hb/L blood × 0.30
  *$Cvo_2 = 56$ mL $O_2$/L blood

  *The %$O_2$ saturation value is entered into the equation as a fraction or decimal value and not as a percent.

According to the Fick equation, originally published by Adolph Fick in 1870, total body oxygen consumption is dependent on two factors: oxygen delivery via blood flow ($\dot{Q}$) and the total amount of oxygen extracted by the body for metabolic processes (arterial-venous oxygen difference [a – v$O_2$ diff]). **Cardiac output**, or $\dot{Q}$, is the total amount of blood (in liters) circulated through the cardiovascular system per minute. It serves as an excellent measure of blood-flow dynamics and overall cardiac performance in the body.

The **(a – v)$O_2$ difference** is the difference between $Cao_2$ and $Cvo_2$. The difference reflects the oxygen extracted and consumed by bodily tissues; however, it mostly represents skeletal muscle oxygen uptake versus other tissues during increasing exercise intensity. To better understand the Fick equation concept, calculate oxygen consumption using some physiological values.

### DOING THE MATH:

Your male client has a resting arterial and mixed venous blood oxygen saturation of 98% and 73%, respectively, and a hemoglobin concentration of 160 g Hb/L blood. His resting cardiac output is 5 L blood/min. During exercise, his cardiac output increases to 10 L blood/min and his mixed venous blood oxygen saturation decreases to 50%. Calculate his oxygen consumption ($\dot{V}O_2$) at rest and during exercise.

**\*Resting condition**
**First, calculate $CaO_2$.**

  *$CaO_2 = 1.34$ mL $O_2$/g Hb × g Hb/L blood × %$O_2$ saturation
  *$CaO_2 = 1.34$ mL $O_2$/g Hb × 160 g Hb/L blood × 0.98
  *$CaO_2 = 210$ mL $O_2$/L blood

**Next, calculate $CvO_2$.**

  *$CvO_2 = 1.34$ mL $O_2$/g Hb × g Hb/L blood × %$O_2$ saturation
  *$CvO_2 = 1.34$ mL $O_2$/g Hb × 160 g Hb/L blood × 0.73
  *$CvO_2 = 157$ mL $O_2$/L blood

**Finally, calculate $\dot{V}O_2$ using the Fick equation.**

  *$\dot{V}O_2 = \dot{Q} \times (a - v)O_2$ diff
  *$\dot{V}O_2 = 5$ L blood/min × (210 mL $O_2$/L blood – 157 mL $O_2$/L blood)
  *$\dot{V}O_2 = 5$ L blood/min × (53 mL $O_2$/L blood)
  *$\dot{V}O_2 = 265$ mL $O_2$/min

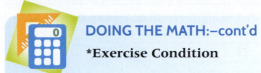

## DOING THE MATH:–cont'd

### *Exercise Condition

For exercise, assume the $CaO_2$ remains the same from rest and only calculate $CvO_2$ during exercise.

$*CvO_2 = 1.34$ mL $O_2$/g Hb $\times$ g Hb/L blood $\times$ %$O_2$ saturation

$*CvO_2 = 1.34$ mL $O_2$/g Hb $\times$ 160 g Hb/L blood $\times$ 0.50

$*CvO_2 = 107$ mL $O_2$/L blood

Next, calculate $\dot{V}O_2$ using the Fick equation.

$*\dot{V}O_2 = Q \times (a - v)O_2$ diff

$*\dot{V}O_2 = 10$ L blood/min $\times$ (210 mL $O_2$/L blood – 107 mL $O_2$/L blood)

$*\dot{V}O_2 = 10$ L blood/min $\times$ (103 mL $O_2$/L blood)

$*\dot{V}O_2 = 1,030$ mL $O_2$/min

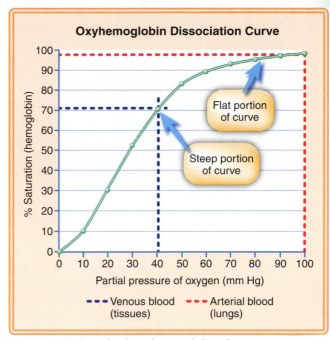

**Figure 6-17.** Standard oxyhemoglobin dissociation curve.

## Hemoglobin-Oxygen Saturation: Oxyhemoglobin Dissociation Curve

The standard oxyhemoglobin dissociation curve is an important instrument for understanding how hemoglobin loads oxygen at the lungs and unloads it to the tissues at various $Po_2$. Thus, the dissociation curve demonstrates the relationship between hemoglobin oxygen saturation (*y*-axis) and the $Po_2$ (*x*-axis; Fig. 6-17). As shown in Figure 6-17, this saturation–partial pressure relationship is not linear. Following the curve from low to high $Po_2$, hemoglobin will more readily bind oxygen at partial pressures associated with the beginning and middle of the curve. Eventually, the curve will slowly reach a plateau as hemoglobin binds its maximum four oxygen molecules to become fully saturated.

Remember, the $Po_2$ provides the driving force to load hemoglobin with oxygen to increase arterial blood oxygen content *at the alveoli*. In contrast, low $PO_2$ *at the tissues* accommodates an unloading of oxygen from hemoglobin. The nonlinear, sigmoidal shape of the oxyhemoglobin dissociation curve in Figure 6-17 provides a few advantages at rest and during exercise at these two exchange sites. To begin with, the curve is fairly level (labeled as "flat portion of curve") for partial pressures greater than 60 mm Hg, a value commonly observed in systemic arterial blood or in the pulmonary capillaries. The application is that oxygen diffusion at the lung, arterial hemoglobin saturation, and arterial blood content will remain relatively stable even in cases when $Po_2$ decreases from 100 to 60 mm Hg (e.g., altitude, aging, mild asthma, maximal exercise in some individuals such as athletes).

Moving from right to left in Figure 6-17, the curve begins a steady and rapid decline (labeled as the "steep portion of curve") below the $Po_2$ of 50 mm Hg, which are values generally observed in systemic veins or in the peripheral tissue capillaries. The application for this portion of the curve is that significant amounts of oxygen can be unloaded to the active tissues more easily in cases of greater demand with only slight changes to the $Po_2$ (e.g., increasing exercise intensity in athletic performance, hypoxia). The ease of unloading is due to a diminishing of the affinity of hemoglobin for oxygen as partial pressure steadily decreases toward 0 mm Hg. Thus, at the steep portion of the curve, smaller changes in partial pressure (approximately between 0 and 50 mm Hg) equal larger comparative changes in hemoglobin oxygen saturation (approximately between 0% and 85%).

Last, by comparing the oxygen saturation value at the uppermost portion of the curve (~98% in arterial blood) with the value at a partial pressure of 40 mm Hg (~70% in venous blood), you can get a sense for the relative amount of oxygen taken up by the tissues at rest (~28%). Observing the curve across this range provides a visual illustration of the a − vO₂ difference that exists across the tissue capillaries. As exercise intensity increases, a decrease in venous oxygen partial pressure should be viewed as a reflection of increased oxygen demand and uptake at the tissues, which will cause a widening of the arterial-venous oxygen difference.

## Factors That Affect Hemoglobin–Oxygen Saturation

The degree of affinity with which hemoglobin binds oxygen can be affected by factors other than the $Po_2$, such as pH, 2,3-bisphosphoglycerate (BPG), temperature, and $Pco_2$. An altered hemoglobin-oxygen affinity will elicit changes in overall blood hemoglobin-oxygen saturation that can be detected by a shifting of the standard oxyhemoglobin dissociation curve in two directions: (1) downward and to the right, and (2) upward and to the left. A shift to the right, called the **Bohr effect**, indicates a decreased affinity of hemoglobin for oxygen (Fig. 6-18). The advantage gained is that, for a given partial pressure (the two vertical lines), the unloading of oxygen (difference between the horizontal lines) is enhanced with this shift. For each example, the oxygen saturation is lower for the right-shifted curve at both higher (>60 mm Hg) and lower (<30 mm Hg) pressures, indicating a greater unloading with the Bohr effect. Exercise is a main contributor to this downward shift and decreased affinity between oxygen and hemoglobin when muscles need a steady oxygen supply the most.

In contrast, a shift to the left, called the **Haldane effect**, indicates an increased affinity of hemoglobin for oxygen (Fig. 6-19). The left-shifted curve represents the opposite effect (i.e., greater affinity between hemoglobin and oxygen, and more difficulty unloading at a given partial pressure) compared with the right shift. In both partial pressure examples, a leftward shift increases oxygen saturation, but more so at lower pressures compared with higher pressures.

The following discussion focuses further on the factors that can alter the dissociation curve. See Table 6-2 and refer back to Figures 6-18 and 6-19 when reading

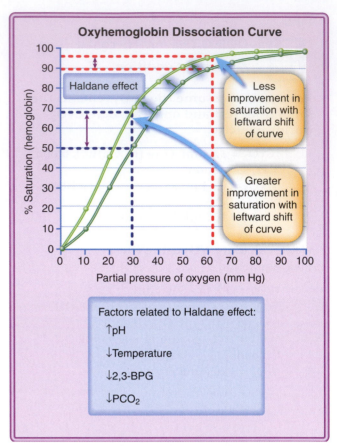

**Figure 6-19.** The oxyhemoglobin dissociation curve shifted to the left, producing the Haldane effect and the factors related to the shifting of the curve.

about each factor to better understand how alterations to each one can affect the oxyhemoglobin dissociation curve and oxygen saturation.

## Blood pH

Proton or hydrogen ion concentration determines blood pH in an inverse manner. When this concentration is elevated, pH decreases and blood becomes more acidic. During conditions such as with increasing exercise intensity and athletic performance, increased hydrogen ion production causes a rightward shift of the oxyhemoglobin curve. Thus, a more acidic environment in the blood causes a decreased affinity of hemoglobin for oxygen and improves the unloading of oxygen at the tissues, which is principally needed during exercise. A decrease in hydrogen ion concentration promotes a more alkalotic environment in the blood, and thereby produces the opposite effect by increasing hemoglobin-oxygen affinity.

## Temperature

A change in temperature caused by varying levels of heat production inversely affects the degree of hemoglobin-oxygen affinity. It has been proposed that hyperthermia (elevated internal temperature) denatures the bond between oxygen and hemoglobin, which will naturally affect affinity. Thus, at a given pH, increased temperature causes a rightward shift in the dissociation

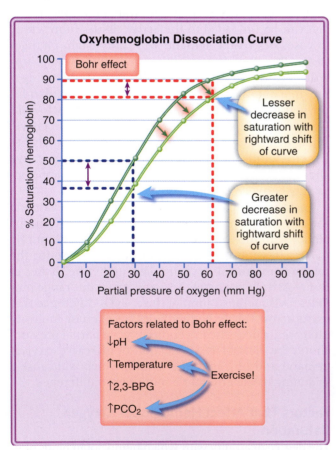

**Figure 6-18.** The oxyhemoglobin dissociation curve shifted to the right, producing the Bohr effect and the factors related to the shifting of the curve.

## Table 6-2. Factors That Influence the Affinity of Hemoglobin for Oxygen

| FACTOR | HIGHER AFFINITY | LOWER AFFINITY |
| --- | --- | --- |
| Temperature | Decreased | Increased |
| Hypoxia (2,3-bisphosphoglycerate) | Decreased | Increased |
| Partial pressure of carbon dioxide | Decreased | Increased |
| pH | Increased (more basic) | Decreased (more acidic) |

curve, again indicating a greater unloading of oxygen to the tissues. Prolonged athletic performance, especially in hot/humid environments, or increasing exercise intensity will promote greater oxygenation of muscle through this mechanism. In contrast, hypothermia (decreased internal temperature) will cause an opposite leftward shift of the curve toward an increasing affinity of hemoglobin for oxygen.

### 2,3-Bisphosphoglycerate

A third factor that affects the oxyhemoglobin dissociation curve is 2,3-BPG. This molecule is an end product created during glycolytic metabolism that occurs primarily within red blood cells and can be bound by hemoglobin. The increased production of 2,3-BPG is an important process during conditions when the $P_{O_2}$ is low, such as in hypoxia elicited by increasing altitude, chronic lung disease, and anemia. High levels of 2,3-BPG shift the oxyhemoglobin curve downward and to the right, which favors decreased affinity and greater unloading of oxygen from hemoglobin to tissues at a given $P_{O_2}$, particularly in cases when oxygen is needed most. A decreased concentration of 2,3-BPG causes an opposite shift to the left and greater affinity between oxygen and hemoglobin.

### Partial Pressure of $CO_2$

The $P_{CO_2}$ is closely and inversely related to the pH level in the blood. High $P_{CO_2}$ commonly coincide with low pH (acidosis); therefore, increased carbon dioxide in the blood affects the oxyhemoglobin curve much like how acidosis does: a rightward shift of the curve favoring unloading of oxygen to tissues (Bohr effect). Also, the binding of carbon dioxide to hemoglobin (see discussion on carbon dioxide transport in blood) facilitates a greater release of oxygen from hemoglobin at the tissue. In cases in which pulmonary ventilation is increased at rest (hyperventilation), low $P_{CO_2}$ in the blood will cause less unloading of oxygen at the tissues and stronger affinity between hemoglobin and oxygen. Hyperventilation, especially when one ascends in altitude for activity or athletic performance, is one way our body can increase or maintain hemoglobin-oxygen saturation. In summary, the $P_{CO_2}$ affects loading and unloading in two separate ways: influencing pH and binding to hemoglobin.

### Role of Myoglobin

**Myoglobin** is also a heme-containing, oxygen-binding protein that is structurally related to hemoglobin, but it is significantly smaller and binds less oxygen than hemoglobin (1 molecule of oxygen compared with 4 for hemoglobin). This protein primarily functions as an intermediate transporter during tissue oxygen exchange, shuttling the gas from hemoglobin in the blood to the mitochondria inside the muscle cell. Myoglobin concentration can be improved through exercise training and is much higher in the muscle fibers of slow-twitch motor units. It also has been viewed as a storage site or reservoir for oxygen because of its higher affinity for oxygen compared with hemoglobin, especially for a given partial pressure less than 60 mm Hg. This property significantly improves capillary–tissue gas exchange and ensures that exchange is unidirectional, principally as the $P_{O_2}$ decreases in the muscle as exercise intensity increases to maximal levels. In addition, the presence of myoglobin in the muscle helps to support oxidative phosphorylation in the mitochondria in cases in which oxygen supply is limited, such as ischemia in the muscle or hypoxia in short-term exposure to altitude.

### Carbon Dioxide Transport in Blood

During rest, bioenergetic pathways in cells, such as the TCA cycle, will produce approximately 200 to 220 mL carbon dioxide per minute, which eventually requires removal by the lungs. Unlike oxygen transport, carbon dioxide can be transported through the blood in *three*

### FROM THEORY TO PRACTICE

You are a personal trainer working with a client who is planning a hiking and camping trip from your near-sea-level city to a much higher elevation (10,000+ feet) in Colorado 3 months from now. Your client has read and heard that the changing atmospheric pressure with increasing altitude will affect the percentage of oxygen in the air, the $PO_2$ in the air, and ultimately the ability of his blood to carry oxygen. He wonders how his body, lungs, in particular, will react to these changes and how he can improve his fitness to do better with his activity at altitude. To create an appropriate exercise program to get him ready for his hiking trip, first consider the effects of altitude on the respiratory system. Given your knowledge of

*Continued*

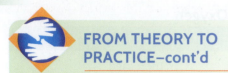

## FROM THEORY TO PRACTICE–cont'd

respiratory system and function, what do you tell him? Consider these questions:

1. What are the effects of increasing altitude on the percent of oxygen in air?
2. What are the effects of increasing altitude on $P_{O_2}$, blood oxygen saturation, and $Ca_{O_2}$?
3. Should your client be concerned about this?
4. How does the respiratory system respond to increasing altitude?
5. What would be the effects of increasing altitude on the oxyhemoglobin dissociation curve, and why would this change be effective for increasing tissue (muscle) oxygenation?

different ways: (1) dissolved in plasma, (2) bound to the protein hemoglobin, and (3) formed as the bicarbonate ion ($HCO_3^-$). The percent contributions of these ways carbon dioxide is transported in the blood are listed in the following subsections and are representative of the total cardiovascular system. Figure 6-20 shows how carbon dioxide is loaded in the blood from the tissues and unloaded from the blood at the lungs.

### Carbon Dioxide Dissolved in the Plasma

It is approximated that 10% of all carbon dioxide transported in the blood is dissolved in the plasma. This is vastly different from oxygen, which has very poor solubility in plasma and is one reason for the much higher pressure gradient for oxygen exchange at the tissue and lung. For comparison, the solubility of carbon dioxide is approximately 20 times greater than that of oxygen. Even so, the majority of carbon dioxide is still not transported in this way.

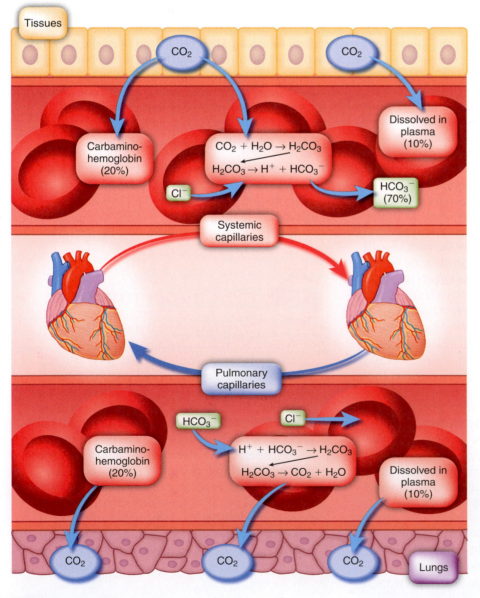

**Figure 6-20.** Carbon dioxide loading at the tissues and unloading at the lungs. The three ways that carbon dioxide is transported through the blood are: (1) dissolved in plasma, (2) bound to hemoglobin to produce carbaminohemoglobin, and (3) in the form of bicarbonate.

## Carbon Dioxide Bound to Hemoglobin

The next form of carbon dioxide transport is via hemoglobin. Approximately 20% of all carbon dioxide in the blood is bound to hemoglobin, forming a compound referred to as **carbaminohemoglobin**. Whereas the binding of oxygen occurs at the site of the heme groups on hemoglobin, carbon dioxide binds directly to the globin proteins on hemoglobin. The major determinant of the affinity that hemoglobin has for carbon dioxide is the overall $P_{O_2}$ in the blood. In states in which the $P_{O_2}$ in the blood is low, as in the veins, carbon dioxide is more tightly bound to hemoglobin. At the lungs, where the $P_{O_2}$ is high in the pulmonary capillaries, carbon dioxide is unloaded more readily because of the decreased affinity between it and hemoglobin.

## Carbon Dioxide in the Form of Bicarbonate Ion

The last means of carbon dioxide transport through the blood is in the form of **bicarbonate**. Bicarbonate is formed on the red blood cell through a reaction catalyzed by the enzyme carbonic anhydrase. Most carbon dioxide is transported from the tissue and back to the lung in this fashion (~70%). At the tissues, carbon dioxide diffuses onto the red blood cell according to its pressure gradient (higher in tissue than blood, as shown in Fig. 6-15) and is combined with water to form carbonic acid in the following reaction:

Reaction proceeds left to right at tissues

$$\longrightarrow$$

$$CO_2 + H_2O \leftrightarrow H_2CO_3 \leftrightarrow H^+ + HCO_3{-}$$

Carbonic anhydrase catalyzes the conversion of carbon dioxide and water to carbonic acid. Once this reaction proceeds, carbonic acid quickly dissociates into a hydrogen ion and bicarbonate ion. The formation of these two ions occurs without the need of an enzyme. Bicarbonate diffuses from the red blood cell into the blood plasma, and hemoglobin binds the hydrogen ion to help maintain blood pH. As bicarbonate leaves the red blood cell, chloride ($Cl^-$) ions must diffuse onto the cell to balance out the positively charged hydrogen ions. This ion exchange process is referred to as the **chloride shift** and is needed to maintain a neutrally charged red blood cell membrane.

At the lungs, the diffusion of carbon dioxide from the blood to the alveoli begins according to the reversed pressure gradient (higher in blood than alveoli, as shown in Fig. 6-15). The re-formation of carbon dioxide occurs because of the reversal of the carbonic anhydrase reaction:

Reaction proceeds right to left at lung

$$\longleftarrow$$

$$CO_2 + H_2O \leftrightarrow H_2CO_3 \leftrightarrow H^+ + HCO_3{-}$$

The binding of oxygen to hemoglobin forces the release of the hydrogen ions previously bound to hemoglobin at the tissues. Bicarbonate diffuses back onto the red blood cell (in exchange for chloride) and combines with the liberated hydrogen ion to form carbonic acid. Carbonic anhydrase dissociates carbonic acid into carbon dioxide and water, and the carbon dioxide diffuses into the alveoli and is expired from the lung.

## Pulmonary Contributions to Acid–Base Balance

From an acid–base viewpoint, the lungs play a critical role in maintaining blood pH at rest and during various intensities of exercise and athletic performance that greatly utilizes anaerobic sources of energy. The pH of the blood is tightly regulated and does not decline to much less than 7.4, even under the most intense exercise conditions. Compared with inside the muscle, the large buffering capacity determined by the bicarbonate concentration in the blood (and minor assistance from the kidney) is a major reason why changes in blood pH are not very significant.

As a review, the combination of hydrogen ions, the concentration of which determines pH in a solution, and bicarbonate forms carbonic acid, and its dissociation provides carbon dioxide and water at the lungs. An increased formation and removal of carbon dioxide by the lungs reduces both the $P_{CO_2}$ and hydrogen ion concentration, thereby raising pH in the blood. Thus, increasing ventilation during exercise and athletic competition is not only helpful for increasing oxygen delivery, but also buffering acidosis through the formation of water and carbon dioxide. This is a relatively fast system to control blood pH compared with the kidneys, which are much slower but have a greater capacity to maintain pH in the long term. In conditions where the lungs are not well ventilated or perfused (e.g., in some respiratory diseases), carbon dioxide is retained, causing higher partial pressures in the blood), hydrogen ion concentration would increase and acidosis will occur, eventually decreasing blood pH.

## *V I G N E T T E  conclusion*

■ Fortunately, most individuals with EIA can continue to enjoy the benefits of regular exercise without significant limitations if proper medical treatment is administered before exercise. Amanda's physician prescribed an inhaled bronchodilator, which is fast acting, simple to use, and convenient. She was instructed to use it about 15 minutes before exercise to reduce asthma symptoms and to improve exercise performance. Amanda's doctor told her that, if her symptoms become more severe, or if her asthma is triggered by other means in addition to exercise, she may need to take additional asthma medications. By properly using her medication and being alert to any changes in her symptoms, Amanda will be able to safely and effectively exercise despite her condition. In fact, individuals like Amanda can enjoy all of the many benefits that come from a properly designed, progressive exercise program.

## CRITICAL THINKING QUESTIONS

1. Exercise conditions such as increasing exercise intensity and prolonged durations of exercise are associated with increasing internal temperature and greater tissue oxygenation. Explain how a greater unloading of oxygen occurs in this case.

2. The FVC and $FEV_1$ (and their ratio) are important clinical measures of respiratory function and are useful for diagnosing and distinguishing between the two main types of lung disease: obstructive and restrictive. With obstructive diseases, the compliance of the lungs is higher than restrictive, but the ability to expel air is reduced because of either poor elastic recoil (emphysema) or airway spasm or collapse (asthma). With restrictive diseases, the compliance of the lungs is much lower than in obstructive disorders, but the ability to exhale air in relation to the total lung volume is preserved or even enhanced. Thus, assuming that FVC is relatively similar between the two diseases, which disease would have a lower **$FEV_1$/FVC ratio**: restrictive or obstructive?

3. One of your beginner clients complains of slightly sore abdominal muscles upon arrival for her training session that day. After inquiring more, she tells you that she spent the previous weekend getting over a nasty cold with coughing fits through the day and night. What is the likely explanation?

4. One of your colleagues asks you about the effects of using supplemental oxygen and better recovery from short-term, intense exercise due to increased blood oxygenation and delivery. Your colleague thinks that it must work because he sees football players using it on the sidelines all the time, but doesn't know for sure. Explain why breathing supplemental oxygen does not help increase oxygen delivery or exchange, and thus is not related to better recovery.

5. Carbon monoxide (CO), which is produced by the combustion of carbon-containing compounds under conditions of limited oxygen (e.g., burning of fireplaces, stoves, furnaces, engine combustion), is a highly toxic and deadly odorless, tasteless, and colorless gas. Although it is produced naturally in the body in tiny amounts and has important biological functions, CO poisoning can occur when a person breathes in the gas at remarkably small quantities (i.e., quantities greater than 50 parts per million of air). CO poisoning can lead to headache, nausea, dizziness, confusion, seizure, coma, and death. How does CO poisoning produce these serious signs and symptoms? In which direction would CO poisoning shift the oxygen-hemoglobin dissociation curve?

## ADDITIONAL RESOURCES

### Websites
American Academy of Allergy Asthma & Immunology (AAAAI). http://www.aaaai.org/home.aspx
American Lung Association: http://www.lungusa.org
Centers for Disease Control and Prevention. General asthma information. http://www.cdc.gov/asthma/links.htm
Centers for Disease Control and Prevention. Asthma action plan. http://www.cdc.gov/asthma/actionplan.html
National Institutes of Health. Asthma action plan. http://www.nhlbi.nih.gov/health/public/lung/asthma/asthma_actplan.pdf

### Books and Articles
Blain GM, Smith CA, Henderson KS, Dempsey JA. Peripheral chemoreceptors determine the respiratory sensitivity of central chemoreceptors to $CO_2$. *J Physiol.* 2010;588(Pt 13): 2455–2471.

Boulpaep EL, Boron WF. *Medical Physiology: A Cellular and Molecular Approach.* Philadelphia, PA: Saunders/ Elsevier; 2009.
Coates El, Li A, Nattie ER. Widespread sites of brain stem ventilatory chemoreceptors. *J Appl Physiol.* 1993;75:5–14.
Duffin J, Ezure K, Lipski J. Breathing rhythm generation: Focus on the rostral venrolateral medulla. *News Physiol Sci.* 1995;10:133–140.
Levitzky M. *Pulmonary Physiology.* 7th ed. Philadelphia, PA: McGraw-Hill; 2007.
West JB. *Respiratory Physiology: The Essentials.* 8th ed. Baltimore, MD: Lippincott Williams & Wilkins; 2008.

## REFERENCES

1. Kline JA, Kubin AK, Patel MM, Easton EJ, Seupal RA. Alveolar dead space as a predictor of severity of pulmonary embolism. *Acad Emerg Med.* 2000;7:611–617.
2. Miller A, ed. *Pulmonary Function Tests in Clinical and Occupational Lung Disease.* Philadelphia, PA: Grune & Sratton; 1986.
3. Dempsey JA, Mitchell GS, Smith CA. Exercise and chemoreception. *Am Rev Respir Dis.* 1984;129(2 Pt 2): S31–S34.
4. Dempsey JA, Hanson PG, Henderson KS. Exercise-induced arterial hypoxaemia in healthy human subjects at sea level. *J Physiol.* 1984;355:161–175.
5. Dempsey JA, Wagner PD. Exercise-induced arterial hypoxemia. *J Appl Physiol.* 1999;87:1997–2006.
6. Powers SK, Martin D, Dodd S. Exercise-induced hypoxaemia in elite endurance athletes. Incidence, causes and impact on VO2max. *Sports Med.* 1993; 16:14–2
7. McCloskey DI, Mitchell JH. Reflex cardiovascular and respiratory responses originating in exercising muscle. *J Physiol.* 1972;224:173–186.
8. Racinais S, Millet GP, Li C, Masters B, Grantham J. Two days of hypoxic exposure increased ventilation without affecting performance. *J Strength Cond Res.* 2010;24:985–991.

9. Harms CA, McClaran SR, Nickele GA, Pegelow DF, Nelson WB, Dempsey JA. Exercise-induced arterial hypoxaemia in healthy young women. *J Physiol.* 1998;507(Pt 2):619–628.

10. Dempsey JA, McKenzie DC, Haverkamp HC, Eldridge MW. Update in the understanding of respiratory limitations to exercise performance in fit, active adults. *Chest.* 2008;134:613–622.

11. Powers SK, Lawler J, Dempsey JA, Dodd S, Landry G. Effects of incomplete pulmonary gas exchange on VO2 max. *J Appl Physiol.* 1989;66:2491–2495.

12. Warren GL, Cureton KJ, Middendorf WF, Ray CA, Warren JA. Red blood cell pulmonary capillary transit time during exercise in athletes. *Med Sci Sports Exerc.* 1991;23:1353–1361.

13. Durand F, Mucci P, Prefaut C. Evidence for an inadequate hyperventilation inducing arterial hypoxemia at submaximal exercise in all highly trained endurance athletes. *Med Sci Sports Exerc.* 2000;32:926–932.

# *Practice What You Know:* Pulmonary Function Under Normal and Chronic Disease Conditions

Performing the following experiments will give you a sense of normal lung function and the impacts of disease on the pulmonary system. The first activity demonstrates the property of surface tension and how surfactant works to decrease this and ease the work of breathing. The next activity will give you experience with how asthma affects breathing at rest and during exercise, and will provide an opportunity for you to compare that with normal breathing. The last activity provides an additional experience with obstructive lung disease. This time we will gain an understanding of emphysema and the breathing difficulties that accompany this disease.

## Surface Tension and Surfactant

Surface tension is force that acts across a liquid surface, like the lining of the alveolar wall. In an alveolus, increasing surface tension will draw all sides together and decrease volume while increasing pressure. A smaller alveolus with high surface tension forces requires a much higher pressure to reinflate during inspiration. As a review from earlier in this chapter, surfactant functions to decrease the work of inspiration by decreasing the surface tension of the round alveoli. Decreasing surface tension will reduce the amount of pressure needed to inflate the lung (increased compliance) by keeping all alveoli stable and open.

### The Work of Breathing Experiment
Equipment

- Two round balloons (the thicker/bigger the balloons, the better the experiment)

Experience

- In the first trial, make an attempt to inflate the balloon with only one deep breath without prestretching it. If you cannot inflate it, that is okay. If you can inflate it, note the difficulty of inflating the balloon.
- In the second trial, pull on the balloon to prestretch it for about 10 to 15 seconds. Then, with one deep breath, inflate the balloon. Note the ease of inflating the second balloon after prestretching as compared with what was experienced during the first trial.

### Take-Home Message
What you have discovered is that one can decrease the surface tension (in this case, the elastic property of the balloon produces the surface tension, much like the lung) by prestretching a balloon before inflation. This is how surfactant works in the alveoli. With surfactant, the lung will inflate with smaller changes in pressure. Without surfactant, as you discovered in the first balloon trial, inflating the lung requires a much greater amount of pressure to overcome the lung's elasticity.

## Asthma

The prevalence of asthma is increasing in the United States, particularly in younger individuals. Asthma impacts quality of life, can limit recreational activities, and increases the burden on our health-care system because of increased hospital visits. Asthma can be managed through lifestyle changes including activity and diet, taking care to avoid environmental triggers (e.g., cold, pollutants, and allergens), and medications. The hallmark characteristic of asthma is a significantly decreased peak expiratory flow rate (i.e., how quickly air can be expired out of the lungs) measured during pulmonary function testing. The main testing measure is to determine the amount of air that can be expired in 1 second. Peak expiratory flow rate can be diminished by the environmental irritants listed earlier and by exercise. On the other hand, medications such as those provided in inhalers can improve peak flow rate and minimize the symptoms of asthma.

**Exercising With Asthma Experiment**
Equipment

- Nose clip or equivalent (to prevent breathing through the nose)
- Straw large enough to breathe through
- Stopwatch

Experience

- Working alone or with a partner, place a nose clip on the nose to ensure mouth breathing at rest and during exercise.
- Using a stopwatch, count the number of breaths taken in 30 seconds at rest by placing a hand on the upper chest or abdominals to assist in counting (i.e., an inhalation and exhalation is one breath). Multiply this number by 2 to calculate the total breaths taken per minute and record this value as "normal rest." In addition, rate the difficulty of breathing on a scale of 0 to 4 using the dyspnea scale at the end of this section.
- Repeat this same activity breathing through a straw, counting the number of breaths in 30 seconds and multiply by 2. Rate the difficulty of breathing using the dyspnea scale. Record these data as "asthma rest." Make sure to keep a tight seal with your mouth around the straw.
- Next, perform 1 minute of aerobic activity (e.g., walking stairs, brisk walking, slow jogging, or biking) at an intensity that produces a modest increase in RR. Immediately following this activity, sit down and count the number of breaths in 30 seconds (again, multiply by 2) and rate breathing difficulty using the dyspnea scale. Record these data as "normal exercise." Rest and recover for a few minutes.
- Last, repeat the same exercise activity while breathing through the straw. Immediately following this activity, sit down and count the number of breaths in 30 seconds (again, multiply by 2) and rate breathing difficulty using the dyspnea scale. Record these data as "asthma exercise." This last exercise may be difficult for you or your subject. If dizziness or light-headedness is experienced, immediately remove the straw and nose clip and breathe normally.
- Compare the data gathered between the two rest trials and then the two exercise trials.

**Asthma Expiratory Flow Rate Experiment**
This simple experiment will give you a general sense of how asthma affects the ability to expire air maximally over a short period. The most accurate way is to measure flow rate over a period of 1 second using a spirometer to measure air flow.

**Equipment**

- Nose clip or equivalent (to prevent breathing through the nose)
- Straw large enough to breathe through
- Stopwatch

**Experience**

- Working alone or with a partner, place a nose clip on the nose to ensure mouth breathing only.
- Start this trial by maximally inspiring air. Once this maximal point is reached, simultaneously start the stopwatch and forcefully expire all of your air. Once you reach the end, stop the time, and record as "normal expiration."

# *Practice What You Know:* Pulmonary Function Under Normal and Chronic Disease Conditions—cont'd

- Complete this trial in the same manner by maximally inspiring and expiring air. The only difference is that you will be breathing out through a straw. Once you reach your peak inspiration, place the straw in your mouth and expire while simultaneously starting the stopwatch. Make sure to keep a tight seal with your mouth on the straw. The end point is similar to the first trial. Record your expiration time as "asthma expiration."
- Compare the times from the two trials and note which one was the longest. What accounts for the differences in expiration durations?

### Take-Home Message

You likely observed large differences between normal and straw breathing for the resting and exercise trials. Most notably, the breathing difficulty was very likely pronounced during the expiration through the straw, especially following exercise and during the expiratory flow rate activity, but not noticed as much with inspiration. This is similar to how asthma feels. With asthma, the bronchioles can become inflamed and narrowed, thus obstructing the flow of air out of the lung. During an acute bout of asthma, individuals will have trouble expiring air and will experience wheezing and shortness of breath because of this obstruction.

## Emphysema

Emphysema is associated with a gradual destruction of lung tissue over time. As the lung loses tissue, it also loses its ability of elastic recoil during expiration. This causes an overinflation of the lungs, which requires greater use of accessory breathing muscles to expire at rest. Shortness of breath is one of the earliest symptoms of emphysema. The severity of shortness of breath becomes greater as the disease continues to progress and is increasingly felt at rest and during normal activities.

### Living With Emphysema Experiment
### Equipment

- Nose clip or equivalent (to prevent breathing through the nose)
- Stopwatch

### Experience

- Working alone or with a partner, place a nose clip on the nose to ensure mouth breathing at rest and during exercise.
- For the first trial, breathe normally at rest for 30 seconds while wearing a nose clip. Count the number of breaths taken within this time frame and multiply by 2 to calculate the number of breaths per minute. After the trial is completed, rate the difficulty in breathing using the dyspnea scale. Record the number of breaths and dyspnea rating as "normal rest."
- The second trial will begin by taking in a deep breath to the very top of your IC. Once there, breathe in and out for 30 seconds, one breath on top of another, without exhaling very much air. You will notice that breathing will be very shallow. Count the number of breaths during this time and, again, multiply by 2. Again, record the number of breaths and dyspnea rating at the end of the trial under the heading "emphysema rest."

### Take-Home Message

You likely observed significant differences in the RRs and dyspnea ratings between the normal and emphysema breathing trials. The goal of this activity was to give you an understanding of what it feels like to have the overinflated lungs of an individual with emphysema. You may have noticed how tired you became and how difficult it was after breathing this way for only 30 seconds. Unlike the asthma experiment, including exercise with the emphysema activity would have been impossible to complete. In addition, you may have felt a significant tightening of the neck muscles (i.e., scalene and sternocleidomastoid) as they worked to elevate the rib cage to assist inspiration in the overinflated lung. Thus, you have experienced firsthand the enormous work of breathing associated with this disease and why the act of breathing is so taxing for individuals suffering from emphysema.

**Dyspnea Scale (0–4)**

| SCORE | LEVEL OF DIFFICULTY BREATHING |
|---|---|
| 0 | No difficulty breathing |
| 1 | Mild; noticeable to patient, not to observer |
| 2 | Some difficulty for patient, noticeable to observer |
| 3 | Moderate difficulty, but patient can continue |
| 4 | Severe difficulty, patient cannot continue |

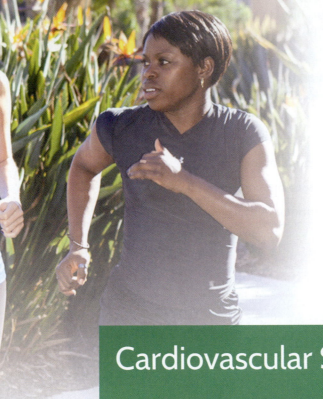

Jeffrey M. Janot, PhD
Gary P. Van Guilder, PhD

CHAPTER 7

# Cardiovascular System

## CHAPTER OUTLINE

# CHAPTER OUTLINE—cont'd

## LEARNING OUTCOMES

1. Describe the roles of the cardiovascular system.
2. Identify the structures of the systemic and pulmonary circuits.
3. Describe the anatomical structures of the heart pump and the cardiac wall.
4. Explain the function of the myocardium and its metabolic demands.
5. Describe the components of blood and their functions.
6. Identify the anatomical features and function of the electrical conduction system and coronary system.
7. Describe the function and features of the normal electrocardiogram.
8. Explain the mechanical events of the cardiac cycle.
9. List the factors that regulate stroke volume at rest and during exercise.
10. Differentiate and calculate various hemodynamic variables (mean arterial pressure, pulse pressure, rate pressure product, cardiac output, total peripheral resistance, ejection fraction) at rest and during exercise.
11. Describe the process of neural and humoral control of the cardiovascular system at rest and during exercise.
12. Compare and contrast sex differences in the cardiovascular system.

## ANCILLARY LINK

Visit Davis*Plus* at http://davisplus.fadavis.com for study and practice resources, including online quizzes, animations that help explain physiological processes, podcasts concerning news and career trends in exercise physiology, and practice references.

## VIGNETTE

■ Early one February morning, 57-year-old Mr. Chu, an overweight, high-strung financial advisor living in Boston, Massachusetts, was struggling to shovel the latest winter snowfall from his driveway. After several minutes of strenuous activity, he became dizzy, short of breath, and extremely tired. Convincing himself that these feelings were of no great concern, he pressed on and continued to overexert himself. However, the physical demand was too much, and he collapsed in the snow, clenching his chest in debilitating pain.

His wife saw what had happened and called 911 immediately. Subsequently, Mr. Chu was rushed to the local hospital in an ambulance.

What do Mr. Chu's signs and symptoms likely indicate?

Every organ, tissue, and cell in the body must have adequate blood flow to carry out its normal physiological function. During resting conditions, many regions of the body (e.g., skin) have a relatively low blood supply because their demand for oxygen is also relatively low. At the same time, other body regions, particularly the kidneys and the liver, are more active and have a higher demand for oxygen that requires a greater blood supply.

During exercise, as the metabolic requirements of certain tissues increase, especially that of skeletal muscle, the supply of blood must be increased to match energy needs. Blood flow delivery to less active tissues is reduced. However, blood flow to critical organs such as the brain and heart must still be maintained or increased because these organs do not tolerate interruptions in flow. The cardiovascular system is responsible for carefully balancing the flow of blood to the tissues. In this chapter, you will gain an appreciation of the cardiovascular system as an elaborate transport system of oxygen, nutrients, and waste products. You will learn the basic structure, organization, and function of this system as it pertains to exercise physiology.

## ROLE OF CARDIOVASCULAR SYSTEM

The cardiovascular system is a complex transport network that consists of the heart, blood, and blood vessels. To ensure that all tissues in the body receive adequate blood delivery, the cardiovascular system acts in a coordinated fashion to maintain **blood pressure (BP)** throughout the circulation. BP is the driving force for blood flow. If the driving pressure for blood flow is sustained, then the transport of oxygen and nutrients to all regions of the body will satisfy the metabolic needs of the tissues, which is especially important during exercise. When the tissues need more oxygen and energy because of greater metabolic activity, the cardiovascular system responds by increasing its output *and* pressure to deliver more blood.

Although the challenge and primary purpose of the cardiovascular system is to maintain BP and deliver adequate oxygen to tissues, it also has an important responsibility to remove metabolic waste products such as carbon dioxide by transporting it to the lungs. By eliminating metabolic waste products and carbon dioxide, the cardiovascular system helps regulate blood pH. In addition, it helps to maintain a constant internal body temperature by regulating blood flow to the periphery, transports fuel and nutrients to working muscle and other tissues, and delivers hormones to their sites of action. Thus, it is important for you to understand that the cardiovascular system and the respiratory system (see Chapter 6) complement one another to maintain adequate oxygen and carbon dioxide levels in the blood.

## ANATOMY OF THE HEART

Key aspects of heart anatomy are the heart pump, cardiac tissue, the pericardium, the cardiac wall, and the myocardium.

### Heart Pump

Figure 7-1 illustrates the structure of the heart. The heart is a four-chambered organ that consists of two atria and two ventricles that work as a dual pump to deliver blood to all body organs and tissues. The right heart pump includes the right atrium and right ventricle, and drives blood through the pulmonary circulation, whereas the left heart pump consists of the left atrium and left ventricle, and drives blood through the systemic circulation. It is important to understand that the right and left heart pumps work in parallel and pump the same amount of blood at the same rate throughout each heartbeat.

A thick muscular wall, the **interventricular septum**, divides the right and left sides of the heart and prevents blood from mixing between the right and left ventricles. To facilitate a continuous unidirectional flow of blood, the heart contains four one-way valves. When these valves are functioning properly, they prevent the retrograde (reverse) flow of blood and play a critical role to ensure that the flow of blood is maintained toward all body tissues.

Two **atrioventricular (AV) valves** separate the atria from the ventricles. They help to ensure that the movement of blood flows from the atria to the ventricles. The right AV valve, also known as the **tricuspid valve**, is located between the right atrium and the right ventricle, whereas the left AV valve is located between the left atrium and the left ventricle. The left AV valve

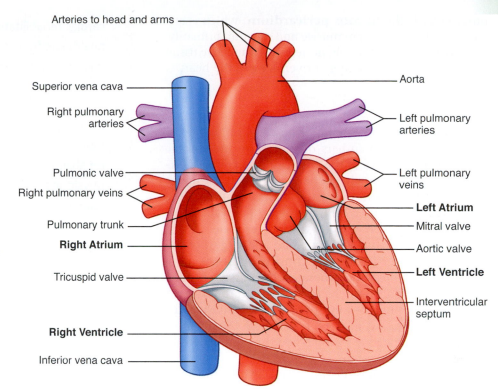

**Figure 7-1.** Structure of the heart. The heart is a dual pump that consists of two atrial chambers and two ventricular chambers separated by the atrioventricular valves. The right ventricle pumps blood to the lungs for oxygenation, whereas the left ventricle pumps blood to peripheral tissues.

is also referred to as the mitral or bicuspid valve. The **semilunar valves**, including the pulmonary valve and the aortic valve, work to direct blood from the ventricles into arteries. The pulmonary valve is located between the right ventricle and the pulmonary artery. It ensures that the flow of blood is directed to the lungs for gas exchange. The aortic valve marks the superior end of the left ventricle, at the base of the aorta. It helps to direct the flow of blood into the aorta and systemic arteries.

## Cardiac Tissue

To quote an old rule of thumb, the heart is roughly the "size of your fist." In the average adult human, the heart weighs about 250 to 350 g and is approximately 12 to 14 cm long. The weight and size of the heart are generally on the lower end of these ranges in women than in men. Therefore, cardiac chamber dimensions, which can affect variables like stroke volume (SV), tend to be smaller in women. As discussed in this chapter, this amazing organ beats continuously throughout the life span (possibly up to 3 billion times!), nourishes itself through its own blood supply, and can beat on its own without prior stimulation, among other unique characteristics.

## Pericardium

Figure 7-2 shows the layers of the heart wall. The **pericardium**, or pericardial sac, serves as a protective covering over the heart and anchors the large blood vessels entering and exiting the heart. The pericardium is composed of two separate layers of tissue. The inner layer is called the **serous pericardium**. It is divided into two

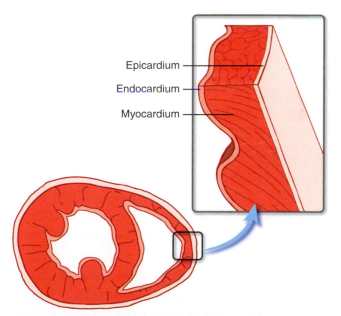

**Figure 7-2.** Layers of the cardiac wall: the endocardium, myocardium, and epicardium. The endocardium is the innermost layer of the heart; the myocardium is the largest layer and is made up of the cardiac muscle; and the epicardium, which contains the coronary blood vessels and cardiac nerves, forms the outer layer.

thin layers of tissue: the **parietal** layer and the **visceral** layer. The parietal layer serves as the inner lining of the fibrous pericardium, and the visceral layer (epicardium) is the outermost lining of the heart wall. The area between the serous layers, called the **pericardial space**, is filled with a small amount of fluid, which reduces friction as the heart contracts within the pericardial sac. The outer layer is the **fibrous pericardium**, which is anchored to the diaphragm muscle and sternum primarily. This layer consists of tough, nonelastic connective tissue that can prevent stretching or overfilling of the heart.

## Cardiac Wall

The **endocardium** is the innermost layer of the heart and lines all the chambers of the heart and cardiac valves. The structure of the endocardium contains endothelial cells and tough, elastic connective tissue under these cells. The connective tissue assists in withstanding great pressures exerted on the endocardial wall during contraction, especially within the left ventricle.

The **myocardium** is the middle and largest of the cardiac wall layers. This layer consists of cardiac muscle, which contracts and generates the pressure needed to eject blood out of the heart. The myocardium layer in the atria is thin (2–3 mm) compared with the ventricles and is largest in the left ventricle (10–15 mm) because of the need to pump blood through the entire systemic vascular system.

The **epicardium** is the outermost layer of the heart and is synonymous with the visceral pericardium. This layer houses the major coronary blood vessels, cardiac nerves, and other small vessels.

cardiac rehabilitation and leadership from allied health and fitness professionals, can participate in daily activities and, in many cases, continue their lives with an improved sense of well-being.

Following surgery, Mr. Chu begins working with Jenna, a physical therapist employed at the hospital-based fitness center who specializes in post-cardiac rehabilitation. Jenna works closely with Mr. Chu's physicians to ensure continuity of care using a teamwork-oriented approach.

## Myocardium

Cardiac muscle shares some similarities with skeletal muscle, but there are distinct differences as well (see Fig. 7-3 and Table 7-1). Cardiac muscle is striated and the fibers contain the contractile proteins actin and myosin within sarcomeres, which allow cardiac muscle to contract like skeletal muscle. In contrast, cardiac muscle functions involuntarily; it has no motor units and *only* type I muscle fibers (slow twitch, aerobic), and its cells contain just one nucleus. One striking difference between cardiac and skeletal muscle is the overall architecture of the muscle itself.

### VIGNETTE *continued*

■ While at the emergency department in the local hospital, Mr. Chu underwent life-saving open-heart surgery to treat a 90% blocked left anterior descending coronary artery. The surgery that was chosen to be the most appropriate for Mr. Chu is known as coronary artery bypass graft surgery (CABG), one of the most common and successful procedures used today to treat victims of coronary artery disease.[1]

During CABG, cardiovascular surgeons obtain healthy arteries or veins from another part of the body to bypass or circumvent blocked arteries in the heart. CABG is successful in relieving chest pain and improving blood flow in regions of the heart that were affected by the blocked vessels. However, once the surgery has been completed, the individual may experience numerous challenges in his or her return to a normal lifestyle. Indeed, surviving a myocardial infarction is just the beginning of a long, challenging process of medically supervised care and rehabilitation. Nevertheless, the majority of victims of myocardial infarction, with proper

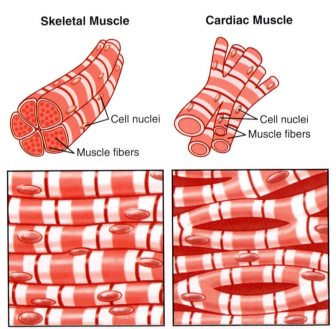

**Figure 7-3.** Cardiac and skeletal muscle fibers. Under electron microscope, the two different types of muscle fibers look similar in that they are both striated. However, the drawing shows a major anatomical difference between skeletal and cardiac muscle. In skeletal muscle, fibers are separated from one another, whereas in cardiac muscle, fibers are interconnected to allow the flow of electrical activity to move from fiber to fiber and throughout the heart.

## Table 7-1. Comparison of Characteristics of Cardiac and Skeletal Muscle Fibers

| CHARACTERISTICS | SKELETAL MUSCLE FIBER | CARDIAC MUSCLE FIBER |
| --- | --- | --- |
| Cell nucleus | Multiple | Single |
| Appearance | Striated | Striated |
| Control | Voluntary | Involuntary |
| Architecture | Nonbranched | Branched |
| Metabolism | Anaerobic/aerobic | Predominately aerobic |
| Motor units | Yes | No |
| Self-excitability | No | Yes |

Skeletal muscle fibers are not interdependent, and their cocontraction is coordinated through control and input from multiple nerves. Cardiac muscle fibers are branched and interconnected to permit electrical impulses to flow directly from one fiber to another; thus, the myocardium has the ability to depolarize and contract as one muscle. This muscle fiber arrangement is an important feature, as discussed later, because the heart's pacing rate is controlled by an area of specialized myocardial cells that conduct impulses one at a time.

The myocardium relies almost exclusively on aerobic metabolism (oxidative phosphorylation) to meet the significantly high energy demands of continuous function.[2] Thus, cardiac tissue has a great number of mitochondria and a very extensive blood supply. These features make the myocardium very resistant to fatigue.

Blockages in the coronary arteries caused by **coronary artery disease** will decrease the amount of oxygen supplied to the myocardium and will force the heart to rely more on anaerobic metabolism. The heart has very little capacity (~10% of total energy supply at most) to derive adenosine triphosphate from anaerobic metabolism to pump efficiently. It is estimated that cardiac muscle cells have only a few minutes (if that) to survive in conditions with limited oxygen supply before irreversible damage occurs. This scenario is the major cause of a heart attack, as you have observed so far in the vignette.

From a fuel standpoint, cardiac muscle can use blood lactate as a source of energy to regenerate adenosine triphosphate when oxygen supply is either adequate or decreased, but sole reliance on this fuel source is inadequate for performing myocardial work under poor oxygen supply conditions. Thus, the major fuel source for cardiac muscle in states of sufficient blood supply is fat (up to 60% of total energy supply) followed by glycogen/glucose and amino acids (up to 40% of total energy supply collectively).

## PULMONARY AND SYSTEMIC CIRCULATION

The cardiovascular system contains two interconnected circulatory networks: the pulmonary circulation and the systemic circulation. Figure 7-4 illustrates a general organization of the cardiovascular system. The **pulmonary circulation** includes the right atrium and ventricle (the right heart pump) and the pulmonary arteries and veins. It delivers oxygen-poor blood (deoxygenated) from the right side of the heart to the lungs through the **pulmonary arteries** for gas exchange (i.e., oxygen is loaded onto the blood and carbon dioxide is released). (See explanatory animation of pulmonary and systemic circulation on the DavisPlus site at http://davisplus.fadavis.com.)

The pulmonary circulation begins as blood enters the right atrium and is passed to the right ventricle through the tricuspid valve. The right ventricle generates the force necessary to pump blood through the pulmonary valve into the pulmonary artery. At this point, blood is transported through the pulmonary circulation to the lungs where it is oxygenated by the respiratory system. Once the blood has been reoxygenated, it travels back to the left side of the heart via the pulmonary veins.

The **systemic circulation** is composed of the left atrium and ventricle (the left heart pump), the aorta, and all other blood vessels. These include arteries, arterioles, capillaries, venules, and veins. The responsibility of the systemic circulation is to deliver fresh oxygenated blood to the peripheral organs and tissues.

Blood that has been loaded with oxygen (oxygenated) in the lungs is returned to the left side of the heart via the **pulmonary veins** into the left atrium. It then is pumped through the left AV valve (bicuspid valve) into the left ventricle. From this point, blood is ejected from the left ventricle through the aortic valve into the aorta, the largest blood vessel. Blood is then distributed from the aorta to the

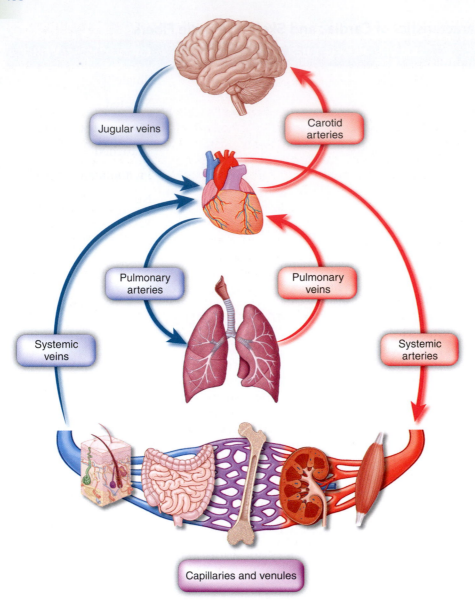

**Figure 7-4.** General organization of the cardiovascular system. The pulmonary circulation includes the pulmonary arteries that perfuse the lungs for gas exchange and the pulmonary veins that return blood to the heart. The systemic circulation is represented by the systemic arteries that supply blood to all other organs and tissues, and veins that return blood back to the heart.

systemic organs and tissues by way of high-pressure systemic arteries. As the systemic arteries approach organs and tissues, they branch extensively and become smaller vessels known as **arterioles**. The extensive branching of the arteries into smaller arterioles causes a large drop in driving pressure that helps to slow down the transport of blood at the tissues. In addition, because the arteriole walls contain a layer of smooth muscle, they can contract and relax. This important function helps to regulate the distribution of blood to specific organs and tissues depending on their metabolic needs.

Arterioles continue to branch and eventually develop into tiny beds of blood vessels known as **capillaries**, the smallest and most numerous of all blood vessels in the body. Capillaries are located at the blood–cell interface and connect the arterioles to the venules. They contain a thin layer of porous endothelial cells that allows for the rapid transfer of gases, nutrients, and waste products to and from the tissues. Oxygen and nutrients from the blood can pass through

the thin porous lining to the tissues, whereas carbon dioxide and waste products can enter the capillary to be removed from the tissues.

As the transfer of substances between the blood and tissues takes place, the capillaries are drained by larger vessels called **venules**. Venules begin the process of returning oxygen-poor venous blood from the systemic organs and musculature to the heart. Venules eventually become larger and merge to form **veins**. Venous blood empties directly into the right side of the heart via the superior and inferior vena cava where the right heart pump begins a new cycle through the pulmonary circulation.

## PRESSURES, VELOCITY, AND CROSS-SECTIONAL AREA

Blood flow through the heart and into the systemic circulation is driven, in part, by a pressure gradient that is established by the left heart pump. For instance, as shown in Figure 7-6 under resting conditions, the average pressure in the left ventricle and aorta is about 120 mm Hg, whereas the pressure in the right atrium is much lower (2 mm Hg), creating a pressure gradient of 118 mm Hg. Therefore, because the pressure is much higher in the aorta, blood will flow to the area of lower pressure (i.e., right atrium). This pressure difference drives blood across the systemic circulation. Table 7-2 outlines the differences in systolic and diastolic pressures between the right and the left heart.

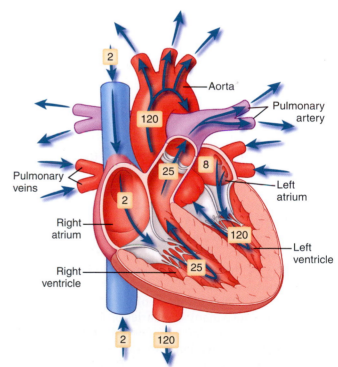

**Figure 7-6.** Average perfusion pressures (mm Hg) inside the heart.* The left heart pump establishes a high-pressure gradient between the aorta and right atrium that helps deliver blood through the systemic circulation. A typical pressure in the aorta during ventricular contraction is 120 mm Hg, which is much higher than the pressure in the right atrium (2 mm Hg), creating a pressure difference of 118 mm Hg. *The pressures denoted in the right and left atrium reflect the average pressure during atrial diastole (relaxation), whereas the average pressures in the right and left ventricles refer to ventricle systole (contraction).

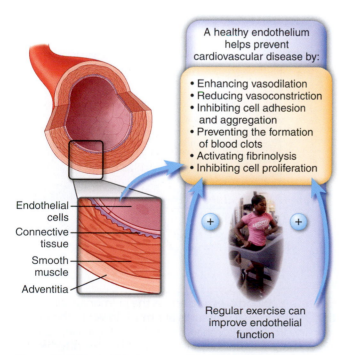

**Figure 7-5.** Favorable impact of exercise on vascular endothelial health.

## Table 7-2. Perfusion Pressures (mm Hg) Inside the Right and Left Heart

| Right atrium | |
|---|---|
| Mean pressure | 2 |
| **Right ventricle** | |
| Mean pressure | 20 |
| Peak systolic | 30 |
| End diastolic | 6 |
| **Left atrium** | |
| Mean pressure | 8 |
| **Left ventricle** | |
| Mean pressure | 100 |
| Peak systolic | 130 |
| End diastolic | 10 |
| **Pulmonary artery** | |
| Mean pressure | 20 |
| Peak systolic | 25 |
| End diastolic | 8 |
| **Aorta** | |
| Mean pressure | 100 |
| Peak systolic | 130 |
| End diastolic | 80 |

Figure 7-7 illustrates the changes in BP, blood flow velocity, and cross-sectional area of vessels across the systemic circulation. Note that a drop in BP begins in small arteries with the largest pressure drop in the arterioles. The small internal diameter of small arteries and arterioles creates a high resistance to blood flow contributing to the sharp decline in BP. Corresponding to the pressure drop is a reduction in blood flow velocity that reaches the slowest velocity in the capillary bed. The velocity of blood flow significantly slows in the capillaries because many capillaries branch off each arteriole, increasing the area of blood distribution in the vascular bed (cross-sectional area). This maximizes the capacity for gas exchange and the transfer of nutrients and metabolic waste products between the capillaries and tissues.

Similarly, the flow of blood through the pulmonary circulation is also a result of a pressure gradient. That is, the systolic pressure is higher in the right ventricle and pulmonary arteries (20 mm Hg) compared with the pulmonary veins (5 mm Hg), creating a driving pressure across the pulmonary circulation of approximately 15 mm Hg. It is important to note, however, that the perfusion pressures of the pulmonary circulation are far less than the systemic circulation, in part because

the pulmonary vessels offer very little resistance to blood flow. This characteristic, along with a large pulmonary capillary cross-sectional area, maximizes gas exchange in the lungs. Figure 7-8 shows the changes in pressure across the pulmonary circulation. Compare the pressure differences with the systemic circulation.

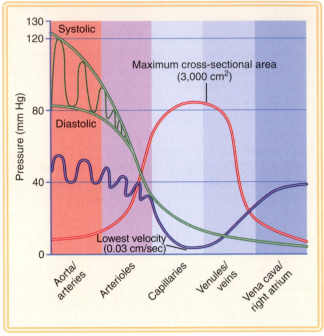

**Figure 7-7.** Blood pressure (green), cross-sectional area (red), and blood flow velocity (blue) across the systemic circulation. Mean arterial pressure declines sharply in the arterioles, along with a slowing of flow velocity because these vessels have a high resistance to blood flow. Cross-sectional area is maximized in the capillaries because of extensive vessel branching in the tissues.

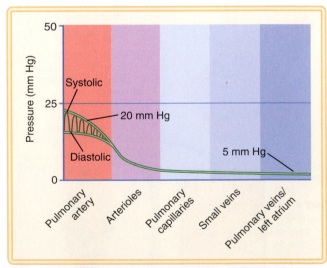

**Figure 7-8.** Blood pressure across the pulmonary circulation. Mean arterial pressures are much lower in the pulmonary circulation compared with the systemic circulation, largely because the blood vessels in the lungs offer very little resistance to blood flow. This characteristic helps to facilitate gas exchange in the lungs.

## CORONARY CIRCULATION

The coronary circulatory system is a special system of blood vessels that supplies the myocardium with blood. The coronary circulation begins with the **right and left main coronary arteries** (Figure 7-9). Each of these main branches starts as small openings in the aortic trunk (ascending aorta) that are situated just above the aortic valve. The right coronary artery runs between the right atrium and the right ventricle and continues on to the posterior portion of the heart. This blood vessel feeds the right atrium, right ventricle, and the inferior/posterior portion of the left ventricle. The left main coronary artery is a very short vessel that eventually branches into two other main coronary vessels: the **left circumflex** and **left anterior descending coronary arteries**. The left circumflex runs between the left atrium and the left ventricle and travels to the lateral and posterior portions of the left ventricle. The left anterior descending artery is the major anterior coronary artery and feeds a large portion of the anterior surface of the heart. The majority of blood flow through the coronary system occurs during *diastole* (when the heart is relaxing). The total amount of blood flow is most influenced by **aortic pressure** during diastole (greater pressure, greater coronary blood flow) and duration of diastole (longer duration, greater coronary blood flow). One condition that can affect both factors is exercise. Exercise will decrease the time that the heart spends in diastole and will increase aortic pressure during the early period of diastole when coronary blood flow is greatest.

In addition to these main coronary arteries are the smaller blood vessels that branch and penetrate the myocardium to create a blood supply network of capillaries within the muscle. The coronary system also contains cardiac veins that drain blood into the right atrium, so that oxygen-poor blood can be recirculated back to the lungs.

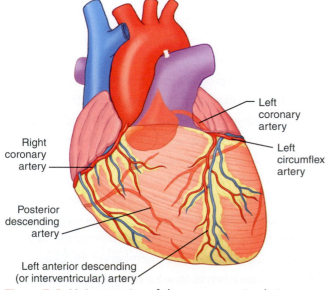

**Figure 7-9.** Major arteries of the coronary circulation.

Right coronary artery

Posterior descending artery

Left anterior descending (or interventricular) artery

Left coronary artery

Left circumflex artery

**VIGNETTE** *continued*

■ The signs and symptoms experienced by Mr. Chu, particularly severe fatigue, nausea, dizziness, and chest pain, indicate that he suffered a myocardial infarction. A myocardial infarction is the result of a blocked coronary artery that causes part of the heart tissue to die (infarct) or become severely damaged. The tissue dies because blood flow and oxygen to the heart muscle is either significantly reduced or stopped entirely, causing major problems in heart function. Other signs and symptoms of a myocardial infarction that a person may experience include severe pain in the jaw, neck, arms, and back. Each year in the United States, about 800,000 people will suffer a myocardial infarction, with 500,000 not surviving this coronary event.[1]

Fortunately, the chances of surviving a heart attack are greater when emergency medical treatment begins as soon as possible, which was the case for Mr. Chu, thanks to his wife, who recognized the early warning signs.

The artery that was predominately blocked in Mr. Chu's heart was a branch of the left anterior descending coronary artery. This artery feeds the front portion of the left ventricle, which is the largest and most active chamber in the heart and is responsible for pumping blood throughout the body. In Mr. Chu's case, an area of tissue in the left ventricle has died. Consequently, this has caused major problems in the function of the left ventricle, particularly the cardiac muscle, which has become very weak and is susceptible to ventricular arrhythmias. These abnormalities will reduce the efficiency of the heart to pump blood by reducing myocardial contraction force, stroke volume, and cardiac output. Thus, Jenna initiates low-intensity cardiovascular training as part of the cardiac rehabilitation program in an effort to increase the strength and efficiency of Mr. Chu's left ventricle to help offset these complications.

## CARDIAC ELECTRICAL CONDUCTION

This section focuses on the flow of electrical impulses (or action potentials) in the heart that triggers the myocardium to contract. Just like with skeletal muscle, cardiac muscle must be stimulated to contract by nerve impulses. These impulses are conducted within the heart from cell to cell during a process termed **depolarization**. Simply put, depolarization involves the exchange of sodium and potassium across the cell membrane. Specifically, these impulses cause the release of calcium into the myocardial cell, which allows the binding of actin and myosin so muscle contraction can proceed. Without calcium present, muscle contraction cannot occur.

A later section will focus on the mechanical or contractile events of one heartbeat and follow the flow of blood through the heart. A key concept to remember is that *electrical events must precipitate mechanical events* in the heart. This means that the myocardium must depolarize (electrical event) first before it can contract (mechanical event), which again is comparatively similar to skeletal muscle contraction. Thus, depolarization and contraction should not be treated as the same physiological event.

## Structures

The important structures of the cardiac conduction system are as follows and are shown in Figure 7-10:
- **Sinoatrial (SA) node**
- AV node and AV bundle
- Right and left bundle branches
- Purkinje fiber network

When the heart's electrical conduction system is functioning properly, electrical impulses are generated by the SA node. The SA node is an area of specialized myocardial cells located in the upper posterior portion of the right atrium. The cells that make up the SA node are autorhythmic cells and can generate their own electrical impulses without prior stimulation (neural or hormonal), a property known as **automaticity**. Because of this property, the SA node is commonly referred to as the "pacemaker of the heart." (See an explanatory animation of the conduction sequence through the heart on the DavisPlus site at http://davisplus.fadavis.com.)

Once the SA node depolarizes, an electrical impulse is propagated throughout the right and left atria that causes the atrial muscle to depolarize. Notably, the impulse does not travel through nerves in the atria (because there are none), but through specialized tracts of myocardial cells. These tracts allow the electrical impulse to move more quickly through the atria versus more slowly if it traveled through the myocardium itself. Once the impulse reaches the bottom or inferior portion of the right atrium, it encounters a second area of specialized myocardial cells called the **AV node**. The AV node serves as the only pathway that the impulse can take into the ventricles to control the rate at which the ventricles are depolarized. The AV node also functions to slow or delay the impulse to give time for the ventricles to fill and atria to provide additional blood to the ventricles before ejection.

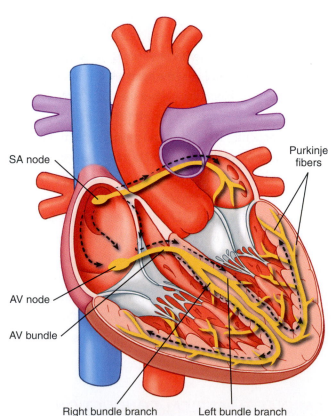

**Figure 7-10.** Cardiac conduction system. Note the pathway of electrical activity that spreads from the sinoatrial node, through the atria, down to the atrioventricular (AV) node/AV bundle, and finally through the two bundle branches and into the Purkinje fibers. Once the impulse reaches the Purkinje fibers, it spreads through the cardiac wall from endocardium to epicardium.

SA node

AV node

AV bundle

Purkinje fibers

Right bundle branch    Left bundle branch

The impulse continues down the conduction pathway and passes through the AV bundle (also known as the bundle of His) located within the interventricular septum. The bundle is the first part of the pathway that is nerve tissue. The AV bundle splits into two separate nerve branches, the **right bundle branch** and the **left bundle branch**, which run down either side of the interventricular septum. These branches help to rapidly transmit the impulse through the ventricles because of the large area of muscle that must be depolarized on time. The branches divide into smaller and smaller fibers until they are spread diffusely beneath the endocardium to form the Purkinje network. These tiny fibers terminate at the myocardium and transmit the impulse to the myocardial cells. From here, the impulse is spread through the myocardial wall from endocardium to epicardium and the ventricles finally depolarize and contract.

## Electrocardiogram

The **electrocardiogram (ECG)** is a recording of the flow of electrical activity that occurs in the heart during one heartbeat. The ECG offers clinical professionals information on the function and structure of the heart at rest and during activity. Function is determined by the heart's ability to conduct impulses (i.e., depolarize) in an organized and uniform manner every heartbeat. Structure is determined by the size and shape of the waveforms on the ECG recording. Cardiac disease can significantly change the function of the electrical conduction system (e.g., arrhythmias) or the structure of the heart (e.g., becomes enlarged or heart attack occurs); the problem can be detected on the ECG by a trained clinical professional. In this way, the ECG is an important diagnostic tool to help determine whether a person has underlying cardiovascular disease.

A normal resting ECG is shown in Figure 7-11. Each waveform on the ECG is related to a specific electrical event during one heartbeat. The P wave signifies atrial depolarization and is the first waveform on the ECG. This wave encompasses the time it takes for the electrical impulse generated by the SA node to travel through the atria to the AV node (see earlier Cardiac Electrical Conduction section for review). The flat line between the end of the P wave and the beginning of the QRS complex refers to the PR segment. It signifies the time it takes for the electrical impulse to travel through the AV node, bundle branches, and Purkinje network. The second waveform of the ECG is the QRS complex that is typically formed by three waves: the Q, R, and S. Collectively, these waves represent the depolarization of the ventricular myocardium. The QRS interval, or width, represents the time required for a depolarization stimulus to spread through the ventricles. Under normal conditions, it takes about 0.1 second or less for the ventricles to depolarize. A slowing of depolarization will widen the QRS interval and may indicate an arrhythmia. The ST segment—measured from the end of the QRS waveform to the beginning of the T wave—signifies the beginning of ventricular repolarization. The ST segment is usually isoelectric (i.e., a flat line on the baseline of the ECG). However, a depressed (negative) or elevated (positive) ST segment indicates that the heart muscle is not receiving adequate blood flow and oxygen (**ischemia**), a condition that can produce a heart attack. The completion of ventricular repolarization is represented by the T wave and is the last waveform on an ECG. Once the ventricles have repolarized, the electrical cycle will repeat beginning with atrial depolarization and another P wave generated by the SA node.

ECGs are also part of graded exercise tests (GXTs), which are administered by health-care professionals (Fig. 7-12). Common information that is gathered during this type of test includes HR, BP, and ECG responses to exercise. The electrodes that are placed on the patient's chest detect the heart's electrical activity. This activity is transmitted to the ECG machine and can be monitored by a trained professional.

## In Your Own Words

You are assisting the medical personnel of a local hospital who are conducting a graded exercise stress treadmill test on a 55-year-old man. The patient reports that he has a history of stable angina but otherwise does not have any immediate health concerns. He mentions that he has never performed such a test.

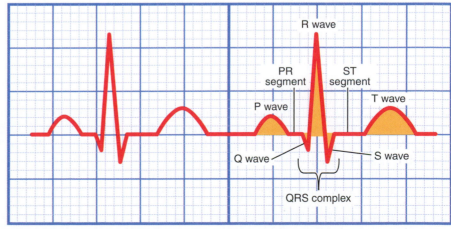

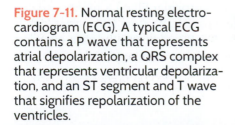

**Figure 7-11.** Normal resting electrocardiogram (ECG). A typical ECG contains a P wave that represents atrial depolarization, a QRS complex that represents ventricular depolarization, and an ST segment and T wave that signifies repolarization of the ventricles.

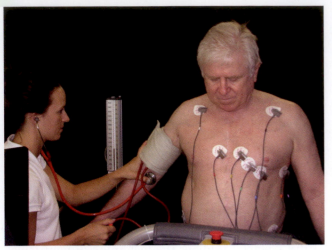

**Figure 7-12.** Graded exercise test (GXT).

Needless to say, he is somewhat apprehensive and does not know what to expect. What would you say to the patient to decrease his anxiety and help him feel more comfortable about performing the stress test?

## VIGNETTE continued

■ After an acute coronary event such as a myocardial infarction, the tissue affected by the blocked artery becomes scarred and electrically inert. The dead tissue is unable to respond to electrical activity from the SA or AV nodes. In conjunction with this problem, there appears to be an increase in sympathetic nervous system activity in the scarred region of the heart. Through a standardized format used to communicate and document health information called SOAP notes (an acronym for *subjective*, *objective*, *assessment*, and *plan for a patient*), Mr. Chu's physician ensures that Jermaine and Brett are aware of this situation, because it can cause potentially life-threatening exercise-induced ventricular arrhythmias. Thus, Jermaine and Brett continually monitor Mr. Chu's heart rate and electrical activity during exercise sessions using an ECG.

## CARDIAC CYCLE

The sequence of electrical and mechanical events that occur during one heartbeat is known as the **cardiac cycle** (Fig. 7-13). It is important to appreciate that this sequence repeats itself beat after beat for an entire lifetime. Earlier, this chapter focused on the electrical events that occur in the heart, such as depolarization and repolarization of the atria and ventricles. Mechanical events refer to contraction and relaxation of the heart's chambers. The relaxation phase is called **diastole**, whereas the contraction phase of the heartbeat is called *systole*. It is important to keep in mind the proper sequencing of electrical and mechanical events: Electrical events will always precede mechanical events. For example, contraction of the atria cannot occur until the atria have depolarized as denoted by the P wave on the ECG. Similarly, ventricular contraction cannot occur until the ventricles have depolarized as shown by the QRS complex. As such, one should not use the terms *depolarization* and *contraction* or *repolarization* and *relaxation* interchangeably because they refer to different types of processes in the heart.

Both atria and ventricles alternate between periods of filling and emptying. The filling phase occurs during diastole (relaxation), whereas the emptying phase occurs during systole (contraction). Therefore, atrial systole occurs during ventricular diastole and vice versa. In other words, the atria contract while the ventricles relax. Likewise, the ventricles contract while the atria relax. The cardiac cycle can be divided into four distinct phases:

Phase 1: ventricular filling
Phase 2: isovolumetric contraction
Phase 3: ventricular ejection
Phase 4: isovolumetric relaxation

Throughout the following discussion, particular attention will be devoted to the flow of blood through the heart, opening and closing of the heart valves, and pressure changes in the atria and ventricles during the four phases of the cardiac cycle. It is important to understand that the same phases of the cardiac cycle occur on the right side of the heart and on the left side.

### Phase 1: Ventricular Filling

The opening of the AV valves (tricuspid and mitral) marks the beginning of phase 1. During this phase, the heart is in diastole. Deoxygenated blood that has been collecting in the right atria passively flows into the right ventricle through the open tricuspid valve. Likewise, on the left side of the heart, oxygenated blood from the pulmonary circulation flows through the open mitral valve to fill the left ventricle. The distinct characteristic of phase 1 is that the two AV valves are *open* while both semilunar valves (pulmonary and aortic) are *closed*. During the first two thirds of diastole, the right and left ventricles fill passively with blood. During the last third of diastole, the atria contract (often referred to as atrial kick). Atrial contraction helps to eject a bit more blood into the right and left ventricles. The contribution of atrial contraction to ventricular filling is highly variable and depends largely on HR. At slow HRs, atrial kick is minimal, but at high HRs, as during intense exercise, the contribution of atrial kick to ventricular filling increases. Classic studies by Wiggers and Katz[13,14] suggest that atrial contraction is responsible for 18% to 60% of

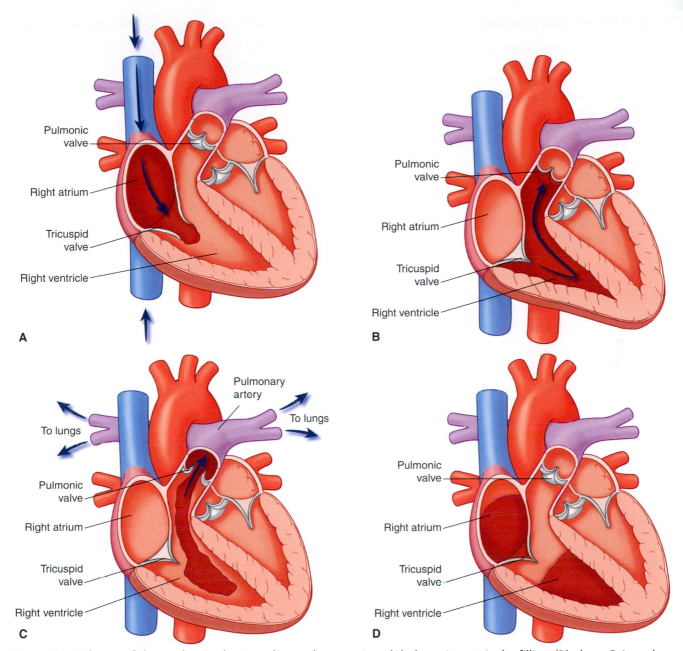

Figure 7-13. Phases of the cardiac cycle. A cardiac cycle comprises: (A) phase 1: ventricular filling; (B) phase 2: isovolumetric contraction; (C) phase 3: ventricular ejection; and (D) phase 4: isovolumetric relaxation. The relaxation phase is called *diastole* and comprises phases 1 and 4, whereas contraction is called *systole* and occurs during phases 2 and 3.

the total ventricular filling volume. Immediately following atrial contraction, the AV valves close, marking the end of phase 1.

## Phase 2: Isovolumetric Contraction

Phase 2 is the beginning of systole and commences when the ventricles depolarize. When the ventricles depolarize, they contract and build up pressure. As the pressure within the ventricles begins to rise, the pressure quickly exceeds right and left atrial pressure, respectively. As a result, the AV valves abruptly close. The semilunar valves are also closed at this time. A distinct

feature of phase 2 is that the ventricles contract with both sets of AV valves and semilunar valves closed. Because the ventricle chambers are closed, the blood has no place to go. Consequently, the ventricles undergo an **isovolumetric contraction** that causes ventricular pressure to rise abruptly and exceed the pressure in the pulmonary artery and aorta, thereby causing the semilunar valves to eventually open. Ventricular contraction proceeds in a very specific direction from the bottom to the top of the heart to ensure that blood moves toward the semilunar valves and can be ejected out of the heart. Opening of the semilunar valves marks the end of phase 2.

## Phase 3: Ventricular Ejection

The opening of the semilunar valves (with both sets of AV valves still closed) at the end of phase 2 marks the onset of ventricular ejection. Ventricular ejection can be subdivided into a *rapid ejection* phase and a *reduced ejection* phase. Rapid ejection is characterized by: (1) a sharp rise in ventricular pressure, (2) a steep increase in aortic pressure, and (3) a reduction in ventricular blood volume as blood flows quickly into the aorta (or pulmonary artery for the right ventricle). During the latter parts of phase 3, the ventricles continue to eject blood but at a much slower pace. This period of reduced ejection is characterized by decreased ventricular and aortic pressures caused by the emptying of most of the blood from the ventricles. Under resting conditions, approximately 70 mL of blood will be ejected from the ventricles during phase 3.

## Phase 4: Isovolumetric Relaxation

The onset of phase 4 marks the end of ventricular systole and the beginning of ventricular diastole. It is represented by abrupt closure of the aortic and pulmonary valves. Because all valves are closed (the AV valves have remained closed since phase 2), no blood can enter the ventricles. As a result, the ventricular myocardium undergoes a period of **isovolumetric relaxation** that is characterized by a decline in ventricular pressure with no change in ventricular volume.

Eventually, ventricular pressure drops below atrial pressure, and the tricuspid and mitral valves open once again. The net effect is the beginning of another cardiac cycle with the reopening of the AV valves and ventricular filling phase (phase 1). The most incredible fact is that the events comprising the four phases of the cardiac cycle are generally completed every second throughout a lifetime.

### V I G N E T T E  *continued*

Two weeks after completing phase I of his cardiac rehabilitation program, Mr. Chu is discharged from the hospital. His physician refers him to a phase II rehabilitation program, a clinically supervised outpatient program designed to restore patients to optimal functional ability within limits of their disease. There, Mr. Chu is introduced to a new physical therapist named Javier, who stays in contact with Jenna regarding Mr. Chu's progress. Javier's goal is to help Mr. Chu recover quickly from surgery and build on the improvements gained while working with Jenna in phase I. Overall, Javier attempts to improve the physical, mental, and social well-being of Mr. Chu, and to stabilize, slow, or reverse the progression of his cardiovascular disease. During his 3 months of working with Mr. Chu, Javier emphasizes safe physical activity to improve conditioning, coupled with risk-factor education and behavior modification.[12]

## REGULATION OF STROKE VOLUME

The amount of blood ejected by the heart in one beat is the ventricular **stroke volume** (SV). Mathematically, SV is the difference between the **end-diastolic volume** (EDV) and **end-systolic volume** (ESV). The EDV is the peak volume of blood that has filled the right and left ventricles during relaxation. The ESV is the volume of blood remaining in the ventricles after ejection. In a healthy human at rest, the amount of blood that fills the heart (EDV) is typically 120 mL, whereas the amount of blood left over after ejection (ESV) is 50 mL. Therefore, the SV would equal 70 mL.

$$SV = EDV - ESV$$

SV can be affected by factors that change EDV or ESV. If EDV increases, then SV will increase. Conversely, if ESV increases, SV will decrease. Many additional factors can influence SV. These include venous return, plasma volume, ventricular filling time, ventricular chamber size, and afterload.

### Venous Return

A primary factor that affects SV is the amount of blood that is returned to the heart from the peripheral veins (i.e., venous return). When venous blood returns and enters the ventricles during diastole, it increases EDV and stretches the myocardium before contraction. The stretch of the muscle tissue is called the **preload**. Increased preload facilitates more optimal alignment of actin and myosin, which helps to form more cross-bridges resulting in a stronger force of contraction (**contractility**). Therefore, a greater amount of blood can be ejected per heartbeat (higher SV). This relationship is known as the **Frank-Starling law of the heart**, an increased stretch of the ventricles (preload) leads to a stronger contraction. In other words, the greater the volume of blood returning to the heart during diastole (EDV), the greater the volume of blood ejected during systole (SV). Figure 7-14 shows the relation among EDV, contractility, afterload, and SV. As the volume of blood is increased in the left ventricle, the amount of blood ejected per heartbeat is also increased to a similar extent according to the middle line. As afterload and contractility increase or decrease, the SV curve is either shifted up or down for a given EDV.

During exercise, the rate of venous return increases, which plays a key role in enhancing SV. How does venous return increase during exercise? First,

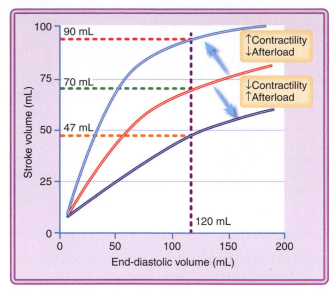

**Figure 7-14.** Influence of end-diastolic volume, afterload, and contractility on stroke volume. The middle line shows that increased filling volume during diastole stretches the left ventricle, leading to a greater force of contraction and stroke volume. This is the basis of the Frank-Starling law of the heart. Based on changes in contractility and afterload, this curve can be shifted up or down. In cases such as exercise, neural and hormonal stimulation increase contractility in the heart at a given end-diastolic volume (in this example, 120 mL blood) and afterload decreases due to vasodilation to increase stroke volume. In cases such as heart failure, contractility is decreased and afterload is increased at a given end-diastolic volume (120 mL blood), which leads to a lower stroke volume.

contraction of skeletal muscles helps to propel blood toward the heart through one-way venous valves. This is known as the skeletal muscle pump. Rhythmic contractions of the skeletal muscles during activity compress veins, causing venous pressure to build. As the pressure increases in the venous vessel during muscle contraction, the one-way valves close abruptly, preventing the backflow of blood away from the heart. However, between contractions when skeletal muscles relax, vessel compression is reduced, which allows the valves to open. Blood is then able to flow toward the heart. Second, the sympathetic nervous system causes smooth muscle in veins to contract. This is referred to as **venoconstriction** and it helps to increase the pressure in veins that drives the blood back to the heart.[15]

## Plasma Volume

A less appreciated factor that influences SV is the plasma volume. Plasma consists mostly of water, electrolytes, and plasma proteins. Dehydration, which lowers plasma volume, has a negative impact on SV. For example, during prolonged exercise in hot and humid environments, sweat rates can be as high as 2 to 3 L/hr. Consequently, plasma volume can be significantly reduced, and a 5% to 20% loss is common for prolonged exercise in the heat. The problem with a significant decline in plasma volume

is that it lowers venous return and ventricular filling pressure. In turn, EDV and preload are reduced, which will lower myocardial stretch and ventricular contractility, producing a lower SV. Conversely, regular exercise training in hot and humid conditions can actually increase plasma volume.[16] As a result, SV is optimized because there is a greater activation of the Frank-Starling mechanism. The importance of maintaining plasma volume during exercise is discussed in detail in Chapter 8.

## Ventricular Filling Time

Another factor that can influence SV and EDV is ventricular filling time. For a normal **resting heart rate** (RHR) of 70 beats per minute (bpm), one cardiac cycle takes 0.8 second, with approximately 0.5 second spent filling the left ventricle during diastole and 0.3 second spent ejecting the blood during systole.[17] At slower HRs, there is more time to fill the left ventricle, resulting in enhanced EDV. However, as HR increases, the time the ventricle is in diastole is reduced. Thus, at high HRs, there is less time to fill the left ventricle leading to a lower EDV. However, an important distinction to understand is that even though there is less ventricular filling time during high HRs, SVs will still be higher than resting conditions because: (1) venous return is increased through the skeletal muscle pump, and (2) the increased force of contraction that occurs through the Frank-Starling mechanism results in more complete emptying of blood. In addition, increased norepinephrine released from sympathetic nerves increases contractility of the myocardium. (Box 7-1 further describes RHR.)

## Ventricular Chamber Size

The size of the left ventricle can also influence SV. Increased ventricular chamber size can accommodate a greater filling volume and, subsequently, a greater SV through the Frank-Starling mechanism. One of the benefits of regular endurance exercise training on

### Box 7-1. Resting Heart Rate

**Heart rate** (HR) is the number of heartbeats per unit time, typically expressed as number of beats per minute (bpm). In a healthy person, a normal RHR typically ranges from 60 to 100 bpm following a period of quiet rest (~10 minutes). A RHR less than 60 bpm is called **bradycardia**, and a rate greater than 100 bpm is called **tachycardia**.[31,32] Under normal circumstances, bradycardia is not a concern and is often seen in many well-conditioned endurance athletes. In fact, it is common for highly trained elite athletes to have RHRs well below 60 bpm, and rates in the 30s or 40s are not surprising. A primary factor that contributes to very low RHRs in well-conditioned athletes is a powerful resting parasympathetic tone.[38]

cardiovascular performance is ventricular chamber enlargement, which helps to increase cardiac output.

## Afterload

The resistance to eject blood out of the heart is known as the **afterload**. The heart must overcome the pressure in the aorta at the end of diastole (diastolic blood pressure [DBP]) to open the aortic valve and eject blood. Increased aortic artery pressure and **total peripheral resistance (TPR)** are the two primary factors that increase afterload. A greater afterload has a negative effect on the SV; that is, an increased afterload will decrease SV. The primary reason for a reduction in SV is because there is less complete emptying of blood resulting in a higher ESV. Therefore, although EDV may not be affected, a greater afterload limits the amount of blood that can be ejected from the left ventricle.

Afterload decreases during cardiorespiratory exercise, which helps to enhance SV and exercise performance. As an individual exercises, the working muscle must be supplied with greater blood and oxygen to match energy demands. To meet this need, the blood vessels vasodilate. This effect reduces the resistance of blood flow to the working muscle and, therefore, reduces the load on the heart. In contrast, resistance exercise tends to increase afterload. The high intramuscular compression associated with the greater muscular effort during resistance training impedes blood flow through the blood vessels, which puts a greater strain on the heart. In addition, resistance training is often associated with a **Valsalva maneuver**—that is, attempting to forcefully exhale while the **glottis** is closed. This increases intrathoracic pressure and places a higher load on the heart. (See an explanatory animation of afterload and preload on the Davis*Plus* site at http://davisplus.fadavis.com.)

## VIGNETTE *continued*

■ During phase II rehabilitation, in addition to promoting the physical well-being of Mr. Chu, Javier seeks to improve the psychological and social aspects as well. Because it is a comprehensive program, phase II rehabilitation utilizes a variety of health-care professionals (e.g., medical doctors, nurses, psychologists, dieticians, physical therapists, health coaches and exercise specialists) who work together to devise a program for the patient. These professionals may counsel the patient and his or her family with respect to proper eating habits, lend emotional support to counteract depression, teach the appropriate use of medications, help the patient make improved lifestyle choices, and provide exercise programming recommendations.

## CARDIAC TERMINOLOGY

To gain a better understanding of the factors that influence the function of the cardiovascular system, it is necessary to become familiar with the concepts of cardiac output, arterial BP, rate-pressure product (RPP), ejection fraction (EF), and TPR. Table 7-3 provides a series of sample calculations that represent typical resting and exercise values for HR, SV, cardiac output, arterial BP, RPP, and TPR in a young, healthy, untrained male subject. Refer to the later Doing the Math section for additional practice.

## Cardiac Output

**Cardiac output ($\dot{Q}$)** is the amount of blood pumped by the heart per unit time (typically expressed per minute) and is equal to the product of SV and HR as shown in the following equation:

$$\dot{Q} \text{ (L/min)} = \text{HR (bpm)} \times \text{SV (mL/beat)}$$

Cardiac output is an excellent reflection of the rate of blood flow through the cardiovascular system. Increases in HR (rate adaptation) and/or SV (volume adaptation) will increase cardiac output, and this is especially important during exercise when blood flow must substantially increase to meet the metabolic demands of the working muscle. Resting $\dot{Q}$ ranges from 5 to 6 L/min, and during exercise it can increase to more than 30 L/min in endurance-trained individuals. Taking into consideration the normal blood volume of 5 L in the cardiovascular system, the heart recirculates this volume once every minute at rest and up to 6 or 7 times that amount per minute during exercise.

## Arterial Blood Pressure

**Systolic blood pressure (SBP)** is the pressure exerted on the systemic arterial walls during the period of ventricular systole (contraction). **Diastolic blood pressure (DBP)** is the pressure exerted during the period of ventricular diastole (relaxation). The mathematical difference between these two pressures is termed the **pulse pressure** (PP). SBP and DBP are reported together as a ratio when measured, with systolic pressure in the numerator and diastolic pressure in the denominator. The ratio is ideally ≤120/80 mm Hg.

The average BP in the cardiovascular system can be estimated by the **mean arterial pressure (MAP)**. MAP is difficult to directly measure in the vascular system. However, data from SBP and DBP can be used to mathematically estimate MAP by the following equation:

$$\text{MAP (mm Hg)} = (\text{SBP} - \text{DBP}) \times 0.33 + \text{DBP}$$

In this manner, MAP is equal to 1/3 of the PP plus the DBP. This is due to differences in the time the heart is in systole and diastole. At rest, the heart is in diastole approximately 60% to 70% of the time during a normal

**Table 7-3.** Sample Calculations That Represent Typical Resting and Exercise Values* for Heart Rate, Stroke Volume, Cardiac Output, Arterial Blood Pressure, Rate–Pressure Product, and Total Peripheral Resistance in a Young, Healthy, Untrained Male Subject[†]

| | HR (BPM) | | SV (ML/BEAT) | | $\dot{Q}$ (L/MIN) |
|---|---|---|---|---|---|
| **Sample $\dot{Q}$** | | | | | |
| Rest | 74 | × | 70 | = | 5.2 |
| Moderate exercise | 140 | × | 90 | = | 12.6 |
| Intense exercise | 180 | × | 100 | = | 19.0 |
| **Sample PP** | | | | | |
| | SYSTOLIC BP (mm Hg) | | DIASTOLIC BP (mm Hg) | | PP (mm Hg) |
| Rest | 120 | − | 80 | = | 42 |
| Moderate exercise | 160 | − | 78 | = | 66 |
| Intense exercise | 180 | − | 80 | = | 82 |
| **Sample MAP** | | | | | |
| | PP (mm Hg) | | DIASTOLIC BP (mm Hg) | | MAP (mm Hg) |
| Rest | 42 | × 0.33 + | 80 | = | 94 |
| Moderate exercise | 66 | × 0.33 + | 78 | = | 100 |
| Intense exercise | 82 | × 0.33 + | 80 | = | 107 |
| **Sample RPP** | | | | | |
| | HR (BPM) | | SYSTOLIC BP (mm Hg) | | RPP (ARBITRARY UNITS) |
| Rest | 74 | × | 120 | = | 8,880 |
| Moderate exercise | 140 | × | 160 | = | 22,400 |
| Intense exercise | 180 | × | 180 | = | 32,400 |
| **Sample TPR** | | | | | |
| | MAP (mm Hg) | | $\dot{Q}$ (L/MIN) | | TPR (ARBITRARY UNITS) |
| Rest | 94 | × | 5.2 | = | 18.1 |
| Moderate exercise | 100 | × | 12.6 | = | 7.9 |
| Intense exercise | 107 | × | 18.0 | = | 5.9 |

*Moderate exercise = 50% maximal oxygen consumption; intense exercise = 75% maximum oxygen consumption.
[†]20 years old with a body weight of approximately 70 kg.
BP, blood pressure; bpm, beats per minute; HR, heart rate; MAP, mean arterial pressure; PP, pulse pressure; $\dot{Q}$, cardiac output; RPP, rate-pressure product; SV, stroke volume; TPR, total peripheral resistance

cardiac cycle; thus, the PP is corrected (using 0.33) in the equation to account for the time discrepancy. At rest, MAP in adults approximates 100 mm Hg (assuming normal SBP and DBP), and during exercise it may reach as high as 110 mm Hg or slightly more.

Current recommendations are to keep SBP and DBP below 120/80 mm Hg to decrease the risk for hypertension. **Hypertension** is diagnosed when an individual's resting BP exceeds 140/90 mm Hg, confirmed by a health professional on two or more occasions.[12] Currently, it is estimated that 33% of the U.S. population has hypertension.[18,19] The danger of progressive and chronic hypertension is its strong association with cardiovascular disease,[20–22] particularly with coronary artery disease and cerebrovascular disease.[21,22] Other complications of high BP entail long-term, harmful effects on the structure and function of the myocardium, as well as damage to peripheral blood vessels and organs. However, regular exercise training is one of the best lifestyle interventions to lower BP and reduce the risk for hypertension. It is not uncommon for regular exercise training to elicit approximately 10-mm Hg reductions in resting BPs in people with mild-to-moderate hypertension.[23]

## Rate-Pressure Product

**Rate-pressure product (RPP)** is the product of HR and SBP:

$$RPP = HR \times SBP$$

It is standard practice not to report units when calculating for RPP. As a noninvasive measurement, it is a good index of myocardial oxygen demand at rest and during activity. Thus, as RPP changes with increases in HR and SBP, the work of the heart and the demand for oxygen also increase. Exercise professionals can use RPP to develop appropriate exercise programs for individuals who suffer from **angina pectoris** (chest pain caused by reduced oxygen delivery to the myocardium). In these cases, it is quite typical to reproduce chest pain events at a similar RPP each time. With this in mind, exercise professionals should set exercise workloads to keep individuals well under the RPP associated with angina to help ensure safe and effective exercise routines.

## Ejection Fraction

**Ejection fraction (%EF)** is the fraction (percent) of blood ejected from the ventricles per heartbeat. The %EF is calculated by dividing SV by EDV:

$$\%EF = SV \ (mL) \ / \ EDV \ (mL) \times 100$$

A normal %EF ranges from approximately 55% to 70% at rest and can increase with exercise (up to 80%). An abnormal or pathological EF is less than 50%.[24,25] An EF at this level is an important clinical measure to determine the severity of myocardial disease.[25] Certainly, if the heart's ability to forcefully contract is diminished because of a myocardial infarction, then the fraction of blood ejected out of the heart will be lower. As a result, ESV will be higher and SV will be reduced.

## HEMODYNAMICS

**Hemodynamics**, the study of factors that contribute to the flow of blood through the cardiovascular system, is tightly regulated by alterations in pressure, flow, and vascular resistance. Recall that blood flow through the systemic circulation is the result of a pressure difference established by the left heart pump. Pressure is highest in the aorta and lowest in the right atrium, creating a high-pressure gradient that drives blood through the systemic circulation. Consequently, changes in BP can have a profound effect on the amount of blood that circulates through the vascular system. In contrast, if HR increases or if the heart contracts more forcefully, the delivery of blood will also increase. Finally, changes in the resistance provided by the circulation can also affect the flow of blood. To properly understand the factors that regulate blood flow, especially during exercise, it is important to appreciate the physical properties of blood and the hemodynamic changes that influence BP, flow, and resistance.

## Blood

A major component of the cardiovascular system is the blood that it transports. The human body normally contains approximately 5 L of blood, which is composed of two primary constituents: **plasma** and cells. Figure 7-15 shows the proportion of plasma and cells in whole blood. Approximately 55% of the blood is plasma. Plasma is the liquid portion of blood that consists mostly of water (90%). Suspended within this watery liquid are electrolytes (e.g., sodium, potassium, chloride, and bicarbonate), proteins (e.g., albumins, globulins, and fibrinogen), and hormones. In addition, plasma is the vehicle that transports other important nutrients and substances to and from the tissues including glucose, amino acids, and urea.

Aside from the plasma, 45% of the blood is made up of "formed elements," or cells. Three important types of cells are contained in blood: red blood cells (RBCs), white blood cells, and platelets. Most of the cells that make up the blood are RBCs, with low concentrations of white blood cells and platelets. The responsibility of RBCs is to carry oxygen from the lungs to other tissues. The oxygen-carrying capacity of RBCs is greatly influenced by the presence of the iron-containing protein **hemoglobin**, a specialized protein that binds oxygen on the surface of RBCs. White blood cells are much less abundant than RBCs, but they have an important function to help prevent infections, whereas platelets play an important role in blood clotting. The fraction of blood that contains cells is known as the **hematocrit**. For example, if the volume of blood occupied by cells

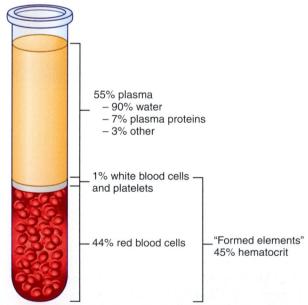

55% plasma
– 90% water
– 7% plasma proteins
– 3% other

1% white blood cells and platelets

44% red blood cells

"Formed elements" 45% hematocrit

**Figure 7-15.** The composition of blood. Blood is mostly composed of liquid called *plasma* (55%). Plasma contains approximately 90% water and a small portion of electrolytes and plasma proteins. Blood also contains a variety of "formed elements" or cells, including red blood cells, white blood cells, and platelets. The cell portion of blood is known as the hematocrit. Blood viscosity is influenced by the number of red blood cells.

is 40% and the remaining 60% is plasma, then the hematocrit is 40%. RBCs are the largest and most abundant cells in the blood, and for this reason they influence the hematocrit more than any other cell. In other words, large changes in the amount of RBCs will cause large changes in the amount of hematocrit.

Blood viscosity, or thickness, can influence the flow of blood through the circulation. Increased blood viscosity will make it more difficult for blood to flow through the vessels, especially through small arteries, arterioles, and capillaries. The concentration of RBCs is the primary factor that influences blood viscosity. A greater concentration of RBCs will increase blood viscosity, whereas reductions in RBCs, as with iron-deficient anemia, will lower viscosity.

## Relation Among Pressure, Cardiac Output, and Vascular Resistance

MAP, cardiac output, and TPR are the primary factors that govern the flow of blood from the heart to peripheral organs and tissues. As described previously, MAP is the average BP within the cardiovascular system. It was calculated as DBP + 0.33 (PP). Another way to calculate MAP is to multiply cardiac output by TPR. This relation is shown in the following equation:

$$MAP = \dot{Q} \times TPR$$

An increase in cardiac output or TPR will increase BP, whereas a decrease in cardiac output or resistance will lower BP. Rearranging the above equation and solving for $\dot{Q}$ demonstrates how changes in pressure and resistance affect blood flow:

$$\dot{Q} = MAP / TPR$$

It should become evident that the rate of blood flow through the circulation is proportional to the pressure, but *inversely* related to the resistance. That is, blood flow will be elevated by either an increase in pressure or a decrease in resistance.

Many factors can contribute to the resistance of blood flow, but the most important factor is the diameter of the blood vessels (Figure 7-16). Reducing the internal radius of a blood vessel (vasoconstriction) increases resistance, whereas increasing the radius (vasodilation) lowers resistance. The arterioles are considered the primary resistance vessels, because they contain a great deal of smooth muscle and can change their radius in concert with the needs of the tissue they supply.

## NEURAL CONTROL OF THE CARDIOVASCULAR SYSTEM

To ensure that all tissues in the body receive adequate blood flow, the heart and vasculature must work in a coordinated fashion to maintain BP throughout the circulation. Regulation of this process occurs primarily through cardiovascular neural control mechanisms that are integrated with sensory information received from the peripheral circulation. In general, control of HR, arterial BP, and ventricular contractility arises from higher brain centers located in the cerebral cortex, referred to as central command. In turn, central command maintains precise control of the cardiovascular system by directing the **cardiovascular control center**.[30]

### Cardiovascular Control Center

Neural impulses arising in the central command regions of the cortex directly influence activity of the cardiovascular control center, which is located in the brainstem above the spinal cord in an area known as the **medulla oblongata**. The medulla is the primary coordinating center that receives sensory input from central command and other brain centers, particularly the hypothalamus, to maintain cardiovascular homeostasis.[17,30] For example, the cerebral cortex and hypothalamus modify the activity of the medulla to adjust HR and BP in response to various forms of stress (e.g., exercise, heat, and emotional stress). The medulla also receives input from various systemic receptors and uses this information to make adjustments in cardiovascular

## SEX DIFFERENCES

Males have a larger blood volume and a greater hematocrit than females. The average hematocrit for a normal male is approximately 42%, whereas that of females is lower, averaging approximately 38%. Thus, males have a greater oxygen-carrying capacity than females, which is one reason that males typically have a higher aerobic capacity than females. One issue that females need to be aware of is iron-deficient anemia. Anemia refers to a loss of RBCs and hematocrit below normal ranges. It can be caused by many factors, but the most common cause is low iron levels in the body. This type of anemia is far more common in women than in men.[26] In premenopausal women, for instance, chronic blood loss because of heavy menstruation may lead to substantial reductions in RBC number and iron levels, especially if iron is not replaced in the diet.[27] Iron is necessary for proper hemoglobin formation. Without it, the ability of hemoglobin to carry oxygen is drastically reduced. Consequently, people may experience several signs and symptoms indicative of low blood oxygen levels (e.g., extreme fatigue, weakness, shortness of breath, and pale skin color) that can affect their ability to perform daily activities and exercise.[27-29]

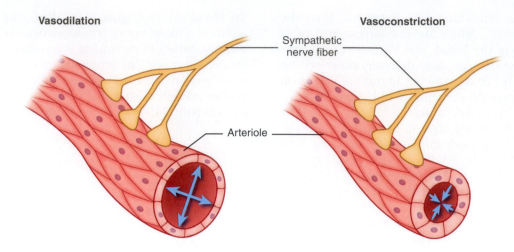

**Vasodilation**

**Vasoconstriction**

Sympathetic
nerve fiber

Arteriole

**Figure 7-16.** Smooth muscle fibers in arterioles are under the control of the autonomic nervous system. Arteriole diameter can be changed to increase or decrease velocity of blood flow based on the needs of tissues. A decrease in vessel diameter is vasoconstriction, which would increase the resistance to blood flow. The opposite effect is an increase in vessel diameter called *vasodilation*, which would decrease the resistance to blood flow through the system.

**DOING THE MATH:**
You are performing an initial screening on a client who is at high risk for cardiovascular disease. After recently joining your medically based fitness center, you discuss and document his pertinent health information, and record his medical history and hemodynamic variables shown in the following table.

| PHYSIOLOGICAL VARIABLE | RESTING VALUE |
|---|---|
| SBP | 160 mm Hg |
| DBP | 90 mm Hg |
| HR | 85 bpm |
| SV | 60 mL/beat |
| EDV | 120 mL blood |

Using this information, complete the following calculations:

1. Calculate ESV.

ESV = EDV − SV
ESV = 120 mL − 60 mL
ESV = 60 mL

2. Calculate SV.

SV = EDV − ESV
SV = 120 mL − 60 mL
SV = 60 mL

3. Calculate %EF.

%EF = SV/EDV
%EF = (60 mL/120 mL) × 100
%EF = 50%

4. Calculate cardiac output ($\dot{Q}$).

$\dot{Q}$ = SV × HR
$\dot{Q}$ = (60 mL/beat × 85 bpm)/1,000
$\dot{Q}$ = 5.1 L/min

5. Calculate PP.

PP = SBP − DBP
PP = (160 mm Hg − 90 mm Hg)
PP = 70 mm Hg

6. Calculate MAP.

MAP = (SBP − DBP) × 0.33 + DBP
MAP = (160 mm Hg − 90 mm Hg) × 0.33 + 90 mm Hg
MAP = (70 mm Hg) × 0.33 + 90 mm Hg
MAP = 23.1 mm Hg + 90 mm Hg
MAP = 113.1 mm Hg

7. Calculate RPP.

RPP = HR × SBP
RPP = 85 bpm × 160 mm Hg
RPP = 13, 600 arbitrary units

## FROM THEORY TO PRACTICE

You are a fitness professional working in an outpatient phase III/IV cardiac rehabilitation program at a local community center that offers medically supervised exercise programs for persons with or at high risk for disease. A middle-aged male client with a recent history of hypertension, coronary artery disease, and myocardial infarction has been assigned to you and will continue the remainder of his rehabilitation at your facility. To create an appropriate exercise program for him to follow, you must consider your client's unique history and the underlying effects that the disease process has potentially rendered on his cardiovascular system. Given your knowledge of central and peripheral cardiovascular hemodynamics and function, list effects that high BP and scar tissue left behind by a myocardial infarction can have on the pumping function and work of the heart, and subsequent blood flow through the system. Consider these variables:

1. Effects of a myocardial infarction and damage on $\dot{Q}$, SV, and HR.
2. Effects of a myocardial infarction and damage on *contractility and preload* to increase force of contraction and blood ejection.
3. Effects of high BP on $\dot{Q}$ *and SV* as they pertain to *afterload*.
4. Effects of existing coronary artery disease and adequate blood flow to the *highly aerobic myocardium*.

function. Figure 7-17 provides a general overview of the neural control of the cardiovascular system. Four primary regions of the medullary cardiovascular control center play important roles in maintaining cardiovascular control:

1. Pressor area: Acts to *increase* BP through vasoconstriction of blood vessels. In response to low-pressure receptors in the aorta and carotid arteries, this area sends signals to increase sympathetic activity to increase HR and BP.
2. Depressor area: Acts to *decrease* BP. In response to increased BP in the aorta and carotid arteries, this area sends impulses to increase parasympathetic activity to lower HR and reduce vasoconstriction of blood vessels.
3. **Cardiac acceleration center:** Acts to increase HR, BP, and ventricular contractility. This center is associated with activation of the sympathetic nervous system.
4. **Cardiac inhibitory center:** Acts to suppress cardiac function, primarily by decreasing HR, SV, and $\dot{Q}$. This center is associated with increased activity of the parasympathetic nervous system.

## Autonomic Nervous System

In response to inputs from the central command center and the periphery, the medulla sends neural output signals to the heart and blood vessels via the **sympathetic** and **parasympathetic** divisions of the autonomic nervous system. These autonomic nerve fibers travel to the heart and blood vessels where they exert control of HR, BP, and ventricular contractility. Generally, the cardiac acceleration and pressor regions are associated with activation of the sympathetic nervous system, and the cardioinhibitory and depressor regions are associated with the parasympathetic nervous system.[18]

## Sympathetic Control

Nerve impulses that arise from the sympathetic nervous system are transmitted by cardiac accelerator nerves (sympathetic nerves) to innervate the heart and blood vessels. In the heart, the accelerator nerves make contact with the SA and AV nodes, and atrial and ventricular myocardial cells. Upon activation from the cardiovascular control center, the nerve endings release the catecholamine **norepinephrine**, which acts to directly increase the pacemaker activity of the SA and AV nodes, thereby increasing HR to rates greater than 100 bpm. Moreover, norepinephrine exerts a powerful effect on myocardial contractility, which helps to increase SV and cardiac output. In the periphery, the sympathetic nerve fibers innervate the adrenal gland to release **epinephrine** and norepinephrine into the blood, which, in turn, increase HR and contractility. This influence is relatively minor compared with direct neural stimulation from the sympathetic nerves. However, during exercise, especially moderate-to high-intensity exercise, the release of epinephrine into the circulation is substantially increased. Epinephrine causes the arterioles to vasodilate. Vasodilation causes vascular resistance to decrease in the arterioles, which increases the supply of blood to the working muscle. Activation of the sympathetic nervous system also constricts pulmonary vessels and constricts vessels in the gastrointestinal regions, skin, kidney, and nonworking muscle. Table 7-4 provides a summary of the effects of sympathetic activation on the cardiovascular system.

## Parasympathetic Control

Nerve impulses that arise from the parasympathetic nervous system are transmitted by the vagus nerve to innervate the SA and AV nodes, and atrial and ventricular myocardial cells. Under resting conditions, the vagus nerve exerts a powerful chronic parasympathetic activity on the heart through the release of **acetylcholine**,

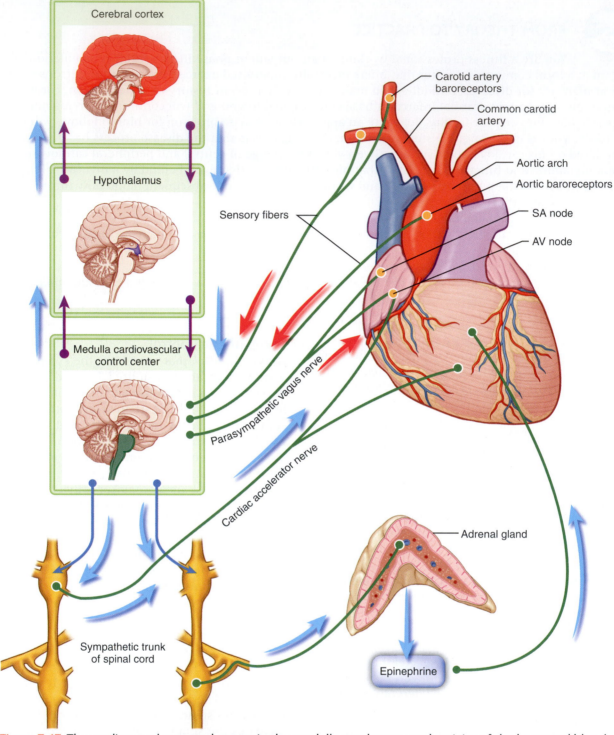

**Figure 7-17.** The cardiovascular control center in the medulla regulates neural activity of the heart and blood vessels through the sympathetic and parasympathetic nervous system. Neural output signals from the medulla are delivered by the vagus nerve (parasympathetic) and the cardioaccelerator nerves (sympathetic).

a neurotransmitter that acts directly on the SA and AV nodes. Acetylcholine suppresses HR by inhibiting pacemaker activity and slowing electrical conduction through the myocardium. Typically, parasympathetic activity keeps HR less than 100 bpm while at rest. This is referred to as **parasympathetic tone**.[15,17] Changes in parasympathetic tone will directly influence HR. For instance, an increase in parasympathetic tone will slow HR (increased

cardioinhibitory activity), whereas a withdrawal of tone (decreased cardioinhibitory activity), which occurs at the initiation of exercise, will elevate HR. Vagal nerve stimulation also reduces myocardial contraction force and dilates blood vessels in the gastrointestinal region, skin, kidney, and muscles.[31,32] Table 7-4 provides a summary of the effects of the parasympathetic system on cardiovascular function.

## Table 7-4. Effects of the Sympathetic and Parasympathetic Nervous Systems on Cardiovascular Function

| FUNCTION | SYMPATHETIC STIMULATION | PARASYMPATHETIC STIMULATION |
|---|---|---|
| Heart rate | Increases | Decreases |
| Myocardial contractility | Increases | Decreases |
| Stroke volume | Increases | Decreases |
| Cardiac output | Increases | Decreases |

## Peripheral Control

The cardiovascular control center receives sensory information from a variety of mechanical, chemical, and thermal receptors located in the peripheral circulation.[17,31–33] These receptors operate by establishing a specific set point to help maintain cardiovascular homeostasis. For instance, mechanical receptors (**mechanoreceptors**) sense changes in BP, blood volume, and muscle tension, whereas chemical receptors (**chemoreceptors**) sense changes in blood gases (i.e., oxygen and carbon dioxide) and blood pH. Thermoreceptors, located throughout the body and in the hypothalamus, sense deviations from the body's temperature set point. Feedback from the internal environment provides the cardiovascular control center with important information with respect to the regulation of a particular cardiovascular parameter (e.g., BP and blood oxygen concentration). Using this feedback, the cardiovascular control center relays signals via the sympathetic and parasympathetic pathways to make changes in the function of the heart and vasculature. An important example of this feedback process involves the control of arterial BP. An increase in resting BP above the set point stimulates pressure receptors (baroreceptors) in the aortic arch and carotid arteries to send information to the cardiovascular control center. To help return BP back to normal, the cardiovascular control center increases parasympathetic tone to the heart and reduces sympathetic activity. The result is a decrease in HR and cardiac output, which lowers BP. The reverse is also true, in that a decrease in resting BP below the set point will result in an increase in HR and cardiac output to elevate BP.[34,35]

## HUMORAL CONTROL OF THE CARDIOVASCULAR SYSTEM

Humoral control of the heart and vasculature involves the release of substances into the circulation that directly or indirectly affect HR and myocardial function, the degree of arteriolar vasodilation or vasoconstriction,

and arterial BP. Some of the most important humoral substances include circulating catecholamines (epinephrine and norepinephrine) released from the adrenal medulla in response to sympathetic nerve stimulation. Moreover, the renin-angiotensin system also plays an important role in the short-term control of arterial BP and blood flow. When BP is lowered, this system produces angiotensin II, a hormone that exerts a powerful vasoconstrictor effect on arteries and veins. It acts to elevate systemic vascular resistance and increase venous return that ultimately raises arterial BP. Other factors include the vasoconstrictor endothelin, which also raises BP by increasing vascular resistance.

Although the sympathetic nervous system stimulates vasodilation of the arterioles that supply blood to exercising muscle, it also decreases blood flow to less active tissues by causing vasoconstriction. That is, it increases vascular resistance to the kidneys, gastrointestinal region, skeletal system, and skin so that more blood can by shunted to the working muscle where vascular resistance is reduced. However, a variety of other factors play an integral role to locally fine-tune blood flow throughout exercise to muscle (see Chapter 8 for a more detailed description of the local factors that increase muscle blood flow during exercise). Local blood flow regulation to the muscle (as well as many other tissues) is intrinsically controlled. This means that muscle has the capacity to regulate its own blood flow in direct proportion to its metabolic demand.[36] Indeed, skeletal muscle has the ability to increase its blood flow within seconds of muscular contraction. The extent of blood flow supply is directly proportional to the number of muscle fibers activated. Strenuous, dynamic exercise elicits large increases in local blood flow, whereas local blood flow changes during low-intensity exercise are proportionally less. What factors contribute to increases in local blood flow during exercise? As exercise begins, changes in the microenvironment of the muscle stimulate the arterioles to vasodilate, which lowers vascular resistance and increases the supply of blood to working muscle. Some of the most important factors that increase blood flow are reduced concentrations of oxygen, increased carbon dioxide concentrations, and decreased blood pH. In addition, working muscle releases a variety of vasoactive metabolites that directly cause the arterioles and small arteries that feed working muscle to dilate. It appears that nitric oxide, adenosine, and prostaglandins are the most important vasodilating metabolites that increase muscle blood flow during exercise. Collectively, the release of epinephrine from the adrenal medulla stimulates blood vessels in the working muscle to vasodilate and causes vasoconstriction of less active tissues during exercise. The net effect is a redistribution of blood to the muscle. In addition, local vasodilating metabolites are released in the microenvironment of contracting skeletal muscle to fine-tune blood flow supply to match metabolic demand.

## V I G N E T T E  *conclusion*

■ The exercise rehabilitation program that Jermaine and Brett develop for Mr. Chu is designed to improve his quality of life so that he can resume normal everyday activities. The goal is to stabilize, slow, or even reverse the progression of cardiovascular disease, thereby reducing the risk for another cardiac event. The exercise program focuses on enhancing Mr. Chu's aerobic fitness capacity and managing his existing cardiovascular risk factors (e.g., hypertension, high cholesterol, insulin resistance, and obesity) through exercise participation and education. Exercise frequency will include participation in sessions most days of the week (4–7 days/week)

at a safe intensity (40%–80% heart rate reserve) for 20 to 60 minutes per session. However, the frequency, intensity, and duration of the exercise program may be impacted by the degree of cardiovascular risk stratification, exercise capacity, and other safety factors (e.g., ischemic threshold, psychological impairment, and musculoskeletal limitations).[1,12,37] By following the guidelines and leadership provided by Jermaine, Brett, and other key healthcare professionals, Mr. Chu resumes his life with the peace of mind that his heart and vasculature are on the right path to becoming disease free.

## CRITICAL THINKING QUESTIONS

1. You are an exercise physiologist in a cardiac rehabilitation program. A patient you are working with experiences significant chest pain and requests to stop exercise. The nurse monitoring the patient's ECG mentions that she sees ST segment changes consistent with an acute myocardial infarction in the anterior portion of the heart and the patient must be transported to the emergency department. What coronary artery is most likely blocked in this situation? Why would myocardial ischemia adversely affect the ST segment?

2. Recall the influence of increased preload on SV. As the volume of blood is increased in the left ventricle, the cardiac muscle stretches, creating more active tension in each cardiac muscle fiber, which produces a greater force of contraction. However, activation of the sympathetic nervous system increases SV through an entirely different mechanism, independent of changes in preload. How does the sympathetic nervous system enhance SV in this manner?

3. A female endurance athlete that you are training recently had the opportunity to participate in a cardiovascular research study at the local university's exercise physiology laboratory. During the test, HR, SV, cardiac output, and maximal oxygen consumption (a direct measurement of maximal cardiorespiratory fitness) were measured. Your client indicates to you that a significantly taller male subject was tested before she was. His maximal oxygen consumption, expressed as milliliters of oxygen consumed per kilogram of body weight per minute (mL/kg/min), was very

similar to hers. However, his maximal SV was higher, but his maximal HR was lower than hers. Intrigued, she wonders how it is possible that maximal fitness capacity can be similar even though maximum HR and SV can be different between men and women. How do you explain this to her?

4. Blood doping has become a popular, albeit highly controversial, method of enhancing exercise performance. In brief, RBCs are removed from a sample of blood, stored for a short period, and then transfused back into the circulation approximately 7 days before an endurance exercise event. Following reinfusion of the stored RBCs, dramatic improvements in RBC count, hemoglobin concentration, and hematocrit levels are observed, which greatly impacts exercise performance. It is possible to enhance aerobic exercise capacity approximately 10% through blood doping. Aside from the positive effects on aerobic capacity, what effect do you think blood doping will have on cardiovascular hemodynamics?

5. Patients who suffer from chest pain (angina) during exercise or activity can experience this symptom at different HRs and SBPs each time; however, angina symptoms usually occur at the same RPP. Why do you think this is the case, and what does RPP generally reflect in the heart?

6. A client whom you have recently begun working with has a personal and family history of hypertension (high BP). The client asks you why it is so bad on the heart to have hypertension and how helpful will it be to lower her BP. What do you tell her?

## ADDITIONAL RESOURCES

Dunbar C, Saul B. *ECG Interpretation for the Clinical Exercise Physiologist.* Philadelphia, PA: Lippincott, Williams & Wilkins; 2009.
Levy MN, Pappano AJ, Berne RM. *Cardiovascular Physiology.* 9th ed. Philadelphia, PA: Mosby Elsevier; 2009.
Mohrman DE, Heller LJ. *Cardiovascular Physiology.* 8th ed. New York, NY: McGraw-Hill, Health Professions Division, 2014.
### Websites
American Heart Association: www.heart.org/HEARTORG
Blaufuss Medical Multimedia Laboratories: www.blaufus.com

Centers for Disease Control and Prevention: www.cdc.gov/heartdisease/index.htm
HeartHub for Patients: www.hearthub.org
### Suggested Readings
Klabunde R. *Cardiovascular Physiology Concepts.* Philadelphia, PA: Lippincott, Williams & Wilkins; 2005.
Quyyumi AA. Endothelial function in health and disease: New insights into the genesis of cardiovascular disease. *Am J Med.* 1998;105:32S–39S.
Tanaka H, Dinenno FA, Monahan KD, Clevenger CM, DeSouza CA, Seals DR. Aging, habitual exercise, and dynamic arterial compliance. *Circulation.* 2000;102:1270–1275.

## REFERENCES

1. American Association of Cardiovascular & Pulmonary Rehabilitation. *AACVPR Cardiac Rehabilitation Resource Manual: Promoting Health and Preventing Disease.* Chicago, IL: Human Kinetics. 2006:xv.
2. Suga H. Ventricular energetics. *Physiol Rev.* 1990;70:247–277.
3. Kraus WE, Torgan CE, Duscha BD, et al. Studies of a targeted risk reduction intervention through defined exercise (STRRIDE). *Med Sci Sports Exerc.* 2001;33:1774–1784.
4. Houmard JA, Tanner CJ, Slentz CA, Duscha BD, McCartney JS, Kraus WE. Effect of the volume and intensity of exercise training on insulin sensitivity. *J Appl Physiol.* 2004;96:101–106.
5. Kraus WE, Houmard JA, Duscha BD, et al. Effects of the amount and intensity of exercise on plasma lipoproteins. *N Engl J Med.* 2002;347:1483–1492.
6. Halbert JA, Silagy CA, Finucane P, Withers RT, Hamdorf PA, Andrews GR. The effectiveness of exercise training in lowering blood pressure: A meta-analysis of randomised controlled trials of 4 weeks or longer. *J Hum Hypertens.* 1997;11:641–649.
7. Dinenno FA, Tanaka H, Monahan KD, et al. Regular endurance exercise induces expansive arterial remodelling in the trained limbs of healthy men. *J Physiol.* 2001;534(Pt 1):287–295.
8. Seals DR, Desouza CA, Donato AJ, Tanaka H. Habitual exercise and arterial aging. *J Appl Physiol.* 2008;105:1323–1332.
9. Seals DR, Walker AE, Pierce GL, Lesniewski LA. Habitual exercise and vascular ageing. *J Physiol.* 2009;587(Pt 23):5541–5549.
10. Van Guilder GP, Hoetzer GL, Smith DT, et al. Endothelial t-PA release is impaired in overweight and obese adults but can be improved with regular aerobic exercise. *Am J Physiol Endocrinol Metab.* 2005;289:E807–E813.
11. Van Guilder GP, Westby CM, Greiner JJ, Stauffer BL, DeSouza CA. Endothelin-1 vasoconstrictor tone increases with age in healthy men but can be reduced by regular aerobic exercise. *Hypertension.* 2007;50:403–409.
12. American College of Sports Medicine, et al. *ACSM's Guidelines for Exercise Testing and Prescription.* 9th ed. Philadelphia, PA: Lippincott Williams & Wilkins; xxi, 380 p. 2014.
13. Braunwald E, Frahm CJ. Studies on Starling's law of the heart: IV. Observations on the hemondynamic functions of the left atrium in man. *Circulation.* 1961;24:633–642.
14. Wiggers CJ, Katz LN. The contours of the ventricular volume curves under different conditions. *Am J Physiol.* 1922;58:439.
15. Guyton AC, Hall JE. *Textbook of Medical Physiology.* 11th ed. Philadelphia, PA: Elsevier Saunders; 2006:xxxv.
16. Gisolfi CV, Cohen JS. Relationships among training, heat acclimation, and heat tolerance in men and women: The controversy revisited. *Med Sci Sports.* 1979;11:56–59.
17. Boron WF, Boulpaep EL. *Medical Physiology: A Cellular and Molecular Approach.* 2nd ed. Philadelphia, PA: Saunders/Elsevier; 2009:xii.
18. Levy MN, Pappano AJ, Berne RM. *Cardiovascular Physiology.* 9th ed. Mosby physiology monograph series. Philadelphia, PA: Mosby Elsevier; 2007:xiv.
19. Mohrman DE, Heller LJ. *Cardiovascular Physiology.* 4th ed. New York, NY: McGraw-Hill, Health Professions Division; 1997:xi.
20. Kenney WL. Parasympathetic control of resting heart rate: Relationship to aerobic power. *Med Sci Sports Exerc.* 1985;17:451–455.
21. Roger VL, Go AS, Lloyd-Jones DM, et al; American Heart Association Statistics Committee and Stroke Statistics Subcommittee. Heart disease and stroke statistics—2012 update: A report from the American Heart Association. *Circulation.* 2012;125:e2–e220.
22. Pescatello LS, Franklin BA, Fagard R, Farquhar WB, Kelley GA, Ray CA; American College of Sports Medicine. American College of Sports Medicine position stand. Exercise and hypertension. *Med Sci Sports Exerc.* 2004;36:533–553.
23. Gu Q, Burt VL, Paulose-Ram R, Yoon S, Gillum RF. High blood pressure and cardiovascular disease mortality risk among U.S. adults: The third National Health and Nutrition Examination Survey mortality follow-up study. *Ann Epidemiol.* 2008;18:302–309.
24. Chobanian AV. Prehypertension revisited. *Hypertension.* 2006;48:812–814.
25. Suri MF, Qureshi AI. Prehypertension as a risk factor for cardiovascular diseases. *J Cardiovasc Nurs.* 2006;21:478–482; quiz 483–484.
26. Chobanian AV, Bakris GL, Black HR, et al. The Seventh Report of the Joint National Committee on Prevention, Detection, Evaluation, and Treatment of High Blood Pressure: The JNC 7 report. *JAMA.* 2003;289:2560–2572.
27. Risk stratification and survival after myocardial infarction. *N Engl J Med.* 1983;309:331–336.
28. Jones RH, McEwan P, Newman GE, et al. Accuracy of diagnosis of coronary artery disease by radionuclide management of left ventricular function during rest and exercise. *Circulation.* 1981;64:586–601.
29. Iron deficiency—United States, 1999-2000. *MMWR Morb Mortal Wkly Rep.* 2002;51:897–899.
30. U.S. National Library of Medicine. What is iron-deficiency anemia? Retrieved from www.nhlbi.nih.gov/health/dci/Diseases/ida/ida_whatis.html March 9, 2014.

31. Brownlie T 4th, Utermohlen V, Hinton PS, Haas JD. Tissue iron deficiency without anemia impairs adaptation in endurance capacity after aerobic training in previously untrained women. *Am J Clin Nutr.* 2004;79:437–443.

32. Haas JD, Brownlie T 4th. Iron deficiency and reduced work capacity: A critical review of the research to determine a causal relationship. *J Nutr.* 2001;131 (2S-2):676S–688S; discussion 688S–690S.

33. Spyer KM. Annual review prize lecture. Central nervous mechanisms contributing to cardiovascular control. *J Physiol.* 1994;474:1–19.

34. Hainsworth R. Reflexes from the heart. *Physiol Rev.* 1991;71:617–658.

35. Marshall JM. Peripheral chemoreceptors and cardiovascular regulation. *Physiol Rev.* 1994;74:543–594.

36. Cowley AW Jr. Long-term control of arterial blood pressure. *Physiol Rev.* 1992;72:231–300.

37. Delp MD, O'Leary DS. Integrative control of the skeletal muscle microcirculation in the maintenance of arterial pressure during exercise. *J Appl Physiol.* 2004;97:1112–1118.

38. American Association of Cardiovascular & Pulmonary Rehabilitation. *Guidelines for Cardiac Rehabilitation and Secondary Prevention Programs.* 4th ed. Champaign, IL: Human Kinetics; 2004:viii.

# *Practice What You Know:* Measuring Heart Rate and Blood Pressure at Rest and During Exercise

## Equipment
- Stopwatch
- Stethoscope (optional)

## Resting Heart Rate

The pulse rate, which in most people is identical to the HR, can be measured at any point on the body where an artery's pulsation is close to the surface. The following are some commonly palpated sites (Fig. 1):

- Radial artery: measured on the thumb side of the wrist, and less commonly, the ulnar artery on the pinky side, which is deeper and harder to palpate (Fig. 1A)
- Carotid artery: located in the neck, lateral to the trachea; more easily palpated when the neck is slightly extended. When using the carotid artery for pulse detection, avoid pushing too hard, because this may evoke a vagal response and actually slow down the HR (Fig. 1B).

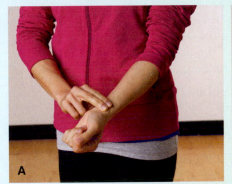
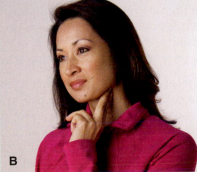

**Figure 1.** Heart rate. (A) Taking the pulse at the radial artery. (B) Taking the pulse at the carotid artery.

True RHR is measured just before an individual gets out of bed in the morning. Thus, in most fitness-training environments, the technician's assessment of RHR will not be entirely accurate. However, this method is an acceptable approach for use in field settings, such as fitness facilities and team coaching environments.

The pulsation heard through auscultation is generated by the expansion of the arteries as blood is pushed through after contraction of the left ventricle. This beat can be quite prominent in leaner individuals. The client should be resting comfortably for several minutes before obtaining the RHR. The RHR may be measured indirectly by placing the fingertips on a pulse site (palpation) or directly by listening through a stethoscope (auscultation).

## Procedure
- Place the tips of the index and middle fingers (not the thumb, which has a pulse of its own) over the artery (typically, radial is used) and lightly apply pressure.
- To determine the RHR, count the number of beats (starting with "one") for 30 or 60 seconds and then correct that score to beats per minute (bpm), if necessary.
- When measuring by auscultation, place the bell of the stethoscope to the left of the client's sternum just above or below the nipple line. (It is important to be respectful of the client's personal space.)

# *Practice What You Know:* Measuring Heart Rate and Blood Pressure at Rest and During Exercise–cont'd

- The client may also measure his or her own RHR before rising from bed in the morning and report back.
- Categorize the client's RHR using the information in Table 1.

### Table 1. Resting Heart Rate Classification

| RESTING HEART RATE | BEATS PER MINUTE |
| --- | --- |
| Sinus bradycardia (slow) | <60 |
| Normal sinus rhythm | 60–100 |
| Sinus tachycardia (fast) | >100 |

## Exercise Heart Rate

Measuring for 30 to 60 seconds is generally difficult. Therefore, exercise HRs are normally measured for shorter periods that are then corrected to equal 60 seconds. Generally, a 10- to 15-second count is recommended over a 6-second count given the larger potential for error with the shorter count.

## Procedure

- Place the tips of the index and middle fingers (not the thumb, which has a pulse of its own) over the artery (typically, radial is used) and lightly apply pressure.
- Count the first pulse beat as "one" at the start of the time interval, then multiply the counted score by either 6 (for a 10-second count) or 4 (for a 15-second count).
- Teaching the client these steps for how to measure his or her own pulse rate during exercise is a worthwhile activity to facilitate self-intensity monitoring.

## MEASURING RESTING AND EXERCISING BLOOD PRESSURE

## Equipment

- Sphygmomanometer (BP cuff)
- Stethoscope
- Chair

BP is defined as the outward force exerted by the blood on the vessel walls. It is generally recorded as two numbers. The higher number, the SBP, represents the pressure created by the heart as it pumps blood into circulation via ventricular contraction. This represents the greatest pressure during one cardiac cycle. The lower number, the DBP, represents the pressure that is exerted on the artery walls as blood remains in the arteries during the filling phase of the cardiac cycle, or between beats when the heart relaxes. It is the minimum pressure that exists within one cardiac cycle. BP is measured within the arterial system. The standard site of measurement is the brachial artery, given its easy accessibility and the ability to hold it level to the heart position.

BP is measured indirectly by listening to the Korotkoff sounds, which are sounds made from vibrations as blood moves along the walls of the vessel. These sounds are only present when some degree of wall deformation exists. If the vessel has unimpeded blood flow, no vibrations are heard. However, under the pressure of a BP cuff, vessel deformity facilitates hearing these sounds. This deformity is created as the air bladder within the cuff is inflated, restricting the flow of blood.

When inflated to pressures greater than the highest pressure that exists within a cardiac cycle, the brachial artery collapses, preventing blood flow. As the air is slowly released from the bladder, blood begins to flow past the compressed area, creating turbulent flow and vibration along the vascular wall. The first BP phase, signified by the onset of tapping Korotkoff sounds, corresponds with SBP. DBP is indicated by the fourth (significant muffling of sound) and fifth (disappearance of sound) phases (Fig. 2).

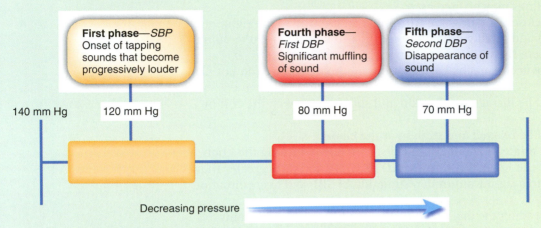

**Figure 2.** Korotkoff sounds and blood pressure phases. DBP, diastolic blood pressure; SBP, systolic blood pressure.

As the cuff is continuously released, BP within the vessel increases and eventually will exceed the pressure within the cuff. At this point, the BP completely distends the vessel wall back to its original shape and the Korotkoff sounds will fade (fourth phase) and then disappear (fifth phase). Typically, in adults with normal BP, the fifth phase is recorded as the DBP. However, in children and adults with a fifth phase below 40 mm Hg, but who appear healthy, the fourth phase may be used.

### Resting Blood Pressure Procedure

- Have the client sit with both feet flat on the floor for 5 minutes. **NOTE:** Crossing the legs may artificially elevate SBP and DBP readings.
- Cuff placement:
- While the right arm is considered standard, many individuals favor placing the cuff on the left arm because of the increased proximity to the heart, which amplifies the heart sounds. **NOTE:** Up to 20% of people will show a significant difference in BP readings between the right and left arms. Such a difference can be clinically significant and should be reported to the person's health-care provider.
- Smoothly and firmly wrap the BP cuff around the arm with its lower margin about 1 inch (2.5 cm) above the antecubital space (i.e., the inside of the elbow). The tubes should cross the antecubital space. **NOTE:** In extremely obese individuals, a more accurate reading may be obtained by placing the cuff on the forearm and listening over the radial artery.
- Because BP cuffs come in a variety of sizes (Table 2), it is important to ensure the correct size is used, because obese or muscular clients may have falsely elevated BP readings, whereas thin, small-framed individuals may have falsely low BP readings with a standard-sized cuff.

### Table 2. Blood Pressure Cuff Sizes Based on Arm Circumference

| ARM CIRCUMFERENCE (CM) | SIZE (CM) | LABEL |
|---|---|---|
| 22–26 | 12 × 22 | Small adult |
| 27–34 | 16 × 30 | Adult |
| 35–44 | 16 × 36 | Large adult |

Data from Kaplan NM, Victor RG. *Kaplan's Clinical Hypertension*. 10th ed. Baltimore, MD: Wolters Kluwer/Lippincott Williams & Wilkins; 2010.

## *Practice What You Know:* Measuring Heart Rate and Blood Pressure at Rest and During Exercise–cont'd

- The client's arm should be supported either on an armchair or by the technician at an angle of 0 to 45 degrees. **NOTE:** Positioning the arm above or below heart level can alter BP readings. If the arm is elevated, BP readings may be reduced; if the arm is too low, BP readings may be increased.
- Turn the bulb knob to close the cuff valve (turning it all the way to the right, no more than finger tight) and rapidly inflate the cuff to 160 mm Hg, or 20 to 30 mm Hg above the point where the pulse can no longer be felt at the wrist.
- Place the stethoscope over the brachial artery using minimal pressure (do not distort the artery).
- The stethoscope should lie flat against the skin and should not touch the cuff or the tubing.
- The client's arm should be relaxed and straight at the elbow.
- Release the pressure at a rate of about 2 mm Hg/sec by slowly turning the knob to the left, listening for the Korotkoff sounds. **NOTE:** Deflation rates greater than 2 mm Hg/sec can lead to a significant underestimation of SBP and overestimation of DBP.
- SBP is determined by reading the dial at the first perception of sound (a faint tapping sound).
- DBP is determined by reading the dial when the sounds become muffled or cease to be heard.
- If a BP reading needs to be repeated on the same arm, allow approximately 5 minutes between trials so that normal circulation can return to the area.
- Share measurements with the client, as well as the classification of values (Table 3).

### Table 3. Classification of Blood Pressure for Adults Aged 18 and Older

| CATEGORY | SYSTOLIC (MM HG) | | DIASTOLIC (MM HG) |
|---|---|---|---|
| Normal* | <120 | and | <80 |
| Prehypertension | 120–139 | or | 80–89 |
| Hypertension† | | | |
| Stage 1 | 140–159 | or | 90–99 |
| Stage 2 | ≥160 | or | ≥100 |

Reading apply to adults not taking antihypertensive drugs and not acutely ill. When systolic and diastolic blood pressures fall into different categories, the higher category should be selected to classify the individual's blood pressure status. For example, 140/82 mm Hg should be classified as stage 1 hypertension, and 154/102 mm Hg should be classified as stage 2 hypertension. In addition to classifying stages of hypertension on the basis of average blood pressure levels, clinicians should specify presence or absence of target organ disease and additional risk factors. This specificity is important for risk classification and treatment.
*Normal blood pressure with respect to cardiovascular risk is less than 120/80 mm Hg. However, unusually low readings should be evaluated for clinical significance.
†Based on the average of two or more readings taken at each of two or more visits after an initial screening.
*Note.* For individuals with diabetes or chronic kidney disease, high BP is defined as ≥130/80 mm Hg. High BP numbers also differ for children and tweens.
From Chobanian AV, Bakris GL, Black HR, et al. *JNC 7 Express: The Seventh Report of the Joint National Committee on Prevention, Detection, Evaluation, and Treatment of High Blood Pressure.* NIH Publication No. 03-5233. Washington, DC: National Institutes of Health & National Heart, Lung, and Blood Institute; 2003.

**NOTE:** If abnormal readings result, repeat the measurement on the opposite arm. In fact, many within the medical community are recommending that BP measurements be taken in both arms. If there is a significant discrepancy (>10 mm Hg) between readings from arm to arm, it could represent a circulatory problem, and the client should be referred to his or her physician for a medical evaluation (McManus & Mant, 2012).

## Common Errors in Measuring Blood Pressure
- Cuff deflation that is too rapid
- Inexperience of the test administrator or inability of the test administrator to accurately distinguish Korotkoff sounds and/or read pressure correctly
- Improper stethoscope placement and pressure
- Improper cuff size or an inaccurate/uncalibrated sphygmomanometer
- Auditory acuity of the test administrator or excessive background noise

## Measuring Blood Pressure During Exercise
BP is more difficult to measure during exercise (compared with rest) because of the excessive amount of movement and noise, unless the person is riding a stationary bicycle.

- A sphygmomanometer with a stand and a handheld gauge are better choices for measuring BP during exercise.
  - With exception of the client moving rather than sitting quietly in a chair, the same procedures are performed for measuring BP during exercise.
  - When monitoring BP during exercise, the technician should become familiar with using a sphygmomanometer with a stand and a handheld gauge.
- If SBP drops during exercise, it should immediately be remeasured before terminating the session, just to ensure accuracy in measurement. If the client was anxious before the cardiorespiratory assessment, it is likely that the initial exercise SBP reading will drop.

## Practicum 1: Resting Measures
Working in groups of two or three, elect one group member to be the subject for the experiment.

- Measure the subject's seated RHR for 30 seconds.
- Measure the subject's seated resting BP.
- Repeat the measurements in the standing position.

## Record the Results
- Enter the results into the following table and calculate the difference in each measure between seated and standing.
- Why do these differences exist?

|       | SEATED      | STANDING    | DIFFERENCE  |
|-------|-------------|-------------|-------------|
| RHR   | _____ bpm   | _____ bpm   | _____ bpm   |
| SBP   | _____ mm Hg | _____ mm Hg | _____ mm Hg |
| DBP   | _____ mm Hg | _____ mm Hg | _____ mm Hg |

## Practicum 2: Heart Rate and Blood Pressure Responses to Exercise
Working in the same groups, elect one group member to be the subject for the experiment. The subject will perform two separate, but increasingly intense 2-minute bouts of continuous stepping. His or her standing HR and BP immediately following each bout will be assessed.

## *Practice What You Know:* Measuring Heart Rate and Blood Pressure at Rest and During Exercise–cont'd

Workload 1: Ask the subject to complete the first 2-minute bout at a moderate effort (4 or 5 out of 10) using a 12- to 16-inch step/riser (leading with either foot).
  • At 1:45, ask the subject for his or her **ratings of perceived exertion** (RPE; see Table 4) and measure the subject's 10- to 15-second exercise HR.
  • At 2:00, instruct the subject to stop stepping and measure the subject's standing BP. Allow the individual to lightly walk in place during the measurement to maintain blood circulation.

### Table 4. Ratings of Perceived Exertion

| RATINGS OF PERCEIVED EXERTION | CATEGORY RATIO SCALE |
| --- | --- |
| 6 | 0 Nothing at all |
| 7 Very, very light | 0.5 Very, very weak |
| 8 | 1 Very weak |
| 9 Very light | 2 Weak |
| 10 | 3 Moderate |
| 11 Fairly light | 4 Somewhat strong |
| 12 | 5 Strong |
| 13 Somewhat hard | 6 |
| 14 | 7 Very strong |
| 15 Hard | 8 |
| 16 | 9 |
| 17 Very hard | 10 Very, very strong |
| 18 | *Maximal |
| 19 Very, very hard | |
| 20 | |

*Denotes reaching point of failure to continue exercise.
Data from Borg, G. (1998). *Borg's Perceived Exertion and Pain Scales*. Champaign, Ill.: Human Kinetics.

Chapter 7: Cardiovascular System 195

Workload 2: Ask the subject to complete the second 2-minute bout at moderate-to-vigorous effort (6 out of 10) using the 12- to 16-inch step/riser (leading with either foot) or running in place for 2 minutes.

- At 1:45, ask the subject for his or her RPE (Table 4) and measure the subject's 10- to 15-second exercise HR.
- At 2:00, instruct the subject to stop stepping (or running) and measure the subject's standing BP. Allow the individual to lightly walk in place during the measurement to maintain blood circulation.

## Record and Plot the Results
- Plot HR, SBP, and DBP from the seated resting position (Practicum 1) through Workload 2 (Fig. 3).
- Compare RPE and observe HR discrepancies.
- Explain why the changes observed exist.

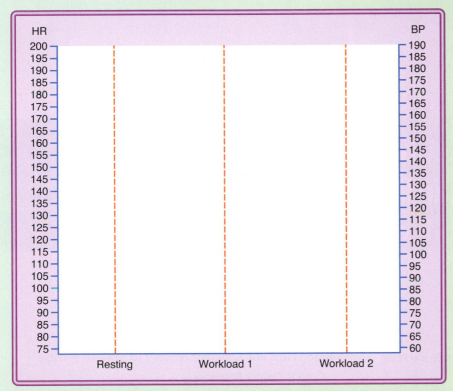

**Figure 3.**

## Application

The relationship between elevated BP and cardiovascular events (e.g., myocardial infarction or cerebrovascular accident) is unmistakable. For individuals 40 to 70 years old, each 20-mm Hg increase in resting SBP or each 10-mm Hg increase in resting DBP above normal doubles the risk for cardiovascular disease (American College of Sports Medicine, 2010). A difference of ≥15 mm Hg between arms increases risk for peripheral vascular disease and cerebral vascular disease, and is associated with a 70% risk for dying of heart disease (McManus & Mant, 2012). If the technician discovers an abnormal BP reading, either at rest or during exercise, it is prudent to recommend that the client visit his or her personal physician.

## REFERENCES

American College of Sports Medicine. *ACSM's Guidelines for Exercise Testing and Prescription* (8th ed.). Philadelphia: Wolters Kluwer/Lippincott Williams & Wilkins; 2010.

McManus RJ, Mant J. Do differences in blood pressure between arms matter? *Lancet.* 2012;379:872–873.

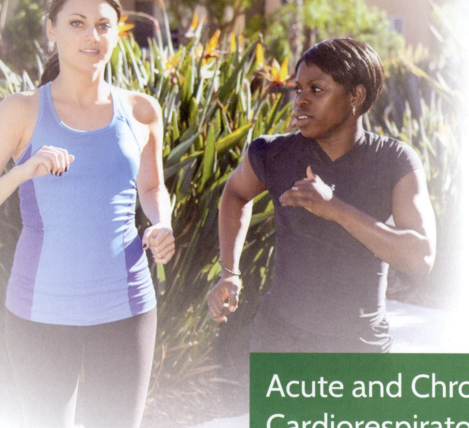

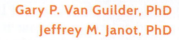

Gary P. Van Guilder, PhD
Jeffrey M. Janot, PhD

CHAPTER 8

# Acute and Chronic Cardiorespiratory Responses to Exercise

## CHAPTER OUTLINE

# CHAPTER OUTLINE—cont'd

# LEARNING OUTCOMES

1. Describe the immediate changes in the cardiovascular and respiratory systems after the start of exercise.
2. Describe the changes in the cardiovascular and respiratory systems during submaximal steady-state exercise.
3. Describe the changes in the cardiovascular and respiratory systems during incremental exercise up to maximum intensity.
4. Describe the changes in the cardiovascular and respiratory systems that occur during recovery from exercise.
5. Compare and contrast common methods to measure ventilatory threshold.
6. Explain the role of receptors that control respiratory and cardiovascular functions during exercise.
7. Identify the factors that regulate the control of peripheral blood flow to the organs and working muscle.
8. Describe the cardiorespiratory adaptations to exercise training that occur at rest.
9. Describe the cardiorespiratory adaptations to exercise training that occur during submaximal and maximal exercise.
10. Describe the acute cardiovascular responses to dynamic and isometric resistance exercise.

# ANCILLARY LINK

Visit Davis*Plus* at http://davisplus.fadavis.com for study and practice resources, including online quizzes, animations that help explain physiological processes, podcasts concerning news and career trends in exercise physiology, and practice references.

## *VIGNETTE*

■ After the first few personal-training sessions with Chris, a previously sedentary man in his late 30s, Rachel recognizes that he seems very concerned about how he feels during workouts. He frequently says things like, "Why is my face so red?" and "I'm starting to feel overheated." As a personal trainer, Rachel recognizes that these are normal responses to physical exertion. Because new clients often have questions about physical exertion, Rachel offers educational fact sheets as part of her comprehensive personal training services. Rachel gives Chris a handout that briefly describes what to expect during a workout.

What else can Rachel do to help alleviate Chris' concerns?

The heart and lungs work together in a coordinated fashion to ensure that all tissues are supplied with enough oxygen-rich blood for metabolic needs. This is especially important during times of increased energy demand, as during exercise, when the oxygen cost of metabolic activity is substantially increased beyond resting conditions. Indeed, exercise places a unique stress on the cardiorespiratory system. Blood flow must be redistributed to sustain increased skeletal muscular work, and waste products of cellular activity must be removed.

Imagine the level of activity the heart and lungs must reach to meet the oxygen demands of a professional road cyclist completing a 120-mile Tour de France stage race in less than 4 hours, or a professional marathoner running 26.2 miles in just over 2 hours. In these highly trained endurance athletes, the cardiovascular and respiratory systems have the remarkable ability to increase the supply of oxygen to working skeletal muscle by 600%! Even in the average recreational athlete or fitness enthusiast, the cardiovascular responses increase 400% to 500% above resting values.

This chapter describes many physiological changes that occur in the cardiovascular and respiratory systems to maximize exercise performance in both untrained and trained individuals. The primary purpose of this chapter is to explain the immediate cardiovascular and respiratory responses to exercise, and the chronic adaptations to training that occur to the cardiorespiratory systems.

## CARDIORESPIRATORY CHANGES AND RESPONSES TO EXERCISE AND RECOVERY

This section discusses the changes that occur with respect to the cardiovascular and respiratory systems immediately after the start of exercise, during submaximal steady-state exercise, and during incremental exercise up to maximum intensity. In general, the immediate changes that occur at the onset of exercise are governed by increased output from the motor cortex in the brain that directs the cardiovascular control and the respiratory control centers located in the medulla.[1,2] These control centers modify the parasympathetic and sympathetic divisions of the autonomic nervous system before, during, and after exercise. The neural and humoral (chemical) factors that fine-tune the cardiorespiratory changes to exercise will be discussed later in this chapter. This section discusses the changes to heart rate (HR), stroke volume (SV), cardiac output ($\dot{Q}$), and blood pressure, as well as changes to the respiratory system during and after exercise.

### Heart Rate

HR is set by the discharge rate of impulses that originate from the sinoatrial (SA) node, the dominant pacemaker of the heart. The electrical function of the SA node must be directly influenced by the autonomic nervous system if HR is to change from rest to exercise. Recall from Chapter 7 that at rest the vagus nerve exerts a powerful chronic parasympathetic activity on the heart through the release of acetylcholine, a neurotransmitter that acts directly on the SA and atrioventricular (AV) nodes to slow HR.[3] Typically, parasympathetic activity keeps the HR at less than 100 beats/min (bpm) while at rest. Upon the initiation of exercise, however, activity of the parasympathetic system is decreased, allowing HR to rise. Activity of the sympathetic nervous system is gradually increased. For comparison, think of a car. For the car to move, we must make sure the brakes are off and the gas pedal is pressed until we reach our desired speed. Physiologically, our nervous system is doing the same thing. For HR to increase, the nervous system releases the "break" (parasympathetic system) and engages the "accelerator" (sympathetic system) to match the metabolic demands for blood flow during exercise.

Even before exercise begins, activity of the cardiovascular system is ramped up.[4] For example, HR and blood pressure are elevated several minutes before the onset of an exercise bout. In general, if the exercise bout is of high intensity or near maximal, or if a person is participating in an emotionally charged exercise event (e.g., cycling race and marathon), then pre-exercise HR and blood pressures are higher. This anticipatory increase in cardiovascular activity is mediated by an increase in sympathetic nervous system activity.[3,5]

Figure 8-1 displays the cardiovascular changes in $\dot{Q}$ (Fig. 8-1A), SV (Fig. 8-1B), and HR (Fig. 8-1C) that occur in the transition from rest to steady-state exercise and into recovery. These changes are rapid and occur

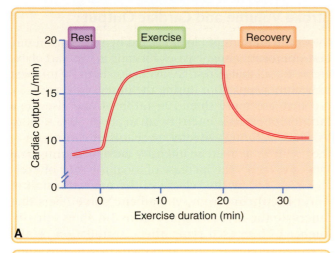

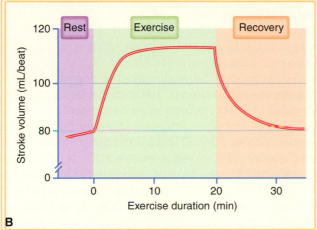

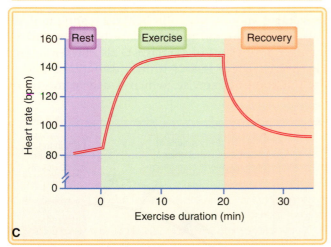

**Figure 8-1.** Cardiovascular changes. Changes in (A) cardiac output ($\dot{Q}$), (B) stroke volume (SV), and (C) heart rate (HR) at rest, during submaximal exercise up to a steady state intensity, and during the post-exercise recovery period.

The cardiorespiratory changes that occur during a prolonged (e.g., greater than 10 minutes) submaximal exercise bout of constant workload are influenced by several factors. These include the duration and intensity of the exercise bout, the type of exercise (e.g., upper body vs. lower body), and whether the exercise is performed in a calm or tumultuous environment (e.g., the effects of wind, temperature, humidity, and altitude). The most important point to keep in mind is that the changes in cardiovascular (and respiratory) parameters precisely match the level of metabolic activity and increase progressively with the intensity of the exercise. For instance, a prolonged submaximal steady-state exercise at 75% maximal oxygen consumption ($\dot{V}O_2$max) will elicit greater increases in cardiorespiratory function compared with a prolonged exercise bout at 50% $\dot{V}O_2$max.

With respect to HR, the initial increase is abrupt and occurs within the first few minutes of activity, primarily by a withdrawal of parasympathetic activity and increased sympathetic activity. If the exercise intensity remains constant and below the lactate threshold, HR will reach a plateau (*steady state*) and remain relatively stable for the duration of a submaximal exercise bout, as illustrated in Figure 8-1C. At this point in the exercise session, the demand for blood, oxygen, and nutrients of the working skeletal muscle is being matched by the output of the cardiovascular system. If the intensity of the exercise bout progressively increases, as with incremental exercise up to maximum intensity, HR continues to rise to match increasing demands for oxygen. Indeed, the demand for oxygen during incremental exercise is relatively proportional to exercise intensity (Fig. 8-2).

## Heart Rate Threshold

Traditionally, the increase in HR during incremental exercise has been thought to be strictly linear with workload and oxygen consumption ($\dot{V}O_2$). However, evidence suggests that *HR is much more likely to respond in a nonlinear fashion during exercise*.[8,9] Hofmann and others observed that most (~86%) subjects in their study demonstrated a nonlinear HR response to exercise. As shown in Figure 8-3, HR exhibits a linear increase until a breakpoint is reached and the rate of increase is slower up to a point of plateau (maximum HR). This breakpoint in HR is termed the **heart rate threshold**.

The breakpoint in HR and the slope response before and after the breakpoint is highly variable between individuals. This may explain the relative error that is associated with using HR to predict $\dot{V}O_2$ during exercise to provide an accurate assessment of exercise intensity. Therefore, to better determine an appropriate exercise intensity, it is recommended to use additional methods (e.g., ratings of perceived exertion or the talk test) instead of relying only on HR,

through neural mechanisms that arise from the cardiovascular control center.[6] Within the first few seconds after muscle begins to contract, HR and SV rise, leading to an increased $\dot{Q}$.[7] As indicated earlier, the increase in HR is mediated by withdrawal of the parasympathetic outflow and increased sympathetic outflow to the heart.

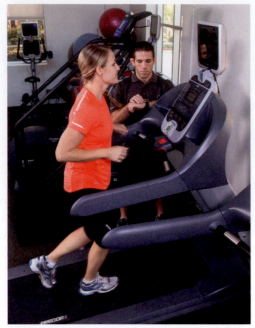

**Figure 8-2.** With incremental exercise up to maximum intensity, heart rate continues to increase to match increasing demands for oxygen.

to decrease intensity prescription error. Previous research also has been devoted to explain the HR breakpoint and relate that point to the occurrence of the lactate threshold.[8,10] To date, research data gathered in this area to elucidate this relation remains unclear because of lack of a strong association between HR and lactate threshold.

## Stroke Volume and Cardiac Output

SV, or the amount of blood ejected by the heart in one beat (mL/beat), also increases abruptly at the start of exercise. Recall that at rest, SV averages about 70 mL/beat in healthy people, but during the onset of exercise, SV can increase more than 100 mL/beat and rises as a function of exercise intensity, up to about 50% to 60% $\dot{V}O_2$max. Although several mechanisms contribute to the rise in SV as exercise intensity increases during prolonged exercise, the increase of SV at the start of exercise is caused by the release of the neurotransmitter **norepinephrine** from sympathetic nerve fibers that innervate the myocardium. Figure 8-4 shows the influence of increased sympathetic stimulation on the heart. Norepinephrine and epinephrine in the blood also enhance the force of contraction of the ventricles (increased contractility), leading to a greater amount of blood ejected out of the heart (greater SV) for any given end-diastolic volume.[3,11]

The increase in SV at the onset of activity will also stabilize during a submaximal exercise bout, typically after the first few minutes of exercise (see Fig. 8-1B). SV increases in proportion to the exercise intensity, but for most people, SV will reach a maximum value at approximately 40% to 60% of $\dot{V}O_2$max. As discussed later in this chapter, SV may continue to increase beyond this level in highly trained endurance athletes.[12]

Recall from Chapter 7 that $\dot{Q}$ is the product of HR and SV ($\dot{Q} = HR \times SV$) and represents the volume (liters) of blood pumped by the heart in 1 minute. It averages about 5 L/min in healthy resting individuals. As you can surmise, because both HR and SV increase at the start of exercise, $\dot{Q}$ also increases (see Fig. 8-1A). There is a 2- to 3-fold increase in $\dot{Q}$ at the initiation of exercise, which is driven mostly by

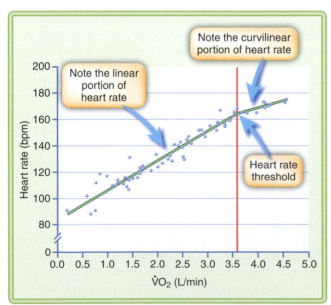

**Figure 8-3.** Heart rate (HR) responses during incremental exercise to maximal oxygen consumption ($\dot{V}O_2$max). The majority of individuals will demonstrate a curvilinear, breakpoint response in heart rate (HR). Also, the HR threshold is clearly identified in this individual.

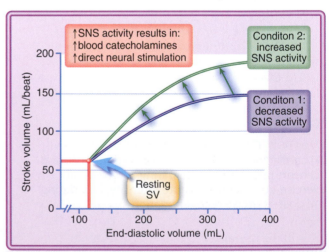

**Figure 8-4.** Influence of sympathetic neural and hormonal stimulation on stroke volume (SV). Increased sympathetic outflow to the heart and catecholamine-mediated stimulation increases cardiac contractility. The result is a greater SV for any given end-diastolic volume. This function aids in increasing SV during exercise. SNS = sympathetic nervous system.

the sharp rise in HR caused by the withdrawal of parasympathetic activity and increased sympathetic stimulation to the heart.

## Factors That Increase Stroke Volume During Exercise

The increase in SV during exercise is influenced by a number of factors that enhance myocardial force of contraction. **Homeometric regulation** includes increased sympathetic nervous system input to the myocardium, as well as circulating catecholamines. **Heterometric regulation** is primarily affected by venous return. The increase in venous return increases end-diastolic volume. This increase in end-diastolic volume (preload) results in an increase in SV via the Frank-Starling mechanism. During exercise, venous return is increased by venoconstriction, the skeletal muscle pump, and the respiratory pump.

### Venoconstriction

Venoconstriction is caused by increased activity of the sympathetic nervous system during exercise. Sympathetic stimulation causes smooth muscle in veins to contract, which causes venous pressure to rise throughout the systemic circulation.[13] The increased venous pressure drives blood back to the heart. As more blood is returned to the heart, end-diastolic volume and preload is increased, which enhances SV.

### Skeletal Muscle Pump

During exercise, the contraction of skeletal muscles helps to propel blood toward the heart through one-way venous valves (Fig. 8-5). This is known as the skeletal muscle pump. Rhythmic contractions of the skeletal muscles during activity compress veins, causing venous pressure to build. As the pressure increases, the one-way valves close abruptly, preventing the backflow of blood away from the heart. However, between contractions when skeletal muscles relax, vessel compression is reduced, which causes the valves to open. Blood is then able to flow toward the heart, and end-diastolic volume, preload, and SV increase.

### Respiratory Pump

Breathing also provides an effective mechanical pump to return venous blood to the heart. During inspiration, pressure inside the thoracic cavity decreases, whereas abdominal pressure increases. This creates a pressure gradient that forces blood to flow from the abdominal region into the thoracic cavity. Blood that has filled veins in the thoracic cavity during inspiration is pumped toward the heart during expiration. Expiration increases the pressure within the thoracic cavity, which compresses the veins. This propels venous blood toward the heart. Abdominal pressure decreases during expiration to allow veins to fill with blood so that it can be delivered into the thoracic cavity on the next inspiratory cycle. Increased rate and depth of breathing during

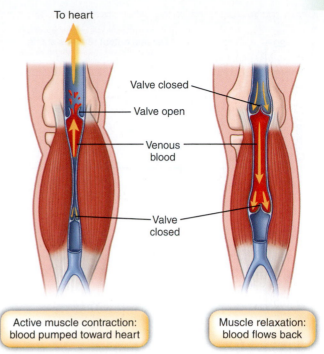

**Figure 8-5.** Skeletal muscle pump. One-way valves in the venous circulation prevent the backflow of blood. During exercise, muscle contractions compress veins, causing some one-way valves to close abruptly, whereas others are forced open. Blood is then forced toward the heart and prevented from flowing away from the heart.

exercise enhances activity of the respiratory pump to return blood to the heart to increase SV.

The traditional interpretation of SV responses during upright, incremental exercise up to maximum are described as a plateau at approximately 40% to 60% $\dot{V}O_2$max. The most common physiological reason to explain this plateau is that very high heart rates shorten ventricular filling time, which reduces end-diastolic volume and, therefore, SV. However, new light has been shed on this interpretation, and research has substantiated a different SV response in endurance-trained athletes compared with less trained individuals. Typical SV responses on maximal effort are approximately 120 to 140 mL/beat for less trained and 180 to 200 mL/beat or more for endurance-trained individuals. For an endurance-trained athlete, current evidence suggests that SV does not plateau with increasing intensity up to $\dot{V}O_2$max. For further explanation of these adaptations, refer to the Research Highlight feature that describes the SV responses in endurance-trained athletes during incremental exercise.

Figure 8-6 demonstrates the changes in $\dot{Q}$ (Fig. 8-6A), SV (Fig. 8-6B), and HR (Fig. 8-6C) during a bout of prolonged submaximal exercise of constant intensity. Notice in the illustration that $\dot{Q}$ remains stable throughout the exercise session. Increases in HR and SV combine to increase $\dot{Q}$ during prolonged exercise. However, Figure 8-5 displays an interesting feature: if the exercise bout continues for a prolonged period, HR slowly rises whereas SV declines, a phenomenon

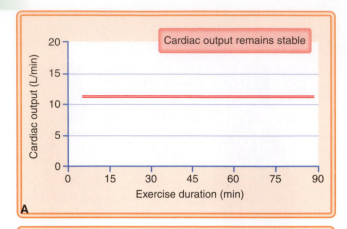

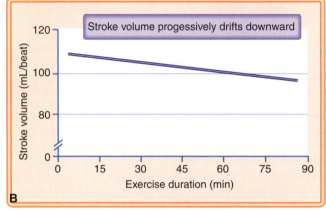

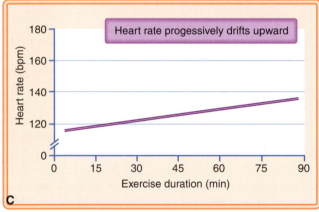

**Figure 8-6.** Influence of increasing exercise duration on (A) cardiac output (Q̇), (B) stroke volume (SV), and (C) heart rate (HR) during a bout of prolonged submaximal exercise of constant intensity.

termed **cardiovascular drift**.[14,15] The progressive increase in HR is required to offset the progressive decline in SV to maintain Q̇.

What mechanisms contribute to the simultaneous decline in SV and rise in HR throughout an exercise bout? It is generally accepted that over the course of a prolonged exercise session, an increased body temperature, coupled with greater sweat rates, dehydration, and blood flow redistribution, reduces plasma volume.[15] A decline in plasma volume lowers venous return, which, in turn, will lower preload and SV. Increased sympathetic nervous system activity to the heart compensates for the decline in SV, and this is the

main reason for the progressive increase in HR over the course of the exercise bout.

As you can imagine, prolonged exercise in a hot, humid environment will amplify cardiovascular drift.[16] For example, it is not uncommon for sweat rates to reach 2 to 3 L/hr and for plasma volume to decline 10% to 20% under hot and humid conditions. Exercise under these environmental stressors can elicit near-maximum heart rates at submaximal exercise intensities. The loss of fluid and electrolytes that occurs through exercise-induced dehydration, coupled with the shift of fluid from the plasma to the tissues, concentrates red blood cells (RBCs) (**hemoconcentration**).[17] Hemoconcentration reflects a relative increase in the oxygen-carrying capacity of the blood without a change in the actual amount of RBCs. Hemoconcentration is beneficial to a person who performs prolonged exercise, especially in the heat or at altitude.

## VIGNETTE *continued*

■ Because Chris has very little experience with physical activity, Rachel decides to devote the warm-up period of his next session to educating him about what happens in the body when exercise begins. As Chris starts to walk on the treadmill, Rachel points out that his HR and SV have both increased. "Can you feel that change in your heartbeat? The HR speeds up to provide more blood and oxygen to your working muscles, enabling you to exercise more vigorously." By pointing out that this is a perfectly normal response to the onset of exercise, Rachel has alleviated some of Chris' fears about what he feels during his workouts. As Chris continues with his warm-up and then the conditioning part of his workout, Rachel continues to explain the changes he feels, such as an increase in respiratory rate (RR) and light sweating for proper thermoregulation. Chris really appreciates the education and seems to be enjoying the exercise instead of becoming stressed and asking questions.

HR, Q̇ and SV, decrease immediately following the cessation of exercise, as illustrated in Figure 8-1. In general, these variables will change rapidly at first and then more slowly during recovery. A host of factors can influence how quickly these variables return to resting levels. The rate of recovery (return to rest) is determined mostly by the intensity and duration of exercise, and the training status of the individual. Recovery time for the cardiovascular variables are proportionally related to intensity, meaning that as intensity increases, so does the steady-state or non–steady-state response

## RESEARCH HIGHLIGHT

### Can Endurance-Trained Athletes Increase Stroke Volume Continuously During Upright, Incremental Exercise to V̇O2max?

The traditional view of SV adaptations to increasing exercise intensity is that it demonstrates a plateau response at approximately 40% to 60% V̇O$_2$max. The reason for this plateau has been attributed to a reduction in diastolic filling time caused by an increased HR during vigorous exercise. The reduced diastolic filling time leads to a smaller end-diastolic volume, which ultimately affects preload and SV. It should be stated that this interpretation does not take into account the training status of the individual, meaning that both relatively untrained and endurance-trained individuals would exhibit the same response in this view. However, within the last 20 years, new research in cardiovascular function has clarified the influence of fitness on SV responses during incremental exercise.[18]

In 1994, Gledhill and colleagues[19] published what has become a classic study providing evidence for a different interpretation of SV changes during exercise in endurance-trained athletes. In this study, SV responses to incremental cycling exercise were compared between two groups of subjects: seven male endurance cyclists and seven active control subjects. Measurements of SV were made at similar HR levels (90, 120, 140, 160, 180, and 190) for both groups. The endurance athletes demonstrated a progressive increase in SV up to maximal exercise, whereas the SV of the active controls plateaued at 40% V̇O$_2$max. The researchers attributed these differing responses to 20% greater ventricular emptying rates and 71% greater ventricular filling rates in the trained athletes. The large improvement in ventricular filling rates was attributed to enhanced diastolic function, where the ventricles of the trained endurance athletes were able to relax faster than the control subjects, thus allowing more time for blood to fill the heart during diastole.

Zhou and others[12] evaluated SV responses during exercise in male participants from three groups of subjects: untrained subjects, recreational runners, and elite runners. The rate of increase in SV during incremental exercise to maximum did not change significantly in untrained participants or recreational runners, indicating a plateau in SV at approximately 40% V̇O$_2$max. In comparison, SV dramatically increased in the elite runners all the way up to V̇O$_2$max. In addition, maximal Q̇ was significantly greater in the elite male participants compared with the other two groups. Maximal HR was similar between groups; thus, the factor most responsible for the maximal Q̇ difference was the variability in SV responses. Hence SV has a much greater influence over improving maximal Q̇ and consequently exercise performance compared with HR.

Zhou B, Conlee RK, Jensen R, Fellingham GW, George JD, Fisher AG. Stroke volume does not plateau during graded exercise in elite male distance runners. *Med Sci Sports Exerc.* 2001;33:1849–1854.

Vella CA, Robergs RA. A review of the stroke volume response to upright exercise in healthy subjects. *Br J Sports Med.* 2005;39:190–195.

Gledhill N, Cox D, Jamnik R. Endurance athletes' stroke volume does not plateau: Major advantage is diastolic function. *Med Sci Sports Exerc.* 1994;26:1116–1121.

and the time it takes to return to rest. Training status is inversely related to recovery time; thus, a more endurance-trained individual will return to resting levels much quicker than a less trained person. In fact, with respect to HR, many athletes and coaches have relied on the time for HR recovery as a marker for training status and possibly as a marker of overtraining (delayed response with overtraining). Finally, as described earlier, cardiovascular drift is a primary determinant of HR recovery time. The greater the drift, the slower the return to resting levels following exercise.

Aside from the factors discussed earlier, certain environmental considerations influence the recovery of the cardiovascular system following exercise. Hot and humid conditions will delay HR recovery because of an elevated HR response during exercise caused by losses in plasma volume and effects caused by increased body temperature (see previous discussion of cardiovascular drift). In addition, altitude will also delay recovery of HR following exercise because of elevated catecholamine and sympathetic nervous system input elicited by hypoxic conditions. In this environment, steady state heart will be elevated for a given workload compared with sea-level conditions.

## Blood Pressure and Total Peripheral Resistance

At rest, a normal healthy systolic blood pressure (SBP) is considered to be less than 120 mm Hg, and a normal diastolic blood pressure (DBP) is considered to be less than 80 mm Hg (i.e., less than 120/80 mm Hg). However, SBP, mean arterial pressure (MAP), and pulse pressure (PP) increase at the onset of cardiorespiratory exercise, whereas DBP remains stable (approximately 70–80 mm Hg).[20] The initial increase in blood pressure during exercise is necessary to supply enough blood to the working muscles to match the increased metabolic demand for oxygen and nutrients. When the tissues need more oxygen and fuel because of greater metabolic activity, the cardiovascular system responds by increasing its output *and* pressure to deliver more blood. The increase in blood pressure at the start of exercise is driven primarily by: (1) increased sympathetic vasoconstriction of veins and arterioles, (2) reduced parasympathetic activity to the heart and blood vessels, and (3) an abrupt increase in $\dot{Q}$.[14,21]

During steady-state submaximal cardiorespiratory exercise, SBP stabilizes at a new level higher than resting, nonexercise conditions. Similarly, because of SBP increases, MAP and PP also rise to a new level and stabilize during submaximal exercise. For each metabolic equivalent increase in exercise workload, SBP rises approximately 7 to 10 mm Hg and will stabilize at that value as long as exercise intensity remains relatively constant. In contrast with the rise in SPB, DBP may remain stable or slightly decrease. The minimal change in DBP during exercise is primarily due to decreases in total peripheral resistance (TPR) of the vessels within the working muscle. An increase in DBP (i.e., greater than 15 mm Hg) is indicative of an abnormal blood pressure response to exercise and is a key factor used to assess the health and function of the cardiovascular system.

As mentioned earlier, TPR decreases during exercise to help facilitate the delivery of blood and oxygen to the working muscles. Blood vessels that supply working muscles vasodilate, whereas vessels that supply nonexercising muscles and organs vasoconstrict.[5] The decrease in TPR with exercise is directly related to the extent of muscle mass used.[22] For example, exercises that primarily use the legs will lower TPR more than upper body exercise (e.g., arm ergometry). Blood flow redistribution during exercise will be discussed in further detail in later sections of this chapter.

When exercise intensity increases, as during incremental exercise bouts, SBP rises to a new higher level to accommodate the need to deliver more blood flow to muscles that are working progressively harder (Fig. 8-7). In addition, because SBP rises and DBP generally remains stable, MAP also progressively rises with increased exercise intensity. Typical maximal values for SBP range from 160 to 220 mm Hg. Any further increase in SBP during exercise is commonly interpreted as a **hypertensive response**. On the contrary, a failure of SBP to increase normally during exercise is described as a **hypotensive response**. Clinically, both responses may be associated with an underlying risk or presence of cardiovascular disease.

At the cessation of an exercise bout (i.e., both a steady-state submaximal bout and an incremental exercise bout), SBP drops within seconds (primarily because $\dot{Q}$ decreases abruptly) and then gradually returns to or below resting values after several minutes. Similarly, DBP, MAP, and PP also return to resting levels during exercise recovery. SBP may actually be lower during recovery than it was before exercise. This reduction in blood pressure after exercise, which may continue for several hours, is called **post-exercise**

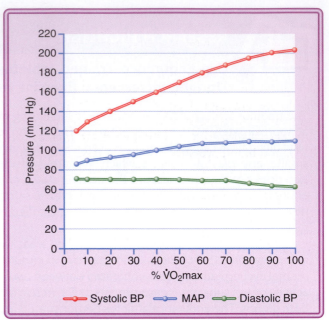

**Figure 8-7.** Systolic, mean arterial, and diastolic blood pressure responses to incremental exercise to maximal oxygen consumption ($\dot{V}O_2$max). Systolic blood pressure increases in a nonlinear fashion because of the need for increasing blood flow during exercise. Mean arterial pressure (MAP) increases slightly as cardiac output ($\dot{Q}$) increases and total peripheral resistance (TPR) decreases. Diastolic blood pressure remains the same or slightly decreases during exercise because of overall vasodilation in the systemic vasculature.

**hypotension.** Post-exercise hypotension, as shown in Figure 8-8, is caused by a sustained decrease in TPR because of overall skeletal muscle vasodilation triggered by nitric oxide–mediated processes.[23] The magnitude

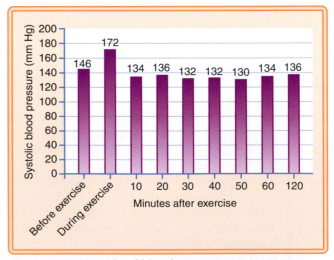

**Figure 8-8.** Example of blood pressure response to a 45-minute, moderate-intensity (60% heart rate reserve) exercise bout and the changes that occur during recovery in a person with hypertension. During exercise, systolic blood pressure (SBP) rises above resting conditions. Once exercise stops, blood pressure drops to levels below pre-exercise conditions. This is known as post-exercise hypotension and is an effective method by which regular exercise can lower blood pressure.

of post-exercise hypotension in the period following exercise appears to be exercise intensity and duration dependent.[23–25] In general, the longer the exercise duration and the higher the intensity, the greater the sustained reduction in blood pressure after exercise. Therefore, regular participation in cardiorespiratory exercise is a great way to prevent high blood pressure and is very effective at lowering blood pressure in people with hypertension.

As the cardiovascular system works to increase HR, SV, $\dot{Q}$, and blood pressure during exercise, the respiratory system also works to increase its output (See explanatory animation of Changes to Heart Rate and Blood Pressure with Exercise on the DavisPlus site at http://davisplus.fadavis.com). Certainly, the respiratory system has tremendous potential to increase gas exchange during exercise, with the utmost goal of intricately balancing the need to supply greater amounts of oxygen to the working muscles with the elimination of carbon dioxide ($CO_2$). To adjust to the extreme stress imposed by exercise, the respiratory system has a remarkable ability to increase pulmonary ventilation (minute ventilation [$\dot{V}_E$]), gas exchange capacity, and pulmonary blood flow so that the demands for oxygen are met with increasing exercise. The following sections will pay particular attention to these changes during and after exercise.

## Pulmonary Ventilation

The change in pulmonary ventilation ($\dot{V}_E$) in the transition from rest to steady state submaximal exercise is illustrated in Figure 8-9. As you can observe, the onset of exercise is characterized by an abrupt and rapid increase in $\dot{V}_E$ that occurs within the first minute of activity followed by a slower increase until steady state is achieved.[26,27] The increase in $\dot{V}_E$ at the onset of exercise is driven by two mechanisms: (1) increased tidal volume ($V_T$), and (2) a slightly increased RR.[28,29] Recall that at rest, a healthy, average-sized man with a $V_T$ of 0.5 L/breath at 15 breaths/min will produce a $\dot{V}_E$ of 7.5 L/min. From rest to steady state exercise, however,

$V_T$ will increase to about 1 to 1.5 L, and RR may reach 15 to 20 breaths/min. Thus, $\dot{V}_E$ may reach 15 to 30 L/min within the first 5 minutes of exercise. As discussed later in this chapter, $\dot{V}_E$ will continue to increase during prolonged submaximal exercise and can reach even greater levels during incremental exercise to maximum intensity. Interestingly, in conjunction with the anticipatory increase in HR before exercise, there is a pre-exercise anticipatory rise in $\dot{V}_E$ (see Fig. 8-9). The increase in $\dot{V}_E$ before exercise is due to increased activity of the respiratory control center in the medulla and other higher brain centers in the cerebral cortex in response to muscle movement.[28]

The increase in $\dot{V}_E$ during submaximal, low- to moderate-intensity exercise is due primarily to a greater depth of breathing and moderate increases in RR.[28,30] Increases in RR contribute more to the increase in $\dot{V}_E$ during high-intensity exercise, whereas changes in $V_T$ affect $\dot{V}_E$ more at lower intensity exercise. Figure 8-10 illustrates the $V_T$ (Fig. 8-10A) and RR (Fig. 8-10B) responses to incremental exercise.

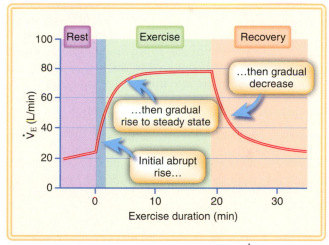

**Figure 8-9.** Changes in minute ventilation ($\dot{V}_E$) at rest, on the start of steady-state, submaximal exercise, and during the post-exercise recovery period.

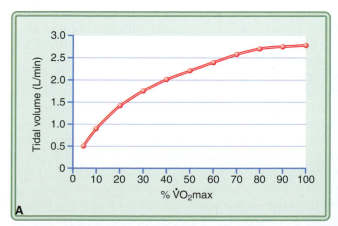

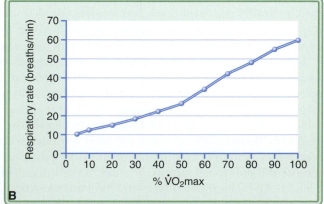

**Figure 8-10.** Tidal volume ($V_T$) (A) and respiratory rate (RR) (B) responses during incremental exercise to maximal oxygen consumption ($\dot{V}O_2max$). Tidal volume is responsible for the early increases in minute ventilation ($\dot{V}_E$), but tends to plateau during higher exercise intensities. At lower exercise intensities (i.e., less than 50% $\dot{V}O_2max$), RR increases linearly. During high-intensity exercise, RR increases nonlinearly and contributes more to changes in $\dot{V}_E$ than $V_T$.

Ventilation can increase to very high levels during exercise in healthy people depending on sex, fitness level, physical stature, intensity of the exercise, and state of the environment in which the exercise is performed. In fact, it is not uncommon for maximal ventilatory rates to exceed 100 to 150 L/min during exercise, and values can be even higher in endurance-trained people. However, certain conditions may limit the capacity to increase $\dot{V}_E$. For instance, at very high exercise intensities, the respiratory muscles may fatigue, limiting maximal endurance performance (Box 8-1). In addition, aging is associated with increased stiffness of the lungs and chest wall, which makes it more difficult to ventilate the lungs.[31-33] See Box 8-2 for a more complete discussion of the age-related changes to the respiratory system.

At the cessation of exercise, $\dot{V}_E$ initially decreases rapidly and then decreases at a much slower rate to resting values (see Fig. 8-8). The initial rapid decrease during recovery likely involves a significant neural component because the change is much too fast to be mediated solely by chemical factors (i.e., $CO_2$ or $H^+$). On the contrary, the slower return of $\dot{V}_E$ to rest appears to be due to chemical factors, particularly the return of blood pH to pre-exercise values.

## Airway Resistance

To facilitate the increased demand for oxygen at the start of exercise, the airways in the conducting and respiratory zones dilate (**bronchodilation**) to bring in more air from the atmosphere. Bronchodilation results in

### Box 8-1. Respiratory Muscle Fatigue

Pulmonary ventilation can increase up to 20 to 25 times above resting values during exercise, compared with only 5-8 times that of rest for $\dot{Q}$. Because of this, many believe that the respiratory system does not limit submaximal and maximal exercise performance in healthy individuals. However, there are some possible exceptions to this theory, particularly near-maximal exercise.

Increasing $\dot{V}_E$ raises the work of breathing and oxygen cost of the respiratory muscles. To meet this increased oxygen demand, more blood must be diverted away from the working muscles used for locomotion or movement and delivered to the muscles that control respiration. During heavy exercise, the inspiratory muscles must overcome the elastic properties (force drawing the lungs in) of lung tissue to inflate the lungs appropriately for gas exchange. Expiratory muscles must work harder to overcome greater airway resistance that can occur at higher airflow rates through the bronchial tree during higher intensities. The nasal passages present an area of high resistance; for that reason, we primarily breathe through the mouth once we reach moderate intensities of exercise. Like any other skeletal muscle, the respiratory muscles are subject to fatigue at vigorous work rates. Thus, respiratory muscle fatigue along with greater demand for oxygen in these muscles could be viewed as limitations to performing maximum exercise.

### Box 8-2. The Respiratory System and Aging

Many structural and functional changes occur in the respiratory system of an older adult that make it more difficult to transport air into and out of the lungs. However, if the lungs remain free of disease, proper gas exchange is maintained across the life span. The most important respiratory changes that occur with aging are decreased lung elastic recoil, a decrease in chest wall compliance, and weakening of the respiratory muscles, including the diaphragm and intercostals.[11,21,31] Thus, advancing age is associated with relatively weak respiratory muscles that must exert greater force on a chest wall that becomes progressively more difficult to expand. As a result, the work of breathing increases in older adults.

In addition to the increased work of breathing, alveolar gas exchange surface area decreases with aging by approximately 20%, although the total number of alveoli available for gas exchange remains relatively constant.[31,32] Part of the reason for the decline in alveolar surface area is that the alveolar ducts and the alveolar spaces increase in diameter. There also appears to be a reduction in the capillary density of the lungs, which contributes to decreased pulmonary blood flow. Each of these factors will influence the efficiency of gas exchange between the alveolar–capillary interface with aging. Another important age-related change in the respiratory system is that the diameter of the bronchioles progressively declines. A narrower airway will make it more difficult to get air into and out of the lungs. Thus, forced vital capacity, or the maximum amount of air that can be eliminated from the lung after a maximal inspiration, is markedly reduced with aging.[33] This decrease is partly due to the reduced respiratory muscle strength, blunted lung elastic recoil, and increased stiffness of the chest wall.[31,32] Consequently, forced expiratory volume during the first second of expiration ($FEV_1$) will be markedly reduced, indicating that airway resistance is increased with aging.

decreased airway resistance, making it substantially easier to deliver air into the lungs. The immediate withdrawal of parasympathetic activity and an acute increase in the release of norepinephrine from sympathetic nerve fibers results in dilation of the smooth muscle of the bronchial tree at the start of exercise.

Additional features of the respiratory system help to decrease airway resistance in the transition from rest to steady-state exercise. First, airway resistance *decreases* at higher lung volumes.[11,29] Thus, at the start of exercise when the lungs expand (increased volume) and $\dot{V}_E$ rises, the airways open up. This helps to lower air-flow resistance, making it easier to increase the delivery of air into the lungs. Second, **alveolar interdependence** (the phenomenon that each alveolus is mechanically tethered to one another and to a neighboring airway, as explained in Chapter 6) allows the alveoli to expand during inspiration. The increased tension in the alveolar walls pulls the airway farther open to reduce airway resistance and facilitates more airflow. As exercise duration increases at a constant workload, bronchodilation and the reduction in airway resistance remain relatively stable.

## Po$_2$ and Pco$_2$

Arterial partial pressure of oxygen (Pao$_2$) and carbon dioxide (Paco$_2$) deviate very little from rest to steady-state exercise. It is common to observe a slight (i.e., less than 1 mm Hg) increase in partial pressure of carbon dioxide (Pco$_2$), and a slight decrease in partial pressure of oxygen (Po$_2$) immediately after the start of exercise. The initial decline in Po$_2$ and very mild increase in Pco$_2$ reflect increased metabolic activity at the start of exercise.[28] Eventually, as $\dot{V}_E$ stabilizes, so do Po$_2$ and Pco$_2$. As explained in Chapter 6, Paco$_2$ is tightly regulated, and under normal circumstances, it is held remarkably constant (40–45 mm Hg), even during intense exercise. Similarly, during lower to moderate intensities of exercise, Pao$_2$ does not change appreciably.

Changes in Pao$_2$ during higher intensity exercise are often observed. Generally, Po$_2$ remains constant up to maximal exercise levels in most people. In some cases, however, Po$_2$ may decrease significantly, a phenomenon known as **exercise-induced hypoxemia**. Exercise-induced hypoxemia may be caused by certain pulmonary diseases that reduce the diffusion of oxygen from the alveoli to the pulmonary capillaries such as emphysema or asthma. Interestingly, this condition is not exclusive to people with pulmonary disease. There is evidence to suggest that some highly trained endurance athletes also exhibit this pattern of hypoxemia at very high exercise intensities, particularly at maximum (see Research Highlight: Exercise-Induced Hypoxemia: Causes and Concerns in Chapter 6 for further explanation). The diffusion limitation in this case could be caused by the rate of blood flow through the pulmonary capillaries (called *increased transit time*) being too rapid for adequate oxygenation secondary to very high cardiac outputs. Also, a possible overventilation and underperfusion of the lung in some areas (called *ventilation-perfusion inequality*) may contribute to exercise-induced hypoxemia.

## Ventilation to Perfusion Equality

For maximum gas exchange to occur, there must be proper matching of pulmonary blood flow to alveolar ventilation. Under normal circumstances (i.e., upright posture at rest), $\dot{V}_E$ is not equally distributed throughout the lung. The top regions (apex) of the lung have a *higher proportion of ventilation to blood flow*, whereas the bottom portions of the lung have a *higher proportion of blood flow to ventilation*. In the transition from rest to steady-state exercise, however, it appears that the balance of $\dot{V}_E$ to pulmonary blood flow is improved.[30,34] This is due to an increased pulmonary blood flow to the top regions of the lung and an overall decrease in pulmonary vascular resistance.

## Ventilatory Drift

During longer duration submaximal exercise of higher intensity (e.g., >75% $\dot{V}O_2$max) and exercise in a hot environment, $\dot{V}_E$ drifts progressively upward (increase in $\dot{V}_E/\dot{V}O_2$ ratio), despite no change in exercise workload. The drifting of $\dot{V}_E$ is primarily due to the increased RRs that accompany higher intensity exercise.[35] One of the primary stimuli for the gradual increase in $\dot{V}_E$ during prolonged exercise is increased circulating catecholamines (epinephrine and norepinephrine) that stimulate the carotid bodies.[16] In addition, increased body temperature that accompanies prolonged exercise may stimulate heat-sensitive receptors in the hypothalamus to increase RR. Ventilatory drift increases the work of breathing and may contribute to sensations of fatigue during exercise in a hot environment.

## Ventilatory Threshold 1 and Ventilatory Threshold 2

Recall that at low-to-moderate exercise intensities, $\dot{V}_E$ gradually increases linearly and stabilizes once steady-state exercise has been achieved. Thus, up to a certain threshold, the change in $\dot{V}_E$ with respect to oxygen uptake is relatively linear (Fig. 8-11). However, as exercise intensity progressively becomes more difficult, $V_E$ increases steeply and breaks from linearity. The point (or exercise intensity) at which $\dot{V}_E$ first breaks from linearity with respect to oxygen uptake (expressed as %$\dot{V}O_2$ max) is termed the **first ventilatory threshold (VT1)**.

In general, for most people, exercise bouts at or below VT1 are considered light-to-moderate exercise intensities and correspond to approximately 40% to 60% $\dot{V}O_2$max. However, exercise intensities corresponding to VT1 can be much higher (e.g., 70% $\dot{V}O_2$max) in well-trained or elite endurance athletes. *The advantage of having a higher ventilatory threshold is the ability to perform steady state*

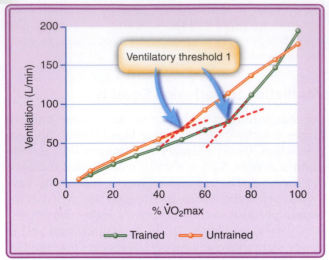

**Figure 8-11.** Differences in the ventilatory threshold 1 (VT1) between an endurance-trained and an untrained individual during incremental exercise to $\dot{V}O_2$max. Ventilation increases in a nonlinear fashion and demonstrates a breakpoint response (VT1) with increasing exercise intensity. Note the differences in the occurrence of VT1 between individuals. In the untrained person, VT1 occurs much earlier (50% $\dot{V}O_2$max) during exercise compared with the endurance-trained individual (70% $\dot{V}O_2$max). In addition, $\dot{V}_E$ is consistently lower for a given $\dot{V}O_2$max in the endurance-trained individual because of positive adaptations to aerobic training.

*exercise at a higher intensity (or speed/pace) with less reliance on anaerobic energy sources.* Having to rely more on anaerobic energy sources at lower workloads can lead to premature fatigue during exercise in untrained individuals.

What factors contribute to the increase in $\dot{V}_E$ up to VT1? It appears that an important factor that influences the breakpoint pattern of VT1 during incremental exercise is increased proton (H+) accumulation derived from metabolic processes such as adenosine triphosphate (ATP) hydrolysis and glycolysis that reduces blood pH. Protons are buffered with bicarbonate, which produces increased levels of $CO_2$, to offset the metabolic acidosis. Peripheral chemoreceptors located in systemic arteries sense the changes in blood pH and increased levels of $CO_2$. In turn, signals from the chemoreceptors are relayed to the central respiratory control center to increase $\dot{V}_E$. This process will lead to greater exhalation of $CO_2$ (i.e., increased $\dot{V}_E$) to support the regulation of metabolic acidosis with increasing exercise intensities.

If a person continues to exercise at progressively higher exercise intensities above VT1, the bicarbonate buffering system is unable to offset metabolic acidosis. Consequently, the respiratory system compensates by substantially increasing $\dot{V}_E$ beyond that of VT1. Eventually, $\dot{V}_E$ continues to increase and reaches a second deviation point, termed the **second ventilatory threshold (VT2)**, often referred to as the **respiratory compensation point**. Therefore, VT2 represents a further disproportionate elevation in $\dot{V}_E$ relative to $\dot{V}O_2$.

## Methods to Identify the Ventilatory Threshold

A variety of laboratory and nonlaboratory methods can be used to identify VT1 and VT2. For example, a more precise laboratory approach that can identify both VT1 and VT2 is to plot the ventilatory equivalents for oxygen ($\dot{V}_E/\dot{V}O_2$) and carbon dioxide ($\dot{V}_E/\dot{V}CO_2$) against exercise workload.[36] In addition, a simple nonlaboratory method is to evaluate the ability of a person to talk during an exercise bout, often referred to as the **"talk test"** method. These methods will be described later in greater detail.

### Ventilatory Equivalent for Oxygen

The **ventilatory equivalent for oxygen** is the amount of $\dot{V}_E$ required to consume 1 L of oxygen. Expressed as a ratio of $\dot{V}_E/\dot{V}O_2$, it provides a good indication of breathing efficiency during exercise and can be used to identify VT1.[36] As shown in Figure 8-12, immediately after the transition from rest to incremental exercise, the $\dot{V}_E/\dot{V}O_2$ ratio decreases, meaning there is a higher degree of oxygen extraction in the working muscles per liter of air ventilated. The ratio will continue a steady decline and eventually it will reach a low point. Immediately after the $\dot{V}_E/\dot{V}O_2$ ratio reaches its lowest point (marked by the arrow on Fig. 8-12), it deviates upward and begins a steady increase as exercise intensity becomes more

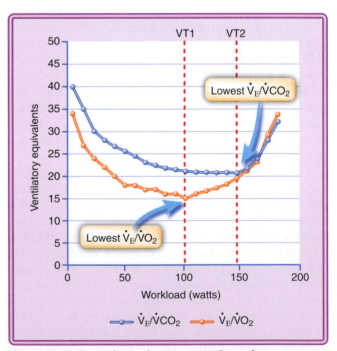

**Figure 8-12.** Typical ventilatory equivalents for oxygen and carbon dioxide ($CO_2$) during incremental exercise. By plotting the ventilatory equivalents for oxygen and $CO_2$, ventilatory threshold 1 (VT1) and ventilatory threshold 2 (VT2) can be identified. VT1 is identified by the lowest $\dot{V}_E/\dot{V}O_2$ ratio, whereas VT2 is identified by the lowest $\dot{V}_E/\dot{V}CO_2$ ratio.

difficult. The first upward deviation point (i.e., the lowest $\dot{V}_E/\dot{V}O_2$ ratio) is the first indication that $\dot{V}_E$ exceeds the rate of $VO_2$ and identifies VT1. Stated another way, VT1 is identified by the workload marked by the lowest $\dot{V}_E/\dot{V}O_2$ ratio.

### Ventilatory Equivalent for Carbon Dioxide

The **ventilatory equivalent for carbon dioxide** is the amount of $\dot{V}_E$ required to expire 1 L of $CO_2$. Recall that $CO_2$, a waste product of cellular metabolism, is increased during exercise. It must be eliminated from the body via exhalation. Similar to the decrease in $\dot{V}_E/\dot{V}O_2$ ratio at the start of exercise, the $\dot{V}_E/\dot{V}CO_2$ ratio also declines, meaning there is a higher degree of $CO_2$ production per liter of air ventilated. While the $\dot{V}_E/\dot{V}O_2$ ratio begins an upward trend at VT1, the $\dot{V}_E/\dot{V}CO_2$ ratio continues to decrease or remains constant (between the dashed vertical red lines in Fig. 8-12). At this point, $\dot{V}_E$ is able to eliminate $CO_2$, which produces a relatively stable $\dot{V}_E/\dot{V}CO_2$ ratio. Eventually and similar to that of the $\dot{V}_E/\dot{V}O_2$ ratio, it will reach its lowermost point (marked by the second arrow on Fig. 8-12). Therefore, VT2 is identified as the workload marked by the lowest $\dot{V}_E/\dot{V}CO_2$ ratio.[36] Immediately after its low point, the $\dot{V}_E/\dot{V}CO_2$ ratio deviates upward and begins a sharp increase as exercise intensity becomes more difficult. The first upward deviation point that follows the $\dot{V}_E/\dot{V}CO_2$ low point is the first indication that rate of $\dot{V}_E$ increases disproportionately to the rate of $CO_2$ production (VT2). Exercise bouts between VT1 and VT2 are considered moderate- to high-intensity exercise (70%–80% $\dot{V}O_2max$). Most people will only be able to withstand exercise sessions at intensities between VT1 and VT2 for 20 to 30 minutes before they fatigue. Exercise intensities above VT2 are considered high to severe and correspond to 80% to 100% $\dot{V}O_2max$.

### Talk Test

Research has demonstrated a practical way to identify the ventilatory threshold by rating ease of speech during exercise using the simple talk test method.[37] Generally, at intensities below the ventilatory threshold, a person is able to talk comfortably while exercising. However, as the intensity of exercise becomes more difficult and approaches levels close to the ventilatory threshold, talking will become more uncomfortable. At this point, talking during the exercise bout requires more effort. The intensity of the exercise bout that reflects the point when talking first becomes uncomfortable identifies VT1 as denoted in Figure 8-13. As exercise intensity progressively becomes harder above VT1, speaking is possible, but it will become even more uncomfortable. The point in the exercise bout when talking is clearly difficult (e.g., gasping for air while trying to talk) identifies VT2. Exercise intensities just below VT2 represent the threshold at which a person can sustain an exercise bout for 20 to 30 minutes. If

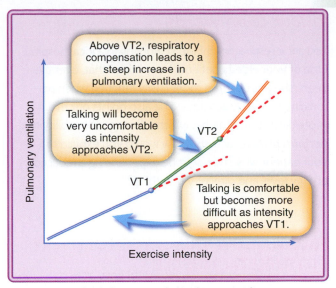

**Figure 8-13.** Identification of the first ventilatory threshold (VT1) and the second ventilatory threshold (VT2) using the talk test. VT1 and VT2, denoted by the circles, can be easily identified by the degree to which talking while exercising becomes progressively more difficult.

exercise intensity rises above VT2, a person will not be able to talk; $\dot{V}_E$ will increase exponentially and an individual will not be able to withstand this intensity level for more than a few minutes. By using the talk test as research indicates, the exercise professional can identify the intensity corresponding to VT1 and VT2 to design a personalized cardiorespiratory exercise program.

## VIGNETTE continued

■ During that same workout, after Chris has completed about 10 minutes of walking on the treadmill at a speed of 4 miles per hour, he mentions that he feels really good and seems to have caught his second wind. Rachel responds by explaining the concept of steady-state exercise: "Your body's response to exercise has now caught up with the demands of the workout. This means that you are providing enough oxygen to the muscles to maintain this level of intensity. As you get in even better shape, you will notice that you are able to handle increasingly difficult workouts. This is one indication that your overall level of cardiovascular fitness is improving. Perhaps more importantly, these improvements experienced during your workouts should translate to better health and function during your everyday life."

## In Your Own Words

You are a respiratory therapist working in a local hospital. One of your elderly patients has noticed that, over the years, she has become more easily fatigued when performing everyday activities. She also points out that it is more difficult to breathe, which influences her ability to perform physical activity. How would you explain to your patient why she might be experiencing a reduced energy level and difficulty breathing?

## BLOOD FLOW AND OXYGEN DELIVERY TO SKELETAL MUSCLE

The metabolic demand for oxygen used to regenerate mitochondrial ATP increases significantly with incremental exercise to maximum. This demand can increase to 15 to 20 times that of rest depending on the intensity that the individual can reach. In particular, blood flow to skeletal muscle must increase proportionally with this demand for exercise performance reasons. A potential limitation of the cardiovascular system is that it contains a finite amount of blood volume (5–6 L) to be circulated. There are three ways the cardiovascular system can overcome this limitation. One strategy is to recirculate blood at a higher rate above resting levels. This takes place with increasing $\dot{Q}$ during exercise. However, increasing $\dot{Q}$ is not enough to meet the high metabolic demands in skeletal muscle with progressive exercise intensity. Therefore, the second strategy is to shunt more blood away from nonactive tissues to active tissues through targeted vasoconstriction. A third strategy is to extract more oxygen from the blood. As described in more detail below, all three strategies help to satisfy the oxygen demands of the working muscle.

### Cardiac Output Responses

As previously discussed, $\dot{Q}$ increases as a function of increases in HR and SV. For less trained individuals, HR contributes more to changes in $\dot{Q}$ during exercise. In contrast, SV contributes more to the increases in $\dot{Q}$ during exercise in trained individuals. Table 8-1 outlines the determinants of $\dot{Q}$ during incremental exercise. Note that, depending on training status, $\dot{Q}$ can increase five to eight times above resting values (25–40 L/min at maximal exercise), which means that the heart can recirculate its total blood volume significantly every minute with increasing exercise intensity. Taken together, increases in $\dot{Q}$ provide the exercising muscle with the blood flow it needs to match its energy demand.

### Redistribution of Systemic Blood Flow

A second strategy to deliver more blood to the working muscle is to redistribute it from less active tissues. To get the most out of our $\dot{Q}$, the sympathetic nervous system and local vasodilators work in concert to redistribute blood flow to where it is needed most: working muscles, heart, and skin. Systemically, there is a sympathetic-mediated (neural and hormonal) vasoconstriction of arterioles that supply blood to the digestive system and kidneys, although this response only reduces the percentage of total $\dot{Q}$ to these areas. In fact, the absolute amount of blood flow to the digestive system and brain remain similar or increase slightly because of an overall increase in $\dot{Q}$ during exercise. Muscle blood flow is mostly increased through local autoregulatory activities (see Chapter 7). Locally, various factors (temperature, $CO_2$, $K^+$, $H^+$), plus the release of the potent vasodilator, endothelium-derived nitric oxide, will contribute to overall vasodilation of arterioles and increase muscle capillary blood flow to match metabolic demand for oxygen. In this manner, the muscle will intrinsically influence its own blood supply.

Figure 8-14 shows the absolute and relative partitioning of $\dot{Q}$ at rest and during exercise near-maximal effort. At rest, approximately 5% (0.25 L/min) and 20% (1 L/min) of $\dot{Q}$ is distributed to cardiac and skeletal muscle, respectively. This leaves roughly 75% of 5 L blood to be divided among the rest of the body. The digestive system receives the largest relative share of $\dot{Q}$ at rest at 25% (1.25 L/min) followed by the kidneys at 20% (1 L/min), brain at 15% (0.75 L/min), bone at 4% (0.2 L/min), and the rest going to the skin and other tissues (e.g., connective tissue and fat).

During maximal exercise, up to 80% to 85% of total $\dot{Q}$ is delivered to skeletal muscle. Along these lines, if maximal $\dot{Q}$ is measured at 30 L/min, then roughly 25 L blood is perfusing skeletal muscle every minute.

**Table 8-1.** Magnitude of Cardiac Output Responses During Exercise as a Function of Heart Rate and Stroke Volume

| VARIABLE | REST | EXERCISE | MAGNITUDE OF INCREASE |
|---|---|---|---|
| Heart rate | 70 beats/min | 200 beats/min | ~2.9 times above rest |
| Stroke volume | 70 mL/beat | 140 mL/beat | 2 times above rest |
| Cardiac output | 4.9 L/min | 28.0 L/min | ~5.8 times above rest |

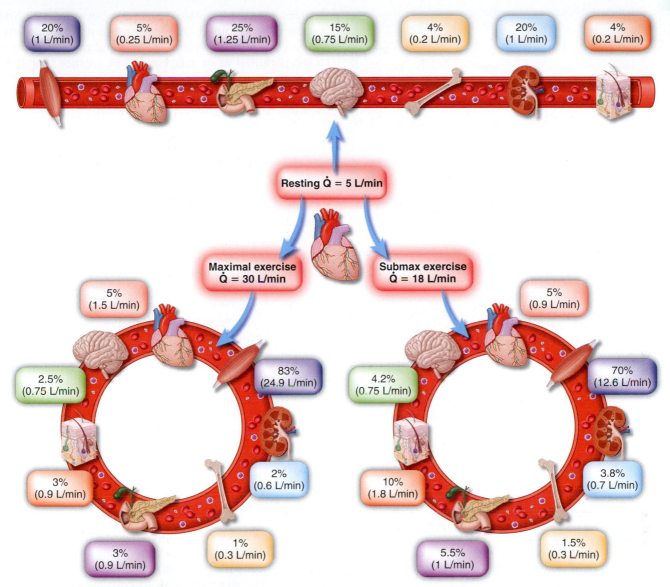

**Figure 8-14.** The changing distribution of blood flow to the major tissues of the body at rest, during moderate intensity, submaximal exercise, and maximal exercise. Both the relative and absolute cardiac output (Q̇) changes are included in the color-coded boxes associated with each tissue. **NOTE:** (1) The relative and absolute change in Q̇ to skeletal muscle (active tissue) from rest to maximal exercise is significant (6-fold increase); (2) the relative and absolute change in Q to the gastrointestinal tract, kidney, and bone decrease (less active tissues); (3) a constant relative and absolute portion of Q̇ is directed to the heart and brain, respectively; and (4) skin blood flow significantly increases up to maximal exercise for thermoregulation purposes and experiences a decrease at maximum to further increase muscle blood flow.

Because of increasing *myocardial* oxygen demand, the heart commands the *same percentage* of Q̇ during exercise to ensure that it gets a progressively increasing quantity of blood flow. This is carried out through progressive vasodilation of coronary vessels. In contrast, the brain requires a *constant or slightly increased amount* of blood flow with increasing exercise intensity, even though the percent contribution of Q̇ to the brain actually decreases. Interestingly, skin (cutaneous) blood flow initially decreases and then gradually increases with exercise intensity because of vasodilation. Increasing blood flow to the skin is for thermoregulation (sweating) reasons and is under the control of the hypothalamus, which overrides the early

sympathetic-mediated vasoconstriction. At maximal exercise, skin blood flow decreases yet again because of vasoconstriction. As a result, the muscles' demand for oxygen and the body's need to maintain arterial blood pressure for muscle blood flow override heat balance during intense exercise.[38]

## Arterial-Venous Oxygen Difference

The arterial-venous $O_2$ (a-v$O_2$) difference increases in a nonlinear fashion with incremental exercise. This reflects enhanced blood flow to and oxygen extraction by the working muscles. Figure 8-15 shows the changes in a-v$O_2$ difference with increasing exercise

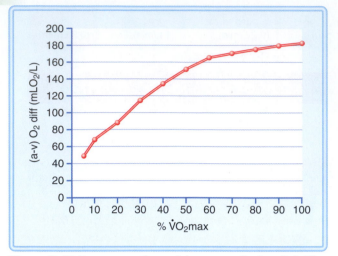

**Figure 8-15.** Response of arterial-venous $O_2$ (a-v$O_2$) difference during incremental exercise to maximal oxygen consumption ($\dot{V}O_2$max). Note the nonlinear increase in a-v$O_2$ difference that reflects the change in whole-body oxygen extraction during exercise as one nears maximal exercise intensities.

intensity. The considerable increase in the a-v$O_2$ difference during incremental exercise is largely the consequence of decreased mixed venous oxygen content as arterial oxygen content stays relatively stable (except in cases of mild-to-severe hypoxemia). Typical maximal

values for this variable can range between 120 and 150 mL $O_2$/L blood. The determinants of the a-v$O_2$ difference response are numerous and reflect the muscles' potential to extract and utilize oxygen: capillary density, proportion of type I motor units within the muscle, mitochondrial mass, oxidative enzyme concentration, and myoglobin concentration.

# CARDIORESPIRATORY CONTROL DURING EXERCISE

Certainly, the cardiorespiratory system must be under precise regulation to maintain the delivery of oxygen to the tissues at rest and to match the increased oxygen demand and removal of $CO_2$ during exercise. The major components involved in the control of the respiratory and cardiovascular systems during *resting* conditions were discussed in detail in Chapters 6 and 7, respectively. The factors working together to maintain cardiorespiratory activity under exercising conditions are the subject of this section.

In brief, both the cardiovascular and respiratory systems function as a coupled unit. Thus, their control is very similar and each system is precisely regulated by higher brain centers located in the cerebral cortex. The cerebral cortex provides the initial drive to increase $\dot{Q}$ and $\dot{V}_E$ at the start of exercise. These areas of the brain

## DOING THE MATH:

A local triathlete is preparing for a race and is in your exercise physiology laboratory today to get a general sense for his current fitness level and test his potential responses running in a hot environmental condition. The testing will consist of resting and exercise measures for the following variables: $\dot{V}O_2$, SV, HR, $V_T$, RR, and blood lactate. The exercise sessions consisted of 60 minutes of exercise at 7 mph on a treadmill at 4% grade under normal conditions and then again under hotter conditions in an environmental chamber. Following are the data table and other pertinent information:

| TESTING VARIABLE | RESTING | NORMAL CONDITION | HOT CONDITION |
|---|---|---|---|
| Oxygen consumption ($VO_2$) (mL/min) | 233 | 2,192 | 2,141 |
| Stroke volume (mL/beat) | 90 | 155 | 120 |
| Heart rate (beats/min) | 55 | 140 | 160 |
| Tidal volume (mL/breath) | 600 | 2,200 | 1,900 |
| Respiratory rate (breaths/min) | 10 | 35 | 45 |
| Lactate (mmol/L blood) | 1 | 2.4 | 3 |
| **Other Laboratory Variables** | | | |
| % $O_2$ saturation (v) | 75 | 50 | 45 |
| % $O_2$ saturation (a) | 97 | 97 | 97 |
| Hemoglobin (g/L blood) | 160 | 160 | 160 |

### DOING THE MATH:–cont'd

For a review of the following calculations, see Doing the Math features in Chapters 6 and 7:
- Calculate $\dot{Q}$ and $\dot{V}_E$ at rest and during both exercise conditions.
- Calculate the content of oxygen in arterial ($CaO_2$) and venous ($CvO_2$) blood at rest and during both exercise conditions.
- Calculate $\dot{V}O_2$ using the Fick equation at rest and during the two exercise conditions.

| VARIABLE | RESTING | NORMAL CONDITION | HOT CONDITION |
|---|---|---|---|
| Cardiac output ($\dot{Q}$) | = (90 mL/beat × 55 bpm) / 1,000<br>= 4.95 L/min | = (155 mL/beat × 140 bpm) / 1,000<br>= 21.7 L/min | = (120 mL/beat × 160 bpm) / 1000<br>= 19.2 L/min |
| Minute ventilation ($\dot{V}_E$) | = 0.6 L/breath × 10 breaths/min<br>= 6.0 L/min | = 2.2 L/breath × 35 breaths/min<br>= 77 L/min | = 1.9 L/breath × 45 breaths/min<br>= 85.5 L/min |
| Arterial content ($CaO_2$) | = 1.34 mL $O_2$/g Hb × 160 g Hb/L × 0.97<br>= 208 mL $O_2$/L | = 1.34 mL $O_2$/g Hb × 160 g Hb/L × 0.97<br>= 208 mL $O_2$/L | = 1.34 mL $O_2$/g Hb × 160 g Hb/L × 0.97<br>= 208 mL $O_2$/L |
| Venous content ($CvO_2$) | = 1.34 mL $O_2$/g Hb × 160 g Hb/L × 0.75<br>= 161 mL $O_2$/L | = 1.34 mL $O_2$/g Hb × 160 g Hb/L × 0.50<br>= 107 mL $O_2$/L | = 1.34 mL $O_2$/g Hb × 160 g Hb/L × 0.45<br>= 96.5 mL $O_2$/L |
| Oxygen consumption ($VO_2$) (mL/min) | = 4.95 L/min × (208 – 161 mL $O_2$/L)<br>= 4.95 L/min × (47 mL $O_2$/L)<br>= 233 mL $O_2$/min | = 21.7 L/min × (208 – 107 mL $O_2$/L)<br>= 21.7 L/min × (101 mL $O_2$/L)<br>= 2,192 mL $O_2$/min | = 19.2 L/min × (208 – 96.5 mL $O_2$/L)<br>= 19.2 L/min × (111.5 mL $O_2$/L)<br>= 2,141 mL $O_2$/min |

$\dot{Q}$ **(L/min)** = SV (mL/beat) × HR (bpm)
$\dot{V}O_2$ **(mL/min)** = $\dot{Q}$ (L blood/min) × a-v$O_2$ difference (mL $O_2$/L blood)
$\dot{V}_E$ **(L/min)** = $V_T$ (mL/breath) × RR (breaths/min)
$O_2$ **content in blood** (mL $O_2$/L blood) = 1.34 mL $O_2$/g Hb × [Hb] (g/L blood) × $O_2$ saturation (% fraction)

direct the activity of the cardiovascular control and the respiratory control centers, located in the medulla oblongata. Cardiovascular sensory information (e.g., HR, SV, and blood pressure) and respiratory sensory information (e.g., $\dot{V}_E$, $PO_2$, $PCO_2$, blood pH level, and respiratory muscle activity) are detected by various peripheral and central chemoreceptors located throughout the body and brain.[3,29,39,40] These receptors provide beat-by-beat and breath-by-breath information that is relayed back to the control centers in the brain whereby adjustments are made in cardiovascular and respiratory function so that homeostasis is maintained during exercise. Cardiovascular control is aimed at maintaining blood pressure, whereas respiratory control is aimed at maintaining adequate $\dot{V}_E$ and arterial $PO_2$ and $PCO_2$ levels.

Some of the most important control mechanisms used to fine-tune activity of the cardiorespiratory system during exercise originates from centrally and peripherally located receptors. Although the immediate changes in the cardiorespiratory system at the onset of exercise are regulated by the control centers in the medulla, the receptors fine-tune the system and provide constant feedback throughout exercise. These receptors, which are located within various parts of the body, are mechanoreceptors, chemoreceptors, baroreceptors, thermoreceptors, and other receptors.

### Mechanoreceptors

Mechanoreceptors provide information about muscle length, tension, force of contraction, and joint angle, which is integrated to give information about the position of the body during exercise. One example of an important mechanoreceptor is the **muscle spindle**. A muscle spindle is embedded within a muscle fiber to sense the stretch of the muscle cell during movement. Similarly, the **Golgi tendon organ** is embedded within muscle tendons to sense changes in muscle force or tension. When stimulated, these receptors also send output signals to the cardiorespiratory control centers with regard to the intensity of movement.[29] Aside from the skeletal muscles and tendons, the joints also contain mechanoreceptors that sense changes in joint movement, pressure, and position. When stimulated during exercise, impulses are relayed to the medulla to modify activity of the cardiovascular and respiratory control centers so that $\dot{Q}$ and $\dot{V}_E$ can be regulated during exercise.

Finally, some evidence suggests that the right atrium and ventricle contain mechanoreceptors that sense changes in the size (or volume) of the chamber. During exercise, when $\dot{Q}$ rises, these receptors send impulses to the respiratory control center to stimulate an increase in $\dot{V}_E$ and HR to match the level of activity.[41]

## Chemoreceptors

The primary chemoreceptors that fine-tune activity of the cardiorespiratory system are the **aortic and carotid bodies**, and the central chemoreceptors located in the medulla.[42] The primary goals of the peripheral and central chemoreceptors are to modulate $\dot{V}_E$ by supplying the respiratory control center with continuous breath-by-breath information on $PaCO_2$, $PaO_2$, and blood pH (increased $H^+$ concentrations).[29] With respect to the peripheral chemoreceptors, the carotid bodies, probably because of their unique anatomical location (carotid arteries are the major blood supply vessel for the brain), appear to be more effective at sensing increased $PaCO_2$ and decreased $PaO_2$ than the aortic bodies. Similarly, the central chemoreceptors, located uniquely in the medulla at the interface with the cerebrospinal fluid, are in position to detect rapid increases in $PCO_2$. For example, when the concentration of arterial $CO_2$ increases during exercise, it rapidly diffuses from the blood across the blood–brain barrier and into the cerebrospinal fluid where hydrogen ions increase (decrease cerebrospinal fluid pH). The $H^+$, in turn, stimulates the central chemoreceptors to increase $\dot{V}_E$ (see Chapter 6 for a review of this topic). Carbon dioxide is then exhaled from the body and $PaCO_2$ decreases, leading to a reduction in $H^+$ concentrations (i.e., an increase in blood pH back to normal). Under normal circumstances, $\dot{V}_E$ rises linearly with changes in $H^+$ concentrations up to the ventilatory threshold as previously described.

Animal studies have indicated that the lung may contain specialized chemoreceptors that are activated by the level of $CO_2$.[43–45] It is thought that an increased

$CO_2$ return to the lung stimulates the lung receptors, which send output signals to the respiratory control center to increase $\dot{V}_E$.[28] The net effect would act to return $PaCO_2$ back to normal during exercise. Currently, no evidence has been reported regarding whether these receptors exist in the human lung.

There is also some evidence to indicate that increased blood potassium can stimulate the carotid bodies to increase $\dot{V}_E$.[46,47] Evidence for this lies in the fact that exercising muscle tends to release potassium into the blood, and the increase in blood potassium is directly related to the increase in $PaCO_2$ during exercise. The precise mechanisms responsible for the influence of potassium on the carotid bodies are currently unclear. Nevertheless, changes in blood potassium levels may play a regulatory role in the ventilatory drive during exercise.

## Baroreceptors

Baroreceptors are stretch (pressure) receptors located in the heart, carotid sinus, aortic arch, and other major arteries throughout the circulation. Not to be confused with the chemoreceptors located in the aortic and carotid bodies, these receptors exert control of HR, blood pressure, vascular resistance, and cardiac contractility through negative feedback to the cardiovascular control center.[3] An important example of this process involves the control of arterial blood pressure. An increase in blood pressure above the resting set point stimulates the baroreceptors in the aortic arch and carotid arteries to send information to the cardiovascular control center. To help return blood pressure back to normal, the cardiovascular control center increases parasympathetic tone to the heart and reduces sympathetic activity. The result is a decrease in HR and $\dot{Q}$ plus overall vasodilation, which reduces blood pressure. The activity of the baroreceptors decreases when blood pressure returns to the set-point level.

The opposite effect also occurs. When blood pressure is reduced to less than the set point, activity to the cardiovascular control center is *decreased*, which causes enhanced activity of the sympathetic nervous system to the heart and increased pressure. At the onset of exercise, the blood pressure set point at which the baroreceptors have established is raised from its resting state, allowing blood pressure and HR to increase abruptly. This is termed the **baroreflex**. The baroreflex plays an important role with the rapid increases in cardiovascular activity at the start of exercise.

If the parasympathetic nervous system becomes overactivated, blood pressure may decrease to an abnormal level (hypotension). A precipitating event, such as being stuck with a needle, the presence of blood, or standing up too quickly from a seated or lying position, usually triggers this hypotensive response. In these cases, HR and blood pressure decrease suddenly because of overstimulation of the vagus nerve (parasympathetic nerve innervating the heart), resulting in a decline in blood flow to the brain. This manifests itself as fainting, which leads to increased blood flow to the brain and the person regaining consciousness.

## Thermoreceptors

One of the main functions of the hypothalamus is to regulate core body temperature. One of the stressors imposed by exercise is increased heat from muscular and metabolic activity that causes body temperature to increase. When body temperature rises during exercise, blood flow through the hypothalamus stimulates thermoreceptors that modify the cardiovascular control center, which causes vasodilation of skin blood vessels to dissipate heat from the body.[21] In addition, through a second pathway, the hypothalamus sends output signals to sweat glands in the skin to increase sweat production (Fig. 8-16). In turn, normal body temperature is maintained during exercise.

## Other Receptors

Many other additional *stretch* receptors appear to exist throughout the peripheral areas of the body that act to increase activity of the cardiorespiratory system during exercise. These receptors are sensitive to tissue stretch or to the mechanical deformation that occurs during muscle contractions, or both. Upon activation, these receptors may influence HR, SV, $\dot{Q}$, blood pressure, and $\dot{V}_E$ during exercise.[28,39,48,49] For example,

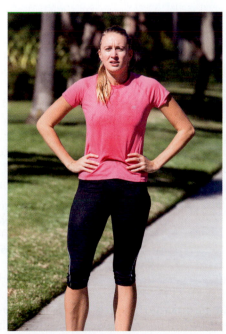

**Figure 8-16.** When body temperature increases during exercise, the hypothalamus sends output signals to sweat glands in the skin to increase sweat production.

stretch receptors are strategically located in the airways and respiratory muscles to monitor lung volumes and muscle length. When the lungs and chest wall inflate rapidly, as during exercise, the walls of the airways are stretched, which activates the receptors to terminate inspiration. In this manner, these receptors may limit the depth and length of the inspiratory cycle so that expiration can proceed. This important function may help to improve the efficiency of breathing during exercise. This is known as the **Hering-Breuer reflex**.

In summary, control of the cardiorespiratory system during exercise is first initiated by higher brain centers in the cerebral cortex that direct activity of the control centers in the medulla. In turn, $\dot{Q}$ and $\dot{V}_E$ are increased to match the level of metabolic activity needed to sustain the exercise task. Activity of the cardiorespiratory system is maintained throughout exercise by a variety of muscle mechanoreceptors, muscle chemoreceptors, central chemoreceptors, lung stretch receptors, arterial baroreceptors, and thermoreceptors that sense changes in skeletal muscle contraction, arterial blood gases and blood pH, RR and depth of breathing, and body temperature. These receptors relay signals to the medullary control centers to precisely adjust cardiorespiratory output to match metabolic demand during exercise.

## SUMMARY OF CARDIORESPIRATORY CHANGES AND RESPONSES TO EXERCISE

A summary of the acute cardiovascular and respiratory changes to exercise are shown in Figures 8-17 and 8-18, respectively. The two systems are separated so that the reader can more clearly see the adjustments that occur within each system. Note that many factors work together to help regulate $\dot{Q}$ to the working muscles. First, increased sympathetic nervous system activity causes HR and SV (because of increased myocardial contractility) to increase. Next, local factors within the working muscle (and sympathetic activity) stimulate vasodilation, which lowers TPR (decreases afterload), which facilitates a greater $\dot{Q}$. Moreover, the respiratory pump, skeletal muscle pump, and venoconstriction help to increase venous return. Venous return enhances end-diastolic volume, which helps to increase SV as exercise intensity increases. Lastly, vasoconstriction of vessels of less active tissues helps to redistribute blood flow to the working muscle. Fine-tuning of the cardiovascular adjustments described earlier is controlled by central and peripheral receptors located throughout the body. These receptors relay signals to the cardiovascular control center to precisely adjust blood flow to match metabolic demand during exercise.

In Figure 8-18, the flow of respiratory adjustments leading to an increase in $\dot{V}_E$ begins with sensory feedback and direct input from central and peripheral

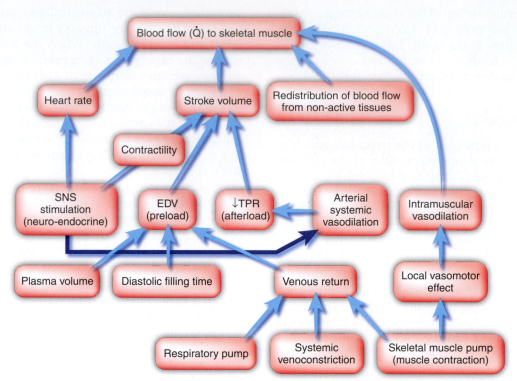

**Figure 8-17.** Summary of acute cardiovascular adjustments to exercise. Dark blue arrow signifies that SNS stimulation not only affects heart rate and stroke volume, but also arterial vasodilation, which may influence blood pressure. All of these systems are interconnected. EDV: end-diastolic volume; SNS: sympathetic nervous system; TPR: total peripheral resistance.

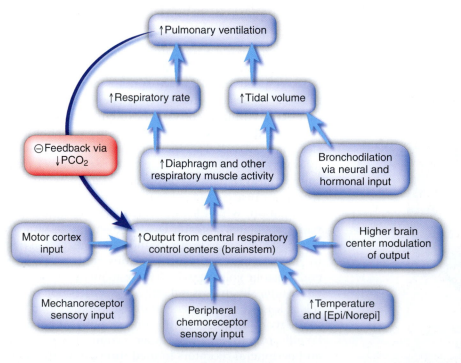

**Figure 8-18.** Summary of acute respiratory adjustments to exercise. The dark blue arrow signifies the interconnectedness of the body systems.

receptors to the respiratory control center. The control center sends signals to the respiratory muscles to contract to increase the rate and depth of $\dot{V}_E$. In addition, the sympathetic system causes the airways to dilate to decrease airway resistance and to enhance pulmonary blood flow. This helps to deliver more air into and out of the lungs during exercise and to ensure that $\dot{V}_E$ is matched with blood flow throughout the lung. Finally, the $PCO_2$ also plays an important role in fine-tuning $\dot{V}_E$. Pulmonary ventilation is stimulated by an increase in $CO_2$ and is reduced when $CO_2$ levels return to normal.

## VIGNETTE *continued*

■ Rachel continues her education efforts during the cool-down phase of Chris' workout by explaining the importance of cooling down and the process by which the body recovers from a bout of exercise. Because Chris has been sedentary until very recently, he requires an extended cool-down, as he will take longer to return to near-resting levels than a more trained individual. Rachel tells him that abruptly stopping a workout is not recommended, particularly in the early stages of his new exercise program. "Your heart rate, breathing rate, and body temperature must be slowly reduced toward your resting levels in order to safely end the workout." Chris responds by saying that he had always been nervous in the past whenever he tried to work out on his own because he would still be out of breath long after he finished exercising. He clearly appreciates the effort Rachel has put into making sure he understands the way his body feels before, during, and after his workouts.

## CARDIORESPIRATORY ADAPTATIONS TO AEROBIC EXERCISE TRAINING

Chronic adaptations are those changes that are established within the body after a period of prolonged, progressive training and are lost if the training stimulus is removed. Overall, the cardiovascular system will demonstrate a greater number of chronic changes following training compared with the respiratory system. Table 8-2 summarizes the primary cardiorespiratory adaptations to exercise training at rest and during exercise.

The following section details the cardiorespiratory changes that occur at rest and during submaximal and maximal exercise after a period of aerobic endurance training.

### Heart Rate, Stroke Volume, and Cardiac Output

Table 8-3 provides a closer look at the central cardiovascular differences between trained and untrained individuals at rest and during maximal exercise. Consistent participation in aerobic exercise decreases resting HR, often to less than 60 bpm. There are some reports of highly trained individuals with resting HRs in the low 30s. The change in resting HR following training is attributed to an increase in vagal tone (parasympathetic) and reduced sympathetic nervous system activity. The autonomic pathways have influence over

the SA node and can modify the discharge rate of impulses from that area to control HR. Although resting HR is reduced with training, resting SV is increased to maintain $\dot{Q}$. A lower resting HR allows more time for ventricular filling. This factor, combined with a larger ventricular chamber size, is a primary reason for greater resting SVs at rest in endurance athletes. Resting $\dot{Q}$ does not change following chronic aerobic exercise training largely due to increased resting SV.

For a given submaximal exercise intensity, HR will be lower (Fig. 8-19A), SV will be higher (Fig. 8-19B), and $\dot{Q}$ (Fig. 8-19C) will be higher in a trained person compared with an untrained person. However, the rate of increase in HR during incremental exercise, as denoted in Figure 8-17, will be lower following training. Indeed, because SVs are higher, the heart is able to beat slower during submaximal exercise following training.

Referring back to Table 8-3, maximal HR remains relatively unchanged after training and may slightly decrease in elite-trained individuals. Maximal SV is substantially increased following training because of a number of factors. First, left ventricular chamber enlargement and increased plasma volume combine to significantly increase end-diastolic volume. Second, increased end-diastolic volume enhances preload, which increases myocardial contractility. Third, training helps to lower TPR (afterload), which facilitates ventricular emptying. Finally, endurance training improves diastolic filling. This is characterized by a more rapid filling of the ventricles to maintain end-diastolic volume, even in the face of very high HRs.[19] Greater maximal SV contributes to increasing maximal $\dot{Q}$ following endurance training.

### Blood Pressure

Regular cardiorespiratory exercise training has been widely recognized to favorably modify resting blood pressure. Generally, the blood pressure–lowering effects of regular exercise are more pronounced in people with higher resting blood pressures and in people with hypertension.[50,51] Importantly, the benefits of exercise on blood pressure can be achieved by following current exercise participation recommendations. Indeed, leading organizations have indicated that if a person engages in regular exercise training of appropriate frequency (i.e., most days of the week), intensity (i.e., 40%–60% HR reserve), and duration (i.e., 30 minutes per day), the likelihood of developing high blood pressure will be substantially reduced.[52]

A variety of proposed mechanisms are shown in Figure 8-20 by which regular cardiorespiratory exercise favorably modifies blood pressure. The simplest explanation is that exercise training reduces the workload placed on the heart and blood vessels by reducing TPR. The reduction in TPR appears to be directly related to a lower sympathetic nervous system activity and increased parasympathetic nervous system activity following training. Decreases in sympathetic activity will

**Table 8-2.** Chronic Cardiorespiratory Changes Due to Aerobic Training at Rest and During Submaximal and Maximal Exercise

| VARIABLE | REST | SUBMAXIMAL EXERCISE | MAXIMAL EXERCISE |
|---|---|---|---|
| **Respiratory** | | | |
| Minute ventilation | No change | Decrease | Increase |
| Respiratory rate | Decrease | Decrease | Increase |
| Tidal volume | Increase | Increase | Increase |
| $Pao_2$ | — | No change | Slight decrease or more |
| $Paco_2$ | — | No change | Slight decrease |
| **Cardiovascular** | | | |
| Cardiac output | No change | No change | Increase |
| Stroke volume | Increase | Increase | Increase |
| Heart rate | Decrease | Decrease | No change or decrease |
| Blood pressure | No change/ Decrease | Decrease | Increase/Decrease/No change |
| a-v$O_2$ difference | Increase | Increase | Increase |
| Plasma/blood volume | Increase | — | — |
| Total hemoglobin/red blood cell volume | Increase | — | — |
| Hematocrit | Decrease | — | — |
| Cardiac size | Increase | — | — |
| Muscle blood flow | No change | Decrease | Increase |
| Capillary density | Increases | — | — |

—, not applicable.

a-v$O_2$ difference, arterial-venous $O_2$ difference; $Paco_2$, arterial partial pressure of carbon dioxide; $Pao_2$, arterial partial pressure of oxygen.

**Table 8-3.** Differences in Cardiac Efficiency Between Untrained and Aerobically Trained Individuals at Rest and During Maximal Exercise

| | HEART RATE (BEATS/MIN) | STROKE VOLUME (ML/BEAT) | CARDIAC OUTPUT (L/MIN) |
|---|---|---|---|
| **Rest** | | | |
| Untrained | 72 | 70 | 5.04 |
| Trained | 50 | 100 | 5.00 |
| **Maximal Exercise** | | | |
| Untrained | 200 | 120 | 24.0 |
| Trained | 190 | 280 | 34.2 |

reduce constriction of blood vessels. Furthermore, exercise training has been shown to improve vasodilation of blood vessels[53,54] and increase arterial diameter.[55] In addition to reduced resting blood pressure, blood pressure is lower for a given submaximal workload following a period of aerobic exercise training.[56] The reason for decreased blood pressure during exercise is that there is reduced output of the sympathetic nervous system for a given submaximal workload following training. Thus, the workload placed on the heart is significantly lessened because of the reduced exercise blood pressure.

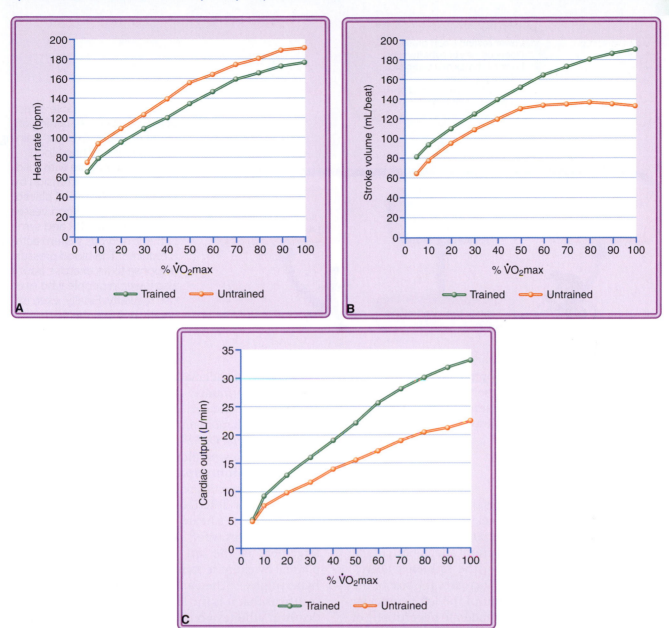

**Figure 8-19.** Differences in heart rate (HR), stroke volume (SV), and cardiac output (Q̇) responses between an endurance-trained individual and an untrained individual. (A) Note that the rate of increase and nonlinearity in HR response in these individuals is relatively similar up to a plateau at maximum. However, HR is lower for a given percentage maximal oxygen consumption (%V̇O₂max) in the trained individual because of normal training adaptations (e.g., increased SV) to aerobic exercise. (B) This graph shows the plateau response in SV that occurs normally in less trained individuals during incremental exercise. The SV response in the endurance-trained individual has major implications for maximizing Q̇ and improving aerobic exercise performance. (C) Note that the trained individual responds in a nonlinear fashion as maximal exercise is approached, with the untrained individual demonstrating a near-plateau response. This graph illustrates the variability that can occur with Q̇ changes during incremental exercise.

Recall that the acute pattern of blood pressure to incremental exercise is a curvilinear increase for SBP and no change or slight decrease for DBP (see Fig. 8-7). The effects of aerobic training on maximal blood pressure responses to dynamic exercise can vary from no change to a slight increase or decrease for a given bout of exercise.[52] For example, individuals with hypertension exhibit reduced maximal blood pressure (systolic and diastolic) responses following exercise training[56] as a result of lower TPR. In contrast, in a person with normal resting blood pressure, the blood pressure achieved at maximum exercise intensity may be higher compared with before training. Given that maximum cardiac outputs substantially rise with training, the increase in maximum blood pressure is necessary to deliver greater volumes of blood to the working muscle.

Regular participation in cardiorespiratory exercise is a powerful lifestyle strategy to lower resting and

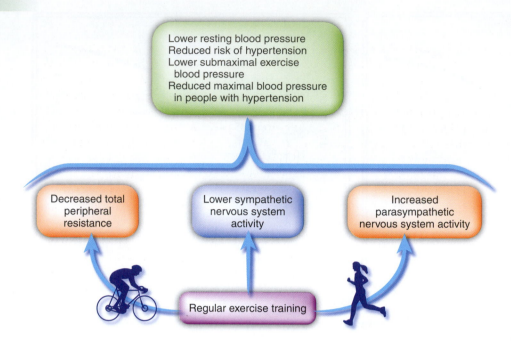

**Figure 8-20.** Favorable effects of regular exercise training on blood pressure. Exercise training can decrease resting blood pressures in people with mild-to-moderate hypertension by lowering the workload placed on the heart and blood vessels, in part because TPR and sympathetic nervous system activity is reduced. The blood pressure response to an exercise bout is also lower in people who exercise regularly. Finally, exercise greatly reduces the risk for development of hypertension.

exercise blood pressures in people with hypertension. The risk for development of hypertension is also significantly reduced with regular exercise. These favorable benefits can be achieved by following current exercise programming guidelines.

## Cardiac Hypertrophy

Figure 8-21 displays the changes that occur to the heart in response to chronic endurance exercise training often referred to as the athlete's heart. See Box 8-3 for a more complete discussion of the structural adaptations of the heart with exercise training, or the "athlete's heart." Generally, endurance training increases the size of the heart, primarily by enlargement of the left ventricular chamber volume and mild-to-moderate hypertrophy of the left ventricular myocardium. Increased left ventricular chamber size is a normal adaptation of the heart to accommodate the training-induced expansion of blood volume that occurs with regular endurance exercise.

These favorable adaptations can substantially enhance exercise performance. Indeed, a larger heart that can accommodate greater left ventricular filling volumes combined with more muscle mass will produce a greater SV and maximal $\dot{Q}$.[57,58]

More serious medical conditions, such as **hypertrophic cardiomyopathy** (Fig. 8-22), can occasionally mimic some of the otherwise normal adaptations to exercise as described earlier. Not to be confused with the athlete's heart, hypertrophic cardiomyopathy is a genetic disorder associated with abnormal enlargement of the left ventricle that cannot be explained by exercise training or other factors related to hypertrophy.[63] The danger of hypertrophic cardiomyopathy is that it is the leading cause of sudden cardiac death in athletes younger than 30 years. One of the main distinguishing factors between athlete's heart and hypertrophic cardiomyopathy is the pattern of left ventricular enlargement. In athlete's heart, the enlargement is symmetrical, meaning that the wall

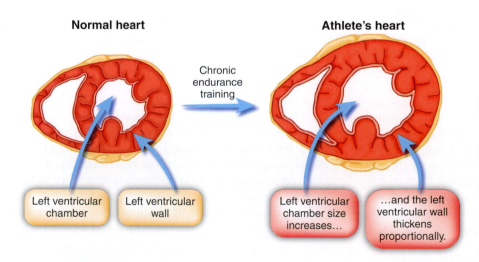

**Figure 8-21.** Changes in the left ventricle following chronic endurance exercise training (i.e., the "athlete's heart"). Generally, the athlete's heart is characterized by an enlarged left ventricular chamber and a proportional increased thickness of the left ventricular wall. These changes greatly increase maximal stroke volume (SV) and maximal cardiac output ($\dot{Q}$) to enhance exercise performance.

## Box 8-3. The Athlete's Heart

The enlargement (or hypertrophy) of the ventricular wall and chambers, most notably the left ventricle, is a normal adaptation that can occur because of long-term aerobic and resistance (usually higher intensity) exercise training. The term **athlete's heart**, or **athletic heart syndrome**, is often used medically to describe this enlargement (as shown in Fig. 8-21). The presence of athlete's heart can be evaluated using a diagnostic test called an **echocardiogram**, which provides an image of the heart that can then be visually inspected by a medical professional. In general, athlete's heart is benign and requires no medical treatment on diagnosis. The type of adaptation that occurs with aerobic training involves an increase in left ventricular chamber size in conjunction with a proportional increase in ventricular wall thickness.[59] The advantage of having an enlarged left ventricle is that it can accommodate more blood during diastole, which results in a greater SV and Q̇. This increases the amount of oxygen delivered to working muscles and improves exercise performance. Thus, the trained aerobic athlete will possess *a bigger and stronger heart muscle that can pump out a greater volume of blood at a much faster rate or velocity* compared with less trained individuals.[60]

Chronic changes to the left ventricle caused by resistance training are slightly different than those elicited by aerobic exercise. Most studies using resistance training have shown an increase in left ventricular wall thickness, but little or no enlargement of left ventricular volume.[61] The magnitude of increase in the thickness of the left ventricular wall is related to the overall intensity and duration of training. In a study by Adler and colleagues,[62] resistance-trained individuals, who were involved in intense resistance training before the study, demonstrated good systolic (ability to contract) and diastolic (ability to relax) function at rest and during isometric exercise. However, the volume of blood pumped out per heartbeat was not improved with training.

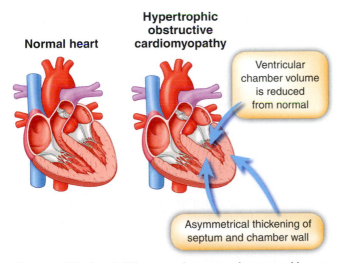

**Normal heart**

**Hypertrophic obstructive cardiomyopathy**

Ventricular chamber volume is reduced from normal

Asymmetrical thickening of septum and chamber wall

**Figure 8-22.** Visual differences between the normal heart and a heart with hypertrophic obstructive cardiomyopathy. Note that the heart on the left has a normal left ventricular chamber size and wall thickness. Hypertrophic obstructive cardiomyopathy is characterized by decreased left ventricular chamber size combined with increased asymmetrical left ventricular wall thickness.

thickness is similar throughout the ventricular chamber. In hypertrophic cardiomyopathy, the enlargement is asymmetric, and an abnormal thickness of the interventricular septum is typically seen with normal wall thickness elsewhere. The mechanism of sudden cardiac death in this condition is abnormal electrical conduction leading to lethal arrhythmias. Thus, it is common for individuals with this disorder to have a cardiac pacemaker implanted to control the heart if arrhythmias occur.

## Blood: Plasma and Other Factors

One of the more important physiological changes that can significantly impact SV at rest and during exercise is the expansion of plasma volume. Typically, plasma volume can be increased up to 500 mL or more due to training. With a greater plasma volume, end-diastolic volume and preload will be augmented, providing more stretch on the myocardium before blood ejection. This will increase the force of contraction, enhance SV, allow for a decrease in HR, and permit the heart to be more efficient at maintaining Q̇ at rest. Total hemoglobin and RBC volume (number of RBCs) may also be improved with training, but the overall concentration of hemoglobin and hematocrit are lower because increased plasma volume dilutes the blood. Upon detraining, losses in central cardiovascular function (SV) are primarily due to rapid changes in blood volume.[68]

## Arterial-Venous Oxygen Difference and Muscle Blood Flow

Training leads to a better capacity to extract oxygen from the blood during exercise (increased a-vO$_2$ difference). Exercise training increases capillary density in the muscle, which improves local blood flow and the surface area for gas exchange. These factors increase oxygen extraction for a given submaximal workload.

As discussed earlier, working skeletal muscles receive the highest amount of blood flow of any tissue, especially during heavy exercise. Much of the increased blood flow to muscle during near-maximal or maximal conditions are due to preferential shunting of blood to the muscle and vasoconstriction of less active areas.

## SEX DIFFERENCES

There are important sex differences that impact the cardiorespiratory response to exercise. First, the heart, primarily the right and left ventricular chamber size, is smaller in women compared with men. As a result, ventricular filling capacity (i.e., end-diastolic volume) is generally lower in women. However, an interesting difference is that despite smaller end-diastolic volumes, ejection fraction tends to be slightly higher in women regardless of differences in chamber size.[64,65] Another difference that affects cardiorespiratory exercise relates to body size.[66] Because women are generally smaller than men, total blood volume is less. The lower body mass combined with smaller ventricular chamber sizes contribute to reduced resting and exercise SVs and cardiac outputs in women. Consequently, maximum cardiorespiratory fitness is lower. Sex can also influence the function of the pulmonary system during exercise.[67] Men have been shown to have greater vital capacities and maximal expiratory flow rates during exercise because of greater lung volume and increased airway diameters. A greater surface area for gas exchange (alveoli–capillary interface) exists in men when matched for age and height compared with women.

## FROM THEORY TO PRACTICE

You are a personal trainer working at a fitness facility that offers exercise programming for persons of all ages and abilities. A 38-year-old female client is interested in working with you to create an aerobic exercise program to improve her cardiorespiratory fitness level. Your client has no personal history of cardiovascular, pulmonary, or metabolic disease other than mild hypertension. Otherwise, she is apparently healthy. A quick exercise history reveals an inconsistent exercise regimen over the last 15 years. Your client desires to begin a running program to compete in local 5K races, run faster without feeling "winded," and "lose a few pounds in the process to help her blood pressure." She has been doing some reading on the excellent cardiovascular and metabolic benefits of interval or "threshold" training and wants to know more about the specific effects of this type of training on her cardiorespiratory system. To help herself in her program, she purchased an HR monitor to help gauge intensity, but isn't sure what more she can do to monitor intensity during her training program. She also expresses an interest in beginning a resistance training program, but heard that it makes your blood pressure go up at rest, which is something she "wants to avoid."

1. Consider simple ways she can monitor intensity during exercise (other than HR) for interval training purposes.
2. Explain why she would feel "winded" during exercise when she tries to run faster.
3. Given your knowledge of the effects of aerobic exercise on the cardiovascular and respiratory systems, list the effects of exercise on the function of these systems to arm her with some health and fitness information.
4. Consider information you would give her regarding the short-term effects of moderate-intensity, dynamic resistance training on blood pressure. Does she need to worry?

Exercise training increases the capacity to redistribute blood flow to the working muscle more effectively. One factor that helps to redistribute blood flow during exercise is local vasodilation of muscle blood vessels. Vasodilation lowers vascular resistance to exercising muscle, which improves the delivery of oxygen and nutrients.[22] Combined with improved oxidative capacity and capillary density, the trained muscle will be more effective at extracting and utilizing greater amounts of oxygen during heavy exercise. Thus, maximal a-vO$_2$ difference will be increased following training.

## Pulmonary Ventilation

Compared with the cardiovascular system, the respiratory system does not experience significant changes at rest following training. The functional structures of lung tissue related to airflow and gas exchange are not influenced by training. Resting $\dot{V}_E$ remains unchanged following training, although RR may be lower and V$_T$ higher at rest because of increased parasympathetic control.

The ventilatory response for a given submaximal workload following training is significantly lower (up to 20%–30%) compared with pretraining levels. Similarly, $\dot{V}_E$ will be lower during incremental exercise up to maximum intensity following a period of aerobic exercise training. Reduced $\dot{V}_E$ during exercise is partly attributed to lower RRs during exercise and increased V$_T$. Indeed, increased strength and endurance of the respiratory muscles with training helps to lower $\dot{V}_E$ during exercise. For example, trained individuals are able to decrease their end-expiratory volume of air (exhale more air) and increase the end-inspiratory volume of air (inhale more air).

In summary, most of the training effects of endurance exercise can be attributed to improved performance and

## RESEARCH HIGHLIGHT

### Respiratory Muscle Training and Endurance Exercise

Although recent advancements indicate that the respiratory muscles are highly oxidative and fatigue-resistant skeletal muscles, it is now generally accepted that both significantly prolonged endurance exercise (in this case, more than 2 hours), and high-intensity exercise (greater than 80% $\dot{V}O_2$max) contributes to respiratory muscle fatigue, which can limit endurance exercise performance[30,69] (see Box 8-1). However, it appears that the same benefits in locomotor muscles that are induced by endurance exercise also occur in the respiratory muscles. Indeed, whole-body aerobic exercise training can improve the work capacity of the ventilatory muscles by enhancing the oxidative capacity of the diaphragm and upper airway muscles.[35,70] As a result, a greater ventilatory demand can be maintained before the induction of respiratory muscle fatigue, which is especially important for a competitive endurance athlete performing very high-intensity exercise (e.g., 10-km running race, 20-km cycling time trial).

Studies have also demonstrated that specific training of the respiratory muscles can delay respiratory fatigue and enhance exercise performance. Holm and colleagues[71] investigated the impact of respiratory muscle training on cycling endurance performance in 10 experienced cyclists ($\dot{V}O_2$max 56.0 mL/kg/min). The cyclists were instructed to complete a 40-km cycling time trial (indoor cycle ergometer) before and after 4 weeks of respiratory muscle endurance training (20, 45-minute rapid breathing sessions through a mouthpiece against a predetermined resistance). Six additional cyclists participated in the control group with no respiratory muscle training over the 4-week time frame. The study demonstrated that respiratory muscle training significantly improved respiratory muscle endurance capacity. Moreover, the improvement in respiratory muscle endurance was associated with enhanced cycling performance. Indeed, the time to complete the 40-km cycling time trial decreased by 4.75% (from 47 minutes before training to 45 minutes after training) in the subjects who completed the respiratory muscle training protocol. There were no changes in cycling performance in the control group. Subjects who participated in the respiratory muscle training program could maintain a markedly higher $\dot{V}_E$ ($\dot{V}_E$ after: 96 L/min) during the time trial compared with pretraining values ($\dot{V}_E$ before: 80 L/min).[71]

Thus, it appears that respiratory muscle–trained cyclists are able to breathe greater volumes of air during intense exercise without increased feelings of breathlessness. The mechanisms that contribute to improvements in respiratory muscle endurance and exercise performance are currently not completely clear. However, notably, the type, frequency, and duration of the respiratory muscle training program, mode and intensity of the exercise bout, and environmental/laboratory conditions in which the exercise bout is performed can influence whether any performance-enhancing benefits are observed. It has been speculated that delayed respiratory muscle fatigue, a redistribution of blood flow from respiratory to locomotor muscles, and a decrease in exercise dyspnea may be responsible for improved exercise performance.[35,72]

efficiency of the cardiovascular system. HR is lower whereas SV is higher at rest and during exercise following training. Combined with increased left ventricular chamber volume, increased plasma volume associated with training helps to increase maximal SV to improve maximal $\dot{Q}$. In addition, training leads to greater blood flow redistribution to the working muscle and better oxygen extraction. With respect to the respiratory system, exercise training lowers $\dot{V}_E$ at any level of exercise intensity. Improved ventilatory efficiency is attributed to increased strength and endurance of the respiratory muscles (improved respiratory muscle oxidative capacity), and improved regulation of blood pH.

## ACUTE CARDIORESPIRATORY RESPONSES TO RESISTANCE TRAINING

The cardiorespiratory responses to resistance exercise can be dramatic depending on the resistance intensity, the total amount of motor units recruited to perform the exercise, the number of repetitions completed, and

the rest periods between exercise sets. The two types of resistance exercise discussed in this section are dynamic and isometric (static), and their effects on HR and blood pressure (Fig. 8-23). These variables are among the most affected through an acute bout of resistance exercise, and both are related to a phenomenon called the *pressor response*. This response and the acute changes in HR and blood pressure to resistance exercise will be discussed further.

## Pressor Response

The **pressor response** is a neural mechanism that helps to regulate HR and blood pressure during exercise. It is composed of both central and peripheral mechanisms. The central mechanism is directly related to the motor control and voluntary effort, which is located in the motor cortex region of the brain. The peripheral influence is driven by the buildup of metabolites (e.g., increased $H^+$, reduced pH, and increased adenosine diphosphate) within the muscles as a result of reduced blood flow secondary to intramuscular compression

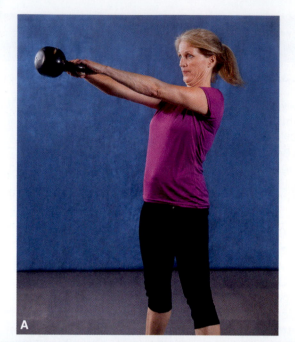

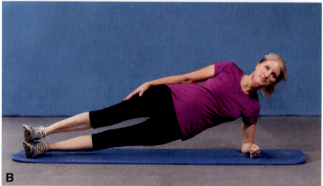

**Figure 8-23.** Examples of types of resistance exercise. (A) Dynamic. (B) Isometric.

## Dynamic and Isometric Resistance Exercise

There is substantial variation in the blood pressure responses to dynamic upper body and lower body resistance exercise (Fig. 8-24). Systolic pressures are generally higher for a given bout of lower body dynamic exercise compared with upper body exercise. Diastolic pressures may slightly decrease in both conditions, with greater reductions often observed during lower body exercise given the larger leg muscle mass used. During high-intensity, dynamic resistance exercise utilizing lower body musculature as in a leg press, SBPs have been measured near 300 mm Hg. Although DBPs will not typically reach that high during heavy dynamic resistance exercise, it is not uncommon for values to approach 150 mm Hg. *Keep in mind that these pressures were elicited by very high-intensity resistance exercise, and most individuals engaging in resistance exercise will not approach these numbers.*[74,75] In fact, most individuals have SBP and DBP responses during resistance training that are very similar to those attained during aerobic exercise.

Figure 8-25 shows typical blood pressure responses to isometric exercise. Isometric exercise has been associated with greater increases in SBP *and* DBP compared with dynamic resistance exercise. Even sustained isometric contractions performed at a relatively low load of 20% maximal voluntary contraction (MVC) can produce rapid increases in HR and

during contraction.[73,74] As a result, the buildup of metabolites activates mechanoreceptors and chemoreceptors in the skeletal muscle to elevate blood pressure and HR to higher levels. By increasing blood pressure and HR, a pressor reflex occurs in an attempt to increase $\dot{Q}$ and skeletal muscle blood flow. Often, the pressor response that occurs during resistance exercise can induce sudden elevations in SBP and DBP that may not closely match the amount of metabolic work performed. Moreover, individuals engaging in heavy resistance exercise often perform, sometimes unwittingly, a breathing maneuver commonly known as the **Valsalva maneuver**. This involves a forceful exhalation against a closed glottis, which does not allow air to be exhaled out of the mouth and nose. This maneuver will greatly increase intrathoracic pressure, which subsequently adds more to the exaggerated blood pressure response during resistance training. The danger is that the magnitude of this response can be harmful to individuals with cardiovascular disease through an increase in myocardial work and pressure within the blood vessels.

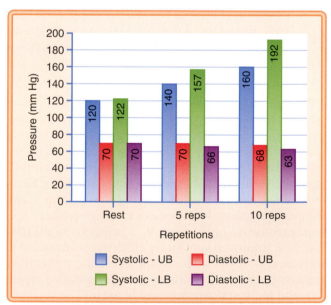

**Figure 8-24.** Systolic and diastolic blood pressure responses to dynamic upper body (UB) and lower body (LB) resistance exercise. Systolic pressure increases in both types of exercise, with LB eliciting the highest increase. Note that diastolic pressure decreases in both conditions, but decreases more with LB exercise because of greater vasodilation, which is related to the larger muscle mass used.

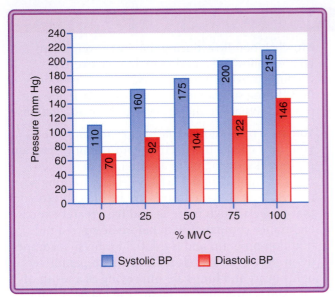

**Figure 8-25.** Systolic and diastolic blood pressure responses to increasing intensity of isometric hand grip exercise. Intensity in this graph is measured as percentage maximal voluntary contraction (%MVC). Note that both systolic and diastolic pressure increase significantly with increasing %MVC.

blood pressure. If the intensity of isometric exercise becomes more difficult by, for example, increasing the duration of contraction or the amount of muscle mass used, HR and blood pressure responses become even more exaggerated.

## In Your Own Words

Your grandfather wants to begin a resistance training program so that he can get stronger and do things more easily around the house. How would you explain to him that older individuals should approach isometric exercises with caution?

Chronic resistance training can lower the HR and blood pressure response to a given workload compared with pretraining levels. An increase in muscular strength lowers the absolute and relative (as a % of MVC) force that the muscle has to generate in response to a given resistance load. This will minimize the magnitude of the pressor response. Therefore, it is possible for an individual to lower cardiovascular stress when performing normal activities that involve strength if they engage in a regular resistance program. When performed correctly at the appropriate intensity, and the pressor response imposed by isometric exercise is minimized, resistance exercise is safe and does not stress the cardiovascular system more than aerobic exercise, even for older adults and those with cardiovascular disease.

## VIGNETTE conclusion

■ After 8 months of working with Rachel, Chris has seen dramatic improvements in his overall health and has lost more than 30 pounds. Rachel has continued her practice of educating Chris on his body's responses to exercise, both within a single session and in terms of the improvements he has made as a result of his ongoing participation in a structured exercise program. He now knows what to expect during a workout and better understands the specific improvements he has made to his overall health. By quickly recognizing a potential exercise barrier early in her relationship with Chris—and by tailoring her training style to the personality and needs of the client—Rachel was able to develop tremendous rapport with Chris and create an environment that will foster long-term adherence to the exercise program.

## CRITICAL THINKING QUESTIONS

1. Bill Jones is 58 years old and still enjoys running 5K to 10K road races. He has noticed that despite putting in the same number of training miles per week, his performance has decreased significantly compared with when he was younger. He recently had a $\dot{V}O_2$max test and was informed that his aerobic capacity was 40 mL/kg/min. When he was 28 years old, his $\dot{V}O_2$max was measured at 57 mL/kg/min. Explain to Bill some of the normal physiological changes that accompany healthy aging that are contributing to his decline in performance.

2. Over the past few years your best friend has experienced moderate asthma symptoms during exercise (e.g., wheezing, shortness of breath, and coughing) while living in the Midwest. These symptoms have made it significantly more difficult for her to perform at her best during competitive exercise events. However, during a recent Nordic skiing event in the Colorado Rockies (an altitude of approximately 9,000 feet), your friend indicated that she performed remarkably well and explained to you that her asthma symptoms were virtually gone while at altitude. Discuss the positive and negative effects of increased altitude on endurance exercise performance in a person who has asthma.

3. Describe the cardiovascular adjustments during recovery from exercise. What determines the rate of recovery in these variables and, in particular, what is the advantage of eliciting a post-exercise hypotensive response in individuals with high blood pressure?

## CRITICAL THINKING QUESTIONS–cont'd

4. The ventilatory threshold has also been used as a less invasive way to evaluate the metabolic state of the cell compared with the lactate threshold. What factors are attributed to the occurrence of the ventilatory threshold during incremental exercise?

5. The redistribution of blood flow during incremental exercise is a very important function of the cardiovascular system. Remembering back, what tissue received the most blood flow during incremental exercise, what organ receives a constant percentage of total $\dot{Q}$ and why, and what organ receives a constant or slightly increased amount of total $\dot{Q}$? Also, skin blood flow decreases during near-maximal exercise. Why is that?

6. Describe the HR, $\dot{Q}$, and SV responses to incremental aerobic exercise in relation to $\dot{V}O_2$ or workload. Are these responses the same from person to person, or is there variability in these responses?

7. Muscle blood flow during maximal exercise increases following a period of aerobic exercise training. In contrast, a decrease in muscle blood flow during submaximal exercise occurs following training. What are the reasons for both adaptations?

8. You are a professional triathlon coach and one of your new clients has been in your training program for 4 weeks, engaging in a combination of swimming, cycling, running, and resistance training activities. With much enthusiasm, he indicates to you that he feels much more fit and has greater exercise endurance compared with before he started the triathlon program and is excited for his first competition. However, he has no idea which parameters of his heart and lungs are improving as a result of his exercise training. What are the major chronic cardiorespiratory adaptations to exercise training that he is experiencing as a result of your program? What laboratory tests could you perform on your client to document his improved exercise capacity?

## ADDITIONAL RESOURCES

Brooks G, Fahey T, Baldwin K. *Exercise Physiology: Human Bioenergetics and Its Applications.* 4th ed. New York: McGraw-Hill Companies. 2005.
2008 Physical Activity Guidelines for Americans. Physical Activity Guidelines Advisory Committee Report, 2008.
**Websites**
Washington, DC: U.S. Department of Health and Human Services, 2008. http://www.health.gov/paguidelines
President's Council on Physical Fitness and Sports: http://www.presidentschallenge.org
Administration on Aging: http://www.aoa.gov
**Suggested Readings**
Beck K, Randolph LN, Bailey KR, Wood CM, Snyder EM, Johnson BD. Relationship between cardiac output and oxygen consumption during upright cycle exercise in healthy humans. *J Appl Physiol.* 2006;101:1474–1480.
Dempsey JA, McKenzie DC, Haverkamp HC, Eldridge MW. Update in the understanding of respiratory limitations to exercise performance in fit, active adults. *Chest.* 2008;34:613–622.

Haverkamp HC, Dempsey JA, Pegelow DF, et al. Treatment of airway inflammation improves exercise pulmonary gas exchange and performance in asthmatic subjects. *J Allergy Clin Immunol.* 2007;120:39–47.
Laughlin MH. Cardiovascular response to exercise. *Am J Physiol.* 1999;227(pt 2):S244–S459.
Mayo JJ, Kravitz L. A review of the acute cardiovascular responses to resistance exercise of healthy young and older adults. *J Strength Cond Res.* 1999;13:90–96.
Rowland T. Endurance athletes' stroke volume response to progressive exercise: A critical review. *Sports Med.* 2009;39: 687–695.
Schultze-Werninghaus G. Effects of high altitude on bronchial asthma. *Pneumologie.* 2008;62:170–176.
Voy R. The US Olympic Committee experience with exercise-induced bronchospasm. *Med Sci Sports Exerc.* 1984;18:328–330.
West JB. Respiratory system under stress. In: *Respiratory Physiology: The Essentials.* 8th ed. Baltimore, MD: Lippincott Williams & Wilkins; 2008.

## REFERENCES

1. Rowell LB. What signals govern the cardiovascular responses to exercise? *Med Sci Sports Exerc.* 1980;12: 307–315.
2. Eldridge FL, Millhorn DE, Kiley JP, Waldrop TG. Stimulation by central command of locomotion, respiration and circulation during exercise. *Respir Physiol.* 1985;59: 313–337.
3. Levy MN, Pappano AJ, Berne RM. *Cardiovascular Physiology.* 9th ed. Mosby physiology monograph series. Philadelphia, PA: Mosby Elsevier; 2007:xiv.
4. Herd JA. Cardiovascular response to stress. *Physiol Rev.* 1991;71:305–330.
5. Joyner MJ, Lennon RL, Wedel DJ, Rose SH, Shepherd JT. Blood flow to contracting human muscles: Influence of increased sympathetic activity. *J Appl Physiol.* 1990;68: 1453–1457.

6. Spyer KM. Annual review prize lecture. Central nervous mechanisms contributing to cardiovascular control. *J Physiol.* 1994;474:1–19.
7. Williamson JW, Nóbrega AC, Winchester PK, Zim S, Mitchell JH. Instantaneous heart rate increase with dynamic exercise: Central command and muscle-heart reflex contributions. *J Appl Physiol.* 1995;78:1273–1279.
8. Hofmann P, Pokan R, von Duvillard SP, Seibert FJ, Zweiker R, Schmid P. Heart rate performance curve during incremental cycle ergometer exercise in healthy young male subjects. *Med Sci Sports Exerc.* 1997;29: 762–768.
9. Vella CA, Roberds RA. Non-linear relationships between central cardiovascular variables and VO2 during incremental cycling exercise in endurance-trained individuals. *J Sports Med Phys Fitness.* 2005;45:452–459.

10. Conconi F, Ferrari M, Ziglio PG, Droghetti P, Codeca L. Determination of the anaerobic threshold by a noninvasive field test in runners. *J Appl Physiol*. 1982;52: 869–873.

11. Guyton AC, Hall JE. *Textbook of Medical Physiology*. 11th ed. Philadelphia, PA: Elsevier Saunders; 2006:xxxv.

12. Zhou B, Conlee RK, Jensen R, Fellingham GW, George JD, Fisher AG. Stroke volume does not plateau during graded exercise in elite male distance runners. *Med Sci Sports Exerc*. 2001;33:1849–1854.

13. Monos E, Berczi V, Nadasy G. Local control of veins: Biomechanical, metabolic, and humoral aspects. *Physiol Rev*. 1995;75:611–666.

14. Brengelmann GL. Circulatory adjustments to exercise and heat stress. *Annu Rev Physiol*. 1983;45:191–212.

15. Coyle EF, Gonzalez-Alonso J. Cardiovascular drift during prolonged exercise: New perspectives. *Exerc Sport Sci Rev*. 2001;29:88–92.

16. Powers SK, Howley ET, Cox R. A differential catecholamine response during prolonged exercise and passive heating. *Med Sci Sports Exerc*. 1982;14:435–439.

17. Montain SJ, Coyle EF. Influence of graded dehydration on hyperthermia and cardiovascular drift during exercise. *J Appl Physiol*. 1992;73:1340–1350.

18. Vella CA, Robergs RA. A review of the stroke volume response to upright exercise in healthy subjects. *Br J Sports Med*. 2005;39:190–195.

19. Gledhill N, Cox D, Jamnik R. Endurance athletes' stroke volume does not plateau: Major advantage is diastolic function. *Med Sci Sports Exerc*. 1994;26:1116–1121.

20. Griffin SE, Robergs RA, Heyward VH. Blood pressure measurement during exercise: A review. *Med Sci Sports Exerc*. 1997;29:149–159.

21. Boron WF, Boulpaep EL. *Medical Physiology: A Cellular and Molecular Approach*. 2nd ed. Philadelphia, PA: Saunders/Elsevier; 2009:xii.

22. Laughlin MH, Roseguini B. Mechanisms for exercise training-induced increases in skeletal muscle blood flow capacity: Differences with interval sprint training versus aerobic endurance training. *J Physiol Pharmacol*. 2008;59(Suppl. 7):71–88.

23. Smelker CL, Foster C, Maher MA, Martinez R, Porcari JP. Effect of exercise intensity on postexercise hypotension. *J Cardiopulm Rehabil*. 2004;24:269–273.

24. Jones H, George K, Edwards B, Atkinson G. Is the magnitude of acute post-exercise hypotension mediated by exercise intensity or total work done? *Eur J Appl Physiol*. 2007;102:33–40.

25. Pescatello LS, Guidry MA, Blanchard BE, et al. Exercise intensity alters postexercise hypotension. *J Hypertens*. 2004;22:1881–1888.

26. Bennett FM, Reischl P, Grodins FS, Yamashiro SM, Fordyce WE. Dynamics of ventilatory response to exercise in humans. *J Appl Physiol*. 1981;51:194–203.

27. Grucza R, Miyamoto Y, Nakazono Y. Kinetics of cardiorespiratory response to dynamic and rhythmic-static exercise in men. *Eur J Appl Physiol Occup Physiol*. 1990;61:230–236.

28. Dempsey JA, Vidruk EH, Mitchell GS. Pulmonary control systems in exercise: Update. *Fed Proc*. 1985;44:2260–2270.

29. Levitzky MG. *Pulmonary Physiology*. 4th ed. New York, NY: McGraw-Hill, Health Professions Division; 1995:xvi.

30. Dempsey JA, Johnson BD, Saupe KW. Adaptations and limitations in the pulmonary system during exercise. *Chest*. 1990;97(3 Suppl.):81S–87S.

31. Oyarzun GM. [Pulmonary function in aging]. *Rev Med Chil*. 2009;137:411–418.

32. Janssens JP, Pache JC, Nicod LP. Physiological changes in respiratory function associated with ageing. *Eur Respir J*. 1999;13:197–205.

33. Waterer, G.W., Wan JY, Kritchevsky SB, et al. Airflow limitation is underrecognized in well-functioning older people. *J Am Geriatr Soc*. 2001;49:1032–1038.

34. Hammond MD, Gale GE, Kapitan KS, Ries A, Wagner PD. Pulmonary gas exchange in humans during exercise at sea level. *J Appl Physiol*. 1986;60:1590–1598.

35. Powers SK, Coombes J, Demirel H. Exercise training-induced changes in respiratory muscles. *Sports Med*. 1997;24:120–131.

36. Mezzani A, Hamm LF, Jones AM, et al; European Association for Cardiovascular Prevention and Rehabilitation; American Association of Cardiovascular and Pulmonary Rehabilitation; Canadian Association of Cardiac Rehabilitation. Aerobic exercise intensity assessment and prescription in cardiac rehabilitation: a joint position statement of the European Association for Cardiovascular Prevention and Rehabilitation, the American Association of Cardiovascular and Pulmonary Rehabilitation, and the Canadian Association of Cardiac Rehabilitation. *J Cardiopulm Rehabil Prev*. 2012;32:327–350.

37. Persinger R, Foster C, Gibson M, Fater DC, Porcari JP. Consistency of the talk test for exercise prescription. *Med Sci Sports Exerc*. 2004;36:1632–1636.

38. Johnson JM, et al. Regulation of the cutaneous circulation. *Fed Proc*. 1986;45:2841–2850.

39. Marshall JM. Peripheral chemoreceptors and cardiovascular regulation. *Physiol Rev*. 1994;74:543–594.

40. McCloskey DI, Mitchell JH. Reflex cardiovascular and respiratory responses originating in exercising muscle. *J Physiol*. 1972;224:173–186.

41. Lloyd TC Jr. Effect on breathing of acute pressure rise in pulmonary artery and right ventricle. *J Appl Physiol*. 1984;57:110–116.

42. Dean JB, Nattie EE. Central $CO_2$ chemoreception in cardiorespiratory control. *J Appl Physiol*. 2010;108: 976–978.

43. Banzett RB, Coleridge HM, Coleridge JC. I. Pulmonary-$CO_2$ ventilatory reflex in dogs: effective range of $CO_2$ and results of vagal cooling. *Respir Physiol*. 1978;34: 121–134.

44. Green JF, et al. Effect of pulmonary arterial $PCO_2$ on slowly adapting pulmonary stretch receptors. *J Appl Physiol*. 1986;60:2048–2055.

45. Trenchard D, Russell NJ, Raybould HE. Non-myclinated vagal lung receptors and their reflex effects on respiration in rabbits. *Respir Physiol*. 1984;55:63–79.

46. Paterson DJ. Potassium and ventilation in exercise. *J Appl Physiol*. 1992;72:811–820.

47. Busse MW, Maassen N, Konrad H. Relation between plasma K+ and ventilation during incremental exercise after glycogen depletion and repletion in man. *J Physiol*. 1991;443:469–476.

48. Piepoli M, Clark AL, Coats AJ. Muscle metaboreceptors in hemodynamic, autonomic, and ventilatory responses to exercise in men. *Am J Physiol*. 1995;269 (4 Pt 2):H1428–H1436.

49. Estavillo JA. Cardiac receptors evoke ventilatory response with increased venous $PCO_2$ at constant arterial $PCO_2$. *J Appl Physiol*. 1990;68:369–373.

50. Whelton SP, Chin A, Xin X, He J. Effect of aerobic exercise on blood pressure: A meta-analysis of randomized, controlled trials. *Ann Intern Med*. 2002;136: 493–503.

51. Cornelissen VA, Fagard RH. Effects of endurance training on blood pressure, blood pressure-regulating mechanisms, and cardiovascular risk factors. *Hypertension*. 2005;46:667–675.

52. Pescatello LS, Franklin BA, Fagard R, Farquhar WB, Kelley GA, Ray CA; American College of Sports Medicine. American College of Sports Medicine position

stand. Exercise and hypertension. *Med Sci Sports Exerc.* 2004;36:533–553.

53. DeSouza CA, Shapiro LF, Clevenger CM, et al. Regular aerobic exercise prevents and restores age-related declines in endothelium-dependent vasodilation in healthy men. *Circulation.* 2000;102:1351–1357.

54. Kingwell BA. Nitric oxide-mediated metabolic regulation during exercise: Effects of training in health and cardiovascular disease. *FASEB J.* 2000;14:1685–1696.

55. Dinenno FA, Tanaka H, Monahan KD, et al. Regular endurance exercise induces expansive arterial remodelling in the trained limbs of healthy men. *J Physiol.* 2001;534(Pt 1):287–295.

56. Pitsavos C, Chrysohoou C, Koutroumbi M, et al. The impact of moderate aerobic physical training on left ventricular mass, exercise capacity and blood pressure response during treadmill testing in borderline and mildly hypertensive males. *Hellenic J Cardiol.* 2011;52:6–14.

57. Ginzton LE, Conant R, Brizendine M, Laks MM. Effect of long-term high intensity aerobic training on left ventricular volume during maximal upright exercise. *J Am Coll Cardiol.* 1989;14:364–371.

58. Seals DR, Hagberg JM, Spina RJ, Rogers MA, Schechtman KB, Ehsani AA. Enhanced left ventricular performance in endurance trained older men. *Circulation.* 1994;89:198–205.

59. George KP, Gates PE, Birch KM, Campbell IG. Left ventricular morphology and function in endurance-trained female athletes. *J Sports Sci.* 1999;17:633–642.

60. Caselli S, Di Pietro R, Di Paolo FM, et al. Left ventricular systolic performance is improved in elite athletes. *Eur J Echocardiogr.* 2011;12:514–519.

61. Effron MB. Effects of resistive training on left ventricular function. *Med Sci Sports Exerc.* 1989;21:694–697.

62. Adler Y, Fisman EZ, Koren-Morag N, et al. Left ventricular diastolic function in trained male weight lifters at rest and during isometric exercise. *Am J Cardiol.* 2008;102:97–101.

63. Ho CY. Hypertrophic cardiomyopathy. *Heart Fail Clin.* 2010;6:141–159.

64. Chung AK, Das SR, Leonard D, et al. Women have higher left ventricular ejection fractions than men independent of differences in left ventricular volume: The Dallas Heart Study. *Circulation.* 2006;113:1597–1604.

65. Yamada AT, Campos Neto Gde C, Soares J Jr, et al. Gender differences in ventricular volumes and left ventricle ejection fraction estimated by myocardial perfusion imaging: Comparison of Quantitative Gated SPECT (QGS) and Segami software programs. *Arq Bras Cardiol.* 2007;88:285–290.

66. Charkoudian N, Joyner MJ. Physiologic considerations for exercise performance in women. *Clin Chest Med.* 2004;25:247–255.

67. Harms CA. Does gender affect pulmonary function and exercise capacity? *Respir Physiol Neurobiol.* 2006;151:124–131.

68. Coyle EF, Hemmert MK, Coggan AR. Effects of detraining on cardiovascular responses to exercise: Role of blood volume. *J Appl Physiol.* 1986;60:95–99.

69. Babcock MA, Pegelow DF, Johnson BD, Dempsey JA. Aerobic fitness effects on exercise-induced low-frequency diaphragm fatigue. *J Appl Physiol.* 1996;81:2156–2164.

70. Sheel AW. Respiratory muscle training in healthy individuals: Physiological rationale and implications for exercise performance. *Sports Med.* 2002;32:567–581.

71. Holm P, Sattler A, Fregosi RF. Endurance training of respiratory muscles improves cycling performance in fit young cyclists. *BMC Physiol.* 2004;4:9.

72. Vincent HK, et al. Adaptation of upper airway muscles to chronic endurance exercise. *Am J Respir Crit Care Med.* 2002;166:287–293.

73. Smith SA, Mitchell JH, Garry MG. The mammalian exercise pressor reflex in health and disease. *Exp Physiol.* 2006;91:89–102.

74. Mayo JJ, Kravitz N. A review of the acute cardiovascular responses to resistance exercise of healthy young and older adults. *J Strength Cond Res.* 1999;13:90–96.

75. Karlsdottir AE, Foster C, Porcari JP, Palmer-McLean K, White-Kube R, Backes RC. Hemodynamic responses during aerobic and resistance exercise. *J Cardiopulm Rehabil.* 2002;22:170–177.

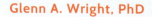

Glenn A. Wright, PhD

CHAPTER 9

# Structure and Function of Muscle and the Nervous System

## CHAPTER OUTLINE

## LEARNING OUTCOMES

1. Compare and contrast the three different types of muscle tissue in the human body.
2. Describe the structural organization of skeletal muscle.
3. Explain the role of the myofilaments actin and myosin in muscle contraction.
4. Describe the structural organization and function of connective tissue.
5. Compare and contrast the different types of skeletal muscle fibers.
6. Explain the process of muscle contraction as described by the sliding filament theory.
7. Describe the role of excitation-contraction coupling as it relates to muscle contraction.
8. Explain the significance of motor unit recruitment in the development of bodily movement.
9. Describe the determining factors of skeletal muscle growth and atrophy.
10. Outline the organization of the different divisions of the nervous system.
11. Identify the primary structures of the nervous system.
12. Explain the basic processes involved in the transmission of nerve impulses throughout the body.
13. Describe the nervous system structures related to, and the processes involved in, proprioception.
14. Explain the basic concepts of motor coordination and movement.

## ANCILLARY LINK

Visit DavisPlus at http://davisplus.fadavis.com for study and practice resources, including online quizzes, animations that help explain physiological processes, podcasts concerning news and career trends in exercise physiology, and practice references.

## VIGNETTE

■ Angela is a physical therapist working as part of the health-care team at a hospital-based fitness facility. Her newest client is Marci, a 67-year-old retiree who is recovering from a stroke. In addition to addressing Marci's cardiac limitations and balance issues, Angela is working with Marci's doctors to develop a plan to manage the spasticity she is experiencing in her left hand, which leaves her with constantly contracted arm musculature, resulting in a permanently clenched fist and bent elbow.

What are some strength-training considerations that Angela must keep in mind when working with Marci? What can she do to help address the spasticity in Marci's left hand?

The body's ability to create muscular force that results in either joint movement (mobility) or joint stiffness (stability) is dependent on the interaction of the skeletal muscles and the nervous system. Muscles rely on messages from nerves to carry out their many important functions. This chapter provides information on the fundamental properties of muscle and nerve tissue, and how these structures interact to function as the body's means of support and movement.

Sometimes called the *neuromuscular system*, the combined structures of the muscular and nervous systems are responsible for the coordinated, efficient movement of the body as it accepts and reacts to the forces present in daily activities. The neuromuscular system is the connection of the muscles to the brain and spinal cord through a network of nerve circuits that direct the ebb and flow of muscular energy.

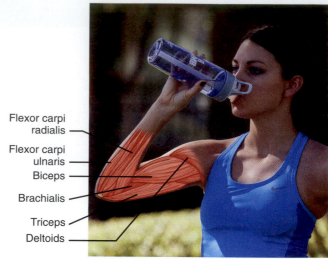

**Figure 9-1.** Example of an action involving muscle under voluntary control.

## MUSCULAR SYSTEM

The muscular system, which is composed of more than 600 individual skeletal muscles, is responsible for movement of various body parts. Although we discuss the three types of muscle tissue in this chapter, most of our attention is focused on the muscular system, made up of only skeletal muscle. Muscle tissue is characterized by its function and whether it is controlled voluntarily or involuntarily. For example, the heart muscle has a specific function of contracting repeatedly. The heart is under involuntary control. Thigh muscles, in contrast, are primarily consciously controlled and function to support body weight and assist in movement of the lower extremity. One property that all muscle tissue has in common is its ability to contract and develop force, which is sometimes referred to as muscular tension.

There are three types of muscle tissue—**skeletal muscle**, **smooth muscle**, and **cardiac muscle** (Table 9-1). Skeletal muscle attaches to the skeleton and, by means of contraction, exerts force on the bones to produce movement at the joints. Because skeletal muscle is under conscious control, it is considered voluntary muscle. For example, a simple task such as picking up a glass of water requires a series of contractions of skeletal muscles in the upper extremity (Fig. 9-1).

This action is consciously controlled as the brain sends nervous signals to the muscles to bring about the intended movement.

Skeletal muscle is also known as **striated** muscle because when it is viewed under a microscope, there is an appearance of alternating light and dark bands (Fig. 9-2A). These striped bands consist of structures that combine to make up the functional contractile unit of skeletal muscle, the **sarcomere**.

In contrast with skeletal muscle, smooth muscle and cardiac muscle are not under conscious control and as such are considered involuntary muscle tissue. Smooth muscle is found in the walls of hollow organs such as the stomach, intestines, and blood vessels, and functions to regulate the movement of materials through the body. Smooth muscle is so named because from a microscopic view it lacks the striated appearance of skeletal muscle (Fig. 9-2B).

Cardiac muscle is a specialized tissue that functions to maintain the constant pumping action of the heart. Cardiac tissue, also called **myocardium**, makes up the four chambers of the heart and is striated in appearance, similar to skeletal muscle (Fig. 9-2C). Two myocardial networks are formed: the atrial myocardium and the ventricular myocardium. Each network of myocardial cells is unique in that its cells interconnect in

## Table 9-1. Types of Muscle Tissue

| TISSUE | NERVOUS SYSTEM CONTROL | FUNCTION |
|---|---|---|
| Skeletal muscle (striated) | Voluntary | Exerts force on the bones to produce movement at the joints |
| Smooth muscle (nonstriated) | Involuntary | Regulates the movement of materials through the hollow organs of the body (e.g., stomach, intestines, and blood vessels) |
| Cardiac muscle (striated) | Involuntary | Specialized tissue that functions to maintain the constant pumping action of the heart |

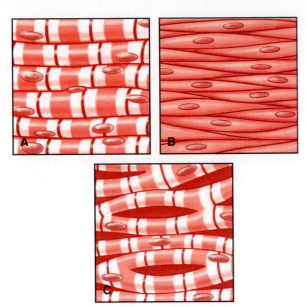

**Figure 9-2.** Microscopic images of three different types of muscle tissues: (A) skeletal muscle (striations), (B) smooth muscle (lack of striations), and (C) cardiac muscle (striations). The main difference between skeletal and cardiac muscle observed in these images is the branching of muscle fibers in the heart, which does not occur in skeletal muscle.

a latticework configuration so that when the stimulus for the heart to contract is received, all the myocardial cells within each network function together as a unit. This allows both atria to contract together and both ventricles to contract together in an alternating fashion.

Because the focus of this chapter is on the structure and function of skeletal muscle and its relationship to the nervous system, the remainder of this discussion excludes smooth and cardiac muscles.

## In Your Own Words

A client you are training is curious about how skeletal muscle is different from cardiac muscle. She asks, "If my heart is essentially a muscle, why can't I control the beating of my heart like I can control my biceps muscles during an arm curl?" How would you answer this client's question?

### Structural Organization of Skeletal Muscle

Muscle fibers, or muscle cells, are held in place by thin sheets of connective tissue membranes called **fasciae** (singular = **fascia**). The fascia that encases the entire muscle is known as the **epimysium**. Within the epimysium are bundles of muscle fibers grouped together in a fibrous sheath of fascia known as the **perimysium**. Within the perimysium are individual muscle fibers wrapped in a fascia called **endomysium** (Fig. 9-3).

A muscle fiber contains a vast network of interconnecting structures and organelles that make muscle contraction possible. The sarcomere, which was introduced previously as the basic contractile unit of muscle, contains the key elements of muscle structure that actually produce movement when stimulated. Each muscle

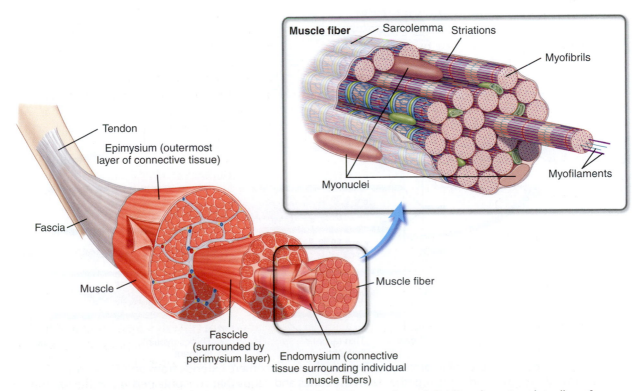

**Figure 9-3.** General organization of muscle, starting with whole muscle and dividing down into bundles of muscle fibers (fascicles), single muscle fibers, myofibrils, and myofilaments (actin is blue, and myosin is purple).

fiber contains several hundred to several thousand threadlike **myofibrils** that run parallel to each other and extend lengthwise like rods throughout the cell. Each myofibril contains many repeating sarcomeres lined up end to end, or in series (Fig. 9-4). Within each sarcomere are overlapping protein filaments, called **myofilaments**, that are arranged in such a way that gives the muscle fibers their striated (or striped) appearance.

The striations in muscle fiber are a result of alternating dark and light bands, which run the length of the cell. The dark areas, called *A bands*, contain the thick filament, which are made up primarily of the protein **myosin**. The light areas, or *I bands*, are where the thin filament is located, made up mostly of the **actin** proteins. Thin filaments also extend into the A bands, where they overlap with the thick filaments.

The A band has a lighter center region called the *H zone* that contains only thick filaments. This region is lighter in color because thin filament does not extend into this area and the thick filament contains only myosin tails in this middle section. In the center of the H zone is the M line, which holds the myosin tails in proper orientation within the middle of the sarcomere. The H zone is only visible in a muscle fiber at resting length. Crossing the center of each I band is a dense Z line that divides the myofibrils into sarcomeres. Thus, the sarcomere is the portion of a myofibril that is found between two Z lines. Thin filaments attach directly to the Z lines.

## Thick and Thin Filaments

The thin filament extends toward the center of the sarcomere from the Z line. The thin filament is actually a combination of three protein molecules: actin, **tropomyosin**, and **troponin**. The actin protein forms the backbone of the filament, whereas the tropomyosin and troponin molecules are situated in a spiral pattern around the actin chain. In conjunction with calcium, tropomyosin and troponin are important in maintaining the relaxation or contraction of a myofibril and, as a result, are referred to as regulatory proteins of the thin filament. Each thin filament is equipped with receptor sites, called *active sites*, to which myosin can bind (see Fig. 9-4).

The thick filament is composed of two myosin protein strands that are twisted together. Another protein, called *titan*, attaches at the Z line and at either end of the thick filament to keep it centered in the sarcomere. Arranged at intervals along the thick filament are tiny projections, called *myosin heads*, that bind with the active receptor sites on the actin filament to create a cross-bridge, linking the two myofilaments together. This connection is essential for muscle contraction.

## Connective Tissue

Connective tissue is made up of dozens of proteins, including **collagen**, the most abundant protein in the body. The two major physical properties of collagen

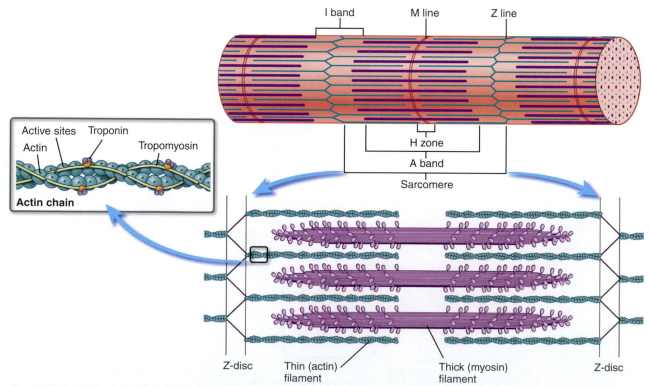

**Figure 9-4.** Microscopic features of a sarcomere. The length of a sarcomere extends from one Z line to another. The myofilaments, myosin and actin, together form the zones and bands that are contained within the sarcomere. The bottom image shows a more detailed view of the relationship between actin and myosin, and provides a closer look at the regulatory proteins, troponin and tropomyosin.

fibers are their tensile strength and relative inextensibility. As a result, structures that contain large amounts of collagen tend to limit motion and resist stretch. Thus, collagen fibers are the main constituents of tissues such as ligaments and tendons that are subjected to a pulling force. Figure 9-5 illustrates the composition of collagen fiber.

Connective tissue within the muscle is also made up of elastic fibers that are responsible for determining the possible range of extensibility of muscle cells. A large amount of elastic fibers are found in the connective tissue that surrounds the sarcomere. Elastic fibers provide a number of roles in skeletal muscle that include:
- Disseminating mechanical stress
- Enhancing coordination
- Maintaining tone during muscular relaxation
- Defending against excessive forces

Elastic fibers are almost always found together with collagen fibers. These two connective tissues work together to support and to facilitate joint movement.

Although various forms of connective tissue are found throughout the body, the structures related most to the practical applications of fitness training are **tendons**, **ligaments**, and fasciae (Table 9-2). Tendons are tough, cordlike tissues that connect muscles to bones. Their primary function is to transmit force from muscle to bone, thereby producing motion. A secondary function of tendons is to resist movement in one direction (i.e., the direction opposite of the force of transmission that produces joint motion). Tendons consist of wavy bundles of collagenous fibers that are usually oriented toward the direction of normal physiological stress. The bundles of collagen straighten when a low level of stretch force is applied.

Further stretch results in deformation of the tendon that is linearly related to the amount of tension applied. If stretched within a certain range (less than 4% of resting length), tendons will return to their original lengths when unloaded. Stretching the tendon beyond its "yield point" results in permanent length changes and microtrauma to the tendon's structural integrity.

Ligaments function primarily to support a joint by attaching bone to bone. Unlike tendons, ligaments take on various shapes, such as cords, bands, or sheets, depending on their location. Ligaments possess a greater mixture of elastic and fine collagenous fibers woven together than their tendinous counterparts. This interwoven structure results in a tissue that is pliant and flexible, and allows freedom of movement, but is also strong, tough, and inextensible so as not to yield easily to applied forces. Whereas tendons provide approximately 10% of the resistance experienced during joint movement, the ligaments and joint capsule (a saclike structure that encloses the ends of bones at a joint) contribute about 47% of the total resistance to movement.[1]

Intramuscular fascia (deep fascia) within a muscle is directly related to flexibility and range of motion at a joint. Its three main functions are to:
- provide a framework that ensures proper alignment of muscle fibers, blood vessels, and nerves.
- enable the safe and effective transmission of forces throughout the whole muscle.
- provide the necessary lubricated surfaces between muscle fibers that allow muscles to change shape during contraction and elongation.

During a passive stretching movement, fascia contributes 41% of the total resistance to joint range of motion.[1] Thus, fascia is second only to the joint capsule (ligaments) in terms of resistance to movement (Table 9-3).

## In Your Own Words

Your client canceled his workout session because he recently sprained his ankle. His doctor told him that the lateral ligaments of his right ankle have been damaged and that he needs to keep the ankle supported and braced for a period of time. In simple terms, describe for your client the function of the ligaments of the ankle and the reason why his doctor recommended keeping the ankle immobilized.

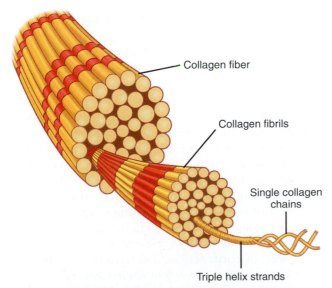

**Figure 9-5.** General organization of a collagen fiber. Single fibers are composed of collagen fibrils and triple-helix strands made up of single collagen chains. This protein is an extremely important one for maintaining the health of connective tissue in the body.

Collagen fiber

Collagen fibrils

Single collagen chains

Triple helix strands

## MUSCLE FUNCTION

The importance of the contribution of skeletal muscle action to normal bodily function cannot be overstated. The primary functions of skeletal muscle are to:
- facilitate locomotion and breathing by generating force.

## Table 9-2. Connective Tissues of the Neuromuscular System

| TISSUE | CHARACTERISTICS | FUNCTION |
| --- | --- | --- |
| Tendons | Cordlike tissues that connect muscles to bones | Transmit force from muscle to bone, thereby producing motion; resist movement in the direction opposite of the force that causes joint movement |
| Ligaments | Attaches bone to bone at the joints | Support the joints by allowing freedom of movement, but are also strong, tough, and inextensible so as not to yield easily to applied forces |
| Fasciae | Sheathlike substance that encases body cavities, muscles, and organs | Perform various functions throughout the body, including supporting innermost body cavities and organs, enabling the safe and effective transmission of forces within the body, and providing lubricated surfaces between muscle fibers that allow muscles to change shape during contraction and elongation |

## Table 9-3. Soft Tissue Structures That Contribute to Joint Resistance

| TISSUE | RELATIVE CONTRIBUTION TO JOINT RESISTANCE |
| --- | --- |
| Joint capsule | 47% |
| Fascia (including muscle) | 41% |
| Tendon | 10% |
| Skin | 2% |

- support posture through static and dynamic force generation.
- produce heat by causing shivering during periods of cold stress.

A muscle's fiber-type composition and the neuromuscular system's ability to recruit muscle fibers for action are characteristics that, in part, determine muscle contraction force and duration.

## Muscle-Fiber Types

Skeletal muscle can be divided into two general categories based on how quickly it shortens: **fast-twitch muscle fibers** and **slow-twitch muscle fibers**. Slow-twitch fibers (also called *slow-oxidative* or *type I muscle fibers*) contain relatively large amounts of **mitochondria** and are surrounded by more **capillaries** than fast-twitch fibers. In addition, slow-twitch fibers contain higher concentrations of **myoglobin** than fast-twitch fibers (also called *type II muscle fibers*). The high concentration of myoglobin, the large number of capillaries, and the high mitochondrial content make

slow-twitch fibers resistant to fatigue and capable of sustaining aerobic metabolism.

As the name implies, slow-twitch fibers shorten more slowly than fast-twitch fibers, such that the speed of shortening and tension development in fast-twitch fibers is three to five times faster than in slow-twitch fibers.[2] Furthermore, slow-twitch fibers create lower force outputs and are more efficient than fast-twitch fibers. As a result, these characteristics of slow-twitch muscle fibers, such as the ability to sustain aerobic metabolism for longer durations because of the higher levels of capillaries, mitochondria, and myoglobin, and the greater efficiency of slow-twitch fibers, are ideal to contribute to the performance of endurance exercise. In contrast, fast-twitch fibers with fast shortening speeds and high-force production are better for activities that require these characteristics, such as sprinting or weight lifting. The characteristics of different types of skeletal muscle fibers are outlined in Table 9-4.

The ability of skeletal muscle to contract depends on three performance characteristics: maximal force production, speed of contraction, and muscle-fiber efficiency.

- **Maximal force production** is expressed by how much force the fiber produces per unit of fiber cross-sectional area. Researchers have found that fast-twitch muscle fibers produce 10% to 20% more force than slow-twitch muscle fibers because fast-twitch fibers contain more myosin cross-bridges per cross-sectional area of fiber.[5]
- The maximal shortening speed of muscle fibers, or **speed of contraction**, is determined by the rate of cross-bridge movement (called *cross-bridge cycling*). Fast-twitch fibers exhibit a high maximal shortening velocity, whereas slow-twitch fibers contract more slowly. This appears to be due to the biochemical properties of muscle fiber, such that

## RESEARCH HIGHLIGHT

### Changing Views on Fast-Twitch Muscle Fibers

It is generally agreed that there are two subtypes of fast-twitch fibers, identified as type IIx and IIa. Traditionally, the fastest type of skeletal muscle fiber in humans has been called the *type IIb fiber*. However, research in the late 1980s led to the discovery of new properties in the skeletal fast-twitch muscle fibers of both rodents and humans, which has prompted scientists to relabel these fastest fibers as type IIx.[3] Type IIx muscle fibers (sometimes called *fast-glycolytic fibers*) contain a relatively small amount of mitochondria, and as a result have a limited capacity for aerobic metabolism and fatigue more easily than slow-twitch (type I) fibers. In fact, these fibers cannot sustain their effort for more than a few seconds. However, they possess a high number of glycolytic enzymes, which provide them with considerable anaerobic capacity. Type IIx fibers are the largest and fastest, and are capable of producing the most force of all the skeletal muscle fibers, but are notably less efficient than slow-twitch fibers.[4] A second subtype of fast-twitch muscle fibers is the type IIa fiber (also called *intermediate* or *fast-oxidative* **glycolytic** *fibers*). These fibers possess speed, are fatigue resistant, and have force-production characteristics somewhere between slow-twitch and type IIx fibers. They are also used for strength and power activities but can sustain an effort for longer than the type IIx fibers—up to 3 minutes in highly trained athletes. Type IIa fibers are unique in that they are highly adaptable. That is, with endurance training, they can increase their oxidative capacity to levels similar to those observed in slow-twitch fibers.

Pette D. Historical perspectives: plasticity of mammalian skeletal muscle. *J. Appl. Physiol.* 2001;90:1119–1124.
Shoepe T, Stelzer JE, Garner DP, Widrick JJ. Functional adaptability of muscle fibers to long-term resistance exercise. *Med. Sci. Sports Exerc.* 2003;35:944–951.

## Table 9-4. Characteristics of Different Types of Skeletal Muscle Fibers

| SLOW-TWITCH (TYPE I, OXIDATIVE) | FAST-TWITCH (TYPE II, GLYCOLYTIC) |
|---|---|
| Contract slowly | Contract rapidly |
| Contract less forcefully | Contract forcefully |
| Fatigue resistant | Fatigue quickly |
| Primary energy system is aerobic | Primary energy system is anaerobic |
| Used in endurance activities | Used in short-term activities that require strength and power Fast-twitch fibers are further classified into type IIa and type IIx.<br>• Type IIa fibers are slightly more oxidative than type IIx.<br>• It is possible to increase either the oxidative qualities or the glycolytic qualities of type IIa fibers through training. |

fibers that contain high levels of a fast form of myosin ATPase (the enzyme required for the breakdown of **adenosine triphosphate [ATP]**) are able to contract with higher speed. Accordingly, fast-twitch fibers possess a faster rate of ATPase activity than slow-twitch fibers.

- **Muscle fiber efficiency** is determined by a measure of the fiber's economy; that is, an efficient fiber requires less energy to perform a given amount of work than a less-efficient fiber. Slow-twitch fibers are more efficient than fast-twitch fibers because of their higher concentrations of myoglobin, larger numbers of capillaries, and higher mitochondrial enzyme activities. In other words, slow-twitch fibers are more efficient at using oxygen to generate more ATP to fuel continuous muscle contractions for extended periods.

A muscle's fiber-type composition is typically an equal mixture of fast- and slow-twitch fibers, although some muscle groups tend to be made up of primarily one or the other. For example, slow-twitch fibers are primarily responsible for the maintenance of body posture and skeletal support. These fibers are able to generate tension for longer periods. In contrast, fast-twitch fibers proliferate in muscles that are used to create greater amounts of force for shorter periods, such as the gastrocnemius and vastus lateralis. The percentage of specific fiber types within skeletal muscle may be influenced by genetics and hormones.

Fiber composition of skeletal muscles is thought to play an important role in sport and exercise performance. It is commonly believed that successful power athletes, such as jumpers and sprinters in track and field, possess a relatively large percentage of fast-twitch fibers, whereas endurance athletes generally have a large percentage of slow-twitch fibers. Researchers have shown that weight lifters and power athletes can exhibit a significant enlargement of muscle fibers, especially fast-twitch fibers,[4,6] whereas endurance athletes tend to develop relatively less increase in muscle size with training, with an emphasis on enlarged slow-twitch fibers.[7] However, considerable variation exists in the percent distribution of different fibers within a muscle. Research on training in sports suggests that athletes with a wide range of different fiber types in their muscles can be successful in the same athletic event.[8] Thus, estimating the fiber-type distribution of muscles (such as is done during certain muscle biopsy procedures) and using these data as a screening procedure for predicting athletic success is discouraged. It should be noted that muscle-fiber composition is only one variable that determines success in overall physical performance. Proper, consistent exercise training is one of the most important variables in the development of a high level of performance.

## In Your Own Words

The fitness facility at which you train enrolls two new members. The new members are good friends who enjoy physical activity and who are interested in beginning a weight-training program together. In college, both men were athletes. John was a long jumper and sprinter. Matt was a long-distance runner. John and Matt often comment about the fact that, even though they were both track and field athletes, John's physique appears to maintain more muscle, whereas Matt's body seems leaner with less muscle mass. How would you explain to John and Matt the possible reasons for the differences in their appearance?

## Muscle Contraction

Although muscle contraction is a complex process that involves many neural and biochemical processes, the ultimate result is the mechanical action of the thin filament sliding over the thick filament to bring about a change in the length of the muscle fiber as a whole. During the resting, nonstimulated state of the muscle fiber, myosin heads are not in contact with the thin filament, since binding sites on the thin filaments for the myosin heads are blocked by tropomyosin. Excitation of the muscle requires the removal of the inhibition by tropomyosin.

### Excitation

Before changes in length of the muscle fiber can take place, the fiber must be stimulated by a nerve impulse at the junction of the alpha motor nerve from the spinal cord and the sarcolemma of the muscle cell, referred to as the **neuromuscular junction**.

The nerve impulse, or electrical signal, that starts the sequence of events that ultimately produces muscle contraction is called an **action potential**. Sent from the brain or spinal cord, an action potential travels along the motor nerve until it reaches the neuromuscular junction. As shown in Figure 9-6, the action potential causes the release of a **neurotransmitter** called **acetylcholine** from the end of the motor neuron into the **synaptic cleft** of the neuromuscular junction (step 1). Once in the synaptic cleft, acetylcholine "excites" (or depolarizes) the muscle fiber, which produces an action potential on the sarcolemma that travels down the transverse tubules (T-tubules) deep into the muscle fiber (step 2). The arrival of the action potential to the T-tubules is the signal to release calcium from the **terminal cisternae** of the sarcoplasmic reticulum (step 3). The calcium then binds to troponin, which causes tropomyosin to shift its position, exposing binding sites on the thin filament (step 4). This sequence of events that leads to exposure of the binding sites is typically referred to as the excitation phase.

### Sliding Filament Theory

Once the binding sites are exposed, the myosin heads from the thick filament attach to the exposed binding sites on the thin filaments and cross-bridges are formed. This is referred to as the "attachment." After the formation of cross-bridges, the **power stroke** occurs, when movement of the myosin head pulls the thin filament to slide over the thick filament toward the center of the sarcomere, leading to a shortening of the sarcomere (i.e., the Z lines are pulled closer together and the H zone is shortened or disappears). Because all of the sarcomeres within a fiber shorten simultaneously, the overall length of the muscle fiber shortens, generating force. Figure 9-7 illustrates the sliding filament theory of muscle contraction. Also see explanatory animation of the sliding filament theory on the DavisPlus site at http://davisplus.fadavis.com.

The power stroke must be performed repeatedly for any significant change in muscle length to occur. After a power stroke, the myosin head must release from its binding site on the thin filament, to reset itself. Detachment of the myosin head from the binding site is accomplished by the replacement of a "fresh" ATP to the myosin head. The ATP is split into adenosine diphosphate (ADP) and inorganic phosphate (Pi) by an enzyme called *ATPase* that is found on the myosin head, releasing a small amount of energy that allows a resetting of the head to its "ready" position (also referred to as "energized" myosin heads). ADP and Pi remain bound to the myosin head in the energized position. When the myosin head reattaches to the next binding site, the release of the Pi initiates the energy release for the power stroke (movement takes place) and then ADP is released from the myosin head. Another "fresh" ATP must be provided to cause detachment and allow the cross-bridge cycle to continue.

One cross-bridge cycle (or one power stroke) results in a very small change (only a 1% decrease) in the muscle from its resting length. Because some muscles can shorten up to more than 50% of their resting

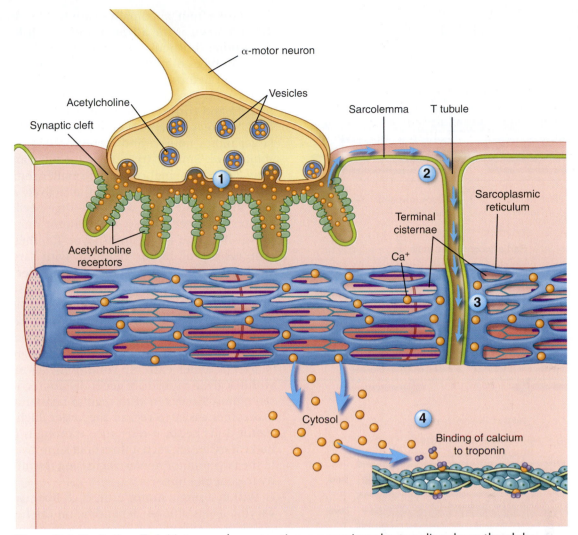

**Figure 9-6.** Excitation. To initiate muscle contraction, a nerve impulse traveling down the alpha motor neuron must cross over the synaptic cleft at the neuromuscular junction. The neurotransmitter acetylcholine is released from the end of the nerve fiber and crosses the synaptic cleft and binds to acetylcholine receptors on the muscle to transmit the impulse down into the muscle (step 1). The impulse spreads across the sarcolemma and enters the muscle through the T-tubules (step 2). Once the impulse reaches the "triad region" and depolarizes, the terminal cisternae of the sarcoplasmic reticulum, calcium is released (step 3). Calcium then binds to troponin, which shifts tropomyosin off of the active binding site on actin (step 4). Now, muscle contraction can begin.

length, the power stroke must repeat over and over again for a meaningful shortening to happen. For repeated cross-bridge cycles to occur, multiple action potentials must reach the neuromuscular junction and stimulate the muscle membrane, which, in turn, maintains the high calcium levels in the muscle and exposed binding sites, which allows the myosin cross-bridges to repeatedly be in a strong binding state, ultimately shifting and pulling on the thin filament until the action potentials stop or complete shortening has taken place. The term for this entire sequence of events from stimulation through shortening is called the **excitation-contraction coupling**. Repeated power strokes can continue as long as there is sufficient calcium in the sarcoplasm and as long as ATP is available and broken down to release the energy required for continued contraction. Figure 9-8 illustrates the sequence of events for muscle contraction.

## Motor Unit Recruitment

As described earlier, movement is created when skeletal muscles receive impulses from motor nerves to contract. The functional unit of movement, the **motor unit**, consists of one motor nerve that originates in the spinal cord and all of the specific muscle fibers it innervates (Fig. 9-9). The number of muscle fibers that a motor nerve innervates varies from motor unit to motor unit and from muscle to muscle, thereby influencing the amount of force production possible within each muscle. Each motor unit consists of muscle fibers that are all the same fiber type (type I, type IIa, or type IIx); therefore, motor units are named by the fiber type that makes up the motor unit. Motor unit size is determined by the number of fibers innervated by the motor neuron.

Type I motor units typically have a relatively small number of fibers per motor neuron (<300 fibers/neuron)

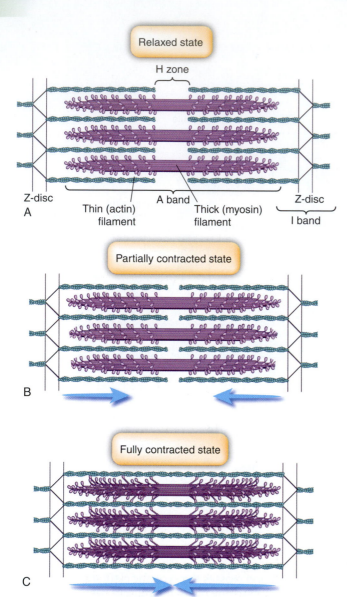

**Figure 9-7.** Sliding filament theory of muscle contraction. (A) Actin and myosin in a relaxed state, (B) a partially contracted state, and (C) a fully contracted state. As the actin slides across the myosin with muscle contraction, the H zone disappears because of the shortening of the sarcomere as Z lines are pulled closer together.

compared with the type II motor units (>300 fibers/neuron). Muscles that are involved with fine motor control that require precise movements consist of small motor units that have relatively few muscle fibers per motor nerve. For example, the extraocular muscles that control very precise eye movement may have motor units that contain only 23 muscle fibers per motor nerve. In contrast, large muscles that are involved with more gross movement and require more force production, such as muscles of the thigh, may have varying sizes of motor units that consist of a mixture of motor unit types where small motor units (type I) may have 100 to 200 fibers and large motor units (type II) may have 1,000 to 2,000 muscle fibers per motor nerve along with other motor units in between these values. When activated, all of the muscle fibers

in a motor unit maximally contract simultaneously. This is known as the **all-or-none principle**.

Another distinguishing characteristic between the different types of motor units is the size (diameter) of the motor neuron that innervates the fibers within the motor unit. Type I motor units have a smaller motor neuron and corresponding soma found in the spinal cord, whereas the type II motor units have a relatively larger motor neuron and corresponding soma in the spinal cord. Smaller (type I) motor units are easier to activate at the spinal cord. The smaller somas require fewer stimuli (a lower threshold) to activate and, therefore, are recruited first with low-force needs. Because greater force needs arise, more motor units and progressively larger motor units (type IIa, then type IIx) that consist of motor neurons with larger somas (higher threshold) are recruited. Thus, **recruitment** order is typically determined by size of the soma of the motor nerve. This is typically referred to as the "size principle of motor unit recruitment." The extent of the number and size of motor unit recruitment is determined primarily by the force needs of the muscle.

Except under extreme conditions, all motor units within a given muscle are generally not recruited at the same time. However, with regular resistance training, it becomes easier to recruit the larger, high-threshold motor units because resistance training is thought to make it easier to reach a threshold stimulus, especially in the larger motor nerves, increasing the muscle's ability to generate force.

Within a single motor unit, each fiber can produce varying levels of force depending on the frequency at which it is stimulated. Remembering that within a motor unit, all fibers are stimulated by the same motor nerve, the response from a single stimulus from the motor nerve to the neuromuscular junction of each of these fibers is termed a **twitch**. A twitch is the smallest amount of force that can be generated by a single fiber, or more typically, by a single motor unit. Also recall that it is typical for the muscle fibers to receive multiple stimuli to shorten. The frequency that these stimuli reach the neuromuscular junction is referred to as **"rate coding,"** and as the rate coding increases, the fibers do not have time to return to full relaxation after an initial stimulus. A series of multiple stimuli in rapid sequence, before relaxation from the first stimulus, results in even greater force production. In other words, when successive electrical stimulation is applied to a muscle, it does not have time to relax between stimuli and there is an additive nature to the amount of force produced. This process is termed **summation**. Continued stimulation at even higher frequencies can lead to a plateau in force production, where, if the stimulatory rate to the neuromuscular junction increases further, no further increase in force will take place. This plateau is known as **tetanus**, and results in peak force production of the motor unit. The body relies on tetanic muscular contractions to produce smooth muscular movement.

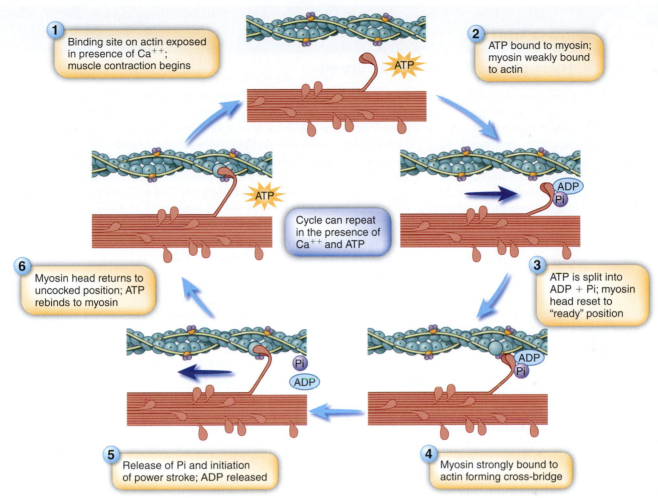

**Figure 9-8.** Sequence of events for muscle contraction. Contraction cycling can begin when the active site is exposed on myosin (1). ATP is bound to myosin (2) and split by the enzyme myosin ATPase to release energy to put the myosin head into the "ready" position (3). Myosin strongly binds actin (4) and the myosin head moves with the release of inorganic phosphate (Pi) to produce the power stroke action of the cross-bridge (5). The end of the movement places myosin back into the uncocked position, and another ATP is needed to provide energy to return it to the "ready" position (6). The continuation of this process also requires the presence of calcium.

Rate coding describes the process by which the force production of a given motor unit varies from that of a twitch to that of tetanus by increasing the frequency of stimulation at the neuromuscular junction (Fig. 9-10; also see explanatory animation of Rate Coding on the *DavisPlus* site at http://davisplus .fadavis.com.). Rate coding may increase with resistance training, which would result in an increase in the frequency of discharge of the motor units and allow for a faster time-to-peak force production for the trained muscle. Rapid movement or ballistic (explosive) training may be particularly effective in provoking increases in rate coding.

## Muscle Growth

Muscle growth, or **hypertrophy**, is responsible for the strength gains experienced after a prolonged period of resistance training (Fig. 9-11). Chronic hypertrophy is associated with structural changes in the size of existing individual muscle fibers (fiber hypertrophy), in the number of muscle fibers (fiber **hyperplasia**), or both.

Muscle fiber hypertrophy is most likely the result of one or more of the following:

- An increased number and thickening of myofibrils
- A greater number of thick and thin filaments
- More sarcoplasm
- Increased connective tissue

An increase in muscle protein synthesis stimulated by resistance training appears to be the mechanism responsible for fiber hypertrophy in trained individuals.

Research on the type of resistance training that evokes the most muscle hypertrophy suggests that training programs should include moderate-to-heavy loads (6–15 repetition maximums [RM]) and moderate volume (3–4 sets) for optimal increases in muscle mass.[9] Further, the frequency of this training should be two to three training sessions per week.[10]

## RESEARCH HIGHLIGHT

### Hyperplasia's Role in Muscle Growth

Most evidence points to muscle fiber hypertrophy as the primary cause of increased muscle size associated with resistance training. However, fiber hyperplasia may also contribute to the muscle growth related to resistance training. It is thought that individual muscle fibers may have the capacity to split into two daughter cells, each of which can develop into new muscle fibers. Located within each muscle fiber are dormant satellite cells, which are myogenic stem cells involved in the generation of new muscle fibers. Stress to the muscle in the form of stretch, injury, immobilization, or intense training (especially eccentric action) stimulates satellite cells to migrate to the damaged region to possibly fuse existing muscle fibers or produce new fibers, or both. This proliferation of satellite cells to the damaged area can last for up to 48 hours after the stressful event.[11] Even though hyperplasia is established as a viable process for increasing muscle growth, hypertrophy of existing muscle fibers represents the greatest contribution to increases in muscle size from a progressive overload resistance-training program.

Hawke TJ, Garry DJ. Myogenic satellite cells: physiology to molecular biology. *J. Appl. Physiol.* 2001;91:534–551.

---

A resistance-training program that induces the stimulation of protein synthesis, and thus muscle growth, naturally increases levels of testosterone and growth hormone. It is presumed that growth hormone increases the availability of amino acids for protein synthesis. Growth hormone also stimulates the release of **insulin-like growth factor I (IGF-I)** and **insulin-like growth factor II (IGF-II)** from skeletal muscle, which works together with growth hormone to stimulate muscle cell growth. IGF-I causes proliferation and differentiation of satellite cells, and IGF-II is responsible for proliferation of satellite cells. A progressive overload resistance-training program can cause a substantial increase in IGF-I levels, resulting in skeletal muscle hypertrophy.[2] Testosterone promotes the release of growth hormone from the pituitary gland and interacts with the neuromuscular system to stimulate protein synthesis as well.[6]

A training program that stresses and manipulates the endocrine system to bring about increases in these muscle-building (i.e., **anabolic**) hormones includes large-muscle-group or multijoint exercises (e.g., dead lift, power clean, and squat) performed at high intensities with short rest intervals between sets. Serum testosterone levels are increased when heavy resistance (85%–95% of **one-repetition maximum [1 RM]**) is used, multiple sets or multiple exercises are performed, or short rest intervals (30–60 seconds) are incorporated.[12] Growth hormone levels are increased when high-intensity (e.g., 10 RM) exercises are performed for multiple sets with short rest periods (e.g., 60 seconds).[13] Consuming adequate amounts of carbohydrate and protein before and after a training session is also important for optimizing the anabolic effects of resistance training.

## Muscle Atrophy

Just as skeletal muscles have the potential for growing larger, they can become smaller under certain circumstances as well. The two main reasons for muscle **atrophy** (or loss of muscle size and strength) are disuse and aging. Prominent causes of disuse atrophy are a result of unloading the muscles, which include periods

## SEX DIFFERENCES

The differences between men and women in their ability to develop muscle strength are essentially based on body weight (muscle mass) and hormone variations. When measured without regard for body weight and body composition (i.e., **absolute strength**), women are approximately 40% to 60% weaker than men in their upper-body strength and 25% to 30% weaker in their lower-body strength.[14] However, when body weight is factored into the comparison, the difference diminishes such that women are only 5% to 15% weaker in their lower-body strength. Further, when lower-body strength among the sexes is compared relative to fat-free mass, the difference disappears altogether.[15] Upper-body strength among the sexes differs significantly even when body weight and fat-free mass are included in the comparison. This is most likely because women have a lower percentage of muscle mass located in their upper body in comparison with their male counterparts.[1] In addition, men show a greater ability for muscular hypertrophy, and thus strength, than women as a result of naturally having blood testosterone levels 20 to 30 times higher than that of women.[16]

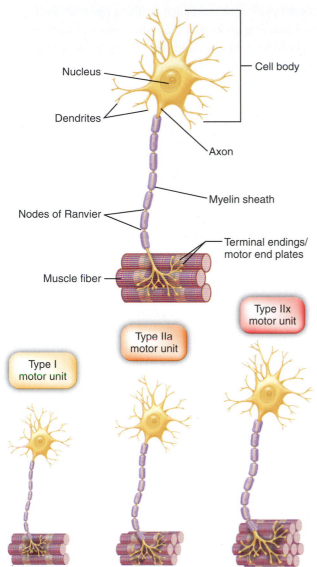

Figure 9-9. Types of motor units. Type I motor units are composed of smaller neuron cell bodies and axons, but have lower motor neuron-to-fiber ratios, which provides more fine motor control. Type IIa and IIx motor units have larger neuron cell bodies and axons, and greater motor neuron-to-muscle fiber ratios. This provides for less fine motor control, but this and other properties give these muscle fibers the ability to contract forcefully and powerfully.

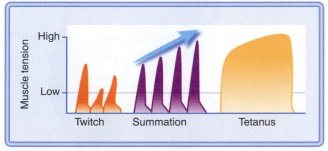

Figure 9-10. By increasing the frequency of impulses to the muscle, the rate coding increases. This will lead to greater force production in the muscle through summation and tetanus.

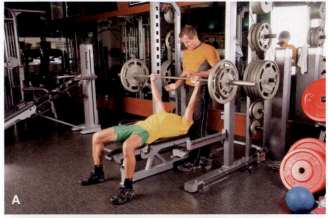

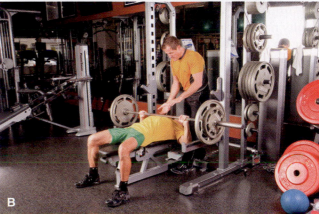

Figure 9-11. Heavy resistance training can lead to greater increases in muscle hypertrophy and strength compared with lighter resistance loads. (A) Starting and ending position. (B) Midrange position.

of prolonged bedrest, immobilization of a limb (such as in casting an extremity for the treatment of a broken bone), or the reduced loading of muscle that occurs during space flight, as well as a lack of adherence to an exercise program. A reduction in protein synthesis is the major process involved during the first few days of muscle disuse, followed by subsequent increased muscle protein breakdown after longer periods of disuse.[17] Both muscle mass and strength are lost with disuse atrophy, but they can be regained by returning the muscle to normal use. Beginning, or returning to, a resistance-training program can be effectively implemented as a rapid means for restoring muscle size and function after a period of muscle disuse for the reasons described in the previous section.

The normal process of aging also contributes to the loss of skeletal muscle mass and strength. In fact, humans can lose up to one third to one half of their muscle mass and strength between the ages of 25 and 80 years.[18,19] Atrophy caused by the aging process is called **sarcopenia**. The cause of sarcopenia may be related to the decreased ability for the **motor unit end plate** to continuously repair and reconstruct with advancing age. Normal repair and reconstruction of motor nerve end-plate structures is called *motor unit remodeling* and causes a selective denervation of muscle fibers, followed by the sprouting of new nerve axons from adjacent motor units. In old age, however, motor unit remodeling becomes less effective, leading to an irreversible degeneration of muscle fibers (particularly type II fibers) and end-plate structures. This deterioration process is called **denervation muscle atrophy**, and it occurs even in healthy, physically active older men and women. The result of sarcopenia is loss of muscle mass and strength accompanied by a proportionate increase in type I muscle fibers as type II muscle fibers are diminished. The aging process, together with relative disuse of skeletal muscle because of the lack of physical activity common in older adults, is related to limited mobility and decreased fitness status among this population.

Fortunately, regular resistance training among older adults has been shown to decrease the effects of sarcopenia and slow the inevitable loss of strength associated with aging.[20,21,22] An increase in both type I and type II muscle fibers can be achieved along with significant increases in muscle strength, bone density, dynamic balance, and overall functional status in older men and women as a result of a moderate-intensity resistance-training program (Fig. 9-12).[23,24] These findings have implications for the positive impact that regular exercise can have on reducing frailty, preventing orthopedic injury, and improving performance of activities of daily life, and, ultimately, the quality of life for the aging population.

## In Your Own Words

Your new client, Henrietta, is a 72-year-old grandmother who enjoys spending time being physically active with her grandchildren. She has noticed in recent years that tasks such as lifting her grandkids and standing up from a chair have become increasingly difficult. How would you explain to Henrietta the possible cause of her progressive weakness?

## NERVOUS SYSTEM

The overall function of the nervous system is to collect information about conditions in relation to the body's internal and external state, analyze this information, and initialize appropriate responses to fulfill specific needs. In other words, the nervous system gathers information, stores it, and controls various bodily systems in response to this input.

### Neural Organization

The nervous system is separated into various divisions based on either structural or functional characteristics. Keep in mind that these divisions—which are called *nervous systems* themselves—are still part of a single, overall nervous system. In terms of structure, the nervous system is divided into two parts: the **central nervous system (CNS)** and the peripheral nervous system (PNS).

### Central Nervous System and Regions of the Brain

The CNS consists of the brain and spinal cord, which are both encased and protected by bony structures—the skull and the vertebral column, respectively. The CNS is responsible for receiving sensory input from the PNS and formulating responses to this input. This makes the CNS the integrative and control center of the nervous system. Although the brain is an extremely complex organ, breaking it down into four major areas is helpful when considering its role in producing movement: cerebrum, diencephalon, cerebellum, and brainstem (Fig. 9-13).

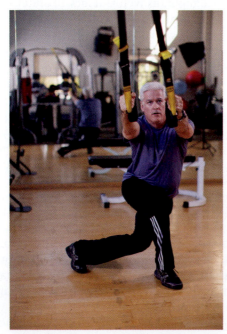

**Figure 9-12.** Participation in strength training can contribute to maintaining strength and function during activities of daily living for older adults.

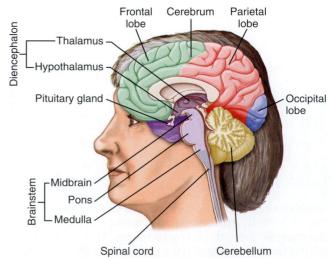

**Figure 9-13.** The major regions and outer lobes of the brain.

## Cerebrum

The largest portion of the brain is called the *cerebrum*. It is a dome-shaped structure that is separated into right and left hemispheres. The two hemispheres are connected to each other through bundles of fibers (or tracts) referred to as the corpus callosum. Encasing the entire cerebrum is a dense outer area called the *cerebral cortex*. Intellectual function, awareness of sensory stimuli, and voluntary motor control are all associated with the cerebral cortex, which is also known as the "conscious brain." The cerebrum can be further divided into four outer lobes: frontal, temporal, parietal, and occipital. Each lobe is responsible for its own general functions (Table 9-5).

## Diencephalon

Another important brain area that is related to the body's response during exercise is the diencephalon. This structure is deep within the brain and houses the thalamus and hypothalamus. The thalamus is considered the "gateway to the cerebral cortex" and acts as an integration center as it regulates the sensory input, including sight, equilibrium, sound, pain, pressure, heat and cold, that is sent to the conscious brain, which makes the thalamus essential for motor control. Located directly below the thalamus in the diencephalon is the hypothalamus. The hypothalamus is the major control center of the autonomic nervous system and neuroendocrine system. It is involved in essential functions that maintain homeostasis such as regulating metabolic rate and body temperature, along with the release of many of the hormones that maintain homeostasis of our body.

## Cerebellum

In terms of coordinated motor control for complex and rapid muscular movements, no other brain structure is as important as the cerebellum. It is located posterior to the brainstem and, like the cerebrum, consists of two hemispheres. Through its connections to the motor area of the cerebral cortex, brainstem, and spinal cord, the cerebellum helps to smooth out motor activities that would otherwise be jerky and uncoordinated.

### Table 9-5. General Functions of the Brain's Outer Lobes

| LOBE | FUNCTION |
| --- | --- |
| Frontal | General intellect and motor control |
| Temporal | Auditory sensory input and its interpretation |
| Parietal | General sensory input and its interpretation |
| Occipital | Visual sensory input and its interpretation |

Peripheral sensors in the skeletal muscles, tendons, joints, and skin send information to the cerebellum. In addition, the cerebellum receives input from the visual, auditory, and vestibular organs. Once received, sensory information is compared, evaluated, and integrated by the cerebellum. Furthermore, after a planned movement is performed, the cerebellum compares the information from the cerebrum about the intended movement with the sensory information from the proprioceptors about the actual movement that took place and relays these data to higher centers of the brain so that a corrective action can be undertaken. Ultimately, the cerebellum functions to regulate posture, locomotion, equilibrium, perceptions of speed of body movement, and other various reflex actions associated with movement.

## Brainstem

Located at the base of the skull, connecting the brain to the spinal cord, the brainstem is responsible for many metabolic functions, cardiorespiratory control, and various highly complex reflexes. This area of the brain is the site of origin for 10 of the 12 sets of cranial nerves. The brainstem consists of three main structures: midbrain, pons, and medulla oblongata (see Fig. 9-13). This region also serves as a junction that relays information between the brain and spinal cord via sensory and **motor neurons**. The brainstem contains a series of specialized neurons called the *reticular formation* that receives and integrates information from all regions of the CNS and works with higher brain centers in controlling muscular activity. The reticular formation receives signals from **proprioceptors** in the joints and skeletal muscles, pain receptors in the skin, and sensory receptors in the eyes and ears. Once activated, the neurons within the reticular formation produce either an inhibitory or facilitatory effect on other neurons, which is necessary for functions such as control of locomotion and maintaining postural tone. Thus, damage to any portion of the brainstem results in impaired movement control.

## Peripheral Nervous System

The PNS is composed of all the nervous structures located outside of the CNS, namely, the nerves and **ganglia** (nerve cell bodies associated with the nerves). In part, the PNS is made up of pairings of nerves that branch out from the brain and spinal cord from different regions. Encased by the vertebrae, the spinal cord consists of ascending and descending nerve tracts that act as the major conduit for the two-way flow of information from the skin, joints, and muscles to the brain. Communication throughout the body is accomplished via spinal nerves of the PNS that exit the spinal cord through small openings between the vertebrae. The ascending nerve tracts carry sensory information, such as signals from receptors in the skin, skeletal muscles, and joints, from the periphery to the brain. These fibers are situated in the **ventral** (front) portion of the spinal cord and are called

**afferent** nerve fibers. The descending nerve tracts, in contrast, are located in the **dorsal** (back) region of the spinal cord and contain motor (or **efferent**) nerve fibers that transmit signals from the brain to target organs, such as skeletal muscles and glands.

Consisting of 43 pairs of nerves (12 pairs of cranial nerves that originate from the brain and 31 pairs of nerves that arise from the spinal cord), the PNS is responsible for carrying sensory information to the CNS and relaying signals from the CNS to the muscles, organs, and other tissues. Named for the region of the spine where they originate and the vertebral level from which they emerge, the paired spinal nerves are classified as 8 cervical, 12 thoracic, 5 lumbar, 5 sacral, and 1 coccygeal (Fig. 9-14). The spinal nerve roots and the muscles they innervate are presented in Table 9-6.

Similar to the CNS, the PNS contains both afferent and efferent neurons. The PNS is separated into two major components: the sensory division and the motor division (Fig. 9-15).

## Sensory Division

Afferent neurons of the sensory division carry signals toward the CNS from receptors in areas such as the internal organs, specialized sense organs (e.g., tongue, nose, ears, and eyes), skin, skeletal muscles, and tendons. In other words, afferent sensory data are incoming information. Depending on the sensory information, the PNS directs the signals to either the brain or the spinal cord where the data can be evaluated and integrated with other incoming information. There are five primary sources of sensory information: mechanoreceptors, thermoreceptors,

**nociceptors**, photoreceptors, and chemoreceptors. Table 9-7 outlines these receptors and the types of information provided by each one.

## Motor Division

After the CNS interprets incoming sensory information from the afferent neurons of the PNS, efferent neurons within the motor division of the PNS handle the outgoing information and can be divided into the somatic and autonomic nervous systems. The somatic nervous system is mostly under voluntary control and carries nerve impulses from the CNS to the skeletal muscles. In some instances, such as reflex contraction in response to receptor information, skeletal muscle contractions are not consciously controlled (e.g., pulling your hand away from a hot stove). In addition to voluntary muscle control, the motor division is also responsible for the body's internal involuntary functions, which it accomplishes through the autonomic nervous system. The autonomic nervous system is made up of nerves that transmit impulses to the smooth muscles, cardiac muscle, and glands. These visceral motor impulses generally cannot be consciously controlled. The autonomic nervous system is categorized into two major divisions: the sympathetic and parasympathetic nervous systems. Most organs are innervated by both sympathetic and parasympathetic neurons, which play an opposing role to each other; that is, the sympathetic nervous system tends to activate an organ, and the parasympathetic nervous system tends to inhibit the activity of an organ.

Perhaps better known as the fight-or-flight system, the sympathetic nervous system prepares the body for

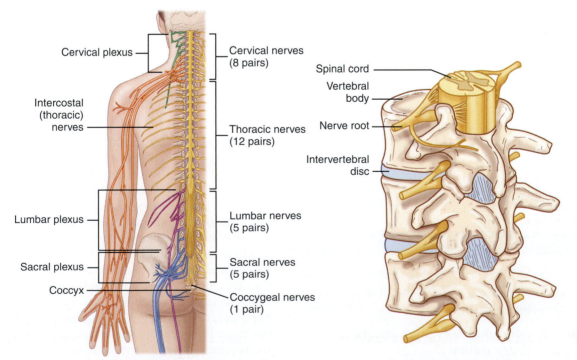

**Figure 9-14.** Spinal cord and branching spinal nerves (posterior view). The spinal column is protected by the vertebral column and distributes peripheral branches of nerves that run through the intervertebral foramen to the rest of the body.

## Table 9-6. Selected Spinal Nerve Roots and Major Muscles Innervated

| NERVE ROOT | MUSCLES INNERVATED |
|---|---|
| C5 | Biceps brachii, deltoid, supraspinatus, infraspinatus |
| C6 | Brachioradialis, supinator, extensor carpi radialis longus and brevis, extensor carpi ulnaris |
| C7 | Triceps brachii, flexor carpi radialis, flexor carpi ulnaris |
| C8 | Extensor pollicis longus and brevis, adductor pollicis longus |
| T1 | Intrinsic muscles of the hand (lumbricals, interossei) |
| L2 | Psoas major and minor, adductor magnus, adductor longus, adductor brevis |
| L3 | Rectus femoris, vastus lateralis, vastus medialis, vastus intermedius, psoas major and minor |
| L4 | Anterior tibialis, posterior tibialis |
| L5 | Extensor hallucis longus, extensor digitorum longus, peroneus longus and brevis, gluteus maximus, gluteus medius |
| S1 | Gastrocnemius, soleus, biceps femoris, semitendinosus, semimembranosus, gluteus maximus |
| S2 | Gluteus maximus, flexor hallucis longus, flexor digitorum longus |
| S4 | Bladder, rectum |

From American Council on Exercise. *ACE's Essentials of Exercise Science for Fitness Professionals*, 2010. San Diego: American Council on Exercise.

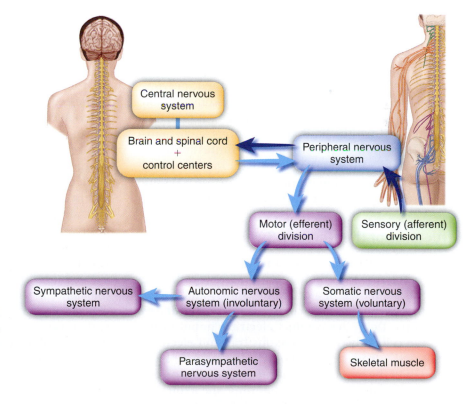

**Figure 9-15.** Organization of the nervous system from the central nervous system (brain, spinal cord, and control centers) to the divisions of the peripheral nervous system. Light blue arrows depict neural messages going out from the central nervous system to peripheral tissues. Dark blue arrows depict neural input coming back to the central nervous system from sensory nerves in the periphery.

physical activity during a stress-related event. The following physiological changes occur due to stimulation by the sympathetic nervous system to facilitate motor function:

- Heart rate and the force of heart contraction increase.
- Arteries that nourish the heart dilate (vasodilation) to supply the cardiac tissue with more blood to meet its increased demands.

- Peripheral arteries that supply the skeletal muscles dilate to allow more blood to these active tissues.
- Visceral arteries constrict (vasoconstriction) to ensure that more blood is diverted to the active skeletal muscles.
- Blood pressure increases to improve blood perfusion within the skeletal muscles and to increase venous return.

## Table 9-7. Sources of Sensory Information Within the Peripheral Nervous System

| SENSORY RECEPTORS | INFORMATION PROVIDED BY RECEPTORS |
|---|---|
| Mechanoreceptors | Signals that relay information about mechanical forces such as pressure, touch, vibrations, or stretch |
| Thermoreceptors | Signals related to changes in body temperature |
| Nociceptors | Signals that provide information about painful stimuli |
| Photoreceptors | Signals corresponding to data involving light to allow vision |
| Chemoreceptors | Signals related to chemical stimuli such as from foods, odors, and concentrations of gases, nutrients, or electrolytes in the blood or tissues |

- Bronchial tubes dilate to increase gas exchange during respiration.
- Metabolic rate increases to provide the body with the energy needs associated with increased physical activity.
- Mental activity and awareness increase to allow enhanced perception of incoming sensory information.
- The liver releases more glucose into the bloodstream to keep up with the increased energy demands of physical activity.

Conversely, the parasympathetic nervous system, sometimes called the "rest-and-digest system," is the primary autonomic branch most active when the body is in a calm and resting state. The parasympathetic nervous system acts to oppose the sympathetic nervous system. It is associated with lower energy consumption and normal bodily maintenance, including stimulating digestion and waste elimination. Actions such as increased digestion in the stomach and intestines, decreased heart rate, constriction of the heart's blood vessels, and constriction of the respiratory airways are stimulated by the parasympathetic nervous system.

## Structures of the Nervous System

The most basic structural and functional component of the nervous system is the neuron (or nerve cell). The neuron is composed of a cell body (soma) and one or more processes—fibrous extensions called **dendrites** and **axons**. Dendrites conduct electrical impulses toward the cell body, whereas axons transmit electrical signals away from the cell body. Neurons may have hundreds of the branching dendrites, depending on the neuron type, but each neuron has only one axon. For an electrical impulse to travel through the nervous system, it must be passed from one neuron to the next. Most neurons do not have direct contact with each other.

Instead, neurons remain separated from each other by a small space called a **synapse**. To transmit the impulse across the synapse from one neuron to the other, the first neuron releases a chemical neurotransmitter substance that attaches to receptors located on the membrane of the second neuron.

Most axons are covered with a fatty substance called **myelin**, which insulates the axon and keeps the electrical current from migrating outside of the neuron. A nerve is made up of the processes of many neurons held together by connective tissue sheaths. Sensory nerves carry impulses to the CNS, whereas motor nerves carry nerve impulses from the CNS to the PNS. Motor neurons form a synapse, called the *neuromuscular junction*, with the skeletal muscles they supply.

## Transmission of Nerve Impulses

Electrical activity is the basis for communication between the different structures of the nervous system. At rest, all cells (including neurons) have a negative electrical charge inside the cell relative to the outside of the cell, which has a positive electrical charge. This difference in electrical charge between inside and outside of the cell is called **resting membrane potential**. The cell is polarized when this difference in electrical charges exists.

Electrical charges are carried by **ions**, which are elements with a positive or negative electrical charge. Potassium ($K^+$) and sodium ($Na^+$) are two important positively charged ions involved in the transmission of electrical impulses throughout the nervous system. At rest, $K^+$ is more highly concentrated inside the cell and $Na^+$ is more highly concentrated outside the cell. An imbalance in the number of ions inside and outside the cell causes the resting membrane potential described earlier. Gates in the cell's membrane change the permeability of the cell, allowing $K^+$ or $Na^+$ to move more freely into and out of the cell. At rest, most of the $Na^+$ gates are closed, whereas a few of the $K^+$ gates are open. Thus, the resting membrane is more permeable to $K^+$ than $Na^+$. This leads to more $K^+$ ions leaving the cell than $Na^+$ ions entering the cell. The result is a net loss of positive charges from inside the cell, making the resting membrane potential negative. Neurons generally have a resting membrane potential of about −70 millivolts (mV).

For a neural message to be generated and travel through the nervous system, a stimulus of sufficient strength must reach the neuron's membrane. Stimulation allows $Na^+$ gates in the membrane wall to open and allow Na⁺ ions to diffuse into the cell, making the inside of the cell more and more positively charged. The process of making the inside of the cell less negative relative to the outside of the cell is called **depolarization**. There is a depolarization threshold at which the increasingly positive charge inside the cell reaches a critical value, typically a depolarization of 15 to 20 mV, which results in all the sodium gates opening wide for a brief moment. Because of the large concentration gradient of Na⁺ between the inside and the outside of the membrane, there is a rapid influx of Na⁺ that results in a spike in positive electrical charge inside the cell once the depolarization threshold is reached.

Figure 9-16 illustrates the sequence of events involving depolarization and repolarization. Na⁺ gates close shortly (a few milliseconds) after opening and Na⁺ influx ceases. At this point, the resting membrane potential has gone from –70 mV to approximately +35 mV. When voltage peaks, the slower K⁺ gates become wide open. A rapid efflux of K⁺ takes place because of the large concentration gradient between the inside and outside of the neural membrane, returning the membrane potential to near resting charge. This spike in positive charge (depolarization) followed by a return to resting membrane potential (repolarization) is called an *action potential*, or nerve impulse.

Once an action potential has been generated, it is carried along the myelinated nerve axon by a series of ionic exchanges at structures called the *nodes of Ranvier*. The impulse travels the entire length of the axon with the same strength (voltage) as it was at the initial point of stimulation. This is referred to as the **all-or-none law of action potentials**. That is, after an action potential is created, it will not stop until it reaches the end of the axon. In concept, this law is similar to the all-or-none principle of motor unit recruitment that was presented in an earlier section. Recall that when activated, all of the muscle fibers in a motor unit maximally contract simultaneously. Thus, once a motor unit is stimulated, it will not deactivate until the muscle contraction has occurred.

When a nerve impulse reaches the neuromuscular junction, the neurotransmitter acetylcholine is released into the synaptic cleft. Acetylcholine binds to receptors on the muscle fiber and opens the Na⁺ gates in the muscle cell membrane, causing the process of depolarization to begin in the muscle cell as well. This process sets the stage for muscle contraction as described in detail earlier in this chapter.

## Proprioception

The sense of knowing where the body is in relation to its various segments and the external environment is called **proprioception**. The sensory information gathered to achieve this kinesthetic awareness comes from structures called **proprioceptors**, which are receptors located in the skin, in and around the joints and muscles, and in the inner ear (Table 9-8). Cutaneous receptors are located in the skin and send sensory information regarding pressure, touch, and movement of the hairs on the skin. Joint receptors are located in the joint capsules and the surrounding ligaments. They transmit sensory information relating to positions, velocities, and accelerations occurring at the joints. In addition, pressure receptors within the joints provide added information about pressure changes that is used for important postural adjustments and normal gait.

**Pacinian corpuscles** are receptors located deep within the skin and the joint capsule that are sensitive to pressure. **Meissner's corpuscles** are receptors located in the superficial layers of the skin that are responsive to light touch. Although these skin receptors do not play a large part in proprioception, it is believed that injured individuals who have experienced joint and ligament receptor damage benefit from increased reliance on cutaneous receptors for proprioception. **Golgi-Mazzoni corpuscles** are located within the joint capsule and are responsive to joint compression. Thus, any weight-bearing activity stimulates these receptors.

## Motor Coordination and Movement

Another type of proprioceptor, the musculotendinous receptor, is involved in muscular control and coordination. There are two such types of receptors: the **Golgi tendon organ (GTO)** and the **muscle spindle**. Connected to approximately 15 to 20 muscle fibers and located between the muscle belly and its tendon, the GTO senses increased tension within its associated muscle when the muscle contracts or is stretched. One of the GTO's functions when it senses a muscle contraction of higher than typical tension is to cause an inhibition of motor unit recruitment (**autogenic inhibition**), thereby decreasing tension in the muscle from which the GTO signal originated. In addition, GTO activation results in an enhanced contraction of the opposing (**antagonist**) muscle group. Both of these properties have important implications in flexibility because a muscle can be stretched more fully and easily when the GTOs have inhibited the muscle's contraction and allowed the antagonistic muscle group to contract more readily. It has been theorized that this function adjusts muscle output in response to fatigue.

A second type of musculotendinous receptor, the muscle spindle, is located mostly in the muscle belly and lies parallel to the muscle fibers. This arrangement causes the muscle spindle to stretch when the muscle itself experiences a stretch force, thereby exciting the muscle spindle and causing a reflexive contraction in the muscle known as the stretch reflex. The muscle spindle's reflex contraction of its associated muscle simultaneously causes the antagonist muscle group to relax (**reciprocal inhibition**). For example, if the gastrocnemius is stretched rapidly (Fig. 9-17), the muscle spindles within the muscle belly cause it to contract to prevent a rapid lengthening of the muscle, which may lead to injury. At the same time, if the opposing muscle group (anterior

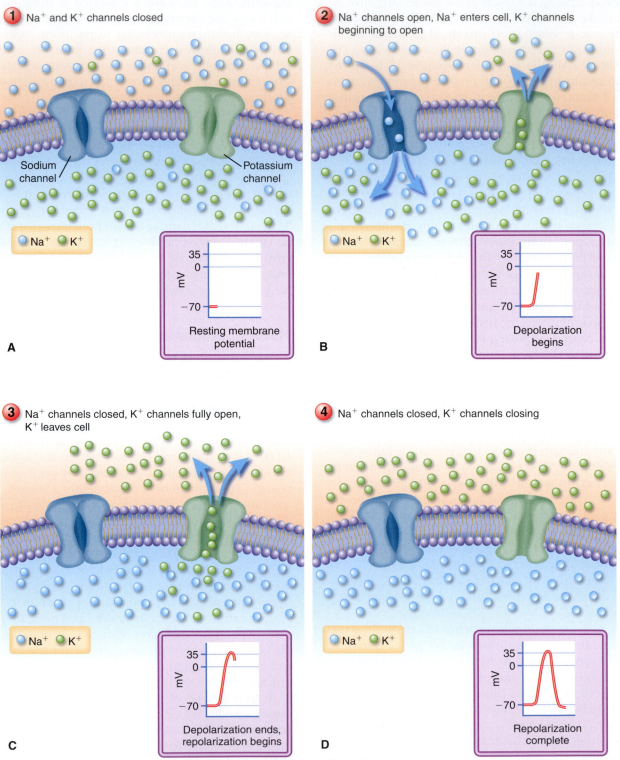

**Figure 9-16.** Sequence of events involving depolarization and repolarization. At rest, the cell membrane is polarized at –70 mV, and sodium and potassium channels are closed (A). At the start of depolarization, sodium channels open and sodium enters the cell (B). During repolarization, sodium channels are closed and potassium is leaving the cell (C). At the end of repolarization, both channels close and the cell membrane charge resets to –70 mV (D).

## Table 9-8. Proprioceptors of the Neuromuscular System

| RECEPTOR | LOCATION | FUNCTION |
|---|---|---|
| Pacinian corpuscles | Deep within the skin and the joint capsule | Detect pressure sensations |
| Meissner's corpuscles | Superficial layers of the skin | Detect light touch sensations |
| Golgi-Mazzoni corpuscles | Joint capsule | Are responsive to joint compression associated with weight-bearing activity |
| Golgi tendon organ | Between the muscle belly and its tendon | Promotes autogenic inhibition and an enhanced contraction of the antagonist muscle group |
| Muscle spindle | Muscle belly | Promotes the stretch reflex and reciprocal inhibition of the antagonist muscle group |

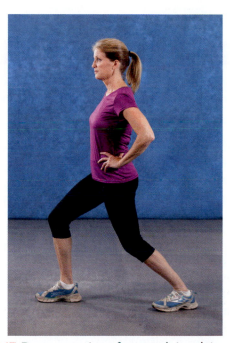

Figure 9-17. Demonstration of a stretch involving the gastrocnemius. If this is performed rapidly, there is a reflex action by the muscle spindle to contract the muscle and prevent further stretch. If the stretch is performed slowly, the muscle spindles are not activated, and the muscle length can be increased.

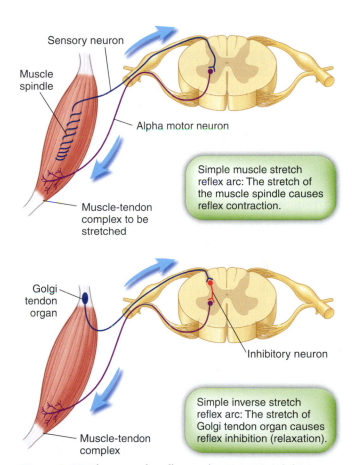

Figure 9-18. The stretch reflex and autogenic inhibition.

tibialis) is contracting, the muscle spindle reflex causes it to relax. The muscle spindles and the GTOs work together through their reflexive actions to regulate muscle stiffness and, therefore, contribute largely to the body's sense of postural control. Figure 9-18 illustrates the stretch reflex and autogenic inhibition. (See explanatory animation of Sensory Motor Integration on the Davis*Plus* site at http://davisplus.fadavis.com.)

The body relies on the **vestibular system** for sensory information related to the position of the head in space and sudden changes in the directional movement of the head. Located in the inner ear, the vestibular system is composed of three fluid-containing semicircular canals that lie at right angles to each other. Each canal contains sensory hair cells that detect the movement of the fluid in the canals. When the angular position of the head changes, fluid rushes over the hair cells and causes them to bend. This response signals to the CNS the direction of the head's rotation and the position of the head during movement. The vestibular system functions to coordinate many motor responses and helps to stabilize the eyes to maintain postural stability during stance and locomotion.

A common dysfunction of the vestibular system is called *vertigo*. Vertigo is characterized by the feeling of dizziness or motion of the body when one is actually stationary. Many times this condition leads to difficulty standing and walking because of an inability to balance. At times the dizziness and disorientation can be so severe that it leads to nausea and vomiting.

## VIGNETTE *conclusion*

■ The key to helping Marci cope with the spasticity in her hand is to have her perform range-of-motion exercise at least daily, because loss of motion causes muscle contractions or shortening. At the outset, Angela should lead Marci through passive range-of-motion exercises to ensure that she learns the proper technique. Once she has mastered these

movements, she can either do them on her own or have a family member help her through them. In the case of severe spasticity like what Marci is experiencing, these exercises can be difficult and rather painful, and should be performed carefully to prevent tissue damage. It is absolutely essential that Angela continues to work closely with Marci's health-care team and adhere to their specified guidelines to avoid exacerbating her condition. That said, it is clear that Angela can have a tremendously positive impact on Marci's post-rehabilitative exercise success and overall well-being.

## CRITICAL THINKING QUESTIONS

1. Two athletes who compete in the same sport and who work out together are similarly matched in height, weight, and body composition. However, they show a significant difference in their ability to produce strength. That is, one athlete is consistently stronger than the other in the bench press and leg press exercises. What is a potential cause for this strength difference?

2. According to the all-or-none principle of muscle contraction, when an action potential is delivered, all of the muscle fibers in a motor unit maximally contract simultaneously. This remains true whether an exerciser is lifting a 5-pound (2.3-kg) dumbbell or a 50-pound (23-kg) dumbbell. How does the neuromuscular system control muscular force production when it is required to lift different weight loads, given that the motor unit will follow the all-or-none principle?

3. Your client, Joe, recently had a cast removed from his forearm after fracturing his wrist 6 weeks ago. His recently healed arm is much smaller and weaker than his noninjured arm. How would you explain the differences between the arms to Joe, and what would you do to help him regain strength in his post-rehabilitative training?

4. Certain neuromuscular diseases, such as myasthenia gravis, occur as a result of a malfunction at the neuromuscular junction and problems with the normal uptake of acetylcholine. Based on the essential characteristics of acetylcholine and its association with the neuromuscular system as described in this chapter, what might be some of the symptoms of an acetylcholine deficiency?

## ADDITIONAL RESOURCES

*Medicine & Science in Sports & Exercise* (**American College of Sports Medicine Position Statements; http://acsm-msse.org**):
Mazzeo RS, Cavanagh P, Evans WJ, et al. ACSM Position Stand: exercise and physical activity for older adults. *Med. Sci. Sports Exerc.* 1998;30:992–1008.
Pollock ML, Gaesser GA, Butcher JD, et al. ACSM Position Stand: the recommended quantity and quality of exercise for developing and maintaining cardiorespiratory and muscular fitness, and flexibility in healthy adults. *Med. Sci. Sports Exerc.* 1998;30:975–991.
Ratamess NA, Alvar BA, Evetoch TK, et al. ACSM Position Stand: progression models in resistance training for healthy adults. *Med. Sci. Sports Exerc.* 2009;34:364–380.
**Websites**
http://www.strokeassociation.org/STROKEORG/LifeAfterStroke/RegainingIndependence/PhysicalChallenges/Spasticity_UCM_309770_Article.jsp

## REFERENCES

1. Johns RJ, Wright V. Relative importance of various tissues in joint stiffness. *J. Appl. Physiol.* 1962;17:824–828.
2. Fiatarone MA, Ding W, Manfredi TJ, et al. Insulin-like growth factor I in skeletal muscle after weight-lifting exercise in frail elders. *Am. J. Physiol.* 1999;277:E135–E143.
3. Pette D. Historical perspectives: plasticity of mammalian skeletal muscle. *J. Appl. Physiol.* 2001;90:1119–1124.
4. Shoepe T, Stelzer JE, Garner DP, Widrick JJ. Functional adaptability of muscle fibers to long-term resistance exercise. *Med. Sci. Sports Exerc.* 2003;35:944–951.
5. Bottinelli RM, et al. Myofibrillar ATPase activity during isometric contractions and isomyosin composition of rat single skinned muscle fibers. *J. Physiol.* 1994;481:663–675.
6. Thorstensson A. Muscle strength, fiber types and enzyme activities in man. *Acta Physiol. Scand. Suppl.* 1976;443:1–45.
7. Edstrom L, Ekblom B. Differences in sizes of red and white muscle fibers in vastus lateralis of musculus quadriceps of normal individuals and athletes: relation to physical performance. *Scand. J. Clin. Lab. Invest.* 1972;30:175.
8. Gollnick PD, Matoba H. The muscle fiber composition of skeletal muscle as a predictor of athletic success. An overview. *Am. J. Sports Med.* 1984;12:212–217.
9. Booth FW, Criswell DS. Molecular events underlying skeletal muscle atrophy and the development of effective countermeasures. *Int. J. Sports Med.* 1997;18:S265–S269.
10. Rhea M, Burkett A, Burkett L. A meta-analysis to determine the dose response for strength development. *Med. Sci. Sports Exerc.* 2003;35:456–464.
11. Hawke TJ, Garry DJ. Myogenic satellite cells: physiology to molecular biology. *J. Appl. Physiol.* 2001;91:534–551.
12. Kraemer WJ, Gordon SE, Fleck SJ, et al. Endogenous anabolic hormone and growth factor responses to heavy resistance exercise in males and females. *Int. J. Sports Med.* 1991;12:228–235.
13. Kraemer WJ, Marchitelli L, Gordon SE, et al. Hormonal and growth factor responses to heavy resistance exercise. *J. Appl. Physiol.* 1990;69:1442–1450.
14. Morrow J, Hosler W. Strength comparisons in untrained men and women. *Med. Sci. Sports Exerc.* 1981;13:194–198.
15. Schantz P, Randall-Fox E, Hutchison W, Tydén A, Astrand PO. Muscle fibre type distribution, muscle cross-sectional area and maximal voluntary strength in humans. *Acta Physiol. Scand.* 1983;117:219–226.
16. Janssen I, Heymsfield SB, Wang ZM, Ross R. Skeletal muscle mass distribution in 468 men and women aged 18–88 yr. *J. Appl. Physiol.* 2000;89:81–88.
17. Bird S, Tarpenning K, Marino F. Designing resistance training programmes to enhance muscular fitness: a review of the acute programme variables. *Sports Med.* 2005;35:841–851.
18. Booth FW, Weeden S. Structural aspects of aging human skeletal muscle. In: Buckwalter JA, Goldberg VM, Woo SL-Y, eds. *Musculoskeletal Soft-tissue Aging: Impact on Mobility.* Rosemont, IL: American Academy of Orthopedic Surgeons; 1993.
19. Lexell J, Taylor CC, Sjöström M, et al. What is the cause of ageing atrophy? Total number, size, and proportion of different fiber types studied in whole vastus lateralis muscle from 15- to 83-year-old men. *J. Neurol. Sci.* 1988;84:275.
20. American College of Sports Medicine. ACSM Position Stand on exercise and physical activity for older adults. *Med. Sci. Sports Exerc.* 1998;30:992.
21. McCartney N. Acute responses to resistance training and safety. *Med. Sci. Sports Exerc.* 1999;31:31.
22. Pollock ML, Gaesser GA, Butcher, JD, et al. The recommended quantity and quality of exercise for developing and maintaining cardiorespiratory fitness, strength, and flexibility in healthy adults. *Med. Sci. Sports Exerc.* 1998;30:975–991.
23. American College of Sports Medicine. *ACSM's Guidelines for Exercise Testing and Prescription.* 8th ed. Philadelphia: Wolters Kluwer/Lippincott Williams & Wilkins; 2010.
24. McArdle WD, Katch FI, Katch VL. *Exercise Physiology.* 5th ed. Philadelphia: Lippincott Williams & Wilkins; 2001.

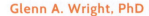

Glenn A. Wright, PhD

## CHAPTER 10

# Acute and Chronic Neuromuscular Responses to Exercise

## CHAPTER OUTLINE

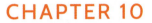

## LEARNING OUTCOMES

1. Explain the reflex response and its association with motor activity.
2. Describe sensory-motor integration and the receptors responsible for proprioception.
3. List the nervous system's contributions to the acute responses during a bout of physical activity.
4. Describe possible neural mechanisms for acute muscle fatigue.
5. Define *delayed-onset muscle soreness* and explain its possible causes.
6. Explain neural adaptations experienced by skeletal muscle as a result of chronic exercise.
7. Describe neuromuscular adaptations that occur after the cessation of a regular resistance training program.

## ANCILLARY LINK

Visit Davis*Plus* at http://davisplus.fadavis.com for study and practice resources, including online quizzes, animations that help explain physiological processes, podcasts concerning news and career trends in exercise physiology, and practice references.

## VIGNETTE

■ Oscar is a 40-year-old father of three who has put off being physically active his entire adult life. He has come to the gym to start lifting weights after deciding to get in better shape to keep up with his very active children.

As part of his New Year's resolution, Oscar has decided to take on the task of improving his upper-body strength by performing free-weight exercises. His first exercise is a chest press performed on a flat bench with 25-pound (11.4-kg) dumbbells. Because he has never tried this movement before, his effort appears uncoordinated and awkward.

During his first set of chest press exercises, Oscar's neuromuscular system transmits a series of electrical impulses to and from the brain and skeletal muscles. Some of these impulses are consciously controlled by Oscar, whereas others involve subconscious reflex activity. With continued practice, the awkwardness of his first set of chest presses will be a thing of the past as Oscar's neuromuscular system learns the new exercise movement and allows him to perform it with efficiency and coordination. If Oscar continues to engage in safe and effective regular strength exercise, he will benefit by increasing the strength of muscles, tendons, and ligaments; enhancing bone density; decreasing the risk for musculoskeletal injury; and improving muscular tone.

How would continuing to engage in safe and effective strength exercise benefit Oscar in the long run, not only in terms of muscular strength, but also via changes in the strength of connective tissues, increased bone density, and injury prevention?

At the beginning of each year, professionals working in the fitness industry prepare for the typical increase in business opportunities as new customers resolve to start a regular exercise program. According to the International Health, Racquet and Sportsclub Association (IHRSA), one third of new gym members in a given year are added between January and March.[1] An influx of new, deconditioned exercisers can be seen in fitness facilities nationwide as they are eager to begin their New Year's resolutions related to getting in better shape. Consequently, those individuals who are introduced to resistance training as part of their fitness programs will encounter a series of neuromuscular responses and adaptations that will essentially change the inner workings of their nervous system and muscle structures.

The interplay between the nervous and muscular systems is ultimately what brings about the enhanced performance and appearance characteristics that many individuals seek when they begin a resistance training program. The specific physiological responses that occur during a bout of exercise call on the body's various systems (e.g., nervous, cardiorespiratory, endocrine, and thermoregulatory) to ensure that the transitions from rest to activity, and then from activity to rest, are efficient. After repeated bouts of exercise, the body adapts to become even more efficient at these transitions. Together with the muscular system, the nervous system ensures that bodily movement is carried out appropriately during acute bouts of activity and adapts to consistent exercise demands over time. Furthermore, the voluntary and involuntary actions that produce the movements involved in all types of physical activity are directed by the nervous system. This chapter explores the contribution of the nervous system to the control of skeletal muscles during movement.

## REFLEX RESPONSES AND MOTOR ACTIVITY

A **reflex** is a response to a certain stimulus that is not under conscious control. Most simple reflexes are dealt with at the level of the spinal cord, whereas more complex responses are processed by the higher brain centers (i.e., cerebral cortex, cerebellum). **Proprioception** (i.e., knowing where the body is in relation to its various segments and the external environment) is largely a result of reflexive responses. The sensory information gathered to achieve this kinesthetic awareness comes from structures called **proprioceptors**, which are sensory receptors located in the skin, in and around the joints and skeletal muscles, and in the inner ear.

### Reflex Arc

A typical reflex arc in the body consists of a nerve pathway from a sensory receptor to the central nervous system (CNS) and from the CNS along a motor pathway to an effector organ (Fig. 10-1). Contracting the skeletal muscle in response to a stimulus may or may not involve the brain. In a simple motor reflex response to a pain stimulus, for example, the reaction is to rapidly move the affected limb away from the source of pain. The pathways for this reflex arc are as follows:

1. A sensory pain receptor (nociceptor) sends an impulse to the spinal cord.
2. Structures that relay sensory information within the CNS, called **interneurons**, are stimulated and, in turn, excite motor neurons.
3. The stimulated interneurons cause **depolarization** of specific motor neurons, which control the skeletal muscles necessary to withdraw the limb from the pain stimulus.

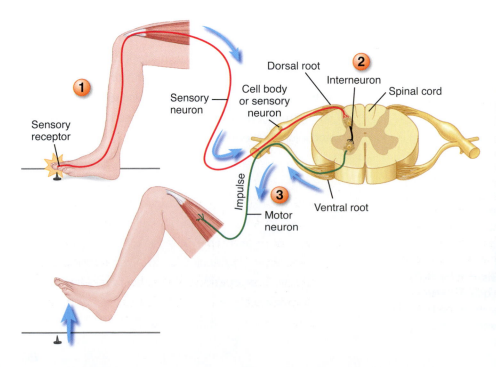

**Figure 10-1.** A reflex arc stimulated by pain and used to remove the limb from the stimulus. (1) A sensory receptor in the foot detects a painful stimulus and sends an impulse to the spinal cord via a sensory neuron. (2) The impulse enters the spinal cord through the dorsal root and the sensory neuron synapses with an interneuron, which, in turn, synapses with a motor neuron. (3) The motor neuron carries an impulse through the ventral root of the spinal cord to the quadriceps muscle. The impulse stimulates contraction of the quadriceps muscle to remove the limb away from the pain stimulus.

These steps describe a motor reflex that occurs extremely fast. The rapidity of the motor reflex is possible because the impulse does not need to travel up to the brain before the skeletal muscle action occurs. Because the brain is not involved, only one option is possible and no other movements need to be planned or considered. In other words, no conscious decisions are made during this reflex response.

## Sensory–Motor Integration

Somatosensory receptors are nervous system structures that report afferent feedback required to perform movement. These receptors include **muscle spindles**, **Golgi tendon organs (GTOs)**, joint receptors, cutaneous mechanoreceptors, and thermal sensors. Sensory information traveling in afferent neurons to the CNS can result in a local reflex at the spinal cord level, or the information can be sent on to the upper regions of the spinal cord or to the brain. The area within the CNS at which the sensory information terminates (whether in the spinal cord or brain) is referred to as an integration center. This area is where the sensory input is interpreted and linked to the motor system.

When sensory impulses terminate in the spinal cord, the response is a simple motor reflex such as the pain withdrawal response described earlier. Termination in the lower brainstem results in more complex subconscious motor responses such as those associated with postural control. When afferent sensory information terminates in the cerebellum, there is also a subconscious motor response, but these responses are more complex than those initiated from the lower brainstem and deal with the coordination of both fine and gross motor movements. Sensory impulses that make it up to the thalamus are distinguishable as sensations by the conscious brain. Lastly, if a sensory signal terminates at the cerebral cortex, the conscious brain recognizes it and uses this information to plan a coordinated response.

Efferent signals sent from the CNS to the peripheral nervous system (PNS) with the purpose of producing skeletal muscle contractions are carried along structures called alpha (α) motor neurons. The cell bodies of the α motor neurons, which are housed within the gray matter of the spinal cord, extend **axons** outward toward the skeletal muscle fibers they innervate to make an intact **motor unit** (see description in Chapter 9). Nerve cells conduct impulses in one direction only; thus, once an α motor neuron is stimulated, it will transmit its signal away from the CNS to its associated muscle fibers.

Whereas an α motor neuron is relatively large in diameter, a gamma (γ) efferent motor neuron is smaller. Neurons that make up γ efferent fibers are about half the diameter of the α motor fibers. These specialized nerve fibers connect with specific stretch sensors located within skeletal muscle, which detect minute changes in muscle fiber length (i.e., muscle spindles).

### FROM THEORY TO PRACTICE

The nervous system's reflexive action to withdraw from a painful stimulus is a means to protect the body from further injury. This type of response can be observed in a runner who sprains his ankle. Immediately after the runner twists his right ankle on an uneven patch of terrain, his attempts to put weight on the injured extremity will result in a quick and powerful withdrawal reflex of the flexor muscles in his right hip and thigh.

In situations when a weight-bearing joint is signaling intense afferent pain impulses to the CNS, a pattern of ipsilateral (same-side) flexion and contralateral (opposite-side) extension occurs when the runner tries to step on his injured extremity. The hip flexors and hamstrings of the right thigh produce hip flexion and knee flexion, respectively, to lift the leg off the ground and prevent further injury caused by weight-bearing. At the same time, the hip extensors and quadriceps of the left side produce hip extension and knee extension, respectively, of the left lower extremity to support the body's weight on the opposite, uninjured limb.

Although the pain withdrawal response is a powerful reflex, the CNS does have the ability to inhibit this response in favor of actions that are more appropriate to the situation. For example, if the runner sprained his ankle on a busy roadway and needed to quickly move on his two feet to escape oncoming traffic, the reflex response would be inhibited by higher brain centers dealing with the more emergent lifesaving task of avoiding being hit by a speeding vehicle.

### VIGNETTE (continued)

■ Oscar's intention to perform his first chest-press exercise was a conscious thought that originated in the cerebral cortex of his brain. He had seen fellow gym members performing this exercise, so although he had never tried it before, he had a visual representation of what he wanted to achieve. The electrical impulses responsible for Oscar's first repetition of the chest press traveled from his brain down to the muscles of his chest, shoulders, and triceps through efferent neurons.

Feedback from receptors in the skeletal muscles, joints, and skin of his upper extremity about the execution of his movement was sent to Oscar's brain through afferent neurons. This two-way communication between the CNS and PNS will help Oscar eventually master the exercise.

## Muscle Spindles

Muscle spindles are receptors found within skeletal muscle that constantly monitor length or changes in length (e.g., stretch) in the muscle. Found in the connective tissues between the fascicles and lying parallel with skeletal muscle fibers, muscle spindles consist of a middle portion that acts as the stretch receptor and the ends made up of **intrafusal fibers**. In contrast, skeletal muscle fibers are called **extrafusal fibers** because they lie outside the muscle spindle capsule (Fig. 10-2A). Intrafusal fibers contain both afferent and efferent pathways, meaning that they are capable of sending sensory information to the CNS and receiving impulses from the CNS, respectively. This complex structure allows muscle spindles to participate in a reflex response that permits the maintenance of normal muscle tone and posture for executing movements.

Because of the muscle spindle's location and connective tissue attachment within muscle, when a muscle fiber is stretched, the central region of the muscle spindle is also stretched. Information about the extent and quickness of the stretch is sent from the muscle spindle to the spinal cord via primary **afferent (Ia) pathways**. Once in the spinal cord, the afferent neuron forms a **synapse** with an α motor neuron (**efferent pathway**), which adds excitatory stimuli to the α motor neuron that summates with a voluntary stimulus for movement that may come from the higher brain centers. The summation of stimuli from voluntary and afferent sources may lead to increased ability to recruit more and larger motor units within the motor unit pool of the muscle, facilitating force production (such as in plyometric jump training; Fig. 10-3). Muscle spindles are sensitive to rapid stretch and may act as protective stretch receptors that trigger a reflexive muscle contraction (in the same skeletal muscle that was just stretched) without involvement from the brain. This reflex, in theory, prevents those muscles from further lengthening to prevent possible injury. Overall, the CNS interprets afferent information from the muscle spindles and sends an impulse to the α motor neurons to increase force production within the same muscle. Thus, by detecting rapid changes in muscle length, the muscle spindle enhances muscle force production.

When the muscle spindle's sensory excitatory impulses arrive at the spinal cord, the signal stimulates

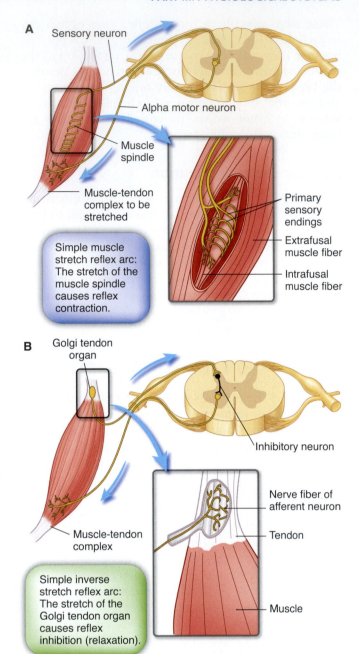

**Figure 10-2.** Muscle spindle and Golgi tendon organ. These proprioceptors are engaged for different purposes to protect the muscle from harm. A, Muscle spindles are used to elicit muscle contraction and protect the muscle from damage caused by rapid stretch. B, Golgi tendon organs are used to relax the muscle and protect it from damage caused by excessive force generation.

a reflex contraction of the muscle where the signal originated at the same time. Also, a branch of the sensory neuron simultaneously stimulates an inhibitory interneuron that innervates an α motor neuron of the **antagonist** muscle group. This leads to a decrease in force production of the antagonist (referred to as **reciprocal inhibition**). Reciprocal inhibition also occurs during voluntary movement where the inhibitory signal then comes from the higher brain centers that

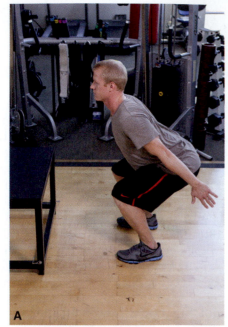

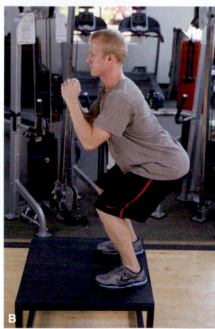

**Figure 10-3.** Plyometric box jump. This counter movement jump is effective at producing rapid stretch in the large muscles of the leg. **A)** Beginning of jump. **B)**. End of jump. During the descent (counter movement), the rapid stretch sensed by the muscle spindles can be used to generate more force during the jumping movement. When the jump is performed immediately after the rapid stretch, greater force is produced during the concentric component of the jump.

cause antagonist muscles to relax as agonist muscles contract. Together, the excitatory signal to the agonist muscle and the inhibitory signal to the antagonist are referred to as the **stretch reflex**. Inhibiting the antagonist muscles is necessary so that the **agonist** muscles can produce reflexive joint movement without being limited by opposing muscle force on the other side of

the joint. The stretch reflex is essential in controlling movement and maintaining posture at the subconscious level.

Intrafusal fibers are actually a collection of 4 to 20 small, specialized skeletal muscle fibers. Because of the lack of intrafusal fibers located in the middle portion of the muscle spindle, the central region cannot contract, it can only be stretched. It is this central region of a muscle spindle that sends sensory information to the CNS. In contrast, each end of a muscle spindle has more concentrated intrafusal fibers, which allows its end regions to slightly shorten. The end regions of a muscle spindle are innervated by the γ motor neurons (Fig. 10-2B). When the α motor neurons are stimulated to cause muscle contraction, the γ motor neurons are also activated (called alpha-gamma coactivation), which causes the ends of the intrafusal fibers to contract. This slight contraction results in the maintenance of the sensitivity of the stretch receptor, even as the extrafusal muscle fibers shorten. If not for the shortening of the intrafusal fibers when the extrafusal fibers shorten, the spindle would become slack. The shortening of the ends of the intrafusal fibers keeps the central region of the spindle taut, maintaining the sensitivity of the spindle as a monitor of the change of length within a muscle.

## Golgi Tendon Organs

Named for the Italian anatomist (Camillo Golgi) who first described them in the late 1800s, GTOs produce an inhibitory reflex action in the muscles they supply. GTOs are capsules located near the muscle fibers' attachments to the tendon at the insertion of a muscle (see Fig. 10-2B). Approximately 15 to 20 muscle fibers are contained within each capsule, but their sensitivity is so great that GTOs can detect changes in tension in a single muscle fiber. When a change in tension occurs within a muscle fiber, the collagen fibers surrounding the GTO are pinched, causing distortion and depolarization of the membranes of the primary (Ib) afferent sensory endings, which sends action potentials indicating the level of tension in the muscle to the CNS. During physical activity, when excessive tension is detected in the musculotendinous unit, either from a stretch force or a contraction force, the afferent signals from the Ib nerve fibers from the GTO synapse with inhibitory interneurons in the spinal cord that innervate α motor neurons. This leads to an inhibition of motor unit recruitment, which effectively decreases force production in the muscle fibers that are experiencing the tension (agonists). Inhibition of the agonists is called **autogenic inhibition**. It has been suggested that these sensory receptors provide a protective function by reducing the risk for injury to the agonist muscle fibers by limiting their force production to prevent undue strain.

## FROM THEORY TO PRACTICE

### ■ NEUROLOGICAL PROPERTIES OF STRETCHING: STATIC VERSUS DYNAMIC STRETCHING

In recent years, studies have demonstrated that static stretching before certain activities may have a negative effect on performance.[2,3] During **static stretching** it is usually recommended to hold a stretch at the greatest range of motion of a joint for 15 to 30 seconds (Fig. 10-4A). This length of time allows the activity of the muscle spindles in the muscle being stretched to desensitize and avoid the reflexive increase in tension while holding the stretch. This concept has been referred to as stress relaxation. Holding the stretch long enough for stress relaxation to occur allows a greater range of motion of the joint, which allows a greater stretch of the muscle and connective tissue of the joint. Holding the stretch beyond 15 seconds also places stresses along the **collagen** fibers, remodeling them as they pull apart (plastic deformation) and lengthening the tissue. The lengthening that occurs when a stretch force is applied is called **creep**. Reductions in tension (stress-relaxation response) and creep are possible explanations for the increases in range of motion observed after an acute static-stretching session; however, two problems arise when static stretching is practiced before activities that require high force and velocity of contraction. First, when creep increases the length of the connective tissues and muscle fibers, the length–tension relationship (see further discussion later in this chapter) at any given joint angle is compromised to some degree; second, the desensitization of the muscle spindle may produce a temporary decrease in reflexive force production in the muscle. Both of these mechanisms have been proposed to explain the common finding of the negative effects of static stretching on power-based activities.[2]

In contrast, during **dynamic (or active) stretching**, which is an attempt to increase the range of motion at the joint using dynamic muscle contractions of the antagonist (opposite) muscle group(s) of the muscles to be stretched (target muscles), these issues are not thought to occur (Fig. 10-4B). Muscle contractions of the opposite muscles use reciprocal inhibition of the α motor neurons going to the target muscles.[4] For example, if the hamstring muscle group is the target muscle to be stretched, a person can lie supine on her back, slowly raise her straight leg off the ground as far as possible toward her head, contracting the hip flexors (flex the hip) and quadriceps (extend the knee). Once the joint has been actively moved to its greatest range of motion, further assistance is added to increase the range of motion a few more degrees, while continuing to contract the opposite muscles. This is held for 2 to 5 seconds and repeated a number of times. Contraction of these muscle groups allows the reciprocal inhibition of muscle tension in the gluteal and hamstring muscle groups to allow a greater range of motion during hip flexion, ultimately improving the range of motion while stretching the hamstrings using the reflexive action within the neuromuscular system.

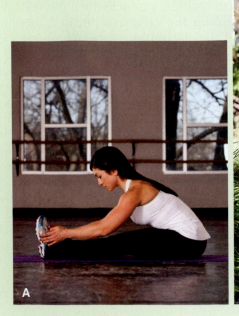
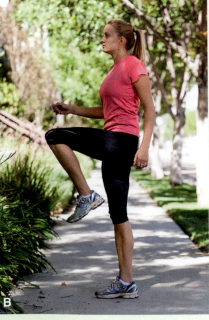

**Figure 10-4.** Static and dynamic stretching. A, Static stretching activity used to improve joint range of motion. B, Dynamic stretching used to increase the range of motion at the joint using dynamic muscle contractions of the antagonist (opposite) muscle group(s) of the muscles to be stretched (target muscles).

## In Your Own Words

You are working out with a friend and spend 10 minutes working on flexibility with static stretching. Your friend says that she is able to stretch farther on the third repetition of a flexibility exercise compared with the first repetition. How would you explain her increased range of motion during the latter sets of stretching?

### Joint Receptors

Joint receptors are located in the joint capsules and the surrounding ligaments. They transmit sensory information relating to positions, velocities, and accelerations that occur at the joints. In addition, pressure receptors within the joints provide added information about pressure changes that is used for important postural adjustments and normal gait. **Pacinian corpuscles** are joint receptors that detect changes in movement or pressure and are located close to the GTOs. When Pacinian corpuscles experience compression or deformation from joint movement, they signal the CNS about the change. They do not, however, provide information about the magnitude of movement or the amount of pressure applied within the joint. **Golgi-Mazzoni corpuscles** are located within the joint capsule and are responsive to joint compression. Thus, any weight-bearing activity stimulates these receptors. **Free nerve endings** are another type of joint receptor. These sensors are nociceptive, which means they detect painful stimuli. Free nerve endings are sensitive to abnormal joint stress or to chemical agents.

## ACUTE NEUROMUSCULAR RESPONSES TO EXERCISE

Up to this point in the discussion, the focus has been on presenting the foundation for understanding specific structures of the nervous system and how they contribute to motor control. This section explores how the neuromuscular system responds during an acute bout of exercise. The focus is on the ability of the neuromuscular system to regulate force production for the levels necessary for movement and participation in different intensities of activity.

### Contractile Characteristics of Motor Units

The function of the motor units that make up a skeletal muscle is to produce force. A motor unit is defined as an α motor neuron and all of the skeletal muscle fibers it innervates. Functional characteristics of the motor units are determined by the type of muscle fibers they contain. Fiber types have been identified by two general methods. One method uses small cross-sectional slices of muscle obtained by the muscle biopsy technique to perform histochemical staining. This method classifies the fiber type by the speed of contraction (or "twitch" speed) that is estimated by the myofibrillar-ATPase reaction within the different fibers within the slice of muscle. ATPase is the enzyme that splits **adenosine triphosphate (ATP)** on the myosin head, and there seems to be a different rate of ATPase activity in the different fiber types. Typically, type I fibers contain an ATPase that splits ATP at a slower rate than the ATPase in type II fibers. Generally, the faster the ATPase is splitting the ATP on the myosin head, the faster the power stroke of the cross bridge cycle can take place. A second method uses single muscle fibers and a process called *electrophoresis* that identifies the proteins of the myosin heavy chain (MHC) isoforms that make up the thick filament in a muscle fiber. Studies have shown that these two classification methods correlate well,[5] and often the names of fiber types from these two methods are used interchangeably.

On the basis of these methods of fiber typing, three common skeletal muscle fiber types have been identified. Type I fibers contain the MHC isoforms that are typically related to "slow twitch" fibers; they tend to have slow contractile speed determined by ATPase activity and use oxidative metabolic characteristics. Type IIa fibers contain MHC isoforms of one subtype of the "fast twitch" fibers that are known to have fast contractile characteristics, fast ATPase enzyme activity, and use a combination of oxidative and glycolytic metabolic characteristics. Lastly, type IIx fibers contain MHC isoforms of the other subtype of the "fast twitch" fibers that also have fast contractile characteristics with even faster ATPase activity, but primarily glycolytic metabolic characteristics.[6]

A motor unit may have between less than 10 to more than 1,000 muscle fibers innervated by the same α motor neuron.[7] All muscle fibers within a motor unit are of the same fiber type; therefore, when a motor unit is activated to contract, all of the fibers contained therein will react similarly in terms of speed of contraction and the ability to produce and maintain force.

Motor units are classified by the type of muscle fibers that are innervated by the α motor neuron. Characteristics of the different motor units are discussed in Chapter 9. As a refresher, type I or a **slow twitch motor unit** consist of an α motor neuron with a relatively small cell body and a small-diameter axon. In addition, type I motor units typically innervate fewer muscle fibers (i.e., ≤300). In contrast, a type II or **fast twitch motor unit** is made up of an α motor neuron with a larger cell body and a large-diameter axon that innervates ≥300 muscle fibers.[8] Small but important differences are observed between type IIa and IIx motor units. For instance, motor neurons that innervate IIx fibers have larger cell bodies than those motor neurons that innervate IIa fibers, and the diameter of the axons of these motor neurons are slightly larger in the IIx motor units. Motor unit size (fibers per motor neuron) varies within the type II motor units; however, both type II motor unit subcategories are characterized by having more fibers per motor unit than the type I motor units. This arrangement means that when a single type I motor unit is stimulated to contract, far fewer muscle fibers are activated than when a single type II motor unit is called on to perform its function.

Other differences between the motor unit types play a role in the force production. Typically, the fibers in type II motor units reach peak tension more rapidly than fibers found in type I motor units because of the faster isoforms of MHC content and faster myosin ATPase activity. Overall, type II motor units are also capable of producing more force than type I motor units primarily because there are more muscle fibers in each type II motor unit than in a typical type I motor unit. However, although more force is typically produced by type II motor units, type I motor units are more fatigue resistant; that is, type I motor units are capable of maintaining maximal force for a much longer period. Slight differences in force-producing properties also exist between type IIa and type IIx. Type IIx motor units generate greater force at a slightly faster velocity of shortening than type IIa, whereas type IIa fibers are more fatigue resistant and easier to recruit than type IIx.

## Regulation of Force Production

Skeletal muscle is capable of generating a wide range of muscular force production for tasks ranging from physical activity for everyday life all the way up to intense participation in sporting activities. Two mechanisms describe a muscle's ability to vary its contractile force production. Both of these tasks are functions of the nervous system. First, the CNS regulates force production by determining the number and size of the motor units that are activated to participate in the force production within the muscle. This is referred to as **motor unit recruitment**. Second, once recruited, the firing rate going down the motor neuron to the fibers within the motor unit can be adjusted by the CNS, leading to an adjustment in force production within the motor unit. This phenomenon is referred to as **rate coding**. Together, recruitment and rate coding determine the amount of force that a muscular contraction can produce (Fig. 10-5).

## Motor Unit Recruitment

Motor unit recruitment requires the soma (or cell body) of the α motor neuron in the spinal cord to receive a threshold stimulus. The stimuli to the soma of the α motor neuron may likely come from the higher brain centers that stimulate voluntary movement, but may also receive stimuli from the different receptors in the muscle (i.e., muscle spindles and GTOs) that may be excitatory or inhibitory. Action potentials from excitatory neurons must exceed the influence of the inhibitory neurons to reach threshold and, as a result, stimulate the soma of the α motor neuron.

As mentioned earlier, the somas of different motor unit types are different sizes (type I < type IIa < type IIx).

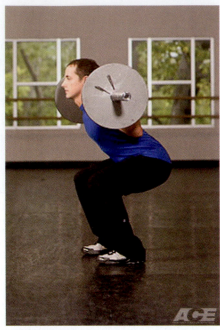

**Figure 10-5.** A heavy back squat exercise requires the central nervous system to increase motor unit recruitment in the muscles of the hip and knee and adjust the rate of impulses through rate coding to increase force development.

Size refers to the diameter, surface area, and capacitance of the soma of the α motor neuron.[9] Many researchers believe that the order in which motor units within a motor unit pool are recruited depends on force needs and is related to the size of the soma of the motor neuron. This is referred to as the **size principle** of motor unit recruitment.

Because type I motor units have the smallest somas, it is easier to reach threshold and they are considered "low threshold" motor units. Large type II motor units have relatively large somas and are considered "high threshold" motor units, with IIx having larger somas than IIa. Therefore, type IIx motor units have the highest threshold and need the greatest stimulus for recruitment of these motor units.

To understand the following discussion, it must be mentioned that, within the nervous system, as the intensity of a stimulus increases, the firing rate of the neurons increase. This means that waves of action potentials with long time intervals between represent a light stimulus, and waves of action potentials with shorter time intervals produce strong responses.

Voluntary movement begins in the brain as a stimulus to move is developed. The CNS delivers the stimulus from the brain to the motor units in the spinal cord responsible for the movement. The variability of the stimulatory rate of the neural impulses traveling down the spinal cord via descending pathways to the motor unit pool determine the motor unit recruitment. The greater the stimulus (greater force needs), the faster action potentials are sent by the brain to the somas of the motor neurons. Summation of the neurotransmitter substances released by the neurons of the descending motor pathways in the spinal cord determine the extent of stimulation to the soma of any α motor neuron within the motor unit pool to a muscle. As a result, at a low stimulatory rate, low threshold motor units are recruited, but only the fastest stimulatory rates will allow summation of the impulses to the α motor neurons to reach threshold in the motor neurons that activate the highest threshold motor units. Stimulatory rates in between will recruit motor units responsive to that level of stimulatory rate. As stimulatory rates change, motor units are dismissed in a predictable order—the motor unit recruited last when the force needs increase is the first unit deactivated when the force begins to decrease.

When an activity requires increasing amounts of force production from working muscles, more and more motor units are stimulated. When little force is required, only a few motor units are activated. Consequently, following the size principle, skeletal muscle contraction involves a progressive recruitment of type I and then type II muscle fibers during activities that necessitate increasing force demands. Specifically, motor units are recruited in the following order: type I, type IIa, and type IIx.

## VIGNETTE (continued)

■ To ensure the appropriate amount of force production to properly execute the chest-press exercise, Oscar's nervous system recruited certain motor units within the pectorals, deltoids, and triceps muscles. He performed three consecutive sets with a 5-pound increase in weight with each set. In the first set, smaller, type I motor units along with some of the lower threshold type IIa motor units were recruited to perform the movement, because the weight load was relatively light. As he continued to perform each set, the weight load increased incrementally, which required Oscar's brain to recruit larger, more powerful, higher threshold type IIa and IIx motor units with each successive set. When a weight load is progressively increased such that it causes the recruitment of multiple type II motor units, and when it is done on a consistent basis (e.g., 2 days per week for at least 12 weeks), motor unit activation improves and the likely result is an eventual hypertrophy of those muscle fibers recruited during training. Consequently, increased strength and the appearance of firm muscles are associated with muscle hypertrophy due to a progressive resistance training program.

## Rate Coding

When a single, threshold stimulus is received, the motor unit is recruited and responds by producing a response called a simple **twitch**. Immediately following the stimulus, there is a short latent phase that lasts a few milliseconds that likely allows for the excitation process (of the excitation-contraction coupling) to occur. The second phase of the twitch is the contraction phase where cross-bridge attachment and sarcomere shortening creates tension in the muscle fibers. If no further stimulus is received, the relaxation phase of the twitch takes place as the cross bridges detach and tension is reduced back to resting levels.

Typically, when a motor unit is stimulated via an α motor neuron, it receives a wave of successive **action potentials** (or nerve impulses). If the action potentials are received before the relaxation phase of the previous stimulus is completed, the tension produced by successive twitches builds on each other (a process called **summation**). Gradual increases in the rate of discharge of action potentials to an α motor neuron results in linear increases in force production. Maximal discharge rates differ across all motor units and depend on the force needs of the task being performed. In activities that require gradual increases in force, maximal discharge rates range from 20 to 60 pulses per second (pps), whereas maximal discharge rates can reach up to 100 pps during rapid, brief contractions.[10,11] The degree of overlap between successive twitches is determined by the rate at which the action potentials are generated. **Rate coding** is a term that describes the regulation of the nervous system's control over the rate at which α motor neurons discharge action potentials. For a more detailed explanation of rate coding, see Chapter 9.

As the force needs of the muscle increase, the stimulus strength increases (increased rate coding); as a result, force production within a motor unit increases as these twitches summate with faster and faster firing rates, up to a point. All motor units have a maximal firing rate where no faster delivery of action potentials will produce a greater force production. When the twitches summate to the point of maximal force production, the muscle experiences **tetanus**. For many motor units within the muscles, when motor units are activated at 80 to 100 pps, they typically reach maximal force production.[12] When motor units are stimulated at firing rates faster than a tetanic rate, no greater force is typically produced; however, an increase in the rate of force development occurs, such that the maximal force is reached sooner after the initial stimulus.

Recall that both motor unit recruitment and rate coding determine muscular force production. These two neural processes work concurrently to ensure the achievement of bodily movement during physical activity. Researchers have determined that contraction speed is controlled for the most part by rate coding, whereas the power produced during muscular contraction is more related to motor unit recruitment.[13]

## Types of Muscle Contraction and Action

In muscle physiology, a contracting muscle is not necessarily shortening, even though many times we describe a "muscle contraction" as shortening of the sarcomeres within a muscle fiber. Muscle contraction actually refers to when the muscle is producing tension within the fibers of motor units recruited. During muscle contraction, the muscle fibers may be producing tension that allows the muscle to stay the same length (an isometric contraction) or the length of the muscle may get longer or shorter. If you attempt to do a leg press with more weight than you are capable of moving, once you put your feet on the platform and push as hard as you can, but the platform does not move, you are performing an isometric contraction. Although your muscles are producing tension through interaction between the thick and thin filaments at the sarcomere level in the muscle fibers recruited, that tension is being absorbed by the elastic components of the muscle as the force produced is not great enough to cause movement.

When the muscle length changes, there are a number of different terms for this, the most common being an isotonic contraction. However, isotonic contraction refers to a muscle that remains under relatively constant tension while its length changes. Many physiologists disagree with this terminology because, when an intact muscle shortens or lengthens, the tension within the muscle actually changes as a result of the mechanical influences at the joint. Some suggested terms to better describe the muscle contraction as the muscle changes length are dynamic contraction, iso-inertional contraction, or dynamic constant external resistance movement. When muscles change length as they produce tension, the actions that take place are referred to as either **concentric** or **eccentric muscle actions**. In concentric muscle actions, a muscle shortens as it produces enough force to overcome the resistance on the leg-press machine and push it away from you, straightening your legs (Fig. 10-6). As you continue the repetition on the leg-press machine, to lower the weight requires less force than the concentric action, yet tension is required to make sure the weight is lowered under control. As the weight is lowered, tension in the muscle is produced by the interaction between the thick and thin filaments; however, now the sarcomeres are lengthening and this is referred to as an eccentric action of the muscle.

In summary, during an isometric contraction, the muscle develops tension without changing length because either the external resistance that needs to be overcome is the same as the tension in the muscle or the muscle is not strong enough to move a fixed or heavy object. During a dynamic contraction, changes in length take place while tension is produced. In concentric actions, muscles shorten as they produce tension that exceeds the external resistance; and in eccentric actions, muscles lengthen as they produce

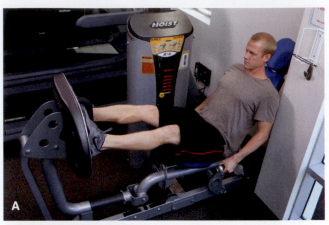

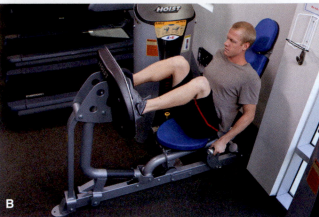

**Figure 10-6.** A leg-press exercise demonstrates the use of both concentric and eccentric movements. A, Pushing the weight up requires the use of concentric movement. B, Lowering the weight under control requires greater eccentric movement demands.

less tension than the external resistance that must be overcome.

## Length–Tension Relationship

A critical factor that determines the force produced when a muscle contracts is related to the length of the muscle. There is an optimal length for the greatest amount of force that a muscle fiber can produce. The relationship between the length of the fiber and force production is a function of the overlap between the thick and thin filaments of the sarcomeres during muscle contraction (Fig. 10-7). For the greatest force production within a fiber, the length of the fiber should allow the greatest amount of cross-bridge attachment to take place. When a muscle fiber is stretched, there is limited ability for cross-bridge attachment because there is less overlap between the thick and thin filaments. In contrast, when the muscle is shortened to approximately 60% of its length, the thin filaments overlap, restricting further cross-bridge attachment. The optimal length is found between 100% and 120% of the muscle's resting length, where the ends of the thin filaments are near the center of the thick filament, because this position produces the greatest overlap and allows the maximum number of cross-bridge attachments.

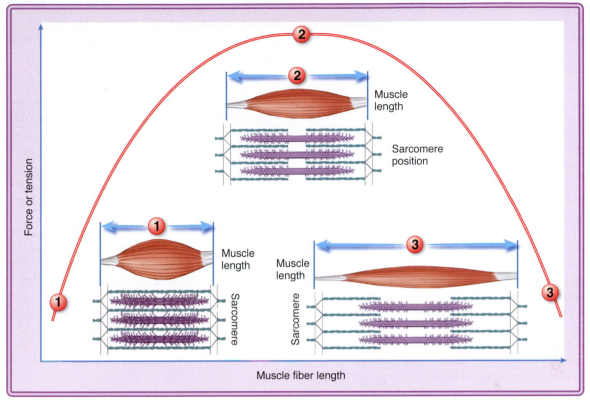

**Figure 10-7.** Length–tension relationship in muscle. In example 1, the muscle is shortened, and myosin and actin cross-bridging is not optimal to produce force or tension. In example 2, the muscle is lengthened optimally, and cross-bridging between actin and myosin is maximized. Thus, force generation is also maximized. This occurs at a fiber length corresponding to 100% to 120% of normal resting length. In example 3, the muscle is overstretched and cross-bridging is less than optimal; thus, force generation is decreased.

## Force–Velocity Relationship

The ability to develop force is also related to the velocity of muscle contraction. In a concentric muscle action, an inverse relationship between force produced and velocity of shortening (i.e., as the velocity of shortening increases, the force production decreases) is known as the **force–velocity relationship** (Fig. 10-8). At faster shortening velocities, the limitation of force production is linked to the inability of the cross-bridge cycle to keep up with the shortening sarcomere. This limits the ability for attachment of the myosin head to the binding site on the actin protein of the thin filament while the filaments slide over one another. The rate of cross-bridge cycling has been attributed to a strong relationship with the maximum rate of splitting of ATP within the contractile system, the function of the myosin ATPase within the muscle fibers. This shows that although force production in the muscle requires extensive cross-bridge attachment, the maximum speed of shortening does not depend on the number of cross-bridges that are able to attach to the thin filament. Slower shortening velocities allow the time for greater numbers of cross-bridge attachments, explaining why in the force–velocity relationship, maximal force is produced at the slowest shortening speeds. This is followed with isometric contractions producing greater forces than

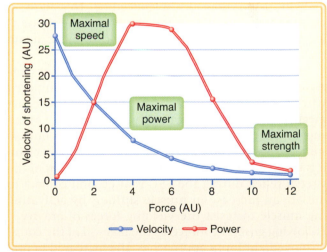

**Figure 10-8.** Force–velocity relationship, which includes power generation. As velocity of contraction or shortening of the muscle decreases, the ability of the muscle to produce force greatly increases. Power output also peaks at low levels of force generation and gradually decreases as force requirements increase. AU = arbitrary units.

concentric actions, reasoning that zero velocity gives plenty of time for cross-bridge cycling to take place. However, the force developed during an eccentric action of the muscle, where the fibers are lengthening, exceeds even isometric contractions by 50% to 100%

because a greater force must be applied to the muscle to detach the cross-bridges during the lengthening of the sarcomere.[6]

## Stretch-Shortening Cycle

In real life, it is not possible to identify movement simply as an isometric or dynamic muscle contraction or eccentric or concentric muscle action. The natural way that muscles function is typically a stretch or lengthening of a muscle followed closely by a shortening of the muscle, and with most forms of movement, this pattern is repeated over and over. Hence this naturally occurring combination of muscle actions is referred to as the **stretch-shortening cycle (SSC)**, where an eccentric action is followed immediately by a concentric action. This is apparent in many forms of locomotion such as walking, running, and hopping.

The SSC is believed by some to involve many interacting features of the mechanical structure of the muscle, as well as neural mechanisms to explain how involvement of the SSC leads to an improvement in muscle performance compared with when the activity is performed by concentric force production alone.

Many researchers believe that greater performance produced in SSC movements is related to a return to resting length of the elastic tissues in the muscle after the stretch and increased muscle activation due to the stretch reflex stimulated by the stretching of the muscle spindles.[14] Some researchers[15] also propose that a rapid movement during the eccentric portion of the SSC allows the stretched muscles to increase the fraction of attached cross-bridges, thus increasing force production, before the start of shortening. This allows a greater work output over the first part of the shortening distance compared with a pure concentric action that begins from a static start.

Evidence also shows that the SSC involves increased neural responses from the CNS compared with strict concentric actions, although the exact mechanisms are not thoroughly understood.[16] Many suggest that the stretch reflex involving the muscle spindles has a primary role in the SSC. Others claim it is involved, but that the greatest involvement of the stretch reflex during the SSC is at ground contact to initiate an increase in muscle stiffness by activating the muscle to resist the yielding forces of gravity.[16] Following ground contact, as the take-off of the countermovement jump approaches, the increased neural input subsides.[16]

"Plyometric" exercises use the SSC in an attempt to improve power production and reactive abilities in the muscles. Training the reactive abilities within the neuromuscular system improves muscle stiffness, rate of force development, and peak velocity of muscle contraction.

An example of the benefit of the SSC is seen comparing two different types of in-place jumps: the countermovement jump and the squat (static) jump. A countermovement jump starts in a standing position.

When the jump commences, the person lowers to a partial squat position rather quickly (eccentric or lengthening of the muscle), followed immediately by a maximal jump vertically (concentric or shortening of the muscle). The squat jump begins in a static partial squat position. When the jump commences, only the maximal concentric movement takes place to jump vertically. Differences in jump height between these two styles of jumps are typically greater than 18% to 20%,[14] as the countermovement jump is typically higher than the squat jump.

Although many proposed mechanisms explain how the SSC increases jump height between the countermovement and squat jumps,[15] it appears the difference is primarily that the countermovement allows greater force production at the start of the concentric action of the jump than starting from a static position. This results in higher ground reaction forces, which lead to greater jump heights when the countermovement is used. The possible mechanisms, such as recovery of the stored elastic energy in the muscle and tendons, and activation of the stretch reflex, appear to play a secondary role in the enhanced performance produced by the SSC.[15]

## Neuromuscular Fatigue

A prominent factor in declining performance capabilities during exercise is skeletal muscle fatigue. In exercise physiology, muscle fatigue is defined as an exercise-induced reduction in the ability of muscle to maintain force or power.[12] There are several theories about the cause of muscle fatigue, which range from energy pathway alterations within the exercising muscle (e.g., glycogen depletion and metabolic by-products) to neural mechanisms. This section focuses on some of the nervous system's potential influences on muscle fatigue during physical exertion.

Similar to skeletal muscle fibers, neurons in the cerebral cortex need nourishment during exercise. A lack of blood glucose (hypoglycemia) during sustained exertion not only disturbs muscle function, but also interferes with the motor output of the cerebral cortex. In one study, cyclists who exercised for 3 hours showed improved cerebral cortex metabolism when they were allowed to supplement with carbohydrates versus cyclists in the same study who did not supplement.[17] This translated to improved performance in muscle strength tests in the cyclists who were able to prevent hypoglycemia through carbohydrate feeding and preserve function of the cerebral cortex.

A chemical disturbance involving ammonia may also be to blame for muscle fatigue during sustained exercise, especially during exercise in the heat. Active muscles release ammonia into the bloodstream, which can cross the blood–brain barrier and alter essential processes such as cerebral blood flow, energy metabolism, synaptic transmission, and the regulation of some **neurotransmitters**.[18] In combination with low blood glucose, excess ammonia in the blood supply could impair an endurance exerciser's ability to sustain muscle activation.[6]

Another neuromechanism that could be responsible for muscle fatigue is related to the conscious perception of effort of the exerciser. A person's subjective judgment of the intensity of the outgoing motor command associated with performing a submaximal contraction is called the **sense of effort**. It has been shown that sustained submaximal exertion, even when performed by a motivated individual, will result in an increase in the sense of effort from when the task began compared with when it ended.[19] For example, a person walking home from the market carrying a shopping bag that weighs 10 pounds (4.5 kg) will experience the bag as feeling heavier by the time he or she makes it home, even though the force production required to carry the bag has not changed. In this case, the increasing sense of effort toward the end of the walk home was independent of the ability of the muscles to exert the desired force to hold the bag. This phenomenon does not appear to be present during high-force, maximal contractions. Thus, the excitation delivered from the higher brain centers to motor neurons can be impaired during prolonged muscle contractions. Consequently, from individuals performing daily activities involving physical activity to endurance athletes training intensely for their sport, most people perceive the discomfort of muscular fatigue before the onset of a physiological limitation within the muscle. It has been speculated that this intolerance for feelings of fatigue is the CNS's way of slowing the exercise pace to a more tolerable level to protect the athlete.[7]

## Delayed-Onset Muscle Soreness

Although many theories have been proposed to explain the occurrence of **delayed-onset muscle soreness (DOMS)**, evidence suggests that it is likely caused by tissue injury from excessive mechanical force, particularly eccentric force, exerted on muscle and connective tissue (Fig. 10-9).[20–22] DOMS is defined as muscle soreness that generally appears 24 to 48 hours and peaks between 2 and 3 days after strenuous exercise. Muscle soreness subsides gradually over the next day or two after peak soreness.

Although not completely understood, the following series of events is thought to lead up to DOMS:

1. First, structural damage to muscle and connective tissue occurs as a result of strenuous eccentric muscle actions.
2. As a result, calcium leaks out of the sarcoplasmic reticulum and collects in the **mitochondria** to the extent that ATP production is halted.
3. Next, the buildup of calcium activates enzymes that break down cellular proteins, including contractile proteins.
4. This breakdown of muscle proteins causes an inflammatory process. The accumulation of histamines, potassium, prostaglandins, and edema

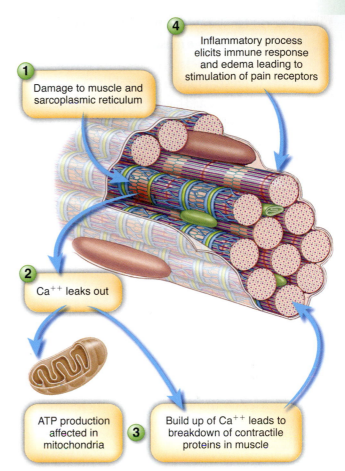

1 Damage to muscle and sarcoplasmic reticulum

4 Inflammatory process elicits immune response and edema leading to stimulation of pain receptors

2 $Ca^{++}$ leaks out

ATP production affected in mitochondria

3 Build up of $Ca^{++}$ leads to breakdown of contractile proteins in muscle

**Figure 10-9.** Proposed mechanism for delayed-onset muscle soreness.

surrounding muscle fibers stimulates free nerve endings (i.e., pain receptors), which results in the sensation of DOMS.

Efforts to prevent DOMS should include beginning a new training program gradually, starting at a very low intensity and progressing slowly through the first few weeks (e.g., 5–10 training sessions). Further, because eccentric exercise is associated with greater suffering from DOMS, attempts should be made to minimize eccentric actions early in the program. Activities that involve strenuous eccentric actions (e.g., dead lifts) can be introduced later in the program after muscles have had a chance to adapt to the new stress of exercise.

### V I G N E T T E  (continued)

■ By the end of Oscar's third set of chest presses, his muscles were suffering from the discomfort of fatigue. His intention of completing 12 repetitions was not realized, as Oscar decided to stop the set at the tenth repetition. It is common for individuals who are new to the discomforts of exercise to have a low tolerance for muscle fatigue. In Oscar's case, his lack of familiarity with the burning sensation associated with acute muscle fatigue led him to consciously (or voluntarily) cease the exercise activity to prevent further discomfort. Essentially, Oscar's muscles could have continued to produce force and complete the 12-repetition set because they had not reached true muscle failure, but his conscious brain directed him to quit at repetition number 10. Unbeknownst to Oscar, his decision to stop the exercise prematurely probably saved him from a certain increased degree of future neuromuscular discomfort (i.e., DOMS).

## CHRONIC NEUROMUSCULAR ADAPTATIONS TO EXERCISE

Up to this point, the acute adjustments of the neuromuscular system in response to a single bout of physical activity have been discussed. The remainder of this chapter focuses on the adaptations of the neuromuscular system to the stress associated with long-term physical activity.

### Muscle Strength

The two main factors attributed to changes in contractile strength are muscle size and neural properties. About 50% of the strength differences among individuals can be accounted for by muscle size, such that muscle fibers with the greatest surface area are capable of producing the most force.[23] Although muscle size is a significant contributor to force production, there is a dissociation between increases in strength and increases in muscle size, especially in the beginning stages of muscle conditioning. Studies have shown that in the beginning stages of a resistance-training program, increases in muscle force precede muscle hypertrophy.[24-26] Thus, it is possible to achieve an increase in strength without a noticeable increase in cross-sectional area in muscle. The initial gains in muscular strength without the increase in cross-sectional area are related to neural adaptations.

Neural adaptations appear to make their biggest contributions to strength gains in the first 8 to 10 weeks of conditioning (Fig. 10-10). After about 10 weeks of resistance training, hypertrophy becomes a more prominent factor in strength improvements. Although the specific neural adaptations responsible for increases in muscle strength are unknown, increases in neural drive to the exercising muscle, changes in the coordination of the muscles involved in the task, and **synchronization** of motor unit activation could explain early strength gains.

After repeated performances of a specific task, increased activation of the trained muscles has been

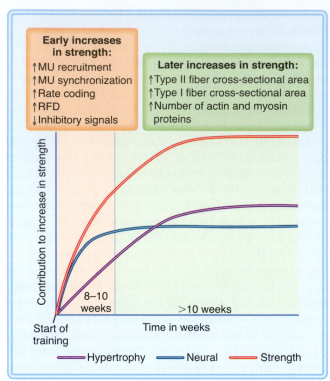

**Figure 10-10.** Relative contributions of neural and muscular adaptations to increasing strength with training over time. Strength increases early during training because of rapid improvements in neuromuscular function and very gradual improvements in hypertrophy. Once neural adaptations are maximized, further increases in hypertrophy are responsible for long-term improvements in muscular strength. Strength increases gradually over time and begins to plateau at a similar time period as the plateau in hypertrophy. MU = motor unit; RFD = rate of force development.

demonstrated in many studies.[27] Evidence of increased activation may exist as a number of different ways of nervous system adaptation. One of the more well-known ways that activation is increased is the improved ability to recruit larger threshold motor units, those that take the greatest stimulus to activate. The ability to recruit the high threshold motor units is important for strength development because these motor units contain the largest number of muscle fibers and typically contain the fiber types that create the most force, the type IIx fibers.

Increased activation may also appear as the result of an increased firing rate of action potentials (**rate coding**) to the muscle once the motor unit has been recruited. Rate coding allows the motor units to vary the force produced, with slow firing rates producing relatively low levels of force and tetanic levels of rate coding producing maximal amounts of force. Training may increase firing rates consistently high enough in the motor unit to produce maximal forces whenever recruited.

A third way that training produces an increase in neural activation is also related to rate coding; however, this one does not lead to increases in force, but it increases the rate of force development. Because tetanic firing rates that travel down the motor neuron to the fibers it innervates produce maximal force in the motor unit, it is possible that even faster rates lead to greater activation of the muscle; however, greater force production is not the result. The result is a shorter period to reach maximal force in that motor unit. During ballistic contractions (i.e., muscular movements that are brief and are performed at maximal velocity), motor units begin firing at very high frequencies, allowing rapid force production to accelerate quickly through a motion, such as throwing or jumping. Gradations of force produced by ballistic contractions have been proposed to be produced by a combination of the recruitment of additional motor units and by an increase in the rate of firing of the motor units.[28]

A reduction in inhibitory signals to the motor units has also been proposed as an adaptation that increases force production following chronic resistance training. A reduction in inhibition to the motor units leads to more motor units activated and/or a higher frequency of discharge of the involved motor units. These inhibitory signals have been suggested to come from GTOs[6] and/or other neural pathways or circuits from the motor cortex or cerebellum that lead to the recruitment of motor units that do not have anything to do with the intended motor task.[29,30] Strength training may improve performance by reducing the extent of cortical activation and, therefore, the activation of neural elements that interfere with the optimal execution of movement.[29]

Another possible adaptation within the nervous system following training involves the distribution of activation among the muscles involved in a specific motor task. When movement occurs at a joint, a coordinated effort between the agonist and antagonist muscles, referred to as coactivation, must exist to allow for joint stability and stiffness. Coactivation varies with factors such as the intensity and type of contraction, movement speed, the amount of fatigue, and the level of training.[31] Coactivation is quite common during joint movement, especially when the agonist contraction is strong, rapid, or both (Figure 10-11).

The relative activation of agonist and antagonist muscles during a strength task can influence the force produced because the opposing torque developed by the antagonist would decrease the net torque produced in the intended direction.[27] Therefore, the level of coactivation must be adjusted by the nervous system to improve agonist muscle performance. It is thought that coactivation may be modified through training. Evidence has been reported that trained athletes exhibit reduced coactivation of the hamstrings muscles compared with untrained subjects when performing isokinetic knee extensions.[27,32] However, this reduction in coactivation does not appear to contribute significantly to improvements in strength.[32,33]

Increased motor unit synchronization (of firing) has been demonstrated following strength training.[27,34]

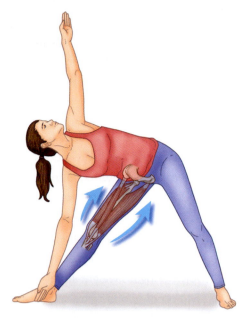

**Figure 10-11.** Coactivation of agonist and antagonist muscles occurs in many activities where joint stability is required. In this yoga pose activity, the quadriceps muscle and hamstrings muscle contract together to prevent the knee from hyperextending to maintain proper body alignment and to prevent a potential injury to the joint.

Although this must be related to changes within the nervous system as a result of the strength training, it is not clear whether synchronous firing increases peak force in maximal contractions. At high stimulation frequencies, there appears to be similar force produced using synchronous and asynchronous firing rates. However, a more synchronous *onset* of discharge of recruited motor units is more likely to increase the rate of force development, rather than maximal force production. Within a given muscle, even if a synchronous onset of discharge takes place, once the recruited motor units begin firing, almost immediately they would be firing asynchronously because of different firing rates.[34] For example, weight lifters typically demonstrate a synchronous pattern of motor unit firing, which aids in the rate of force development and the capability to exert steady forces.[35,36]

## In Your Own Words

After 1 month of participating in a twice-weekly circuit-training routine, your client remarks that he is encouraged by his noticeable increase in muscle strength. However, he expresses frustration at the fact that, although his strength has improved, he has not noticed any significant changes in appearance. He is curious to learn why he is consistently able to lift more weight, but does not have a corresponding increase in muscle mass. How would you explain the reason for this apparent discrepancy between strength and muscle size?

## VIGNETTE (continued)

■ After 8 weeks of resistance training, Oscar is noticeably more proficient at performing free-weight exercises. Not only is he able to lift heavier weights than he could in the first week of his program, he is also able to produce the movements with more fluidity and less awkwardness. Oscar's nervous system has fine-tuned his exercise movements so that more motor units are recruited in a synchronous fashion with each lift. Furthermore, the muscles paired on the opposing sides of his joints now activate more cooperatively during his weight-lifting movements. This coactivation of opposing muscles ensures a more coordinated and graceful motion, even when he progressively increases the weight.

## Muscle Fiber Adaptations

The nervous system's ability to recruit and control different motor unit firing patterns during physical activity influences both the motor skill and the type of exertion required. Recall that single motor units contain only one type of muscle fiber: either type I or type II. The principle of specificity is apparent when looking at how certain types of training cause adaptations in muscle fibers. Although it is well-known that resistance training results in an increase in cross-sectional area of all fiber types, most research demonstrates that the type II motor units hypertrophy to a greater relative amount than type I units.[37,38] Because the "size principle"

suggests that all motor unit types are recruited with relatively heavy loads, the greater hypertrophy in type II fibers may reflect the greater relative involvement of these fibers to produce the muscular force necessary during training.[6] The increased cross-sectional area of the muscle fibers in response to resistance training is attributed to an increase in the myofibrillar number and myofibrillar area as a result of adding actin and myosin proteins, increasing the number of thick and thin filaments.[6]

A conversion of fiber type from one form to another resulting from training has been demonstrated. Until recently, fiber type adaptations were thought to only take place from the type IIx to IIa; however, a change from type I to type IIa has been observed using sprint training[39] and resistance training using ballistic bench-press throws and SSC (stretch shortening cycle) pushups.[40] These studies give evidence of a possible bidirectional transformation of fiber types from type I and type IIx to IIa. However, some researchers suggest using caution when interpreting past and present research results in this area because the histochemical methods in fiber typing techniques have improved. There are likely more than the accepted three different fiber types (types I, IIa, and IIx) with a possibility of hybrid MHC isoforms,[5] which makes interpretation of results complicated (see later Research Highlight feature).

In contrast, a program of aerobic-endurance training causes type I fibers to increase in size. Accordingly, with aerobic training, type II fibers do not show an increase in size because they are typically not recruited to the same extent during endurance activities. In some instances, long-duration exercise (e.g., a 20-week program of aerobic-endurance training) may eventually recruit type IIa fibers and even cause some type IIx fibers to take on the characteristics of the more oxidative type IIa fibers.

## RESEARCH HIGHLIGHT

### Can Muscle Fiber Types Change Because of Chronic Training?

For some time, it has been known that elite endurance athletes tend to have a high percentage (60%–70%) of "slow twitch" fibers (type I) and elite sprinters have a high percentage (~80%) of "fast twitch" fibers (type II).[41] In addition, elite weight lifters and power lifters have been found to have a significantly higher percentage of "fast twitch" fibers (~60%) than endurance athletes (~40%).[42] Although these findings may suggest a relationship between muscle fiber type and athletic performance, the real question may be: Do athletes choose sports and events in which their physiological makeup (i.e., muscle fiber type) allows them to be successful performers, or can the observations of specific fiber type differences in elite athletes be explained by changes in fiber type because of chronic training? The second part of this question has been debated by many over the years.

Until recently, it was generally accepted the fiber type conversion was only possible between the type II (fast) fiber types. Interestingly, both endurance training and strength training produced a shift of type IIx fibers to type IIa fibers. Many studies have shown that sedentary people have higher amounts of type IIx fibers than fit people, and other studies have shown high correlation between the percentage of type IIa fibers and activity levels in people. As a result, some have considered the type IIx fiber a "default" fiber type that changes once activity commences, no matter the type of activity.

## RESEARCH HIGHLIGHT–cont'd

An understanding of muscle fiber typing techniques is needed to answer the debated question about fiber type changes caused by training. Many of the early studies that classified muscle fiber types and investigated the possibility of fiber type conversion used the histochemical staining technique for myosin ATPase. The contractile speed of muscle is primarily determined by the function of its myosin protein (of the thick filament), which has been shown to correlate with the myosin ATPase activity[43]; therefore, this technique can differentiate differences in the phenotype of muscle fibers. This technique identifies three classifications of muscle fibers–type I, type IIa, and type IIx in humans–using the shade of color the staining produces of the fiber cross-sectional view of a muscle sample under a microscope.

Newer techniques to determine muscle fiber types and changes caused by training have focused on the MHC isoform composition of fibers, that is, the protein makeup of the myosin protein itself. Each myosin protein is made up of two MHC protein strands that are known to have the following pure fiber types. Type I fibers are made up of two MHC Iβ and the two fast fiber types in humans, type IIa is made of two MHCIIa, and type IIx is made from two MHCIIx.[5,6] The two MHCs that make up the myosin protein are arranged similar to the way two wires would be twisted together, with the tails of each MHC twisted together and the protein heads sticking out (Fig. 10-12). The process to identify the different MHCs of a muscle fiber is called *gel electrophoresis*. Electrophoresis separates the MHC isoforms of the muscle sample by the size (molecular weight) and charge of their protein content where similar-size molecules produce distinct bands in the gel.

There are two ways to use gel electrophoresis to determine fiber typing. One is to homogenize a sample of mixed muscle fibers, which grinds and mixes all the different fibers of the muscle sample and loads them into a sample well of gel. This method is able to determine the different MHCs of a number of fibers from the sample and can tell you the percentage of different MHCs (I, IIa, and IIx) of the muscle sample, similar to the myosin ATPase information. The other way to use gel electrophoresis is to use single muscle fibers in each well of the electrophoresis device, rather than using a homogenized mixture of a number of muscle fibers. The advantage of the single-fiber technique is the separation of the MHCs is on a per fiber basis. This technique has identified not only the three pure fiber types (types I, IIa, and IIx) that make up the myosin protein, but also mixtures of the MHCs referred to as hybrid fiber types.[44] In hybrid fiber types, the two MHCs that make up the myosin protein are made up of two different MHCs and have been identified to exist as a continuum between the "pure" myosin proteins, that is, a myosin protein with two MHCs that are the same. Hybrid fiber types identified in humans include MHC I/IIa (found in the continuum between types I and IIa) and MHC IIa/IIx (found between types IIa and IIx). They generally exist in a hierarchal fashion along the continuum of human muscle fiber types.[44]

The purpose of understanding the techniques for determining muscle fiber types has to do with the original controversial debate: Can muscle fiber type change with chronic training? Changes in muscle fiber type from IIx to IIa and vice versa have been found in many studies over the years using ATPase stains and using gel electrophoresis with homogenized muscle samples. Because these studies have shown little evidence of fast (type II) to slow (type I) fiber conversion, it was accepted that changes were only possible within the fast fiber types. Because fewer studies have identified changes from slow to fast or fast to slow, the possibility of this conversion is a topic of debate by muscle physiologists. A likely explanation for the few studies that have observed the conversion from fast to slow or slow to fast is that the hybrid fiber type found in the continuum from slow to fast may be moldable to the type of training being performed to cause changes from slow to fast. For example, Andersen et al.[39] observed a decrease in the fibers that contain only MHC type I and an increase in the fibers that contain only MHC type IIa after 3 months of intensive strength and sprint training. Liu et al.[40] also found that strength training with a combination of methods that included heavy lifting on one day, ballistic strength training another day, and stretch shortening cycle training on a third day of the week during a 6-week training program produced decreases in type I with increases in IIa and no significant change in IIx fibers. The group who trained with heavy lifting 3 days per week was found to only convert IIx fibers to IIa with no significant change in type I. These two studies indicate that high-velocity movements may provide a stimulus to change slow fibers to fast fibers. Although the methods for detecting the hybrid fiber types have only recently been developed,[44] it might be that there was an abundant number of type I/IIa fibers (a hybrid of one MHC type I and one MHC type

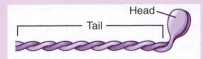

**Figure 10-12.** Two myosin heavy chains and the architecture used to make up a myosin protein.

*Continued*

## NEUROMUSCULAR ADAPTATIONS AFTER CESSATION OF RESISTANCE TRAINING

Individuals involved in a resistance training program occasionally must reduce training or stop altogether for many reasons, including injury, work-related travel, or just a busy lifestyle. During these periods of training cessation, the principle of training reversibility, or detraining, suggests that the stoppage or marked reduction of training leads to a partial or complete reversal of training-induced adaptations.[17] On such occasions, it is helpful to know the quantity of training necessary to maintain strength levels when time is limited.

It has been demonstrated that following at least 10 weeks of strength training, three times per week, where strength gains were documented, if training frequency was reduced to only one training session per week, strength can be maintained for at least 12 weeks.[45] It is important to mention that training mode, duration, and especially intensity must be maintained in the training program to maintain the strength gains over this period of reduced training. Therefore, it appears that missing an exercise session periodically or reducing training frequency for up to 3 months will not adversely affect muscular strength as long as other training variables (i.e., intensity) are maintained.

With complete cessation of strength training, the degree of strength loss appears to depend on training experience, the length of the cessation period, and age. Strength-trained athletes who have chronically trained for many years take longer to lose strength than those who have only strength-trained for a few months.[45,46] Strength-trained athletes likely retain strength for a longer period because of the greater gains in muscle mass over long training periods. Although significant muscle mass loss in the type II muscle fibers has been shown to occur following 14 days of detraining in strength-trained athletes,[46] strength does not appear to be affected until after longer periods of training cessation.[47] It has been proposed that following 4 weeks of training cessation, neural training adaptations are significantly lost, whereas following 8 to 12 weeks, a significant loss of muscle fiber size in both type I and type II muscle fibers contributes to the losses in muscular strength in strength-trained athletes.[47]

Differences in the response to complete training cessation appear to be different when the strength gains are recently acquired and may vary by age as well. During short-term training programs (usually 8–12 weeks), rapid increases in strength take place by previously untrained individuals. Younger (20–30 years old), untrained men and women tend to increase strength more than older (65–75 years old) men and women in short-term training programs.[48] During detraining, the older population appears to experience a greater decrease in absolute strength (how much weight can be lifted); however, relative to the gains seen in the initial training program, there is little difference in the percent of strength loss seen after 12 weeks of no training. If training continues to be neglected, however, the older population tends to see both greater absolute and relative strength losses than the younger population. Therefore, strength gains are maintained equally well in young and old men and women for up to about 12 weeks following complete training cessation; however, changes during longer periods of detraining may be affected by age.

## VIGNETTE Conclusion

■ As many as half of all new exercisers drop out of their routines within the first 6 months of participation. Oscar's dedication to performing his new workout plan will certainly be challenged as he strives to juggle the family, work, and social aspects of his busy life. However, if Oscar can continue to maintain his weight-lifting routine, and eventually add in aerobic exercise and stretching, the overall health and fitness benefits of being a regular exerciser will far outweigh the time or perceived inconvenience of committing to such a program.

Fitness professionals can assist individuals like Oscar in maintaining exercise adherence and progressing properly through their programs by providing sound education on the benefits of being physically active and by designing safe and creative workout programs. Understanding the neuromuscular mechanisms behind the acute responses and chronic adaptations to exercise helps fitness professionals communicate the myriad changes that occur in the musculoskeletal system because of regular training in a way that can be motivating and applicable to all exercisers.

## CRITICAL THINKING QUESTIONS

1. How would you explain the difference in reaction times between a simple reflex arc (such as withdrawal from a painful stimulus) and a planned motor response (such as deciding to step out of the way of an oncoming vehicle)?

2. After 2 months of working with a very athletic client on strengthening his lower extremities for recreational sports participation, you introduce stiff-leg dead lifts into his weight-training routine. Three days after the workout, your client reports to you that his legs, specifically his hamstrings, are extremely sore and he has not experienced this type of discomfort until now. What could be the reason for this client's new degree of post-workout muscle soreness, considering he is a conditioned recreational athlete and has been consistently exercising his lower extremities for the past 2 months?

3. Explain why it is important to stretch a muscle slowly while stretching, no matter whether you are using static or dynamic stretching exercises.

4. A client you have been training for the last 6 months has made significant improvements in strength and muscle mass. He is concerned that all of his training in recent months will be wasted because he has a business trip scheduled with no access to exercise equipment for a 10-day period. What can you tell him to ease his mind that he will be able to take his business trip and not lose any significant progress made over the last 6 months?

## ADDITIONAL RESOURCES

Enoka RM. *Neuromechanics of Human Movement*. 4th ed. Champaign, IL: Human Kinetics; 2008.
Shumway-Cook A, Woollacott MH. *Motor Control: Translating Research Into Clinical Practice*. 4th ed. Baltimore, MD: Wolters Kluwer/Lippincott Williams, & Wilkins; 2011.

International Health, Racquet and Sportsclub Association: www.ihrsa.org.
American Council on Exercise: www.acefitness.org.

## REFERENCES

1. International Health, Racquet & Sportsclub Association. The IHRSA Health Club Consumer Report: The Story Behind Members and Their Health Clubs. 2013. Boston, MA: International Health, Racquet & Sportsclub Association.
2. Guissard N, Duchateau J. Neural aspects of muscle stretching. *Exerc Sport Sci Rev*. 2006;34:154–158.
3. Behm DG, Chaouachi A. A review of the acute effects of static and dynamic stretching on performance. *Eur J Appl Physiol*. 2011;11:2633–2651.
4. Bandy WD, Irion JM, Briggler M. The effect of static stretch and dynamic range of motion training on the flexibility of the hamstring muscles. *J Orthop Sports Phys Ther*. 1998;27:295–300.
5. Pette D, Staron RS. Myosin isoforms, muscle fiber types, and transitions. *Microsc Res Tech* 2000;50:500–509.
6. Brooks GA, Fahey TD, Baldwin KM. *Exercise Physiology: Human Bioenergetics and Its Applications*. 4th ed. New York, NY: McGraw Hill; 2005.
7. Wilmore JH, Costill DL, Kennedy WL. *Physiology of Sport and Exercise*. 4th ed. Champaign, IL: Human Kinetics; 2008.
8. Close R. Properties of motor units in fast and low skeletal muscles of the rat. *J Physiol*. 1967;193:45–55.
9. Binder MD, Heckman CJ, Powers RK. The physiological control of motor neuron activity. In: Rowell LB, Shepherd JT, eds. *Handbook of Physiology: Sec. 12. Exercise: Regulation and Integration of Multiple Systems* (pp. 3–53). New York, NY: Oxford University Press; 1996.
10. Van Cutsem M, Duchateau J, Hainaut K. Neural adaptations mediate increase in muscle contraction speed and change in motor unit recruitment behavior after dynamic training. *J Physiol*. 1998;513:295–305.
11. Van Cutsem M, Feiereisen P, Duchateau J, Hainaut K. Mechanical properties and behavior of motor units in the tibialis anterior during voluntary contractions. *Can J Appl Physiol*. 1997;22:585–597.
12. Enoka RM. *Neuromechanics of Human Movement*. 4th ed. Champaign, IL: Human Kinetics; 2008.
13. Petit J, Giroux-Metges MA, Gioux M. Power developed by motor units of the peroneus tertius muscle of the cat. *J Neurophysiol*. 2003;90:3095–3104.
14. Bosco C, Viitasalo J, Komi P, Luhtanen P. Combined effect of elastic energy and myoelectrical potentiation during stretch-shortening cycle exercise. *Acta Physiol Scand*. 1982;114:557–565.
15. Bobbert M, Gerritsen K, Litjens M, Van Soest A. Why is countermovement jump height greater than squat jump height? *Med Sci Sports Exerc*. 1996;28:1402–1412.
16. Taube W, Leukel C, Gollhofer A. How neurons make us jump: The neural control of stretch-shortening cycle movements. *Exerc Sport Sci Rev*. 2012;40:106–115.
17. Nybo L. CNS fatigue and prolonged exercise: Effect of glucose supplementation. *Med Sci Sports Exerc*. 2003;35:589–594.
18. Felipo V, Butterworth RF. Neurobiology of ammonia. *Progr Neurobiol*. 2002;67:259–279.
19. Jones LA, Hunter IW. Effect of fatigue on force sensation. *Exp Neurol*. 1983;81:640–650.
20. Clarkson P, Sayers S. Etiology of exercise-induced muscle damage. *Can J Appl Physiol*. 1999;24:234–248.
21. Friden J, Lieber R. Structural and mechanical basis of exercise-induced injury. *Med Sci Sports Exerc*. 1992;24:521–530.
22. Smith L. Acute inflammation: The underlying mechanism in delayed onset muscle soreness. *Med Sci Sports Exerc*. 1991;23:542–551.
23. Leiber RL, Fridén J. Functional and clinical significance of skeletal muscle architecture. *Muscle Nerve*. 2000;23:1647–1666.
24. Akima H, Takahashi H, Kuno SY, et al. Early phase adaptations of muscle use and strength to isokinetic training. *Med Sci Sports Exerc*. 1999;31:588–594.

25. Häkkinen K, Kraemer WJ, Newton RU, Alén M. Changes in electromyographic activity, muscle fiber and force production characteristics during heavy resistance/power strength training in middle-aged and older men and women. *Acta Physiol Scand.* 2001;171:51–62.

26. Rutherford OM, Jones DA. The role of learning and coordination in strength training. *Eur J Appl Physiol.* 1986;55:100–105.

27. Sale DG. Neural adaptation to strength training. *Med Sci Sports Exerc.* 1988;20:S135–S145.

28. Desmedt JE, Godaux E. Ballistic contractions in man: Characteristic recruitment pattern of single motor units of the tibialis anterior muscle. *J Physiol.* 1977;264:673–693.

29. Carroll TJ, Riek S, Carson RG. Neural adaptations to resistance training: Implications for movement control. *Sports Med.* 2001;31:829–840.

30. Chalmers G. Do Golgi tendon organ really inhibit muscle activity at high force levels to save muscles from injury, and adapt with strength training? *Sports Biomech.* 2002;1:239–249.

31. Duchateau J, Enoka RM. Neural adaptations with chronic activity patterns in able-bodied humans. *Am J Phys Med Rehabil.* 2002;81(11 Suppl.):517–527.

32. Amiridis IG, Martin A, Morlon B, et al. Co-activation and tension-regulating phenomena during isokinetic knee extension in sedentary and highly skilled humans. *Eur J Appl Physiol.* 1996;73:149–156.

33. Carolan B, Cafarelli E. Adaptations in coactivation after isometric resistance training. *J Appl Physiol.* 1992;73:911–917.

34. Sale DG. Neural adaptation to strength training. In: Komi P, ed. *Strength and Power in Sport.* 2nd ed. Oxford, United Kingdom: Blackwell Publishing; 2003.

35. Duchateau J, Semmler JG, Enoka RM. Training adaptations in the behavior of human motor units. *J Appl Physiol.* 2006;101:1766–1775.

36. Edgerton VR, et al. The matching of neuronal and muscular physiology. In: Borer KT, et al., eds. *Frontiers of Exercise Biology.* Champaign, IL: Human Kinetics; 1991.

37. Staron RR, Malicky ES, Leonardi MJ, Falkel JE, Hagerman FC, Dudley GA. Muscle hypertrophy and fast fiber type conversions in heavy-resistance-trained women. *Eur J Appl Physiol.* 1990;60:71–79.

38. Tesch PA, Hakinen K, Komi PV. The effect of strength training and detraining on various enzyme activities. *Med Sci Sports Exerc.* 1985;17:245.

39. Andersen JL, Klitgaard H, Saltin B. Myosin heavy chain isoforms in single fibres from m. vastus lateralis of sprinters: Influence of training. *Acta Physiol Scand.* 1994;151:135–142.

40. Liu Y, Schlumberger A, Wirth K, Schmidtbleicher D, Steinacker JM. Different effects on human skeletal myosin heavy chain isoform expression: Strength vs. combination training. *J Appl Physiol.* 2003;94:2282–2288.

41. Costill DL, Daniels J, Evans W, Fink W, Krahenbuhl G, Saltin B. Skeletal muscle enzymes and fiber composition in male and female athletes. *J Appl Physiol.* 1976;40:149–254.

42. Widrick J, Stelzer J, Shoepe T, Gardner D. Functional properties of human muscle fibers after short term resistance exercise training. *Am J Physiol.* 2002;283:R408–R416.

43. Barany M. ATPase activity of myosin correlated with speed of muscle shortening. *J Gen Physiol.* 1967;50:197–218.

44. Galpin A, Raue U, Jemiolo B, et al. Human skeletal muscle fiber type specific protein content. *Anal Biochem.* 2012;425:175–182.

45. Graves JE, Pollack ML, Leggett SH, Braith RW, Carpenter DM, Bishop LE. Effect of reduced training frequency on muscular strength. *Int J Sports Med.* 1988;9:316–319.

46. Hortobágyi T, Houmard JA, Stevenson JR, Fraser DD, Johns RA, Israel RG. The effects of detraining on power athletes. *Med Sci Sports Exerc.* 1993;25:929–935.

47. Mujika I, Padilla S. Muscular characteristics of detraining in humans. *Med Sci Sports Exerc.* 2001;33:1297–1303.

48. Lemmer J, Hurlbut D, Martel G, et al. Age and gender responses to strength training and detraining. *Med Sci Sports Exerc.* 2000;32:1505–1512.

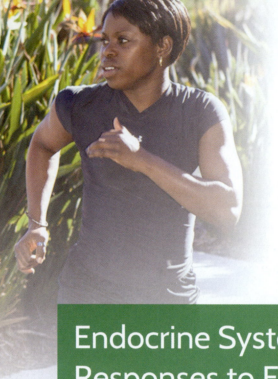

Glenn Wright, PhD
Sabrena Merrill, MS

CHAPTER 11

# Endocrine System and Hormonal Responses to Exercise

## CHAPTER OUTLINE

## LEARNING OUTCOMES

1. List the main structures of the endocrine system and the hormones that they produce.
2. Explain the basic actions of the hormones released by the major endocrine glands.
3. Compare and contrast the two major classes of hormones (steroid vs. nonsteroid hormones).
4. Explain the negative feedback system as it relates to endocrine system control of physiological functions.
5. Describe the hormonal regulation of metabolism during exercise, including the hormones involved and how they influence the availability of carbohydrates and fats for energy during prolonged exercise.
6. Describe the hormonal regulation of fluid balance during exercise.
7. Explain the major endocrine system adaptations experienced as a result of chronic exercise training.

## ANCILLARY LINK

Visit Davis*Plus* at http://davisplus.fadavis.com for study and practice resources, including online quizzes, animations that help explain physiological processes, podcasts concerning news and career trends in exercise physiology, and practice references.

## *VIGNETTE*

■ As long as Perla can remember, she has dreamed of becoming a competitive gymnast. At the age of 6, Perla's parents enrolled her in her first tumbling class at a local gymnastics center, and she has been continuously involved with the sport since that time. At the age of 13, Perla began competing on a national level and showed promise as an Olympic hopeful. During the transition from regional to national competition, Perla experienced her first menstrual period (menarche) and grew increasingly concerned about her appearance and body weight. To deal with her body-image concerns, Perla focused intently on increasing her practice hours in the gym and decreasing her caloric intake. These alterations in lifestyle directly affected Perla's endocrine system to the point that she stopped menstruating. At first, Perla was pleased with not having to deal with monthly cycles, but she soon learned from her physical education teacher that not menstruating could lead to serious health problems.

How might Perla's lack of menstrual periods affect her long-term health and performance?

The integration and regulation of bodily operations is in large part facilitated by the endocrine system. Almost all aspects of human function are influenced by biochemical messengers called **hormones** that are produced by endocrine glands and tissues. Hormones regulate growth, metabolism, sexual development and function, and responses to stress. Because of their involvement in the regulation of metabolism and stress, hormones play a significant role in the body's responses to acute exercise and chronic physical training.

as fuel mobilization and metabolism to provide energy for cell function, hydration status, and protein synthesis for repair of tissues following exercise. Having no ducts, endocrine glands release their hormones directly into the extracellular spaces around the tissues, where the hormones diffuse into the bloodstream for transport to **target tissues**, that is, tissues (or cells) where the hormones perform their function. Table 11-1 lists the major endocrine glands involved with the response to exercise and summarizes some selected effects of their associated hormones.

## STRUCTURAL OVERVIEW OF THE ENDOCRINE SYSTEM

Many of the endocrine glands and other tissues that release hormones regulate many of the responses to exercise. During exercise, hormones regulate such things

## Hypothalamus and Pituitary Gland

The **pituitary gland** is often referred to as the "master gland," because of its regulatory effect on several other endocrine glands and its importance in controlling a number of diverse bodily functions. No larger than a

**Table 11-1.** The Endocrine Glands, Their Hormones, Target Cells, Controlling Factors, and Functions

| ENDOCRINE GLAND | HORMONE | TARGET CELLS | STIMULUS | FUNCTION |
|---|---|---|---|---|
| Anterior Pituitary | Growth hormone (GH) | All cells of the body | Hypothalamus-GH-releasing hormone, GH-inhibiting hormone (somatostatin) | Stimulates growth of the skeletal system and general growth of muscle and other tissues; increases rate of protein synthesis, mobilizes fats for use of fat as energy fuel; decreases carbohydrate use for a fuel |
| | Thyroid-stimulating hormone (TSH) | Thyroid gland | Hypothalamus-thyrotropin-releasing hormone (TRH) | Stimulates the release of thyroxin ($T_4$) and triiodothyronine ($T_3$) released by thyroid gland |
| | Adrenocorticotropic hormone (ACTH) | Adrenal cortex | Hypothalamus-corticotropin-releasing hormone (CRH) | Regulates the release of glucocorticoids from the adrenal cortex |
| | Follicle-stimulating hormone (FSH) | Ovaries, testes | Hypothalamus-gonadotropin-releasing hormone (GnRH) | Initiates release of the follicles and promotes secretion of estrogen in the ovaries in women; stimulates sperm production in men |
| | Luteinizing hormone (LH) | Ovaries, testes | Hypothalamus-gonadotropin-releasing hormone (GnRH) | Causes follicle to rupture, stimulating ovulation; promotes secretion of estrogen and progesterone; causes testes to secrete testosterone |

## Table 11-1. The Endocrine Glands, Their Hormones, Target Cells, Controlling Factors, and Functions–cont'd

| ENDOCRINE GLAND | HORMONE | TARGET CELLS | STIMULUS | FUNCTION |
|---|---|---|---|---|
| Posterior Pituitary | Antidiuretic hormone (ADH) | Kidneys | Hypothalamus-secretory neurons as result of dehydration | Assists in controlling water reabsorption by the kidneys, constricts blood vessels, which helps regulate blood pressure |
| | Oxytocin | Uterus, breasts | Hypothalamus-secretory neurons | Controls uterus contraction during childbirth; milk secretion |
| Thyroid | $T_4$ and $T_3$ | Most cells of the body | TSH from anterior pituitary | Increases rate of cellular metabolism; for body temperature regulation |
| | Calcitonin | Bones | Increased plasma calcium concentrations | Decreases calcium concentration in the blood by increasing osteoblast activity |
| Parathyroid | Parathyroid hormone (PTH) | Bones, intestines, kidneys | Low plasma calcium concentrations | Increases calcium concentration in the blood by increasing osteoclast activity; also increases calcium absorption from intestines and kidneys |
| Adrenal Medulla | Catecholamines (epinephrine and norepinephrine) | Most cells of the body | Sympathetic nervous system activity | Stimulates glycogen catabolism in the liver and skeletal muscle, and mobilizes triglycerides from the adipose tissue and skeletal muscle; increases blood flow to muscle; constricts most arterioles and venules in body, increases blood pressure; increases heart rate and contractility; increases metabolic rate |
| Adrenal Cortex | Aldosterone | Kidneys | Renin-angiotensin mechanism; increased plasma potassium concentrations | Increase sodium retention and potassium excretion through the kidneys; helps maintain plasma volume |

*Continued*

**Table 11-1.** The Endocrine Glands, Their Hormones, Target Cells, Controlling Factors, and Functions—cont'd

| ENDOCRINE GLAND | HORMONE | TARGET CELLS | STIMULUS | FUNCTION |
|---|---|---|---|---|
| | Cortisol | Most cells in the body | ACTH from anterior pituitary | Controls metabolism of carbohydrates, catabolism of proteins, and mobilization of fats; exerts anti-inflammatory effects |
| | Small amounts of testosterone and estrogens | Ovaries, breasts, and testes, muscle and adipose tissue | ACTH | Assist in development of female and male sex characteristics (see Testes and Ovaries later in table) |
| Pancreas | Insulin | Most cells of the body | Increased plasma glucose and amino acid concentrations | Decreases blood glucose levels; increases use of glucose as fuel or storage as glycogen; increases storage of fat in adipose tissue, increases uptake of amino acids |
| | Glucagon | Primarily liver | Low blood glucose concentrations; sympathetic stimulation | Stimulates gluconeogenesis and glycogenolysis in the liver and lipolysis in adipose tissue to maintain blood glucose levels |
| Testes | Testosterone | Sex organs, skeletal muscle, bone, and others | LH | Promotes male reproductive organ growth and other male sex characteristics, promotes skeletal muscle growth, sperm production, libido |
| Ovaries | Estrogens | Many tissues including adipose, bone, uterus | FSH | Promotes female reproductive growth and development, regulates menstrual cycle and pregnancy; maintains bone mineral content; distributes fat in adipose tissue |
| | Progesterone | Uterus, breasts | | Regulates menstrual cycle and pregnancy, prepares breasts for lactation |

pea, the pituitary gland is located at the base of the brain beneath the **hypothalamus** and is divided into anterior and posterior lobes (Fig. 11-1).

Working together with the hypothalamus, the anterior lobe of the pituitary gland has a widespread influence throughout the body. The hypothalamus is linked to the anterior pituitary lobe through a specialized circulatory system, which functions to transport specific hormones called **releasing factors** and **inhibiting factors** from the hypothalamus to the anterior pituitary lobe. Releasing factors are hormones that function to control the release of other hormones by stimulating the pituitary; that is, before the release of an anterior pituitary hormone, the anterior pituitary must be stimulated by the hypothalamus. Input from the nervous system about stimuli such as anxiety, stress, and physical exertion controls the output of releasing factors from the hypothalamus. Inhibiting factors perform the opposite function by inhibiting pituitary hormone release. Thus, although the pituitary gland has been called the "master gland," it is really the hypothalamus that is controlling its functions.

The anterior portion of the pituitary gland releases six hormones that affect various important bodily functions: **follicle-stimulating hormone (FSH)**, **luteinizing hormone (LH)**, **thyroid-stimulating hormone (TSH)**, **adrenocorticotropin hormone (ACTH)**, **growth hormone (GH)**, and **prolactin**. Of these six hormones, four are tropic hormones (i.e., FSH, LH, TSH, and ACTH) and the remaining two (i.e., GH and prolactin) are nontropic.

**Tropic hormones** are substances that stimulate other endocrine organs to secrete their own hormones. For example, FSH and LH are called *gonadotropins* because of their effects on the gonads (ovaries and testes). These substances control the secretion of **estrogen** and **progesterone** in the ovaries and the production of **testosterone** in the testes. TSH stimulates the synthesis and release of triiodothyronine ($T_3$) and thyroxine ($T_4$) (known together as the "thyroid hormones") from the thyroid gland. ACTH controls the secretion of glucocorticoid hormones (cortisol) in the adrenal gland that influence the metabolism of carbohydrates and maintenance of blood glucose levels.

**Nontropic hormones** stimulate target cells directly to induce effects. GH specifically stimulates growth of the skeletal system, but also general growth of muscle and other tissues. Because it promotes cell division and cellular proliferation throughout the body, GH plays a major role in protein synthesis. By facilitating amino acid transport through the cell membrane into the cells, GH acts as a potent anabolic agent. GH also supports the action of cortisol by decreasing glucose uptake by the tissues, increasing **free fatty acid (FFA)** mobilization to the blood, and enhancing **gluconeogenesis** (the formation of glucose from noncarbohydrate sources) in the liver. The net effect of these actions of GH is to preserve blood glucose concentration in the blood for use by the nervous system and muscle cells.

Lastly, prolactin is involved in mammary gland development along with the initiation and maintenance of breast-milk production and secretion during and after pregnancy in females.

The hormones secreted by the posterior pituitary are actually produced by neurons that originate in the hypothalamus and terminate in the posterior lobe of the pituitary. These hormones actually move down the axons and are essentially stored in the posterior pituitary gland. These hormones are then released into circulation as needed by stimulation of a neural reflex to the hypothalamus.

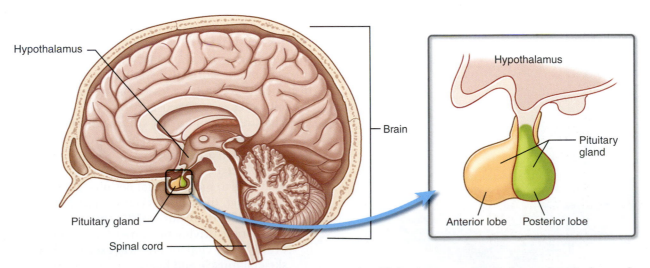

**Figure 11-1. Pituitary gland.** Often referred to as the "master gland," the pituitary gland is located at the base of the brain beneath the hypothalamus and is divided into anterior and posterior lobes.

The posterior lobe releases a hormone called **antidiuretic hormone (ADH)**, which is also called *vasopressin*. ADH acts on the kidneys and is considered an **antidiuretic** (i.e., a substance that inhibits urine production, thereby aiding in the retention of bodily fluid). In essence, ADH controls water loss by the kidneys by increasing the water permeability of the kidney's collecting ducts, facilitating the conservation of water in the blood. The posterior portion of the pituitary also releases **oxytocin**, a hormone that stimulates the smooth muscles of the reproductive organs and intestines. In new mothers, oxytocin contracts the uterus during childbirth and stimulates milk production after childbirth.

## Thyroid Gland

Often called the "major metabolic hormones," $T_3$ and $T_4$ are iodine-containing hormones that are released by the thyroid (Fig. 11-2) to regulate the metabolic rate, thereby increasing the body's oxygen consumption and heat production. The thyroid hormones also act permissively (its presence improves the function of other hormones) with other hormones, especially to assist in the metabolism of carbohydrates, proteins, and lipids. Some of the permissive effects of $T_3$ and $T_4$ are to improve:

- Protein and enzyme synthesis
- Rapid cellular uptake of glucose
- **Glycolysis** and gluconeogenesis
- Lipid mobilization, increasing FFAs for use in aerobic metabolism

The third hormone released by the thyroid gland, calcitonin, decreases blood calcium and phosphate levels by accelerating the absorption of calcium by the bones. The skeleton is in a constant state of remodeling whereby old bone is cleaved away by cells called **osteoclasts** and new bone is laid down by cells called **osteoblasts**. Calcitonin

inhibits bone removal by the osteoclasts while simultaneously promoting bone formation by the osteoblasts.

## Parathyroid Glands

The **parathyroid glands** are four structures—sometimes more depending on a person's anatomy—located on the posterior surface of the thyroid gland. These glands release parathyroid hormone (PTH), which is primarily responsible for controlling the levels of calcium and phosphate in the blood through its actions on the kidneys, skeleton, and small intestine. When blood calcium levels are low, PTH increases bone **resorption** (i.e., stimulates osteoclasts), which functions to break down bone mineral (calcium and phosphate) for its release into the blood. PTH also signals the kidneys to reabsorb calcium so that it is not lost in the urine, and excrete phosphate. PTH also provokes increased calcium absorption by the intestinal wall and works synergistically with vitamin D to maintain the body's calcium levels.

## Adrenal Glands

The **adrenal glands** are two pyramid-shaped organs located close to the superior border of each kidney (Fig. 11-3). Each gland consists of two distinct parts: the **medulla** (inner portion) and the **cortex** (outer portion). The adrenal medulla and the adrenal cortex are so distinct that each portion is, in effect, its own distinct endocrine organ. The adrenal medulla is part of the sympathetic nervous system and produces two hormones: **epinephrine** (adrenaline) and **norepinephrine** (noradrenaline). Collectively, these substances are called **catecholamines** and they function cooperatively to prepare the body for emergencies or stressful events. They exert widespread effects on the organ systems that are critical for exercise performance. This readying process is often referred to as the fight-or-flight response and consists of preparing the body for strenuous physical activity in the face of an emergency or stressful situation.

Epinephrine is the primary hormone (75%–80%) released by the adrenal medulla. Under the influence of epinephrine (and to a lesser extent, norepinephrine), the following responses occur:

- The strength of cardiac contraction increases, resulting in increased cardiac output due to a greater stroke volume.
- Generalized vasoconstriction in most tissues in the body acts to increase total peripheral resistance. Combined, these effects cause an increase in systolic blood pressure (SBP), thus ensuring an appropriate driving pressure to force blood to the organs most vital for physical exertion, that is, skeletal muscle and heart.
- Vasodilation of heart and active skeletal muscle blood vessels occurs.
- Epinephrine dilates the respiratory passages to aid in moving air into and out of the lungs, and

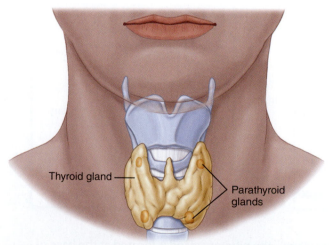

**Figure 11-2.** Thyroid gland and parathyroid glands. The thyroid gland is located anterior to the upper part of the trachea. The parathyroid glands are located on the posterior surface of the thyroid gland.

Thyroid gland

Parathyroid glands

## RESEARCH HIGHLIGHT

### Depressed Thyroid Function Is Not a Clear Cause for Obesity

The increasing prevalence of obesity in the United States and other developed nations has led to an increase in research investigating the causes and comorbidities associated with obesity. Because the thyroid secretes the major metabolic hormones ($T_3$ and $T_4$), it has been the focus of various studies on obesity given that abnormal thyroid function affects metabolic rate. For example, abnormally high $T_4$ secretion can raise basal metabolic rate up to four times greater than normal, resulting in rapid weight loss. In contrast, depressed thyroid function (**hypothyroidism**) can lead to weight gain. Other common symptoms of hypothyroidism include:

- Fatigue
- Puffy face
- Cold intolerance
- Joint and muscle pain
- Constipation
- Dry, thinning hair
- Decreased sweating
- Heavy or irregular menstrual periods and impaired fertility
- Depression
- Slowed heart rate

A direct correlation of obesity with deficient thyroid function is uncertain because the medical literature provides conflicting conclusions. For example, a moderate increase of TSH concentration, which is an endocrine system response to depressed thyroid function, has been found in obese children.[1,2] However, researchers have concluded that elevated TSH levels seem to be a consequence rather than a cause of obesity because weight loss leads to a normalization of increased thyroid hormone levels.

Adding to the uncertainty among the connection between obesity and thyroid function is the fact that weight gain in individuals with hypothyroidism is complex and not always related to excess fat accumulation. According to the American Thyroid Association, most of the extra weight gained is due to an excess accumulation of salt and water.[3] Furthermore, massive weight gain is rarely associated with hypothyroidism. Generally, only 5 to 10 pounds of body weight may be attributable to the thyroid, depending on the severity of the hypothyroidism. Lastly, if weight gain is the only symptom of hypothyroidism that is present, it is less likely that the weight gain is solely due to the thyroid.

Considering that hypothyroidism is prevalent in only 3.7% of the U.S. population,[4] and that obesity occurs at a much higher rate (approximately one third of U.S. adults are obese),[5] thyroid dysfunction is not a common cause of obesity. If a fitness professional encounters an obese client who reports weight gain along with other common symptoms of hypothyroidism, the client should be referred to his or her health-care professional for evaluation.

Aoki Y, Belin RM, Clickner R, Jeffries R, Phillips L, Mahaffey KR. Serum TSH and total T4 in the United States population and their association with participant characteristics: National Health and Nutrition Examination Survey (NHANES 1999-2002). *Thyroid.* 2007;17:1211–1223.

American Thyroid Association. Thyroid and Weight Patient Brochure. 2005. www.thyroid.org/patients/brochures/Thyroid_and_Weight.pdf

Flegal KM, Carroll MD, Ogden CL, Curtin LR. Prevalence and trends in obesity among US adults, 1999-2008. *J Am Med Assoc.* 2010;303:235–241.

Grandone A, Santoro N, Coppola F, Calabrò P, Perrone L, Miraglia del Giudice E. Thyroid function derangement and childhood obesity: An Italian experience. *Biomed Central Endocr Disord.* 2010;10:8. www.biomedcentral.com/1472-6823/10/8

Marras V, Casini MR, Pilia S, et al. Thyroid function in obese children and adolescents. *Horm Res Paediatr* 2010;73:193–197.

reduces digestive activity and bladder emptying during exercise.

- Blood glucose concentration is also influenced by the release of epinephrine.

In general, epinephrine stimulates the mobilization of stored carbohydrates and fats for the purpose of making them available as energy to fuel muscular work.

- Specifically, epinephrine stimulates the release of liver glycogen (**glycogenolysis**) and provides the substrates for production of glucose in the liver (gluconeogenesis). It also stimulates glycogenolysis in skeletal muscles.
- Epinephrine also increases blood fatty acid levels by promoting **lipolysis** (the breakdown of triglycerides in adipose tissue to FFAs and glycerol).
- Epinephrine affects the central nervous system by promoting a heightened state of arousal and increased alertness to permit "quick thinking" to help cope with the impending stressor (or exercise activity).

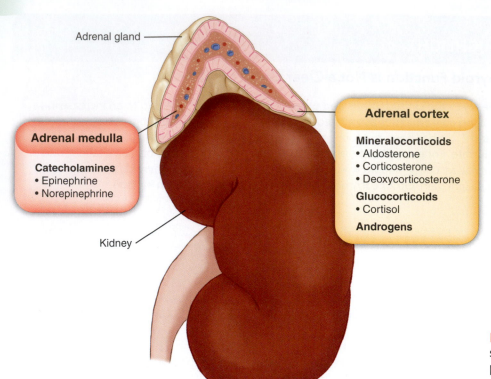

Figure 11-3. Adrenal glands and secretions. The adrenal are two pyramid-shaped organs located close to the superior border of each kidney.

The adrenal cortex secretes mineralocorticoids and glucocorticoids primarily. **Mineralocorticoids** are a group of hormones released from the adrenal cortex that play an important role in regulating extracellular electrolyte balance. Aldosterone is the major mineralocorticoid released from the adrenal cortex and accounts for most (at least 95%) of all mineralocorticoid activity. Aldosterone affects electrolyte balance by promoting the reabsorption of sodium in the kidneys, which results in overall retention of bodily sodium. Water follows sodium such that an increase in sodium also results in fluid retention within the body and an increase in blood pressure. In addition, sodium retention causes potassium excretion, which means that aldosterone also affects potassium balance. Thus, the following factors stimulate aldosterone release:

- Decreased plasma sodium
- Increased plasma potassium
- Decreased blood volume
- Decreased blood pressure
- Increased sympathetic stimulation to the kidneys

Together with ADH, aldosterone works to conserve the body's fluid content. This helps to minimize plasma volume loss, maintain blood pressure, and prevent dehydration.

**Glucocorticoids**, stimulated as a result of low blood glucose levels, are a group of hormones released from the adrenal cortex that facilitate the regulation of plasma glucose concentrations and mobilization of fatty acids. Cortisol (also called *hydrocortisone*) is the major glucocorticoid released from the adrenal cortex; it accounts for approximately 95% of all glucocorticoid presence in the body. Cortisol contributes to FFA mobilization from adipose tissue, glucose synthesis in the liver (i.e., gluconeogenesis), and a decrease in the rate of glucose utilization by the cells. Its effect is slow, however, allowing other faster acting hormones, such as epinephrine and glucagon, to primarily regulate with glucose and FFA mobilization. Besides glucose control, cortisol also acts to stimulate protein catabolism (breakdown) to release amino acids for use in repair and energy production, works as an anti-inflammatory agent, depresses immune reactions, and works synergistically with epinephrine to increase vasoconstriction.

Lastly, the adrenal cortex also releases a small amount of **gonadocorticoids**. Gonadocorticoids are primarily androgens, of which testosterone is most common. Small amounts of estrogens and progesterone are also produced by the adrenal cortex. These amounts, however, are insignificant compared with production in gonads. In women, the androgens account for the low levels of testosterone found in the blood.

## Pancreas

The pancreas is situated behind and slightly below the stomach. In addition to its role in producing digestive enzymes (an exocrine function), the pancreas serves as an endocrine gland that produces hormones involved in regulating carbohydrate metabolism (Fig. 11-4). The islets of Langerhans within the pancreas secretes insulin from the **beta cells (β cells)**

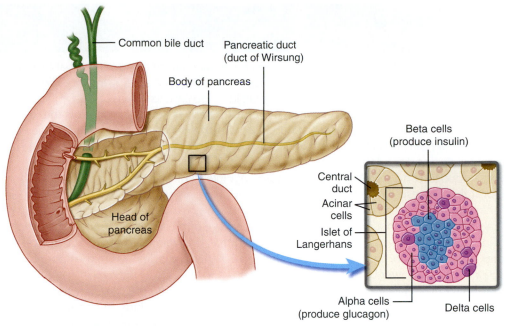

**Figure 11-4.** Pancreas. The pancreas produces digestive enzymes and serves as an endocrine gland that produces hormones involved in regulating carbohydrate metabolism.

and glucagon from the **alpha cells (α cells)**, which work in opposition to control the amount of glucose circulating in the blood.

**Insulin** acts to facilitate the uptake and utilization of glucose (blood sugar) by cells, thereby lowering blood glucose when elevated, such as after a meal that contains carbohydrates. Increased glucose uptake attenuates the breakdown of **glycogen** (the storage form of glucose) in the liver and muscle. Insulin also plays a role in lipid and protein metabolism, as it favors lipid formation and storage, and facilitates the uptake of amino acids into cells.

**Glucagon** generally opposes the actions of insulin. Glucagon stimulates an almost instantaneous release of glucose from the liver and is part of a negative feedback loop in which low blood glucose levels stimulate its release. In other words, one of glucagon's primary roles is to facilitate an increase in blood glucose concentration. Glucagon maintains blood glucose by stimulating the breakdown of liver glycogen (glycogenolysis) and production of glucose from amino acids in the liver (gluconeogenesis). Glucagon also appears to play a secondary role in stimulating lipolysis in adipose, which provides fatty acids as a fuel for cells, and glycerol for gluconeogenesis, conserving glucose in the blood during times of fasting or during long-duration exercise.

In addition to the effect that blood glucose has on stimulating insulin release when glucose levels are high and stimulating glucagon release when glucose levels are low, the sympathetic nervous system and catecholamine levels also regulate release of these pancreatic hormones. Therefore with exercise, as the intensity of exercise increases, the increase in the sympathetic stimulus tends to increase glucagon levels in the blood and inhibit insulin release.

## Gonads

The gonads are the endocrine glands that produce hormones that promote sex-specific physical characteristics and regulate reproductive function. The sex hormones testosterone and estrogen are found in both males and females, but in varying concentrations. In males, testosterone is produced in the testes and regulated by LH from the anterior pituitary. Following secretion from the testes in men and small amounts from the ovaries and adrenal cortex in women, testosterone travels through the circulation bound to transport proteins until binding to target tissues. At the target tissue, testosterone must be released from the transport protein before crossing the cell membrane and ultimately binding to the receptor in the nucleus of the cell, causing an increase in protein synthesis (transcription). Testosterone's **anabolic** (tissue-building) function contributes to the male-female differences in muscle mass and strength that first appear during puberty (see later Sex Differences feature). Testosterone also acts to initiate sperm production (together with FSH), and stimulate the development of the secondary sex characteristics in males.

In females, the ovaries are the primary source for the production of estrogens and progesterone during the menstrual cycle. Estrogens (primarily **estradiol**) regulate follicle maturation and ovulation, menstruation, the physiological adjustments during pregnancy, and the appearance of female secondary sex characteristics. Furthermore, estrogen affects most cells in the female body including the bones, blood vessels, adipose, lungs, liver, and intestines. In females, progesterone primarily prepares the uterus for pregnancy after ovulation takes place and regulates the second half of the menstrual cycle.

## SEX DIFFERENCES

Anthropometric differences between men and women are clearly distinguishable in terms of body size and composition. In early childhood, these differences are minimal, but starting in early adolescence girls begin to accumulate more body fat than boys, and boys begin to increase lean mass at a significantly higher rate than girls. The endocrine system is mainly responsible for these changes because it controls the release of the gonadotropic hormones that begin the process of puberty. In both sexes, the anterior pituitary lobe significantly increases its secretion of FSH and LH, which provokes the ovaries to develop and regulate estrogen release in girls and the testes to develop and regulate sperm production in boys.

Testosterone production and secretion from the testes in adolescent males results in increased bone formation and increased protein synthesis. Consequently, adolescent boys are larger and more muscular than girls, which are physiological characteristics that remain throughout adulthood. The distribution of muscle mass also differs between males and females such that men carry a higher percentage of muscle mass in the upper body compared with women. Findings from Janssen and colleagues[6] revealed that, on average, total skeletal muscle mass in men was 36% greater than in women, and that women exhibited 40% less muscle mass in the upper body and 33% less muscle mass in the lower body compared with men.

Estrogen that is produced and released from the ovaries in adolescent girls stimulates a broadening of the pelvis, breast formation, and increased fat deposition in the thighs and hips. Estrogen also has a significant influence on the growth rate of bone, allowing the final bone length to be achieved within 2 to 4 years after the onset of puberty. This results in a rapid growth spurt in girls around the time of puberty. In contrast, males have a longer growth phase, which can ultimately allow them to attain a greater height than females.

On average, these anthropometric differences between adult males and females mean that women:
- Are approximately 5 inches (13 cm) shorter than men
- Weigh about 30 to 40 lb (14–18 kg) less than men
- Have 40 to 50 lb (18–22 kg) less fat-free mass than men
- Have 7 to 13 lb (3–6 kg) more fat mass than men
- Maintain 6% to 10% more relative body fat than men

## VIGNETTE *continued*

■ When Perla was 16, she suffered a severe tibial fracture from landing incorrectly during one of her gymnastics floor routines. Upon further evaluation and testing, Perla's physician noticed that her bone mineral density was below average for a female of Perla's age. This provoked the physician to ask Perla about her dietary habits and the regularity of her menstrual cycles. Perla replied that she was in constant fear of gaining weight, which led her to eat two small, low-calorie meals each day. She also informed her doctor that she had not had a menstrual period since shortly after she experienced menarche, about 3 years ago. The physician referred Perla to a certified eating disorders specialist and directed her to refrain from any type of high-impact physical activity until after her fracture had fully healed and she had completed thorough rehabilitation of her lower leg.

## CLASSIFICATION OF HORMONES

Hormones are chemical substances produced by endocrine tissues that generally fit into one of two categories: steroid-derived hormones and nonsteroid hormones. The chemical makeup of hormones determines how they interact with target sites throughout the body. (See explanatory animation showing the actions of steroid and non-steroidal hormones on the DavisPlus site at http://davisplus.fadavis.com.)

Most **steroid hormones** are manufactured from cholesterol, which makes them soluble in water and allows them to diffuse rather easily through cell membranes. The adrenal cortex, ovaries, testes, and placenta secrete steroid hormones.

**Nonsteroid hormones** are subdivided further into those made from protein, or **peptide** hormones (made of short amino acid chains of more than two amino acids), and those produced from single amino acids. Nonsteroid hormones are soluble in blood plasma, but because they are derived from an amino acid(s) and not lipid, they cannot cross the cell membrane. As a result, nonsteroid hormones interact with specialized receptors on the cell membrane and not inside the cell. The thyroid gland and adrenal medulla secrete amino acid hormones, whereas all other nonsteroid hormones are made from protein or peptide hormones. The major endocrine organs and the types of hormones they produce are presented in Table 11-2.

Substances called **prostaglandins** are often considered to be a third class of hormones, although technically they are not. Prostaglandins are biologically active lipids found in the plasma membrane of most cells. Typically, prostaglandins *act* as local hormones, meaning that they exert their effects on the immediate area where they are produced and released. However, some can remain intact long enough to circulate in the bloodstream and affect other more distant tissues. Prostaglandins have many functions, but the function most related to the scope of this chapter is their action on blood vessels. Prostaglandins are important mediators of the inflammation response because they increase vascular permeability (which promotes swelling) and vasodilation. In addition, they sensitize nerve endings of pain receptors, making prostaglandins a contributor to both inflammation and pain.

## FROM THEORY TO PRACTICE

Ibuprofen is an over-the-counter (OTC) **NSAID** that is taken to control pain, fever, and inflammation. Common trade names include Advil and Motrin. Ibuprofen works by inhibiting an enzyme called *cyclooxygenase* (COX), which promotes the synthesis of prostaglandins. Thus, the inflammation and pain invoked by the secretion of prostaglandins are blocked when COX is prevented from synthesizing prostaglandins.

Ibuprofen's analgesic (pain-relieving) and anti-inflammatory properties make it an effective drug for the treatment of muscle pain and soft-tissue injury. Headaches, backaches, toothaches, and menstrual pain are also effectively treated with ibuprofen.[7,8,9] In addition, ibuprofen acts as an antipyretic (fever-reducing) medication, so its use for easing the symptoms of the common cold is also common.[10,11]

However, common adverse effects include nausea, indigestion, gastrointestinal ulceration and bleeding, diarrhea, nose bleed, headache, dizziness, fluid retention, and high blood pressure. Long-term use of ibuprofen and other NSAIDs can also lead to acute, reversible renal insufficiency caused by the inhibition of renal vasodilatory prostaglandins.[12]

Because ibuprofen is an effective OTC medication for muscle pain and inflammation, it is often recommended for the discomfort associated with sore muscles after a bout of vigorous exercise and for the treatment of overuse injuries. Fitness professionals should avoid advising their clients to take ibuprofen (or any other medications) and should never offer clients pain relievers before, during, or after their exercise sessions. Recommending any medication (whether OTC or prescription) or nutritional supplement is outside the scope of practice for professionals working in the fitness field. If clients have questions regarding taking a medication for pain relief, they should be referred to their health-care providers to assure the safety of ibuprofen and other NSAIDs, and to minimize adverse effects of their use.

## Table 11-2. Major Endocrine Organs and the Types of Hormones They Produce

| STEROID HORMONES | PEPTIDE-DERIVED HORMONES | AMINO-DERIVED HORMONES |
|---|---|---|
| **Adrenal Cortex** <br> Aldosterone Cortisol | **Hypothalamus** <br> Corticotropic-releasing hormone <br> Gonadotropin-releasing hormone <br> Thyrotropin-releasing hormone | **Adrenal Medulla** <br> Epinephrine <br> Norepinephrine |
| **Gonads** <br> Estrogens <br> Progesterone <br> Testosterone | **Posterior Pituitary** <br> Antidiuretic hormone <br> **Anterior Pituitary** <br> Adrenocorticotropic hormone <br> Follicle-stimulating hormone <br> Thyroid-stimulating hormone <br> Growth hormone <br> **Pancreas** <br> Glucagon Insulin | **Thyroid Gland** <br> Thyroxin <br> Triiodothyronine |

# HORMONE INTERACTIONS WITH TARGET CELLS

Hormones are secreted in response to a need to maintain homeostasis and, as a result, function to return the body's physiology back into normal range. When hormones are released into the bloodstream, they are carried to a specific organ or tissue containing target cells where they must bind to a specific receptor before they can perform their intended functions. Two critical factors determine the strength of the effects of the hormone at the target cells: (1) the plasma concentration of the hormone in the blood, and (2) the number of receptors available to bind to in the cell or on the cell membrane.

Hormone concentration in the plasma is determined by the rate of release of the hormone from its endocrine gland. The rate of release is determined by the incoming input from chemical changes in the plasma, other hormones, and/or the nervous system. The input received comes in as either inhibitory or excitatory information. The net result of the combination of inhibitory or excitatory input determines whether the hormone release will happen, and if it does, the rate at which it will be released.

Hormone concentration in the plasma is also determined by the rate at which the hormone is metabolized (inactivated) or removed from the plasma by the kidneys or liver. Within the blood, hormones circulate either freely or attached to carrier proteins specifically for this purpose. For example, thyroid and steroid hormones require a carrier protein because steroid hormones are not soluble in plasma. Freely circulating hormones remain active for less than an hour, and sometimes only for a few minutes. Hormones bound to carrier proteins may be bound for long durations of time, possibly up to several weeks; however, only unbound hormones can bind to receptors, making the bound hormones somewhat of a reserve that is circulating in the blood. The amount of unbound hormone is determined by the quantity of carrier protein available and the ability of the hormone and carrier protein to bind to each other. The greater number of carrier proteins available allows less "free" hormone concentration in the plasma, decreasing the likelihood of the hormone-receptor binding to take place. This will likely decrease the effect of the hormone, even though there may be a high concentration of the total (free + bound) hormone in the plasma.

Changes in plasma volume during exercise tend to increase the plasma hormone concentration without a change in the rate of secretion or metabolism of the hormone. During exercise, changes in plasma volume occur with fluid shifts caused by changes in blood pressure, metabolite changes, and dehydration caused by sweating.

The target cell's ability to respond to the influence of a hormone depends on the number of target cell receptors that occur either on the cell's membrane (for nonsteroid hormones) or within the cell's interior (for steroid hormones). Hormones connect with their appropriate target cells through a lock-and-key arrangement in which the lock (receptor) can only be opened by a specific key (hormone) (Fig. 11-5). As the circulating hormone travels through a tissue, there are three possibilities for the hormone to determine whether the hormone will have an effect on that cell, and it is determined by the receptors found in the cells of the tissue. Again, referring to the lock-and-key relationship, the three possibilities are:

- The key will not fit the lock (no effect).
- The key will fit the lock, but not turn (no effect, and also blocks the binding site).
- The key will fit the lock and turn (effect).

Cells typically have 2,000 to 10,000 hormone receptors. However, the number of receptors can be altered to increase or decrease the cell's sensitivity to the hormone based on physiological demand. A process called **downregulation** occurs when an increased amount of a specific hormone decreases the number of receptors available to it, making the cell less sensitive to the hormone. This occurs as a physiological mechanism to prevent target cells from over-responding to persistently high hormone levels. Downregulation can be seen in individuals with obesity, because there appears to be a reduction in the number of cells responsive to insulin. Because of the increased levels of blood glucose in an obese individual, the $\beta$ cells in the pancreas must release more insulin than usual to meet the demand and return the blood to homeostatic levels. This near-constant elevation in blood insulin levels can cause target cells to downregulate and decrease the number of receptors for insulin, increasing the subject's resistance by decreasing sensitivity to this hormone. Obese individuals with chronic insulin resistance (or insulin insensitivity) are at risk for the development of type 2 diabetes, because blood glucose remains high despite high insulin levels.

In contrast, **upregulation** describes a state in which target cells develop a greater number of receptors in response to decreasing hormone levels. With upregulation, the greater number of receptors allows the cells to increase sensitivity to the lower concentration of hormone present. Upregulation improves the chance that the little bit of hormone available will bind to a receptor and cause an effect. For example, exercise increases the sensitivity of insulin receptors on the skeletal muscles in individuals with diabetes when insulin levels are chronically low, such as in the case of type 1 diabetes.[13]

Once binding of hormones to receptors takes place, hormones can affect the target cells in one of four ways:

- Modify cellular protein synthesis
- Alter the rate of cellular enzyme activity
- Change plasma membrane permeability
- Promote secretory activity

Hormones can also exert both direct and indirect cellular effects. For example, insulin release prompts muscle

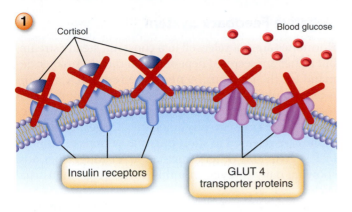

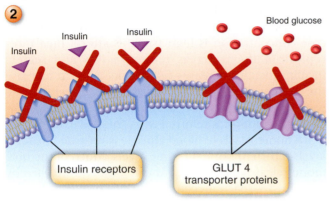

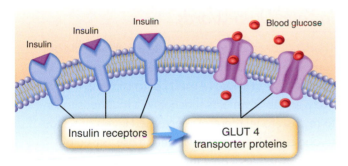

**Figure 11-5.** Relation between hormone and physiological function. Hormones connect with their appropriate target cells through a lock-and-key arrangement in which the lock (receptor) can only be opened by a specific key (hormone). (1) Key will not fit the lock (no effect). In this case, the hormone cortisol (i.e., the key) will not bind to insulin receptors (i.e., the lock). Accordingly, there is no effect; that is, there is no signal provided to GLUT-4 transporter proteins to facilitate blood glucose uptake into the skeletal muscle. (2) Key will fit lock but will not turn (no effect). In this case, the hormone insulin (i.e., the key) cannot bind to insulin receptors (i.e., the lock) because the binding sites are locked. This scenario commonly occurs in obese individuals and is called *insulin resistance*. Similar to (1), there is no blood glucose uptake (i.e., no effect). (3) Key will fit lock and turn (effect). In this case, the hormone insulin (i.e., the key) binds to insulin receptors (i.e., the lock). Subsequently, GLUT-4 transporter proteins are activated and these proteins facilitate blood glucose uptake from the plasma to the skeletal muscle (i.e., the effect).

fibers to take up glucose, which is a primary effect. In conjunction with glucose uptake, muscle fibers increase the synthesis of glycogen, which is a secondary effect. Together, these primary and secondary insulin effects work to maintain fuel **balance** during a bout of exercise.

## Steroid Hormone Activity

Because steroid hormones are lipid based, they pass easily through the cell membrane. Once inside the cell, steroid hormones bind with specific receptors, forming a hormone–receptor complex, which then enters the cell's nucleus and binds with the cell's **deoxyribonucleic acid (DNA)** to activate certain genes. This process is called *direct gene activation* and it causes **messenger ribonucleic acid (mRNA)** to be synthesized within the nucleus. The mRNA is the template for protein synthesis because it carries instructions from the nucleus to the cytoplasm to manufacture new proteins (Fig. 11-6). The proteins may be used for creating enzymes that affect cellular processes, developing structural proteins to be used for tissue growth or repair, or making regulatory proteins that can change enzymatic function.

## Nonsteroid Hormone Activity

Nonsteroid hormones cannot cross the cell membrane, so they must interact with specific receptors on the cell

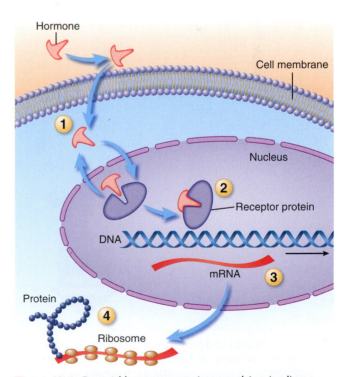

**Figure 11-6.** Steroid hormone action resulting in direct gene activation. (1) The steroid hormone enters the cell and migrates to the cell's nucleus. (2) Within the cell's nucleus the steroid hormone binds with the cell's DNA, resulting in gene activation. (3) mRNA is synthesized within the nucleus. (4) mRNA serves as the template for protein synthesis elsewhere in the cell.

membrane. Thus, it takes two sets of messengers to deliver the signals required to carry out the intended action of the hormone. First, a nonsteroid hormone binds with its receptor on the cell membrane. This triggers a sequence of enzymatic reactions that leads to the creation of a second messenger, which is a molecule inside the cell that transmits signals from the first messenger (hormone) to the target cell. For example, hormone–receptor binding on the cell membrane activates the enzyme adenylate cyclase, which then converts adenosine triphosphate (ATP) to **cyclic adenosine monophosphate (cAMP)**. cAMP is a pervasive second messenger that activates a series of reactions that ultimately has an effect on the cell, activating enzymes for metabolism (Fig. 11-7).

In addition to altering enzyme activity, nonsteroid hormones can either facilitate or inhibit the uptake of certain substances by the cells. For example, insulin facilitates glucose transport into the cell. In contrast, epinephrine inhibits insulin release by the pancreas, thereby slowing glucose uptake by the cells.

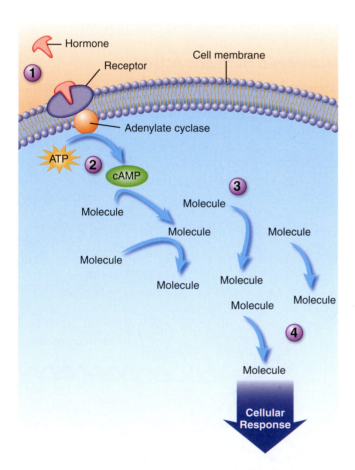

**Figure 11-7.** Nonsteroid hormone action with an intracellular second messenger. (1) A nonsteroid hormone (the first messenger) binds with a receptor on the cell membrane. (2) The nonsteroid hormone–receptor complex activates cyclic adenosine monophosphate (cAMP) within the cell. (3) cAMP acts as a second messenger by activating a sequence of enzymatic reactions. (4) The series of reactions ultimately elicits a cellular response (i.e., the effect).

## Negative Feedback System

Hormones are not released in a constant, steady stream, but rather are secreted depending on the physiologic demand for their actions. A **negative feedback system** is used to regulate the secretion of most hormones such that the release of a specific hormone is increased or decreased in response to physiological changes. Some hormones are released in short bursts in periods of an hour or less, whereas others fluctuate over longer periods, showing daily or even monthly cycles (e.g., menstrual cycles).

The regulation of plasma glucose concentration is an example of how the endocrine system uses negative feedback to maintain homeostasis. When plasma glucose concentration is high (such as after a meal), receptors in the pancreas recognize this and secrete insulin. Insulin increases cell permeability to increase the uptake of glucose, which reduces blood glucose back to homeostatic levels. The return of homeostasis after a disruption is referred to as "negative feedback." Once homeostasis of blood glucose is returned, insulin levels return to normal resting levels. Much of the hormone release in the endocrine system is controlled by negative feedback mechanisms. Cells of the endocrine organs monitor hormone levels and concentrations of ions, nutrients, and even water in the blood and respond accordingly.

## In Your Own Words

There has been extensive coverage in the media of competitive athletes who use anabolic steroids as ergogenic aids to improve sports performance. In the body, anabolic steroids function in a manner similar to testosterone; therefore, increased levels of testosterone exist during anabolic steroid use. Based on your knowledge of how the endocrine system uses a negative feedback system to regulate physiological processes, explain to a friend how regular anabolic steroid use affects a male athlete's testosterone levels in the blood and, as a result, endogenous (internal) testosterone production.

## HORMONAL RESPONSES TO ACUTE EXERCISE

Up to this point, the discussion has focused primarily on the general structure and function of the endocrine system. Normal bodily function depends on the timely release and inhibition of a variety of hormones as they work together to bring about important actions at their target organs. The endocrine system plays a significant role in controlling physiological functions during exercise as well. The significant hormonal actions that are most responsive to an acute bout of exercise are presented in this section.

Two examples of the maintenance of homeostasis by the endocrine system during exercise include the maintenance of blood glucose and the maintenance of plasma volume. Most of the study of acute hormone response to resistance exercise has centered on the anabolic/catabolic responses for changes in muscle mass and body composition.

## Blood Glucose Maintenance

Carbohydrate and fat metabolism maintain ATP production in the muscles during prolonged exercise. Exercise rapidly increases glucose uptake by skeletal muscle, which may increase 7 to 20 times over the values observed at rest.[14] Without a way of maintaining glucose in the blood during exercise, the levels would plummet, leading to hypoglycemia and decreases in performance of the muscles and, more importantly, nervous system function because the primary fuel for brain and nerve cells is blood glucose.

FFAs typically contribute less to the energy needs of the muscles during endurance exercise than carbohydrates; however, mobilization and utilization of FFAs helps to maintain blood glucose by providing an alternate fuel source in the muscles for ATP production. Oxidation of FFA provides more energy during prolonged, low- to moderate-intensity exercise, especially during the later stages of longer duration exercise. Overall, the extent of FFA utilization, and therefore glucose sparing, is dependent on the mobilization of FFA from the adipose (lipolysis) tissue.

A number of hormones regulate glucose and FFA content in the blood during exercise. Despite the large increase in glucose utilization during prolonged, moderate-intensity exercise, blood glucose levels stay surprisingly constant during exercise. The breakdown of stored liver glycogen to glucose (liver glycogenolysis) and the production of glucose in the liver from lactate, amino acids, and glycerol (gluconeogenesis) are primarily responsible for maintaining blood glucose during exercise.

Recall from earlier in this chapter that the increase in liver glycogenolysis is mediated by increases in glucagon. As shown in Figure 11-8, glucagon increases in the blood almost immediately on commencement of exercise, releasing glucose from the liver at the onset of exercise. As a result, it is not uncommon to see a small increase in blood glucose early in a prolonged exercise bout.

Increased muscular activity also stimulates the sympathetic nervous system to increase catecholamine release to further increase liver glycogenolysis. Catecholamine release is rapid at the beginning of exercise (see Fig. 11-8), sometimes showing small, but significant increases as an anticipatory response before exercise begins. Following the initial rise, catecholamine

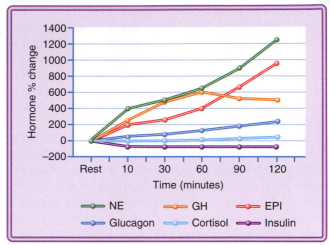

**Figure 11-8.** Percent change in plasma concentrations of selected hormones during 120 minutes of prolonged exercise. *(Data from Kolkhorst, FW and Buono MJ. Virtual exercise physiology laboratory. Baltimore: Lippincott Williams & Wilkins, 2004; and Viru, A and Viru, M. Biochemical monitoring of sport training. Champaign, IL: Human Kinetics Publishers, 2001.)*

release gradually increases throughout the exercise bout and is dependent on exercise intensity. Relatively high-intensity exercise (>60% maximal oxygen consumption [$\dot{V}O_2$max]) shows a large increase in epinephrine,[15] whereas response to low-intensity exercise may be minimal. Activation of the sympathetic system during exercise also suppresses insulin release from the pancreas, decreasing insulin in the blood.[16] This decrease in insulin reduces glucose uptake by the nonworking muscles, thus helping to maintain blood glucose.

During moderate-intensity prolonged exercise, it appears that blood glucose is maintained primarily by the increase in glucagon and decrease in insulin, with the catecholamines playing a more secondary role. During very strenuous exercise, the greater release of glucose from the liver is likely caused by large increases in sympathetic stimulation to increase liver glycogenolysis. Therefore, catecholamines likely play a greater role than the increase in glucagon and decrease in insulin with high-intensity exercise.

Gluconeogenesis in the liver (production of glucose) also provides glucose to the blood during exercise; however, this is more likely a significant factor during lower intensity exercise that takes place for a long duration, and/or after liver glycogen stores are approaching very low levels or have been depleted. The process of gluconeogenesis requires noncarbohydrate substrates (i.e., amino acids, glycerol, and lactate) to be delivered to the liver, where glucose is produced and released into the blood. Recall that cortisol and glucagon both play a role in providing amino acids and glycerol for gluconeogenesis in the liver. Cortisol release is not significantly elevated until later in an exercise bout (>45 minutes), and glucagon levels tend to increase further after liver glycogen has been depleted (see Fig. 11-8). Blood flow to the liver decreases at higher intensity exercise, limiting the extent of the assistance gluconeogenesis may provide during exercise, except at low intensities. Gluconeogenesis likely contributes the most to increases in blood glucose following prolonged exercise if intake of carbohydrate is delayed.

Maintaining blood glucose levels depends on being able to use a mixture of fuels for energy production during prolonged exercise. During the early phases of endurance exercise bouts, carbohydrates are the primary fuel of choice, coming from both muscle glycogen stores and blood glucose. However, gradually over time, prolonged endurance exercise depletes the body's glucose reserves and requires that muscle fibers rely more heavily on the oxidation of FFAs to produce energy for contraction. The greater utilization of FFA as a fuel source serves to conserve blood glucose and, therefore, liver glycogen as well.

FFAs are stored in adipose and muscle tissue as triglycerides. For muscle cells to access these fats stored in the adipose tissue, they must first be broken down and released (mobilized) into the circulation. FFAs are a primary fuel source both at rest and during the later stages of endurance exercise. During physical exertion, the rate at which FFAs are mobilized increases over time to keep up with the muscular demand. Once released, the higher concentration of FFAs in the blood causes an increase of FFA uptake by the muscle cells.

Many of the same hormones that regulate blood glucose are also responsible for the mobilization of FFAs for use as fuel during exercise. These include insulin, catecholamines, glucagon, and cortisol together with GH. Because insulin inhibits FFA mobilization, the decrease in circulating insulin levels during exercise is a major factor that prompts the secretion of the other hormones to begin their function to mobilize FFAs. Notice in Figure 11-8 that the hormones involved with FFA mobilization either take some time to reach peak levels (catecholamines, glucagon, GH) or have a delayed response (cortisol). It is likely that the delayed mobilization of FFA reduces the utilization of FFA for fuel until later in the exercise bout because it takes time for the optimal levels of the lipolytic hormones to reach significance. Once catecholamines, glucagon, GH, and cortisol reach high enough levels, mobilization of FFA from the adipose tissue to the plasma increases to provide an alternate fuel source to the active muscles.

## Plasma Volume Maintenance

The maintenance of plasma volume during exercise is critical for optimal function of the cardiovascular, metabolic, and thermoregulatory systems of the body. When exercise begins, there is a fluid shift from the plasma to the interstitial and intracellular fluid compartments. This is a result of the increase in hydrostatic pressure (blood pressure) that pushes fluid from the plasma, combined with the formation of metabolites that create an increase in osmotic pressure, which pulls fluid from the plasma to these other compartments. During exercise, sweating also increases the movement of fluid out of the plasma and creates further plasma volume losses when the environment (heat and humidity) leads to increased sweat rates during exercise. To counteract the plasma volume shifts during exercise, ADH from the posterior pituitary and aldosterone from the adrenal cortex influence the kidneys to conserve more water, therefore reducing the amount of urine produced. Although both hormones have similar overall effects of maintaining plasma volume, they go about it in difference ways.

ADH is released when osmoreceptors, found in the hypothalamus, determine that the blood has high plasma **osmolality** (high solute concentration) or as a result of low plasma volume caused by improper fluid replacement (Fig. 11-9). There is also evidence to support that exercise is a potent stimulus for ADH secretion.[17,18] ADH release is intensity dependent such that, at intensities greater than approximately 60% $\dot{V}O_2max$, ADH release increases exponentially. Once ADH is secreted from the posterior pituitary, it binds to receptors in the collecting duct and distal convoluted tubule of the kidneys, influencing a greater reabsorption of water to the blood.

Aldosterone release is through a somewhat complicated system, known as the **renin-angiotensin mechanism**, which is related to the regulation of blood pressure. Plasma volume is a major determinant of bloodpressure; that is, when plasma volume decreases, so does blood pressure. There are specialized cells in the kidneys that secrete an enzyme called *renin* in response to low blood pressure in the kidney and direct sympathetic stimulation to the kidney, such as with exercise of increasing intensity. Renin activates a plasma protein called angiotensinogen to angiotensin I, which is, in turn, converted to angiotensinogen II by angiotensin-converting enzyme (ACE) in the lung. Angiotensin II is a very potent vasoconstrictor (which increases blood pressure) and also causes the release of aldosterone from the adrenal cortex. Aldosterone promotes sodium reabsorption in the renal tubule, which increases water content of the plasma (Fig. 11-10) and blood pressure.

The effects of ADH and aldosterone are at work during exercise and persist for up to 12 to 48 hours after a bout of exercise, leading to a reduction in urine production during this time frame. Longer elevations of ADH and aldosterone are related to greater hormone responses created by high-intensity exercise, greater levels of dehydration, or both.

## *FROM THEORY TO PRACTICE:* FAT BURNING AND HIGH-INTENSITY ENDURANCE EXERCISE

You should remember that lipolysis and mobilization of FFA from adipose tissue is influenced most notably by exercise responses of catecholamines, glucagon, GH, and cortisol. The release of each of these hormones is dependent on exercise intensity; that is, the higher the intensity of exercise, the greater the release of these hormones into the blood. It has also been mentioned that the use of FFAs as a fuel source for exercise is dependent on the concentration of FFA in the blood. Then why is it that when prescribing exercise for the purpose of "burning fat," recommendations usually are to exercise at lower intensities? Wouldn't we increase the lipolytic hormones more and mobilize more fat if we exercised harder?

The answers to these questions are that we would indeed increase the circulation of these hormones, because it is true that higher exercise intensity leads to greater release of these hormones into the blood.

However, mobilization of FFAs (and glycerol) from the adipose tissue requires adequate blood flow to the adipose tissue to carry the mobilized FFAs to the muscle. Unfortunately, with higher intensity exercise, blood flow to the adipose tissue is decreased as the need for more blood to the active skeletal muscles increases. The increase in sympathetic stimulation and resulting increases in catecholamines with increases in intensity cause vasoconstriction to tissues that are not as vital to the circulation. With the decrease in blood flow through the adipose tissue during higher intensity exercise, less mobilization of FFA is possible.

Another factor related to the decrease in mobilization of FFAs during high-intensity endurance exercise is blood lactate levels. As intensity increases, blood lactate levels also increase. The lactate in the blood that is received by the adipose tissue is thought to be converted to glycerol phosphate, the form of glycerol necessary to store FFAs as triglycerides in the adipose cells. So, although lipolysis may be stimulated by higher levels of the lipolytic hormones in the blood, the circulating lactate increases the concentration of glycerol in the adipose cells to such a high concentration that as soon as FFAs are released from glycerol, new triglycerides are formed before they can leave the adipose cell.[22] Therefore, to increase the mobilization of FFAs to be utilized as a fuel in the muscle during exercise, the intensity must be high enough to increase the release of the lipolytic hormones into the blood, but not so high that blood flow to the adipose is restricted and blood lactate levels are not much higher than resting levels. Moderate-intensity exercise is typically recommended to realize the greatest utilization of FFAs during prolonged exercise.[23]

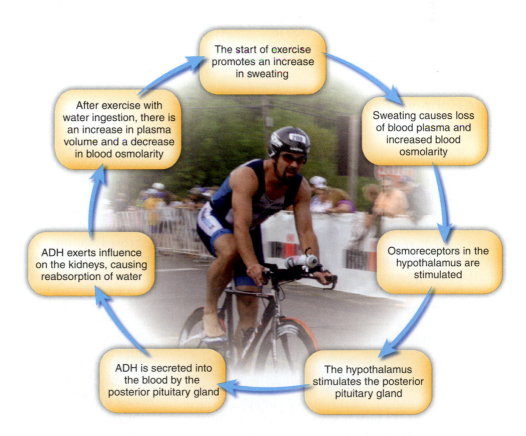

The start of exercise promotes an increase in sweating

Sweating causes loss of blood plasma and increased blood osmolarity

Osmoreceptors in the hypothalamus are stimulated

The hypothalamus stimulates the posterior pituitary gland

ADH is secreted into the blood by the posterior pituitary gland

ADH exerts influence on the kidneys, causing reabsorption of water

After exercise with water ingestion, there is an increase in plasma volume and a decrease in blood osmolarity

**Figure 11-9.** Influence of antidiuretic hormone on the conservation of body water during exercise. *(Photo courtesy of Craig Durant.)*

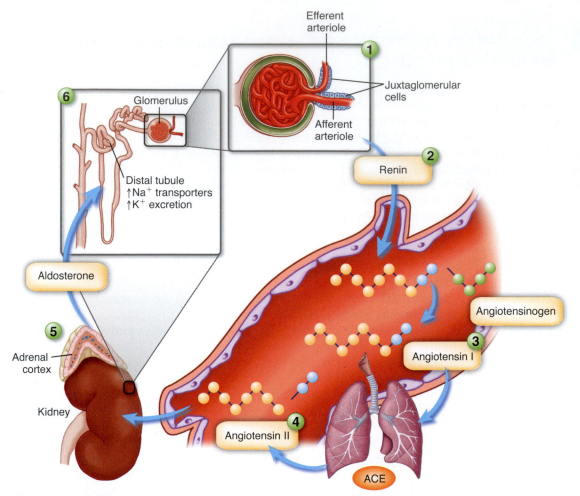

**Figure 11-10.** Influence of aldosterone on the conservation of body water during exercise. The six key steps involved in the renin-angiotensin mechanism are shown. (1) Sweating reduces plasma volume and blood flow to kidneys. (2) Reduced renal blood flow stimulates release of renin. (3) Renin induces formation of angiotensin I. (4) Angiotensin I is converted to angiotensin II by angiotensin-converting enzyme. (5) Angiotensin II stimulates the release of aldosterone. (6) Aldosterone promotes sodium reabsorption, leading to increased water content in the plasma.

## Acute Hormone Response to Resistance Training

Because of the role in promoting protein synthesis and increasing muscle mass, the hormones most studied regarding resistance exercise include testosterone, GH, and cortisol. Hormonal responses to resistance exercise are similar to prolonged aerobic exercise in that the intensity and volume of exercise play an important role in the overall response of the different hormones. However, more training variables play a role when describing the hormone response to resistance training. Training variables that influence hormone release include:

- Exercise choice
- Exercise order
- Volume (total reps)
- Intensity (load)
- Rest between sets

The acute hormone response depends on the many different combinations of the above variables, which makes it difficult to give a simple description of the response to resistance exercise. The following is a summary of what is known to produce the greatest hormone response for the selected hormones that influence protein synthesis resulting in muscle hypertrophy.

### Testosterone

Exercise choice and relative intensity (**percent one repetition max [%1RM]**) are important training variables that regulate testosterone release during resistance exercise. Increases in testosterone levels in the blood are noticed immediately after exercise when training includes exercises that use large muscle groups (total body exercises such as squats, deadlifts, Olympic lifts, etc.) at relatively high loads (>80%–85% 1RM). Resistance exercise sessions with too high of an intensity may limit testosterone release, because very high intensities (approaching 100% 1RM) may limit the amount of volume that can be performed in a training session. Very high volume during a resistance exercise session is likely to reduce the expected testosterone response; lower rest time between sets (~1 minute) has also produced higher testosterone release during an exercise bout.[19]

Testosterone levels in women are approximately 10% that of men, with some variance between women. In general, testosterone levels in women do not change significantly with resistance exercise training[20]; however, this may also vary because some women release greater concentrations of testosterone from the adrenal glands.

## Growth Hormone

Acute GH response to resistance exercise is dependent on a number of training variables. Large muscle mass exercises using high relative loads are important; however, as with testosterone release, too high of intensities may limit the total amount of work performed in an exercise session. Total volume of work completed seems to be a critical variable in seeing elevated GH release. Short rest periods (~1 minute) between sets and exercises also seem to be important for increasing GH in the blood.

Human GH administration has been banned by many sporting organizations, but this has been difficult to enforce. Human GH is naturally occurring and increases with exercise training and competition. It is administered by athletes because of its purported role in stimulating protein synthesis and aiding in the recovery of muscles after strenuous training or competition. Not a lot of science has tested these claims; so much of the claims of what human GH administration can do are anecdotal. Problems stem from such unanswered questions as, what adverse effects are likely, at what dosages, and how much human GH administration is enough to receive the benefits without adverse effects? In addition, for those adverse effects that may be observed, which ones are reversible and which ones are not? For these reasons, GH administration has been banned, but not enforced well primarily because, different from other performance-enhancing drugs and hormones, a blood test is required to detect GH use. Other "drug testing" has been done using urine samples, which are less invasive and easier to obtain than blood samples.

## Cortisol

Like GH, cortisol increases during resistance training when workouts include large muscle mass exercises, high-volume training with short rest periods between sets. Cortisol response to resistance exercise seems to coincide with the anaerobic metabolic load, which is probably why large-muscle, total body–type exercise provides the greatest stimulus for cortisol release.

Cortisol is typically referred to as a catabolic hormone because of its role in protein turnover, lipolysis, and providing substrates for gluconeogenesis. As a result of cortisol's role in muscle protein degradation, many researchers and coaches have attempted to attenuate the release of cortisol through recommending carbohydrate intake during and after exercise.[21] Given the role of cortisol in tissue remodeling, cortisol may be important for breaking down tissue protein to rebuild new proteins following training. It is also likely that increased cortisol following high-intensity resistance training may be exerting its anti-inflammatory effects necessary for any muscle damage triggered by the resistance exercise session. In both of these cases, low-to-moderate acute elevations of cortisol following resistance exercise may actually be an important part of the recovery process.

## HORMONAL ADAPTATIONS TO CHRONIC EXERCISE TRAINING

In general, the hormonal response to a given absolute exercise load declines with chronic exercise training (Fig. 11-11). This increased efficiency may result from improved target tissue sensitivity (upregulation) or responsiveness, or both, to a given amount of hormone. In addition, as changes in physiology (adaptations) take place with chronic training, similar absolute workloads (e.g., km/hr, Watts, kg) following training become lower relative workloads (e.g., % $\dot{V}O_2$max, %1RM) and, therefore, produce less overall stress to the body's physiological systems. This is demonstrated by a reduction of sympathetic nervous system stimulation at similar absolute workloads following training. As a result, the hormones that are regulated at least partially by intensity of exercise (most of them) show much lower secretion rates following training. In addition, at maximal levels following training, many of the hormones discussed previously are secreted at a greater rate. Table 11-3 outlines a selection of hormones and their general responses to endurance-exercise training. Resistance training also

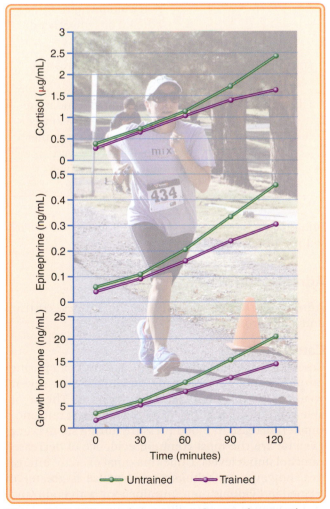

Figure 11-11. Hormonal responses of cortisol, epinephrine, and growth hormone during prolonged exercise in untrained and trained individuals.

## Table 11-3. Hormone Responses to Endurance Exercise and Training

| HORMONE | ACUTE EXERCISE RESPONSE | CHRONIC EXERCISE ADAPTATION | SIGNIFICANCE |
|---|---|---|---|
| Growth Hormone (GH) | Increase with increasing exercise intensity | Lesser response in trained subjects | Increase in fatty acid mobilization and gluconeogenesis |
| Adrenocorticotropic Hormone (ACTH) | Increase with increasing exercise intensity | Unknown | Increases availability of cortisol and other glucocorticoids |
| Thyroxin (T$_4$) | Little or no change | Increase of T$_4$ turnover without toxic effects | Unknown |
| Cortisol | Increases with duration and intensity | Increases less for the same work rate, may increase more with exhaustion | Increases glycogen storage, liver gluconeogenesis, lipolysis, and some anti-inflammatory effect |
| Epinephrine | Increases with intensity, especially >50% maximal oxygen consumption ($\dot{V}O_2$max) | Increases less for same absolute work rate | Increases blood glucose, muscle blood flow, heart rate, contractility |
| Norepinephrine | Increases with intensity beginning at lower intensities than epinephrine; difficult to determine whether adrenal or sympathetic nerves the source | Increases less for same absolute work rate | Blood pressure regulation, increases heart rate, and contractility |
| Insulin | Decreases with increasing work rates | Increases less for same absolute work rate | Reduces the stimulus to utilize blood glucose |
| Glucagon | Increases initially and more significantly with longer duration; decreases after initial increase with short-duration, high-intensity exercise | Increases less following training period | Increases blood glucose by stimulating glycogenolysis and gluconeogenesis |

brings about hormonal response alterations, particularly with testosterone, GH, and cortisol.

## Adrenal Hormones

Adrenal hormones include catecholamines, cortisol, and aldosterone.

## Catecholamines

Catecholamine (i.e., epinephrine and norepinephrine) output declines significantly during the first several weeks of submaximal endurance training. The favorable training adaptations of a lowered heart rate and a smaller increase in blood pressure during submaximal exercise are the most common evidence of decreased catecholamine levels. Under maximal exercise intensities, however, catecholamine response is greater in trained individuals than untrained for both endurance and resistance exercise, likely because trained individuals can perform at higher absolute intensities.

## Cortisol

Circulating cortisol levels tend to decrease slightly as a result of exercise training, likely because of the trained individual being better at preserving blood glucose. However, with acute increases in training volume, trained individuals may experience elevated resting cortisol levels, possibly indicating a state of overreaching or overtraining.

## Aldosterone

Aldosterone levels also tend to be lower at the same absolute workloads following endurance and resistance training. Because sympathetic nervous system response is lower at the same workloads following training, and one stimulus of the cells that release renin from the kidney to set off the renin-angiotensin mechanism is the sympathetic response, there are fewer stimuli for the release of aldosterone from the adrenal cortex during exercise following training.

However, hot and humid environmental conditions may increase aldosterone response to dehydration regardless of the workload.

## Pancreatic Hormones

Individuals who participate in regular endurance exercise maintain blood levels of insulin and glucagon during exercise that are closer to resting values. In addition, insulin receptor sensitivity is improved following training. This is important because the trained state requires less insulin at any specific point from rest through submaximal-intensity exercise. Less sympathetic stimulation following training releases less glucagon and inhibits the release of insulin to a lesser extent. In addition, the combination of resistance exercise and endurance training improves active muscles' insulin sensitivity more than endurance training alone.[24] Thus, individuals with blood glucose regulation problems (i.e., those with metabolic syndrome or diabetes) stand to benefit from both modes of exercise training (Fig. 11-12).

## Growth Hormone

Endurance-trained individuals show a smaller increase in circulating GH levels at a given exercise workload than their untrained counterparts. However, GH release is also stimulated by volume of work done; therefore, if the trained individual increases training volume, such as running a greater distance and or at a higher absolute training intensity (running faster), GH can also be expected to rise with training. Similarly, increased resistance training volume (greater sets, reps, and total amount of weight lifted per workout) and intensity (heavier loads) augments GH release (via increases in testosterone) and interacts with nervous system function to increase muscle force production, especially in men.[25,26]

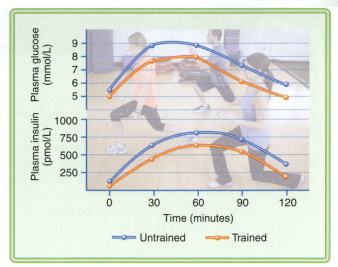

**Figure 11-12.** In response to an oral glucose challenge, both plasma glucose and plasma insulin levels are attenuated following chronic exercise training. This physiological adaptation is beneficial for those individuals at risk for metabolic syndrome and type 2 diabetes.

## Testosterone

In addition to GH, testosterone is a primary hormone that affects resistance-training adaptations. Heavy resistance exercise (i.e., 85%–95% of 1 RM), or moderate- to high-volume training with multiple sets and/or exercises with less than 1-minute intervals, together with training larger muscle groups, leads to an increase in testosterone release.[20] Following long-term resistance training in men, resting testosterone levels increase, which is associated with strength improvement over time.[27]

## In Your Own Words

You are concerned that your 72-year-old grandmother is less stable on her feet than she used to be. Explain to her why she is at greater risk for balance problems and falling.

---

## SEX DIFFERENCES

Both relative and absolute strength comparisons between men and women reveal that men are stronger.[28,29,30] This means that even when total body weight is taken into consideration, men still exhibit more muscular strength than women. In fact, differences in muscle mass and strength between men and women predispose older women to a greater risk for balance problems and falling.[31] Part of the difference can be accounted for by the fact that for a given body weight, most men have a higher fat-free mass than their female counterparts. Lower testosterone levels in women (one tenth of the levels found in men) contribute to women having less overall muscle mass than men, which is the main factor that explains the difference in muscle strength between the sexes.[32]

Despite the muscle mass and strength differences between women and men, women can achieve muscle hypertrophy, and thus influence body composition by increasing fat-free mass, through exercise. Similar to the magnitude of gains in men, women can significantly increase strength by up to 20% to 50% by engaging in a program of regular strength training.[33]

## RESEARCH HIGHLIGHT

### Influence of Hormones on Amenorrhea in Athletes

A condition called the **female athlete triad** has been observed in women, particularly young women, who engage in chronic intense training and who emphasize weight loss. The female athlete triad is a collection of three conditions: (1) disordered eating, (2) **amenorrhea** (menstrual irregularities), and (3) **osteoporosis**.

Of particular importance to female athletes is the influence of the endocrine system on the maintenance of bone. Estrogen provides a protective effect on bone such that from the time a female starts menstruating to the time she experiences menopause, estrogen produced and secreted from the ovaries acts to slow down the body's process of breaking down bone. The following functions illustrate estrogen's role in bone health:

- Increases calcium absorption in the intestines
- Reduces excretion of calcium by the kidneys
- Inhibits bone resorption
- Decreases bone turnover

Certain female athletes are at risk for the development of **primary amenorrhea** (the absence of menarche in females ≥16 years old) or **secondary amenorrhea** (the absence of menstruation for longer than 3 months after normal menstrual function), both of which indicate menstrual dysfunction. Sports such as figure skating, gymnastics, ballet, bodybuilding, diving, distance running, and cycling are associated with higher rates of female athletes who have amenorrhea.

Menstrual dysfunction is a concern because cessation of menstruation removes estrogen's protective effect on bone. This leads to increased calcium loss from the skeleton with a concomitant decrease in bone mass. Extended periods of amenorrhea result in an increased risk for osteoporosis, a condition wherein bones fracture easily because of decreased bone mineral density.

Although high-intensity and/or high-volume training was once thought to be the main cause of menstrual dysfunction in female athletes, it seems that inadequate nutrition is the more plausible explanation. The key factor in secondary amenorrhea appears to be caloric restriction (either in the presence or the absence of exercise training) that ultimately causes significant hormonal alterations in women. Reduced caloric intake is associated with a decreased secretion of LH and $T_3$, both of which are involved in normal menstrual function. These alterations, and the resultant decrease in estrogen because of the cessation of menstruation, are responsible for the disruption of normal bone formation in athletes with amenorrhea.[34,35] Because eating disorders are often associated with an energy deficit due to caloric restriction, fitness professionals should pay attention to any signs or symptoms of disordered eating patterns in their clients. If any signs or symptoms of disordered eating patterns are noticed, referral to a certified eating disorders specialist should be made.

Louckes AB, Thuma JR. Luteinizing hormone pulsatility is disrupted at a threshold of energy availability in regularly menstruating women. *J Clin Endocrinol Metab.* 2003;88:297–311.

Redman LM, Louckes AB. Menstrual disorders in athletes. *Sports Med.* 2005;35:747–755.

## VIGNETTE *conclusion*

■ It took several months for Perla's fracture to heal and for her to complete a comprehensive rehabilitation program for her lower leg. By the end of rehabilitation, Perla had regained normal menstrual function and, with the help of a registered dietitian, had begun to eat an adequate, balanced diet. During the period of healing and rehabilitation when Perla could not perform gymnastics training, she chose other exercise modalities like swimming, cycling, and lifting weights. After her leg cast was removed and rehabilitation was complete, Perla worked with a post-rehabilitation exercise specialist to help her relearn proper movement patterns so that she could effectively carry out activities of daily living and exercise- and sports-related activities without fear of reinjuring her leg. She now has a more appropriate view of fitness and nutrition, and has decided to pursue other sport and recreational activities. Perla perceived her leg fracture as an early warning sign of the perils of osteoporosis. Her main concern now is that she build and maintain as much bone density as possible throughout her young adult and midlife years.

## CRITICAL THINKING QUESTIONS

1. Each hormone has a specific function within the body. How does a hormone carry out its focused action as it travels in the circulatory system throughout the entire body? How does the body ensure that only the intended tissues are targeted?

2. Which two hormones are important for preventing excessive dehydration during exercise, and how do they act to facilitate water conservation?

3. Highly conditioned endurance athletes show an enhanced physiological ability to mobilize FFAs for use as fuel during prolonged exercise. Which hormones are responsible for this glycogen-sparing effect, and how does it aid in the exerciser's performance?

4. Testosterone is released by the testes in men, but women also have circulating testosterone. Where does testosterone come from in women? Compared with men, how much testosterone do women have in circulation? How does this relate to the ability of women to develop big muscles from an exercise program, such as resistance training?

## ADDITIONAL RESOURCES

Endocrine Society—Hormone science to health. http://www.endocrine.org/
Hormone Health Network: www.hormone.org
Kohrt WM, Bloomfield SA, Little KD, Nelson ME, Yingling VR. Physical activity and bone health. *Med Sci Sports Exerc.* 2004;36:1985–1996.

Nattiv A, Loucks AB, Manore MM, Sanborn CF, Sundgot-Borgen J, Warren MP. (2007). ACSM Position Stand: The female athlete triad. *M Sci Sports Exerc.* 2007;39:1867–1882.

## REFERENCES

1. Grandone A, Santoro N, Coppola F, Calabrò P, Perrone L, del Giudice EM. Thyroid function derangement and childhood obesity: An Italian experience. *BMC Endocrine Disord.* 2010;10:8.
2. Marras V, Casini MR, Pilia S, et al. Thyroid function in obese children and adolescents. *Hormone Res Paediatr.* 2010;73:193–197.
3. American Thyroid Association. Thyroid and Weight Patient Brochure. 2005. www.thyroid.org/patients/brochures/Thyroid_and_Weight.pdf
4. Aoki Y, Belin RM, Clickner R, Jeffries R, Phillips L, Mahaffey KR. Serum TSH and total T4 in the United States population and their association with participant characteristics: National Health and Nutrition Examination Survey (NHANES 1999-2002). *Thyroid.* 2007;17:1211–1223.
5. Flegal KM, Carroll MD, Ogden CL, Curtin LR. Prevalence and trends in obesity among US adults, 1999-2008. *J Am Med Assoc.* 2010;303:235–241.
6. Janssen I, Heymsfield SB, Wang Z, Ross R. Skeletal muscle mass and distribution in 468 men and women aged 18-88 yr. *J Appl Physiol.* 2000;89:81–88.
7. Jain AK, Ryan JR, McMahon FG, et al. Analgesic efficacy of low-dose ibuprofen in dental extraction pain. *Pharmacotherapy.* 1986;6:318–322.
8. Noyelle RM, et al. Ibuprofen, aspirin, and paracetamol compared in a community study. *Pharm J.* 1987;238:561–564.
9. Pearce I, et al. Ibuprofen, a prostaglandin synthetase inhibitor compared to paracetamol, a peripheral analgesic, on classical migraine. *Practitioner.* 1983;227:465–467.
10. Czaykowski D, Fratarcangelo P, Rosefsky J. Evaluation of the antipyretic efficacy of single dose ibuprofen suspension compared to acetaminophen elixir in febrile children. *Pediatr Res.* 1994;35:829 (Abstract).
11. Winther B. The therapeutic effectiveness of ibuprofen on the symptoms of naturally acquired common colds. *Am J Rhinol.* 2001;15:239–242.
12. Bennett WM, Henrich WL, Stoff JS. The renal effects of nonsteroidal anti-inflammatory drugs: summary and recommendations. *Am J Kidney Dis.* 1996;28:(Suppl 1):S56–S62.
13. Goodyear L, Kahn B. Exercise, glucose transport, and insulin sensitivity. *Ann Rev Med.* 1998;49:235–261.
14. Felig P, Wahren J. Fuel homeostasis in exercise. *N Engl J Med.* 1975;293:1078–1084.
15. McArdle WD, Katch FI, Katch VL. *Exercise Physiology.* 5th ed. Baltimore, MD: Lippincott Williams & Wilkins; 2001.
16. Bloom SR, Edwards AV. The release of pancreatic glucagon and inhibition of insulin in response to stimulation of the sympathetic innervation. *J Physiol.* 1975;253:157–173.
17. Sutton JR, et al. Plasma vasopressin, catecholamines and lactate during exhaustive exercise at extreme stimulated altitude: "Operation Everest II." *Can J Appl Sport Sci.* 1986;11:43.
18. Wade CE. Response, regulation and actions of vasopressin during exercise: A review. *Med Sci Sports Exerc.* 1984;16:506–511.
19. Kraemer WJ, Marchitelli L, Gordon SE, et al. Hormonal and growth factor responses to heavy resistance exercise protocols. *J Appl Physiol.* 1990;69:1442–1450.
20. Kraemer WJ. Endocrine responses to resistance exercise. *Med Sci Sports Exerc.* 1988;29:S152–S157.
21. Bird SP, Tarpenning KM, Marino FE. Liquid carbohydrate/essential amino acid ingestion during a short-term bout of resistance exercise suppresses myofibrillar protein degradation. *Metabolism.* 2006;55:570–577.
22. Powers S, Howley E. *Exercise Physiology: Theory and Application to Fitness and Performance.* 7th ed. New York, NY: McGraw Hill; 2009.

23. Hawley JA. Fat burning during exercise: Can ergogenics change the balance? *Phys Sportsmed.* 1998;26:56–63.

24. Cuff DJ, Meneilly GS, Martin A, Ignaszewski A, Tildesley HD, Frohlich JJ. Effective exercise modality to reduce insulin resistance in women with type 2 diabetes. *Diabetes Care.* 2003;26:2977–2982.

25. Davis SN, Galassetti P, Wasserman DH, Tate D. Effects of gender on neuroendocrine and metabolic counterregulatory measures responses to exercise in normal man. *J Clin Endocrinol Metab.* 2000;85:224–230.

26. Kraemer WJ, Fleck SJ, Maresh CM, et al. Acute hormonal responses to a single bout of heavy resistance exercise in trained power lifters and untrained men. *Can J Appl Physiol.* 1999;24:524–537.

27. Hakkinen KA, Pakarinen A, Kraemer WJ, Newton RU, Alen M. Basal concentrations and acute responses of serum hormones and strength development during heavy resistance training in middle-aged and elderly men and women. *J Gerontol A Biol Sci Med Sci.* 2000;55: B95–B105.

28. Leyk D, Gorges W, Ridder D, Wunderlich M, Rüther T, Sievert A, Essfeld D. Hand-grip strength of young men, women and highly trained female athletes. *Eur J Appl Physiol.* 2007;99:415–421.

29. Ford LE, Detterline AJ, Ho KK, Cao W. Gender- and height-related limits of muscle strength in world weightlifting champions. *J Appl Physiol.* 2000;89: 1061–1064.

30. Miller AE, McDougall JD, Tarnopolsky MA, Sale DG. Gender differences in strength and muscle fiber characteristics. *Eur J Appl Physiol Occup Physiol* 1993;66:254–262.

31. American Geriatrics Society; British Geriatrics Society and American Academy of Orthopaedic Surgeons Panel on Falls Prevention. Guideline for the prevention of falls in older persons. *J Am Geriatr Soc.* 2001;49:664–672.

32. Mittendorfer B, Rennie MJ. Swings and roundabouts for muscle gain and loss: Differences between sexes? *J Appl Physiol.* 2006;100:375–376.

33. Hubal MJ, Gordish-Dressman H, Thompson PD, et al. Variability in muscle size and strength gain after unilateral resistance training. *Med Sci Sports Exerc.* 2005;37: 964–972.

34. Louckes AB, Thuma JR. Luteinizing hormone pulsatility is disrupted at a threshold of energy availability in regularly menstruating women. *J Clin Endocrinol Metab.* 2003;88:297–311.

35. Redman LM, Louckes AB. Menstrual disorders in athletes. *Sports Med.* 2005;35:747–755.

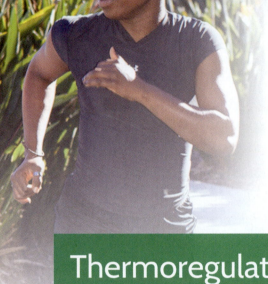

Fabio Comana, MA, MS

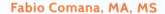

CHAPTER 12

# Thermoregulatory System and Thermoregulatory Responses to Exercise

## CHAPTER OUTLINE

## CHAPTER OUTLINE—cont'd

## LEARNING OUTCOMES

1. Describe thermal balance within the body and the mechanisms of thermoregulatory control.
2. Identify environmental factors that influence the thermoregulatory mechanisms within the body.
3. Describe the thermoregulatory differences between men and women, and between adults and children.
4. Define the challenges faced when exercising in hot environments, and how the body adapts both acutely and chronically to these conditions.
5. Define the challenges faced when exercising in cold environments, and how the body adapts both acutely and chronically to these conditions.
6. Identify the differences between the major heat illnesses with regard to causes, symptoms, and treatment.
7. Provide strategies to help individuals acclimate to hot and cold environments.

## ANCILLARY LINK

Visit Davis*Plus* at http://davisplus.fadavis.com for study and practice resources, including online quizzes, animations that help explain physiological processes, podcasts concerning news and career trends in exercise physiology, and practice references.

## *VIGNETTE*

■ On August 20, 2008, Max Gilpin, a Kentucky high-school football player, collapsed during practice with a body temperature of 107°F (42°C). Three days later, he died as a result of what experts believed to be primarily heat illness. Although stories of athletes collapsing or even dying on the field surface from time to time, what made this story so tragic was that the boy's death was completely preventable.

Five months later, in January 2009, Gilpin's head coach was arraigned on a reckless homicide charge because it was alleged that he denied the athlete water throughout practice. In addition, a lawsuit filed by Gilpin's parents alleged that six of the team's coaches were negligent in their actions, because more than 20 minutes had passed after the teenager collapsed before one of the coaches called EMS.

Although the head coach was acquitted of the criminal charges, there are lessons to be learned from this tragedy. In fact, the team's coaches broke several of the most important rules of dealing with heat illnesses, some in terms of prevention and others in terms of their response.

How could a basic understanding of exercise physiology, thermoregulation, and heat stress have helped to prevent Max Gilpin's early and tragic death?

Humans exhibit a tremendous ability to not only survive, but thrive in a variety of different environments. This is attributed, in part, to the efficiency of our physiological systems and how they quickly learn to adapt to environmental stressors. One such system is our thermoregulatory system, which maintains our body temperature within certain boundaries regardless of the environment. In fact, the efficiency of the human thermoregulatory system makes it one of the most efficient among mammals.

Humans are **homeothermic**; that is, regardless of the environment in which people exist or the effects of other influences that may alter body temperature (e.g., heat generated during activity or exercise), humans possess the capacity to maintain a relatively constant internal or **core body temperature**. This homeostatic function involves various mechanisms that respond acutely to temperature changes and allow people to adapt chronically to preserve or remove heat more efficiently. Unfortunately, the possibility also exists that these stressors may overwhelm the body's thermoregulatory control, potentially reducing performance and inducing harm. Without any regulatory control mechanisms to remove this heat, it is estimated that the body's core temperature would increase by 1.0°C every 5 minutes.

The human body is inefficient in using energy. Only 25% of all energy expended in the body is actually used to perform physiological work (e.g., muscle contraction), whereas the balance is generated as heat that must be removed.[1,2] Although much of this heat is produced in the deeper tissues of the body, it must be transported to the periphery (e.g., skin) for removal. Because the thermal properties of water are approximately 26 times greater than air, heat is transported and removed from the body faster through water than through air.[1] For example, standing in a 70°F (21.1°C) room does not feel as cold as immersion in water at the same temperature. Consequently, the blood, which is composed primarily of water, provides an effective means of shuttling heat from the core to the periphery.

## THERMOREGULATORY MECHANISMS WITHIN THE BODY

Humans normally maintain a core body temperature that ranges between 97°F and 100°F (36.1°C and 37.8°C), fluctuating by several degrees throughout the day in response to internal and external factors such as activity, diet, emotions, and the external environment.[3] Core body temperatures are generally lowest during sleep and highest during exercise or with exposure to hot environments. A person's core body temperature is generally warmer than his or her skin temperature, but it varies significantly depending on environmental temperatures (varying by up to 35°F [20°C]).

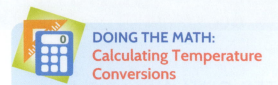

**DOING THE MATH: Calculating Temperature Conversions**

**Converting °C to °F**

(°C × 1.8) + 32 = °F
Example—converting 20°C to °F:
- (20°C × 1.8) + 32 = °F
- 36 + 32 = 68°F

**Converting °F to °C**

(°F − 32)/1.8 = °C
Example—converting 72°F to °C:
- (72°F − 32)/1.8 = °C
- 40/1.8 = 22°C

Within specific limits, humans possess a great capacity to tolerate temperature extremes and survive in a variety of different climates. People can briefly tolerate core temperatures that decline to 80.5°F (26.9°C) or increase to 105.8°F (41.0°C), or active muscle tissue temperatures greater than 107.4°F (41.9°C) (Fig. 12-1).[4,5] At higher temperatures, cells start to die, because many proteins within the cell begin to unravel.

## VIGNETTE continued

■ Max Gilpin's body temperature when he collapsed on the field was approximately 107°F (42°C), which places him in the temperature range associated with heat stroke. Although humans may be able to briefly tolerate this condition, a quick response is necessary to prevent death.

True core temperature is difficult to measure given how it differs by location and how it is influenced locally by internal and external factors. Common measurement sites used to estimate core temperature include the rectum, eardrum (tympanic temperature), esophagus, sublingual (under the tongue), axillary (under the armpit), and more recently, using a forehead scan. Skin temperatures also vary by location, but mean skin temperature denotes a weighted average of temperature readings taken at several locations around the body. Given the discrepancies between core and surface temperatures, an estimate of average body temperature is determined using the following equation:

$$\text{Average body temperature} = (\text{core temperature} \times 0.6) + (\text{mean skin temperature} \times 0.4)$$

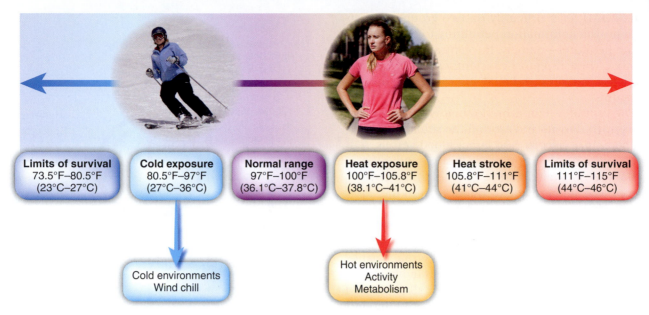

**Figure 12-1.** Core temperature tolerance ranges. Note the normal temperature range maintained by the human body and the various extremes tolerated on either end of the spectrum when exposed to extreme cold and heat, respectively. *(Photo on left courtesy of Crystal Taylor.)*

Basic mercury thermometers have long been a standard tool for measuring core temperature, whether placed in the mouth or under the armpit. Tympanic (ear) temperatures became standard practice 10 to 15 years ago, essentially replacing oral thermometers in many circumstances. As the device does not directly touch the tympanic membrane, it actually reads ear canal temperature, which is assumed to match core temperature. More recently, temporal (forehead) temperature readings are becoming common practice to determine core temperature in medical practices. Scanners or strips designed to measure heat are placed on the forehead at the location of the temporal artery. If a patient's blood flow is normal, the readings can be fairly accurate; but the reality is that these readings can be influenced by solar radiation, by any changes in blood flow to the skin, and by skin temperature, which is impacted by the environment.

Rectal temperature requires insertion of a thermometer or recording device into the rectum. This method is still widely used in research because it is considered one of the most accurate methods for measuring core body temperature. Esophageal temperature is a less popular method used to assess core temperature because of the difficulty associated with inserting the thermistor (a special resistor made from a ceramic or a polymer material whose resistance varies significantly with temperature) into the esophagus. Furthermore, this method can irritate the mucous passages (e.g., nasal passages), and subjects often experience significant discomfort during monitoring. Ingestible thermometers represent the latest technology for assessing core temperature during exercise or for sustained periods. The thermometer is generally designed as a pill that is ingested and passes slowly through the gastrointestinal tract. The pill transmits recordings to an external device and will continue to do so until it is passed from the body. Although accurate and convenient, expense is a key limitation as each pill is designed for single use only.

The **preoptic/anterior hypothalamus (POAH)** in the brain is the coordinating center for temperature regulation and acts much like an internal thermostat.[6] Unlike a thermostat, however, this center does not turn off heat production within the body, but instead initiates responses to reduce increases in core body temperature. This is because the body is constantly undergoing a physiological process (i.e., keeping you alive), and thus cannot stop producing heat.

- When the body perceives heat, it strives to increase heat loss through peripheral **vasodilation** of blood vessels, which redistributes blood carrying heat toward the periphery. It can also increase sweat rates and decrease heat production via reduced muscle tone and a reduction in voluntary activity.
- When the body perceives cold, it strives to decrease heat loss through peripheral **vasoconstriction** of blood vessels, which redistribute blood toward the core. It can also increase heat production via shivering (nonmetabolic **thermogenesis**) and increases in voluntary activity. The POAH can also facilitate increases in the levels of specific hormones that facilitate heat production and muscle action.

The POAH relies primarily on two groups of receptors to provide information pertaining to core and surface temperatures—namely, the central and peripheral receptors. These receptors constantly monitor core and surface temperatures, and relay information to the control centers.

- The central receptors are located within the **hypothalamus** and around the spinal cord, abdominal **viscera**, and larger blood vessels.
- The peripheral receptors are located under the skin, sensing temperature changes in the environment, and provide feedback to both the hypothalamus and the **cerebral cortex**.

The central receptors monitor blood temperature as it circulates throughout the core of the body and serve as the major system for maintaining thermal balance. They are extremely sensitive to changes in blood temperature and can detect changes as small as 0.018°F (0.01°C). The peripheral receptors, in contrast, monitor changes in skin temperature, which are influenced by the external environment. These receptors also send information to the cerebral cortex, which controls conscious or voluntary action (i.e., perform voluntary movement, reduce exposed body surface area by curling up during cold exposure, or reduce voluntary movement during heat exposure). The peripheral receptors act as an early warning system to the POAH to help regulate impending thermal challenges to the body's core temperature. Collectively, these receptors monitor changes in core temperature attributed to metabolic heat production and the influence of the environment.

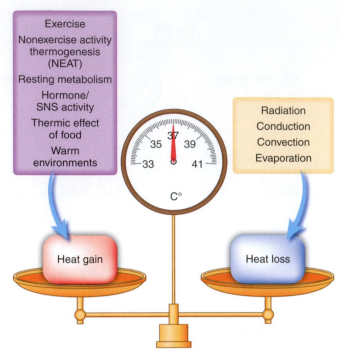

**Figure 12-2.** Various factors that influence metabolic heat gain and heat loss. Heat loss must match heat gain to maintain a constant core temperature. SNS = sympathetic nervous system.

## FACTORS THAT AFFECT HEAT GAIN

Internal and external factors influence body temperature. The body generates heat through various metabolic actions that can increase significantly during exercise and activity, or it may gain heat from the external environment when it is warmer than the body's core temperature. Mechanisms for heat gain within the body include (Fig. 12-2):

- Resting metabolism—represents the energy expended to maintain all physiological function and generally accounts for approximately 60% to 75% of all the energy expended by the body in 1 day.
- Muscle activity—represents the energy expended to perform work to move the body during activity or exercise, and generally accounts for approximately 15% to 30% of all the energy expended by the body in 1 day.
- Hormone and nervous activity—represents the energy expended by various physiological systems within the body due to increased activation of these systems (i.e., **sympathetic nervous system** [SNS] stimulation of the fight-or-flight response).

- Thermic effect of food—represents the energy expended to chew, digest, absorb, and store food throughout the day and generally accounts for approximately 10% of all energy expended by the body in 1 day.
- Nonexercise activity thermogenesis—represents the energy expended to perform a variety of low-intensity, short-duration actions or movements that accumulate throughout the day (e.g., postural changes, fidgeting, tapping a pencil). The energy expended in 1 day via nonexercise thermogenesis varies tremendously among individuals.
- Warm environments—represents heat that moves into the body from environments that are warmer than the body's core temperature.

## FACTORS THAT AFFECT HEAT LOSS

Various forms of heat exchange exist between the body and the surrounding environment. The predominant method that functions at rest involves dry heat exchange, implying that heat transfer moves along a thermal gradient that exists between two surfaces, mediums, or objects (i.e., heat moves from warmer objects to cooler objects). **Conduction**, **convection**, and **radiation** all function via dry heat exchange, whereas **evaporation**, generally the predominant thermoregulatory method used during exercise, does not (Fig. 12-3).

Resistance to dry heat exchange is called insulation, which traps warm air between surfaces. Examples of insulation include the enclosures used in homes

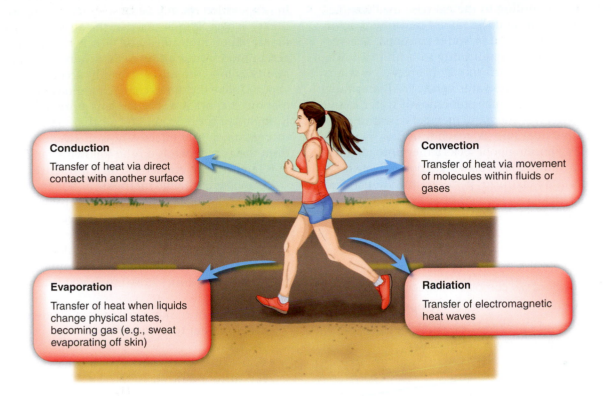

**Conduction**
Transfer of heat via direct contact with another surface

**Convection**
Transfer of heat via movement of molecules within fluids or gases

**Evaporation**
Transfer of heat when liquids change physical states, becoming gas (e.g., sweat evaporating off skin)

**Radiation**
Transfer of electromagnetic heat waves

**Figure 12-3.** The body's thermoregulatory mechanisms that primarily protect against overheating at rest and during exercise.

(e.g., walls, roofs), clothing (certain fabrics, dark clothing that absorbs heat), layers of clothing, and the thin blanket of warm air that envelopes a person's body and becomes trapped within the hairs on his or her skin.

Heat loss is accomplished by:
- Conduction
- Convection
- Radiation
- Evaporation
- Excretion, albeit insignificant to the body

(See explanatory animation of the mechanisms of heat loss on the Davis*Plus* site at http://davisplus .fadavis.com.)

## Conduction

Conduction involves the exchange or transfer of heat from warmer objects to cooler objects via direct molecular contact. It functions in all three physical states (i.e., solid, liquid, and gas), although this means of heat transfer occurs primarily through solid and liquid states. The transfer of heat via conduction depends on the following variables:
- The thermal gradient (i.e., the temperature difference between the two surfaces)
- The thermal properties of the two surfaces, objects, or mediums in contact

For example, compare the difference between a glass and a Styrofoam cup when both are filled with hot coffee.

The glass gets much hotter to the touch, because it is a better conductor of heat than the Styrofoam cup.

In the body, heat passes via conduction from the core to the periphery through direct contact between cells, tissues, and fluid mediums. Heat may also pass between the body and external objects with which the body comes into contact (e.g., immersion into water or placing a hand on a cold countertop). Although the role of conduction at rest varies by situation and environment (i.e., air or water), its contribution to heat dissipation during land-based exercise is small considering the amount of body surface area that makes contact with solid objects and the short duration of this contact (e.g., foot contact with the ground or equipment). However, its contribution to heat removal when the body is immersed in water is significant.

## Convection

Convection involves the exchange or transfer of heat across a surface by the movement of molecules within the fluids or gases. The keys to heat removal via convection are the movement between the two surfaces and the thermal gradient. Greater movement and larger thermal gradients exchange heat more rapidly. For example, air currents from a fan will remove blankets of warm air from the skin surface, and heat moves rapidly out of the body when a person treads water lightly as opposed to standing still in water.

The contribution from convection to heat loss during exercise varies according to the exercise medium (i.e., land or water based) and the rate of movement across the body (i.e., wind speed or water currents). Convection contributes more significantly to heat loss during land-based exercises performed on breezy or windy days. Although treading water lightly facilitates rapid heat loss given the thermal properties of water, active swimming generates adequate metabolic heat to offset this convective heat loss. A coach training his or her athletes in a swimming pool seeks a thermoregulatory-neutral temperature that reduces additional thermoregulatory costs and maximizes performance. Researchers estimate that ideal pool temperatures for training range between 75°F and 82°F (23.9°C and 27.8°C).[7]

## In Your Own Words

A parent of a child enrolled in your swimming program asks why her child complains of becoming cold quickly in the pool, even though the temperature is the same as that of the air outside. What explanation would you provide to answer her question?

## Radiation

Radiation involves the passage of electromagnetic heat waves moving along a temperature gradient from a warm or hot object into a cooler object (e.g., the sun's rays warming the Earth at sunrise or heat waves rising off the tarmac on a hot day). The human body constantly radiates heat through skin into the surrounding cooler environment and any objects surrounding the body, while simultaneously receiving heat from warmer objects surrounding it.

## Evaporation

Evaporation is the transfer of heat when a liquid changes physical states by becoming gas, a process that requires energy to vaporize the liquid. The energy required to change physical states is provided by heat, a form of energy in the body. As the vapor (gas) leaves the skin surface, so too will the heat. Because water is an excellent conductor of heat, sweat (which is composed mostly of water) has the capacity to hold significant quantities of heat. The average adult body contains approximately two to four million heat-activated sweat glands (**eccrine glands**) that have the ability to release large volumes of sweat, a hypertonic saline containing water and valuable **electrolytes** such as sodium, chlorine, potassium, magnesium, and calcium. The water in sweat is removed from the skin surface as water vapor, while the electrolytes can crystallize on the skin and leave a white, salty residue.

Water vapor suspended in the air has weight and exerts pressure that is commonly referred to as relative humidity, which is a measure of how much vapor the air can actually hold before it condenses into a liquid

and falls as rain. This pressure plays an important role in evaporative cooling because when the relative humidity is high, it indicates that the air already contains many vapor molecules and has a limited ability to accept more water from sweat. When the relative humidity is low, the air can readily accept more water vapor. Unlike the dry exchange methods for heat elimination, evaporation is dependent more on the relative humidity of the surrounding air than on the temperature gradient. The effectiveness of sweat evaporation from the skin depends on the following factors:

- Temperature gradient, which influences the three dry heat exchange methods: in hot environments, as the temperature gradient becomes smaller, the efficacy of the dry heat exchange mechanisms is reduced; therefore, individuals will need to sweat to thermoregulate
- The relative humidity of the surrounding air, which determines how much water vapor it can accept
- The amount of skin surface area exposed to the environment to facilitate sweat removal from the body
- Convective air currents that lift the vapor into the surrounding air

Sweat must evaporate for heat to leave the body. For each liter of sweat lost, the body removes approximately 580 kcal (2,428 kJ) of heat.[8] Sweat dripping off the body or remaining in the clothes does not contribute to cooling but does contribute to fluid losses and potential **dehydration**. Not all sweat is lost to the environment (i.e., some will always drip off the body). Hence people tend to sweat volumes larger than what is truly needed to dissipate the heat generated. For example, a 165-lb (75-kg) man generating 750 kcal of heat each hour during a 2-hour training session would

**DOING THE MATH:**
**Calculating True Sweat Weight**

Using the previous example:

165-lb (75-kg) man generating 750 kcal of heat per hour for 2 hours

- If 580 kcal = 1,000 mL:
- 750 kcal/hour = 1,300 mL + sweat dripping off body
- Assuming some sweat is dripping off, his sweat rate = ~1,600–1,700 mL/hr or 3,200–3,400 mL water lost in 2 hours

Remember: 1 kg water or sweat = 1 L or 1,000 mL and 1 kg = 2.2 lb:

- 3.2–3.4 kg × 2.2 = 7.0–7.5 lb lost in 2 hours

Percentage loss of body weight:

- (7.0 lb/165 lb) × 100 = 4.2%
- (7.5 lb/165 lb) × 100 = 4.5%

need to sweat approximately 1.3 L/hr to remove this heat. However, given how some sweat drips off the body, a more accurate estimate would be a sweat rate closer to 1.6 to 1.7 L/hr, representing 7.0 to 7.5 lb water lost in 2 hours, or 4.2% to 4.4% of his body weight.

The body relies predominantly on the dry heat exchange methods (i.e., conduction, radiation, and convection) to remove heat produced within the body at rest (Table 12-1). However, during exercise, when metabolic heat production increases significantly, the efficacy of the dry heat exchange mechanisms becomes limited. The body generates approximately 1.0 to 1.5 kcal of heat per minute at rest, but this can increase to 20 to 25 kcal/min during intense exercise.[9] Consequently, sweating becomes the most efficient thermoregulatory mechanism to remove any excess heat produced during exercise. Sweating can begin with the anticipation of exercise or within 3 minutes of initiating exercise and tends to plateau within 30 minutes, at which point it reaches a balance related to exercise load and heat production. In addition to noticeable sweat losses, the average adult also loses approximately 350 mL each day through unnoticed sweating that occurs at rest (defined as insensible perspiration, or fluid seepage through the skin).[2]

## Excretion

**Excretion** involves the loss of heat via any materials excreted from the body, whether in the gaseous (air exhalation), liquid (urine), or solid (feces) states, and generally contributes negligibly to heat removal from the body. Excretion does account for significant fluid removal from the body considering daily urine output, fluid volume contained in feces, and the estimated additional 300 mL of fluid lost through the mucous membranes of the respiratory passages. Because evaporation depends on the availability of adequate amounts of fluid within the body, fluid lost to excretion may influence sweat rates.

## FACTORS THAT INFLUENCE THERMOREGULATION

Several factors influence thermoregulation, including sex, age, body size and composition, conditioning level, hydration status, clothing, and environmental factors.

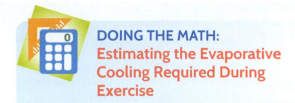

**DOING THE MATH:**
**Estimating the Evaporative Cooling Required During Exercise**

Step 1: Compute total oxygen consumption ($\dot{V}O_2$) for exercise bout—$\dot{V}O_2$ (L/min × time)

- Example: 2.0 L/min × 60 min = 120 L

Step 2: Convert $\dot{V}O_2$ to energy expenditure (1 L/min $O_2$ consumed = approximately 5.0 kcal)

- Example: 120 L = 600 kcal

Step 3: Calculate heat production (assume 22%–25% mechanical efficiency in humans; therefore, estimate 75%–78% heat production)

- Example (using 25% mechanical efficiency): 600 kcal × 0.75 = 450 kcal

Step 4: Calculate evaporation needs (sweating accounts for 80% of heat elimination during heavy exercise)

- Example: 450 kcal × 0.8 = 360 kcal
- 360 kcal/580 kcal = 0.62 L, or almost 22 oz (1.375 lb)

*Remember, 1 L water = 580 kcal.

## Age

Despite having higher concentrations of sweat glands than adults, children sweat at lower rates because of smaller quantities of body water; therefore, children cannot utilize evaporative cooling as efficiently as adults. In addition, lower quantities of subcutaneous fat and larger surface area/body mass ratios result in reduced insulation and, subsequently, heat leaving a child's body rapidly in cold environments. These differences predispose children to greater risk for thermoregulatory problems,

## Table 12-1. Thermoregulation at Rest and During Exercise

| THERMOREGULATORY MECHANISM | REST | EXERCISE |
|---|---|---|
| Conduction and convection | 20% of total | 10%–15% of total |
| Radiation | 55%–60% of total | 5% of total |
| Evaporation | 20% of total | 80% of total |
| Excretion/lungs | 5%–10% of total | <2% of total |

## SEX DIFFERENCES

Although females possess greater densities of sweat glands than males, they generally begin sweating at higher core temperature thresholds and produce less sweat for three key reasons[10]:

- Females have less lean mass than men.
- Females have less body water than males.
- Females have larger surface area/body mass ratios (i.e., more fat mass, less lean mass), which favors the dry heat exchange methods (i.e., conduction, radiation, and convection).

However, **subcutaneous** fat tissue is also an insulator, hampering the body's ability to effectively remove heat via the dry heat exchange methods. Because **adipose tissue** contains less water than muscle, it offers greater insulation against heat loss than muscle tissue. Therefore, heavier women who lose the ability to thermoregulate via the dry heat exchange methods may need to rely more heavily on sweating. In addition, during the **luteal phase** of menstruation, core temperatures normally increase, which requires a greater need to thermoregulate.[11]

which can be accentuated by their general lack of awareness of the symptoms of hot or cold stress on the body.[12]

Older adults are also more susceptible to the hot and cold stress, given their greater tendencies toward the following conditions[7]:

- Dehydration (because of a diminished sense of thirst and general tissue dehydration)
- Loss of subcutaneous fat tissue to insulate
- Loss of muscle tissue to generate heat
- Potential cognitive losses associated with aging or disease that reduce awareness to environmental stress
- Changes within the skin layer
- Reduced thermoregulatory efficiency
- Medication usage that can affect hydration status and blood distribution

## VIGNETTE continued

■ Because youth cannot utilize evaporative cooling as effectively as adults, Max Gilpin's age—he was 15 years old at the time of his death—likely influenced the speed with which his body overheated. Age is an important risk factor of which coaches and exercise leaders must be aware.

## Body Size and Composition

Although muscle tissue is capable of generating more heat, peripheral muscle mass and body fat both offer some resistance to heat loss via insulation. Although larger surface areas generally dissipate heat more rapidly, those with less muscle tissue generate less heat and may lose heat rapidly, increasing their risks for **hy-thermia** in colder environments. Body composition [is des]cribed in detail in Chapter 23.

## Conditioning Level

More conditioned individuals are capable of performing more work, and are therefore able to generate more heat. Consequently, the body undergoes several adaptations with training to improve thermoregulatory efficiency to allow it to remove heat more effectively. Some of these adaptations, which are discussed in greater detail later in this chapter, include increases in blood volume, improved redistribution of blood to the skin surface during exercise, increased sweat rates, and reduced core temperature thresholds at which sweating is initiated.

## In Your Own Words

A friend is curious why she sweats more than her girlfriend when they both work out together at the local health club. Although she believes she is better conditioned than her friend, they are approximately the same size and work out at similar intensities. What answer would you offer to explain the possible differences in their sweat rates?

## Hydration Status

It is estimated that the sensation of thirst in adults younger than 50 years normally begins when a person reaches approximately 1% loss of body weight. For example, if a 180-lb (81.8-kg) man lost 1.8 lb (0.82 kg), this would initiate the sensation of thirst. Aging is associated with a gradual reduction in the mechanisms that drive the sensation of thirst. A dehydrated state causing a 2% loss of body weight can begin to negatively impact performance by increasing heart rate and **cardiac output** (because of a reduced blood volume associated with exercise and sweating), and elevating core body temperature.[2] For example, a 175-lb (79.5-kg) man needs to lose 1.6 L water (1.6 kg or 3.5 lb) to lose 2% of his body weight before becoming dehydrated. Therefore, individuals should attempt to maximally hydrate before commencing exercise, as adequate hydration levels allow for more efficient **thermoregulation** and preservation of a normal core temperature (Fig. 12-4). It is not uncommon, however, for athletes to lose up to 6% to 10% of body weight via sweating during exercise.[13]

## V I G N E T T E  *continued*

■ Denying athletes access to water–as Max Gilpin's coaches are accused of doing–is a serious error in judgment that coaches or exercise leaders can make, especially when working outdoors in a hot, humid environment. Without adequate hydration, an exerciser's thermoregulation processes will become ineffective and his or her core temperature will steadily increase, leading to heat illness and, as in Gilpin's case, eventual death.

## Clothing

Clothing insulates the body and reduces conductive, convective, and radiant heat-loss efficacy (i.e., clothing retards radiant heat gain from the environment). In colder environments, this proves beneficial to preserving the body's core temperature. The mesh pattern in clothing fibers trap and warm air to insulate the body, creating a barrier of air between the material and the skin. Loose-fitting clothing or moisture-wicking fabrics (e.g., Cool-max®, DryLite®) promote movement of water vapor through the fabric to transfer moisture from the skin to the environment more efficiently. Moisture-wicking

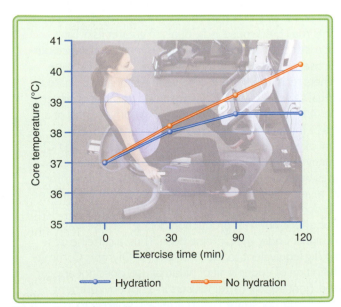

**Figure 12-4.** Effect of hydration on core temperature during prolonged exercise.

clothing also promotes heat preservation in cold environments by keeping the skin dry. Football gear and non-breathable materials, in contrast, impair the body's ability to dissipate heat effectively.

## V I G N E T T E  *continued*

■ The padding worn by a football player provides insulation against effective heat loss, effectively trapping the warm air against the athlete's body and preventing evaporative cooling. This has been a contributing factor in several on-field incidents and deaths, most likely including that of Max Gilpin. If a workout or practice is being held on a hot, humid day, coaches should consider having athletes remove their padding for at least a portion of the practice session to allow the athletes to effectively cool down.

In cold environments, layering creates greater insulation to protect against heat loss, but it is important to note that wet clothing loses up to 90% of its insulating properties given water's high thermal properties. Therefore, it becomes very important to remove wet layers from the skin in cold environments. The efficacy of clothing as an insulator is influenced by various factors, including the following:

- Wind speed accelerates the removal of the insulated layers of warm air.
- Darker colors absorb more radiant heat from the environment.
- Body movement will disrupt any blanket of air formed between the skin and clothing.
- Loose-fitting clothing will ventilate air trapped against the body more easily.
- Having more surface area exposed to the environment (i.e., less skin covered by clothing) promotes greater heat removal, although it can predispose the body to radiant heat gain in hot environments, as well as sunburn.
- Fibers capable of wicking moisture away from the skin faster keep it dry and can prevent excessive heat loss. Conversely, any resistance to removing water vapor offered by some fabrics (e.g., rubberized suits) reduces the efficacy of evaporative cooling.[14]

## Environmental Factors

The environment greatly influences the body's ability to remove heat during exercise. In cooler environments, where temperature gradients between the body and the environment are significantly large, the body relies on the dry heat exchange methods to dissipate heat and less on evaporative cooling, thereby preserving body water. One example of this environmental impact involves an individual who does not sweat much when running at a moderate intensity on a brisk or cold day.

In hotter, dry environments where the temperature gradient between the body and environment is small, the dry heat exchange methods become less efficient, increasing the body's reliance on evaporative cooling. For example, an individual would need to sweat more profusely when running at the same moderate intensity on a hot day. If environmental temperatures exceed the body's core temperature during exercise (i.e., temperatures that exceed 100°F [37.8°C]), environmental heat may actually enter the body, thereby creating a greater reliance on sweating.

In hot, humid environments, none of the body's thermoregulatory mechanisms works effectively, given the loss of a thermal gradient and the air's inability to accommodate more water vapor. In this situation, the body will continue to sweat in an attempt to remove heat, but because the sweat cannot vaporize and thereby remove heat, the individual becomes susceptible to heat illnesses. Exercising in these environments requires additional means to cool the body, such as consumption of cool fluids, removal of insulating layers,

## VIGNETTE *continued*

■ The high humidity that August afternoon likely impeded Gilpin's ability to effectively lower his core temperature through evaporative cooling (i.e., sweating). It is essential that coaches and exercise leaders are aware of the environmental conditions and modify the practice or exercise session accordingly. Armed with this knowledge, they can provide more frequent water breaks or lower the intensity or duration of the workout.

and the application of cool/cold water, either in the form of wet towels or by wetting the person's clothes.

Wind is another environmental factor that influences the thermoregulatory mechanisms. In warmer environments, wind improves the efficacy of convection by moving molecules of hot air away from the body. In colder environments, it may induce cold stress by removing the insulating blanket of hot air around the body. The effects of temperature, wind, and humidity on the body are discussed further later in this chapter.

## RESEARCH HIGHLIGHT

### Energy Drinks and Thermoregulation

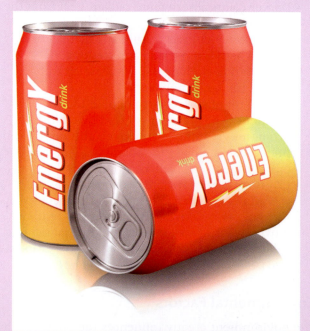

The consumption of caffeinated beverages such as energy drinks among youth and adults, athletes (competitive or recreational), and military populations has increased in recent years. It has been proposed that consumption of excessive amounts of caffeine in conjunction with exercise in hot environments may predispose individuals to greater risks for development of heat illnesses.[17] To examine heat balance during exercise in a hot environment after consuming caffeine, researchers recruited 10 men who were not heat acclimated or habitual caffeine users. They consumed dosages of either caffeine (4.1 mg/lb body weight; 9 mg/kg body weight) or a placebo before completing a 30-minute cycle at 50% maximal oxygen consumption ($\dot{V}O_2max$) in a 105°F (40°C), 25% relative humidity environment. Core and surface temperatures were recorded, as were ratings of thermal comfort. Results revealed increased mean temperatures in the caffeine group before the start of exercise, attributed to caffeine's thermogenic effect, but heat production during exercise was only slightly higher under the caffeine dose. Thus, a caffeine dose of 9 mg/kg (equivalent to the International Olympic Committee's definition of upper limit of habitual use) does not appear to appreciably alter heat balance during work with nonacclimated, nonhabitual caffeine users in a hot environment. According to the researchers, the small increase in body temperature demonstrated with caffeine is unlikely to increase physiological strain on the body to sufficiently impact endurance performance or the risk for heat illness.

Ely BR, Ely MR, Cheuvront SN. Marginal effects of a large caffeine dose on heat balance during exercise-heat stress. *Int J Sport Nutr Exerc Metab.* 2011;21:65–70.

## THERMOREGULATION IN HOT ENVIRONMENTS

Warmer skin surface temperatures are detected by the peripheral receptors that stimulate both the POAH and cerebral cortex. The response from the cortex may take the form of a voluntary action to reduce movement and heat generation, or a move to a cooler, shaded area. However, it is the increase in blood temperature identified by central receptors that activates SNS responses from the POAH.[6] Surface **arteriole** and sweat gland responses are far more sensitive and receptive to temperature changes detected by the central receptors than by the skin receptors. The POAH stimulates a SNS response to the smooth muscles that encircle the surface arterioles to vasodilate and bring more blood (which is carrying heat) to the skin's surface. At the eccrine glands, the POAH stimulates a SNS response to initiate sweat production in the coiled portion of the gland. The general response to increasing core temperatures follows the sequence outlined in Figure 12-5.

With rising core temperatures, the body needs to expend additional energy beyond the demands of working muscles to thermoregulate. Many physiological systems in the body experience acute adaptations that facilitate the body's ability to meet the energy demands of exercise and thermoregulation. For example, blood is redistributed away from the liver, kidneys, and other organs toward the muscles and skin to meet their increased demands. **Hemoglobin** is also capable of releasing more oxygen to muscle cells as blood temperature rises, increasing oxygen availability to produce additional energy.

### Physiological Responses to Heat Stress

During exercise in warmer environments, two competing cardiovascular demands exist:

- The need for oxygen and nutrient delivery to the exercising muscles
- The need for peripheral blood flow to the skin to remove heat

The added cost of thermoregulation during exercise increases the burden on the **cardiovascular system**, as it now needs to transport blood to both the exercising muscles and the skin surface. This essentially creates competition for the body's blood volume. This increased demand for cardiac output is met by increasing heart rate and heart contractility to ensure appropriate circulation to these two regions and by redistributing blood away from nonessential organs and systems (e.g., gastrointestinal tract, liver, and kidneys; Table 12-2). These acute changes are mediated by SNS activity that produces vasoconstriction in nonessential organs and vasodilation of vessels in the exercising muscles and near the skin surface. At rest, in moderate environments, approximately 6% of all blood flow reaches the skin, whereas this value declines to approximately 2% in colder environments because of peripheral vasoconstriction that redirects blood to the core for heat preservation.[15,16] During lower

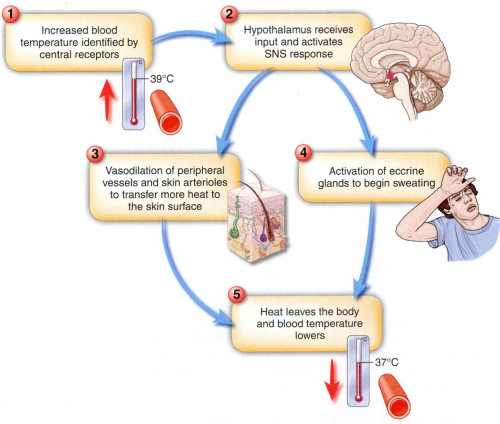

**Figure 12-5.** Thermoregulatory response sequence to increasing core temperatures.

**Table 12-2. Blood Flow Distribution to Essential and Nonessential Organs at Rest and During Exercise**

| ORGAN | REST | EXERCISE |
| --- | --- | --- |
| Muscles | 15%–20% | 70%–85% |
| Liver/gastrointestinal tract | 20%–25% | 3%–5% |
| Heart | 4%–5% | 4%–5% |
| Skin | Moderate environments: 6%<br>Cold environments: 2% | Light-intensity exercise: 14%–15%<br>Moderate-intensity exercise: 12%<br>High-intensity exercise: 2% |
| Brain | 14%–15% | 3%–4% |
| Kidneys | 20%–22% | 2%–4% |
| Other | 7% | 3% |

intensities of exercise, reduced muscle demand facilitates greater blood distribution to the skin and efficiency in thermoregulation. However, during heavier exercise intensities, during which metabolic heat production increases, competition for blood between the exercising muscles and the skin exists. Ultimately, blood distribution to the skin will decrease in favor of delivery to the exercising muscles, which potentiates the risk for thermal stress and heat illness.

These changes cannot continue indefinitely. Eventually, the demands of exercise and thermoregulation will exceed the cardiovascular system's ability to meet these demands. When the body reaches this point, it becomes unable to regulate against an increasing core temperature. When core temperatures increase to 104°F to 105.8°F (40°C–41°C), it usually signals the brain to begin to cease exercise.

Prolonged cardiovascular and thermoregulatory stress, and increases in core temperature elevate circulating levels of epinephrine, the hormone generally associated with higher intensity exercise. **Epinephrine** enhances **glycogen** utilization, which increases the potential for increased **lactate** production, exhaustion, and fatigue. A temporary adjustment made in the blood can retard the onset of fatigue under rising core temperatures. This adjustment involves a shift in the oxygen dissociation curve to increase the amount of oxygen unloaded from hemoglobin and improve its uptake into the muscle cells, a phenomenon known as the **Bohr effect**.[1,17]

Figure 12-6 illustrates the differences between hot and thermoneutral environmental effects on heart rate, cardiac output, stroke volume, and core temperature.

Loss of water and electrolytes in sweat triggers hormonal responses meant to reduce these losses and preserve water volume (blood volume) and electrolyte concentrations (predominantly sodium).

- **Antidiuretic hormone (ADH)**, also known as **arginine vasopressin** or **vasopressin**, is a hormone released from the posterior pituitary gland in response to decreased blood volume and blood pressure. Its function is to preserve blood volume by stimulating water **reabsorption** from the kidney tubules back into the blood.[1]
- **Aldosterone** is a hormone released from the adrenal cortex gland in response to reduced blood sodium concentrations, and decreased blood volume and blood pressure. Aldosterone stimulates reabsorption of sodium (and the chlorine that moves with it) from the kidney tubules back into the blood to preserve blood concentration.[1] This, in turn, will improve the body's ability to retain water.

Aldosterone also functions at the sweat ducts. Sweat is formed within the coiled secretory portion of the eccrine glands and contains concentrations of electrolytes similar to those found in the blood, given that **plasma** is the major contributor to sweat (Fig. 12-7). As it passes up through the uncoiled portion of the gland (i.e., the duct), aldosterone reabsorbs sodium and chlorine out of sweat, moving it into the surrounding tissue, where it ultimately moves back into the blood. Therefore, the concentrations of sodium and chlorine in sweat are generally lower (hypotonic) than those in plasma by the time sweat reaches the skin surface. During light sweating, the body has time to reabsorb these electrolytes from sweat ducts, but during heavy sweating, when sweat moves through the ducts at faster rates, there is less time for reabsorption. Consequently, the electrolyte concentration of sweat increases during exercise. Although present in lower concentrations, other minerals such as potassium, calcium, and magnesium are not reabsorbed out from the sweat duct and remain the same regardless of sweat rates. Sweat concentration and the efficiency of this reabsorption process is primarily determined by genetics and controlled locally by aldosterone. Improvements in conditioning status, however, will enhance aldosterone's efficacy for reabsorbing electrolytes out of sweat. As listed in Table 12-3, with improved aldosterone efficacy, acclimated or conditioned individuals can reabsorb more sodium back out of sweat.

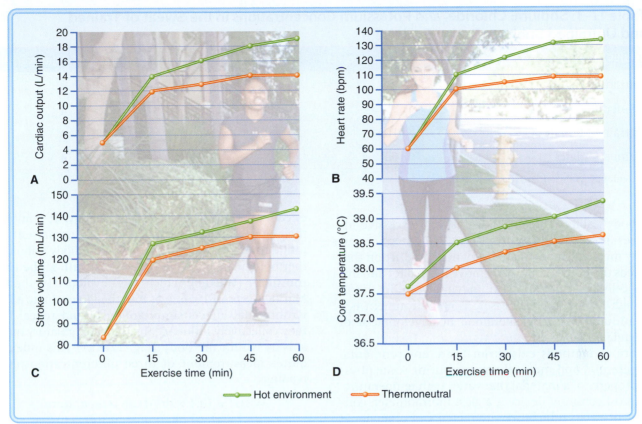

**Figure 12-6.** Physiological responses to moderate-intensity exercise across cardiac output (A), heart rate (B), stroke volume (C), and core temperature (D) in both a hot environmental condition (35°C) and a thermoneutral condition (20°C).

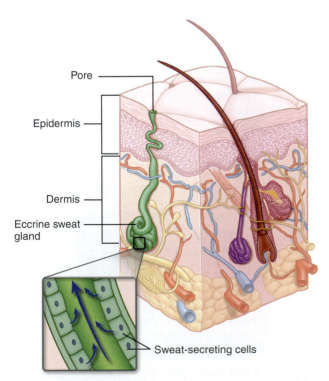

**Figure 12-7.** The skin and key underlying anatomical features involved in forming sweat.

Sweat rates generally range between 0.5 and 1.5 L/hr during light- to moderate-intensity exercise, but can increase to 3.0 to 4.0 L/hr in well-conditioned, large male athletes who have acclimatized to hot environments.[2] Rates of fluid loss from sweat vary among individuals and according to environmental factors, but generally a person can expect to lose fluid as follows:

- Sweat rates at rest:
  - 0.05 L/hr (1.7 fluid oz/hr) at 80°F (26.7°C)
  - 0.6 L/hr (20.3 fluid oz/hr) at 110°F (43.3°C)
- Light activity:
  - 0.2 L/hr (6.8 fluid oz/hr) at 80°F (26.7°C)
  - 1.0 L/hr (33.8 fluid oz/hr) at 110°F (43.3°C)
- Moderate activity:
  - 0.4 L/hr (13.5 fluid oz/hr) at 80°F (26.7°C)
  - 1.5 L/hr (50.7 fluid oz/hr) at 110°F (43.3°C)
- Heavy activity:
  - 0.6 L/hr (20.3 fluid oz/hr) at 80°F (26.7°C)
  - 2.0 L/hr (67.6 fluid oz/hr) at 110°F (43.3°C)

## Evaluation of the Environment

Circulatory blood flow to muscle tissue takes precedence over temperature regulation. When exercising in warmer climates, this may ultimately compromise

**Table 12-3.** Sodium, Chloride, and Potassium Concentrations in the Sweat of Trained and Untrained Subjects During Exercise

| SUBJECTS | SWEAT $NA^+$ (mmol/L) | SWEAT $CL^-$ (mmol/L) | SWEAT $K^+$ (mmol/L) |
|---|---|---|---|
| Untrained males | 90 | 60 | 4 |
| Trained males | 35 | 30 | 4 |
| Untrained females | 105 | 98 | 4 |
| Trained females | 62 | 47 | 4 |

$Cl^-$, chloride; $Na^+$, sodium; $K^+$, potassium.

the body's ability to control against any excessive increases in core temperature. Despite the thermoregulatory mechanisms available, any heat production that exceeds the body's ability to remove it can alter and impair cellular function, and inevitably inflict harm through heat-related illnesses. The environment is a key influence on the likelihood of development of heat-related illnesses.

Various methods exist to measure environmental temperature, and most rely on measuring some physical property of a material that varies with temperature. The most common device is a glass thermometer, consisting of a glass tube filled with mercury or other liquid such as alcohol (mix with a colored dye as alcohol is clear) that has expansion and contraction properties (i.e., it shrinks when cold; expands when warmed). Mercury is more accurate than alcohol because it expands more evenly across most temperatures, but it cannot be used at temperatures less than –40°C (–40°F) because it freezes.

Thermocouples consist of two conductors of different materials (usually metal alloys) that produce a voltage near the point of contact of the two conductors. This voltage is dependent on, although not necessarily proportional to, the difference in temperature between the junction and other parts of these conductors.

You'll recall that thermistors are resistors made from a ceramic or a polymer material whose resistance varies significantly with temperature. A pyrometer is a noncontacting device that intercepts and measures thermal radiation and can be used to determine the temperature of an object's surface.

Infrared light is electromagnetic radiation with longer wavelengths than visible light. This range of wavelengths includes most thermal radiation emitted by objects near room temperature. Infrared light is emitted or absorbed by molecules when they change their rotational-vibrational movements.

However, to better understand how the environment can impact and reduce thermoregulatory efficiency, it is important to note that it is not air temperature alone that influences the body's ability to remove heat; humidity, air currents, and thermal radiation all contribute to heat stress or retard heat removal from the body.

A heat index is a commonly used system that provides an overall impression of these environmental effects on thermoregulatory efficiency. It combines their effects into a single index score that represents the influence the environment has on the body's ability to thermoregulate effectively. The **wet-bulb globe thermometer (WBGT)**, which was developed by the U.S. Marine Corps in 1956, was intended to evaluate all environmental effects simultaneously and reveal how they collectively influence the thermoregulatory mechanisms within the body (Fig. 12-8).[18] This index requires measurement of three different atmospheric readings:

$$WBGT = (0.1 \times \text{dry-bulb temperature}) + (0.7 \times \text{wet-bulb temperature}) + (0.2 \times \text{globe temperature})$$

The components of the WBGT are as follows:
- **Dry-bulb temperature** is the actual air temperature.
- **Wet-bulb temperature** considers the amount of moisture in the air and reflects the cooling effect of evaporation. This thermometer has its

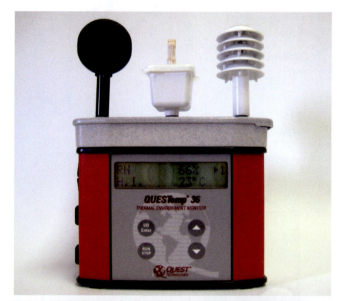

**Figure 12-8.** A wet-bulb globe thermometer (WBGT) evaluates all environmental effects simultaneously and reveals how they collectively influence the thermoregulatory mechanisms within the body. *(Reprinted with permission from Miller M, Berry D. Emergency response management for athletic trainers. Baltimore: Wolters Kluwer/Lippincott Williams & Wilkins; 2011.)*

bulb wrapped in cloth and kept wet with water via wicking action. As water evaporates from this bulb, it lowers the measured temperature reading, which reflects the cooling effect of sweat evaporating from the skin into the ambient environment. On days with higher humidity, this cooling effect is lowered as less water evaporates into the environment. Note that in the formula, the coefficient for the wet-bulb temperature measurement is highest, reflecting the importance of evaporation to heat exchange with the environment.

- **Globe temperature** reflects radiant heat and is normally higher than the dry-bulb temperature. To measure this effect, a thermometer is placed inside a black rubber globe, which will absorb radiant heat energy, providing a good indicator of the environment's radiant heat load.

## Risks Associated With Heat Stress

Information gathered from WBGT technology has helped researchers create the **heat stress index**, which evaluates the combined effect of air temperature and relative humidity to determine an apparent temperature, or how hot it actually feels (Fig. 12-9).[19] The chart is also very easy to use for the general public, as the necessary information can be obtained from the local weather service. Based on apparent temperatures, guidelines have been established to caution people to exposure and define the risk for development of heat-related illnesses.

Prolonged exposure to hot environments or excessive metabolic heat production can lead to heat-related illnesses (**hyperthermia**) that vary in symptomology and severity. The sequence of these illnesses progresses from **heat cramps**, to **heat syncope**, to **heat exhaustion**, and ultimately to **heat stroke** (Fig. 12-10). The onset and symptoms experienced can vary among individuals.

## Heat Cramps

Heat cramps are characterized by severe and painful cramps within the larger skeletal or lower extremity muscles.[20] Causes include the sodium losses and dehydration that accompany high sweat rates with inadequate or inappropriate rehydration, or both. Cramps may also occur frequently when someone is wearing a heavy sweatshirt or in those individuals who have high

**A**

| | Air temperature (°F) | | | | | | | | | | |
|---|---|---|---|---|---|---|---|---|---|---|---|
| | 70 | 75 | 80 | 85 | 90 | 95 | 100 | 105 | 110 | 115 | 120 |
| | Heat sensation (°F) | | | | | | | | | | |
| 0% | 64 | 69 | 73 | 78 | 83 | 87 | 91 | 95 | 99 | 103 | 107 |
| 10% | 65 | 70 | 75 | 80 | 85 | 90 | 95 | 100 | 105 | 111 | 116 |
| 20% | 66 | 72 | 77 | 82 | 87 | 93 | 99 | 105 | 112 | 120 | 130 |
| 30% | 67 | 73 | 78 | 84 | 90 | 96 | 104 | 113 | 123 | 135 | 148 |
| 40% | 68 | 74 | 79 | 86 | 93 | 101 | 110 | 123 | 137 | 151 | |
| 50% | 69 | 75 | 81 | 88 | 96 | 107 | 120 | 135 | 150 | | |
| 60% | 70 | 76 | 82 | 90 | 100 | 114 | 132 | 149 | | | |
| 70% | 70 | 77 | 85 | 93 | 106 | 124 | 144 | | | | |
| 80% | 71 | 78 | 86 | 97 | 113 | 136 | | | | | |
| 90% | 71 | 79 | 88 | 102 | 122 | | | | | | |
| 100% | 72 | 80 | 91 | 108 | | | | | | | |

(Relative humidity — row labels)

| <90°F | No discomfort |
| 90°F–104.9°F | Heat cramps—possibility |
| 105°F–129.9°F | Heat cramps, heat exhaustion—likely; heat stroke—possibility |
| 130°F+ | Heat stroke—high risk |

**B**

| | Air temperature (°C) | | | | | | | | | | |
|---|---|---|---|---|---|---|---|---|---|---|---|
| | 21 | 24 | 26.5 | 29.5 | 32 | 35 | 38 | 40.5 | 43 | 46 | 49 |
| | Heat sensation (°C) | | | | | | | | | | |
| 0% | 18 | 20 | 23 | 25 | 28 | 30 | 32 | 35 | 37 | 39 | 41 |
| 10% | 18 | 21 | 24 | 26 | 29 | 32 | 35 | 37 | 40 | 43 | 46 |
| 20% | 19 | 22 | 25 | 28 | 30 | 34 | 37 | 40 | 44 | 48 | 54 |
| 30% | 19 | 23 | 25 | 29 | 32 | 35 | 40 | 45 | 50 | 57 | 64 |
| 40% | 20 | 23 | 26 | 30 | 34 | 38 | 43 | 50 | 58 | 65 | |
| 50% | 20 | 24 | 27 | 31 | 35 | 41 | 48 | 57 | 65 | | |
| 60% | 21 | 24 | 28 | 32 | 37 | 45 | 55 | 64 | | | |
| 70% | 21 | 25 | 29 | 34 | 41 | 51 | 62 | | | | |
| 80% | 21 | 25 | 30 | 36 | 45 | 57 | | | | | |
| 90% | 21 | 26 | 31 | 39 | 50 | | | | | | |
| 100% | 22 | 26 | 32 | 42 | | | | | | | |

(Relative humidity — row labels)

| <32°C | No discomfort |
| 32°C–39.9°C | Heat cramps—possibility |
| 40°C–53.9°C | Heat cramps, heat exhaustion—likely; heat stroke—possibility |
| 54°C+ | Heat stroke—high risk |

**Figure 12-9.** A) Fahrenheit, and B) Celsius. The heat stress index evaluates the combined effect of air temperature and relative humidity to determine an apparent temperature, or how hot it actually feels.

sodium concentrations in their sweat. Prevention and treatment normally involve cessation of exercise, proper hydration and sodium replacement, and transfer of individuals suffering from cramps to cooler locations to administer fluid and saline solutions.

## FROM THEORY TO PRACTICE

High humidity prevents sweat from evaporating. And remember, sweat that does not evaporate does not cool the body. Use the heat stress index to determine the risk of exercising at various combinations of temperature and humidity. Whereas a 90°F outdoor temperature is relatively safe at 10% humidity, the heat stress of 90°F at 50% humidity is the equivalent of 96°F. When the heat stress index increases to more than 90°F, you may want to consider postponing your exercise session until later in the evening. Or, plan ahead and beat the day's heat by working out early in the morning.

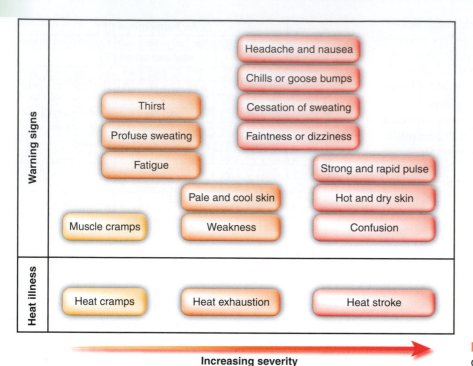

**Figure 12-10.** Heat-related illness categories and warning signs.

## VIGNETTE *continued*

■ Clearly, it is important to recognize the warning signs of impending heat illness. The body exhibits signs long before heat stroke or even heat exhaustion occurs. Had Max Gilpin's coaches recognized his symptoms earlier–and responded appropriately by providing fluids and allowing him an opportunity to effectively cool down–his heat illness likely would have been treated at the stage of heat cramps or heat exhaustion, and he never would have experienced the heat stroke that killed him. Coaches and exercise leaders must be well-versed in the warning signs of heat illness, and that knowledge must be coupled with an appropriate response that helps to alleviate the situation.

## Heat Syncope

Heat syncope is identified by symptoms of fatigue and weakness, profuse sweating and thirst, light-headedness and syncope (partial or complete loss of consciousness), and sometimes pallor (pale color).[20] Causes are generally attributed to peripheral vasodilation, **hypotension**, and possible **hypohydration** associated with prolonged heat exposure, continued sweating, and inadequate fluid replacement. Prevention and treatment normally involve cessation of exercise, fluid replacement and **hyperhydration**, transfer of individuals to cooler locations, and acclimatization to exercise and environment.

## Heat Exhaustion

Heat exhaustion is characterized by more severe symptoms, including fatigue and exhaustion, dizziness, fainting and syncope, diarrhea, nausea, headaches and vomiting, profuse sweating and chills, a weak and rapid pulse, and elevated core temperatures.[20] Causes include an inability of the cardiovascular system to adequately meet the body's needs for blood distribution to the muscles and skin because of dehydration and blood volume loss. In such cases, the thermoregulatory mechanisms cannot remove heat adequately, which creates confusion within the cardiovascular system regarding where to distribute blood. Consequently, these individuals may sweat profusely and may appear either cool and pale or hot, red, and flushed. This illness usually occurs with increasing core temperatures or in nonacclimated individuals exposed to hot environments. Prevention and treatment normally involve halting exercise and moving the individual into cooler environments, and assuming a **supine**, legs-elevated position to facilitate blood return to the heart. It is important to remove any restrictive clothing and attempt to cool the body using fans or the application of wet towels. If the individual is conscious, administer fluids immediately; however, if the individual is unconscious, medically supervised intravenous administration is necessary.

## Heat Stroke

Heat stroke is identified by extreme hyperthermia, where the body's thermoregulatory system fails, which is life-threatening.[20] This situation mandates immediate medical attention because if left untreated, heat stroke will progress to a coma, death, or both. It is characterized by core temperatures exceeding 104°F (40°C); complete cessation of sweating; rapid pulse rates and weak pulse pressures; rapid and shallow breathing; confusion,disorientation, and most likely a state of unconsciousness; and very red, flushed, dry, hot skin. Treatment normally involves immediate immersion in a bath of cool or ice water, or wrapping the body in cold, wet sheets or towels while fanning the body vigorously. Medically supervised intravenous administration is critical for survival.

## Exertional Heat Stroke: Position Statements

The American College of Sports Medicine released a position statement on exertional heat illness in 2007.[21] This statement identifies that exertional heat illness can affect athletes during high-intensity or long-duration exercise and result in activity withdrawal or collapse during or after activity. Maladies include exercise-associated muscle cramping, heat exhaustion, or exertional heat stroke (EHS). Although some are more prone to heat illness (i.e., unacclimated, on certain medications, dehydrated, or recently ill), EHS can affect all athletes, even in relatively cool environments. They define EHS as a rectal temperature greater than 40°C (104°F) accompanied by symptoms or signs of organ system failure, most frequently occurring within the central nervous system.

Early recognition and rapid cooling strategies are critical to reducing morbidity and mortality associated with EHS. Clinical changes associated with EHS can be subtle and may be missed if supervisory personnel or athletes do not maintain conscious awareness and monitor at-risk athletes closely. Fatigue during exercise occurs more rapidly as heat stress increases, and it represents the most frequent causes of exercise cessation. If and when athletes collapse from exhaustion in hot conditions, the term heat exhaustion is often applied. Heat exhaustion is generally resolved with symptomatic care and oral fluid administration. Muscle cramping, in contrast, usually responds to rest and replenishment of lost fluids and sodium.

In the National Athletic Trainers' Association Position Statement (NATA) on prevention of sudden death in sports, NATA intentionally includes EHS and exertional hyponatremia (Box 12-1).[5] The position statement for athletes includes recommendations on prevention, recognition, and treatment. To prevent potential heat

## Box 12-1. Hyponatremia: Can Athletes Drink Too Much Water?

Hyponatremia is an electrolyte imbalance in which the sodium concentration in serum (liquid part of blood without the clotting agents) is lower than normal (<135 mEq/L). In most cases, it occurs as a result of excess body water diluting serum sodium (i.e., overhydration), although the condition can be caused by excessive loss of sodium because of vomiting, diarrhea, or even sweating.[33] Sodium losses in the body typically reduce fluid volumes because as the body loses its primary solute (substance), it loses a means to retain fluid. This signals the release of ADH. As a result of ADH-stimulated water retention, blood sodium becomes diluted and hyponatremia may result.

It can also occur as a result of a combination of losing excess sodium and overhydrating, and may sometimes occur during exercise when one rehydrates with water but fails to replace lost electrolytes. Exercise-associated hyponatremia, however, is not uncommon; in fact, it was estimated that 13% of the athletes who finished the 2002 Boston Marathon were in some form of hyponatremic condition.

This condition, however, gained widespread notoriety recently because of several deaths associated with excessive water intake, a condition also known as water intoxication. In 2007, a radio station in California ran a contest in which the winner would receive a Nintendo Wii gaming system. The goal of the contest was to see how much water contestants could drink without going to the bathroom. The contest was aptly called "Hold Your Wee for a Wii." Contestants were given 2 minutes to drink an 8-ounce bottle of water and then given another bottle after a 10-minute break. The eventual winner drank 2 gallons of water. However, she called in sick to work, and was found dead in her home 5 hours after the contest. She died of hyponatremia.

Water intoxication or "water torture" has also been identified as the cause of death of students at Chico State University and Southern Methodist University in recent years. As part of fraternity hazing rituals, students were forced to drink as much as water as they could before vomiting. In one case, the estimated amount of water consumed was as much as 15 L. Both students died of hyponatremia.

When sodium levels in the serum and extracellular fluids in the body become low, water is pulled inside the cells of the body to try to restore the normal intracellular/extracellular sodium concentration. When this happens in the cells of the brain, the brain swells. Because the brain is encased in the skull, this swelling causes excessive pressure on the brain, resulting in seizures and death.

Hyponatremia can also occur in athletes competing in long-lasting endurance events, especially on hot days. The loss of sodium in sweat coupled with a high intake of water dilutes the body fluids and can lead to hyponatremia. To prevent hyponatremia, it is recommended that for endurance events (e.g., running, cycling) that last longer than 45 to 60 minutes, athletes consume a "sports drink" that contains adequate amounts of electrolytes. One of the factors that make hyponatremia difficult to diagnosis is that the symptoms are similar to those of dehydration and heat illness. Those symptoms can include confusion, fatigue, headache, muscle cramps, nausea, and vomiting. Correctly identifying the cause of these symptoms and getting immediate treatment for the condition is imperative for a positive outcome.

illness, NATA recommends a thorough prescreening for a history of heat illness or potential risk factors; giving special consideration to athletes wearing protective equipment during periods of high environmental stress; gradual acclimation of athletes over a period of 1 to 2 weeks; proper hydration (euhydration) and fluid replacement after activity; and appropriate education to supervisory personnel.

Unlike the American College of Sports Medicine, which recognizes EHS at a rectal temperature of 40°C, NATA diagnoses EHS at a core (rectal or gastrointestinal) temperature greater than 104°F to 105°F (40.0–40.5°C) plus central nervous system dysfunction (e.g., disorientation, confusion, dizziness, loss of consciousness, collapse). According to NATA, treatment must be to reduce core temperature to no less than 102°F (38.9°C) as soon as possible to limit risk for morbidity and mortality. NATA advocates cold-water immersion (35°F–59°F [1.5–15.0°C]) as the most effective method, but also suggests water dousing or wet ice-towel rotations as effective alternatives.

## Adaptations to Heat Stress

Repeated exposure to hot environments results in relatively rapid improvements in the body's tolerance for heat and in its ability to dissipate heat. These adaptations involve physiological adjustments and structural changes within the cardiovascular and thermoregulatory systems that allow the body to perform work at lower core temperatures (Fig. 12-11). This process of acclimation to hot environments normally occurs within 9 to 14 days, although well-conditioned individuals usually require less time to acclimate.[22] To optimize one's ability to acclimate to hot environments, individuals should

reduce their normal training volume and intensity initially, training at intensities less than 70% $\dot{V}O_2$max for durations lasting between 20 and 60 minutes.[22]

With appropriate exposure to hot environments, the cardiovascular system will undergo several important adaptations:

- A progressive expansion of blood volume, increasing over the first 10 days
- This occurs predominantly because of an improved ability to reabsorb sodium from the kidneys, which increases blood and interstitial volumes by 10% to 15%.
- More effective cardiac output and blood distribution to the skin in light of the expanded blood volume
- Improved cutaneous blood flow within the peripheral regions

With appropriate exposure to hot environments, the **thermoregulatory system** will undergo several important adaptations:

- Increased sweat rates to remove more heat
- Decreased sweat thresholds (i.e., the temperature at which sweating initiates)
- More effective distribution of sweat over the surface of the skin
- Decreased electrolyte concentrations in sweat, given improvements in the efficiency in reabsorbing these electrolytes from sweat
- Sweat glands may take 7 to 10 days to sensitize to the effects of aldosterone, which increases sodium and chlorine reabsorption but does not alter the small losses of potassium.[23]

Although these adaptations are rapid and remain as long as the individual continues to be exposed to the hot environments, they can be lost within 2 to 4 weeks after returning to more moderate environments.

## Oral Rehydration Therapy

Oral rehydration therapy is a simple dehydration treatment developed for the World Health Organization and the United Nations International Children's Emergency Fund to rehydrate individuals suffering from conditions like severe diarrhea or from diseases like cholera or rotavirus.[24] It contains a specific ratio of salt, sugar, and water ingested by mouth and saves millions of children's lives each year from death due to diarrhea associated with many third world diseases. The original formula contained 2.5 mL salt, 30 mL glucose, and 1 L water, creating a concentration slightly more concentrated than human blood, thus forcing the body to retain more water (311 vs. 298 mmol/L in blood). The oral rehydration therapy formula has since been reformulated to reduce the solution's concentration (osmolarity) slightly to reduce the incidence of vomiting. The new formula now contains salt (2.6 g/L), glucose (13.5 g/L), potassium chloride (1.5 g/L), and trisodium citrate (2.9 g/L) mixed with 1 L of water.[24] The importance of these formulas is that they have served as the basis for the development of the multibillion-dollar sports drink industry that exists today.

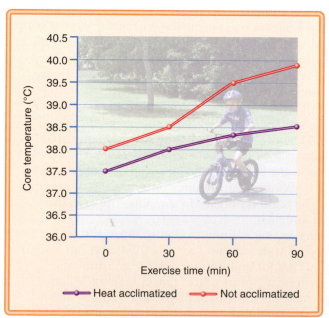

**Figure 12-11.** Adaptations to heat stress involve physiological adjustments and structural changes within the cardiovascular and thermoregulatory systems that allow the body to perform work at lower core temperatures.

## RESEARCH HIGHLIGHT

### Can Drinking "Slushies" Prolong Exercise in the Heat?

Exercising in the heat poses serious challenges to the thermoregulatory mechanisms of the body, and evidence supports the notion that once a critical level of core temperature is attained, fatigue and termination of exercise quickly follow. Studies have shown that cooling the body before exercise lowers core temperature and can increase the heat storage capacity of the body. This can prolong the period it takes to reach that critical core temperature, thereby prolonging exercise duration. Studies have tried external cooling options (e.g., cold-water immersion or wearing ice jackets), but neither of these options is practical in a competitive setting.[4,25] Precooling by ingesting cold fluids has also been shown to decrease core temperature before exercise, resulting in significant improvements in cycling performance.[9] Researchers in Australia conducted a study that compared the effects of drinking cold water with drinking ice slurries ("slushies") on pre-exercise rectal temperature and subsequent exercise performance.[26] The thought was that because the body would have to use more internal heat to convert the slushie from a solid to a liquid, core temperature would be lowered, thereby delaying the time it took to reach a critical level. This would theoretically result in better exercise performance.

Results of the study supported their hypothesis. Pre-exercise core temperature was 0.4° C lower after slushie ingestion compared with drinking cold water, and subjects were able to exercise 19% longer. The subjects' ratings of thermal overload and perceived exertion were also lower throughout the slushie trial. Therefore, it was concluded that ingesting a slushie before exercise is a tasty, practical, and effective way to hydrate the body before exercise in the heat.

Siegel R, Maté J, Brearley MB, Watson G, Nosaka K, Laursen PB. Ice slurry ingestion increases core temperature capacity and running time in the heat. *Med Sci Sports Exerc.* 2010;42:717–725.

## Effective Strategies for Exercising in the Heat

Given the potential for development of heat illnesses, coaches, trainers, and health practitioners should always strategize to avoid potential complications that will impair performance and compromise individual health. The following list provides general guidelines that exercise leaders can follow to ensure a safe and effective exercise experience.

- Be attentive to the environment and avoid exercising outdoors if possible when the WBGT reading exceeds 82.4°F (28°C) or if the heat index value is greater than 105.
- Dress appropriately by selecting fabrics, layers, and colors best suited for efficient thermoregulation.
- Consume fluids before, during, and after exercise or activity.
  - Attempt to avoid dehydration ≥2% of body weight.
  - Measure pre-exercise and post-exercise weights to evaluate the efficacy of current hydration strategies and determine whether a hydration deficit exists.
  - Because the sensation of thirst is usually only experienced at 1% dehydration, begin drinking water in an obligatory fashion or at regular intervals for the 24 hours preceding an event.
  - Consume 500 to 600 mL (17–20 oz) 2 hours before the event or training session.[4]
  - Top off hydration reserves during the warm-up phase by consuming 200 to 300 mL (7–10 oz) every 10 to 20 minutes.[4]

- For events lasting less than 60 minutes, water is usually all that the body requires unless the individual sweats profusely or has high sweat concentrations, or if the environmental conditions prove to be extreme.
- For events lasting more than 60 minutes, a sports beverage containing water, electrolytes, and some **carbohydrates** may be more appropriate.
  - Consume 200 to 300 mL (7–10 oz) every 15 minutes and, if the beverage contains carbohydrates, select a 5% to 8% **glucose** solution (contains 12.5–20 g per 240 mL or 8-oz serving).
- During the post-exercise period, replace lost fluids with a quality sports drink at 100% to 125% of the weight lost, or with water at 120% to 150% of the weight lost.
  - The additional amounts account for the volume of fluid that will be lost to urine.
  - When consuming water versus a quality sports drink, more fluid will be lost to urine.

### Newer Technology: Body Cooling Systems

If you conduct an Internet search on body cooling systems, the results will yield more than 30 different brands selling either body ventilation systems or body cooling systems ranging from vests, neck bands, and leg chaps to gloves and handheld cooling devices. These devices have gained popularity since the early 1990s, thanks in part to the demand from military personnel working in the line of duty in the deserts of Iraq and Afghanistan while carrying packs weighing 100 to 125 lb (45.5–56.8 kg). Their own physiological survival and ability to combat their enemies depend on their ability to maintain safe core temperatures.

Researchers examined the effectiveness of superficial cooling vests on core body temperature and skin temperature in 10 hypohydrated, hyperthermic male participants.[27] After completing exercise in a heated environment that elevated core temperatures to 38.7°C (101.6°F) and produced body weight losses of more than 3.0%, subjects then recovered in thermoneutral environments with or without cooling vests until their core temperature returned to baseline. Although the time to return to baseline was 22.6% faster with the cooling vest, the researchers concluded that we should not use them if we need to rapidly reduce elevated core temperatures. They suggest that cold- or ice-water immersion should continue to remain the standard of care for rapidly cooling, severely hyperthermic individuals until more effective cooling systems are developed.

Cooling the neck is believed by some to improve exercise capacity in hot environments by either physically lowering core temperature or by dampening perceived levels of thermal strain, thereby allowing individuals to override their inhibitory signals to stop. Using a cooling collar, researchers examined time to volitional exhaustion, heart rate responses, rectal temperature, neck skin temperature, ratings of perceived exertion, and thermal sensation and feeling scale in subjects exercising at approximately 70% $\dot{V}O_2$max.[28] Results demonstrated that the cooling collar prolonged time to exhaustion (13.5% increase) and enabled participants to tolerate higher rectal temperatures and heart rates at the point of termination. These researchers concluded that cooling the neck with devices like a cooling collar can have significant positive impacts on athletic performance.

## THERMOREGULATION IN COLD ENVIRONMENTS

The importance of thermoregulation in cold environments is often overlooked, considering how infrequently individuals experience this exposure in comparison with heat stress. Given the high rates of metabolic heat production during exercise and the fact that most outdoor training is performed in more moderate environments, this is understandable. But for those individuals participating in water or winter sports, or sweating in cold or cooler environments, cold stress is important and can provoke significant harm if ignored.

### Physiological Responses to Cold Stress

The effects of cold stress are dependent on the environmental temperature, the individual's **metabolism**, and the resistance to heat loss provided by insulation, whether it be from peripheral adipose or muscle tissue

or from clothing. The peripheral receptors are the first to sense cold environmental temperatures, acting as an early-warning system to prevent a decline in core temperature. This sensory information travels to the POAH and the cerebral cortex.

- The cerebral cortex controls voluntary actions by creating movement, initiating the act of adding layers of clothing, or curling the body up into a ball to preserve heat.
- The POAH activates a sympathetic nervous response via the **neurotransmitter norepinephrine** to stimulate the smooth muscle encircling surface arterioles to vasoconstrict and redirect blood away from the periphery toward the core.[6] Core temperature can be preserved through vasoconstriction when skin temperatures decrease to approximately 68°F (20°C), but any further reductions in surface temperature must be controlled by metabolic regulation.

The first form of metabolic regulation that occurs within the body is called **nonshivering thermogenesis**, which increases the body's internal heat production by 100%. This response, which is regulated by the POAH and mediated through norepinephrine, involves small, temporary increases in metabolic rate. However, if this mechanism proves insufficient in maintaining core temperature, the body turns to skeletal muscle to provide a more significant source of heat production. The POAH activates the brain centers that control muscle tone to stimulate shivering, a low-grade, rapid, and involuntary sequence of contractions and relaxations in skeletal muscle. This mechanism is effective in generating heat without inducing muscle fatigue, as the intensity of the muscle action is insufficient for physical work, but effective for generating heat, increasing the body's rate of heat production threefold to fivefold over rest.

Any further need for heat preservation relies on voluntary muscle action from movement or exercise that can elevate metabolic rates 20 to 25 times greater than at rest. In theory, it is estimated that the heat generated during intense exercise can sustain a relatively constant core temperature in ambient environmental temperatures that decrease to less than –20°F (–28.8°C) without a need for additional insulation.[11] Prolonged cold exposure stimulates increases in the levels of specific hormones circulating in the body. Norepinephrine and epinephrine (**catecholamines**) from the adrenal gland and thyroxin from the thyroid gland accelerate metabolic rates in cells up to 100%, further increasing heat production. As illustrated in Figure 12-12, the body has a sequence of mechanisms it will activate when it needs to preserve heat to maintain core temperature.

Prolonged exposure to cold stress can negatively affect exercise performance. Sustained exercise normally mobilizes **free fatty acids**, increasing their availability for use in the muscle cells for energy, a process mediated by the catecholamines. Although cold stress increases catecholamine levels, free fatty acid levels do

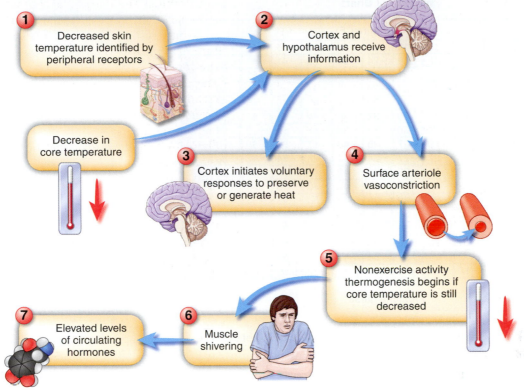

**Figure 12-12.** Thermoregulatory response sequence to decreasing core temperatures.

not rise in proportion because of peripheral vasoconstriction of the vessels supplying the skin and subcutaneous fatty tissue. A reduction in free fatty acid availability forces increased reliance of glycogen and blood glucose that may accelerate the onset of fatigue. Reductions in core temperature also alter the physiological function of nerves and muscles by altering normal muscle fiber–recruitment patterns, decreasing muscle-shortening speed, and reducing the muscle's force-generating capacity, all of which reduce strength and power output from the muscle. Reduced core temperatures also have a gradual slowing effect on the heart's **sinoatrial (SA)** node, reducing the ability to elevate heart rates.

## Evaluation of the Environment

Ambient air temperature and wind induce cold stress on the body by reducing the temperature gradient and increasing convective heat loss, both of which accelerate heat loss. The **wind chill index**, originally developed in 1945 and amended in 2001, is a measure of the apparent temperature felt on exposed skin because of these combined effects (Fig. 12-13).[27,29] The wind chill index will always be lower than the air temperature. Based on the apparent temperatures, guidelines have been established to caution people to exposure and their risk for hypothermia and adverse effects such as frostbite and death.

$$\text{Wind chill (°F)} = 35.74 + 0.6215T - 35.75$$
$$(V^{0.16}) + 0.4275(V^{0.16})$$

where T represents air temperature (°F) and V represents wind speed (miles/hr).

## Risks Associated With Cold Stress

Hypothermia is a condition that occurs when the body loses heat faster than it is able to produce it, reducing core body temperatures to less than 95°F (35°C). At this temperature, the hypothalamus begins to lose its ability to thermoregulate effectively and the metabolism begins to slow down. For every 18°F (10°C) decrease in core (and cellular) temperature below normal, metabolism slows by approximately 50%.[30,31] Hypothermia usually manifests itself from exposure to low temperatures or from any condition that decreases heat production, increases heat loss, or impairs thermoregulation. Signs and symptoms of hypothermia vary by core temperature and are categorized by three stages of severity:

- Mild hypothermia: Core temperatures decline to 90°F to 95°F (32.2°C–35.0°C).
  - This condition involves SNS activation demonstrated by symptoms that include vasoconstriction, shivering, hypertension, tachycardia (accelerated heart rate), rapid breathing, cold diuresis (urine output), and mental confusion.
- Moderate hypothermia: Core temperatures decrease to 82°F to 90°F (27.8°C–32.2°C).
  - This condition is characterized by violent shivering, impaired muscle coordination, as evidenced by slow and labored movement, and stumbling, although the individual may appear alert.

**Wind Chill Chart**

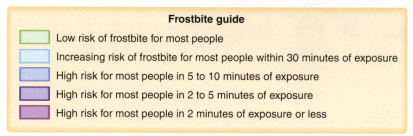

| | | | | | Temperature (°F) | | | | | | | | |
|---|---|---|---|---|---|---|---|---|---|---|---|---|---|
| Calm | 5 | 0 | −5 | −10 | −15 | −20 | −25 | −30 | −35 | −40 | −45 | −50 | |
| 5 | 4 | −2 | −7 | −13 | −19 | −24 | −30 | −36 | −41 | −47 | −53 | −58 | |
| 10 | 3 | −3 | −9 | −15 | −21 | −27 | −33 | −39 | −45 | −51 | −57 | −63 | |
| 15 | 2 | −4 | −11 | −17 | −23 | −29 | −35 | −41 | −48 | −54 | −60 | −66 | |
| 20 | 1 | −5 | −12 | −18 | −24 | −30 | −37 | −43 | −49 | −56 | −62 | −68 | |
| 25 | 1 | −6 | −12 | −19 | −25 | −32 | −38 | −44 | −51 | −57 | −64 | −70 | |
| 30 | 0 | −6 | −13 | −20 | −26 | −33 | −39 | −46 | −52 | −59 | −65 | −72 | |
| 35 | 0 | −7 | −14 | −20 | −27 | −33 | −40 | −47 | −53 | −60 | −66 | −73 | |
| 40 | −1 | −7 | −14 | −21 | −27 | −34 | −41 | −48 | −54 | −61 | −68 | −74 | |
| 45 | −1 | −8 | −15 | −21 | −28 | −35 | −42 | −48 | −55 | −62 | −69 | −75 | |
| 50 | −1 | −8 | −15 | −22 | −29 | −35 | −42 | −49 | −56 | −63 | −69 | −76 | |
| 55 | −2 | −8 | −15 | −22 | −29 | −36 | −43 | −50 | −57 | −63 | −70 | −77 | |
| 60 | −2 | −9 | −16 | −23 | −30 | −36 | −43 | −50 | −57 | −64 | −71 | −78 | |
| 65 | −2 | −9 | −16 | −23 | −30 | −37 | −44 | −51 | −58 | −65 | −72 | −79 | |
| 70 | −2 | −9 | −16 | −23 | −30 | −37 | −44 | −51 | −58 | −65 | −72 | −80 | |
| 75 | −3 | −10 | −17 | −24 | −31 | −38 | −45 | −52 | −59 | −66 | −73 | −80 | |
| 80 | −3 | −10 | −17 | −24 | −31 | −38 | −45 | −52 | −60 | −67 | −74 | −81 | |

*Wind (mph)* is the left axis.

**Frostbite guide**

- Low risk of frostbite for most people
- Increasing risk of frostbite for most people within 30 minutes of exposure
- High risk for most people in 5 to 10 minutes of exposure
- High risk for most people in 2 to 5 minutes of exposure
- High risk for most people in 2 minutes of exposure or less

**Figure 12-13.** The wind chill index is a measure of the apparent temperature felt on exposed skin.

- Surface blood vessels undergo additional vasoconstriction to preserve heat to the vital organs, whereas the peripheries (lips, ears, fingers, toes) experience reduced blood flow and may become blue.
- Severe hypothermia: Core temperatures decline to less than 82°F (27.8°C).
  - This condition involves a cessation of shivering, difficulty with speech and cognitive processing, amnesia, incoherent or irrational behavior, an inability to use or control extremity movement, and cellular metabolic processes that begin to shut down, initiating clinical death.
  - Pulse and respiration rates generally decrease, although ventricular tachycardia and atrial fibrillation can occur. As the core temperatures decrease further, the physiological systems falter and the individual ultimately succumbs to death.
  - At these temperatures, the hypothalamus has lost all its ability to thermoregulate.

Exposure to cold can cause damage to the skin surface in a variety of ways:
- Trench foot (immersion foot) occurs with repetitive exposure to wet, nonfreezing temperatures.
- Frostnip represents superficial cooling of the tissue without cellular destruction.
- Chilblains are superficial ulcers of the skin that occur with repeated exposure to cold.
- Frostbite involves the freezing and destruction of tissue.

Alcohol consumption can also increase the risk for hypothermia via its action as a vasodilator. Although it enhances blood flow to the extremities, providing a sensation of feeling warm, it will accelerate heat loss and increase the likelihood of hypothermia in cold or cooler environments. In fact, alcohol complicates approximately 50% of reported cases of hypothermia.[8]

## Adaptations to Cold Stress

Initial adaptations to repeated bouts of cold exposure lasting 30 to 60 minutes reduce the physiological stress and discomfort on the body. This results in a dampening of the physiological responses to cold, with perhaps the most noticeable change being a delayed onset of shivering because of the improved efficacy of heat generation from nonshivering thermogenesis. Longer, repeated exposures lasting between 3 hours and 14 days in environments ranging between 41°F and 59°F (5°C and 15°C) produce hypothermic habituation. Hypothermic habituation is a physiological adaptation that involves small shifts in normal core temperatures coupled with slight reductions in the body's metabolic response to cold stress.[11,32]

Because heat loss in water is more rapid than in air, repeated cold-water exposure causes a slightly different acclimation response that involves blunted vasoconstriction of peripheral vessels and an improved ability to maintain slightly higher peripheral skin temperatures.

## RESEARCH HIGHLIGHT

### Is It Possible to Freeze Your Lungs by Running in Extremely Cold Weather?

A common myth is that running in cold weather is dangerous and can actually "freeze your lungs." There is absolutely no evidence to support this concept, as people have been known to safely exercise in places as forbidding as Antarctica. Although other reasons may exist to avoid exercise outdoors in freezing temperatures, they have nothing to do with the possibility of freezing lung tissue. When air is inhaled, it is warmed and humidified as it passes through the nose and mouth and goes down the airways into the lungs. By the time the air reaches the lungs, it is completely warmed to body temperature. Air as cold as –0°F (–40°C) is 100% warmed and humidified by the time it reaches the lungs, and it has been estimated that even air as cold as –148°F (–100°C) would not pose a problem.[32] A possible complication of this warming and humidification is that the airways may dry out as they lose water to humidify the incoming air. In some individuals, this may cause a dry cough, or even exercise-induced asthma. The cold air itself can also be irritating to the airways. These effects are not long-lasting and have not been shown to result in any long-term adverse effects.

When exercising in these extreme temperatures, it may be wise to cover the mouth with a scarf, balaclava, or face mask, which will help to trap some of the water vapor from being exhaled and prevent the irritation caused by cold air coming into direct contact with the airways. A more serious problem associated with exercising in the cold is frostbite. Exposed skin begins to freeze at temperatures less than 32°F (0°C), and this effect becomes magnified when there is significant wind (refer to Figure 12-13). Wearing a face mask or balaclava helps to minimize the amount of exposed skin, in addition to helping humidify and warm the inhaled air.

Castellani JW, Young AJ, Ducharme MB, Giesbrecht GG, Glickman E, Sallis RE. Prevention of cold injuries during exercise. *Med Sci Sports Exerc.* 2006;38:2012–2029.

## Effective Strategies for Exercising in the Cold

Appropriate clothing and layering of clothing that minimizes exposed skin surface helps prevent hypothermia. Synthetic fabrics and wool fibers are superior to cotton, because they provide better insulation and tend to dry more quickly after getting wet. Some synthetic fabrics (e.g., polyester) are designed to wick perspiration away and minimize heat losses from the body. Layering clothing creates multiple blankets of warm air, but is only effective if each layer remains dry. Individuals not wearing wicking fabrics must remove the wet layers quickly to avoid excessive heat loss.

Cold, dry air accelerates dehydration from the mucous membranes located in the conducting zones of the respiratory system. It is important to maintain adequate levels of fluid intake to offset dehydration and consume warm beverages to help warm the body. Pre-exercise and post-exercise weight measurements provide an effective means to gauge the adequacy of current hydration practices. Use sunscreens or sun blocks to protect against solar radiation.

## VIGNETTE conclusion

■ The tragedy of Max Gilpin's death may have been averted had his coaches adhered to accepted practices for exercising in the heat and humidity. The strategies presented in this chapter must be followed, with a particular focus on hydration guidelines before, during, and after exercise. Of all the mistakes allegedly made that hot August afternoon, withholding water, as the coaches have been accused of doing, was arguably the biggest contributing factor to Gilpin's death. Perhaps more troubling, though, is the lack of response once his heat-related illness had clearly taken hold. If none of the coaches acted within 20 minutes of Gilpin's collapse, as has been alleged, this certainly would have contributed to his death 3 days later. Acting appropriately—and quickly—is of the utmost importance when responding to heat illness.

# CRITICAL THINKING QUESTIONS

1. You are the coach of a high-school football team. It is 4 days before your first game of the season. You wake up and the temperature is predicted to be 90°F with 60% relative humidity at the time when practice is scheduled. You really need for your team to practice and get ready for your first game. What steps could you take to ensure a safe practice environment for your athletes?

2. You are a participant in a 10K road race. A runner "goes down" in front of you. Her face is red, she is sweating profusely, and she is confused about what happened. What do you suspect is going on, and what can you do to help this individual?

3. You are going to go on a cross-country ski outing to a lake up in the mountains. The distance to the lake is approximately 15 miles. The goal is to have a picnic at the lake and then ski back down. The temperature is 20°F and there is no wind. How would you dress for this outing, and what could you bring along to ensure a safe and comfortable trip?

4. You are a highly competitive runner. You are going to run a challenging (hilly) half marathon (13.1 miles). The day of the race is rather warm and there is a slight breeze. How would you properly hydrate for this event, and what would you wear during the race?

## ADDITIONAL RESOURCES

Gatorade Sports Science Institute (GSSI): www.gssiweb .com. The GSSI is committed to helping athletes optimize their health and performance through research and education in hydration and nutrition science.

Armstrong LE, Casa DJ, Millard-Stafford M, Daniel S, Pyne SW, Roberts WO. Exertional heat illness during training and competition. *Med Sci Sports Exerc*. 2007;39: 556–572.

Casa DJ, Giskiewicz KM, Anderson SA, et al. National Athletic Trainer's Association Position Statement: Preventing sudden death in sports. *J Athl Train*. 2012;47:96–118.

**Research Articles**

Armstrong LE, Casa DJ, Millard-Stafford M, Moran DS, Pyne SW, Roberts WO. Exertional heat illness during training and competition. *Med Sci Sports Exerc*. 2007; 39:556–572.

Castellani JW, Young AJ, Ducharme MB, Giesbrecht GG, Glickman E, Sallis RE. Prevention of cold injuries during exercise. *Med Sci Sports Exerc*. 2006;38:2012–2029.

Maughan RJ, Shirreffs SM. Preparing athletes for competition in the heat: Preparing an effective acclimatization strategy. *Sports Sci Exchange*. 1997;10(2).

Medicine and Science in Sports and Exercise (American College of Sports Medicine Position Statements): www.acsm-msse.org

Sawka MN, Burke LM, Eichner R, Maughan RJ. Exercise and fluid replacement. *Med Sci Sports Exerc*. 2007; 39:377–390.

## REFERENCES

1. American College of Sports Medicine. *ACSM's Advanced Exercise Physiology*. Philadelphia, PA: Lippincott Williams & Wilkins; 2006.

2. Gisolfi CV, Wenger CB. Temperature regulation during exercise: Old concepts, new ideas. *Exerc Sport Sci Rev*. 1984;12:339–372.

3. Cooper KE. Some historical perspectives on thermoregulation. *J Appl Physiol*. 2002;92:1717–1724.

4. Casa DJ, Armstrong LE, Hillman SK, et al. National Athletic Trainers' Association: Position statement: Fluid replacement for athletes. *J Athl Train*. 2000;35:212–224.

5. Casa DJ, Giskiewicz KM, Anderson SA, et al. National Athletic Trainer's Association Position Statement: Preventing sudden death in sports. *J Athl Train*. 2012; 47:96–118.

6. Becker KL. *Principles and Practice of Endocrinology and Metabolism*. 3rd ed. Philadelphia, PA: Lippincott Williams & Wilkins; 2001.

7. Kenney WL, Munce TA. Aging and human thermoregulation. *J Appl Physiol*. 2003;95:2598–2603.

8. Maughan RJ. Temperature regulation during marathon competition. *Br J Med*. 1984;18:257–260.

9. Fregly MJ, Blatteis CM. *Handbook of Physiology*. New York, NY: Oxford University; 1996.

10. Stephenson LA, Kolka MA. Thermoregulation in women. *Exerc Sports Sci Rev*. 1993;21:231–262.

11. Horvath SM. Exercise in a cold environment. *Exerc Sport Sci Rev*. 1981;9:221–263.

12. Bar-Or O. Children's responses to exercise in hot climates: Implications for performance and health. *Sports Sci Exchange*. 1994;7:1–4.

13. American College of Sports Medicine. Exertional heat illness during training and competition. *Med Sci Sports Exerc*. 2007;39:556–572.

14. Godek SF, Bartolozzi A, Godek J, Roberts W. Sweat rate and fluid turnover in American football players compared with runners in a hot and humid environment. *Br J Sports Med*. 2005;39:205–211.

15. Johnson JM. Physical training and the control of skin blood flow. *Med Sci Sports Exerc*. 1998;30:382–386.

16. Johnson JM. Regulation of the cutaneous circulation. *Fed Proc*. 1986;45:2841–2850.

17. American College of Sports Medicine. *ACSM's Resource Manual for Guidelines for Exercise Testing and Prescription*. 5th ed. Philadelphia, PA: Lippincott Williams & Wilkins; 2005.

18. Department of Army. *Prevention, treatment and control of heat injuries*. Technical Bulletin Medical 507. 1980:1–21.

19. Cheung SS, Mclellan TM. Heat acclimation, aerobic fitness, and hydration effects on tolerance during uncompensable heat stress. *J Appl Physiol*. 1998;84: 1731–1739.

20. American College of Sports Medicine. *ACSM's Guidelines for Exercise Testing and Prescription*. 8th ed. Philadelphia, PA: Lippincott Williams & Wilkins; 2010.

21. Armstrong LE, Casa DJ, Millard-Stafford M, Daniel S, Pyne SW, Roberts WO. Exertional heat illness during training and competition. *Med Sci Sports Exerc.* 2007; 39:556–572.

22. Armstrong LE. Heat acclimatization. In: TD Fahey, ed. *Encyclopedia of Sports Medicine and Science.* Internet Society for Sport Science. March 10, 1998. http:// sportsci.org.

23. Pilardeau P, Vaysse J, Garnier M, Joublin M, Valeri L. Secretion of eccrine sweat glands during exercise. *Br J Sports Med.* 1979;13:118–121.

24. UNICEF: *New formulation of Oral Rehydration Salts (ORS) with reduced osmolarity.* www.unicef.org/media/media_31825.html. Accessed October 1, 2012.

25. White AT, Davis SL, Wilson TE. Metabolic, thermoregulatory, and perceptual responses during exercise after lower vs. whole body precooling. *J Appl Physiol.* 2003;94:1039–1044.

26. Siegel R, Maté J, Brearley MB, Watson G, Nosaka K, Laursen PB. Ice slurry ingestion increases core temperature capacity and running time in the heat. *Med Sci Sports Exerc.* 2010;42:717–725.

27. Lopez RM, Cleary MA, Jones LC, Zuri RE. Thermoregulatory influence of a cooling vest on hyperthermic athletes. *J Athl Train.* 2008;43:55–61.

28. Tyler CJ, Sunderland C. Cooling the neck region during exercise in the heat. *J Athl Train.* 2011;46:61–68.

29. National Weather Service. *Windchill temperature index.* Washington, DC: Office of Climate, Water and Weather Services; 2001.

30. McArdle WD, Toner MM, Magel JR, Spinal RJ, Pandolf KB. Thermal responses of men and women during cold-water immersion: Influences of exercise intensity. *Eur J Appl Physiol.* 1992;65:265–272.

31. Moran DS, Castellani JW, O'Brien C, Young AJ, Pandolf KB. Evaluating physiological strain during cold exposure using a new cold strain index. *Am J Physiol.* 1999;272:R556–R564.

32. Castellani JW, Young AJ, Ducharme MB, Giesbrecht GG, Glickman E, Sallis RE. Prevention of cold injuries during exercise. *Med Sci Sports Exerc.* 2006;38:2012–2029.

33. Schrier RW. Does asymptomatic hyponatremia exist? *Nat Rev Nephrol.* 2010;6:185–188.

## *Practice What You Know:* Determining Your Own Sweat Rate

Knowing your sweat rate can help you to determine your fluid replacement needs following exercise. Sweat rate can easily be found by measuring your body weight before and after exercise, and taking into account the amount of fluid in ounces taken in during exercise. Sweat rate can be calculated using the following equations:

Weight of fluid lost = (pre-exercise weight − post-exercise weight) + weight of fluid consumed during exercise (16 oz = 1 lb)

Amount of fluid lost = weight of fluid lost × 16 oz/lb

Sweat rate = amount of fluid lost/exercise time (in hours)

**To practice this exercise:**
- Record pre-exercise body weight after voiding*
- Exercise for a certain period
- Record the amount of fluid consumed during exercise
- Record post-exercise body weight after voiding*

**Example for 2 hours of exercise:**
- Pre-exercise weight (voided): 145 lb
- Post-exercise weight (voided): 142 lb
- Fluid consumed during exercise: 24 oz (1.5 lb)
  - Weight of fluid lost = 3 lb body weight lost + 1.5 lb fluid consumed = 4.5 lb
  - Amount of fluid lost = 4.5 lb × 16 oz/lb = 72 oz
  - Sweat rate per hour = 72 oz/2 hr (36 fluid oz/hr)

### Variations:

To determine sweat rates under different conditions, try the following:

- Exercise at different intensities
- Exercise with a fan blowing on you
- Exercise in a hotter (and/or more humid) or colder environment

*Always weigh yourself under the same conditions (e.g., without clothes or wearing the same, dry clothes)

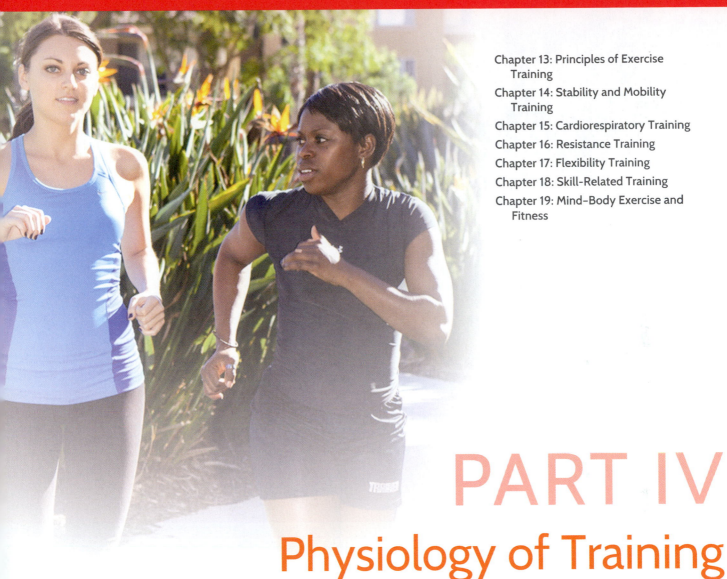

# PART IV
# Physiology of Training

Part IV of this textbook focuses on the practical application and incorporation of many of the principles presented in earlier chapters. Chapter 13 presents general training principles that can be applied to any of the areas described in the subsequent chapters. Chapters 14 through 19 then present the most current research-based training strategies for stability and mobility training (Chapter 14), cardiorespiratory training (Chapter 15), resistance training (Chapter 16), flexibility training (Chapter 17), skill-related training (Chapter 18), and mind–body exercise (Chapter 19). Each of these chapters provides the scientific background related to each type of training, the most up-to-date training guidelines in each of these areas, and specific recommendations on how to systematically design a safe and effective program for clients.

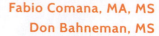

Fabio Comana, MA, MS
Don Bahneman, MS

CHAPTER 13

# Principles of Exercise Training

## CHAPTER OUTLINE

## LEARNING OUTCOMES

1. Explain the need for an integrated approach to training.
2. Identify the various parameters of physical fitness that should be considered when designing exercise programs.
3. Identify key training principles that apply to all exercise programs.
4. Describe a general programming model incorporating macrocycles, mesocycles, and microcycles.
5. Explain Hans Seyle's general adaptation syndrome and its application to exercise.
6. Describe the concepts of overtraining and fatigue, and their physiological impact on the systems of the body.
7. Identify key physiological adaptations associated with exercise.

## ANCILLARY LINK

Visit Davis*Plus* at http://davisplus.fadavis.com for study and practice resources, including online quizzes, animations that help explain physiological processes, podcasts concerning news and career trends in exercise physiology, and practice references.

## VIGNETTE

■ Ashley is a college sophomore who recently started an exercise regimen but lacks a strong understanding of the science behind exercise programming and behavioral change. Her knowledge is limited to her own exercise history, ideas shared by friends, and what she has read in consumer magazines (e.g., celebrity workouts). Consequently, Ashley's program emphasizes aerobic exercise with little resistance training, and the weight training she does perform involves high-volume, muscle isolation–type workouts at lower intensities out of fear of bulking up. Ashley has struggled with her weight for several years, and has started and stopped multiple weight-loss efforts in the past. Once again, she started out enthusiastically, anticipating a quick drop in weight and improvement in her appearance, but after 6 weeks, she has lost very little weight. She is disappointed and reluctant to continue exercising. She decides to hire Sam, a personal trainer at her university's athletic center, to help her develop a program and keep her on track.

What are some of the physical and psychological barriers that are inhibiting Ashley's success, and how can Sam help her overcome them?

Ashley's experience with exercise training is a common one. At the root of her problem is a lack of sound foundational principles on which to base exercise training programs. This lack of understanding often originates, or is compounded by, the wealth of misinformation printed in consumer publications, produced for TV infomercials, or posted on Internet websites.

Whether programming for function, health, fitness, or performance, all cardiopulmonary and resistance training programs follow key training principles that are introduced in this chapter and described in greater detail in the following chapters. This chapter also includes discussions on the principles of overload, specificity, progression, diminishing returns, and reversibility and justification for an integrated approach to training that considers all parameters of physical fitness. Furthermore, this chapter presents an overview of a periodized programming model built on the understanding of the body's adaptation to stress and the effects of overtraining and fatigue on the body.

## OVERVIEW OF PROGRAMMING

Successful exercise programs follow a comprehensive, systematic, and integrated approach to maximize opportunities to achieve optimal results. Although volumes of research exist on the benefits of integrated training, an ever-increasing gap continues to exist between research and practical application. Exercise programs must have functionality. In other words, there needs to be specific carryover of

the gains made in a gym or health club into the activities of daily living (ADL), where we spend the majority of our time and where we are most likely to get hurt. Currently, many exercise programs still focus primarily on aesthetics (i.e., building muscle, trimming fat), training the body and muscle groups in isolation, and fail to emphasize functionality through an integrated, multijoint, multiplanar, and proprioceptively enriched approach (Fig. 13-1).[1] Following are brief descriptions of these aspects of programming:

- **Integration** involves training all parameters of physical fitness addressed previously in Chapter 2 to improve functional strength (capacity to perform ADLs) and neuromuscular efficiency (reduce injury potential by improving the capacity of the neuromuscular system to produce force, reduce force, and dynamically stabilize the kinetic-chain body segments during movements.[2] For example, rather than following a resistance training program simply aimed at building muscle size, an individual would participate in a program that included resistance training, but also incorporated exercises and drills to improve balance, mobility (moving joints through full ranges of motion needed for one's ADLs), stabilization (controlling movement with good technique), and power (moving explosively).

- **Multijoint movements** and exercises are those that incorporate the whole body (kinetic-chain) as opposed to single, isolated joints. For example, a triceps push-down exercise represents an isolated exercise, whereas a push-press (squat

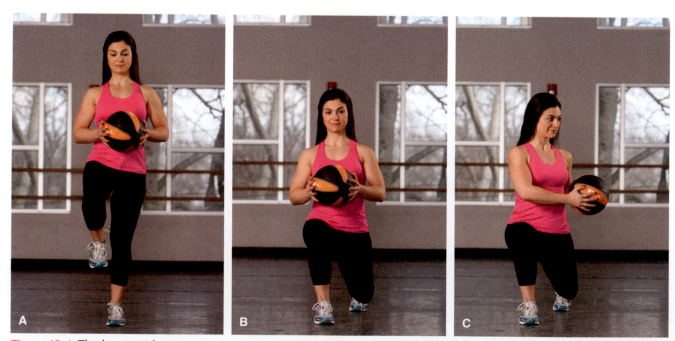

**Figure 13-1.** The lunge with torso rotation is an example of a common multiplanar exercise. A, Initiating the lunge. B, Lunge. C, Torso rotation.

coupled with an overhead press) represents a multijoint movement. These types of exercises better reflect our ADLs, train the body to function as one continuous unit to create and tolerate forces, and will also help to burn additional calories as more muscles groups work simultaneously.

- **Multiplanar training** creates movements in all three planes to reflect the movements of our ADLs more accurately.[3] For example, when performing a standing dumbbell (Db) shoulder press, rather than simply completing repetitions pushing overhead, the individual may complete some repetitions in this fashion but include repetitions in which the direction of movement is changed (i.e., include a rear rotational press pushing the Db upward and behind—rotating the trunk backward—and a front rotational press pushing the Db upward and across the front of the body—rotating the trunk forward). Traditional exercise programs tend to emphasize the sagittal plane and often neglect the frontal and transverse planes that account for more injuries.[4,5] Key differences between a traditional, muscle-based program and a movement-based, multiplanar program are highlighted in Tables 13-1 and 13-2.
- **Proprioceptively enriched environments** are unstable, yet controllable situations in which exercises or movements are performed in

such a manner that they place demands on the body to use its balance and stabilization mechanisms. Basic examples by which proprioception can be challenged include sitting or standing on unstable surfaces like wobble boards or inflated air bladders or even performing ground-based exercises where the body's stability is challenged (e.g., single-leg squat with a reach to a target, single-leg cable press).

In addition to these key functional aspects of programming, another critical consideration when starting or designing an exercise program is to evaluate appropriate levels of stability and mobility through the entire **kinetic chain**. The term *kinetic chain* is used to describe the relationship or connection between your nerves, muscles, and bones that function together to produce movement. For example, when performing a standing bicep curl, it is the muscles, nerves, and structures not only in your upper arm, but also in your shoulders, trunk, and hips that must all function together to stabilize the body while producing elbow flexion; if not, you may fall forward.

Chapter 14 presents the concepts of joint stability and joint mobility as an integral component to achieving efficient movement, whether through an exercise or a complex movement.[6] It is important for health and fitness professionals to rethink training in terms of movement rather than as exercises. Although the functional aspects of programming should

## Table 13-1. Common Exercises Used in a Traditional Muscle-Based Program

| EXERCISE | PRIMARY MUSCLE GROUP(S) | PRIMARY JOINTS INVOLVED IN MOVEMENT | MOVEMENT PLANE(S) OF THE JOINT(S) |
|---|---|---|---|
| Squats | Lower extremity, trunk | Hips, knees, ankles, lumbar and thoracic spine | Sagittal* |
| Lunges | Lower extremity, trunk | Hips, knees, ankles | Sagittal* |
| Leg extensions | Quadriceps | Knee | Sagittal* |
| Leg curls | Hamstrings | Knee | Sagittal* |
| Standing calf raises | Calves | Ankle | Sagittal* |
| Bench press | Chest, shoulders | Shoulder, elbow | Transverse, sagittal* |
| Incline dumbbell press | Chest, shoulders | Shoulder, elbow | Transverse |
| Seated high row | Back | Shoulder, elbow | Transverse |
| Bent-over dumbbell row | Back | Shoulder, elbow | Sagittal* |
| Military press | Shoulders, triceps | Shoulder, elbow | Frontal, sagittal* |
| Lateral dumbbell raises | Shoulders | Shoulder | Frontal |
| Dumbbell curls | Biceps | Elbow | Sagittal* |
| Preacher curls | Biceps | Elbow | Sagittal* |
| Lying triceps extensions | Triceps | Elbow | Sagittal* |
| Cable press downs | Triceps | Elbow | Sagittal* |
| Crunches | Trunk | Hips, lumbar spine | Sagittal* |
| Leg raises | Trunk | Hips, lumbar spine | Sagittal* |
| Supine oblique crunches | Trunk | Trunk | Transverse |

*Heavy emphasis on sagittal plane: 14 of 18 exercises (78%) move in sagittal plane; 4 of 18 (22%) move in transverse plane (no hips); 2 of 18 (11%) move in frontal plane (shoulders only, no lower extremity or trunk).

Lack of balance in program: 2 exercises emphasize ankles; 4 emphasize knees; 4 emphasize hips; 4 emphasize trunk; 6 emphasize shoulders; 8 emphasize elbows.

## 13-2. Common Exercises Used in a Balanced Multiplanar Program

| EXERCISE | PRIMARY MUSCLE GROUP(S) | PRIMARY JOINTS INVOLVED IN MOVEMENT | MOVEMENT PLANE(S) OF THE JOINT(S) |
|---|---|---|---|
| Squat | Lower extremity, trunk | Hips, knees, ankles, lumbar and thoracic spine | Sagittal* |
| Front lunge | Lower extremity, trunk | Hips, knees, ankles | Sagittal* |
| Side lunges | Lateral hip | Hips, knees, ankles | Frontal |
| Rear rotational lunges | Lower extremity, trunk | Hips, knees, ankles, trunk | Transverse, sagittal* |
| Standing low cable hip abduction with external rotation | Lower extremity, trunk | Hips, trunk | Frontal, transverse |
| Lateral step up | Lower extremity, lateral hip | Hips, knees, ankles | Frontal |
| Resistance band— external rotations | Rotator cuff muscles | Shoulder | Transverse |
| Bench press | Chest, shoulders | Shoulder, elbow | Transverse, sagittal* |
| Close grip chin up | Back, biceps | Shoulder, elbow | Sagittal* |
| Incline dumbbell press | Chest, triceps | Shoulder, elbow | Transverse, sagittal* |
| Wide-grip pull-up | Back, biceps | Shoulder, elbow | Frontal |
| Standing dumbbell lateral raises | Shoulders | Shoulder | Frontal |
| Bird-dogs | Core | Trunk, hip, shoulder | Sagittal* |
| Crunches | Trunk | Hips, lumbar spine | Sagittal* |
| Stability ball lateral trunk bends | Core, trunk | Trunk | Frontal |
| Side plank | Core, trunk | Trunk | NA |
| Standing horizontal cable rotations | Trunk | Trunk | Transverse |
| Heavy ball rotational lifts | Hips, trunk | Hips, trunk | Sagittal,* transverse |

*More balanced approach: 9 of 18 exercises (50%) move in sagittal plane; 7 of 18 (39%) move in transverse plane; 6 of 18 (33%) move in frontal plane.

More balance in program: 5 exercises emphasize ankles; 5 emphasize knees; 4 emphasize elbows; 7 emphasize shoulders; 9 emphasize hips; 9 emphasize trunk.

be applied to program design, they are implemented with a common goal: to achieve, maintain, or promote desired levels of stability and mobility needed by the body. In basic terms, **stability** defines the ability to control the position or movement of a joint and should never compromise mobility. Moving a joint in one plane while controlling undesirable movement in other planes defines stability (e.g., allowing the knee to flex and extend while walking, while controlling against unwanted movement in the other planes). To achieve optimal stability, logic would dictate that we immobilize a joint, but in doing so, we lose mobility. **Mobility**, in contrast, defines the degree of unrestricted or functional movement needed at a joint and should never compromise stability.[7]

The analogy of a building may help illustrate this point: Before making any modifications to a building, one must evaluate the integrity (stability) of its foundation. If this foundation lacks adequate stability, then the building will develop weak links that lead to structural deficiencies. Much like a building, the human body also requires appropriate levels of stability to withstand the effects of gravity and the external forces we place on it through our ADLs and training programs. Without this stability, the body is more vulnerable to injury. However, unlike a building that does not need to move, the human body is also designed to move and develops in response to the stresses placed on it through movement, gravity, and other external forces. If the body lacks the appropriate levels of stability and mobility throughout its kinetic chain, these same weak links may develop that lead to deficiencies in joint loading or movement.[8] These deficiencies always impact the neuromuscular and skeletal systems initially, but will ultimately have negative effects on the other systems in the body.

A different analogy is to view the body's movement system as you do a computer. The hardware is our muscles and skeleton, whereas the software that drives the computer's actions is our nervous system. If a system's software becomes faulty, then at some

point it will inflict damage on the hardware. This occurs within the body in much the same way. The cumulative effects of poor posture, sustained awkward positions, repetitive movements, and dysfunctional movement from lifestyle and occupation alter our nervous system's function, which, in turn, can affect our hardware. Within the human body, this manifests as pain and possible injury.[3] That being said, when starting an exercise program, the question that should be raised is whether any evaluation of the existing structures has been conducted beforehand to identify potential weak links.

This relationship of stability and mobility within the human body is unique and serves as a foundation to all programs. If appropriate levels of each are achieved, restored, or maintained at each joint, then movement efficiency is ensured and the exercise experience can only be positive. Although all joints and regions require some levels of stability and mobility, as illustrated in Figure 13-2, some require greater levels of one over the other according to their functional roles within the body.[9,10]

For example, gait (walking) is our default movement pattern (Fig. 13-3). If we briefly examine the body's need to complete this task, we discover:

- The foot, with 26 bones, is generally stable to accept the load of the body as a foot strikes the ground with each step, and to provide a solid surface to push and propel the body forward.
- The ankle is considered a mobile joint, allowing movement in multiple planes (pronation/supination, dorsiflexion, and plantarflexion) to facilitate heel strike, shock absorption, and

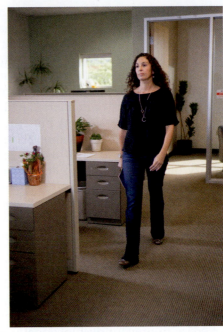

Figure 13-3. Gait is the body's default movement pattern.

toe-off (when the toes leave the ground) to propel the body forward.
- The knee is considered a stable joint moving primarily in one plane (sagittal) as part of gait, minimizing movement into the remaining planes that can lead to injury.
- The hips are considered a mobile joint, moving in all three planes to allow leg swing forward and backward, rotating the hips as the leg swings, and also shifting the hips in the frontal plane over each stance leg (support leg) to avoid falling.
- The lumbar spine is considered a stable joint, controlling the movement and position of the trunk over the hips that move three-dimensionally during movement; this helps protect the low back from injury.
- The thoracic spine is considered a mobile joint, enabling greater multiplanar movements in the upper extremity (this concept is illustrated in the From Theory to Practice feature on page 336).
- The scapulothoracic region is considered a stable region because it provides the stable platform (much like at the foot) from which you can create push-pull movements with your arms.
- The glenohumeral joint is considered a mobile joint, allowing you the opportunity to place your hands just about anywhere in space.

Typically, when one joint (e.g., hip) lacks adequate levels of mobility, the adjacent, more stable joints (e.g., low back and knees) will compromise some stability to assist in providing the needed mobility. This renders these stable joints more vulnerable to injury. In fact, if one examines the most commonly

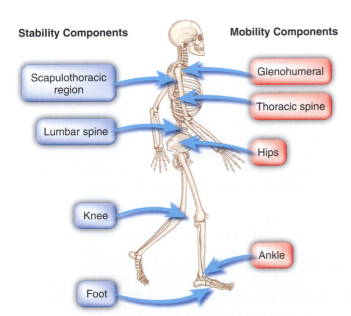

**Stability Components**

Scapulothoracic region

Lumbar spine

Knee

Foot

**Mobility Components**

Glenohumeral

Thoracic spine

Hips

Ankle

Figure 13-2. The stability–mobility relationship during basic walking (gait).

injured regions of the body—the low back, knee, and shoulder (scapula-thoracic) regions—they all happen to be more stable joints. So, is this coincidence, a general lack of stability within those regions, or a lack of mobility in adjacent regions? Although it cannot be stated with complete certainty, the prevailing thought among practitioners leans toward a lack of mobility (i.e., low-back pain may not be caused by weak trunk muscles, but may be attributed to a lack of appropriate mobility needed in the hips and thoracic spine).[11] This may help explain why sedentary office workers who develop tight hip flexors and a bent-over posture (thoracic kyphosis) often complain of low-back pain. This should help you understand the concept of the entire kinetic chain, whereby muscles, nerves, and joint action at one segment of the body may impact function at another segment.

Although Chapter 14 will cover the concept of restoring stability and mobility within the kinetic chain in more detail, it is extremely important to develop a training philosophy built on the notion that movement efficiency precedes exercise to prevent dysfunctional movement and potential injury movement. Although a trainer aims to instruct an exercise correctly, he or she must first understand that a body that lacks the appropriate levels of stability and mobility may never be able to physically complete the exercise flawlessly. Given the prevalence of musculoskeletal injuries, this concept represents an emerging trend in training, with some programs shifting toward emphasizing a more movement-centered approach rather than an exercise-driven approach.

## In Your Own Words

Now that you have been introduced to the concept of stability and mobility and its application to walking, explain in your words why fitness professionals should consider shifting a training philosophy toward one that emphasizes movement quality, at least initially.

Now that you have had an opportunity to consider a shift in your programming philosophy toward movement as a pre-requisite to programming, the next set of concepts to understand are the programming principles that one manipulates when designing an exercise program.

## GENERAL TRAINING PRINCIPLES

As illustrated in Figure 13-4, most exercise programs, regardless of intent, are designed around two key variables: volume (i.e., the amount of work performed) and intensity (i.e., the level of work performed).[12] Generally, with cardiorespiratory programs, **volume** refers to the frequency and duration of an exercise bout, whereas with resistance exercise, volume is defined by the number of sets × repetitions (reps), and often includes the **time under tension** (i.e., the amount of time spent completing a full repetition). **Intensity** in cardiorespiratory programs refers to the level of work performed that is reflected through speed, grade, watts, or intensity level on cardiorespiratory equipment. With resistance training, intensity generally refers to the amount of weight lifted.

Although load and intensity are the two primary variables manipulated in an exercise program, they fall under general training principles that apply to all forms of physical training, whether aerobic conditioning or resistance training. These include:

- Overload
- Specificity
- Progression
- Diminishing returns
- Reversibility

Having a solid understanding of these principles provides great insight into the design of safe and effective programs.

## FROM THEORY TO PRACTICE

Standing with your feet spaced about the width of your hips, drive your left arm across the front of your body and upward as you rotate your entire body to the right. Repeat this movement in the opposite direction and perform two to three repetitions in each direction in a controlled manner.
- Notice how far you reach with each arm.
- Notice the movement in your feet (mobile joint) in multiple planes as you reach upward.
- Notice the movement in your hips (mobile joint) in multiple planes as you reach upward.
- Notice the movement in your thoracic spine (mobile joint) in multiple planes as you reach upward.

Now repeat this movement, but restrict any movement in your feet and notice the difference in the quantity of movement (i.e., how far you can reach).

Repeat this movement, but restrict any movement in your hips and notice the difference in the quantity of movement (i.e., how far you can reach).

Hunch forward, flexing your thoracic spine, and repeat this movement and notice the difference in the quantity of movement (i.e., how far you can reach).

Notice how mobilization of multiple joints along the entire kinetic chain helps promote greater movement?

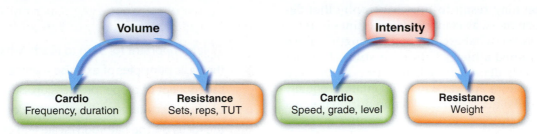

Figure 13-4. Volume and intensity variables of programming. Reps, repetitions; TUT, time under tension.

## Overload

To enhance physiological improvements and stimulate adaptations to training, the program variables must be manipulated to impose a continual physical **overload** on the system or systems being trained (i.e., exercises or workouts performed are greater than those to which the systems—muscles, cardiorespiratory—are accustomed). Overload can be applied with volume (e.g., increasing the duration of a cardiorespiratory bout or performing more repetitions) and intensity (e.g., training harder with more resistance or running faster).

## Specificity

**Specificity** determines the outcome of a specific type of training program, implying that the specific training adaptation or outcome is determined by the method of training.[13] For example, to strengthen the chest muscles, a program that incorporates heavier intensities and lower volume on bench press and other chest exercises should be followed. The acronym SAID *(specific adaptations to imposed demands)* is used interchangeably with this principle, suggesting that the body will undergo physiological adaptations specific to the stresses applied through the variables of program design. The manipulation of volume and intensity under this principle should be guided by the desired training outcomes.

## Progression

**Progression** is the systematic application of overload to promote long-term benefits or prepare an athlete or individual for a specific event. This implies the manipulation of training variables to elicit greater itensities or volumes of training. An important consideration of progressive overload is that the increased physical demands placed on the physiological systems must be applied gradually and systematically over time to allow for appropriate training stimuli, recovery, and adaptation, and to avoid overtraining, burnout, and potential injury.[6] Therefore, progression should consider all physiological, psychological, and emotional parameters. The manipulation of volume and intensity generally follow an inverse relationship in which, when intensity increases, the training volume decreases somewhat proportionally. Progressions to a program can be made *quantitatively* by changing the actual amount of external resistance lifted and/or *qualitatively* by changing the nature of the exercises to challenge the neural and structural components to adapt to a new movement or motor skill.[14]

## Diminishing Returns

Individuals' responses to training vary according to a person's unique genetic composition and conditioning level. Regardless of the training program, some individuals respond more effectively than others, demonstrating great variance in the potential to achieve training outcomes. Typically, individuals who are starting a new program demonstrate significant gains, whereas those who have been consistently training for a period of time show smaller margins of improvement over time. This implies that the rate of fitness improvement diminishes over time as an individual approaches his or her genetic potential. This is sometimes confused with a plateau effect in training where an individual fails to progress his or her program variables appropriately. As a result, the individual experiences a leveling off in training performance.

## Reversibility

**Detraining** is defined as a loss (partial or complete) of any training-induced adaptation that occurs as a result of a decrease in a training stimulus. These physiological losses are often associated with a decrease in training volume or intensity, and the quantity of detraining experienced may differ by the duration of the training cessation.[15]

Furthermore, the various parameters of fitness (e.g., endurance and speed) will demonstrate losses at differing rates. Detraining, however, differs from tapering, which is defined as an intentional reduction in the training volume or intensity for short periods, designed to prepare the body for competition.

Detraining may result in muscle atrophy that decreases muscle mass, as evidenced by declines in muscle fiber cross-sectional area in both strength-trained and sprint-trained athletes.[15] In their study, Lemmer and colleagues[16] demonstrated that strength-induced training adaptations appeared to be maintained equally in younger and older men and women during the first 12 weeks of detraining, but then demonstrated more significant losses thereafter. Detraining-induced losses of flexibility and cardiorespiratory fitness appear to be greater than losses in muscular strength. However, it also appears that maintaining some form of minimal muscle stimulation is important to reduce the rates of detraining. After 3 months of strength training three times a week, individuals who cut back to one session per week were successfully able to maintain most of the strength gains attained during the 3-month training period. Likewise, to maintain cardiorespiratory fitness, a maintenance program of three sessions per week is generally recommended.[17] This reinforces the notion of maintenance training once goals are attained to prevent any unwanted losses. Therefore, a simple guideline to participate in a least one resistance-training workout each week and at least three cardiorespiratory sessions each week can minimize detraining effects and is fairly consistent with the American College of Sports Medicine guidelines for exercise.[12] For individuals pressed for time, circuit-training formats present an excellent option that may satisfy both cardiorespiratory and resistance training simultaneously.

## PROGRAMMING CONSIDERATIONS

Understanding the application of progression by manipulating individual training variables is critical to

### VIGNETTE continued

■ It is important for Sam to teach Ashley some of the basic principles of exercise training, particularly the concept of proper progression. But first, Sam can help her with a goal-setting process that takes the focus off the bathroom scale and onto more meaningful objectives. The idea is to explore *why* Ashley wants to lose weight. Is it simply to improve her appearance, or are there health-related reasons for her desire to get fit? Does her motivation for change come from within, or do other individuals hassle her about her weight fluctuations? Understanding the true impetus behind why Ashley hired him will allow Sam to help her set goals that can serve as steppingstones of success. Once those goals are established, Sam and Ashley can work together to develop a progressive exercise program that will allow Ashley to experience multiple successes along the way.

programming success, but additional considerations are also essential. These include attention to safety and identification of needs and desires. Effective exercise programming must first include a comprehensive health risk assessment (i.e., assess risk vs. benefits of exercise, presence of exercise contraindications); then collect information pertaining to one's health-exercise history and lifestyle preferences that

## RESEARCH HIGHLIGHT

### Training and Detraining of Resistance and Endurance Training

This study investigated changes in body composition, body size, muscle strength, and maximal oxygen consumption ($\dot{V}O_2$max) after 24 weeks of resistance or endurance training and 24 weeks of detraining in young men. Thirty healthy college-aged men were assigned to a resistance or endurance group that participated in three training sessions per week under supervision, or to a control group. $\dot{V}O_2$max, upper and lower body strength, body fat, lean body mass, and body circumference were measured before, after 24 weeks, and following detraining. As expected, after training the exercise groups demonstrated significant increases in the measured parameters. However, after detraining, it was the resistance-trained group that maintained their training adaptations (strength, lean mass) for more prolonged periods than the adaptations gained by the endurance-trained group. However, after detraining, both groups maintained conditioning levels greater than baseline (beginning of the study). The applications from this study appear to be consistent with current consensus: (1) detraining losses do not necessarily return people back to pretraining levels; and (2) with detraining, aerobic gains are lost to a greater extent than the gains made from resistance training.[18]

Lo MS, Lin LLC, Yao WJ, Ma MC. Training and detraining effects of the resistance vs. endurance program on body composition, body size, and physical performance in young men. *J Strength Cond Res*. 2011;25:2246–2254.

consider past or existing injuries and individual wants, needs, and desires. Furthermore, a needs assessment of the individual and activity is always suggested for effective programming. This entails gathering information on the demands of the desired sport or selected activity (e.g., energy systems, movement patterns) and an evaluation of the overall strengths and weaknesses of the individual.

## General Adaptation Syndrome

A key principle behind progression in program design is derived from the understanding of how the body responds to the application of stress through volume or intensity. This understanding has paved the way for strategic manipulation of volume, intensity, and other variables over time, while allowing for adequate recovery, to optimize adaptation and performance. This concept became known as **periodization**, which is an important principle to grasp within program design. This chapter introduces the body's response to stress and the concept of periodization.

**Stress** is a nonspecific response by the body to any stimulus that overcomes, or threatens to overcome, the body's ability to maintain homeostasis (the equilibrium between the body's internal biological mechanisms). This includes the stress of exercise. When the body experiences an acute bout of stress, it stimulates the release of key hormones such as epinephrine and norepinephrine as part of the fight-or-flight response. This response is designed to help humans survive and involves a complex set of interactions within the body's organs and systems. The autonomic nervous system is responsible for this response, activating the sympathetic nervous system, via the action of the hypothalamus. Under this stress, the hypothalamus directs the pituitary gland to initiate the hypothalamic-pituitary-adrenocortical axis and hypothalamic-pituitary-gonadal axis to release a variety of hormones that are critical to managing stressors, and to help the body adapt and overcome. Although the fight-or-flight response is critical to survival during times of acute physical stress, it can have unhealthy consequences if the stress is sustained for prolonged periods.

Stress pioneer Dr. Hans Selye developed the theory of general adaptation as a result of his research on the physiological effects of chronic stress on animals. He observed that the body responds to an external source of stress with a predictable biological pattern in an attempt to maintain and restore the body's internal homeostasis. Selye theorized that this pattern of change occurs in reaction to any kind of stress, and that this pattern eventually leads to disease conditions, such as ulcers, arthritis, hypertension, arteriosclerosis, or diabetes. He called this pattern the **general adaptation syndrome (GAS)**. For decades, researchers have studied his syndrome, and his theories have held up to all levels of scientific scrutiny.[19] His model essentially explains the physiological manner in which a body responds to stress by moving through specific stages, or phases (Fig. 13-5).[20]

### Alarm or Shock Stage

When a stressor occurs, the body's initial response is through the fight-or-flight response, which prepares the body for physical activity. However, this initial response can exact a toll on the body that may decrease the effectiveness of the immune system, rendering the person more susceptible to illness and injury. Traditionally, with exercise, individuals initially feel fatigued, weak, and sore, and experience a decline in performance during this stage that may last a few days to several weeks.[13]

### Resistance or Adaptation Stage

If the stressor continues, the body must adapt or perish; therefore, it mobilizes its internal resources in an effort to return to a state of homeostasis. Homeostasis begins restoring balance through a period of adaptation (recovery, repair, and renewal) that involves changes that occur at many levels to reduce the effect of the stressor(s). Essentially the body responds by altering its physiological structures. An applicable example is with resistance training where after the initial shock phase (4–6 weeks in adults and 2–3 months in older adults), muscle adaptation becomes evident through noticeable increases in muscle size (cross-sectional area) and strength (improved motor unit synchronization and firing).[13] This early part of this stage is characterized by the return of the muscle's normal function after the losses experienced during the alarm phase. However, problems may begin to manifest when the body is not afforded adequate levels of recovery, which may move it into the final stage.

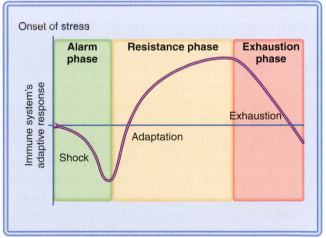

**Figure 13-5.** General adaptation syndrome. This model explains the physiological manner in which a body responds to stress by moving through specific phases.

## Exhaustion Stage

In the final stage, prolonged exposure to the stress without adequate recovery depletes the body's resources and its tolerance of the stressor(s). This implies that the immune system gradually declines or collapses and the body's ability to resist illness or injury is compromised or depleted, which can become a health threat. It is difficult to maintain a state of wellness when a significant portion of the body's energy resources are channeled into coping with a stressor. This adversely affects the body's physiological systems like the autonomic nervous system, contributing to disease as the body fails to maintain normal function. In exercise, this is commonly associated with excessive training and burnout, and is called **overtraining**.

## Overtraining

Overtraining is attributed to inadequate recovery that compromises the body's immune function and its ability to continue adapting, and is characterized by the following general signs and symptoms:

- Decreased performance over a 1- to 2-week period
- Increased resting heart rate or blood pressure, or both
- Decreased body weight
- Reduced appetite or loss of appetite
- Nausea
- Disturbed sleep patterns and inability to attain restful sleep
- Muscle soreness and fatigue
- General irritability and altered moods

These symptoms are the same as those experienced when becoming ill and are indicative of an immune system that is overwhelmed. Bear in mind, however, that all stressors manifest themselves physiologically within the body; therefore, although an exercise program may be appropriate, it may be compounding effects of additional stressors (e.g., finances and relationships) that may be overwhelming the body's immune function. Therefore, it is important to constantly monitor changes in performance and overall wellness during a training program. Typically, when overtraining is experienced, it is recommended that the training volume and intensity be decreased or stopped for a period of 1 to 2 weeks to allow opportunities for full recovery. The suggestion to decrease the intensity and volume of exercise is driven out of the understanding that moderate-intensity exercise has an immune-boosting effect, whereas intense exercise has a temporary immune-suppressing effect.

## Periodization

An understanding of Selye's GAS served as a programming basis for many prominent physiologists who systematically manipulated training variables to create manageable training periods or planned cycles called **macrocycles**, **mesocycles**, and **microcycles**. Each can be defined chronologically or by outcome. They offer greater opportunities to maintain focus on goals, to evaluate progress, to avoid burnout or loss of motivation, and to provide chances to revisit and modify the desired outcomes. These models of manipulating training variables organized into planned cycles were first proposed by Leo Matveyev, a Russian sports physiologist, in the 1960s and termed *periodization* (Fig. 13-6).

Although Matveyev's model was proposed for elite strength and power athletes to prepare them for competition, his approach to training has since transcended many populations, whether sport specific, resistance based, or for general conditioning. This original model was considered linear; volume and intensity changed in a reciprocal manner throughout the training macrocycle (i.e., as volume decreases, intensity increases). More recently, nonlinear or undulating models have been introduced that involve more frequent fluctuations in volume and intensity, and other variables. Both appear

---

### SEX DIFFERENCES

Research on the human fight-or-flight response has been disproportionately based on male studies, due, in part, to the natural, cyclical variations in hormonal and neuroendocrine responses in females that make results difficult to interpret. Research supported by the National Institute of Mental Health formulated a theory that characterizes female responses to stress by a pattern termed "tend-and-befriend" rather than by fight-or-flight.[21] The research supports the premise that female stress responses have evolved to maximize survival of both self and offspring. This "tend-and-befriend" pattern involves offspring nurturance under stress to protect them from harm (tending), and befriending (creating and joining social groups for the exchange of resources and protection). These findings are supported in literature that substantiates how females prefer to affiliate, or make close connections under stress, a response that is sex linked to different neuroendocrine responses between men and women, and to different social and cultural roles between the sexes. Unfortunately, the implications of this research to the applications of exercise stress are still unclear. Generally, it is still believed that females should follow similar training methods as men, with special considerations for sex-specific differences (e.g., greater Q-angles at the knee that increase knee instability).

## FROM THEORY TO PRACTICE

Have you ever noticed that, after taking a brief break from your typical training program, you feel recharged and refreshed when returning back to exercise? This may reflect the needed bout of additional recovery to allow your body to fully recover.

If you are currently exercising, get in the habit of measuring and recording your resting heart rate, taken first thing in the morning two to three times a week. Track any noticeable changes that may occur over a period of 1 to 2 weeks. As conditioning levels improve, resting heart rate should decrease and not increase, which is indicative of illness, injury, or overtraining. Next, keep an active log of your exercise performance and note any noticeable decreases in performance over a 1- to 2-week period.

If any symptoms of overtraining are detected, take a quick inventory of your life and the stressors your encounter on a daily basis. If you identify any additional excessive stressors, plan to reduce your exercise intensity and volume (frequency of training, sets, reps, duration) for a period of 1 week as you attempt to cope and adjust to these new stressors. When returning to your regular training, track any positive changes you may experience.

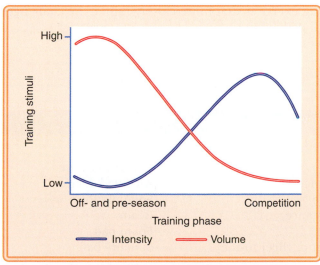

**Figure 13-6.** Matveyev's linear periodization model. Periodization involves skillfully modifying program variables over time to effectively transition a program from a more generalized approach toward one that addresses the specific needs, demands, and desires of an individual.

to be equally effective in promoting improvements in strength and performance,[22] but the nonlinear method is believed to impose greater levels of stress on the body, given the more frequent bouts of alarm or shock

that may compromise immune function and trigger potential overtraining.[23]

The application of linear and nonlinear (undulating) models is discussed in greater detail in Chapter 16. Periodization, therefore, is the art of skillfully modifying program variables over time to effectively transition a program from a more generalized approach toward a program that addresses the specific needs, demands, and desires of an individual.

### Macrocycles

The largest division of time is termed the *macrocycle*, which can constitute an entire training program ranging from a few months to a few years. This is the defined time period in which an individual strives to achieve the desired outcomes. Examples of shorter macrocycles include losing 20 lb (9.1 kg) before a wedding or bulking up to add 10 lb (4.5 kg) before an upcoming rugby season in 6 months. An example of a longer macrocycle might be that of an Olympian who has enjoyed some much-needed recovery after the 2012 London Olympics and is now planning to prepare for the 2014 World Championships and the 2016 Olympics in Rio de Janeiro.

### Mesocycles

Within each macrocycle are two or more smaller time periods called *mesocycles*, each lasting several weeks to several months. The duration of a mesocycle is generally determined by the time identified to achieve a distinct training objective. Mesocycles are organized into weeks or months as dictated by the training goal, by one's competition schedule, or even one's work/home-life demands. For example, a university strength coach may spend time building muscle mass (hypertrophy) as a mesocycle, then progress his or her athletes into a 5-week strength mesocycle to increase force production, before progressing again into a 4-week power mesocycle to increase the athlete's explosiveness.

### Microcycles

Within each mesocycle are two or more smaller time periods called *microcycles*, each lasting between a few sessions to several weeks. They represent the smallest period for organizing programming variables and denote daily or weekly training variations. For example, within a hypertrophy mesocycle, a client might move from machine-based training to using free weights between one week and the next.

Training programs often have multiple goals or desired outcomes, and thus may have several mesocycles occurring simultaneously (e.g., core, cardio, and flexibility) as illustrated in Figure 13-7. However, it is important for the practitioner to understand how these individual mesocycles will need to fit coherently within the available time to exercise within a session or within a week. Occasionally, time limitations may necessitate a need to prioritize training goals and mesocycle design

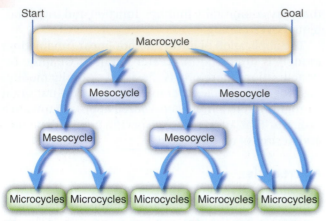

*Mesocycles frequently overlap due to different training modalities being performed simultaneously (for example, cardio exercise and resistance training).

**Figure 13-7.** Relationships among the three programming phases. Training programs often have multiple goals or desired outcomes; therefore, they may have several mesocycles occurring simultaneously (e.g., core, cardio, and flexibility).

to devote adequate training time to achieve a desired training outcome.

## Additional Programming Considerations

Although exercises and movements should always be safe, yet challenging, and implemented in a systematic and progressive nature that ultimately includes activity- or movement-specific exercises that mimic the desired outcome(s), other considerations should be made that lead to optimal program design. Traditionally, individuals limit their considerations to the basic variables that include frequency, intensity, duration, sets, repetitions, tempo, rest intervals, and recovery periods (between workouts), and often neglect other variables that can significantly impact training success (Table 13-3).

The order or sequence in which exercises are performed is an important consideration that can impact both injury and performance. Generally, power-type (explosive) exercises and heavy-strength exercises should be performed at the beginning of the workout after an appropriate warm-up, when energy and concentration levels are highest and fatigue level is lowest. Performing these exercises later in a workout when higher levels of fatigue are more likely may increase the risk for injury.[24]

Perform primary or linear exercises at the beginning of a workout, whereas assistance or rotary exercises should be performed later in the workout. Primary or linear exercises are those that involve multiple joints where many segments of the body move together in a similar plane. Examples of linear exercise include squats, lunges, shoulder presses, and bench presses (Fig. 13-8).

Assistant or rotary exercises target single joints with more isolated movements, moving around one joint. Examples of rotary exercises include leg extensions, hamstrings curls, and biceps curls. As illustrated in Figure 13-9, fitness professional should also consider other factors when sequencing exercises into a program. The general progression represented in this illustration is one that moves from more isolated and supported exercises for deconditioned individuals toward more integrated and unsupported exercises for more conditioned individuals, representing exercises that more closely mimic the challenges of daily living.

## Table 13-3. Integrated Training Variables

| PLANE OF MOTION/BODY POSITION | BASE OF SUPPORT | SURFACES |
|---|---|---|
| Sagittal<br>Frontal<br>Transverse<br>Combination of all | **Static:**<br>• Hip-width<br>• Narrow-stance<br>• Wide-stance<br>• Staggered-stance<br>• Split-stance<br>• Tandem-stance (heel-to-toe)<br>• Single-leg | Ground/floor<br>Bench/machine<br>Air-filled device<br>Solid platform<br>Beam<br>Foam pad<br>Stability ball |
| **BODY POSITION** | **BASE OF SUPPORT** | **EXTREMITY MOVEMENTS** |
| Supine<br>Prone<br>Sitting<br>Standing | **Dynamic:**<br>• Stepping<br>• Lunging<br>• Jumping<br>• Bounding<br>• Hopping | Bilateral (two)<br>Unilateral (single) |

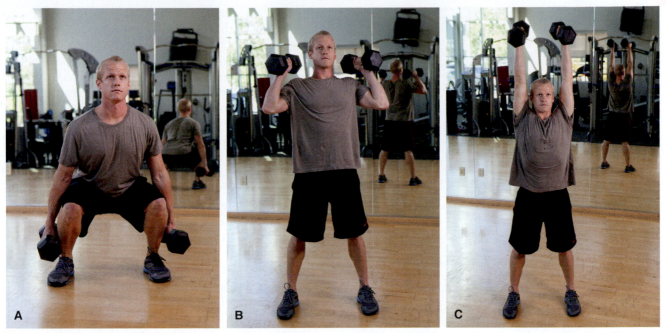

**Figure 13-8.** The push-press squat with overhead press is an example of a multijoint, linear exercise. A, Lowered squat position. B, Completed squat concentric movement. C, Overhead press position.

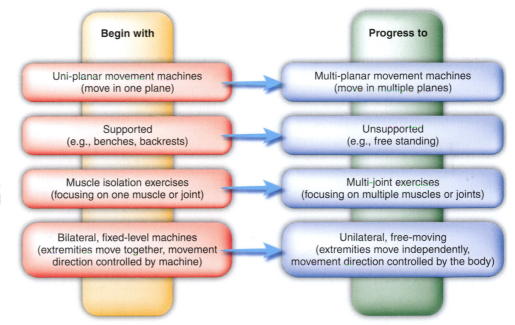

**Figure 13-9.** Appropriate program progressions. The general progression represented in this illustration is one that moves from more isolated and supported exercises for deconditioned individuals toward more integrated and unsupported exercises for more conditioned individuals, representing exercises that more closely mimic our challenges of daily living.

| Begin with | Progress to |
| --- | --- |
| Uni-planar movement machines (move in one plane) | Multi-planar movement machines (move in multiple planes) |
| Supported (e.g., benches, backrests) | Unsupported (e.g., free standing) |
| Muscle isolation exercises (focusing on one muscle or joint) | Multi-joint exercises (focusing on multiple muscles or joints) |
| Bilateral, fixed-level machines (extremities move together, movement direction controlled by machine) | Unilateral, free-moving (extremities move independently, movement direction controlled by the body) |

## FATIGUE

**Fatigue** describes a decrease in performance that is experienced during sustained effort (Fig. 13-10). This decrease represents a body's or system's inability to maintain the desired or required work intensity and is typically felt as a sensation of being "tired." Contrary to popular belief, this sensation is not necessarily due to the accumulation of lactate, although it is one of several possible contributing factors. The reality is that fatigue is probably multifactorial and attributed to many causes: peripheral factors (within muscles), central factors (within the nervous system), or other factors not directly associated with the exercising muscles (e.g., cardiopulmonary system, thermoregulatory system, tolerance for discomfort, and mental toughness).

## Energy Systems

Energy depletion, or the inability to sustain energy supply that meets current exercising demands, is perhaps the most logical explanation for fatigue. Whether aerobic or anaerobic, both systems rely on substrate to continue fueling activity. As discussed in Chapter 4, the phosphagen system composed of adenosine triphosphate (ATP) and phosphocreatine (PCr) depletes quickly. Although ATP

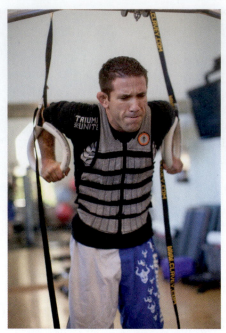

**Figure 13-10.** An exerciser experiencing the multifaceted phenomenon of fatigue.

molecules are generated from multiple sources (e.g., glucose, fatty acids, and PCr), it is their creation from the rapid breakdown of PCr near the myosin heads that sustains this energy pathway for short-duration, high-intensity bouts of exercise. As the muscle's stores of PCr deplete, this system's ability to quickly regenerate ATP diminishes, thus inevitably reducing the body's ability to sustain this intensity of exercise (Fig. 13-11).

Fatigue attributed to limitations within the fast glycolytic pathway is unique and is associated more with metabolic by-products than with fuel depletion. Subsequently, they will be discussed later in this section. Whether anaerobic or aerobic, carbohydrates

can contribute significantly or exclusively to the manufacture of ATP to fuel exercise. During higher intensity, sustained bouts of exercise, glycogen levels can deplete more rapidly in comparison with when they are utilized aerobically through the Krebs cycle and electron transport chain. Glycogen depletion rates are controlled primarily by exercise intensity and, to a lesser degree, by the muscle fiber type and exercise duration.

Glycogen depletion from either type I or type II fibers depends on exercise intensity. During lower intensity, endurance-type events, the type I fibers will deplete glycogen faster than the type II fibers, which may not even be recruited to do work. As the intensity of the endurance event increases, glycogen utilization from the type II(a) and ultimately type II(x) fibers will increase.

Based on muscle fiber type, function, and the activity performed, certain muscles may fatigue faster than others. The gastrocnemius, for example, has a higher concentration of type II fibers than the soleus muscle, and thus is best suited for explosive or forceful movements.

## Metabolic By-products

The accumulation of hydrogen ions in muscle tissue results in acidosis or a decrease of tissue pH. A decline in tissue pH impacts various events within the metabolic pathways that ultimately trigger fatigue because of a decrease in the muscle's ability to produce energy. These include:
- Decreased glycolytic-enzyme activity
- Reduction in myosin-ATPase activity (enzyme that splits ATP)
- Increased pain receptor sensitivity in muscle tissue
- Decreased ability to release and reabsorb calcium from the sacroplasmic reticulum
- Interference with calcium's ability to bind to troponin

## Neural Fatigue

As described in Chapters 9 and 10, neurotransmitters play an integral role in relaying the nerve impulse across the neuromuscular junction. Acetylcholine (Ach) is the neurotransmitter involved in voluntary muscle action. After its release from the presynaptic membrane, it is quickly degraded to acetic acid and choline by the enzyme acetylcholinesterase, ensuring that it only executes a specific function. This enzyme may become hyperactive, therefore preventing Ach from binding to the post-synaptic membrane and inhibiting muscle activation, or it may become hypoactive, thereby allowing Ach to accumulate on the post-synaptic receptors and inhibit muscle relaxation.

## Thermoregulatory Stress

Exercise in the heat or any form of exercise that elevates core temperature necessitates the expenditure of

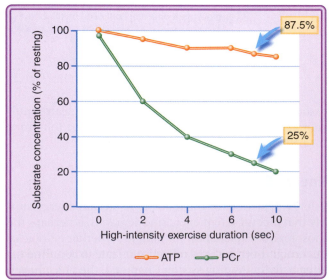

**Figure 13-11.** The decline in concentrations of phosphocreatine (PCr) associated with short-duration, high-intensity exercise.

additional energy to cool the body. Although increases in core temperature shift in oxygen-dissociation curve downward to release more oxygen to fuel this additional work, it also increases the utilization of carbohydrates that may accelerate glycogen depletion and fatigue. Thermoregulation is described in Chapter 12.

## Cardiopulmonary Fatigue

The muscles involved in passive respiration consume approximately 2% of the body's total oxygen uptake; but during active inspiration (exercise) when additional muscles become involved, this number may increase to 11% and compromise the amount of available oxygen for the exercising muscles. During sustained exercise where sweat losses become significant, a decrease in blood volume compromises blood flow and nutrient/oxygen delivery to various organs or tissues. Heart rate may increase to offset reductions in stroke volume to maintain circulation, which also demands additional oxygen that may be limited or unavailable. This offers one explanation why your heart rate may gradually increase during a cardiorespiratory session where the exercise intensity is fixed. The inability to sustain cardiopulmonary efficiency decreases nutrients and oxygen delivery to and metabolic by-product removal (hydrogen ions and carbon dioxide) from the tissue, imposing more stress on the muscular system.

## Tolerance for Discomfort and Mental Toughness

The use of intrinsic (e.g., power words and self-talk) and extrinsic motivators (e.g., verbal encouragement from coaches, cheering crowds, and music tempo) does provide adequate distraction to enable an individual to dig a little deeper, push a little harder, or last a little longer. Although not fully understood, these motivators may negate or blunt an individual's conscious or subconscious sensations of fatigue and desire to stop, and allow them to tolerate greater levels of discomfort.

From the information presented earlier, it appears that fatigue cannot be attributed exclusively to one factor, but perhaps is better viewed as a multisystem event. Increasing one's resistance to fatigue therefore necessitates a program in which all systems are overloaded appropriately, either in isolation or via integration, but in a manner that permits the body the opportunity to adapt and resist the onset of fatigue. Furthermore, it is also important for practitioners to remember that the overall exercise experience is perhaps one of the most critical determinants to exercise adherence.[25] Ekkekakis et al.[25] examined 33 research articles published between 1999 and 2009 that investigated the relationship between exercise intensity and emotional responses. They discovered evidence of a dose–response relationship where higher intensities of exercises were associated with lower levels of enjoyment. They also discovered that when exercise intensities are self-selected,

rather than imposed, they foster greater tolerance to higher levels of intensity. This information provides a rationale for examining the impact that current exercise guidelines may have on adherence. Besides effectiveness and safety, it is becoming increasingly clear that programs should also account for the overall experience and consider how the programming variables impact the emotional and cognitive domains that influence participation.

## VIGNETTE continued

After a few months of working with Sam, Ashley has begun to experience her first real success with an exercise program. With Sam's encouragement, she is eating better, has lost some weight, and perhaps most importantly, reports an improved, more active quality of life. She has added a second workout on her own each week and uses that time to complete a total-body resistance-training circuit. After Sam taught her the truth about the myth of women bulking up from weight training, Ashley felt comfortable enough to add this element to her program. She has really enjoyed her workouts, and loves seeing her strength improve and the changes in her body's shape. It is clear to Sam that Ashley's self-esteem and self-efficacy have improved dramatically.

In addition to this positive feedback, Ashley also reports to Sam that during her more recent resistance-training sessions, she quit several of the exercises because of "fatigue." She describes the fatigue as a shakiness in her arms when the weights feel too heavy to move. After talking to her about the weight loads she is using, Sam feels that this is not a case of physiological fatigue, but a lack of mental toughness on Ashley's part. She is simply giving up on the set of lifts as soon as it becomes a bit difficult. Sam decides to teach Ashley some techniques to help her overcome these barriers, including tips on how to use self-talk to push herself through a difficult set.

## MUSCLE SORENESS

Although overload and muscle damage (especially from eccentric training) provide a strong stimulus for growth, they also lead to muscle soreness. Acute muscle soreness, evident during intense exercise, the latter stages of exercise, and the immediate recovery period, is generally the result of an accumulation of waste products (e.g., hydrogen ions) or a temporary fluid shift exerting pressure on pain receptors. This soreness usually disappears within minutes or hours following exercise. **Delayed-onset muscle soreness (DOMS)** however, is normally experienced between 12 and 72 hours after exercise. Mechanical stresses placed on the muscle during training result in microtrauma or microtears within the myofibrils that cause disarrangement of the sarcomeres.[6,26] This is believed to trigger an immune response releasing histamines and prostaglandins into that local area, causing edema or fluid accumulation inside the muscle compartment. Both events stimulate the local nociceptors (pain) receptors. This occurrence falls in line with Hans Selye's alarm or shock phase. During this phase and until adequate repair has occurred, some of the muscle's physiological and functional capabilities are compromised:

- Reductions in the muscle's force-generating capacity: the physical disruption of the myofibrils reduces the excitation-coupling and contraction process between actin and myosin, and also creates a loss of some contractile protein
- Impaired muscle glycogen synthesis commencing 6 to 12 hours after exercise, compromising the muscle's potential to store energy reserves
- Structural damage, evident by the presence of specific muscle enzymes and myoglobin in the blood following training
- Impaired calcium homeostasis that interferes with troponin binding

Although DOMS is inevitable when beginning a resistance training program or making significant overload changes within a program, several strategies exist whereby the magnitude of DOMS can be controlled or minimized:

- Reduce the initial volume of time in eccentric training (i.e., the time under tension performing the eccentric portion of the rep).
- Start training at lower intensities, increasing gradually.

- Control exercise volume (sets × reps and tempo). Because muscle typically does not show any significant growth for 4 to 6 weeks (2–3 months in older adults), it raises the question why one would impose unnecessary muscle soreness upon beginners? Although multiple sets may burn a few more calories, the associated DOMS may negatively impact the overall exercise experience and adherence. A recommendation is to consider starting with one set for the first 1 to 2 weeks, then progressing the number of sets gradually thereafter.

## In Your Own Words

Your friend has just started resistance training and is now experiencing muscle soreness to the point at which he is becoming discouraged from continuing with his workout regimen. In your own words, briefly explain DOMS and suggest some strategies he could implement to help manage his muscle soreness.

## VIGNETTE conclusion

■ With a greater understanding of programming principles and behavioral change, Ashley was able to successfully integrate an exercise program into her lifestyle for the first time. Consequently, she dismissed some preconceived training myths and has adopted a training program that is better suited to her needs and desires, and enables her to meet her goals. Ashley credits Sam's teachings with allowing her to have a program with greater structure and purpose, thereby improving her overall experience and increasing the likelihood of her continuing to exercise.

## CRITICAL THINKING QUESTIONS

1. You have been asked to present on the foundational principles of program design to a group of dieticians who have studied exercise science in theory, but now seek ideas on how to apply their knowledge into practice. Using the information provided in this chapter, draft eight key talking points that you believe would help illustrate the application of scientific principles.

2. You are training an 18-year-old athlete who is preparing to play competitive sports on a scholarship at college (university) that begins in 8 weeks. Over the past 2 weeks you have noticed that his performance has decreased; he has lost 5 lb (2.3 kg) and has consistently demonstrated higher levels of

fatigue than normal. Using your understanding of Hans Seyle's GAS and the general principles of training, what recommendations would you make at this juncture that would allow him some much-needed recovery, yet not allow him to suffer from excessive detraining before he reports to his team?

3. Mike is a 38-year-old salesman and ex-college recreational runner who is now 10 lb (4.5 kg) heavier than what he was during his mid-twenties. He currently plays golf with business clients two to three times per month and plays the occasional recreational game of pick-up basketball every second weekend with his friends at the local park. He

is tired of being this deconditioned and would like to improve his overall fitness, which may also improve his games of golf and basketball. To help motivate him to start training, he has registered for a one-on-one basketball tournament and a charity golf tournament that are both 4 months away. Although his work schedule is somewhat tight, he is committed to exercising three to four times per week, each for 60 minutes.

Using the information provided, design his program macrocycle and mesocycles that follow the training model phases provided in this chapter to prepare him for both events. Keep in mind that he has a 1-week work conference 6 weeks from today and a 1-week family vacation scheduled in 12 weeks from today that will need to be considered in your program layout.

## ADDITIONAL RESOURCES

American Council on Exercise. *ACE Personal Trainer Manual.* 5th ed. San Diego, CA: American Council on Exercise; 2014. Chapters 5 and 9.

Baechle TR, Earle RW, eds. *Essentials of Strength Training and Conditioning.* Champaign, IL: Human Kinetics; 2008. Chapter 19.

Clark MA, Lucett SC. *NASM Essentials of Sports Performance Training.* Baltimore, MD: Lippincott Williams & Wilkins; 2010. Chapter 1.

## REFERENCES

1. Clark, MA, Sutton, BG, and Lucett, SC (Editors). *NASM Essentials of Personal Fitness Training, (4th edition revised).* Burlington, MA: Jones & Bartlett Publishing, 2014.
2. Clark MA. *Integrated Training for the New Millennium.* Thousand Oaks, CA: National Academy of Sports Medicine; 2000.
3. Sahrmann S. *Diagnosis and Treatment of Movement Impairment Syndromes.* St. Louis, MO: Mosby; 2002.
4. Ford KR, Myer GD, Hewett TE. Valgus knee motion during landing in high school female and male basketball players. *Med Sci Sports Exerc.* 2003;35: 1745–1750.
5. Fredericson M, Cookingham CL, Chaudhari AM. Hip abductor weakness in distance runners with iliotibial band syndrome. *Clin J Sports Med.* 2000;10: 169–175.
6. American Council on Exercise (ACE). *ACE Personal Trainer Manual.* 5th ed. San Diego, CA: ACE; 2014.
7. Houglum PA. *Therapeutic Exercise for Musculoskeletal Injuries.* 2nd ed. Champaign, IL: Human Kinetics; 2005.
8. Kendall FP, McCreay EK, Provance PG, Rodgers MM, Romani WA. *Muscles Testing and Function with Posture and Pain.* Baltimore, MD: Lippincott, Williams & Wilkins; 2005.
9. Cook G, Jones B. *Secrets of the Hip and Knee.* 2007. www.functionalmovement.com
10. Cook G, Jones B. *Secrets of the Shoulder.* 2007. www.functionalmovement.com
11. Clark MA, Lucett SC. NASM *Essentials of Sports Performance Training.* Baltimore, MD: Lippincott Williams & Wilkins; 2010.
12. American College of Sports Medicine. *ACSM's Guidelines for Exercise Testing and Prescription.* 9th ed. Baltimore, MD: Lippincott Williams & Wilkins; 2014.
13. Baechle, TR and Earle, RW (Editors). *Essentials of Strength Training and Conditioning* (3rd edition), Champaign, IL: Human Kinetics, 2008.
14. Kraemer W, Zatsiorsky V. *Science and Practice of Strength Training.* 2nd ed. Champaign, IL: Human Kinetics; 2006.
15. Mujika I, Padilla S. Detraining: Loss of training-induced physiological and performance adaptations. Part I: Short term insufficient training stimulus. *Sports Med.* 2000;30:79–87.
16. Lemmer JT, Hurlbut DE, Martel GF, et al. Age and gender responses to strength training and detraining. *Med Sci Sports Exerc.* 2000;32:1505–1512.
17. Hickson RC, Foster C, Pollock ML, Galassi TM, Rich S. Reduced training intensities and loss of aerobic power, endurance and cardiac growth. *J Appl Physiol.* 1985;58:492–499.
18. Lo MS, Lin LLC, Yao WJ, Ma MC. Training and detraining effects of the resistance vs. endurance program on body composition, body size, and physical performance in young men. *J Strength Cond Res.* 2011;25:2246–2254.
19. Garhammer J. Periodization of strength training for athletes. *Track Tech.* 1979;73:2398–2399.
20. American Council on Exercise (ACE). *ACE's Essentials of Exercise Science for Fitness Professionals.* San Diego, CA: ACE; 2010.
21. National Institute of Mental Health. *A Neuroendocrine Model Explains Gender Differences in Behavioral Response to Stress.* June 7, 2001. http://nih.gov. Retrieved, March, 2013.
22. Baker D, Wilson G, Carlyon R. Periodization: The effect on strength on manipulating volume and intensity. *J Strength Cond Res.* 1994;8:235–242.
23. Plisk SS, Stone MH. Periodization Strategies. *J Strength Cond Res.* 2003;25:19–37.
24. Fleck SJ, Kraemer WJ. *Designing Resistance Training Programs.* 3rd ed. Champaign, IL: Human Kinetics; 2003.
25. Ekkekakis P, Parfitt G, Petruzzello SI. The pleasure and displeasure people feel when they exercise at different intensities: Decennial update and progress towards a tripartite rationale for exercise intensity prescription. *Sports Med.* 2011;41:641–670.
26. Proske U, Allen TJ. Damage to skeletal muscle from eccentric exercise. *Exerc Sports Sci Rev.* 2005;33:98–104.

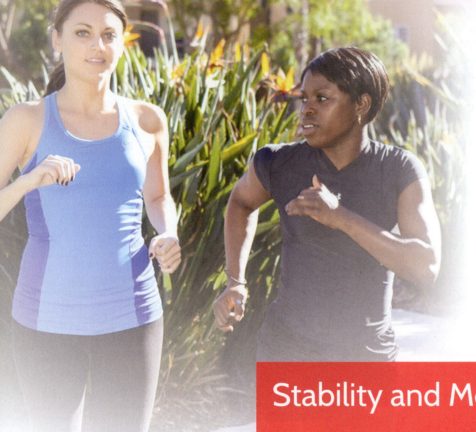

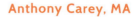
Anthony Carey, MA

CHAPTER 14

# Stability and Mobility Training

## CHAPTER OUTLINE

## LEARNING OUTCOMES

1. Explain the role of stability and mobility in movement and in preventing injury.
2. Identify which joints require an emphasis on mobility and which require an emphasis on stability.
3. Describe the differences between active and passive stability.
4. Explain the importance of stability and mobility to posture and postural control.
5. Identify the benefits of muscle balance.
6. Describe the consequences of muscle imbalance on neuromuscular function and movement efficiency.
7. Explain how to manipulate key training variables to design effective corrective exercise programs.
8. Demonstrate stability and mobility exercises for specific regions of the body.

## ANCILLARY LINK

Visit Davis*Plus* at http://davisplus.fadavis.com for study and practice resources, including online quizzes, animations that help explain physiological processes, podcasts concerning news and career trends in exercise physiology, and practice references.

## VIGNETTE

■ Ken is a software engineer for a large corporation who spends the majority of his workday seated in front of his computer. Although he manages to visit his local health club three times a week to participate in cardiovascular exercise, weight training, and some light stretching, he has been struggling with almost constant pain in his shoulders and neck. In addition, he has been having some pain and tightness in the front of his hips. Ken tells his doctor that he has begun skipping his after-work exercise sessions because of headaches and is concerned about becoming too inactive and too reliant on painkillers. Ken's doctor refers him to an occupational physiologist, who suggests that the design of Ken's workstation may be at least partially to blame for his chronic pain.

What adjustments can be made to Ken's work environment to help alleviate his symptoms? In addition, how might Ken's exercise program be modified to meet his current needs?

In its ideal state, the human body strives to tolerate the effects of all stressors placed on it and maintain some balance between these stressors. This is certainly true of the neuromusculoskeletal system. When referring to this system, we focus on two key stressors that are necessary for our survival: the ability to maintain specific postures and positions; and the ability to move, or, more specifically, *stability* and *mobility*.

This chapter explores these concepts in greater detail, including the relationship between stability and mobility, how they individually and collectively impact movement efficiency, and how to restore an optimal relationship when it has been altered to improve overall movement efficiency and quality of life.

First, we consider components of the kinetic chain and how it functions as one integrated unit (where movement or forces at one joint affect successive joints), and the effects of stability and mobility on the chain. We also examine the need for stability to prevent injury and to act as a platform for generating force within the body (e.g., why we need to tighten our core when pushing a heavy load). Next, we discuss four key anatomical components that contribute to good posture and efficient movement: the passive, active, control, and actively passive components. Finally, we consider training principles and exercises that help increase stability and mobility.

This knowledge will serve as a critical foundation for all exercise programming that includes movement. Considering how technology has facilitated human lives, but also rendered humans more stationary, the potential for developing muscle imbalances and dysfunctional movement continues to increase. Thus, health and fitness professionals need to include a thorough evaluation of the consequences of inactivity on the skeletal structure, the neuromuscular system, and the ability to move the body efficiency.

## FUNDAMENTAL CONCEPTS

**Stress** is defined as a nonspecific response to any stimulus that overcomes, or threatens to overcome, the body's ability to maintain **homeostasis** (equilibrium of the body's internal biological mechanisms). Stressors may originate from many different sources but manifest themselves physiologically within the body. Sources include physical (e.g., gravity or ground reactive forces), physiological (e.g., pain, vigorous exercise, glycogen depletion, or dehydration), environmental (e.g., hot or cold), nutritional (e.g., inadequate caloric intake, nutrient deficiencies, or skipped meals), psychological or emotional (e.g., sorrow, fear, or anxiety), chemical (e.g., blood acid–base imbalance or low oxygen supply), or social sources (e.g., life events or personal conflicts).

**Stability** may be defined as the capacity to control the position or movement of a joint or series of joints, whereas **mobility** may be defined as the capacity to create the appropriate quantity of movement around and across joint(s). Using a building analogy, stability improves when the individual structures and foundation are more fixed and allow for less movement. Thus, by definition, these terms appear to be in competition with one another; that is, increasing joint stability appears to decrease joint mobility and vice versa.

However, the reality in humans is that both are critical to move efficiently and safely. For example, controlling spinal movement in one plane (e.g., flexion or extension) may promote greater intervertebral and spinal stability, but comes at a cost of reducing or sacrificing spinal mobility in the frontal or transverse planes. However, if the spine lacks overall stability (e.g., evident with poor core function), then any movement may be altered or compromised, and increase the potential for injury. Therefore, although stability at the joint should not compromise mobility, and although mobility at that joint should not compromise stability, efficient movement at joints and throughout the entire body, or the entire kinetic chain, is derived from an optimal balance between the two.

## INTEGRATED KINETIC CHAIN CONCEPTS AND CONSEQUENCES

Most movements the human body makes involve the coordinated interaction of nerves, muscles, and connective tissue spanning multiple joints that produce the desired movement. These actions are not limited to nerves instructing muscles to contract concentrically (shortening) or eccentrically (lengthening) against bones to move the joint (Fig. 14-1A and 1B), but also involve nerves instructing other muscles to contract isometrically (no change in muscle length) to hold a joint position (Fig. 14-1B).

Holding joint positions is important because it may serve as a platform for movement at other joints or serve as the foundation to tolerate reactive forces being transferred to the body by gravity or external forces (e.g., dumbbells in a chest press). Furthermore, as muscles contract, they also develop tension in connective tissue that spans the surrounding area, proving additional stability. For example, when placing your hand on another person's chest and pushing against them, muscles acting across the shoulder and elbow joints produce force and movement, whereas muscles around the shoulder blade, trunk, hips, and legs (down to the feet) generate tension at the joints and within the tissue to stabilize body segments and prevent the body from falling backward.

### Fundamental Movement

To continue developing the understanding of the relationship between stability and mobility in the human body, this section briefly examines the body's design

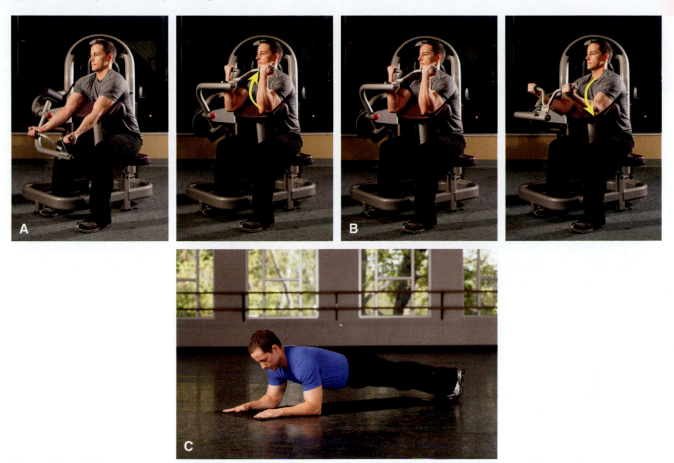

**Figure 14-1.** Different types of muscle contractions. A, Concentric contraction of the biceps. B, Eccentric contraction of the biceps. C, Isometric contraction of the tricep, anterior deltoid, pectoralis major, abdominals, and glutes.

## FROM THEORY TO PRACTICE

### ■ KINETIC CHAIN EFFECT

Standing upright with your feet together, place both hands on the back of your partner's shoulders. Close your eyes, relax your entire body, and then attempt to give your partner a push. Notice how you moved backward as you pushed him or her away and how you did not produce much force in the push? Next, return to your starting position, placing both hands back on your partner's shoulders, but this time, tighten your core muscles (trunk and hips) and position your legs in a split-stance (walking step) position to stabilize your lower extremity. Repeat the push action, but notice the difference in your body movement and the amount of force produced.

This integrated or whole-body function called the **kinetic chain** can be considered as the interplay of components, where the body is essentially a system of interdependent segments linked together. The idea behind the kinetic chain is that every part of the human body, including muscles, joints, nerves, and tissue, works together to produce movement.

The analogy of a computer can be used to further illustrate the functionality of the human body's integrated system. The muscles, ligaments, bones, and fascia represent the hardware, whereas the central and peripheral nervous systems represent the software. As with a computer, the body's hardware relies on quality information being received from the software to execute a function (i.e., efficient movement in humans). Corrupted software, however, will deliver bad information and lead to hardware malfunctions (i.e., altered movement).

Unlike computers, in the human body, the hardware (i.e., muscles) is also capable of changing function and altering the information being fed back to the software (i.e., nervous system). Consequently, the nervous system will need to develop an alternate plan to execute movement. The problem with this alternate plan or movement strategy is that it will come at some cost to the body, which is termed *dysfunctional*. Essentially, this implies a movement compensation that ultimately leads to additional stress placed on the body that typically results in pain or an injury.

*Continued*

## FROM THEORY TO PRACTICE–cont'd

For example, a sprained knee will cause a person to limp in an effort to avoid placing further stress on the damaged ligaments. This limp alters the body's mechanics at the ankle, hip, and spine. If this individual continues to walk on the injured knee and does not receive proper therapy, ligament healing is prolonged. In the interim, the body is learning to incorporate a new walk to avoid pain, therefore developing new neural pathways to the muscles to execute this new walk. Eventually, when the ligaments do heal, while the person should resume normal walking, the software (influenced by the hardware) now communicates poor or dysfunctional information. The limp compensation has taught the nervous system (software) to develop an alternate strategy over time.

This is an important concept to appreciate as it relates to stability and mobility. As an interdependent system, lack of mobility or stability at one or more segments will have an effect on adjacent segments, as well as segments farther removed. Much like with a building, if a segment of the foundation is unstable or weak, it will impact the entire structure, increasing its potential to collapse. In the human body, for instance, a loss of ankle mobility will affect the hip joint and ultimately the lumbar spine.[1]

## VIGNETTE continued

■ Amy is Ken's occupational physiologist, and she visits Ken's office to evaluate the ergonomics of his workstation. She immediately recognizes that his computer monitor is too low, causing Ken to bend his neck downward while working. Ken also sits with his shoulders rounded forward, which helps explain the tightness in his chest and fatigue in his upper back. Amy provides Ken with a series of exercises to help with his posture and recommends he stand, stretch, and move about more frequently throughout the day. Amy also recommends that he include a daily walk during his lunch hour. These activities will help manage the tightness and discomfort he experiences throughout the day while at work. Amy also discovers that Ken's company offers a corporate wellness program, so she arranges a meeting with Tricia, the company's employee fitness director.

and function during the most fundamental of movements: walking. The foot acts as the platform from which the body propels itself forward (heel-lift and toe-off phases) and accepts load (heel strike) after completing a leg-swing movement. Furthermore, the foot must also tolerate the downward force exerted by gravity and any ground reactive forces moving upward through the body from the ground at contact (Newton's third law of motion). The foot is generally considered a stable structure, although it actually consists of 26 bones and 33 smaller joints.

The ankle, in contrast, moves through various movements during walking; in the sagittal plane (vertical plane moving front to back), the ankles move through:
- Supination (ankle rolling outward) at heel strike and pronation (ankle rolling inward) as the

foot makes full contact with the ground (see Fig. 14-2A)
- Flexion at heel strike (called *dorsiflexion*) and a form of extension as one pushes off (called *plantarflexion*; see Fig. 14-2B)

This movement in multiple planes qualifies the ankle as a more mobile joint.

The knee moves between flexion (bending) and extension (extending) in the sagittal plane during walking, and normally controls against undesirable action into any other plane at the knee (i.e., the knee collapsing inward or rotating inward). As defined previously, the ability to control movement in a specific plane defines stability; thus, the knee is considered stable during walking.

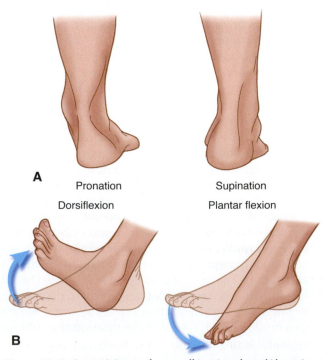

**A**    Pronation    Supination

Dorsiflexion    Plantar flexion

**B**

**Figure 14-2.** An activity such as walking involves (A) supination and pronation, and (B) dorsiflexion and plantarflexion of the foot from heel strike to the push-off phase.

The hips demonstrate movement in all three planes as one moves from the heel-strike phase on one leg through a complete stride to where that same heel strikes again; this qualifies the hips as a mobile joint. At heel strike, the hip of the front (leading) leg is tilted forward (i.e., facing downward), a position called *hip flexion* (sagittal plane). At the same time, the hip is slightly rotated away from the leading leg, creating movement into the transverse (rotational) plane. To illustrate this position, extend one leg out in front as if taking a giant step and observe the direction of your hips and umbilicus (belly button)—they should rotate and orientate away from forward. As you continue walking and lift one leg off the ground to swing it forward, your hips need to shift left and right over the supporting (stance) leg to prevent falling. This movement from left to right occurs in the frontal plane. Consequently, the hips move in all three planes during the practice of walking, qualifying them as a mobile joint.

Although only the lower extremity has been discussed, the stability–mobility relationship across the body's segments appears to follow an alternating pattern that should be understood as a guiding principle when working to restore movement efficiency throughout the body's kinetic chain.

## Transfer of Loads and Forces Throughout the Body

To generate force, the body requires a stable point from which to create an action and tolerate a reaction. Typically, this represents a fixed anchor point (e.g., ground, bench, wall, and backrest of a chair) that allows the body to express the energy it has stored in the muscles, tendons, and fascia as force. When standing and pushing upward to press dumbbells overhead (Fig. 14-3), the forces generated from the ground must pass from the foot through all the segments that lead to the hand(s). This could include the ankle, knee, hip, spine, scapulothoracic (shoulder blade) region, glenohumeral (arm socket) joint, and elbow. If there is instability at one or more of the segments leading to the hand(s), some force will be lost or dissipated; this can be referred to as an energy "leak." The greater the force needed, the greater the reaction force needed from the ground or other object to push back. Imagine attempting to perform a maximal vertical jump from a small, inflatable children's raft floating in a pool. As you push off the raft to jump, the raft would sink deeper into the pool, diluting much of the energy you needed to explode upward. This is a simplified analogy of what could happen at any joint(s) in the body during a movement.

## Injury Prevention

With more than 230 joints in the body, stability is a top priority. If the joints in the body are not stable, the surrounding soft-tissue structures and even the bones themselves could be injured. Stable joints help prevent

### FROM THEORY TO PRACTICE

Although this textbook provides a conceptual overview of the stability–mobility relationship throughout the kinetic chain, it is important to experience the movements for yourself.

- Stand in a staggered stance (walking position) with your right foot forward.
- Lift the ball of your right foot while maintaining contact with the heel to mimic the initial phase that follows a leg swing while walking. Notice the ankle position (dorsiflexion and supination).
- Allow the ball of the foot to slowly fall forward to touch the ground, noticing how your foot moves slightly into pronation (collapsing inward) during the process.
- Observe the position of your knee and hips as the foot falls forward (knee flexion and hip flexion). As the foot is placed flat, observe the direction of your hips and umbilicus (slightly rotated away from the lead leg because of your position).
- As you shift your body forward over your support (stance) leg, notice how your hips and knee move into extension (extend).
- As the rear foot and ankle prepare to lift off and swing forward, observe how the ankle is moving toward plantarflexion.
- As the leg lifts off the ground, your hips will start to shift left in preparation for the left leg striking the ground.
- As your rear leg swing forward, notice how your hips rotate with the leg swinging forward.

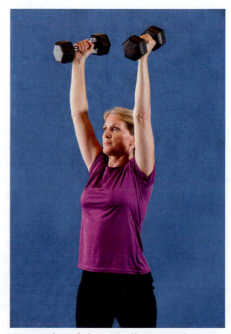

**Figure 14-3.** Overhead dumbbell press. This exercise requires full-body joint stabilization to perform with appropriate technique and force development.

both **macrotrauma** (acute injury such as a sprain or fracture) and repetitive **microtrauma** (chronic injury caused by overuse or repetitive poor form). Macrotrauma occurs when a force is placed on the body or joint and it exceeds the stability level or ability to maintain stability within the joint. Examples include sporting accidents where impact forces from the ground or from collisions with opponents are large and result in an injury. However, it may also occur because of the body's inability to tolerate the forces imposed on the body during an activity (e.g., throwing out the back while lifting). Here the activity demanded more stabilization than what the body's stabilizing system could provide.

Repetitive microtrauma is a more challenging issue to specifically identify in comparison with macrotrauma. It is attributed to the fact that the injury that occurred to the body could have resulted from weeks, months, or even years of repeatedly applying a small stress on a body segment that went unnoticed until the accumulation results in an injury. Repetitive microtrauma is also defined as a low-grade, persistent stress placed on the body and represents the majority of the pain and discomfort a person experiences. Adding to the complexity of this type of stress is that the stability issue may be far removed from the area of the body where the injury itself has manifested. Think of a dentist who is bent over her patients for 8 hours a day and after several weeks of playing tennis she develops inflammation in her elbow or "tennis elbow." This condition may be the result of the poor stability she developed within her shoulder complex because of her bent-over posture during work. Over time, imbalances between her chest and anterior shoulder muscles, and her thoracic (back) extensor muscles and scapular muscles affected the mechanics in her shoulder. This may have reduced the normal movement within her thoracic spine and shoulder, creating compensated movements as she tried to generate forces in the elbow to strike the tennis ball. This may have ultimately contributed to her injury.

## STABILITY SYSTEMS

Stability within the body can be classified in two ways[2]: local stability and full-body or global stability. **Local stability** refers to stability provided by each individual joint within the body, whereas **full-body stability** refers to the overall stability of the body, which is a sum of all the local stability links in the kinetic chain. A local instability will have repercussions on overall force production throughout the entire kinetic chain because it will limit the body's ability to transfer forces efficiently through that one particular joint. This concept applies whether one is producing force (e.g., throwing a punch) or absorbing force (e.g., landing from a jump).

The human body is also a master of compensation. Although a person may have some local instability, they may have been able to develop a compensation strategy

to mask this instability. Such compensations will always have consequences because the unstable joint that is compensating can produce postural misalignment and movement issues at that location or even within areas far removed from that particular joint. For example, for a person suffering from some shoulder discomfort when raising his right arm overhead, he may compensate by leaning his trunk to the left or arching his low back to help move that arm overhead. This places additional stresses on the lumbar spine that over time may lead to losses in stability, postural misalignment, movement issues, and even pain in that region.

Panjabi[3] developed a conceptual model for spinal stabilization and his principles have since been applied to all of the joints in the body. His model includes three separate, but interdependent components or systems as he defined them that the body uses to promote stability: the passive, the active, and the control systems. However, a fourth component, the actively passive system, will also be discussed in this section.[4]

### Passive System

The **passive system** relies on structures that essentially remain consistent in their size, shape, and length, which all contributes to the stability within that joint. For example, if you compare the ball and socket joints of the hip and shoulder, the acetabulum (socket) of the hip is much deeper than the glenoid fossa (socket) of the shoulder. The depth of the acetabulum allows the femoral head to sit deeper within the socket, thus surrounded by more surface area, which adds to its stability. In contrast, the glenoid fossa is much shallower, providing less surface area for contact with the humeral head, and thus decreasing the joint's stability. This trade-off on stability, however, does allow the shoulder joint greater movement or mobility than the hip. Ligaments and the joint capsule (connective tissue surrounding a joint) also contribute to the passive stability of the joint. These nonelastic components help preserve the structural integrity of the joint while assisting in guiding joint motion.

### Active System

The **active system** consists of the muscular system. Muscles actively contract and provide necessary stiffness to a joint by creating tension to aid in stabilization. This mechanism typically consists of a cocontraction of muscles that cross a joint from all angles. For example, the chest and posterior shoulder muscles cocontracting will help stabilize the shoulder joint. The amount of contraction from each contributing muscle varies by the task at hand (e.g., heavier loads require more force production by the muscles). Researchers sometimes discuss the muscular system in terms of local and global muscles.[5] The reference applies to the geographic location of the muscles in relation to the joint.

- A **local muscle** is typically defined as a deep muscle located directly next to the joint and it generally crosses only one joint. Examples of local muscles might include the multifidus or subscapularis, each with a primary responsibility of providing local stability (Fig. 14-4A).

- **Global muscles** are larger muscles that are located more superficially and generally cross two or more joints. They are more responsible for bigger, gross motor movements like the biceps brachii in elbow flexion (Fig. 14-4B).

A familiar training scenario today is observed with general exercisers who spend too much time focused on training the global muscles, usually for aesthetic reasons, and fail to address the local muscles. This leads to a general lack of stability within these deeper muscles, which is needed to tolerate loads and volumes of work placed on the global muscles, ultimately resulting in the potential for injury.

## Control System

The **control system** refers to the aforementioned software of the body or the neurological contribution to stability. The control system depends on interpreting the incoming sensory information (afferent) and then formulating a plan to execute an action or response (efferent). The afferent information is received via the various proprioceptors in the body (muscle spindles, Golgi tendon organs, joint mechanoreceptors, cutaneous, vestibular, and visual).

The message sent to the muscular system to provide any needed stability can be done consciously or unconsciously (reflexive). For example, our core muscles function reflexively to stabilize the trunk in preparation for any spinal loading.[6] We can also consciously prepare our body in anticipation of loads. Imagine a person holding a large box who appears to be struggling with the weight of the box. He walks toward you and asks you to hold it for him while he ties his shoe. In anticipation of the heavy box being placed in your arms, you will consciously stiffen your hips, spine, and shoulders to stabilize these joints. In other words, you will proactively prepare the body by stabilizing in advance.

Most of what the body does for stabilization is done unconsciously without having to be processed consciously in the brain. This provides a rapid process, reacting within 54 to 126 milliseconds to protect joints against unexpected loads and forces, and to avoid injury.[6] For example, you are walking down a dark, unfamiliar hallway and you do not see a step down in front of you. As your foot drops lower than you expected and abruptly hits the ground, the muscles around the knee must fire in less than 70 milliseconds to stabilize the knee and protect it from damage. If it were necessary for you to consciously think and process this response, your response would be too slow and injury would occur.

## Actively Passive System

A fourth component can be added to Panjabi's model: the **actively passive system**. The actively passive system is composed of the fascial tissue and how it is arranged throughout the body. Although previously defined, fascia constitutes a form of connective tissue that is different from the traditional collagen and elastin tissue found in muscle, but it does contain myofibroblasts, which are specialized muscle cells that can undergo contraction and shortening.[7]

Fascia also contains many mechanoreceptors (specialized sensory receptors sensitive to mechanical stimuli or changes such as tension, stretching, vibration and pressure) that provide proprioceptive (positioning) information in the same manner as they do in a joint capsule, muscle, or ligaments.[8] Fascia is continuous around the body and is present in multiple levels within the body, separating tissue, muscles, and body compartments, and even serving as attachment areas for muscles to bones (Fig. 14-5).

However, unlike muscle tissue that is sectional (i.e., spans one or several joints), the continuous nature of fascia surrounding the entire body makes it unique. This continuous sheath of tissue spanning the body helps provide stabilization through tension (stretching and lengthening) rather than having to create compression or contraction as found with muscle. Through this tension, the fascial system helps the body meet its stability requirements and does so using far less energy than one has with muscular contractions. Given this ability, this chapter refers to the fascia as actively passive. Consequently, both the muscular and the fascial systems work together to contribute to the body's stabilization needs.[9]

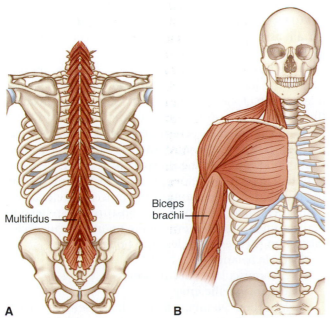

Multifidus

Biceps brachii

**A**  **B**

**Figure 14-4.** The geographic location of muscles in relation to the joint. A, Example of a local muscle. B, Example of a global muscle.

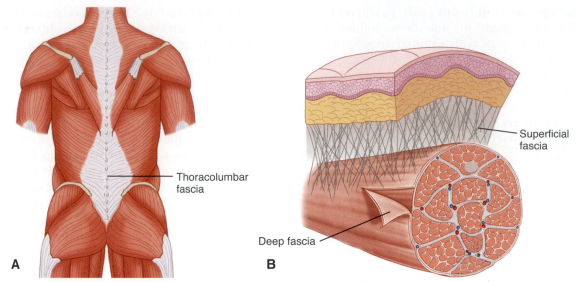

**Figure 14-5.** Fascia is continuous around the body and is present at multiple levels within the body, separating tissue, muscles, and body compartments, and attaching muscles to bones. A, Superficial fascia in the human body. B, The architecture of fascia as it exists under the skin and around muscle.

## ROLE OF POSTURE IN THE STABILITY–MOBILITY RELATIONSHIP

**Static posture** (how an individual stands) is one fundamental way to gather information on the relationship between stability and mobility, as postural alignment demonstrates balance between opposing muscle groups at each joint (Fig. 14-6). Each joint is surrounded by muscles that normally function in all three planes of motion; when a proper relationship exists among these muscles, that joint is free to move

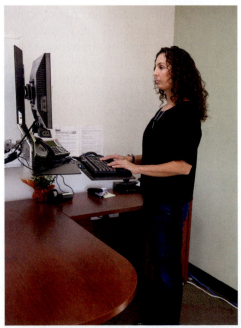

**Figure 14-6.** Static posture is a fundamental way to gather information on the relationship between stability and mobility, as postural alignment demonstrates balance between opposing muscle groups at each joint.

through its designed range of motion (ROM) without restriction. Proper joint alignment also reduces susceptibility of the joint surfaces to excessive wear and tear because the surfaces are moving congruently (smoothly) on each other the way they were designed to function. This spreads the forces placed on the joint across the entire surface area.

For example, if the glenoid fossa (shoulder socket) and humeral head (ball of the humerus) are properly aligned, then movement allows these surfaces to move congruently with each other and distribute forces over the surfaces evenly (e.g., from a compression force occurring during an overhead dumbbell press as the arm rotates upward). However, if these surfaces are not properly aligned, the structures can fail to move congruently, which places more stress on certain areas of the joint surfaces and accelerates wear and tear.

If the muscle or connective tissue, or both, on one side of the joint pull more than the other, the proper relationship of the two sides is not maintained. Instead, the ROM in one direction becomes greater and the ROM in the other direction decreases. This alters the mechanics within the joint and may increase the distribution of forces acting on specific areas of the joint. Standing posture therefore presents a snapshot of how the individual components of the musculoskeletal system function cohesively. Static posture is a reflection of three important elements of the neuromusculoskeletal system (nerves, muscles, and bones):

- Muscle balance
- Neuromuscular coordination
- Mechanical efficiency

Each of these elements is interdependent, and each is essential to the functional stability–mobility relationship of the musculoskeletal system. Figure 14-7 provides examples of good and poor posture.

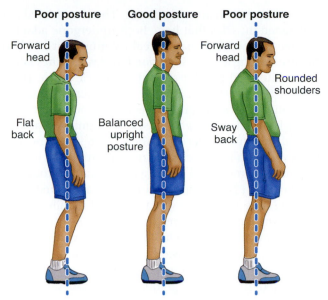

**Figure 14-7.** Examples of good and poor posture. The two examples of poor posture demonstrate a head-forward and flat-back position and head forward with rounded shoulders and a sway back (locked knees, hips forward, increased backward lean through mid-torso, significant rounding of thoracic spine, head-forward position). Both of these postures put the body outside of normal alignment.

## Muscle Balance

Each muscle in the body performs specific functions, and each muscle has a counterpart, commonly called the **antagonist** (i.e., produces the opposite movement—biceps and triceps). In other words, if a muscle or group of muscles flexes a joint, then a muscle or group of muscles extends the joint. As mentioned briefly in the previous section, with proper postural alignment, these opposing muscle groups have a mutually respectful

arrangement. They maintain an equal degree of pull on either side of a joint and share the essential information from the nervous system. This allows the joint to move with equal efficiency and freedom in all directions.

Imbalances in this relationship are reflected in muscles that become posturally lengthened or posturally shortened (see discussion in the next section). These imbalances alter the position of the joint, which results in abnormal movement and abnormal loading (wear and tear) on various structures within the body. It is important to understand that these changes to length within muscles and muscle groups associated with poor posture do not occur overnight, but may occur over the course of a few weeks, months, and years.

Abnormal movement usually begins with neurological changes that control movement because of changing muscle function, and this begins to negatively affect movement. This is generally followed by structural changes within the muscle cells occurring within the sarcomere, impacting the length–tension relationship that governs force production. A posturally lengthened muscle will adapt by adding additional sarcomeres in series (at the ends), whereas a posturally shortened muscle will adapt by removing sarcomeres in series.[10] Figure 14-8 illustrates force production curve within a sarcomere, demonstrating how slight stretching beyond normal resting length increases the spatial arrangement between the muscle's contractile proteins (actin and myosin) and increases its force-generating capacities.[11] However, additional stretching of sarcomeres beyond optimal lengths reduces the potential for contractile protein binding and decreases the muscle's force-generating capacities. Likewise, shortening the muscle creates overlap between the contractile fibers and also reduces its force-generating capacity. Refer to Chapter 9 for a detailed explanation of muscle contraction and the actions of actin and myosin.

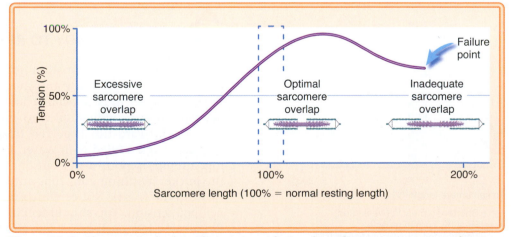

**Figure 14-8.** Changes in the length–tension relationship of a sarcomere according to the alignment of actin and myosin. From left to right, the ability to produce tension or force in the muscle is maximized with optimal overlap or connection between actin and myosin. Maximal tension occurs at and just above 100% of normal resting length. Beyond this point of maximal tension, actin and myosin are pulled apart and overlap is no longer optimized. Thus, the ability of the muscle to produce tension is reduced.

Biologically, muscles adapt to the stresses placed on them (e.g., undergoing growth with resistance training) and when lengthened or shortened indefinitely because of poor posture, prolonged awkward positions (e.g., seated for long periods), or any other cause of muscle imbalance (e.g., poor training program design), they will adapt to increase their force-generating capacity in this new position. This adaptive change is to either add or remove sarcomeres in series and shift that muscle's length–tension curve.[10,12]

Muscles can shorten in as little as 2 to 4 weeks when held in passively shortened positions without stretching or use through a full or functional ROM (e.g., continuous bouts of sitting without hip extension activity can shorten the hip flexors).[11,13] In addition, with prolonged inactivity, our fascia begins to adapt to conform to the limited lines of length, which further adds to adaptive changes within the tissue.[4]

As illustrated in Figure 14-9, a healthy muscle that gradually becomes shortened (e.g., hip flexors from excessive sitting) will lose sarcomeres, shifting its curve to the left. This increases sarcomere strength in the shortened position (i.e., the position in which the muscle is predominantly held—below 100% of normal resting length).[13] Conversely, a healthy muscle that gradually becomes lengthened (e.g., rhomboids from excessive forward rounded shoulders) will add sarcomeres, shifting its curve to the right. This increases sarcomere strength in the lengthened position (i.e., the position in which the muscle is predominantly held—above 100% of normal resting length).[13]

Figure 14-9 demonstrates how positioning the joint back into a good postural position (e.g., pulling shoulder blades back to neutral) or performing some quick stretches on tight muscles does not resolve the problem that involves a structural change. The lengthened and shortened muscles that have both undergone adaptive changes are weaker than a healthy muscle at 100% of healthy resting length (illustrated by dashed lines falling below the solid line for a healthy muscle at the 100% mark). Thus, restoring healthy resting length and normal muscle force-generating capacity is not as simple as a quick stretch to a tight muscle. It requires a physiological adaptation accomplished over time and best achieved by: (1) consciously repositioning the joint in optimal alignment and keeping this position throughout the day, and (2) participating in a program aimed at improving muscle stability (strength) and mobility (flexibility) in the normal resting length positions. For example, when an individual exhibits forward-rounded shoulders, conscious awareness of shoulder position plus a passive stretching program of the shortened (tightened) muscles will gradually add more sarcomeres back in series and help restore the muscle's normal resting-length and length-tension relationship.

In addition, performing high-back rows to strengthen the posterior muscles (rhomboids, posterior deltoids) using full ROM exercises is not recommended initially. Because the rhomboids are weak in the good postural position, but strong in the lengthened position, momentum generated during a full ROM row (starting with arms extended to farthest point away from the body, with shoulder rounded forward), will carry the movement through the weaker region, essentially bypassing the ROM where the muscle needs strengthening the most. A more appropriate approach is to perform this same exercise initially with either an isometric contraction in a good postural position or using a limited ROM that avoids excessive lengthening where the muscle is already strong.

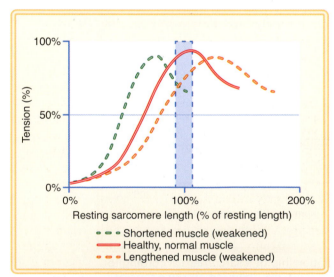

**Figure 14-9.** Alterations to the length–tension relationship of a sarcomere. When muscle is tight and shortened or weakened through excessive lengthening at rest, the ability of that muscle to produce tension or force is reduced.

### FROM THEORY TO PRACTICE

Given the information just acquired on sarcomere lengthening and shortening, how can proper muscle balance and function be restored in an individual who exhibits an anterior (forward-tilted) pelvis? Imagine your hips as a bucket filled with water. While standing, attempt to pour water out of the front of the bucket by tilting your hips anteriorly (toward the front). Notice which muscles developed tension. You should feel it in the hip flexors and low back extensors. Next, attempt to pour water out the back of the bucket by tilting your hips posteriorly (toward the back). Notice which muscles developed tension. You should feel tension in the abdominals, hamstrings, and glutes.

## VIGNETTE continued

■ Ken, Amy, and Tricia discuss Ken's concerns and agree to a plan: Ken will use his company's wellness center twice each week and continue with his cardiovascular and flexibility program; but instead of performing resistance training on his own, Ken will begin working with Tricia once each week to evaluate and potentially redesign his program.

During their first session, Tricia performs a postural assessment and conducts some basic movement screens. She suggests that Ken stop resistance training temporarily and focus instead on specific stability and mobility exercises with minimal or no resistance to address his postural misalignments and some minor muscular imbalances, in particular, his rounded shoulders. Although Ken was initially reluctant about "taking a step back" in his program, he sees the value in addressing his postural concerns and agrees to participate in this program. After 2 weeks of participation, he notices a difference in his physical sensations, feeling less muscle fatigue and soreness throughout the day, and is now enjoying his exercise program.

## Neuromuscular Coordination

In motor control terms, **neuromuscular coordination** applies to the relationship between input and output. *Input* is the information that the body gathers about the position of its parts in space relative to one another, the location of its center of gravity and external environment. This information is gathered through the somatosensory system (e.g., muscle spindles, Golgi tendon organs, joint mechanoreceptors, and cutaneous receptors) and vestibulo-ocular and visual mechanisms (ears and eyes). With faulty postural alignment, these information-gatherers become biased toward inappropriate positioning of the body segments. In other words, over time the body sets a new baseline for what it considers normal as its point of reference.

*Output* is reflected in either movement or the stabilization strategy that the body uses in response to input. It would be the result of how one processes the input and executes the movement response. That means coordinating certain muscles to work as the prime movers, others to assist (synergists), others to neutralize, and others to potentially turn off and do absolutely nothing. Furthermore, output also involves timing, intensity, and duration of muscular activity that proves critical to efficient stability and mobility.[14]

As an example, the quadriceps muscles during gait function as primary stabilizers of the knee joint during leg swing (i.e., holding a slight knee-bent position for ground clearance), at heel strike (i.e., slowing down knee extension and holding the extended position to strike the ground), and through the weight-bearing portion of the walk cycle (i.e., maintaining knee extension as a support leg). If the quadriceps were to contract concentrically too soon during the leg swing, the knee would extend prematurely and the person would catch his or her toes on the ground and trip. If the quadriceps contracted too much, then the knee joint would be excessively compressed, locking the knee into hyperextension. If the quadriceps remained contracted too long, they would interfere with the ability of that knee to flex as it lifts off the ground, and impede the action of the opposite leg to function to continue walking.

Remember, in the presence of muscle imbalances, nerve function is altered, thereby changing muscle performance. When this chapter makes reference to a shortened muscle, it often describes the muscle as tight or under tension. Think of when you last received a massage and the therapist discovered tight muscles in your back and neck that appeared tense. A shortened muscle experiences increased tonicity (*hypertonicity*: hyper = increased, tonicity = muscle tone or tension) from the nervous system because of that nerve's altered function. This implies that the muscle now requires only a smaller or weaker nerve impulse to activate a contraction (also called *lowered irritability threshold*). As detailed in Chapter 9, nerves subscribe to the "all-or-nothing" principle where a specific strength of stimulus is needed in the nerve to generate an action potential that results in muscle activation. With a lowered irritability threshold, the strength of stimulus needed to generate an action potential in a nerve that results in muscle activation is lowered.[15]

Normally, when one activates a muscle (agonist) at a joint, one also simultaneously innervates the opposite muscle (antagonist) to create movement. Termed **reciprocal inhibition**, this is the action whereby the central nervous system sends an impulse to the agonist muscle to contract while simultaneously partially or completely inhibiting (relaxing) the antagonist muscle, to enable and control movement.[16] However, if the antagonist is shortened and hypertonic (i.e., reduced irritability threshold), then this muscle may become prematurely activated before the agonist (target muscle) and actually inhibit the action of the agonist that one is attempting to activate, essentially reversing the normal reciprocal inhibition process (i.e., prematurely activating the antagonist will result in inhibition of the agonist). Therefore, hypertonic muscles appear to decrease the normal neural effect of reciprocal inhibition. For example, if a person exhibited shortened (tight) hip flexors and attempted to activate the gluteus maximus for hip extension, the normal activation process would activate that muscle while simultaneously inhibiting the hip flexor. However, in this case, the hypertonic hip flexor will fire prematurely and prevent activation of the gluteus maximus.

Although both muscles on either side of the joint demonstrate weakness because of their altered length–tension relationship, this phenomenon of reciprocal inhibition contributes to further weakening of muscles that cannot be activated because of reduced neural input and perpetuates the existing muscle imbalance. In this situation, the body must call on other muscles at the joint (called *synergists*) to assume the role of becoming the prime mover to move the joint, referred to as **synergistic dominance**.

Continuing with the previous example, the tight hip flexor inhibits and weakens the gluteus maximus, thereby forcing the hamstrings (a synergist) to assume a greater role in hip extension. Unfortunately, the hamstrings are not designed for this function and may suffer from overuse or overload, increasing their likelihood for tightness and injury. Furthermore, the hamstrings do not offer the same degree of movement control of the femoral head during hip extension as the gluteus maximus does, and this limitation increases the likelihood for dysfunctional movement and injury to the hip. This would be an example of microtrauma, whereby the hip joint undergoes abnormal mechanics as a result of the hamstrings substituting for the gluteus maximus. This would ultimately lead to reduced mobility at the hip as a result of long-term stability compensation.

Figure 14-10 presents a chronological overview of the collective neural and muscle changes that occur within the body as a result of a muscle imbalance associated with poor posture, awkward positions, or poor exercise program design. The shortened muscle develops a lowered irritability threshold that will impact movement at the joint it crosses. Any desired muscle action of its antagonist is subject to this altered neural action (reciprocal inhibition) that will necessitate the action of synergists to help create the movement (synergistic dominance).

## Mechanical Efficiency

**Mechanical efficiency** applies to any system of moving parts; its goal is to minimize mechanical stress and energy expenditure. This can be seen in the engineering of some of the finest automobiles in the world through their aerodynamic design, transfer of power from engine to drive train, shock absorption, and so on. Compare that with the design of the old steam engine locomotive, for example, where most of the available energy was lost and it took long distances to speed up and slow down. When looking at the human body, we can see many ways in which it is designed to maximize efficiency. Muscles act on bones, which serve as levers to create movement or overcome resistance. The design of the joints and shapes of the bones create optimal paths of motion, and the articulating cartilage (cartilage on the surface of the bones) and arrangement of connective tissue are designed to minimize stress. With

proper mobility and stability at any given joint, optimal motion and, therefore, mechanical efficiency can be achieved.

A mechanical term that serves to help this discussion is **vectors**. Vectors are physical quantities that include both magnitude and direction. For example, if one force is applied in a vertical direction and a second force is applied in a horizontal direction, the net force or vector would move in a diagonal direction. Similarly, if a big force was applied in a vertical direction and a smaller force was applied in a horizontal direction, the net movement would be more toward the vertical force. In the human body, vectors function to create all movement. Understanding vectors is important when observing movement because muscles never work in isolation, but function as integrated groups. Many muscles function by providing opposing, directional, or contralateral pulls at joints (termed *force-couples)* to achieve efficient movement or to provide the necessary counterforce to control motion in an opposing direction.

For example, maintaining a neutral pelvic position in the sagittal plane is achieved via opposing force-couples among four major muscles, all having attachments on the pelvis. As shown in Figure 14-11, various muscles act across the joint to control its position and movement:

- The rectus abdominis pulls upward on the anterior (front), inferior (lower) pelvis, whereas the hip flexors pull downward on the anterior, superior (upper) pelvis.
- On the posterior surface, the hamstrings pull downward on the posterior, inferior pelvis, whereas the erector spinae group pulls upward on the posterior, superior pelvis.

When these muscles demonstrate good balance, the pelvis holds optimal alignment; however, when one muscle becomes tight or over-dominant, it alters this relationship and changes the alignment of the pelvis. Changes to pelvic position will affect the position of the spine above and femur below, therefore altering posture and the loading on the joints along the kinetic chain.

A common scenario that affects people in today's society is tight hip flexors. In part, this is a consequence of the large amounts of time spent sitting, which shortens the hip flexors. As a result, the pelvis tilts forward as the shortened hip flexors rotate the front of the pelvis downward. The tight hip flexors neurologically inhibit the antagonists at this joint (hamstrings, gluteus maximus, and abdominals) as these muscles become posturally lengthened.

From a stability-mobility standpoint, this altered position of an anterior-tilted pelvis and its associated lumbar extension generates higher compressive forces on the articulating surfaces of the lumbar spine (the bony surfaces that connect with each other). This creates limitations in mobility with hip extension and flexion of the lumbar spine.

Another example of a force-couple occurs at the glenohumeral (arm socket) joint during arm abduction (action of moving the arm away from the midline of

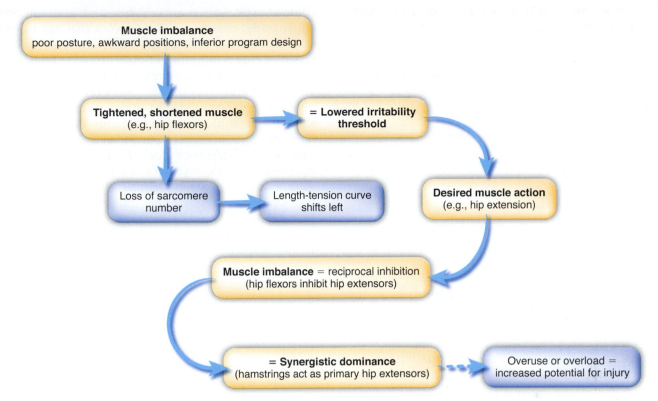

Figure 14-10. Development of synergistic dominance. This problem is initiated through muscle imbalances that can produce tightened, shortened muscles, among other problems. This imbalance will elicit an inhibition of important prime movers during activity. In this example, tight hip flexors override the function of gluteus muscles (hip extensors), which shifts the responsibility of producing hip extension to the hamstrings. This can lead to overuse injury.

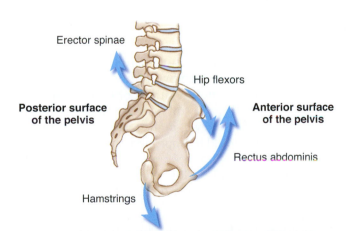

Figure 14-11. Maintaining neutral pelvic position is determined by force-coupling of opposing muscles around the hip. When either of these muscles is tight or weakened, they affect the position of the pelvis and alter the function of the remaining stabilizing muscles.

cuff muscles pulling the head downward and inward before the deltoids engage, the humeral head would not be able to glide inferiorly (slide downward) before rotation occurs (Fig. 14-12). This is critical to rotation because it provides space for the humeral head to rotate upward under the action of the deltoids, which also pull the head upward. Thus, the initial force-couple action of this movement involves an inferior glide of the humeral head, timed to precede the upward pull action of the deltoids that if acting alone, would result in the head gliding upward. This would cause

the body to an overhead position). Whereas the deltoids act as the prime mover in arm abduction, it is the collaborative action of the rotator cuff muscles (supraspinatus, infraspinatus, subscapularis, and teres minor), with respect to magnitude and direction, as well as timing of contraction, that counter the direct upward pull of the deltoids to produce rotation. Without the action of the supraspinatus pulling the humeral head inward, and the actions of the three other rotator

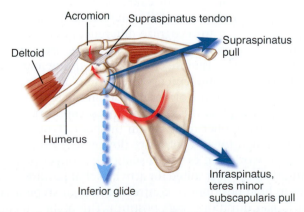

Figure 14-12. During shoulder abduction, the deltoids are the prime movers and the rotator cuff muscles work together to produce rotation of the arm. This is another example of force-coupling between these muscles.

the humoral head to strike the coracoacromial arch, causing an impingement.

## In Your Own Words

Take what you have learned about the role of posture in the stability–mobility relationship and explain to an older adult the importance of proper posture for muscle balance, coordination, and mechanical efficiency.

## TRAINING PRINCIPLES

Most of what we do with movement every day is done unconsciously and automatically. We might initiate the process consciously, but once the action begins, most of it is generally automated. For example, you might see that your shoe is untied and consciously make the decisions to bend down to tie it. But once the voluntary movement starts, there is no need to consciously think about the bending movement from the hip and knee. When learning a new exercise or dance pattern, nearly all of the learning that takes place is provided through visual and auditory information (i.e., the movement is demonstrated using visual and/or spoken cues). The kinesthetic part of learning or learning by feeling works off the existing point of reference, both good and bad, and is not something that can be evaluated in the mirror.[17]

When people learn a new movement, they often miss some critical kinesthetic cues that the body provides, partly because the tendency is to be more concerned with the final *outcome* of the movement rather than the process of getting there. In other words, the focus is more on what needs to be accomplished (i.e., tying your shoe) rather than the quality of the movement (i.e., how to get to tying your shoe). Often, failure to kinesthetically learn may result in learning faulty movements, although it may feel normal. So what can be done about this? First, it is important to understand that the best way to influence the body's stability and mobility strategy is to implement proper positions or movements that can be maintained for sustained periods or repeated with low-intensity activity. For example, the precision and control of corrective exercise movements allows the nervous system to recognize differences between the formerly familiar movements or positions and the corrected ones. This is more effective than trying to implement dynamic movements that essentially generate momentum with the bigger muscles in the body.[18]

To help explain this concept, this section briefly reviews muscle fiber roles within the body. Type I fibers are designed for low-intensity (low grade) muscle activity or work that can be sustained for longer periods; thus, they are best suited for activities that require muscles to hold positions or control movement (repetitive) for longer durations (e.g., posture). This ability to control position or movement defines stability; thus, type I fibers appear synonymously with stability training. In contrast, type II fibers are designed for higher intensity (high-grade) muscle activity or work that can be sustained for shorter periods; thus, they are best suited for activities that require brief bursts of movements (e.g., jumping and bench pressing). Therefore, any corrective exercise program that aims to restore muscle imbalance, neuromuscular coordination, and mechanical efficiency should address the type I fibers rather than the type II fibers initially. For example, an individual with forward-rounded shoulders with weak rhomboids may not necessarily see any improvement in his posture if he spends time at the gym strengthening these muscles with heavy resistance (type II fiber training). A more appropriate approach would be to implement exercises that target the type I fibers in that muscle group (coaching proper positioning and maintaining that position for longer periods or performing a series of low-grade isometric contractions in that position).

### Volume

Volume of training applies to the quantity of work performed and is manipulated by time (i.e., time under tension, the duration of muscle work) or by the total number of repetitions performed (i.e., sets × reps). Time under tension is effectively used with isometric-type exercises where proper postural alignment or positions are held with isometric contractions for longer periods. Both should be considered when designing corrective exercises aimed at improving posture and movement quality.

### Intensity

Load or intensity refers to how hard the body or muscles work and is measured by numerous variables that include subjective interpretations of effort (ratings of perceived exertion), amount of weight lifted, speed, or grade completed. However, in the case of improving stability, the loads should be appropriately matched to target type I fibers as discussed previously. Consequently, the intensity should be limited to light-to-moderate loads (no higher than a 5 or 6 out of 10 effort).

### Guidelines for Restoring Muscle Balance and Stability–Mobility

As a general principle, it is best to restore mobility before addressing stability. Attempting to increase stability at a joint or to a body segment that lacks mobility is more likely to force the body to compensate movement or further limit motion as it attempts to stabilize itself.

### Increasing Mobility

There are three primary ways one can help introduce mobility to the body:

- Myofascial release or self-myofascial release
- Stretching
- Mobilizing movements

Box 14-1 provides exercises for increasing mobility at the ankle, hip, thoracic spine, and shoulder girdle.

## Myofascial Release and Self-Myofascial Release

**Myofascial release** is a technique that involves the use of various tools to reduce adhesions (knots) within fascial (soft) tissue, which, in turn, helps restore tissue extensibility (movement) and reduce muscle discomfort. Common tools used for myofascial release include rollers (foam or other materials); balls of different sizes, shapes, and densities; or hands, knuckles, sticks, or assorted specialty tools (e.g., Thera Cane). Self-myofascial release denotes techniques an individual performs on himself without the assistance of another person or health and fitness professional.

Essentially, this technique involves the application of pressure to the targeted muscle or region demonstrating the greatest levels of discomfort or sensitivity using any myofascial release tool. This discomfort represents adhesions or knots in the fascial tissue where the connective tissue fibers have lost their original orientation because of some form of trauma (acute—injury; chronic—overuse, inactivity, awkward positions). Nerve receptors reacting to this trauma have become overactive and created tension that pulls fibers out of alignment generating that knot. Although myofascial release techniques work, the exact mechanism is not yet fully understood or agreed on. One consensual belief is that myofascial release relaxes the overactive nerve receptors (neurological response), thereby reducing tension within the fibers and any discomfort. Then the action of rolling realigns the fibers into their proper orientation (mechanical response), which then permits more unrestricted movement.

## Box 14-1. Exercises to Increase Mobility at the Ankle, Hip, Thoracic Spine, and Shoulder Girdle

### Ankle
1. Begin in a standing position with your toes elevated and a moderate stretch on the calf.
2. Flex the hip opposite of the one to be stretched to 90 degrees.
3. Immediately extend the flexed hip to the standing position while flexing the torso forward at the waist. The knee of the stretching leg should gently extend more and increase the stretch as a result of the torso coming forward.
4. Extend the torso to return to the starting position.
5. Repeat the motion in a controlled, deliberate tempo.
6. Flex the opposite hip and knee, and hold them flexed at 90 degrees.
7. Bring the flexed leg across the body, causing the foot to roll slightly to the inside border.
8. Bring the flexed leg out to the side, away from the body, causing the foot to roll slightly to the outside.

### Hip
1. Place one foot on a chair with the knee and hip flexed. The back knee is straight, and the foot is toed in slightly about 30 degrees. The torso remains upright as the pelvis is pushed forward, initiating a slight stretch in the anterior hip. Once here, three separate movements are performed with the arms to address mobility of the anterior hip in all three planes.
   a. Lift both hands up and overhead with the elbows straight as the pelvis comes forward.
   b. With arms held out in front at chest level, rotate the upper body, arms, and head away from the back leg.
   c. Lift the same arm as the back leg straight over the head and reach over the top of the head, causing the spine to side bend away from the back leg.

### Thoracic Spine
1. Lie on one side with both knees together. The hips and knees are flexed to 90 degrees.
2. Place extended arms on the floor at a 90-degree angle from your body. The palms are on top of each other and level with the shoulders.
3. Slowly lift the top arm up and over your body toward the floor behind. Turn the head with the arm. The knees must stay together directly stacked. Take deep breaths to relax the body and allow gravity to slowly bring the arm toward the floor.

### Shoulder Girdle
1. Lie on your back with the knees bent and feet flat on the floor. Relax arms at your side.
2. Put your little finger on the floor with palms facing your thighs.
3. Slide the arms up along the floor to shoulder level, keeping the elbows straight.
4. At shoulder level, rotate your arms so that the hands face above the head with the thumb side contacting the floor.
5. Then bring the hands over the head along the floor until palms touch, keeping the elbows straight.
6. Reverse the process on the way down.

Various protocols for myofascial release exist, but perhaps the most common modality is one where the tool is rolled or moved in a linear pattern, moving 3 to 6 inches along the sensitive or tender region for at least 30 seconds (Fig. 14-13), until the tenderness subsides.

## Stretching

Stretching, particularly static stretching, has become a highly debated topic within fitness, especially with respect to its benefit before exercise. The benefits of static stretching following exercise remain consistent: It promotes greater flexibility that can reduce injury.

Static stretching can be either passive or active. Passive stretching involves the assistance of another person or device (e.g., strap, doorframe, or ground) to assist in lengthening the targeted muscle groups, whereas active stretching involves actively contracting the antagonistic (opposite) muscle(s) to the muscle group being lengthened. Both techniques are discussed in further detail in Chapter 17.

## Increasing Stability

As discussed earlier, improving stability is achieved by either positioning the joints in good postural positions followed by a series of isometric contractions (positional isometrics) or through limited ROM exercises in which load and intensity of muscle action are controlled (isolated strengthening). General guidelines for each of these are presented in the following lists. Specific exercises for increasing stability in the knee and lumbar spine are presented in Box 14-2.

To perform positional isometrics, do the following:
1. Position the joint in a good postural or neutral position.
2. Complete one set of four to six repetitions.
3. Hold each isometric contraction for 5 to 30 seconds, with a 2-second recovery interval between each set.
4. The intensity of the contraction can vary, remaining fixed at a specific intensity or progressively increasing with each repetition, but should

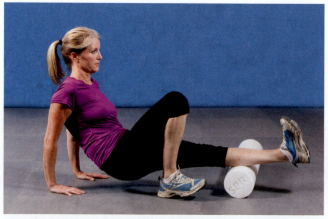

**Figure 14-13.** This person is practicing a traditional foam rolling activity in myofascial release.

### Box 14-2. Exercises to Increase Stability at the Knee and Lumbar Spine

**Knee (Isolated Strengthening)**
1. Step forward into an anterior lunge.
2. As the front ankle, knee, and hip begin to flex, reach forward with both hands and then lean forward with your torso, while maintaining vertical alignment of the knee over the second toe.
3. Slowly decelerate your forward movement, holding this position briefly for 2 seconds before pushing back to your starting position.
4. Repeat.

**Lumbar Spine (Positional Isometrics)**
1. Begin by lying on your side, resting on your elbow that is positioned directly under the shoulder.
2. Rest the palm of your opposite hand on your outer thigh.
3. Extend both legs, aligning both feet in parallel to create a straight line from the ear to the ankle.
4. Lift the hips off of the floor, supporting the body with the elbow/forearm and bottom foot, maintaining that straight alignment for 10 to 30 seconds.

attempt to target type I fibers with intensities ideally no greater than a 5 to 6 out of 10 effort.

To perform isolated strengthening, do the following:
1. Position the joint in a good postural or neutral position.
2. Complete 1 to 2 sets of 10 to 15 repetitions.
3. Perform a controlled concentric contraction, followed by a 4-second eccentric contraction, holding the end range between the two contractions phases for 2 seconds.
4. The intensity of the contractions should be no greater than 50% of maximal effort.

## Mobilizing Movements That Integrate Stability and Mobility

Mobilizing movements are designed to lengthen the muscle and fascial component simultaneously through slow, controlled, rhythmical movements. These movements progressively lengthen tissue across multiple joints. This technique, however, should only be introduced after some flexibility has been restored to individual joints through a stretching program; otherwise, whole-body or integrated movements may suffer from some compromise because of the limitations that occur at one or more joints.

Mobilizing movements are neurologically more complex because they involve both mobility and stability requirements across multiple joints. The two primary mechanisms needed to successfully perform mobilization movements are co-contraction and tensegrity.

**Cocontraction** occurs when muscles surrounding joints (agonist and antagonists) contract together either through dynamic (concentric/eccentric) or isometric action. This creates compression within the joint that brings joint surfaces closer together to reduce any unwanted motion at the involved joint(s) (i.e., improve stability). For example, the action of engaging both the anterior and the posterior muscles around the shoulder joint while raising the arm overhead at an intensity that does not restrict movement improves stability while allowing appropriate amounts of movement.

**Tensegrity**, or "tension-integrity," contributes to stability through tension sharing that occurs between soft tissue and the bones without compression. It produces stability through tension created by the myofascial components pulling in opposing directions.[4] An analogy to help explain this concept is to imagine shrink wrap covering a plate of food. Once the wrap is placed over the plate, you pull it at every edge possible to create tension and secure the food it covers. To illustrate this effect in the human body, examine the cocking phase of a throw. The anterior portion of the glenohumeral joint is stabilized through tension created by lengthening of the anterior muscles and tissue (e.g., pectoralis major, anterior deltoid, and biceps brachii). This creates a pull force at the origin of many of these muscles (muscle attachment closer to the midline of the body or the skeleton), creating more tension to stabilize the body. The action of the arm physically moving backward pulls on the other ends of these muscles (distal attachments), creating tension across the shoulder joint (as these muscles cross the joint and are being pulled in either direction), helping to stabilize it. The illustration provided demonstrates how tension can be created by pull forces from multiple points and how that can create a stable structure (Fig. 14-14).

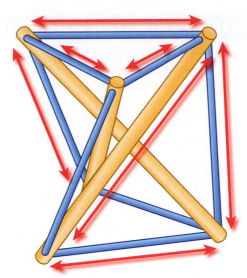

**Figure 14-14.** This model shows how the process of tensegrity works. Arrows show the directions of forces that work in conjunction with each other to supply stability to the model in the figure.

## VIGNETTE conclusion

■ After working with the employee fitness director for 6 weeks and following a stability–mobility program, Ken's frequency and intensity of discomfort has greatly diminished, and he no longer complains of excessive soreness at the end of the workday. Furthermore, he has made some changes to his work habits to spend less time sitting and to take frequent breaks to stretch and move around the office. A follow-up evaluation reveals improved posture and movement efficiency. These changes, coupled with improved ergonomics in his workstation and an understanding of how his previous lifestyle caused his issues, have changed Ken's behavior and greatly improved his quality of life.

## CRITICAL THINKING QUESTIONS

1. You are standing on a chair of normal height. You jump from the chair to land on the ground with both feet at the same time. The ankles, knees, and hips all flex as you hit the ground to stop your descent. Is this an example of stability? Mobility? Both? Please describe.

2. Lower back pain and tightness affects millions of people around the world. A client describes lower back "tightness" as part of her current concerns with exercise. She sits all day at work and regularly stretches the lower back by bringing the knees to the chest when lying supine. While viewing her posture, you note that the lower back is flat and missing the normal lordotic curve. Knowing that the short and tight lower back muscles should increase extension in the lumbar spine (therefore increasing the lordotic curve), is this an issue of true muscular tightness or muscle tension increasing to provide stability? Should this client continue to stretch her lower back?

3. An athlete approaches you with a primary goal to improve his golf game. Specifically, he wants to get stronger as he lacks distance driving the ball off the tee. You ask him to demonstrate his golf swing and note that the ROM of his back swing is very limited. He does not get any turn to bring the club

*Continued*

## CRITICAL THINKING QUESTIONS–cont'd

head back behind him. When designing his exercise program, which of the following do you begin with?

a. Upper body strengthening

b. Lower body strengthening

c. Rotational mobility in the hips and thoracic spine

### ADDITIONAL RESOURCES

American Council on Exercise. *ACE Advanced Health and Fitness Specialist Manual.* San Diego, CA: American Council on Exercise; 2009.

Carey A. *The Pain-Free Program: A Proven Method to Relieve Back, Neck, Shoulder and Joint Pain.* Hoboken, NJ: John Wiley and Sons; 2005.

Cook G. *Movement. Functional Movement Systems: Screening, Assessment and Corrective Strategies.* Santa Cruz, CA: On Target Publications; 2002.

### REFERENCES

1. Wrobel JS, Connolly JE, Beach ML. Associations between static and functional measures of joint function in the foot and ankle. *J Am Podiatr Med Assoc.* 2004;94:535–541.

2. Comerford MJ, Mottram SL. Functional stability re-training: Principles and strategies for managing mechanical dysfunction. In: Beeton KS, eds. *Manual Therapy Masterclasses—The Vertebral Column.* Edinburgh, UK: Churchill Livingstone; 2003:155–175.

3. Panjabi M. The stabilizing system of the spine. Part I. Function, dysfunction, adaptation, and enhancement. *J Spin Disord Tech.* 1992;5:383–389.

4. Myers T. *Anatomy Trains: Myofascial Meridians for Manual and Movement Therapists.* New York, NY: Churchill Livingstone; 2008.

5. Bergmark A. Stability of the lumbar spine. A study in mechanical engineering. *Acta Orthop Scand.* 2000; 6:15–26.

6. Hodges PW, Richardson CA. Inefficient muscular stabilization of the lumbar spine associated with LBP. A motor control evaluation of the TVA. *Spine.* 1996;21:2640–2650.

7. Schleip R, Lehmann-Horn F, Klingler W. Fascia is able to contract in a smooth muscle-like manner and thereby influence musculoskeletal mechanics. In: Liepsch D, ed. *Proceedings of the 5th World Congress of Biomechanics.* Munich, Germany; ISI Current Contents, 2006:51–54. www.isinet.com/isi/ Retrieved March, 2014.

8. Stecco C, Porzionato A, Lancerotto L, et al. Histological study of the deep fasciae of the limbs. *J Bodyw Mov Ther.* 2008;12:225–230.

9. Ingber D. Tensegrity and mechanotransduction. *J Bodyw Mov Ther.* 2008;12:198–200.

10. MacIntosh RR, Gardiner PF, McComas AJ. *Skeletal Muscle, Form and Function.* 2nd ed. Champaign, IL: Human Kinetics; 2006.

11. Sahrmann S. *Diagnosis and Treatment of Movement Impairment Syndromes.* St Louis, MO: Mosby; 2002.

12. De Boer MD. Effect of 5 weeks horizontal bed rest on human muscle thickness and architecture of weight-bearing and non-weight bearing muscles. *Eur J Appl Physiol.* 2008;104:401–407.

13. American Council on Exercise (ACE). *ACE Personal Trainer Manual.* 5th ed. San Diego, CA: ACE; 2014.

14. Loram ID, Lakie M, Di Giulio I, Maganaris CN. The consequences of short-range stiffness and fluctuating muscle activity for proprioception of postural joint rotations: The relevance to human standing. *J Neurophysiol.* 2009;102:460–474.

15. Sahrmann, SA. *Movement System Impairment Syndromes of the Extremities, Cervical and Thoracic Spines,* St. Louis, MO: Mosby; 2010.

16. Salvo S. *Massage therapy: Principles and practice.* Philadelphia, PA: Elsevier, Health Sciences Division; 1999.

17. Shadmehr R, Smith MA, Krakauer, John W. Error correction, sensory prediction, and adaptation in motor control. *Ann Rev Neurosci.* 2010;33:89–108.

18. Boudreau SA, Farina D, Falla D. The role of motor learning and neuroplasticity in designing rehabilitation approaches for musculoskeletal pain disorders. *Man Ther.* 2010;15:410–414.

# *Practice What You Know*

## STABILITY AND MOBILITY RELATIONSHIPS DURING LATERAL FLEXION

The interplay between stability and mobility during various movements can be experienced by performing an action in which one segment of the body is stabilized and then repeating the action while allowing the previously stabilized area to become more mobile.

### Stable Hips and Pelvis Experience

- Stand with your feet together, with both arms straight overhead.
- Keeping your hips and pelvis completely still, side-bend to your left as far as you can.
- Make a mental note of how far you can reach with your fingertips and which muscles are lengthening.

### Mobile Hips and Pelvis Experience

- Next, repeat the side-bend to the same side (left), but allow your hips and pelvis to shift to your right as you bend to the left.
- Note how far you can reach with your fingertips and which muscles you feel lengthening.

### Application

In the first experience, where the hips and pelvis remain stable, the motion occurs at the spine via lateral flexion, upward rotation of the right scapula, and downward rotation of the left scapula, all collectively contributing to the reach with the fingertips. The stretch sensation is felt mainly along the right side of the torso. This example demonstrates that motion and mobility are emphasized at specific segments (torso and scapulae) in the kinetic chain when other segments (hips and pelvis) are fixed with the stabilizers.

In the second experience, right hip adduction and left hip abduction are introduced as the pelvis shifts right and the arms reach left. Although the pelvis is moving in the opposite direction, the ability to bend to the side is greater and the reach is farther. This example demonstrates the critical interplay between stability and mobility. The pelvis shifting to the right calls on the right hip abductors to eccentrically contract as they control the movement of the hip to the right. Accordingly, the stretch sensation is felt lower than in the previous example, toward the outer right hip rather than only in the torso. In other words, some of the burden of the right-side lateral spine flexors was relieved and taken on by the right-side hip abductors.

From these experiences, you can see that the coupled motion of the spine and the hips ultimately creates more mobility in the side-bend movement. As long as the movement is controlled properly by the stabilizer muscles of the hips and pelvis, adding left hip abduction and right hip adduction to the motion effectively creates more ROM. Conversely, in cases where lateral flexion is desired but a stable pelvis is required, because of low-back pain or other dysfunction, side bending can be achieved with a stable, nonmoving pelvis, but the ROM will be reduced.

## *Practice What You Know*

### EXPERIENCING THE KINETIC CHAIN

This chapter describes the body as a continuous kinetic chain where movement at one joint affects the position and function at another joint. The following activities will help you experience important connections throughout the body's kinetic chain.

#### Ankle Pronation and Supination

Because the body is one continuous kinetic chain, the position of the ankle will impact the position of the tibia and the femur. Barring structural differences in the skeletal system (e.g., tibial torsion or femoral anteversion), a pronated ankle position typically forces internal rotation of the tibia and slightly less internal rotation of the femur.

- To demonstrate this point, stand with your shoes off and place your hands firmly on the fronts of your thighs. Notice what happens to the orientation of the knees and thighs when moving between pronation and supination. In addition, notice how the calcaneus everts as the ankle is pronated. Individuals who exhibit excessive pronation or supination in standing and gait are exposing the structures in the body's kinetic chain to forces and wear patterns that can result in pain and injury over time.

#### Thoracic Position and Glenohumeral Mobility

Good shoulder mobility requires that the thoracic spine be in proper, neutral alignment so that the scapulothoracic joint is in the ideal position to allow unimpeded movement of the humeral head in the glenoid fossa.

- To demonstrate this point, stand tall with a neutral spine and the arms resting along your sides. Flex the shoulders to raise both arms overhead. Return the arms to the starting position.
- Next, perform the same overhead arm raise with the thoracic spine flexed forward, or "hunched over." Notice the difference (i.e., reduction) in glenohumeral ROM when the thoracic spine is in proper alignment compared with the flexed-forward position.

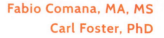

Fabio Comana, MA, MS
Carl Foster, PhD

## CHAPTER 15

# Cardiorespiratory Training

## CHAPTER OUTLINE

## CHAPTER OUTLINE—cont'd

## LEARNING OUTCOMES

1. Describe the importance of performing a pre-exercise health-risk appraisal on all potential exercise participants.
2. Explain how cardiorespiratory exercise affects the muscular, cardiovascular, and respiratory systems.
3. Describe the components of a well-designed cardiorespiratory training session.
4. List general guidelines for cardiorespiratory exercise for health, fitness, and weight loss.
5. Explain various modes of cardiorespiratory exercise.
6. State program design strategies for cardiorespiratory training for participants of various levels of fitness and abilities.
7. Explain the importance of exercise recovery and regeneration between training sessions.

## ANCILLARY LINK

## VIGNETTE

■ Abraham is a 44-year-old cyclist who has been competing for the past 16 years. He is working with his coach, Todd, on developing a workout regimen to help him achieve his goal of finishing in the top 10 in the state championship road race. Abraham will be racing in the 40+ Open category and will be competing against former professional cyclists. To design Abraham's performance training program, Todd asks the following questions:

- How long is the event (time, distance, etc.)? The event is 72 miles.
- What is the course profile (flat, rolling, mountains, etc.)? The course is hilly, so climbing will be the top training priority, in addition to enhancing Abraham's sprinting ability to stick with accelerations and possibly sprint at the finish.
- Will weather be a factor (hot, hot/humid, cold, rain, wind)? Yes, it is a late summer race, so the weather will be hot and humid.
- Where is the event? The event will take place in and around the city of Asheville, North Carolina, a region with a strong road cycling community, so competition will be stiff.

How might Todd approach the development of Abraham's workout regimen? What type of workout will enable Abraham to safely reach his goals?

Humans are designed to move. Since emerging as a distinct species, humans moved (exercised) to secure food, escape from dangerous situations, attract mates, and do a variety of other activities that have allowed the species to thrive. In the small groups of hunter-gatherers who still exist, everyday levels of physical activity are extraordinarily high, essentially equivalent to walking/running 10 to 12 miles/day.[1] The so-called diseases of civilization (e.g., heart disease, diabetes, and many cancers) are uncommon in these groups.[2] Because physical movement is essential for human survival, the organ systems involved in energy metabolism (muscular and cardiorespiratory) function best when subjected to regular physical challenges.

Physical activity leads to improvements in work capacity (e.g., **cardiorespiratory fitness**), the sense of well-being, and overall health, as well as fewer diseases. However, the obligatory need for physical activity is very low in modern society. Most people can do their jobs and feed themselves with a minimum of exertion. Accordingly, the need for people to structure their lives in a way that intentionally includes either higher levels of physical activity or even any exercise at all has increased dramatically.

## HEALTH-RISK APPRAISAL

Research demonstrates the positive impact that exercise and physical activity have on reducing a person's risk for development of cardiovascular, pulmonary, and metabolic diseases, as well as cancer, anxiety, depression, and premature death.[3,4] Although exercise and physical activity promote numerous physiological, psychological, and emotional benefits, there are some inherent risks. In general, moderate levels of exercise and physical activity do not provoke any dangerous cardiovascular or musculoskeletal events in healthy individuals, but there is an increased risk for harm in individuals who are not healthy, or who present with existing disease or are at *risk* for disease.[5] A systematic screening will address an individual's cardiovascular risk factors and identify any signs and/or symptoms of cardiorespiratory disease (Box 15-1). The purposes of the preparticipation screening include[5]:

- Identification of individuals with medical **contraindications** that require exclusion from exercise programs until those conditions have been abated or controlled
- Recognition of individuals with clinically significant disease(s) or conditions who should participate in a medically supervised exercise program
- Detection of individuals who should undergo a medical evaluation and/or exercise testing as part of the health screening process before initiating an exercise program or increasing the frequency and intensity of their current program

Further consideration should be given when assessing an individual's risk as to whether the exercise program is self-directed or is being conducted under the consultation and supervision of a qualified health and fitness professional. With self-directed exercise, a standard

## Box 15-1. Signs and Symptoms of Coronary Artery Disease

Signs or symptoms of coronary artery disease (CAD) are also included in risk stratification, but given the need for specialized training to make a diagnosis, these signs and symptoms must *only* be interpreted by a qualified licensed professional within the clinical context in which they appear. These signs and symptoms include[5]:

- Pain (tightness) or discomfort (or other **angina** equivalent) in the chest, neck, jaw, arms, or other areas that may result from **ischemia**
- Shortness of breath or difficulty breathing at rest or with mild exertion (**dyspnea**)
- **Orthopnea** (dyspnea in a reclined position) or paroxysmal nocturnal dyspnea (onset is usually 2 to 5 hours after the beginning of sleep)
- Ankle **edema**
- **Palpitations** or **tachycardia**
- Intermittent **claudication** (pain sensations or cramping in the lower extremities associated with inadequate blood supply)
- Known heart murmur
- Unusual fatigue or difficulty breathing with usual activities
- Dizziness or **syncope**, most commonly caused by reduced perfusion to the brain

Exercise and fitness professionals should be familiar with each of these conditions and document them in a client's file if: (1) the client has a history of any of these symptoms, or (2) the client develops these signs or symptoms while under the health and fitness professional's supervision.

It is imperative that the client's personal physician be made aware of any signs or symptoms suggestive of CAD that may have been discovered as a result of this prescreening session or during an ongoing exercise program.

questionnaire is completed by the individual with little to no feedback from the health and fitness professional. These questionnaires are designed to provide information regarding existing risks for participation in activity and the need for medical clearance beforehand. A preparticipation screening *must* be performed on all new participants, regardless of age, on entering a facility that offers exercise equipment or services. The screening procedure should be valid, simple, cost- and time-efficient, and appropriate for the target population. In addition, there should be a written policy on referral procedures for at-risk individuals.

Individuals who participate in self-guided activity should at least complete a general health-risk appraisal. The Physical Activity Readiness Questionnaire (PAR-Q) has been used successfully when a short, simple medical/health questionnaire is needed (Fig. 15-1). It is, however, limited by its lack of detail and may overlook important health conditions, medications, and past

Physical Activity Readiness
Questionnaire - PAR-Q
(revised 2002)

# PAR-Q & YOU

## (A Questionnaire for People Aged 15 to 69)

Regular physical activity is fun and healthy, and increasingly more people are starting to become more active every day. Being more active is very safe for most people. However, some people should check with their doctor before they start becoming much more physically active.

If you are planning to become much more physically active than you are now, start by answering the seven questions in the box below. If you are between the ages of 15 and 69, the PAR-Q will tell you if you should check with your doctor before you start. If you are over 69 years of age, and you are not used to being very active, check with your doctor.

Common sense is your best guide when you answer these questions. Please read the questions carefully and answer each one honestly: check YES or NO.

| YES | NO | | |
|---|---|---|---|
| ☐ | ☐ | 1. | Has your doctor ever said that you have a heart condition <u>and</u> that you should only do physical activity recommended by a doctor? |
| ☐ | ☐ | 2. | Do you feel pain in your chest when you do physical activity? |
| ☐ | ☐ | 3. | In the past month, have you had chest pain when you were not doing physical activity? |
| ☐ | ☐ | 4. | Do you lose your balance because of dizziness or do you ever lose consciousness? |
| ☐ | ☐ | 5. | Do you have a bone or joint problem (for example, back, knee or hip) that could be made worse by a change in your physical activity? |
| ☐ | ☐ | 6. | Is your doctor currently prescribing drugs (for example, water pills) for your blood pressure or heart condition? |
| ☐ | ☐ | 7. | Do you know of <u>any other reason</u> why you should not do physical activity? |

## If

## you

## answered

## YES to one or more questions

Talk with your doctor by phone or in person BEFORE you start becoming much more physically active or BEFORE you have a fitness appraisal. Tell your doctor about the PAR-Q and which questions you answered YES.

- You may be able to do any activity you want — as long as you start slowly and build up gradually. Or, you may need to restrict your activities to those which are safe for you. Talk with your doctor about the kinds of activities you wish to participate in and follow his/her advice.
- Find out which community programs are safe and helpful for you.

## NO to all questions

If you answered NO honestly to <u>all</u> PAR-Q questions, you can be reasonably sure that you can:
- start becoming much more physically active — begin slowly and build up gradually. This is the safest and easiest way to go.
- take part in a fitness appraisal — this is an excellent way to determine your basic fitness so that you can plan the best way for you to live actively. It is also highly recommended that you have your blood pressure evaluated. If your reading is over 144/94, talk with your doctor before you start becoming much more physically active.

**DELAY BECOMING MUCH MORE ACTIVE:**
- if you are not feeling well because of a temporary illness such as a cold or a fever — wait until you feel better; or
- if you are or may be pregnant — talk to your doctor before you start becoming more active.

**PLEASE NOTE:** If your health changes so that you then answer YES to any of the above questions, tell your fitness or health professional. Ask whether you should change your physical activity plan.

<u>Informed Use of the PAR-Q</u>: The Canadian Society for Exercise Physiology, Health Canada, and their agents assume no liability for persons who undertake physical activity, and if in doubt after completing this questionnaire, consult your doctor prior to physical activity.

**No changes permitted. You are encouraged to photocopy the PAR-Q but only if you use the entire form.**

NOTE: If the PAR-Q is being given to a person before he or she participates in a physical activity program or a fitness appraisal, this section may be used for legal or administrative purposes.

"I have read, understood and completed this questionnaire. Any questions I had were answered to my full satisfaction."

NAME _____

SIGNATURE _____  DATE_____

SIGNATURE OF PARENT _____  WITNESS _____
or GUARDIAN (for participants under the age of majority)

**Note: This physical activity clearance is valid for a maximum of 12 months from the date it is completed and becomes invalid if your condition changes so that you would answer YES to any of the seven questions.**

**CSEP | SCPE**
THE GOLD STANDARD IN EXERCISE
SCIENCE AND PERSONAL TRAINING

© Canadian Society for Exercise Physiology  www.csep.ca/forms

**Figure 15-1.** Physical Activity Readiness Questionnaire (PAR-Q). Experts recognize the PAR-Q as a minimal, yet safe, pre-exercise screening measure for low-to-moderate, but not vigorous, exercise training. *(Reprinted with permission from the Canadian Society for Exercise Physiology)*

injuries. If an individual answers "No" to all of the questions on the PAR-Q, it is considered safe for him or her to begin a moderate-intensity exercise program and progress the program gradually. An answer of "Yes" to any of the questions requires that he or she see a physician before starting any exercise program.

The process of conducting a health-risk appraisal involves detailed information gathering and a thorough review of the client's health information, medical history, and lifestyle habits, which will enable the health/fitness professional to determine risk stratification or the need for medical examination, as well as develop recommendations for lifestyle modifications and strategies for exercise testing and programming. As such, health and fitness professionals should consider using a more in-depth screening questionnaire for assessing their clients. In 1998, American College of Sports Medicine (ACSM) and the American Heart Association (AHA) published a screening tool that is more comprehensive than the PAR-Q and has undergone several revisions since its conception (Fig. 15-2).[5] The basis for performing a risk stratification before engaging in a physical-activity program is to determine the following[5]:

- The presence or absence of known cardiovascular, pulmonary, and/or metabolic disease
- The presence or absence of cardiovascular risk factors
- The presence or absence of signs or symptoms suggestive of cardiovascular, pulmonary, and/or metabolic disease

---

### AHA/ACSM Health/Fitness Facility Preparticipation Screening Questionnaire

Assess your health needs by marking all *true* statements.

**History**

You have had:

____ A heart attack

____ Heart surgery

____ Cardiac catheterization

____ Coronary angioplasty (PTCA)

____ Pacemaker/implantable cardiac defibrillator/rhythm disturbance

____ Heart valve disease

____ Heart failure

____ Heart transplantation

____ Congenital heart disease

*If you marked any of the statements in this section, consult your physician or other appropriate healthcare provider before engaging in exercise. You may need to use a facility with a **medically qualified staff**.*

**Symptoms**

____ You experience chest discomfort with exertion

____ You experience unreasonable breathlessness

____ You experience dizziness, fainting, blackouts

____ You take heart medications

**Other health issues**

____ You have diabetes

____ You have asthma or other lung disease

____ You have burning or cramping in your lower legs when walking short distances

____ You have musculoskeletal problems that limit your physical activity

____ You have concerns about the safety of exercise

____ You take prescription medication(s)

____ You are pregnant

**Cardiovascular risk factors**

____ You are a man older than 45 years

____ You are a woman older than 55 years, you have had a hysterectomy, or you are postmenopausal

____ You smoke, or quit within the previous 6 mo

____ Your BP is greater than 140/90

____ You don't know your BP

____ You take BP medication

____ Your blood cholesterol level is >200 mg/dL

____ You don't know your cholesterol level

____ You have a close blood relative who had a heart attack before age 55 (father or brother) or age 65 (mother or sister)

____ You are physically inactive (i.e., you get less than 30 min. of physical activity on at least 3 days per week)

____ You are more than 20 pounds overweight

*If you marked two or more of the statements in this section, you should consult your physician or other appropriate healthcare provider before engaging in exercise. You might benefit by using a facility with a **professionally qualified exercise staff** to guide your exercise program.*

____ None of the above is true

*You should be able to exercise safely without consulting your physician or other healthcare provider in a self-guided program or almost any facility that meets your exercise program needs.*

Balady et al. (1998). AHA/ACSM Joint Statement: Recommendations for Cardiovascular Screening, Staffing, and Emergency Policies at Health/Fitness Facilities. *Medicine & Science in Sports & Exercise, 30*(6). (Also in: *ACSM's Guidelines for Exercise Testing and Prescription*, 8th Edition, 2009. Lippincott Williams and Wilkins http://www.lww.com )

www.acsm-msse.org/pt/pt-core/template-journal/msse/media/0698c.htm

**Figure 15-2.** The American Heart Association/American College of Sports Medicine (AHA/ACSM) Health/Fitness Facility Preparticipation Screening Questionnaire. *(Reprinted with permission from The American Heart Association/American College of Sports Medicine (AHA/ACSM) Health/Fitness Facility Preparticipation Screening Questionnaire., pages 1009–1018).*

## In Your Own Words

Are you prepared to manage a situation during an exercise session in which a client shows any of the aforementioned signs or symptoms suggestive of coronary artery disease? Describe to a peer how you would respond to an emergency situation in which a client experiences cardiac distress as a result of exercise training.

Risk stratification is important because someone with only one positive risk factor will be treated differently than someone with several positive risk factors. Risk is categorized as low, moderate, or high.

This process involves three basic steps that should be followed chronologically:

- Identifying **coronary artery disease (CAD)** risk factors
- Performing a risk stratification based on CAD risk factors
- Determining the need for a medical examination/ clearance and medical supervision

Table 15-1 presents clinically relevant CAD health risks that should be used to identify the total number of positive risk factors an individual possesses. Each

**Table 15-1.** Atherosclerotic Cardiovascular Disease Risk Factor Thresholds for Use with American College of Sports Medicine Risk Stratification

| RISK FACTORS | DEFINING CRITERIA | POINTS |
|---|---|---|
| **Positive Risk Factors** | | |
| Age | Men ≥ 45 years<br>Women ≥ 55 years | +1 |
| Family history | Myocardial infarction, coronary revascularization, or sudden death before 55 years of age in father or other first-degree male relative, or before 65 years of age in mother or other first-degree female relative | +1 |
| Cigarette smoking | Current cigarette smoker or those who quit within the previous 6 months, or exposure to environmental tobacco smoke (i.e., secondhand smoke) | +1 |
| Sedentary lifestyle | Not participating in at least 30 minutes of moderate-intensity physical activity (40%–60% $\dot{V}O_2R$) on at least 3 days/week for at least 3 months | +1 |
| Obesity* | Body mass index ≥ 30 kg/m² or waist girth >102 cm (40 inches) for men and >88 cm (35 inches) for women | +1 |
| Hypertension | Systolic blood pressure ≥ 140 mm Hg and/or diastolic blood pressure ≥ 90 mm Hg, confirmed by measurements on at least two separate occasions or currently on antihypertensive medications | +1 |
| Dyslipidemia | LDL cholesterol ≥ 130 mg/dL (3.37 mmol/L) or HDL cholesterol < 40 mg/dL (1.04 mmol/L) or currently on lipid-lowering medication; if total serum cholesterol is all that is available, use serum cholesterol >200 mg/dL (5.18 mmol/L) | +1 |
| Prediabetes | Fasting plasma glucose ≥ 100 mg/dL (5.50 mmol/L), but <126 mg/dL (6.93 mmol/L) or impaired glucose tolerance where a 2-hour oral glucose tolerance test value is ≥140 mg/dL (7.70 mmol/L), but <200 mg/dL (11.00 mmol/L), confirmed by measurements on at least two separate occasions | +1 |
| **Negative Risk Factor** | | |
| High serum HDL cholesterol | ≥60 mg/dL (1.55 mmol/L) | −1 |
| | **Total score:** | |

It is common to sum risk factors in making clinical judgments. If high-density lipoprotein (HDL) is high, subtract one risk factor from the sum of positive risk factors, because high HDL decreases cardiovascular disease risk.

*Professional opinions vary regarding the most appropriate markers and thresholds for obesity; therefore, allied health professionals should use clinical judgment when evaluating this risk factor.

LDL, low-density lipoprotein; $\dot{V}O_2R$, $\dot{V}O_2$reserve.

*Source:* Reprinted from American College of Sports Medicine. *ACSM's Guidelines for Exercise Testing and Prescription.* 9th ed. Philadelphia, PA: Wolters Kluwer/Lippincott Williams & Wilkins; 2014, by permission.

positive risk factor category equals one point. There is also a *negative* risk factor for a high level of **high-density lipoprotein (HDL)**, as a point is subtracted if the individual has an HDL cholesterol score that is equal to or exceeds 60 mg/dL. It is the total number of risk factors and the presence or absence of signs or symptoms that ultimately categorizes an individual's CAD risk during exercise or physical activity, or both.[5] The health and fitness professional should add up the total number of risk factors for a client, subtracting one point for higher HDL cholesterol if appropriate, and use this score to stratify the client's risk (Fig. 15-3A). The classification of risk will dictate any subsequent requirements for medical clearance, additional exercise testing, and level of physician supervision during exercise testing (Fig. 15-3B).

## In Your Own Words

Considering the large portion of the adult population who are sedentary and overweight or obese, it is not uncommon for health and fitness professionals to be tasked with helping individuals who present with several cardiovascular disease risk factors begin an exercise program and lose weight. Explain to a peer how you would recommend to such a client that he or she undergo a medical evaluation and clearance before engaging in vigorous-intensity exercise. How would you respond with a programming option for an individual who would like to begin exercising immediately, even before he or she has a physician's clearance?

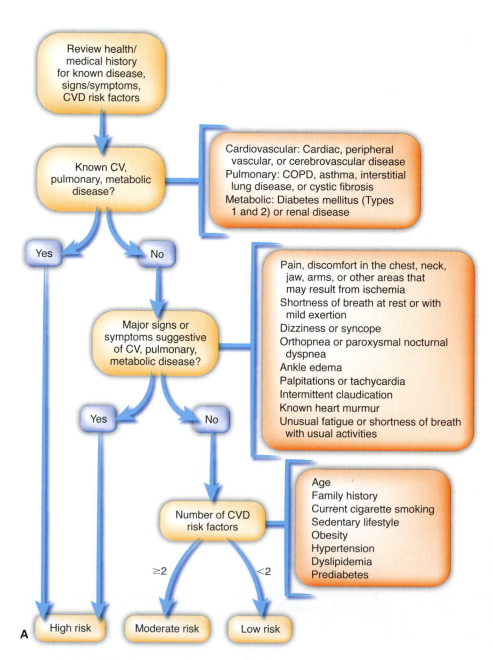

**Figure 15-3.** A, Logic model for classification of risk. CV, cardiovascular; CVD, cardiovascular disease. (Adapted from American College of Sports Medicine. ACSM's Guidelines for Exercise Testing and Prescription. 9th ed. Philadelphia, PA: Wolters Kluwer/Lippincott Williams & Wilkins; 2014, by permission)

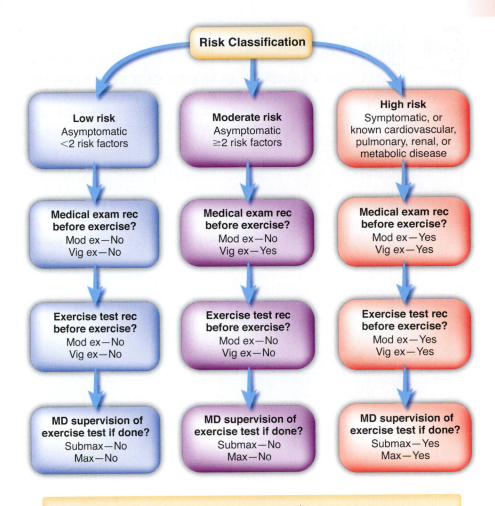

**Risk Classification**

| Low risk<br>Asymptomatic<br><2 risk factors | Moderate risk<br>Asymptomatic<br>≥2 risk factors | High risk<br>Symptomatic, or<br>known cardiovascular,<br>pulmonary, renal, or<br>metabolic disease |
|---|---|---|
| **Medical exam rec before exercise?**<br>Mod ex—No<br>Vig ex—No | **Medical exam rec before exercise?**<br>Mod ex—No<br>Vig ex—Yes | **Medical exam rec before exercise?**<br>Mod ex—Yes<br>Vig ex—Yes |
| **Exercise test rec before exercise?**<br>Mod ex—No<br>Vig ex—No | **Exercise test rec before exercise?**<br>Mod ex—No<br>Vig ex—No | **Exercise test rec before exercise?**<br>Mod ex—Yes<br>Vig ex—Yes |
| **MD supervision of exercise test if done?**<br>Submax—No<br>Max—No | **MD supervision of exercise test if done?**<br>Submax—No<br>Max—No | **MD supervision of exercise test if done?**<br>Submax—Yes<br>Max—Yes |

**Mod Ex:** Moderate intensity exercise; 40%–<60% $\dot{V}O_2R$; 3–<6 METs
"An intensity that causes noticeable increases in HR and breathing."

**Vig Ex:** Vigorous intensity exercise; ≥60% $\dot{V}O_2R$; ≥6 METs
"An intensity that causes substantial increases in HR and breathing."

**Not Rec:** Reflects the notion a medical examination, exercise test, and physician supervision of exercise testing are not recommended in the preparticipation screening; however, they may be considered when there are concerns about risk, more information is needed for the Ex $R_x$, and/or are requested by the patient or client.

**Rec:** Reflects the notion a medical examination, exercise test, and physician supervision are recommended in the preparticipation health screening process.

B

**Figure 15-3.–cont'd** B, Medical examination, exercise testing, and supervision of exercise testing preparticipation recommendations based on classification of risk. Ex Rx, exercise prescription; HR, heart rate; METs, metabolic equivalents; $\dot{V}O_2R$, oxygen uptake reserve. *(Reprinted from American College of Sports Medicine. ACSM's Guidelines for Exercise Testing and Prescription. 9th ed. Philadelphia, PA: Wolters Kluwer/ Lippincott Williams & Wilkins; 2014, by permission)*

Routine exercise testing before initiating a vigorous-intensity physical activity program is recommended only for individuals at high risk for exercise-related complications. Exercise testing is also warranted whenever the health/fitness professional has concerns about an individual's cardiovascular disease risk, the health/fitness professional requires additional information to design an exercise program, or when the exercise participant has concerns about starting an exercise program of any intensity without such testing.

## COMPONENTS OF A CARDIORESPIRATORY WORKOUT SESSION

There are basically three components of any training session: warm-up, the conditioning phase, and cooldown. In some exercise bouts, the intensity of exercise may be very gradually increased, stabilized, and then decreased, so that the components of the session are almost imperceptibly different. For example, going for a run during which the first and last half miles are slower than the middle portion of the run incorporates

## FROM THEORY TO PRACTICE

### ■ ASSESSING CARDIOVASCULAR RISK: CASE STUDY EXAMPLE

Joe is a 49-year-old man who stands 5'11" (1.8 m) and weighs 240 pounds (109 kg). He currently smokes one pack of cigarettes a day and indicates no history of regular physical activity over the past 10 years. He also has a **sedentary** occupation and travels frequently for work. His latest physical examination revealed the following information:

- **Blood pressure** (repeated twice): 138/88 mm Hg
- Total **cholesterol**: 208 mg/dL; HDL cholesterol: 41 mg/dL; low-density lipoprotein (LDL) cholesterol: 134 mg/dL
- No medications
- Fasting blood glucose (last medical examination): 98 mg/dL
- Family history: father diagnosed with CAD at age 62 years; mother diagnosed with **type 2 diabetes** at age 50 years

Questions:

- What are his positive risk factors for heart disease?
- What is his risk stratification according to the ACSM's guidelines?
- What testing and programming guidelines should a personal trainer follow before working with Joe?

### Risk Factors, Defining Criteria and Scores

| RISK FACTORS | DEFINING CRITERIA/COMMENTS | | SCORE |
|---|---|---|---|
| **Positive Risk Factors** | | | |
| Age | 49 years | 45-year-old threshold for men | 1 |
| Family history | Male | None (father diagnosed with CAD at age 62) | 0 |
| | Female | None | 0 |
| Cigarette smoking | Current | 1 pack a day | 1 |
| | Quit in past 6 months | | 0 |
| Physical activity | Sedentary | | 1 |
| Hypertension | SBP | 136 mm Hg | 0 |
| | DBP | 88 mm Hg | 0 |
| | Medications | None reported | N/A |
| Dyslipidemia | Cholesterol | Do not use, as LDL and HDL scores are available | |
| | HDL | 41 mg/dL | 0 |
| | LDL | 134 mg/dL | 1 |
| | Medications | None reported | N/A |
| Impaired fasting glucose | Blood glucose | 98 mg/dL | 0 |
| Obesity | BMI | 33.6 | 1 |
| | Circumference | No measurement at this time | N/A |
| | Body fat | No measurement at this time | N/A |
| **Negative Risk Factor** | | | |
| HDL | Score <60 mg/dL | | 0 |
| | **Total score:** | | 5 |

BMI, body mass index; CAD, coronary artery disease; DBP, diastolic blood pressure; HDL, high-density lipoprotein; LDL, low-density lipoprotein; SBP, systolic blood pressure.

Answers:

- What are his positive risk factors for heart disease? *Age, current smoker, high LDL, high body mass index, and sedentary lifestyle*
- What is his risk stratification according to the ACSM's guidelines? *Moderate because he has no known diagnosis, although he has five positive risk factors*
- What testing and programming guidelines should a personal trainer follow before working with Joe? *Theoretically, he could participate in moderate-intensity activity and submaximal testing without a medical team. However, given his high number of risk factors, Joe should consider getting a medical examination before starting an exercise program.*

all three components of a workout session. In other training sessions, where the conditioning phase may be more challenging, the transitions from warm-up to conditioning to cool-down may be quite distinct.

## Warm-up

The warm-up is a period of lighter exercise preceding the conditioning phase of the exercise bout. The warm-up should last for 5 to 10 minutes for most healthy adults. It should begin with low- to moderate-intensity exercise or activity that gradually increases in intensity.

If higher intensity intervals are planned during the conditioning phase, the latter portion of the warm-up could include some brief higher intensity exercise to prepare the exerciser for the more intense elements of the stimulus phase. As a general principle, the harder the conditioning phase and/or the older the exerciser, the more extensive the warm-up should be (see Part VIII of this textbook for specific recommendations for various populations). However, the warm-up should not be so demanding that it creates fatigue that would reduce performance, especially when working with competitive athletes.

Some controversy exists regarding stretching as part of the warm-up. It probably does no harm to do some brief stretching at the end of the warm-up, although if very high-intensity elements are to be included in the workout, stretching may actually inhibit the ability to achieve full intensity.[6,7] This is attributed to the fact that stretching improves muscle **elasticity** (decreasing tissue viscosity), which lowers the force-generating capacity of the contractile proteins of the muscle. Moreover, the practice of stretching *before* performing any warm-up is not justified and may potentially be harmful. The warm-up may be subdivided into a more general cardiovascular warm-up followed by a more exercise- or event-specific dynamic warm-up (if unique muscular elements are to be performed during the training session).

## Conditioning Phase

The conditioning phase, which must be appropriate for the individual's current fitness level and consistent with his or her training goals, should be planned in terms of frequency, intensity (using steady state or interval training formats), duration, and modality. Although definitive evidence is lacking, empirical evidence suggests that the higher intensity elements of a session should take place fairly early in the conditioning phase, and that the conditioning phase should conclude with more steady-state exercise, even if the intensity is still in the range likely to serve as a stimulus.

When using steady state bouts of exercise, health/fitness professionals should be conscious of **cardiovascular drift**, a cardiovascular phenomenon that represents a gradual increase in heart-rate (HR) response during a steady-state bout of exercise.[8] Causes for this drift include:

- Small reductions in blood volume that occur during exercise because of fluid lost to sweat and fluid moving into the spaces between cells, which results in a compensatory increase in HR to maintain cardiac output, offsetting the small decrease in stroke volume (Cardiac output = HR × stroke volume)
- Increasing core temperature that directs greater quantities of blood to the skin to facilitate heat loss, consequently decreasing venous return to the heart and blood available for the exercising muscles

Aerobic interval training generally involves bouts of steady-state exercise performed at higher intensities for sustained periods (typically a minimum of 3 minutes), followed by a return to lower aerobic intensities for the recovery interval. These intervals often use exercise-to-recovery ratios between 1:2 and 1:1 (e.g., a 4-minute steady-state bout is followed by an 8-minute recovery period at a lower intensity when following a 1:2 exercise-to-recovery ratio).

It should also be noted that higher intensity intervals of 15 to 30 seconds may effectively recruit (and thus stimulate) type II muscle fibers, and are essentially aerobic from the standpoint of the overall metabolic response to training.[9] Assuming that aerobically trained type II muscle fibers may serve as "lactate sinks" (structures that are proficient at using lactate for energy) during hard steady-state exercise, the aerobic training stimulus should include at least some higher intensity segments in programs for individuals with goals that go beyond basic cardiorespiratory conditioning.

## Cool-down

The cool-down should be of approximately the same duration and intensity as the warm-up (i.e., 5–10 minutes of low- to moderate-intensity activity). This phase is directed primarily toward preventing the tendency for blood to pool in the extremities, which may occur when exercise ends. The cessation of significant venous return from the "muscle pump" experienced during exercise can cause blood to accumulate in the lower extremity, reducing blood flow back to the heart and out to vital organs (e.g., the brain, potentially causing symptoms of light-headedness). An active cool-down also helps remove metabolic waste from the muscles so that it can be metabolized by other tissues.

## GENERAL GUIDELINES FOR CARDIORESPIRATORY EXERCISE

The *2008 Physical Activity Guidelines for Americans* released by the U.S. Department of Health & Human Services provides comprehensive science-based recommendations to reduce the risk for many adverse health outcomes. Many of the recommendations are derived from the knowledge that most health benefits occur with at least 150 minutes a week of moderate-intensity physical activity, and that the benefits of physical activity far outweigh the possibility of adverse outcomes. Specific guidelines for adults aged 18 to 64 years include the following:

- Perform 150 minutes per week of moderate-intensity aerobic physical activity or 75 minutes per week of vigorous-intensity aerobic physical activity, or a combination of both.
- Obtain additional health benefits from performing greater amounts of activity than those quantities.
- Perform aerobic bouts that last at least 10 minutes, preferably spread throughout the week.
- Participate in muscle-strengthening activities that involve all major muscle groups at least 2 days per week.

With regard to cardiovascular programming, however, the most widely accepted guidelines for physical activity and basic fitness training are those presented by the ACSM and the AHA. These guidelines frequently use the FITT acronym to discuss cardiovascular programming guidelines.[3,5] This acronym represents frequency, intensity, time (duration), and type (modality), but health/fitness professionals should also consider including an *E* (i.e., FITTE) to represent "enjoyable" or "experience." Exercisers should always enjoy the experience, because this influences the thoughts and emotions that can ultimately dictate participation and **adherence** rates.

Frequency, intensity, and duration collectively represent the exercise volume, load, or magnitude of training that is likely to provoke the physiological adaptations to the training response. A dose–response relationship exists between volume and the health/fitness benefits achieved, implying that greater benefits are achieved with increased volumes. In fact, the newest ACSM guidelines[5] build on the FITT acronym to introduce the FITT-VP principle of exercise prescription or programming, with the V representing volume and the P representing either pattern or progression. These recommendations state that exercisers should target a volume of ≥500 to 1,000 MET-minutes per week or should increase pedometer step counts by ≥2,000 steps/day to reach a daily step count of ≥7,000 steps. Exercising below these volumes may still be beneficial for more deconditioned individuals. In terms of pattern, ACSM guidelines state that exercise can be performed in one continuous session per day or in multiple sessions lasting ≥10 minutes to accumulate the desired duration and volume of daily exercise. Again, very deconditioned individuals may benefit from exercise bouts lasting less than 10 minutes. Finally, all exercisers should have a gradual progression of volume achieved by adjusting duration, frequency, and/or intensity until the desired goal (which should be exercise maintenance) is attained. Programming

with a proper progression may enhance adherence and reduce the risks for musculoskeletal injury and adverse cardiac events.

Health/fitness professionals generally progress their patients' or clients' programs by manipulating these variables. The rate of program progression depends on each individual's health status, exercise tolerance, available time, and program goals. Improvement in cardiorespiratory fitness occurs most quickly from progressive increases in exercise intensity and fades when training intensity is reduced. Changes in fitness are more sensitive to changes in intensity than to changes in the frequency or duration of training.

## In Your Own Words

Clients should enjoy the exercise experience, as this influences the thoughts and emotions that can ultimately dictate participation and adherence rates. People often report that exercising with others makes the task more enjoyable. Describe some examples of family- or community-based activities that new exercisers can incorporate into their lifestyles to promote exercise and increased movement as a shared experience with their loved ones, friends, or both.

## Frequency

Although minimal health benefits can be attained in as little as one to two sessions per week, current guidelines recommend physical activity on most days of the week.[4] ACSM recommendations are presented in Table 15-2. For the beginning adult exerciser, the balance should be in the direction of more moderate-intensity exercise,

## Table 15-2. Cardiorespiratory Recommendations for Healthy Adults

| EXERCISE TYPE | WEEKLY FREQUENCY |
|---|---|
| Moderate-intensity aerobic exercise • 40% to <60% $\dot{V}O_2 R$ or HRR | Minimum of 5 days/week |
| Vigorous-intensity aerobic exercise • ≥60% $\dot{V}O_2 R$ or HRR | Minimum 3 days/week |
| Combination of moderate- and vigorous-intensity aerobic exercise | 3–5 days/week |

HRR, heart-rate reserve; $\dot{V}O_2R$, $\dot{V}O_2$ reserve.
Data from American College of Sports Medicine. *ACSM's Guidelines for Exercise Testing and Prescription.* 9th ed. Philadelphia, PA: Wolters Kluwer/Lippincott Williams & Wilkins; 2014, by permission.

because high-intensity exercise has been associated with a risk for exercise-related complications, injury, and a poor experience in beginning exercisers.[10]

## Intensity

Exercise intensity is arguably the most important element of the exercise program to monitor. At the same time, it is the most difficult element to present quantitatively. There are numerous methods by which the health/fitness professional can program and monitor exercise intensity:

- HR
  - Percentage of maximal heart rate (%MHR)
  - Percentage of MHR reserve; also called the *Karvonen formula*
- Oxygen consumption ($\dot{V}O_2$) or **metabolic equivalent (MET)**
- $\dot{V}O_2$ reserve ($\dot{V}O_2R$)
- Ratings of perceived exertion (RPE)
- Caloric expenditure
- Talk test
- Blood lactate and **second ventilatory threshold (VT2)**

## Heart Rate

One of the simplest ways to prescribe exercise is by using HR. This can be done by calculating a simple percentage of maximal HR (%MHR) or by taking a percentage of the difference between the resting heart rate (RHR) and the MHR. This latter method is called the percentage of heart rate reserve (%HRR) or Karvonen formula. The formulas for both methods are as follows:

**Percentage of MHR**
Target HR (THR) = MHR × % intensity

**Karvonen Method**
THR = (HRR × % intensity) + resting heart rate (RHR)
HRR = MHR − RHR

It is obvious in the Doing the Math feature that the two methods yield very different results. Use of the %MHR formula, although easier to use, systematically underestimates exercise HRs by 10% to 15% compared with the %HRR formula. Thus, when using the %MHR method, it is customary to use higher intensities when calculating THRs (e.g., 60%–80% vs. 50–70%). ACSM provides guidelines for using %MHR (Table 15-3).

An advantage of the %HRR method is that it reduces discrepancies in training intensities between individuals with different resting heart rates (RHRs) and accommodates the training adaptation that decreases RHR, therefore expanding HRR (Fig. 15-5, Table 15-4).

Using %MHR or %HRR is probably the most widely used approach for programming and monitoring exercise intensity, but it is necessary to know an individual's MHR to be at all useful. The only way this can be accurately done is by performing some sort of maximal exercise test. Given the risk associated with

### DOING THE MATH

Joe has an MHR of 180 beats per minute (bpm) and resting HR of 75 bpm. Calculate exercise HRs that correspond to 50% to 70% of %MHR and 50% to 70% of %HRR.

%MHR

Lower limit: 180 × 0.50 = 90

Upper limit: 180 × 0.70 = 126

THR range = 90–126 bpm

%HRR

Reserve = 180 − 75 = 105

Lower limit = 105 × 0.50 = 53; 53 + 75 = 127.5, or 128 bpm

Upper limit = 105 × 0.70 = 73.5; 73.5 + 75 = 148.5, or 149 bpm

conducting a maximal effort test, MHR is normally determined via a variety of mathematical formulas. Although these calculations are usually easy to compute and provide an easy marker from which health/fitness professionals can anchor exercise intensity (e.g., %MHR), estimated MHR is not a very accurate anchor for individual exercise programming and should be questioned because of its inherent error. Numerous variables impact MHR, including the following:

- Genetics
- Exercise modality (e.g., MHR varies between running and cycling because of the involvement of upper-body musculature)
- Medications
- Body size: MHR is generally higher in smaller individuals who have smaller hearts, and hence lower stroke volumes, which explains why female individuals often have higher RHRs than male individuals (Box 15-2)
- Altitude: altitude can lower the MHR reached due to most individuals' inability to train at higher intensities
- Age: MHR does not show a consistent 1-bpm decline with each year in all individuals

Beyond the invalidity of MHR, a significant concern with using a straight percentage of MHR to design and monitor training intensities stems from the fact that discrepancies in individual RHRs are not taken into consideration and may therefore lead the health/fitness professional to overestimate or underestimate appropriate exercise intensities.

Overtraining increases the risk for injury and creates a potentially negative experience, whereas undertraining can quickly disengage the individual from the exercise

## RESEARCH HIGHLIGHT

### Maximum Heart Rate: How Useful Are The Prediction Equations?

In most instances, MHR is not measured but is estimated using prediction equations. The most common equation used to predict MHR is: 220 – age. This equation was introduced in 1971 and was widely accepted by the health/fitness community.[11] However, the validity of the formula has come under attack for several reasons. Most importantly, MHR varies significantly among people of the same age. For example, the formula 220 – age, which was never intended for use with the general population, demonstrates a standard deviation (SD) of approximately 12 bpm.[11] This implies that for 68% of a population (or 1 SD assuming a normal distribution of data), the true MHR would differ from the estimated mathematical calculation by 12 beats on either side of that value (Fig. 15-4). The remaining 32% would fall even further outside of this range (e.g., for 95%, or 2 SDs of the population, the true MHR would fall within 24 beats on either side of the calculated value).

Another concern with the 220 – age formula is the fact that it also tends to overestimate MHR in younger adults and underestimate MHR in older adults (e.g., a 25-year-old may never reach 195 bpm [i.e., 220 – 25], whereas a 60-year-old may exceed 160 bpm [i.e., 220 – 60] quite comfortably).

As a result of the earlier discrepancies, newer equations have been developed and claim to be more accurate. ACSM offers various other commonly used equations for estimating MHR[5]:

- Tanaka equation[12]: MHR = 208 – (0.7 × age)–appropriate for healthy men and women
- Gelish equation[13]: MHR = 207 – (0.7 × age)–appropriate for a broad range of fitness and age levels for both males and females
- Gulati equation[14]: MHR = 206 – (0.88 × age)–appropriate for asymptomatic middle-aged women referred for stress testing

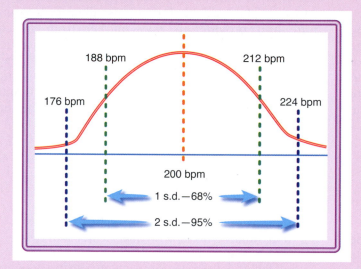

**Figure 15-4.** Standard deviation (s.d.; i.e., 12 beats per minute [bpm]) for the 220 – age maximum heart rate prediction equation for 20-year-olds.

American College of Sports Medicine. *ACSM's Guidelines for Exercise Testing and Prescription.* 9th ed. Philadelphia, PA: Wolters Kluwer/Lippincott Williams & Wilkins; 2014.

Fox SM III, Naughton JP, Haskell WL. Physical activity and the prevention of coronary heart disease. *Ann Clin Res.* 1971;3:404–432.

experience because of boredom and perhaps insufficient challenge. Given that the risk for serious cardiovascular complications during exercise in sedentary individuals is strongly related to inappropriately high exercise intensities,[10] guiding exercise on the basis of a percentage of estimated age-based MHR is strongly discouraged.

### Ratings of Perceived Exertion

Ratings of perceived exertion (RPE) emerged in the late 1970s and early 1980s as a subjective method of gauging exercise intensity. It has since gained wide acceptance as a method of monitoring exercise intensity. There are two versions of the RPE scale: the classical (6–20) scale and the more contemporary category-ratio (0–10) scale, which was developed to remedy inconsistencies with the use of the classical RPE scale (Table 15-5).[15]

Although fully subjective, the RPE scale (in both forms) has been shown to be capable of defining the ranges of objective exercise intensity associated with effective exercise training programs. In simple terms, a rating of "moderate" on the RPE scale is more or less equivalent to 70% of MHR, a rating of "somewhat hard" is more or less equivalent to 80% of MHR, and a rating of "hard" is more or less equivalent to 85% of MHR. Thus, for all practical purposes, RPE ratings of moderate to hard span the range of recommended

## Table 15-3. Recommended Framework for Exercise Intensity for Apparently Healthy Adults

| ACTIVITY/EXERCISE LEVEL | FITNESS CLASSIFICATION | %MHR | %HRR/$\dot{V}O_2$MAX OR $\dot{V}O_2$R |
|---|---|---|---|
| Sedentary: no habitual activity or exercise, extremely deconditioned | Poor | 57%–67% | 30%–45% |
| Minimal activity: no exercise, moderately to highly deconditioned | Poor/fair | 64%–74% | 40%–55% |
| Sporadic physical activity: no or suboptimal exercise, moderately to mildly deconditioned | Fair/average | 74%–84% | 55%–70% |
| Habitual physical activity: regular moderate-to-vigorous intensity | Average/good | 80%–91% | 65%–80% |
| High amounts of habitual activity: regular vigorous-intensity exercise | Good/excellent | 84%–94% | 70%–85% |

MHR, maximal heart rate; HRR, heart-rate reserve; $\dot{V}O_2$max, oxygen consumption maximum; $\dot{V}O_2$R = oxygen consumption reserve.
Adapted from American College of Sports Medicine. *ACSM's Guidelines for Exercise Testing and Prescription.* 8th ed. Philadelphia, PA: Wolters Kluwer/Lippincott Williams & Wilkins; 2010, by permission.

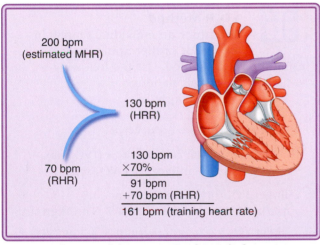

**Figure 15-5.** Use of the Karvonen formula for a 20-year-old man (average shape; resting heart rate = 70 bpm). bpm, beats per minute; HRR, heart-rate reserve; MHR, maximum heart rate; RHR, resting heart rate.

## Table 15-4. Comparing Percentage of Heart Rate Reserve Estimations in Two 30-Year-Olds With Different Resting Heart Rates

| | PERSON A (bpm) | PERSON B (bpm) |
|---|---|---|
| MHR (220 − 30) | 190 | 190 |
| RHR | 50 | 80 |
| HRR (MHR − RHR) | 140 | 110 |
| 60% HRR | 84 | 66 |
| Adding RHR | 84 + 50 | 66 + 80 |
| Training HR | 134 | 146 (12-beat difference) |

bpm, beats per minute; HR, heart rate; HRR, heart-rate reserve; MHR, maximum heart rate; RHR, resting heart rate.

## Box 15-2. Body Position and Resting Heart Rate

There is some debate over the body position in which RHR is measured. The Karvonen formula was created measuring true RHR, taken in the morning in a reclining position. RHR varies by approximately 5 to 10 beats when a person transitions from lying to standing, thereby altering the size of the HRR. Given the concern with some inconsistencies with individuals measuring their own HR, efforts should be made to measure RHR in the body position in which the individual will exercise. This may necessitate the need for two sets of training zones: one for seated/recumbent positions and another for standing activities.

exercise training intensities. The RPE system works well for about 90% of people. Very sedentary individuals often find it difficult to use, as they find any level of exercise fairly hard. However, in the very sedentary, even a small amount of low-intensity exercise is effective in terms of producing some exercise training benefits and improved health outcomes. At the other end of the continuum, individuals who have high muscular strength may under-rate the intensity of exercise if they focus on the muscular tension requirement of exercise rather than on the breathing elements. With practice during cardiorespiratory exercise, these individuals can usually learn to use the scale fairly effectively.

## Table 15–5. Ratings of Perceived Exertion

| RPE | CATEGORY RATIO SCALE |
|---|---|
| 6 | 0 Nothing at all |
| 7 Very, very light | 0.5 Very, very weak |
| 8 | 1 Very weak |
| 9 Very light | 2 Weak |
| 10 | 3 Moderate |
| 11 Fairly light | 4 Somewhat strong |
| 12 | 5 Strong |
| 13 Somewhat hard | 6 |
| 14 | 7 Very strong |
| 15 Hard | 8 |
| 16 | 9 |
| 17 Very hard | 10 Very, very strong |
| 18 | *Maximal |
| 19 Very, very hard | |
| 20 | |

RPE, ratings of perceived exertion.
Data from Borg, G. (1998). *Borg's Perceived Exertion and Pain Scales.* Champaign, Ill.: Human Kinetics.

## $\dot{V}O_2$ or Metabolic Equivalents

The traditional reference standard for exercise intensity is expressed in terms of percentages of maximal oxygen consumption ($\dot{V}O_2$max), which is the maximum amount of oxygen (milliliters) that a person can use in 1 minute per kilogram of body weight. $\dot{V}O_2$max can be estimated and converted to an MET. In cases where $\dot{V}O_2$ is not directly measured during either testing or training, expressing exercise intensity in terms of METs, which are multiples of an assumed average metabolic rate at rest of 3.5 mL/kg/min, is commonplace. This is easy and intuitive for many people to understand (e.g., at 5.0 METs, they are working five times harder than at rest). It is important to recognize, however, that the resting metabolic rate is not exactly 3.5 mL/kg/min in every individual, or even in the same person at all times. Nevertheless, the utility of using METs rather than directly measured $\dot{V}O_2$ is so substantial that it more than makes up for any imprecision (Table 15-6).

The great volume of experimental studies conducted in the 1960s and 1970s suggested that there are minimal improvements in $\dot{V}O_2$max if the intensity of training is below a threshold of 40%/50% of $\dot{V}O_2$max or $\dot{V}O_2$R.[16] While acknowledging that lower intensity exercise can result in improvements in aerobic capacity in very sedentary or unfit individuals, there does appear to be a lower limit intensity below which exercise is of minimal benefit.

## $\dot{V}O_2$R

Similar to the HRR method in its concept, $\dot{V}O_2$R is the difference between $\dot{V}O_2$max and resting $\dot{V}O_2$. Therefore, to calculate $\dot{V}O_2$R, a person's $\dot{V}O_2$max and resting $\dot{V}O_2$ must be provided. The $\dot{V}O_2$ resting value of 3.5 mL/kg/min is commonly used as a factor in this equation.

$\dot{V}O_2$R Method

$$\text{Target } \dot{V}O_2 = ([\dot{V}O_2\text{max} - \dot{V}O_2\text{ rest}] \times \% \text{ intensity}) + \dot{V}O_2 \text{ rest}$$

## Caloric Expenditure

When the human body burns fuel (e.g., **fats**, **carbohydrates**), oxygen ($O_2$) is consumed, which yields calories to perform work. Although the number of calories produced per liter of $O_2$ consumed varies according to the fuel utilized (i.e., 4.69 kcal/L $O_2$ for fats; 5.05 kcal/L $O_2$ for glucose), a value of 5 kcal/L $O_2$ is sufficiently accurate considering the fact that people burn a combination of fuels throughout their daily activities.

- Caloric expenditure is usually calculated in terms of the gross or absolute $\dot{V}O_2$ during an activity

### DOING THE MATH
### $\dot{V}O_2$R Method

Determine an individual's target intensity for cardiorespiratory training using the $\dot{V}O_2$R method. Use the following variables in your calculations.

$\dot{V}O_2$max = 30 mL/kg/min
$\dot{V}O_2$ rest = 3.5 mL/kg/min
Desired intensity = 60% $\dot{V}O_2$R

$\dot{V}O_2$R formula: Target $\dot{V}O_2$ = ([$\dot{V}O_2$max − $\dot{V}O_2$rest] × % intensity) + $\dot{V}O_2$ rest

Target $\dot{V}O_2$ = ([30 mL/kg/min − 3.5 mL/kg/min] × % intensity) + 3.5 mL/kg/min

Target $\dot{V}O_2$ = (26.5 mL/kg/min × % intensity) + 3.5 mL/kg/min

Target $\dot{V}O_2$ = (26.5 mL/kg/min × 0.60) + 3.5 mL/kg/min

Target $\dot{V}O_2$ = 15.9 mL/kg/min + 3.5 mL/kg/min = 19.4 mL/kg/min

Once you have calculated the percent $\dot{V}O_2$R value, convert it to a MET value (using the following formula) to identify physical activities that require similar energy expenditures.

MET conversion formula = $\dot{V}O_2$R value ÷ 1 MET

1 MET = 3.5 mL/kg/min ÷
$\dot{V}O_2$R value = 19.4 mL/kg/min

MET conversion: 19.4 mL/kg/min ÷ 3.5 mL/kg/min = 5.5 METs

## FROM THEORY TO PRACTICE

Selecting an appropriate intensity is always a major challenge for health/fitness professionals who seek proper levels of overload, yet want to create an optimal experience, especially when working with newer, deconditioned individuals, those who are apprehensive about undergoing cardiorespiratory fitness testing, and individuals for whom HR measures are invalid (e.g., those taking beta-blockers).

The "session RPE" was developed as a method of monitoring the combined intensity and duration of an exercise session.[17,18] If an individual is asked to rate the overall intensity of an exercise bout about 30 minutes after the conclusion of that bout using the category-ratio (0–10) scale, and then multiplies this rating by the duration of the bout, a score representing the combined intensity and duration of the bout is generated (i.e., the training load).[19–21] In practice, this daily score can be summated on a weekly basis, generating a weekly training load for self-monitoring purposes. This is an effective programming and monitoring tool that promotes appropriate initial exercise intensities, creates some ownership of programming on the part of the individual, and allows a limited degree of training flexibility to facilitate adherence.

This model can be used exclusively and indefinitely to monitor exercise intensity, or it can be used during only the initial stage of an individual's program, perhaps before conducting any cardiorespiratory tests for aerobic fitness.

Health/fitness professionals should adhere to the following guidelines when using the session RPE model:
- Spend time helping the individual become familiar with the 0 to 10 RPE scale.
- Determine appropriate RPE intensities for each exercise session based on the individual's current activity levels, while providing a small overload challenge (e.g., a 5 out of 10 effort for someone who has been exercising at a 4–4.5 effort).
- Identify the frequency and duration that is appropriate for the individual's current conditioning level and is feasible within his or her schedule (e.g., three times a week for 15 minutes).
- Implement an RPE training volume model (i.e., RPE × frequency × duration).
  - For example, Joe's key goal is to improve his cardiorespiratory fitness, and he and his trainer mutually decide that a feasible start is for him to participate in cardiovascular training sessions three times each week for approximately 20 minutes each, at a 5 out of 10 effort.
  - His total weekly training volume is 3 × 20 minutes = 60 minutes, and his target goal for week one = 60 minutes × RPE of 5 = 300 points.
  - Joe's progression over 3 weeks at a 10% progression rate per week:
    - Week 1 = 300 points
    - Week 2 = 330 points
    - Week 3 = 363 points
  - The trainer can provide Joe options on how he can achieve his target number by manipulating any of the three variables (i.e., intensity, frequency, and duration; Table 15-7). While allowing Joe some flexibility and ownership of his program, the trainer should subscribe to the KISS principle (keep it simple and short) to avoid confusion and potential dropout.

by measuring or estimating the total quantity of $O_2$ consumed per minute and multiplying it by 5 kcal/L $O_2$. If the quantity of $O_2$ consumed is provided or measured in relative terms (i.e., mL/kg/min), this value must first be converted to gross or absolute terms to determine the total amount of $O_2$ consumed before the caloric value can be calculated.

Most pieces of commercial cardiovascular exercise equipment provide estimates of caloric expenditure in this same manner. Although they may not always be 100% accurate, they calculate caloric expenditure by estimating gross or absolute $\dot{V}O_2$ based on the amount of work being performed (i.e., speed, grade, and watts).

If direct measurement of $\dot{V}O_2$ during activity is not available, the health/fitness professional can use published MET estimates for a variety of activities (see Table 15-6). Online caloric-expenditure calculators are available for a variety of physical activities at the American Council on Exercise website (www.acefitness.org/calculators).

### Talk Test

Following up on suggestions from a generation ago, several groups have explored the value of the talk test

**Table 15-6.** Metabolic Equivalent Values of Common Physical Activities Classified as Light, Moderate, or Vigorous Intensity

| LIGHT (<3 METS) | MODERATE (3–6 METS) | VIGOROUS (>6 METS) |
|---|---|---|
| **Walking**<br>Walking slowly around home, store, or office = 2.0*<br>**Household and Occupation**<br>Sitting—using computer, work at desk, using light hand tools = 1.5<br>Standing performing light work, such as making bed, washing dishes, ironing, preparing food, or working as store clerk = 2.0–2.5<br>**Leisure Time and Sports**<br>Arts and crafts, playing cards = 1.5<br>Billiards = 2.5<br>Boating—power = 2.5<br>Croquet = 2.5<br>Darts = 2.5<br>Fishing—sitting = 2.5<br>Playing most musical instruments = 2.0–2.5 | **Walking**<br>Walking 3.0 mph = 3.0*<br>Walking at a very brisk pace (4 mph) = 5.0*<br>**Household and Occupation**<br>Cleaning, heavy—washing windows, washing car, cleaning garage = 3.0<br>Sweeping floors or carpet, vacuuming, mopping = 3.0–3.5<br>Carpentry—general = 3.6<br>Carrying and stacking wood = 5.5<br>Mowing lawn—walk power mower = 5.5<br>**Leisure Time and Sports**<br>Badminton—recreational = 4.5<br>Basketball—shooting around = 4.5<br>Bicycling on flat surface—light effort (10–12 mph) = 6.0<br>Dancing—ballroom slow = 3.0; ballroom fast = 4.5<br>Fishing from riverbank and walking = 4.0<br>Golf—walking pulling clubs = 4.3<br>Sailing boat, wind surfing = 3.0<br>Swimming leisurely = 6.0†<br>Table tennis = 4.0<br>Tennis doubles = 5.0<br>Volleyball—noncompetitive = 3.0–4.0 | **Walking, Jogging, and Running**<br>Walking at very, very brisk pace (4.5 mph) = 6.3*<br>Walking/hiking at moderate pace and grade with no or light pack (<10 pounds, 4.5 kg) = 7.0<br>Hiking at steep grades and with pack 10–42 pounds (4.5–19 kg) = 7.5–9.0<br>Jogging at 5 mph = 8.0*<br>Jogging at 6 mph = 10.0*<br>Running at 7 mph = 11.5*<br>**Household and Occupation**<br>Shoveling sand, coal, etc. = 7.0<br>Carrying heavy loads, such as bricks = 7.5<br>Heavy farming, such as bailing hay = 8.0<br>Shoveling, digging ditches = 8.5<br>**Leisure Time and Sports**<br>Basketball game = 8.0<br>Bicycling on flat surface—moderate effort (12–14 mph) = 8; fast (14–16 mph) = 10<br>Cross-country skiing—slow (2.5 mph) = 7.0; fast (5.0–7.9 mph) = 9.0<br>Soccer—casual = 7.0; competitive = 10.0<br>Swimming—moderate/hard = 8–11†<br>Tennis singles = 8.0<br>Volleyball—competitive at gym or beach = 8.0 |

*On flat, hard surface.

†MET values can vary substantially from person to person during swimming as a result of different strokes and skill levels.

MET, metabolic equivalents; mph, miles per hour.

*Source:* Reprinted from American College of Sports Medicine. *ACSM's Guidelines for Exercise Testing and Prescription.* 9th ed. Philadelphia, PA: Wolters Kluwer/Lippincott Williams & Wilkins; 2014, by permission; adapted and modified from Ainsworth BE, Haskell, WL, & Whitt, MC. Compendium of physical activities: An update of activity codes and MET intensities. *Med Sci Sports Exerc.* 2000;32(Suppl): S498–S504.

as a method of monitoring (and controlling) exercise training intensity.[22–27] The physiological basis of the talk test is presented in Chapter 8. The usual experience with the talk test is that if two people are exercising and having a conversation, one of them will eventually turn to the other and say something like, "If we are going to keep talking, you are going to have to slow down." The talk test works on the premise that at about the intensity of the **first ventilatory threshold (VT1)**, the increase in ventilation is accomplished by an increase in breathing frequency. One of the requirements of comfortable speech is to be able to control breathing frequency. Thus, at the intensity of VT1, it is no longer possible to speak comfortably.

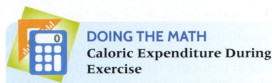

**DOING THE MATH**

**Caloric Expenditure During Exercise**

Caloric expenditure = ($\dot{V}O_2$ [mL/kg/min] × body weight [kg]/1,000) × 5 kcal/L/min

If Mary weighs 154 lb and exercises for 25 minutes and maintains an average $\dot{V}O_2$ of 35 mL/kg/min, what would be her total caloric expenditure for the entire exercise bout?

- Convert 154 lb to kilograms by dividing by the conversion factor of 2.2 (1 kg = 2.2 lb):
  - 154 lb/2.2 = 70 kg
- Mary's relative $\dot{V}O_2$ = 35 mL/kg/min. To calculate her gross or absolute $\dot{V}O_2$, multiply her $\dot{V}O_2$ by her body weight:
  - 35 mL/kg/min × 70 kg = 2,450 mL/min or 2.45 L/min
- If Mary consumes 5 kcal/L $O_2$, her caloric expenditure each minute is calculated as follows:
  - 2.45 L/min × 5 kcal/L = 12.25 kcal/min
- If Mary exercised for 25 minutes, her total caloric expenditure during the entire exercise bout is calculated as follows:
  - 12.25 kcal/min × 25 minutes = 306 kcal

Studies in a variety of populations (e.g., healthy individuals, cardiac patients, and athletes) have demonstrated that the talk test is a very good marker of VT1. Typically, below the VT1, people will respond to any of a number of speech-provoking stimuli (e.g., normal conversation, a structured interview, or reciting a standard paragraph) by stating that they can speak comfortably. Above VT1, but below a second metabolic marker called the *VT2*, they will be able to speak, but not comfortably. VT2 represents the point at which high-intensity exercise can no longer be sustained given the accumulation of lactate that begins to overwhelm the blood's buffering capacity. Above the intensity of the VT2, speech is not possible, other than single words.

The talk test has several advantages as a method of programming and monitoring exercise compared with a given %$\dot{V}O_2$max or %MHR, because it is based off of an individual's unique metabolic or ventilatory responses. Thus, for most people, training at intensities at which the answer to the question, "Can you speak comfortably?" becomes less than an unequivocal "Yes" may represent the ideal training intensity marker. Therefore, the talk test is an appropriate marker to use for many individuals, especially for those seeking to lose weight or develop their aerobic efficiency. At VT1, fats continue to contribute significantly to the number of calories burned (caloric quality). In addition, training at or near this intensity (unique to the individual's own metabolism) increases the likelihood of a better exercise experience. Higher intensity training for those individuals with performance goals can be regulated in terms of the VT2.

**Table 15-7. Training Progression and Options Using Frequency × Duration × Intensity (Ratings of Perceived Exertion)**

|  | FREQUENCY | DURATION | INTENSITY (RPE) | TOTAL POINTS |
|---|---|---|---|---|
| **Week One Goal** |  |  |  | 300 |
| Options | 3 sessions | × 20 | × 5 | **= 300** |
|  | 2 sessions | × 20 | × 5 | = 200 |
|  | 1 session | × 18 | × 5.5 | = 99 |
|  |  |  |  | **299** |
|  | 2 sessions | × 16 | × 5 | = 160 |
|  | 2 sessions | × 13 | × 5.5 | = 143 |
|  |  |  |  | **303** |
| **Week Two Goal** |  |  |  | 330 |
| Options | 3 sessions | × 22 | × 5 | **=330** |
|  | 2 sessions | × 22 | × 5 | = 220 |
|  | 1 session | × 18 | × 6 | = 108 |
|  |  |  |  | **328** |
|  | 2 sessions | × 19 | × 4 | = 152 |
|  | 2 sessions | × 16.5 | × 5.5 | = 181 |
|  |  |  |  | **333** |

RPE, ratings of perceived exertion.

## VIGNETTE continued

■ Abraham needs to focus on developing his endurance to ride 72 miles and be strong throughout. His longest training rides should be about 25% longer than this distance (i.e., 90–100 miles). The workout plan will also enhance his ability to climb with sustained and very intense efforts and to accelerate both in flat-terrain sprints and while going uphill.

First, Todd conducts field assessments to determine Abraham's HR at VT1 and VT2. His program's training time will break down as follows:

- ~80% of time below VT1 (warm-ups, cool-downs, long rides, recovery rides)
- ~10% between VT1 and VT2 (longer intervals/ sustained efforts on harder climbs)
- ~10% at or above VT2 (sprints and hill sprints/ accelerations)

## Duration

Exercise duration generally refers to the amount of time spent performing the physical activity, or it can be expressed in terms of exercise quantity (e.g., run 2 miles, take 5,000 steps, or burn 250 kcal). ACSM[5] presents guidelines on recommended intensities that reduce the risks for **mortality** and **morbidity**, and improve overall fitness. However, health/fitness professionals should consider the following points:

- The quantity of exercise or physical activity may be performed in one continuous bout, or be performed intermittently and accumulated throughout the day in bouts lasting a minimum of 10 minutes each.
- Although the guidelines provide recommended quantities to improve overall health/fitness, the needs of the individual should always be considered first. Health/fitness professionals should select suitable durations and progressions that fit each individual's current conditioning level, tolerance, and availability, and aspire only to attain the recommendations when appropriate.

## RESEARCH HIGHLIGHT

### Which Is Better: High Intensity or Low Intensity?

The debate concerning high- versus low-intensity exercise continues, and although a significant amount of more recent research has focused on the aerobic benefits of high-intensity interval training (HIIT), experts cannot reach any single conclusion regarding its efficacy, because it all depends on the perspective from which they approach the argument. Research has revealed that HIIT results in similar improvements in $\dot{V}O_2max$ and mitochondrial density as bouts of lower-intensity exercise (LIE), but which form of exercise is more appropriate for a sprint athlete versus the overweight business executive simply seeking to improve health? Certainly, some research demonstrates how HIIT increases levels of free fatty acids (FFA) in the blood because of greater levels of circulating epinephrine, which is supposed to drive greater aerobic metabolism in the cells. But research also demonstrates that the increased levels of blood lactate that follow HIIT begin to inhibit hormone-sensitive lipase activity, the enzyme responsible for mobilizing fats. Furthermore, increased lactate levels act as a precursor for glycerol 3-phosphate, promoting the re-esterification of those FFAs into triglycerides within adipocytes (fat cells) if the FFAs are not taken into the muscle cells, but instead remain in the blood. HIIT builds ventilatory power, or the speed and magnitude with which individuals move air into and out of the lungs. LIE, in contrast, builds ventilatory endurance, or the capacity of the endurance muscles to sustain work and resist fatigue. Both are critical to ventilation and the delivery of adequate levels of oxygen to the muscle cells.

Perhaps the most popular form of HIIT is what many term *Tabata training*, coined after the researcher who, together with his colleagues, challenged conventional thinking back in 1996 and introduced training methods for improving aerobic fitness (i.e., $\dot{V}O_2max$). In their study using 14 physically fit, young, male subjects, Tabata and colleagues compared two training methodologies and examined improvements in both aerobic and anaerobic fitness.

- In experiment one, seven subjects performed steady state exercise five times per week on cycle ergometers, with each session performed at 70% of $\dot{V}O_2max$ for 60 minutes (total of 300 minutes per week).
- In experiment two, seven subjects performed HIIT five times per week on cycle ergometers, with four sessions performed at workloads equivalent to 170% of $\dot{V}O_2max$. The subjects completed seven to eight reps, with the workload progressing by 11 watts on subsequent sessions when nine intervals could be attained. Each set involved a 20-second work interval followed by a 10-second recovery interval, totaling approximately 4 minutes of work per session. On the fifth day, the subjects completed a 30-minute interval at 70% of $\dot{V}O_2max$, followed by only 4 sets at 170% of $\dot{V}O_2max$.

After 6 weeks, aerobic capacity in experiment one increased by 9% (52.9 to 58 mL/kg/min), whereas anaerobic capacity did not increase. However, after 6 weeks, aerobic capacity in experiment two increased by 13% (48.2 to 55 mL/kg/min), whereas anaerobic capacity improved by 28%. The results of this study demonstrated that

## RESEARCH HIGHLIGHT—cont'd

steady-state moderate-intensity aerobic training that improves maximal aerobic power does not improve anaerobic capacity, whereas HIIT may improve both anaerobic and aerobic capacity in a more time-efficient manner. Unfortunately, the nature and results of this study have largely been misinterpreted by many fitness professionals who market Tabata training to the public. Although the study used 14 physically fit, young, male subjects exercising on bicycle ergometers, this form of training is now performed with many different population groups (e.g., deconditioned individuals, females, and older adults) and includes other forms of cardiorespiratory exercise (e.g., treadmill, elliptical, and sprints), and even resistance training (e.g., body weight and externally loaded resistance), none of which can truly be completed at 170% of $VO_2$max. The unfortunate reality is that the only real similarity of these programs to Professor Tabata's research is the 2:1 work-to-recovery ratios. Although the results achieved and the efficiency with which those results are gained are impressive, a health and fitness professional should always examine the appropriateness of such practices with each individual client.

Another more recent training method follows the research by Gunnarsson and Bangsbo in 2012, called the 10-20-30 Training Concept, more commonly known as the Copenhagen method.[28] In this study, 18 moderately trained runners (6 females, 12 males) were divided into a high-intensity training (10-20-30) group and a control group to compare the effects of both methods on the health profile, muscular adaptations, $VO_2$max, and running performance of the study participants. While the control group continued their normal training methods during the seven-week study, the 10-20-30 group implemented a format of 30 seconds of low-intensity running at less than 30% of maximal intensity, 20 seconds of moderate-intensity running at less than 60% of maximal intensity, and 10 seconds of high-intensity running at more than 90% of maximal intensity (i.e., a 60-second interval). This interval was repeated five times (i.e., 5 minutes of continuous exercise) before taking a 2-minute recovery, and the entire circuit was repeated three to four times. At the conclusion of the study, $VO_2$max in the 10-20-30 group was 4% higher, and performance in a 1,500-m and a 5-km run improved by 21 and 48 seconds, respectively. Furthermore, in the 10-20-30 group, systolic blood pressure was lower by 5 mm Hg, and total and LDL cholesterol were lower by 0.5 and 0.4 mmol/L, (19.3 and 15.5 mg/dL) respectively, in comparison with the control group. The results demonstrated that this method of training, with short, near-maximal bouts (e.g., 10 seconds), can improve health, fitness, and performance despite large reductions in training volume. This format of training with slightly longer recovery intervals is generally better suited for most individuals contemplating HIIT.

A prevailing mentality is to exercise hard and maximize total caloric expenditure in a session to effectively promote weight loss (concept of caloric *quantity*). While this method largely ignores the overall exercise experience (an influential driver of exercise adherence), it also fails to consider the concept of caloric *quality* (i.e., what fuel is being burned). Which is more important: quality or quantity? The debate continues, and based on individual research design, experts draw different conclusions. In a perfect world, exercisers want to achieve both caloric quantity (total number of calories) and caloric quality (absolute calories, not percentage, coming from fat). In endurance athletes, this spares glycogen and saves unwanted muscle breakdown, helping them finish their race. Training hard burns carbohydrates and creates adaptations that improve an individual's glycolytic storage and utilization capabilities, as well as the ability to better tolerate and reconvert lactate back to usable forms of energy efficiently. The adaptation of increased muscle glycogen storage pulls approximately 2.5 g of water for each stored gram of glycogen. "Expanding the tank" is great for an athlete, but is this what an individual seeking weight loss or an exerciser seeking to simply improve health and fitness wants or needs?

HIIT is also believed to contribute more significantly than LIE to increasing excess post-exercise oxygen consumption (EPOC), which may accelerate weight loss. A study by Knab and colleagues[29] investigated the contribution of EPOC to overall caloric expenditure. The details of their research are presented in Chapter 4, but in brief, their study demonstrated that 45 minutes of vigorous exercise that expended 519 kcal increased EPOC for 14 hours, totaling 190 kcal, or an average of 13.6 kcal/hr. This represents 37% of the kcal expended in energy. Although this may have serious implications for weight loss, it is important to remember that this study used 10 young, well-conditioned men who could perform sustained, vigorous-intensity exercise. Research consistently supports larger EPOCs with higher intensity and longer duration exercise. Regardless, with weight loss, every kilocalorie counts, so even smaller EPOCs will contribute to weight loss.

Although diet has the greatest influence on what fuel is burned, providing an appropriate training stimulus can influence fuel utilization at rest and during exercise.[30] Therefore, LIE may initially help the body adapt to utilizing fats more efficiently, while simultaneously offering a better experience. So what is the consensus or take-away message? Contrary to popular opinion, which waivers back and forth over time (i.e., in the 1980s, LIE was popular; in the 2000s, HIIIT is more popular), the reality is that most individuals probably need, and benefit from, both types of training.

Gunnarsson TP, Bangsbo J. The 10-20-30 Training Concept improves performance and health profile in moderately trained runners. *J Appl Physiol.* 2012;113:16–24.

Tabata I, Nishimura K, Kouzaki M, et al. Effects of moderate-intensity endurance and high-intensity intermittent training on anaerobic capacity and $VO_2$max. *Med Sci Sports Exerc.* 1996;28:1327–1330.

Benefits gained from exercise and physical activity are dose related (i.e., greater benefits are derived from greater quantities of activity). For example, physical activity expending ≤1,000 kcal/week generally only produces improvements to health (e.g., lower blood pressure and cholesterol). This is considered a minimal recommendation for activity, whereas greater quantities expending ≥2,000 kcal/week promote effective weight loss and significant improvements to overall fitness.

Exercise guidelines for adults aged 18 to 64 call for the following[4]:

- Moderate-intensity exercise or activity performed for at least 30 minutes a session, a minimum of 5 days per week for a total of 150 minutes per week, or
- Vigorous-intensity exercise or activity performed for at least 20 to 25 minutes a session, a minimum of 3 days per week for a total of 75 minutes per week, or
- A combination of both (e.g., 20–30 minutes of moderate-to-vigorous exercise or activity performed 3–5 days per week)

Specific guidelines for overweight and obese individuals or those seeking to manage their weight include the following:

- Perform 50 to 60 minutes of moderate-intensity exercise or activity each day, 5 to 7 days a week, for a total of 300 minutes, or
- A total of 150 minutes of vigorous exercise or activity per week, performed a minimum of 3 days a week, or
- A combination of both

Specific guidelines for children and adolescents aged 6 to 17 include the following:

- Perform at least 60 minutes of moderate-to-vigorous physical activity every day
- Include vigorous-intensity activity a minimum of 3 days per week
- Participate in muscle-strengthening and bone-strengthening activity a minimum of 3 days per week

Health/fitness professionals must bear in mind that novice exercisers will generally not be able to complete 30 minutes of moderate-intensity cardiorespiratory exercise, nor will they be capable of achieving the recommended frequency (Table 15-8).

## In Your Own Words

Many individuals who are new to exercise have a difficult time piecing together all of the necessary components (e.g., frequency, intensity, duration, and type) of a well-rounded training program. How will you make your exercise recommendations to your clients practical and applicable to their individual circumstances?

## Exercise Progression

While exercise needs to create an enjoyable and positive experience for participants, the health/fitness professional will need to determine how to progress each individual's program. Progression follows some basic training principles, including the following:

- The principle of **overload** states that when additional stresses are placed on the organs or systems (e.g., cardiorespiratory or muscular) in a timely and appropriate manner, physiological adaptations and improvement will occur. The rate of progression in a program depends on the individual's current conditioning level, program goals, and tolerance for the slight discomfort associated with increasing training load or volume.
- The principle of **specificity** states that the physiological adaptations made within the body are specific to demands placed on the body—sometimes referred to as the SAID principle: specific adaptations to the imposed demands. This implies that if an individual's goals are consistent with running a half marathon, the training program should progress to mimic the demands of that activity, to provide the specific stimuli that elicit appropriate adaptations within the body. The decision to progress to event- or sports-specific modalities should be made with consideration for the individual's skills and abilities, as well as his or her current conditioning level.
- √ Even among aerobic exercises, the transfer of benefits from one type of exercise to another

## Table 15-8. Recommendations for Exercise Duration and Quantity

| PHYSICAL FITNESS CLASSIFICATION | WEEKLY EXPENDITURE (Kcal) | DURATION/DAY (min) | WEEKLY DURATION (min) |
|---|---|---|---|
| Poor | 500–1,000 | 20–30 | 60–150 |
| Poor-fair | 1,000–1,500 | 30–60 | 150–200 |
| Fair-average | 1,500–2,000 | 30–90 | 200–300 |
| Average-good | >2,000 | 30–90 | 200–300 |
| >Good-excellent | >2,000 | 30–90 | 200–300 |

*Source:* Adapted from American College of Sports Medicine (2010). *ACSM's Guidelines for Exercise Testing and Prescription* (8th ed.) Wolters Kluwer/Lippincott Williams & Wilkins.

is far from 100%. Research demonstrates that activities that use similar muscles (e.g., cycling performed by runners) have about 50% of the value of performing specific training (e.g., running) on a minute-by-minute basis. Muscularly nonsimilar training (e.g., swimming performed by runners) has about 25% of the value of performing specific training on a minute-by-minute basis.[18,31]

Exercise duration is probably the most appropriate variable to manipulate initially, building the exercise session by 10%, or 5 to 10 minutes every week or two over the first 4 to 6 weeks. Thereafter, and once adherence is developed, progressions can be implemented by increasing exercise frequency and then exercise intensity, but the progressions should always remain consistent with the individual's goals.[5] It may be particularly important to include multiple modalities of exercise (e.g., walking, cycling, and elliptical training) and even variations within a modality (e.g., steady-state exercise, interval training, and **Fartlek training**) to limit the risk for boredom, burnout or orthopedic injury from overuse as the volume of exercise builds.

## FROM THEORY TO PRACTICE

Fartlek training was developed in Sweden in the 1930s; its name is derived from a Swedish term that means "speed play." This training format provides a sequence of different intensities that stress both the aerobic and anaerobic systems, something rarely achieved with exclusive steady-state training (aerobic), and different from traditional interval training (anaerobic with specific work-to-rest ratios). Consequently, this training format can be adapted to meet the needs of intermittent-sport athletes by essentially mimicking the changes of pace that occur during these events (e.g., rugby, soccer, football, hockey, and lacrosse).

For example, Fartlek running involves varying the pace throughout the run, alternating between fast segments and slow jogs. Unlike traditional interval training that involves specific timed or measured segments, Fartlek training sessions are less structured. Work–rest intervals can be based on how the body feels. With Fartlek training, the exerciser can experiment with pace and endurance. Many runners, especially beginners, enjoy Fartlek training because it involves speed work but is more flexible than and not as demanding as traditional interval training.

*VIGNETTE continued*

■ A sample set of workouts that Todd developed for Abraham is as follows:

- Monday (optional): recovery ride—40 to 60 minutes, all below VT1, on flat or rolling terrain
- Tuesday: sprint/hill sprint work—60 minutes total; 15-minute warm-up (below VT1) followed by 4 to 6 hill sprints (1 minute near-maximal effort at an RPE of 9), with a 4-minute recovery (below VT1) between intervals. Then cool down (below VT1) for the rest of the ride to complete the hour. Abraham can ride a hilly course or repeat the same hill multiple times. Progress this workout to "sprints" instead of hill sprints during the last 6 to 8 weeks of training to boost leg speed and promote recovery from harder training months.
- Wednesday: recovery ride—40 to 60 minutes, all below VT1, on flat or rolling terrain
- Thursday: longer intervals (below VT2) to improve power and recovery just below VT2—60 minutes total; 15-minute warm-up followed by three or four 5-minute intervals at just below/at VT2 (RPE = 6–7), with 5-minute recovery between intervals (below VT1). Finish with a cool-down (below VT1). *Note:* These intervals should start on flat/rolling terrain and progress to include hills that take approximately 5 minutes to summit. Also, if doing a local race on Saturday, this ride should get scaled back to have only two intervals of 3 to 4 minutes each with 5- to 6-minute recovery intervals.
- Friday: rest day
- Saturday: long ride—start with 2 to 3 hours and progress by approximately 15 to 20 minutes per week until reaching approximately 5 hours. Abraham should reach 5-hour rides several months before the event to allow for time to taper. Most of the ride should be at or below VT1 on varied terrain that includes hills. The intensity can go up to just below VT2 on a few hills and on a few efforts on flat/rolling terrain if riding with a group. As an alternative, Abraham can do a local race as part of his training/assessment.

*Continued*

*VIGNETTE continued*

• Sunday: longer recovery ride—most of the 1.5- to 2.5-hour ride should be performed below VT1. Enjoy the day.

   *Note:* Every third or fourth week should be an easier week to promote harder efforts on other weeks and allow for additional recovery. This can be achieved by cutting intervals on Tuesday and Thursday by one third to one half, then cutting the Saturday ride by 1 hour, and limiting the Sunday ride to 90 minutes.

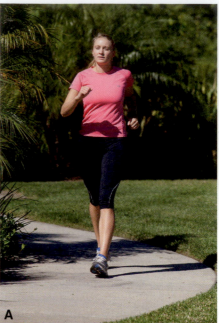

## MODES OR TYPES OF CARDIORESPIRATORY EXERCISE

Virtually any type of activity that involves a large amount of muscle and can be performed in a rhythmic fashion and sustained for more than a few minutes can be classified as cardiorespiratory exercise (Fig. 15-6). If this type of exercise is performed regularly, there are adaptations in the various organ systems (heart, lungs, blood, and muscles) that improve the ability of the person to move around or otherwise perform sustained exercise (i.e., the cardiorespiratory training effect). Because of the unique muscular requirements of ambulatory exercises (e.g., walking, running, cycling, rowing, and skating), these exercises are usually considered to be the primary cardiorespiratory exercises. Other related exercises (e.g., stair climbing, elliptical exercise, and arm cranking) can also be classified as aerobic, or cardiorespiratory, exercise. Even game-type activities, assuming that they require sustained bodily movement, can be considered cardiorespiratory exercise. In this regard, the cardiorespiratory benefit of game-type exercise is proportional to the amount and intensity of ambulatory activity involved. Thus, golf can be beneficial if it involves walking for approximately 3 miles (4.8 km) (the average length of a standard 18-hole course), but it is less beneficial than a steady walk of the same duration (because of the lower intensity of the intermittent walking during golf). Similarly, singles tennis is generally more valuable from the standpoint of cardiorespiratory exercise than doubles, because of the more extensive running required to cover the entire court. Table 15-9 provides a list of physical activities that promote improvement or maintenance of cardiorespiratory fitness.

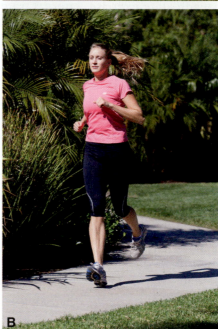

**Figure 15-6.** Examples of cardiorespiratory exercise: (A) walking and (B) jogging.

### Equipment-Based Cardiovascular Exercise

Exercise equipment designed for cardiorespiratory training is a prominent feature in most fitness facilities, as well as in the home exercise market (Fig. 15-7). The aerobic value of any of these equipment-based approaches is largely based on how much muscle mass is dynamically involved in the exercise movement. Sustained moderate-intensity exercise (i.e., more than 10 or 15 minutes in duration) is the key to cardiorespiratory exercise training. Many pieces of higher end exercise equipment have programs designed to estimate the MET or caloric cost of exercise. If they also have an input feature that allows the exerciser to enter body weight, the caloric cost of exercise may be estimated. However, the accuracy

**Table 15-9.** Physical Activities That Promote Improvement or Maintenance of Cardiorespiratory Fitness

| EXERCISE DESCRIPTION | RECOMMENDED GROUP | ACTIVITY EXAMPLES |
| --- | --- | --- |
| Endurance activities that require minimal skill or fitness | All adults | Walking, slow-dancing, recreational cycling or swimming |
| Vigorous-intensity endurance activities that require minimal skill | Adults who participate in regular exercise or have better than average fitness | Jogging, rowing, elliptical training, stepping, indoor cycling, fast-dancing |
| Endurance activities that require higher skill levels | Adults with acquired skill and higher fitness levels | Swimming, cross-country skiing |
| Recreational sports | Adults who participate in regular training with acquired fitness and skill levels | Soccer, basketball, racquet sports |

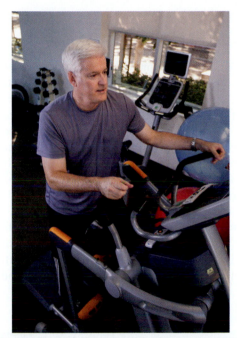

**Figure 15-7.** Elliptical machines are a prominent feature in most fitness facilities. Other common types of exercise equipment in fitness facilities include stair steppers, cycle ergometers, treadmills, rowing machines, and arm ergometers.

of estimates for the MET cost of exercising on a particular device is only as good as the research supporting the equation. In many cases, these data are quite good. In other cases, the numbers are much less reliable. Common sense is required when using the MET or caloric values generated by exercise equipment. In many cases, the data are based on university students who are already fairly fit and are exercising without the benefit of handrail support. Thus, in less-fit individuals, and particularly if handrail support is required, the values suggested by the exercise device may overestimate the actual value attained. It is important to understand that the calorie counts on

exercise machines (or those obtained from formulas) are simply estimates and will never be 100% accurate. Therefore, it is best to use them as rough benchmarks from workout to workout.

## Group Exercise

Group exercise classes have been one of the hallmarks of the exercise industry since the beginning of organized gymnastics programs in Europe a century and a half ago (Fig. 15-8). Group gymnastic routines and calisthenics were once the dominant modes of group exercise. The latter represented a significant portion of the physical fitness exercises of the military in the period beginning before World War I, and its use continues even now. In the early 1970s, with the emergence of choreographed "aerobic dance" programs, the group exercise focus shifted significantly toward using dance-type movements, very often with music, as the dominant mode of group exercise. During the past few decades, an enormous variety of exercise

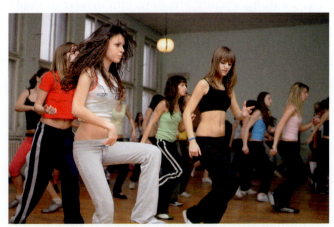

**Figure 15-8.** Group exercise classes have been a common form of cardiorespiratory exercise for more than a century.

types, with almost every focus imaginable, has emerged. Common to all these activities is the use of music to drive the tempo of exercise and to make the exercise more enjoyable. The choreography of group exercise can vary enormously, as can the exercise intensity. Some group exercise programs (e.g., group indoor cycling) can be very strenuous, often requiring workloads that elicit $\dot{V}O_2$ or HR values greater than those achieved during exercise tests. When working with small groups, the health/fitness professional should always keep in mind the effect of music on the exercise intensity. Exercisers will tend to follow the tempo or percussive beat of music. If fast-tempo music is used, the exercise intensity may be higher than intended.

## Circuit Training

Because of the specificity principle of exercise, resistance training programs designed to improve muscular strength and endurance are not intrinsically suited to producing cardiorespiratory training effects. As an adaptation of military training exercises, the concept of circuit weight training emerged in the 1950s and 1960s, based on the premise that sequential exercises using different muscle groups might allow the exerciser to focus on one muscle group while a previously used group is recovering (e.g., squats followed by chest presses, leg extensions, shoulder presses, leg curls, and arm curls). The logic behind this practice was that the overall metabolic rate might remain high enough to allow cardiorespiratory training effects, while still focusing the exercises on muscular components. Early controlled studies of this concept produced disappointing results, with improvements in aerobic capacity averaging only 5% to 7%. In attempts to find a way to improve circuit training, there was a variety of industry-sponsored research studies in the early and mid-1970s. These studies demonstrated that alternating muscular strength and endurance activities with classical aerobic training (e.g., running, cycling, stepping, and rowing) in rapid sequence allowed for significant cardiorespiratory training effects to be observed (i.e., super circuits). Depending on equipment availability, circuit training can be performed either by a single individual or by groups of people rotating in an organized manner through several exercise stations.

## Outdoor Exercise

Over the past few decades, a wide variety of outdoor exercises have emerged out of recreational activities, many with the promise of providing cardiorespiratory fitness. Activities that require a lot of walking or running are, of course, very likely to provide cardiorespiratory training. Other outdoor activities (e.g., climbing and canoeing) are much more variable in their cardiorespiratory training effects and depend almost entirely on how they are conducted.

## Seasonal Exercise

Many activities, particularly outdoor activities, are more seasonal in their application. To the degree that they require the exerciser to perform physical activity, they are likely to have a large cardiorespiratory training effect. Thus, cross-country skiing and snowshoeing in the winter months are similar to walking and running in the warmer months. Although there are clearly highly specific benefits of each type of exercise, the enjoyment and enthusiasm related to performing different types of activities during different seasons, and the underlying commonality of cardiorespiratory fitness, suggests the value of seasonal variation.

## Water-Based Exercise

Aquatic exercise can provide a convenient alternative form of exercise that is pleasant, reduces orthopedic loading, and is capable of training different muscle groups than those used during ambulatory activities (Fig. 15-9). Although the classical water-based exercise is swimming, group classes (e.g., water aerobics) and games (e.g., water polo and water volleyball) can be effective methods of exercise as well. It is important to remember that the energy cost of ambulatory activity in the water (e.g., walking in thigh-deep or chest-deep water) is related to the depth of the water and can increase markedly with only very slight increases in the speed of ambulating in the water. Second, immersion in water causes the blood to be

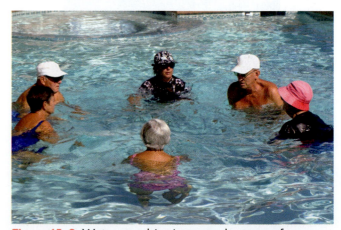

**Figure 15-9.** Water aerobics is a popular type of cardiorespiratory exercise for older or obese persons. In particular, water-based exercise can be valuable for individuals in these populations who may also have orthopedic issues, as the buoyancy provided by the water unloads the traditional targets of ambulatory exercise. *(Photo from Thinkstock)*

redistributed to the central circulation, away from the limbs. In people with compromised circulatory function, this can lead to complications (e.g., breathlessness and heart failure). The energy cost of swimming is highly variable and depends not only on swimming velocity, but on the stroke, technique, and skill of the swimmer.

## Mind–Body Exercise

Mind–body exercises are often performed for reasons other than cardiorespiratory training, but cardiorespiratory training effects may still be achieved. The main concepts behind mind–body exercise are that it is performed with focus, with attempts to control and regulate the breathing, with a conscious intent to follow a specific form, and as a means of linking the physical and emotional aspects of the person (see Chapter 19). As such, mind–body exercise is generally not associated with high-intensity aerobic activity. Nevertheless, as a regular feature of an exercise program, it may provide an intensity comparable with that of walking. **Pilates**, **hatha yoga**, **Nia**, and **tai chi** are representative types of mind–body exercise.

## Lifestyle Exercise

Normally, when people think of exercise, they think of an activity that is a "time-out" from real life, something that they specifically have to plan to do, which their hunter-gatherer ancestors, or even their grandparents who were farmers, did not have to worry about doing. However, it is important to remember that humans once got ample amounts of exercise by simply performing daily chores around the house. The best examples of this are the reports of health variables among the Amish, who, because of their religious beliefs, live a life that is much like that of a 19th-century farmer in the United States. These reports suggest that domestic activities can be more than enough to make people quite fit and contribute to excellent health.[32] Accordingly, activities like working in the yard should be viewed in the context of the total exercise load and be considered comparable with walking for exercise.

## PROGRAM DESIGN FOR CARDIORESPIRATORY TRAINING

The basic concept of program design is to create an exercise program with appropriate frequency, intensity, and duration to fit the individual's current health and fitness, with adequate progressions to help the client safely achieve his or her goals. Exercise intensity can be monitored using a variety of methods that have generally been developed through university-based research that included actual measurement of MHR, $\dot{V}O_2max$, blood lactate concentrations and HR at VT1

and VT2, power output (wattage), and other variables. These assessments provide accurate individualized data for use in exercise programming, but they are often not practical or available to most health and fitness professionals or consumers. As such, health/fitness professionals generally have to rely on submaximal fitness assessments and prediction equations derived from these studies to predict variables such as MHR and $\dot{V}O_2max$, and then use these predicted values to set appropriate training intensities. Exercise guidelines based on predictions of MHR or $\dot{V}O_2max$ can help individuals reach their goals, but they have a lot of room for error that must be accounted for when setting and modifying exercise intensities.

Although the evidence base for percentage of $\dot{V}O_2max$ or $\dot{V}O_2R$ is very deep, the very large range of acceptable percentages creates the concern that a given percentage is not very specific in terms of recommending exercise. Katch and colleagues[33] suggested that the "relative percent concept" was essentially flawed and did not take into account the individual metabolic responses to exercise that might more properly represent the lowest effective training stimulus.

Although contemporary guidelines for exercise training are still presented in terms of the relative percent concept, the two-decades-old comments of Professor Katch are still remarkably convincing. Although experimental evidence is lacking, this lowest effective training intensity at which adaptations might be provoked is probably better defined in terms of VT1. Although training below this threshold may have some benefit, it is highly probable that training very much below this threshold will yield minimal cardiorespiratory fitness benefits.[34] It is arguable that very extensive low-intensity training is important in terms of expending energy in programs designed for weight loss, although there does appear to be a lower limit of exercise intensity that is critical when training for cardiorespiratory fitness. Thus, basing the training program on metabolic or ventilatory responses is much more meaningful than using arbitrary ranges of %$\dot{V}O_2max$ or %$\dot{V}O_2R$.

Training programs based on %$\dot{V}O_2max$ or %$\dot{V}O_2R$ depend on a maximal exercise test to be accurate, or on some estimate of $\dot{V}O_2max$ derived from a submaximal test. Given that maximal tests are rarely available, and that equations for estimating $\dot{V}O_2max$ are not exceedingly accurate, particularly if any handrail support is allowed during treadmill testing or training,[35,36] recommending exercise on the basis of this gold standard technique probably is much less useful than is widely assumed.

The submaximal talk test for VT1 and the VT2 threshold test provide fairly precise HR data that relate directly to the metabolic markers of the VT1 and VT2. The submaximal talk test for VT1 can provide the health/fitness professional with the client's HR at VT1 to use when designing programs for weight loss and improving general fitness. The higher intensity VT2 threshold test allows the health/fitness professional to establish the client's HR at VT2 for use in more advanced programming with clients who have advanced-fitness and endurance sports performance goals.

These two metabolic markers, VT1 and VT2, whether based on respiratory responses or blood lactate responses, provide a convenient way to divide intensity into three training zones that are determined without any use of, or reference to, MHR (Fig. 15-10):
- Zone 1 (relatively easy exercise) reflects HRs below VT1.
- Zone 2 reflects HRs from VT1 to just below VT2.
- Zone 3 reflects HRs at or above VT2.

Stated simply, if an exerciser can talk comfortably, he or she is training in zone 1. If the exerciser is not

sure if he or she can talk comfortably, he or she is working in zone 2. If the exerciser definitely cannot talk comfortably while training, he or she is working in zone 3.

Cardiorespiratory training programs typically consist of exercise sessions designed to fit into one of the following four categories:
- Initial aerobic conditioning
- Aerobic endurance training
- Aerobic and anaerobic training
- Anaerobic training

Exercisers can be placed into a given category based on their current health, fitness levels, and goals. Thus, individualized cardiorespiratory programs can be created for individuals ranging from sedentary to endurance athletes. Programming in each category can be based on a three-zone training model, using HR at VT1 and VT2 to develop individualized programs based on each exerciser's metabolic responses to exercise. It is important to note that various exercise intensity markers, including ones based on predicted values such as %HRR or %MHR, can also be relied on, but the exercise intensities will not be as accurate for individual clients as when they use measured HR at VT1 and VT2 (Table 15-10).

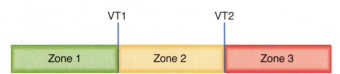

**Figure 15-10.** Three-zone training model. This model can be used to create individualized cardiorespiratory training programs for individuals ranging from sedentary to endurance athletes. VT1, first ventilatory threshold; VT2, second ventilatory threshold.

## Table 15-10. Three-Zone Training Model Using Various Intensity Markers

| INTENSITY MARKERS | ZONE 1 | ZONE 2 | ZONE 3 | ADVANTAGES/LIMITATIONS |
|---|---|---|---|---|
| Metabolic markers: VT1 and VT2* (HR relative to VT1 and VT2)* | Below VT1 (HR < VT1) | VT1 to just below VT2 (HR ≥ VT1 to <VT2) | VT2 and above (HR ≥VT2) | • Based on measured VT1 and VT2<br>• Ideally, VT1 and VT2 are measured in a laboratory with a metabolic cart and blood lactate<br>• Field tests are relatively easy to administer, require minimal equipment, and provide accurate corresponding HRs at VT1 and VT2<br>• Programming with metabolic markers allows for individualized programming |
| Talk test* | Can talk comfortably | Not sure if talking is comfortable | Definitely cannot talk comfortably | • Based on actual changes in ventilation caused by physiological adaptations to increasing exercise intensities<br>• Very easy for practical measurement<br>• No equipment required<br>• Can easily be taught to clients; allows for individualized programming |
| RPE (terminology)* | "Moderate" to "somewhat hard" | "Hard" | "Very hard" to "extremely hard" | • Good subjective intensity marker<br>• Correlates well with talk test, metabolic markers, and measured %V̇O₂max<br>• Easy to teach to most clients |

## Table 15-10. Three-Zone Training Model Using Various Intensity Markers—cont'd

| INTENSITY MARKERS | ZONE 1 | ZONE 2 | ZONE 3 | ADVANTAGES/LIMITATIONS |
|---|---|---|---|---|
| RPE (0–10 scale) | 3–4 | 5–6 | 7–10 | • Good subjective intensity marker<br>• Correlates well with talk test, metabolic markers, and measured $\%\dot{V}O_2max$<br>• 6–20 scale is not as easy to teach to clients as the 0–10 scale<br>• *Note:* An RPE of 20 represents maximal effort and cannot be sustained as a training intensity |
| RPE (6–20 scale) | 12–13 | 14–16 | 17–20 | • Good subjective intensity marker<br>• Correlates well with talk test, metabolic markers, and measured $\%\dot{V}O_2max$<br>• 6–20 scale is not as easy to teach to clients as the 0–10 scale<br>• *Note:* An RPE of 20 represents maximal effort and cannot be sustained as a training intensity |
| $\%\dot{V}O_2R$ | 40%–59% | 60%–84% | ≥85% | • Requires *measured* $\dot{V}O_2max$ for most accurate programming<br>• Impractical because of expensive equipment and testing<br>• Increased error with use of *predicted* $\dot{V}O_2max$ or *predicted* MHR<br>• Relative percentages for programming are population based and not individually specific |
| %HRR | 30%–59% | 60%–84% | ≥85% | • Requires *measured* MHR and RHR for most accurate programming<br>• Measured MHR is impractical for most trainers and clients<br>• Use of RHR increases individuality of programming vs. strict %MHR<br>• Use of *predicted* MHR introduced[5] potentially large error; the magnitude of the error is dependent on the specific equation used<br>• Relative percentages for programming are population based and not individually specific |
| %MHR | 64%–76% | 77%–93% | ≥94% | • Requires *measured* MHR for accuracy in programming<br>• Measured MHR is impractical for most trainers and clients<br>• Use of *predicted* MHR introduces potentially large error; the magnitude of the error is dependent on the specific equation used |

*Continued*

**Table 15-10.** Three-Zone Training Model Using Various Intensity Markers—cont'd

| INTENSITY MARKERS | ZONE 1 | ZONE 2 | ZONE 3 | ADVANTAGES/LIMITATIONS |
|---|---|---|---|---|
| METs | 3–6 | 6–9 | >9 | • Does not include RHR, as is used in %HRR<br>• Relative percentages for programming are population based and not individually specific<br>• Requires *measured* $\dot{V}O_2$max for most accurate programming<br>• Can use in programming more easily than other intensity markers based on $\dot{V}O_2$max<br>• Limited in programming by knowledge of METs for given activities and/or equipment that gives MET estimates<br>• Relative MET ranges for programming are population based and not individually specific (e.g., a 5-MET activity might initially be perceived as vigorous by a previously sedentary client) |
| Category terminology for exercise programming | Low to moderate | Moderate to vigorous | Vigorous to very vigorous | |

*These are the preferred intensity markers to use with the three-zone model when designing, implementing, and progressing cardiorespiratory training programs using the American Council on Exercise Integrated Fitness Training Model.

HR, heart rate; HRR, heart-rate reserve; METs, metabolic equivalents; MHR, maximum heart rate; RHR, resting heart rate; RPE, ratings of perceived exertion; $\dot{V}O_2$max, maximal oxygen consumption; $\dot{V}O_2R$, $\dot{V}O_2$ reserve; VT1, first ventilatory threshold; VT2, second ventilatory threshold.

## FROM THEORY TO PRACTICE

### ■ AMERICAN COUNCIL ON EXERCISE'S INTEGRATED FITNESS TRAINING MODEL

Cardiorespiratory training programs have traditionally focused on steady-state training to improve cardiorespiratory fitness, with progressions based on increased duration and intensity. Intervals have been loosely categorized and have primarily been focused on reducing boredom through higher and lower intensity segments, or training intervals at or near the **lactate threshold (LT)** to improve speed during endurance events. While these methods are effective, they have often been looked at as very different training programs for individuals trying to improve function, health, fitness, or performance. The American Council on Exercise's Integrated Fitness Training Model (ACE IFT Model) provides a systematic approach to cardiorespiratory training that can take an exerciser all the way from being sedentary to training for a personal record in a half marathon. Table 15-11 provides an overview of the cardiorespiratory training phases of the ACE IFT Model. Detailed descriptions are provided that explain the training focus of each stage and strategies for implementing and progressing exercise programs to help individuals reach their goals within the phase, and advance to the next phase if desired. It is important to note that not every person will start in phase 1, because many individuals will already be regularly participating in cardiorespiratory exercise, and only those with very specific performance or speed goals will reach phase 4. In addition, the submaximal talk test for VT1 is recommended for introduction in phase 2, whereas the VT2 threshold test should ideally be introduced during phase 3.

**FROM THEORY TO PRACTICE–cont'd**

**Table 15-11. American Council on Exercise Integrated Fitness Training Model Cardiorespiratory Training Phase Overview**

**Phase 1: Aerobic-Based Training**
- The focus is on creating positive exercise experiences that help sedentary clients become regular exercisers.
- No fitness assessments are required before exercise in this phase.
- Focus on steady-state exercise in zone 1 (below HR at VT1).
- Gauge by the client's ability to talk (below talk test threshold) and/or RPE of 3–4 (moderate to somewhat hard).
- Progress to phase 2 once the client can sustain steady-state cardiorespiratory exercise for 20–30 minutes in zone 1 (RPE to 3–4) and is comfortable with assessments.

**Phase 2: Aerobic Efficiency Training**
- The focus is on increasing the duration of exercise and introducing intervals to improve aerobic efficiency, fitness, and health.
- Administer the submaximal talk test to determine HR at VT1. There is no need to measure VT2 in phase 2.
- Increase workload at VT1 (increase HR at VT1), then introduce low zone 2 intervals just above VT1 (RPE of 5) to improve aerobic efficiency and add variety in programming.
- Progress low zone 2 intervals by increasing the time of the work interval and later decreasing the recovery interval time.
- As client progresses, introduce intervals in the upper end of zone 2 (RPE of 6).
- Many clients will stay in this phase for many years.
- If a client has event-specific goals or is a fitness enthusiast looking for increased challenges and fitness gains, progress to phase 3.

**Phase 3: Anaerobic Endurance Training**
- The focus is on designing programs to help clients who have endurance performance goals and/or are performing ≥7 hours of cardiorespiratory exercise per week.
- Administer the VT2 threshold to determine HR at VT2.
- Programs will have the majority of cardiorespiratory training time in zone 1.
- Interval and higher intensity sessions will be very focused in zones 2 and 3, but will make up only a small amount of the total training time to allow for adaption to the total training load.
- Many clients will never train in phase 3, because all of their noncompetitive fitness goals can be achieved through phase 2 training.
- Only clients who have very specific goals for increasing speed for short bursts at near-maximal efforts during endurance competitions will move on to phase 4.

**Phase 4: Anaerobic Power Training**
- The focus is on improving anaerobic power to improve phosphagen energy pathways and buffer large accumulations of blood lactate to improve speed for short bursts at near-maximal efforts during endurance competitions.
- Programs will have similar distribution to phase 3 training times in zones 1, 2, and 3.
- Zone 2 training will include very intense anaerobic power intervals.
- Clients will generally only work in phase 4 during specific training cycles before competition.

HR, heart rate; RPE, ratings of perceived exertion; VT1, first ventilatory threshold; VT2, second ventilatory threshold.

## Initial Aerobic Conditioning

### Training Focus

The initial aerobic conditioning phase has a principal focus of getting individuals who are either sedentary or have little cardiorespiratory fitness to begin engaging in regular cardiorespiratory exercise of low to moderate intensity with a primary goal of improving health and a secondary goal of building fitness. These clients may have long-term goals for fitness and possibly even sports performance, but they need to progress through this stage first. The primary goal for the health/fitness professional during this phase should be to help the client have positive experiences with cardiorespiratory exercise and to help him or her adopt exercise as a regular habit. The intent of this phase is to develop a stable aerobic base on which the client can build improvements in health, endurance, energy, mood, and caloric expenditure.

The training focus of the initial aerobic conditioning stage is establishing a regular exercise pattern, with relatively low- to moderate-intensity exercise of only moderate duration, to establish an aerobic base. Zone 1 training, where the training HR is below the VT1 level, may not be strenuous enough to provoke significant changes in $\dot{V}O_2$max (the classical definition of the cardiorespiratory training effect), but it will contribute in a general way to improved health. Once regularity of exercise habits is established, the duration of exercise is extended until the exerciser progresses to the next stage and is able to exercise for 30 to 60 minutes on most days with little residual fatigue. This approach to training ensures the safety of exercise, while at the same time allowing some of the potential physiological adaptations and most of the health benefits to occur. In individuals who desire or require higher levels of fitness, higher intensity training may then be incorporated as they progress to the next stage. Within this general design is recognition that the benefit-to-risk ratio of low-intensity zone 1 training is very high for the beginning exerciser, with the possibility for very large gains in health and basic fitness, and almost no risk for either cardiovascular or musculoskeletal injury. As the exerciser develops more ambitious goals, more demanding training (either longer or more intense) can be performed.

The underlying base of most training programs is the development of aerobic power. Indeed, a consensus statement from the World Health Organization in 1968 defined endurance as equivalent to $\dot{V}O_2$max. Based on the large body of controlled training studies performed in the 1970s, the term *training effect* can be thought of as equivalent to the increase in $\dot{V}O_2$max that occurs during the first 3 to 6 months of an aerobic endurance exercise program.

As long ago as the 1950s, the concept of a minimal-intensity threshold for provoking the training effect was articulated by Karvonen,[37] who made the observation that training at intensities of less than 50% of HRR (approximately 60% of MHR) failed to cause reductions in RHR. This concept was confirmed in randomized training studies during the 1970s with $\dot{V}O_2$max as the outcome measure. A variety of studies have shown that there is a larger increase in $\dot{V}O_2$max with more intense training. Thus, the aerobic benefits of training increase markedly with training intensity. However, training is much less comfortable as intensity increases, which means there is an increased risk of individuals dropping out during the first few weeks of training. Furthermore, in previously sedentary adults who might have an underlying risk for cardiovascular disease, more high-intensity exercise is associated with a greater risk for cardiovascular complications. Thus,

an important rule of exercise training for sedentary adults is to start slowly during the beginning weeks of an exercise program. This guideline is sometimes frustrating, because many exercisers are enthusiastic at the beginning of a program and want rapid gains, and the health/fitness professional may want to impress clients with challenging, creative workouts. Restraint, proper education, and careful planning are clearly essential during the early stages of any training program.

Improvements in $\dot{V}O_2$max may continue for 6 to 12 months after the beginning of a regular exercise program. This increase may be accentuated if there is significant weight loss, because the most appropriate expression of $\dot{V}O_2$max is when it is normalized for body weight (e.g., mL/kg/min). Lower intensity exercise programs have been shown to be associated with a variety of beneficial health outcomes, although there may be smaller increases in $\dot{V}O_2$max at low exercise intensities than can be achieved with higher intensity training. Nevertheless, outcomes related to longevity and a reduced incidence of many of the "diseases of civilization" have been well documented with exercise that is not sufficient to cause large increases in $\dot{V}O_2$max.[38] In any case, with any beginning exerciser, this approach will ensure that not only are there significant gains in health and functional status, but there will be a minimum of injuries (i.e., a very high benefit-to-risk ratio).

## Program Design

The primary goal of this phase is to help clients have positive experiences with exercise to facilitate program adherence and success. Cardiorespiratory fitness assessments are not necessary at the beginning of this phase, because they will only confirm low levels of fitness and potentially serve as negative reminders about why the sedentary client with low levels of fitness may not have good **self-efficacy** regarding exercise. All cardiorespiratory exercise during this phase should fall within zone 1 (sub-VT1), so the health/fitness professional can use the client's ability to talk comfortably as the upper exercise-intensity limit. The client can also use the 0 to 10 category ratio scale, while exercising at an RPE of 3 to 4 (moderate to somewhat hard). It is not necessary to conduct the submaximal talk test assessment to determine HR at VT1 until the next phase of training.

As a general principle, exercise programs designed to improve the aerobic base begin with zone 1–intensity exercise, with HR below VT1 performed for as little as 10 to 15 minutes two to three times each week. However, this should be progressed as rapidly as tolerated to 30 minutes at moderate intensity (zone 1; below "talk test" with HR below VT1) performed at least five times each week. Changes in duration from one week to the next should not exceed a 10% increase versus the week prior. Once this level of exercise can be sustained on a regular basis, the primary adaptation of the aerobic base will be complete.

For the most part, early training efforts should feature continuous exercise at zone 1 intensity. Depending on how sedentary a person was before beginning the program, this level of easy exercise may be continued for as little as 2 weeks or for more than 6 weeks. The beginning duration of exercise should match what the client is able to perform. For some, this might be 15 continuous minutes, whereas for others it might be only 5 to 10 continuous minutes. From that point, duration should be increased at a rate of no more than 10% from one week to the next until the client can perform 30 minutes of continuous exercise. Once the client is comfortable with assessments and can sustain steady state cardiorespiratory exercise for 20 minutes in zone 1 (RPE of 3–4), he or she can move on to aerobic endurance training.

## Aerobic Endurance Training

### Training Focus

Aerobic endurance training has a principal training focus of increasing the time of cardiorespiratory exercise while introducing intervals to improve aerobic efficiency, fitness, and health. Clients who exercise sporadically will progress to this phase only after they have become consistent with their cardiorespiratory exercise and can comfortably perform a minimum of 20 to 30 minutes of steady-state cardiorespiratory exercise in zone 1 (RPE of 3–4). During aerobic endurance training, the health/fitness professional will be able to program more variety in terms of exercise frequency and duration. The health/fitness professional can also challenge the client through the introduction of intervals, first in the lower end of zone 2 and eventually in the upper end of zone 2. For the highly motivated exerciser who is interested in progressing toward performance goals, intervals that reach just above VT2 (into zone 3) can be introduced as an advanced challenge, often just before the client moves into phase 3 of cardiorespiratory training.

Once the aerobic base is developed, the exerciser may want to consider the value of additional gains in fitness that will result from increases in exercise intensity, frequency, or duration. However, it is important to understand that after an aerobic base has been achieved, additional gains in fitness will become progressively smaller or will require disproportionately large increases in training intensity, frequency, or duration. This is the time when the health/fitness professional needs to carefully evaluate the goals of each client. What are the client's exercise goals—health and basic fitness benefits, improved appearance, and/or weight-loss benefits? Or does he or she want to complete competitive challenges? Competitive competence at the biological limit of the exerciser requires significantly higher training loads. Athletes may have to train at very high loads for only a 1% to 2% increase in performance, with matching increases in the time requirement of training and the risk for injury.[21]

Within the context of aerobic training, the health/fitness professional must consider the relative proportion of different intensities of exercise. Early studies suggested that training at about the intensity of the "threshold" (i.e., zone 2) was the most effective intensity. Subsequent studies have suggested that very well-trained nonathletes tend to perform a high proportion of their training (approximately 50%) at this intensity.[39,40] Interestingly, much of this training can be categorized by the verbal anchor "hard," or an RPE of 6 on the 0 to 10 scale. Extensive training at this level requires a motivated exerciser, so this phase of training is reserved for the already motivated and committed client. However, once the volume of cardiorespiratory training goes over approximately 7 hours per week, a different pattern of training distribution seems to appear. This training distribution for clients and athletes training ≥7 hours per week is discussed in the next section (see Aerobic and Anaerobic Training).

Aerobic endurance training is the primary cardiorespiratory training phase for regular exercisers in a fitness facility who have goals for improving or maintaining fitness, weight loss, or both. Cardiorespiratory training in this phase includes increasing the workload by modifying frequency, duration, and intensity, with intervals introduced that go into zone 2 and eventually approach HR at VT2. The zone 2 intervals in this phase provide a stimulus that will eventually increase the HR at VT1, resulting in the client being able to exercise at a lower HR when at the same level of intensity, and also allowing the client to exercise at higher intensities while at the VT1 HR.

Clients training in phase 2 who have a one-time goal to complete an event, such as a 10K run, can reach their goal of completing the event within the training guidelines of this phase. Once a client begins working toward multiple endurance goals, trains to improve his or her competitive speed, begins training ≥7 hours per week, or simply wants to take on the challenge of training like an athlete, the client should move on to the next stage of cardiorespiratory training.

For the many clients who never develop competitive goals or the desire to train like an endurance athlete, training in this phase will provide very adequate challenges to help them improve and maintain cardiorespiratory fitness for many years. The workouts in most nonathletically focused group exercise classes fall into this phase.

### Program Design

At the beginning of aerobic endurance training, the health/fitness professional can have the client perform the submaximal talk test to determine HR at VT1. This HR will be used for programming throughout the phase and will need to be reassessed periodically as fitness improves to determine whether the HR at VT1 has increased and training intensities need to be adjusted.

This phase of cardiorespiratory training is dedicated to enhancing the client's aerobic efficiency by progressing the program through increased duration of sessions, increased frequency of sessions when possible, and the introduction of zone 2 intervals. The warm-up, cool-down, recovery intervals, and steady-state cardiorespiratory exercise segments are performed at or just below VT1 HR (RPE of 3–4 on the 0–10 scale) to continue to advance the client's aerobic base. Aerobic intervals are introduced at a level that is just above VT1 HR, or an RPE of 5 (0–10 scale). The goal of these intervals is to improve aerobic efficiency by raising the intensity of exercise performed at VT1, improve the client's ability to use fat as a fuel source at intensities just below VT1, improve exercise efficiency at VT1, and add variety to the exercise program.

As a general principle, intervals should start out relatively brief (initially about 60 seconds), with an approximate hard-to-easy ratio of 1:3 (e.g., a 60-second work interval followed by a 180-second recovery interval), eventually progressing to a ratio of 1:2 and then 1:1. The duration of these intervals can be increased in regular increments, depending on the goals of the exerciser, but should be increased cautiously over several weeks depending on the client's fitness level. As a general principle, the exercise load (calculated from the session RPE or the integrated time in the zone) should be increased by no more than 10% per week. Early in this phase, exercise bouts with a session RPE greater than 5 (e.g., hard exercise) should be performed infrequently. As the client's fitness increases, steady-state exercise bouts with efforts just above VT1 (RPE of 5) can be introduced.

Low zone 2 intervals should first be progressed by increasing the time of each interval and then moving to a 1:1 work-to-recovery (hard-to-easy) interval ratio. As the client progresses, intervals can progress into the upper end of zone 2 (RPE of 6) at a 1:3 work-to-recovery ratio, progressing first to longer intervals and then eventually moving to intervals with a 1:1 work-to-recovery ratio. Well-trained and motivated nonathletes can progress to where they are performing as much as 50% of their cardiorespiratory training in zone 2. Once the well-trained nonathlete reaches ≥7 hours of training per week or develops performance goals, he or she can progress to the next stage of training. Clients with advanced fitness who are training for a one-time event or are preparing to advance to phase 3 can perform brief intervals (30 seconds) that go just above VT2 (RPE of 7) to further develop aerobic capacity and provide additional variety.

It is not necessary to measure VT2 during this phase, because an RPE of 5 to 6 (0–10 scale) can be used to represent intensities in zone 2, and an RPE of 7 (very hard) can be used to identify efforts just above VT2. Programming variables and variety during aerobic endurance training are diverse enough for clients who do not have competitive goals to train in this phase for many years.

## Aerobic and Anaerobic Training

### Training Focus

This stage is designed for clients who have endurance performance goals and/or are performing ≥7 hours of cardiorespiratory training per week. The training principles in aerobic and anaerobic training are for clients who have one or more endurance performance goals that require specialized training to ensure that adequate training volume and appropriate training intensity and recovery are included to create performance changes that help the client reach his or her goals. Clients do not need to be highly competitive athletes to train in zone 3. They need only to be motivated clients with endurance performance goals and the requisite fitness from aerobic endurance training to build on.

A variety of studies with different types of athletes, including Nordic skiers, cyclists, and runners, have suggested that 70% to 80% of training is performed at intensities lower than the VT1 (zone 1).[39,40] These same studies suggest that athletes typically perform 5% to 10% of their training above the VT2 (zone 3). Thus, even though zone 3 training can be effective in terms of provoking improvements, only a small amount is tolerable, even in competitive athletes. Surprisingly, very little training is actually performed in the intensity zone between the two thresholds (zone 2). This intensity has been called "the black hole" (where there is a psychological push to do more, but a physiological pull to do less), because it is the zone where exercise is hard enough to make a person fatigued, but not hard enough to really provoke optimal adaptations.[39]

Most of the studies with training loads have simply observed what athletes spontaneously do during training. In a very well-controlled study of training distribution, researchers randomized cross-country runners into groups, where the total training load was controlled and equalized.[41] High-intensity (zone 3) training was limited to approximately 10% of total training time in both groups. One group increased the amount of easy (zone 1) training from the spontaneous 70% to about 85%, and decreased the amount of moderately hard (zone 2) training from the spontaneous 20% to about 5%. The other group, conversely, decreased zone 1 training from the spontaneous 70% to about 60% and increased zone 2 training from 20% to about 30%. After 5 months, the improvement in performance favored those who had performed more zone 1 training. Despite zone 1 being relatively easier training, the results supported the contention that zone 2 training is essentially a "black hole."[39] It may be that there is an important interaction of the distribution of training with the total volume of training, but the best evidence is that in individuals who are already routinely exercising and who desire to move toward their optimal biological potential, most training (approximately 80%) should be performed at intensities where speech is comfortable (zone 1), and about 10% of training should be performed at intensities above VT2 (zone 3), where the physiological provocation to make large gains is present.

It is currently unclear whether the dominant training intensity within a zone matters. It is easy to speculate that zone 1 training should, for the most part, be performed relatively high in zone 1. Similarly, it would seem to make sense that, except for training designed to augment anaerobic pathways, most zone 3 training should be performed relatively low in zone 3, with progression by duration rather than by intensity. This remains an area in need of controlled studies.

With the increase in training load during phase 3, consideration must also be given to the amount of recovery training. It can be taken as axiomatic that training hard enough to provoke adaptations requires recovery before subsequent training can be performed. Thus, where the regular recreational exerciser in the initial aerobic conditioning phase of training can safely and comfortably perform essentially the same training bout every day, the competitive-level exerciser will need to use a decidedly hard/easy approach to training, or he or she will be at risk for problems from accumulating fatigue and loss of training benefit from the inability to repeatedly do really hard training sessions. Studies have indicated that maladaptations to training (e.g., **overtraining syndrome**) are almost exclusively attributable to a failure to incorporate appropriate recovery days, particularly if they are coupled with extensive travel or other occupational or social stressors.[42] The concept of training monotony is important (not the degree to which training is boring, but the degree to which it does not change on a day-to-day basis). Many illnesses, as well as stagnation of training performances, can be attributed to high training monotony.[43] This is probably only an issue when the training load is fairly high relative to the capacity of the person (30 minutes at moderate intensity performed daily does not create a risk for overtraining for most exercisers).

An example of equivalent training loads performed in a high-monotony manner versus a low-monotony manner is presented in Figure 15-11. Extensive experience relative to preventing illnesses and other subtle markers of overtraining, as well as the results of experimental studies, suggest that alternating "hard" and "easy" training days is more effective than training that is more or less the same every day.[44] In any case, even in the most seriously trained athlete, it is probably not productive to perform more than three or four high-intensity or very long training sessions per week. Interestingly, studies performed with athletes working under the direction of a coach have indicated that athletes almost always work harder and longer than the coach intended for them to on designated recovery days. And because they were not adequately recovered, they almost always trained less hard and for less time than the coach intended on training days.[45] This finding has helped greatly in the understanding of why overtraining syndrome occurs so frequently in athletes (who have the best inherent physical talent) while working under coaches (who are usually very well educated and motivated to enhance the success of their athletes).

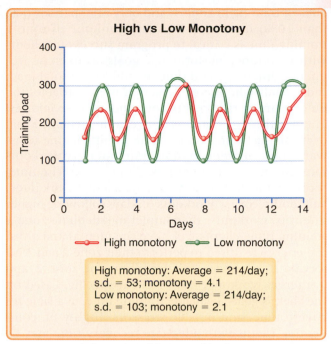

**Figure 15-11.** Schematic of low- and high-monotony training programs with the same average loading per day. In the low-monotony program, the higher standard deviation of training loads leads to a lower calculated training monotony, which is defined by the average divided by the standard deviation (s.d.) during each week. At a given level of training load, programs with lower monotony (e.g., more day-to-day variability in loading) are usually more effective at producing training results and less provocative of maladaptation to training.

## Program Design

Program design during this phase should be focused on helping the client enhance his or her aerobic efficiency to ensure completion of goal events, while building anaerobic endurance to achieve endurance performance goals. Improved anaerobic endurance will help the client perform physical work at or near VT2 for an extended period, which will result in improved endurance, speed, and power to meet primary performance goals. To program effective intervals for improving anaerobic endurance, the health/fitness professional can have the client perform the VT2 threshold test to determine the client's HR at VT2. Once the health/fitness professional has current values for the client's HR at VT1 and VT2, a three-zone model that is specific to the client can be established. For example, if a client's HR at VT1 is 143 bpm and HR at VT2 is 162 bpm, the client's HR zones would be as follows:

- Zone 1 = less than 143 bpm
- Zone 2 = 143 to 161 bpm
- Zone 3 = 162 bpm and above

These HR zones can then be used as intensity markers to help the client stay within the correct zone for the desired training outcome of a given workout.

Training intensity should be varied, with 70% to 80% of training in zone 1, approximately 10% to

20% of training in zone 3, and only brief periods (less than 10%) in zone 2. This large volume of zone 1 training time is critical to program success for clients with endurance performance goals, as exercise frequency, intensity, and time all add to the total load. Individuals who increase each of these variables too quickly are at risk for burnout and overuse injuries. The health/fitness professional can help clients avoid overtraining by distributing zone 1 training time across warm-ups, cool-downs, moderate-intensity workouts focused on increasing distance and/or exercise time, recovery intervals following zone 2 and 3 work intervals, and recovery workouts on days following higher intensity workouts. By completing adequate zone 1 training time, clients will have the mental and physical energy required to perform their zone 2 and 3 intervals as planned. The frequency of zone 2 and 3 interval workouts will be client-specific, based on the client's goals, available training time, available recovery time, and outside stressors. Highly fit, competitive clients with adequate recovery time may be able to successfully complete and recover from three to four workouts with zone 2 or 3 intervals during weeks where the goal is to increase the load. If the client is not highly fit, has minimal recovery time, or is lacking in total training time, the health/fitness professional should design a program that has only one or two total zone 2 or 3 interval days. In recreation-level competitors, almost all of this training is performed in zone 1, with the exception of perhaps a single zone 3 training session per week.

The volume of training should be progressively increased (less than 10% per week) until the total weekly volume reaches a maximum of three times the anticipated duration of the target event for which the exerciser is training. This "rule of threes" is a classic concept from marathon running. Although there is a lack of direct experimental evidence, the concept is generally well supported. Using running events as a model, the volume of high-intensity interval training performed on hard days will vary with the duration of the event. Thus, a person preparing for a 1-mile race might do about 2.5 times the racing distance (e.g., performing 10 × 400 m intervals is a reasonable training load), whereas someone preparing for a 10K might do approximately equal to the race distance in his or her higher intensity intervals (6 × 1 mile intervals may be appropriate). Someone preparing for a marathon might have a multiplier of approximately 0.25 (6 × 1 mile intervals might be appropriate; Fig. 15-12). Obviously, these kinds of volume multipliers are highly empirical, and probably best fit serious competitive athletes. Scaled-down versions, based more on common sense and time available rather than on experimentally derived data, are appropriate for more recreational competitors.

Intervals performed in zone 2 will generally be of longer duration than intervals performed in zone 3. This is due to the inability to sustain long intervals at zone 3 intensities where HR equals or exceeds HR at

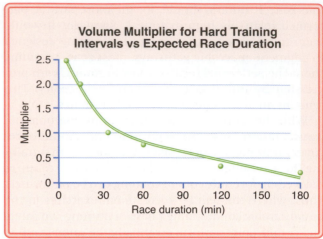

**Figure 15-12.** Schematic volume multiplier for the amount of high-intensity training within a "hard day" in relation to the expected duration of a competitive event. When preparing for a short event (e.g., running 1 mile), it might be appropriate to perform 2.5 times the race distance or duration (with appropriate recovery interval; e.g., 10 reps × 400 m run followed by 400 m walk-jog recovery intervals). For a longer event, such as a marathon (for a 3-hour competitor), the multiplier might be quite low (0.25; e.g., 6 × 1 mile).

VT2 (RPE ≥ 7 on the 0–10 scale), as compared with zone 2 intervals where HR will be between HRs at VT1 and VT2 (RPE of 5 or 6). Higher intensity zone 3 work will also require greater recovery intervals relative to work intervals when compared with those used in zone 2.

If the client begins showing signs of overtraining (e.g., increased RHR, disturbed sleep, or decreased hunger on multiple days), the health/fitness professional should decrease the frequency or intensity, or both, of the client's intervals and provide more time for recovery. Also, if the client cannot reach the desired intensity during an interval, or is unable to reach the desired recovery intensity or HR during the recovery interval, the interval session should be stopped and the client should recover with cardiorespiratory exercise at an RPE of 3, and no more than 4, to prevent overtraining.

## Anaerobic Training

### Training Focus

The fourth phase of cardiorespiratory training focuses on anaerobic power. Only highly fit and competitive clients with very specific goals related to high-speed performance during endurance events will require exercise programming in this phase. Some examples of athletes who might perform phase 4 training include runners and cyclists who compete in events that require repeated sprinting and recovery throughout the race and during the final sprint finish, competitive kayakers who need to paddle vigorously for short periods to navigate through difficult sections of rapids, and athletes in sports such as basketball and soccer where success requires both cardiorespiratory endurance and the ability to sprint repeatedly.

This anaerobic power training phase can essentially be thought of as strength training, although it is specific to the mode of activity (e.g., running and cycling). The intent is to perform very high-intensity training of near-maximal muscular capacity, but with enough recovery to prevent the rapid accumulation of fatigue, so that the muscular system can be taxed maximally.

This is very specialized training intended to be performed by individuals preparing for competition. It is intended to increase the tolerance for the metabolic byproducts of high-intensity exercise, including exercise performed at intensities greater than $\dot{V}O_2max$. Because this kind of training is very uncomfortable and, in older or at-risk individuals, potentially dangerous, it should be performed only after a long period of training accommodation.

The underlying physiological principle of this type of training is that if there is substantial and sustained depletion of the **phosphagen** stores and accumulation of lactate (and other acid metabolites), the body will adapt with a larger phosphagen pool and potentially larger buffer reserves. Studies have suggested that adaptations of this sort can occur but are relatively modest in magnitude (10%).[46] For reasons that are not well understood, men appear to improve their anaerobic capacity more than women. Although there are not a lot of well-controlled studies, it appears that interval training with relatively brief (30-second) high-intensity elements is just as effective in terms of producing gains in anaerobic capacity as longer high-intensity bursts (where phosphagen depletion and lactate accumulation might be larger, and thus be expected to be more provocative of change). Although controlled studies demonstrating the best way to improve anaerobic capacity are not available, it is generally assumed that high-intensity bouts with relatively short recovery periods that provoke larger disturbances in **homeostasis** are preferred. Thus, a training session of $10 \times 70$ seconds at 115% of $\dot{V}O_2max$, with a new repetition beginning every 2 minutes, might be typical. This kind of training session requires an extended warm-up and cool-down, and is tolerable only once or twice weekly.

### Program Design
Most clients will never reach this phase of training, because only clients with very specific goals for achieving high sprinting speed and/or short bursts of very high levels of power for challenges such as short hills will require anaerobic power training. Some health/fitness professionals who work with more highly competitive clients may work with several clients per year who train in this phase, whereas other health/fitness professionals may not work with anyone in this phase for several years. Even elite athletes will spend only part of a given year performing anaerobic training cycles to prepare for specific competitions.

Obviously, this kind of training is designed only for individuals interested in competition, and can be tolerated only on a limited basis. Examples might include $6 \times 100$ m acceleration runs, where the middle 40 m are performed at absolute maximal intensity. There may be 5 minutes of recovery between runs, allowing for full recovery. This type of training should not generally be viewed as cardiorespiratory training. It is entirely supplemental and designed for muscular accommodation.

The total weekly exercise program for a client in training for anaerobic power will look similar to a client training in the previous phase (aerobic and anaerobic training), with 70% to 80% of the training time in zone 1, approximately 10% to 20% of training in zone 3, and only brief periods (less than 10%) in zone 2. The difference will be in the types of intervals performed during some of the zone 3 workout time. Intervals for anaerobic power training will be very short sprints or hill sprints designed to tax the phosphagen stores in the muscles and create a rapid increase in blood lactate levels. These short, highly intense intervals (RPE of 9–10) will be followed by long recovery intervals that may be 10 to 20 times longer than the work intervals. For example, a coach may have an athlete perform $5 \times$ 10-second accelerations while cycling on a relatively flat road with little traffic, with each acceleration followed by a 2- to 3-minute recovery interval. These anaerobic power intervals are supplementary to the full training program performed by a client who has endurance performance goals. As such, these intervals should be performed only once per week as a complement to the full endurance training program.

## RECOVERY AND REGENERATION

As a general principle, training should be periodized. This means that there should be a regular cycle of hard and easy days, hard and easy weeks, and hard and easy months. The point of training is to gradually progress the overload, but then to allow the body to recover and adapt to the changes provoked by hard training sessions. The more challenging the training program, the more that recovery and regeneration become important. A person interested only in basic fitness, who is performing 30 minutes of moderate-intensity training daily, hardly needs to worry about periodization. However, even in these individuals, there is an advantage to periodically adding a hard day, taking a day completely off, or changing the mode of exercise. The biggest mistakes made, once the training load starts to go up to accomplish more ambitious goals, are to take too few recovery days, to try to do something other than recover on recovery days, and to try to progress the training load on recovery days (when it should only be progressed on hard days). The bottom line is that recovery days are for recovery. If a client does not recover fully and properly, he or she will not be able to work hard enough on the hard training days to elicit further adaptations. Although there is a lack of well-controlled data about exactly how to peri-odize training plans, it is fair to say that even in the most serious athletes, there should be no more than four hard-training days per week. Even in this group, there are good data to suggest that it is much better to per-form three really intense workouts per week rather than to do the same workload over 7 days. In less seri-ous competitors, 2 or 3 hard days per week are probably adequate to allow progress toward most goals. How-ever, as mentioned earlier, it is common for athletes to train too hard on days the coach thinks are devoted to recovery. If there is a secret to athletic success, it is in the creative use of rest—that is, really recovering on recovery days.

## VIGNETTE conclusion

■ To assess Abraham's progress with the training program, Todd uses the following two methods:

- Select rolling terrain or a hill that is similar in length and difficulty to the biggest hill of the race (e.g., 2-mile hill). Perform a "timed" effort at VT2

up the hill every 4 weeks to assess power and velocity while riding uphill.
- Select a race every month from about 4 months to 1 month before the event (three to four races total). Abraham needs to get "race legs," get used to being in a racing pack, test himself (mentally and physically) against competition, and practice his race day routine (e.g., food, hydration, and gear). The goal is to see his performance level and sustainability of effort continually improve. Placing well in these races is nice, but not a priority.

The key when working with competitive athletes is to balance proper progression and recovery, and to optimize each client's performance on the day of the race or competition. This is very different from working with typical gym-goers, who are usually interested in improving health and fitness, but without a specific target date in mind.

## CRITICAL THINKING QUESTIONS

1. During an initial meeting with a client, the health and fitness professional measures the client's RHR in the seated position. The health and fitness profes-sional plans on using the RHR value to program a recommended training intensity for the client based on the Karvonen formula. The client will be engaged in walking and running as the primary modes of training for cardiorespiratory exercise. How might the health and fitness professional's choice of the client's body position during the RHR assessment cause inaccuracies in exercise intensity recommendations?

2. A popular fitness website promotes the use of the formula "220 − age" for estimating MHR and then using a percentage of that value to recommend exercise intensity. Several of your clients question

why you use the VT1 test for determining appro-priate cardiorespiratory exercise intensity instead of the aforementioned formula. What is the best response to this question?

3. Tracy is a fitness professional who specializes in high-intensity performance training. Many of her clients are former collegiate athletes. A general problem that Tracy notices among these former athletes is that they tend to want to train at exceedingly high intensities 5 to 6 days per week. In fact, Tracy often feels like these clients try to dictate their own train-ing programs instead of following her individualized programming. What might Tracy say to these clients to educate them about the appropriate frequency and volume of high-intensity exercise training?

## ADDITIONAL RESOURCES

American College of Sports Medicine. *ACSM's Guidelines for Exercise Testing and Prescription*. 9th ed. Philadelphia, PA: Wolters Kluwer/Lippincott Williams & Wilkins; 2014.
American Council on Exercise. *ACE Personal Trainer Manual: The Ultimate Resource for Fitness Professionals*. 4th ed. San Diego, CA: American Council on Exercise: 2010.

Compendium of Physical Activities Tracking Guide. Available at: https://sites.google.com/site/compendiumof-physicalactivities/tracking-guide

## SUGGESTED READINGS

American College of Sports Medicine. *ACSM's Resource Manual for Guidelines for Exercise Testing and Prescription.* 6th ed. Philadelphia, PA: Lippincott Williams & Wilkins; 2009.

Daniels J. *Daniels' Running Formula.* 2nd ed. Champaign, IL: Human Kinetics; 2005.

Edwards S. *The Heart Rate Monitor Book.* Sacramento, CA: Fleet Feet Press; 1993.

Noakes T. *The Lore of Running.* 4th ed. Champaign, IL: Human Kinetics; 2001.

Powers SK, Howley ET. *Exercise Physiology: Theory and Application to Fitness and Performance.* 7th ed. New York, NY: McGraw-Hill; 2008.

Wilmore JH, Costill DL, Kenney WL. *Physiology of Sport and Exercise.* 5th ed. Champaign, IL: Human Kinetics; 2012.

## REFERENCES

1. Booth FW, Roberts CK. Linking performance and chronic disease: Indices of physical performance are surrogates for health. *Br J Sports Med.* 2008;42: 950–953.

2. Booth FW, Lees SJ. Fundamental questions about genes, inactivity, and chronic diseases. *Physiol Genomics.* 2007;28:146–157.

3. Haskell WL, et al. Physical activity and public health: Updated recommendations of the American College of Sports Medicine and the American Heart Association. *Med Sci Sports Exerc.* 2007;39:1423–1434.

4. U.S. Department of Health & Human Services. *2008 Physical Activity Guidelines for Americans: Be Active, Healthy and Happy.* 2008. Retrieved from www.health.gov/paguidelines/pdf/paguide.pdf

5. American College of Sports Medicine. *ACSM's Guidelines for Exercise Testing and Prescription.* 9th ed. Philadelphia, PA: Wolters Kluwer/Lippincott Williams & Wilkins; 2014.

6. Yamaguchi T, Ishii K. Effects of static stretching for 30 seconds and dynamic stretching on leg extension power. *J Strength Cond Res.* 2005;19:677–683.

7. Thacker SB, Gilchrist J, Stroup DF, Kimsey CD. The impact of stretching on sports injury risk: A systematic review of the literature. *Med Sci Sports Exerc.* 2004;36: 371–378.

8. Wilmore JH, Costill D, Kenney WL. *Physiology of Sport and Exercise.* 4th ed. Champaign, IL: Human Kinetics; 2008.

9. Gorostiaga EM, Walter CB, Foster C, Hickson RC. Uniqueness of interval and continuous training at the same maintained exercise intensity. *Eur J Appl Physiol.* 1991;63:101–107.

10. Foster C, Porcari, JP, Battista, RA, et al. The risk of exercise training. *Am J Lifestyle Med.* 2008;10:279–284.

11. Fox SM III, Naughton JP, Haskell WL. Physical activity and the prevention of coronary heart disease. *Ann Clin Res.* 1971;3:404–432.

12. Tanaka H, Monahan KD, Seals DR. Age-predicted maximal heart revisited. *J Am Coll Cardiol.* 2001;37: 153–156.

13. Gellish RL, Goslin BR, Olson RE, et al. Longitudinal modeling of the relationship between age and maximal heart rate. *Med Sci Sports Exerc.* 2007;39:822–829.

14. GULATI, M., Shaw, LJ., Thisted, RA., et al. (2010) Heart Rate Response to Exercise Stress Testing in Asymptomatic Women. *Circulation* 122:130 – 137.

15. Borg G. *Borg's Perceived Exertion and Pain Scales.* Champaign, IL: Human Kinetics; 1998.

16. Foster C, Porcari JP, Lucia A. Endurance training. In: Durstine JL, et al., eds. *Pollock's Textbook of Cardiovascular Disease and Rehabilitation.* Philadelphia, PA: Lippincott Williams & Wilkins; 2008.

17. Herman L, Foster C, Maher MA, Mikat RP, Porcari JP, et al. Validity and reliability of the session RPE method for monitoring exercise training intensity. *South Afr J Sports Med* 2006;18:14–17.

18. Foster C, Hector LL, Welsh R, et al. Effects of specific vs. cross training on running performance. *Eur J Appl Physiol.* 1995;70:367–372.

19. Foster C, Florhaug, JA, Franklin, J, et al. Monitoring exercise training during non-steady state exercise. *J Strength Cond Res.* 2001;15:109–115.

20. Foster C, Daniels J, Seiler S. Perspectives on correct approaches to training. In: Lehmann M, et al., eds. *Overload, Performance Incompetence and Regeneration in Sport.* New York, NY: Kluwer Academic/Plenum Publishers; 1999.

21. Foster C, Daines E, Hector L, Snyder AC, Welsh R. Athletic performance in relation to training load. *Wis Med J.* 1996;95:370–374.

22. Cannon C, Foster, C, Porcari, JP, et al. The talk test as a measure of exertional ischemia. *Am J Sports Med.* 2004;6:52–57.

23. Persinger R, Foster C, Gibson M, Fater DC, Porcari JP. Consistency of the talk test for exercise prescription. *Med Sci Sports Exerc.* 2004;36:1632–1636.

24. Voelker SA, Foster, C, Porcari, JP, et al. Relationship between the talk test and ventilatory threshold in cardiac patients. *Clin Exerc Physiol.* 2002;4:120–123.

25. Recalde PT, Foster, C, and Skemp-Arlt, KM, et al. The talk test as a simple marker of ventilatory threshold. *South Afr J Sports Med.* 2002;9:5–8.

26. Porcari JP, et al. Prescribing exercise using the talk test. *Fit Manage.* 2001;17:46–49.

27. Dehart BM, Foster, C, Porcari, JP, Fater DCW., Mikat R.P. Relationship between the talk test and ventilatory threshold. *Clin Exerc Physiol.* 2000;2:34–38.

28. Gunnarsson TP, Bangsbo J. The 10-20-30 Training Concept improves performance and health profile in moderately trained runners. *J Appl Physiol.* 2012; 113:16–24.

29. Knab, AM, Shanely RA, Corbin KD, et al. A 45-minute vigorous exercise bout increases metabolic rate for 14 hours. *Med Sci Sports Exerc.* 2011 Sep;43(9):1643-8. doi: 10.1249/MSS.0b013e3182118891.

30. Hill-Haas SV, Dawson BT, Coutts AJ, Rowsell GJ. Physiological responses and time–motion characteristics of various small-sided soccer games in youth players. *J Sports Sciences* 2009;27:1.

31. Loy SF, Holland GJ, Mutton DK. Effects of stair climbing vs. run training on treadmill and track running. *Med Sci Sports Exerc.* 1993;25:1275–1278.

32. Bassett DR, Schneider PL, Huntington GE. Physical activity in an Old Order Amish community. *Med Sci Sports Exerc.* 2004;36:79–85.

33. Katch V, Weltman A, Sady S, Freedson P. Validity of the relative percent concept for equating training intensity. *Eur J Appl Physiol.* 1978;39:219–227.

34. Meyer T, Lucía A, Earnest CP, Kindermann WA conceptual framework for performance diagnosis and training prescription from submaximal parameters: Theory and application. *Int J Sports Med.* 2005;26:1–11.

35. Berling J, Foster C, Gibson M, Doberstein S, Porcari J. The effect of handrail support on oxygen uptake during steady state treadmill exercise. *J Cardiopulm Rehabil.* 2006;26:391–394.

36. McConnell TR, Foster C, Conlin N, Thompson NN. Prediction of functional capacity during treadmill testing: Effect of handrail support. *J Cardiopulm Rehabil.* 1991;11:255–260.

37. Karvonen M, Kentala E, Mustala O. The effect of training on heart rate: A longitudinal study. *Ann Med Exp Biol Fenn.* 1957;35:307–315.

38. Booth, FW, Chakravarthy MV, and Spangenburg EE. Exercise and gene expression: physiological regulation of the human genome through physical activity. *J Phys.* 2002;543:399–411.

39. Seiler KS, Kjerland GO. Quantifying training intensity distribution in elite athletes: Is there evidence for an (optimal) distribution? *Scand J Med Sci Sports.* 2006;16: 49–56.

40. Esteve-Lanao J, San Juan AF, Earnest CP, Foster C, Lucia A. How do endurance runners actually train? Relationship with competition performance. *Med Sci Sports Exerc.* 2005;37:496–504.

41. Esteve-Lanao J, Foster C, Seiler S, Lucia A. Impact of training intensity distribution on performance in endurance athletes. *J Strength Cond Res.* 2007;21:943–949.

42. Meeusen R, Duclos ME, Gleeson M. Prevention, diagnosis and treatment of overtraining syndrome. *Eur J Sport Sci.* 2006;6:1–14.

43. Foster C. Monitoring training in athletes with reference to overtraining syndrome. *Med Sci Sports Exerc.* 1998;30:1164–1168.

44. Hansen AK, Fischer CP, Plomgaard P, Andersen JL, Saltin B, Pedersen BK. Skeletal muscle adaptation: Training twice every second day vs. training once daily. *J Appl Physiol.* 2005;98:93–99.

45. Foster C, Heimann KM, Esten PL, Brice G, Porcari JP: Differences in perceptions of training by coaches and athletes. *South Afr J Sports Med.* 2001;8:3–7.

46. Tabata I, Nishimura K, Kouzaki M, et al. Effects of moderate-intensity endurance and high-intensity intermittent training on anaerobic capacity and $\dot{V}O_2$max. *Med Sci Sports Exerc.* 1996;28:1327–1330.

# *Practice What You Know:* Threshold Testing

Threshold testing is based on the physiological principle of changes in ventilation to protect the acid–base balance of the body. As exercise intensity increases, ventilation initially increases in a somewhat linear manner. However, after a certain intensity, there are two distinct deflection points associated with metabolic changes within the body. One point, called the *VT1*, represents a level of intensity where **lactate** begins to accumulate within the blood. To protect from the accumulation of lactate causing metabolic acidosis, the hydrogen ions associated with lactate are buffered by bicarbonate that is in the blood. This neutralizes the potential decrease in pH (increased acidity) and produces extra $CO_2$, which increases ventilation as it is exhaled. The increased ventilation is accomplished primarily through a parallel increase in **tidal volume** and **respiratory rate**. At about the intensity that the first ventilatory threshold occurs, tidal volume no longer increases rapidly. The extra ventilation is largely attributable to an increase in respiratory rate. However, because ability to talk comfortably is largely related to the ability to suppress the respiratory rate, the progressive increase in breathing frequency above VT1 makes comfortable speech difficult.

As the intensity of exercise continues to increase, the buffering of lactate by bicarbonate (designed to protect against decreases in pH) becomes inadequate and the blood becomes more acidic. This change in pH stimulates the ventilatory center in the brain and the VT2, sometimes called the **respiratory compensation threshold (RCT)**, becomes evident. This leads to a very large increase in total ventilation and respiratory rate. At the same time, speech becomes decidedly uncomfortable.

The measurement of VT1 and VT2 is relatively simple in a well-equipped laboratory. However, the majority of health/fitness professionals will not have access to metabolic analyzers and will need valid field tests to identify these markers. This section provides a simple field test for determining VT1 and VT2, which can also be associated with HR and RPE to guide exercise training. This type of testing, based on a field test for estimating the ventilatory thresholds, is an alternative estimation of the LT or the **onset of blood lactate accumulation (OBLA)**.

## CONTRAINDICATIONS

This type of testing is not recommended for:

- Individuals with certain breathing problems (e.g., **asthma** or other **chronic obstructive pulmonary disease (COPD)**)
- Those recovering from a recent respiratory infection

## SUBMAXIMAL TALK TEST FOR FIRST AND SECOND VENTILATORY THRESHOLDS

This test is best performed using either a treadmill or calibrated cycle ergometer. It is crucial to remember that threshold measurements are based on muscular power output. Ventilation and HR are responses to changes in muscular power output. The exercise intensity should start at very comfortable levels of exertion, and the increments need to be small. Although one should definitely not increase the workload based on HR, the increments should be small enough so that the HR at the end of the successive stages does not increase more than 10 bpm. Consequently, this test will require some preparation to determine the appropriate increments that elicit an approximate 10-bpm increase (0.5 mile/hr, 1% incline, or one to two levels on a bike/elliptical trainer are typical). Because the act of speaking itself can change the sense of breathing effort, the stages should be long enough (2 or 3 minutes) so that the talking challenge during the last 30 seconds of each stage is dictated solely by the physiological response to exercise.

Before exercise begins, the subject should recite (out loud) a standard speech-provoking stimulus. The Pledge of Allegiance and the alphabet are good examples. After reciting the paragraph, ask the subject, *"Can you speak comfortably?"* The subject has only three options for replying: "Yes" (a *positive* talk test response), "Yes . . . but" (an *equivocal* talk test response), and "No" (a *negative* talk test response). During the last 30 seconds of each stage, the subject should recite again (out loud) the same paragraph and answer the same questions. At intensities below the VT1, the response will consistently be "Yes." At just about the intensity of the VT1, the response will become equivocal. Subjects will most likely always say, "Yes . . . but" (and then add some qualifier). At just about the intensity of the VT2, the response will become negative ("No"). In conducting the test, it is important not to coach the subject. That is, simply ask the question about being able to speak comfortably and let the subject respond. Just after the talk test is performed, before the workload is increased, HR and RPE should be noted. The test can be terminated at the first point that is equivocal, because few people want to (or need to) train at intensities above VT1. Also, even in older individuals (who may have inadequacy of blood flow to the heart muscle with exercise), the ability to speak comfortably tends to be lost before the heart muscle begins to become **ischemic**. In more advanced exercisers or in athletes who may want to do 10% to 15% of their training above the VT2, the test can be terminated the first time the test becomes negative. In either case, the talk test is a submaximal test.

### Equipment
- Treadmill, cycle ergometer, elliptical trainer, or arm ergometer
- Stopwatch
- HR monitor with chest strap (optional)
- Cue cards, if needed; any 30- to 50-word paragraph will do

### Pre-test Procedure
- Predetermine the testing stages, because this test involves small incremental increases in intensity specific to each individual. The goal is to increase workload in small increments to determine VT1. Large incremental increases may result in the individual passing through VT1, thereby invalidating the test:
  - Recommended workload increases are approximately 0.5 mile/hr, 1% grade, or 15 to 20 watts.
  - The objective is to increase HR at each stage by approximately 10 bpm.
  - Because the stages need to be 2 to 3 minutes long, and because it is critical to start below the VT1, this test often requires approximately 20 to 30 minutes to complete. However, because it is essentially a submaximal test, it can be approached as a normal training session.
- Describe the purpose of this graded exercise test, review the predetermined protocol, and allow the subject the opportunity to address any questions or concerns. Each stage of the test lasts 2 to 3 minutes to allow for stable breathing responses and to allow attainment of stable values for HR.
- Toward the latter part of each stage (i.e., last 20–30 seconds), ask the subject to recite the Pledge of Allegiance or another predetermined passage. The subject's ability to talk without difficulty will be evaluated. Note the HR and RPE before increasing the workload.
- Allow the subject to walk on the treadmill or use the ergometer to warm up and get used to the apparatus. If using a treadmill, avoid holding the handrails. If the subject is too unstable without holding on to the rails, consider using another testing modality, because handrail support changes the increments in muscular power output and will make the test less valid.
- Take the subject through a light warm-up (2–3 out of 10 effort) for 3 to 5 minutes, maintaining a heart rate less than 120 bpm.

### Test Protocol and Administration

- Once the subject has warmed up, adjust the workload intensity so the subject's HR is less than 120 bpm, or an intensity level of 2 to 3 on the 0 to 10 or 10 to 11 on the 6 to 20 scale.
- Ask the subject to recite a standard paragraph out loud.
- Upon completion of the recital or reading, ask the subject to identify whether he or she can speak comfortably.
- If VT1 ("Yes...but") is not achieved, progress through the successive stages, repeating the protocol at each stage until VT1 is reached.
- Once VT1 is identified, the test can be terminated and the subject can progress to the cool-down phase (matching the warm-up intensity) for 3 to 5 minutes.
- The test can also be continued in a similar fashion until VT2 is identified, being sure to always conclude the test with a 3- to 5-minute cool-down.
  - √ The VT1 and VT2 vary with exercise mode (e.g., treadmills and bikes), so it is important to conduct the tests with the exercise modality that the subject uses most frequently.

## Application

The HR at VT1 can be used as a THR when determining exercise intensity. Those interested in sports conditioning and/or competition would benefit from training at higher intensities, but those interested in health and general fitness are well served to stay at or slightly below this exercise intensity. However, even during steady-state training, the ability to speak comfortably is a better marker of the continuing metabolic state than HR.

Well-trained individuals can estimate their own VT2 during their training by identifying the intensity at which speech is definitely not comfortable (e.g., they answer the question with a "No").

The VT1 and VT2 are commonly related to performance. For example, if two athletes with the same $\dot{V}O_2$max are competing, the athlete with the higher VT will likely outperform the other athlete. Elite marathon runners, requiring just more than 2 hours to finish, often race at about the intensity of VT1. Similarly, athletes who race in events that require about 1 hour to complete (10 miles running or 40-km cycling time trials) often race at about the intensity of VT2.

# CHAPTER 16

# Resistance Training

## CHAPTER OUTLINE

# CHAPTER OUTLINE–cont'd

References
Practice What You Know

## LEARNING OUTCOMES

1. List the benefits and key adaptations associated with resistance training.
2. Identify the general guidelines for resistance training provided by various professional and federal organizations.
3. List the three primary types of strength training and explain the purpose of each.
4. Describe the primary components and variables of exercise program design.
5. Define *linear* and *nonlinear periodization*, including the differences between the concepts.
6. Describe the three types of training cycles, including the purpose of each.
7. Identify the primary equipment needed for a strength training program.

## ANCILLARY LINK

Visit Davis*Plus* at http://davisplus.fadavis.com for study and practice resources, including online quizzes, animations that help explain physiological processes, podcasts concerning news and career trends in exercise physiology, and practice references.

## VIGNETTE

■ Marina is a 33-year-old mother of a 4-year-old. She works full time and has joined a health club near her office so that she can exercise during her lunch hour. The last time Marina followed a regular exercise program was before her son was born, when she participated in group fitness classes, such as dance aerobics and indoor cycling, and worked out on cardiovascular equipment two to three times per week. At that time, Marina preferred aerobic exercise because her primary goal was to lose weight and she was interested in burning as much fat as possible.

Recently, Marina has become motivated to restart her exercise program because her company began offering a discounted membership at the health club. The company's new arrangement allows 15 minutes of paid time added to her lunch hour to provide the needed time to complete her workout and return to work. Her primary motivation is to take advantage of this benefit to get into shape and lose the pregnancy weight she gained. She seeks a time-efficient way to "burn fat" (as she states) and improve her muscle definition. Marina understands that resistance (weight) training will "tone" her body but is fearful of becoming too muscular. Marina is considering making an investment in personal training to help her develop a specific fitness program.

How can a personal trainer address Marina's desire to burn fat and improve muscle definition, while allaying her fears about bulking up as a result of resistance training?

Whereas cardiovascular programming appears relatively logical and intuitive, and follows the traditional FITT acronym for frequency, intensity, time, and type, resistance training may seem complex and confusing. Individuals participate in resistance training programs for different reasons, ranging from "toning" and "shaping" to body building and power lifting. A large volume of research studies in this area have helped health and fitness professionals understand how to manipulate specific training variables in a systematic manner to achieve the desired outcome(s).[1]

Load and intensity represent the two basic programming pillars for resistance training. The American College of Sports Medicine (ACSM) and the National Strength and Conditioning Association provide specific guidelines built around frequency, intensity, sets, repetitions, rest intervals, tempo, exercise order, pattern, progression, and selection. Each are discussed in detail throughout this chapter. Furthermore, resistance training programs should be organized in a specific manner that progresses over time to maximize the potential for success. These progressions coincide with Hans Selye's **general adaptation syndrome (GAS)** and are designed to optimize opportunities for adaptation. Linear and nonlinear periodization models (progressions) are two unique methods for exercise program design, each of which is described in detail in this chapter.

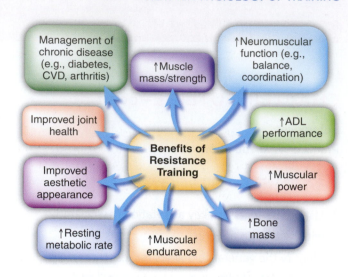

**Figure 16-1.** Benefits of engaging in a regular resistance training program. Many of these improvements (e.g., activities of daily living [ADL] performance, resting metabolic rate, joint and bone health, management of chronic diseases) stem from improvements in muscle mass and neuromuscular function.

## BENEFITS OF RESISTANCE TRAINING

Strength can be defined as the ability to generate maximal muscle tension against an external force, or as the ability of muscles to generate force to overcome the inertia of an object.[2] When skeletal muscles contract, the cumulative tension of each individual muscle fiber produces forces of specific magnitude and direction.

The purpose of resistance training is to impose external loads on the body to improve the strength, size, and functionality of human skeletal muscle. The most effective method of resistance training is to apply external loads that become progressively more challenging over time to elicit changes in muscle tissue structure and improved function of the neuromuscular system. Although a well-designed program may improve physical appearance, function, and performance (e.g., force output), it also provides other benefits that promote good health (e.g., increasing bone mineral density; Fig. 16-1).

### Improved Physical Function

The ability to perform lifestyle, work, or sporting activities can be improved with the appropriate application of resistance training. Adults who fail to follow a resistance training program may experience muscle loss, defined as **atrophy**. The progressive loss of muscle mass associated with the aging process is termed **sarcopenia**. On average, humans can lose 5 lb (2.3 kg) of muscle

mass per decade during adulthood.[3] Key reasons for this loss include reduced anabolic hormone levels (e.g., human growth hormone and testosterone) and an overall decrease in the volume and intensity of exercise specifically for the muscular system.[3] Resistance training is an effective method for slowing the decline of muscle mass.[1,4] Men and women who are interested in maintaining a healthy, active lifestyle and remaining physically independent should make resistance training a regular component of their exercise program.

### Aesthetic Appearance and Body Composition

Although fitness professionals are strong advocates of the functional benefits of resistance training, the reality is that for many noncompetitive adults (i.e., recreational active fitness enthusiasts not currently competing in any particular athletic events), especially younger adults, their primary reasons for participating in a resistance training program is driven by the desire to improve aesthetics, which, in turn, can drive self-esteem and a sense of self-worth.[5] Whereas Generation Y adults (aged 18–31 years in 2013) list "looking better," "losing weight," and "feeling better about themselves" as their primary reasons for participating in resistance and cardiorespiratory training, middle-aged and older adults (Generation X: aged 31–48 years in 2013; Baby Boomers: aged 49–67 years in 2013; and "Eisenhowers," or the "Silent Generation": aged >68 years in 2013) focus more on health and functional benefits, and less on weight loss and aesthetics.[5] Although some women express reservations regarding "bulking up" with weight training and may abstain from this type of exercise, they generally desire a lean, fit physique that results from resistance training. Furthermore, the general consensus among health and fitness researchers, educators, and practitioners is that the inclusion of weight training will improve muscle tone, size, and overall appearance.

## Metabolic Increase

The addition of muscle mass to the body translates into an increased metabolism (resting metabolism) and number of calories expended throughout the day. Studies indicate that the addition of muscle mass can increase resting metabolism by 7%, which can translate to an additional 100 calories a day or the loss of 10.5 lb (4.7 kg) over the period of a year.[6,7] Their estimates are based on studies conducted on adults who had gains in muscle mass between 1 and 2 kg (2.2–4.4 lb). A frequently discussed, yet perhaps nonvalidated topic regarding resistance training involves what many consider to be significant increases in metabolism following resistance training, by elevating the excess post-exercise oxygen consumption (EPOC). In comparison with aerobic exercise, fewer studies have investigated the effects of resistance training on EPOC, but findings do suggest that resistance training elicits a valuable EPOC response for weight loss, weight management, or both.[8,9] Resistance training EPOCs are dictated primarily by intensity, where higher intensity workouts (e.g., heavier loads) generate a greater EPOC.[9] When comparing higher work-rate type workouts (more work, less recovery) that are currently popular versus traditional training with longer rest intervals, higher intensity workouts appear to be superior to lower intensity circuits with respect to EPOCs.[10,11] Thus, today's popular workouts must consider increasing intensity as well as volume (work rate) if they seek to boost the EPOC.

## Reducing Risk for Injury and Chronic Disease

The ACSM and the U.S. Department of Health & Human Services (HHS) recognize additional benefits associated with resistance training that include increased bone mineral density; improved blood lipid profiles, mitochondrial density, and oxidative capacity; lowered blood pressure; improved glucose tolerance, management, or reduction in the risk for development of type 2 diabetes; and various emotional and cognitive benefits such as reduced risk for depression.[1,12] Effective program design can also reduce the risk for injuries associated with poor exercise technique, muscle overuse, and imbalance. A strength training program implementing both upper and lower body exercises with movements in multiple planes of direction can improve balance and coordination, while strengthening the muscles that help avoid falls.[1] In older adults, increased strength also improves abilities to perform activities of daily living (ADL), and can manage or reduce pain associated with arthritis or osteoarthritis.[13]

**VIGNETTE** *continued*

■ Marina hires Geoff as her personal trainer. As part of the initial rapport-building and information-gathering stage, Geoff asks Marina to dig a little deeper into her motivation to exercise, beyond burning fat while avoiding bulking up. He learns that, as a young mother, Marina is motivated by her desire to be a role model for her child. Geoff explains that there are countless benefits of resistance training, many of which are applicable to Marina's situation. For instance, reducing the risk for injury and illness will enable Marina to be a more active, engaged parent. It is important for health and fitness professionals to understand the many benefits of each component of a well-rounded workout regimen and then to apply those benefits to each individual client's objectives. Finding additional sources of motivation will help clients maintain long-term exercise adherence.

## GENERAL GUIDELINES

The HHS and ACSM provide recommendations for Americans regarding the use of resistance training. Resistance training is considered both muscle-strengthening and bone-strengthening, and can be achieved by performing exercises using individual body weight or external resistance (e.g., free weights, weight-lifting machines). The guidelines recommend that muscle-strengthening activities involve the major muscle groups of the body and should be performed at least 2 days a week to optimize benefits. Both organizations also suggest a minimum of 1 set of 8 to 12 repetitions for each exercise, but recognize that 2 to 4 sets per muscle group may be more effective. Researchers have demonstrated that age does not impact exercise intensity progression; thus, all programs should be progressive in nature to continue to provide overload on the musculoskeletal system.[14,15]

ACSM[1] also publishes resistance training guidelines that are rather broad but are based on the application of the variables of exercise program design, specifically frequency, intensity, time, type of exercise, repetitions, and sets, which determine **volume** of training, pattern, and progression, designated by the acronym **FITT-VP** (Table 16-1). A general overview of FITT-VP is as follows:

- *Frequency* refers to the number of times a workout is performed within a specified time frame (e.g., two or three times a week).

**Table 16-1.** The American College of Sports Medicine's Guidelines for Resistance Training (FITT-VP)

| VARIABLE | RECOMMENDED GUIDELINE |
|---|---|
| Frequency | 2–3 days a week per major muscle group |
| Intensity | 60–70% of 1 RM for novice to intermediate exercisers to improve strength |
| | >80% of 1 RM for experienced exercisers to improve strength |
| | 40–50% of 1 RM for older adults and sedentary individuals to improve strength |
| | <50% of 1 RM to improve muscular endurance |
| Time | No specific duration for training effectiveness |
| Type | Exercises should involve all major muscle groups |
| | Multijoint exercises are encouraged for all adults |
| | Single-joint exercises should be used following multijoint exercises |
| | Use a variety of equipment and/or body weight exercises within the program |
| Repetitions | 8–12 repetitions, achieving muscle fatigue by the last repetition |
| Sets | 2–4 sets of the same muscle group per workout |
| | Rest intervals of 2–3 minutes should be used between sets |
| | Recovery of >48 hours is encouraged between exercise sessions |
| Progression | Gradual progression of intensity, repetitions, sets, or frequency is recommended for continuous improvement in training program outcomes (e.g., strength, endurance, power) |

1 RM, one-repetition maximum.

*Source:* Adapted from American College of Sports Medicine. *ACSM's Guidelines for Exercise Testing and Prescription.* 9th ed. Philadelphia, PA: Lippincott Williams & Wilkins; 2014.

- *Intensity* defines amount of resistance or external load that is applied to the muscle and is a primary variable manipulated in resistance training.
- *Time* refers to duration of training. No specific duration has been indicated in research related to effectiveness of the training response.
- *Type* refers to choice of exercise to address each major muscle group in the body. Multijoint exercises are recommended for all adults engaging in resistance training.
- *Repetitions* define the consecutive number of times a movement is performed before taking a rest or recovery interval.

- *Sets* are defined as groups of repetitions.
- *Pattern* refers to rest intervals between sets and between exercise sessions.
- *Progression* refers to strategies to gradually increase intensity, frequency, and volume over the course of a training program.

As a side note, volume (total amount of work performed), which is another primary variable manipulated in resistance-training program design, can be measured in various ways that are discussed later in this chapter. One simple method involves multiplying sets and repetitions (e.g., 2 sets × 12 repetitions = 24). This concept and the individual FITT-VP variables are discussed in greater detail in the following sections.

## SEX DIFFERENCES

Men typically participate in resistance training to build muscle mass, whereas women tend to be more apprehensive about muscle hypertrophy and favor the pursuit of muscle "toning" and "shaping" instead.

Although muscle undergoes the same structural response to training in men and women, it is specific anabolic markers such as testosterone that serve as triggers to initiate the process of muscle growth. Females do produce testosterone in the ovaries and adrenal glands, but at a rate that is 15 to 20 times less than most males.[16] Consequently, a female's fear of "bulking up" is unfounded. Some women, however, do show greater hypertrophy responses than others, particularly in the lower extremities. Interindividual differences in testosterone production, sensitivity, and signaling (to make more muscle) account for these differences. Any woman who does experience greater than desired muscle growth should modify her program accordingly by moving toward more endurance resistance training as opposed to strength or hypertrophy resistance training.

Research demonstrates that although men achieve greater amounts of absolute strength (total amount of strength or force produced), the sexes are more aligned with respect to relative strength (ratio of weight lifted or force produced relative to or divided by body mass). For example, although a 220-lb (100-kg) man may have a maximal bench press of 265 lb (120.5 kg) and a 110-lb (50-kg) woman may have only a maximal bench press of 100 lb (45.5 kg), when their performances are expressed relative to their own body weight (Fig. 16-2), these differences become smaller (i.e., man: 265 ÷ 220 = 1.2; woman: 100 ÷ 110 = 0.91). Women are very capable of making positive adaptations to resistance training and can make significant strength gains from a properly structured and supervised, progressively challenging resistance training program.[17] Exercise program design for men and women does not need to vary at all, and both should follow similar patterns of progression.[14]

One unique area of concern with training women lies with an anatomical difference that exists at the knee. Structurally, women have a wider pelvis to accommodate childbirth. A wider pelvis, accompanied by shorter limbs (i.e., femur), results in an increased Q-angle, defined as the angle formed by a line running from the anterior superior iliac spine at the hip to middle of the patella (knee cap) versus a second line drawn from middle of the patella to the tibial tuberosity (bump on the shin bone beneath the knee). This deviation is illustrated in Figure 16-3 and is generally considered to be approximately 17 to 18 degrees in females versus only 13 degrees in males.[18] What is the significance of this increased Q-angle? Using an analogy of a building, if loads (e.g., structural mass) are placed on joints, optimal support or stability is achieved when the joints are aligned in the same linear plane as the forces (e.g., beams aligned vertically on top of each other). If the beams are offset at an angle, then the integrity of that joint becomes more compromised, increasing the likelihood of damage, or injury in the case of humans.

Researchers in sports medicine have attempted to causally link increased risk for injury to the anterior cruciate ligament during activities such as landing from a jump to an increased Q-angle in females. The theory is that, because the loading mechanics at the knee are less optimal with a greater Q-angle, (specifically when the knee caves inward due to improper neuromuscular control upon landing), the anterior cruciate ligament takes on a greater stress and is more likely to tear. However, other factors such as poor strength, lower extremity flexibility, and overall landing mechanics and proprioception, among others, should also be considered as potential issues increasing the risk for injury.

Females also have smaller bones, ligaments, and muscles that offer less protection to the knee joint from stress or injury, and have greater circulating levels of hormones that make the joints more lax or elastic. These differences are important to consider when training females in any activity, especially resistance training where additional external loads (i.e., resistance) are used. Failure to consider knee mechanics and to improve stability and mobility around the hip, knee, and ankle may increase a female's risk for injury.[19]

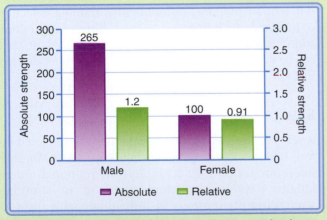

Figure 16-2. Data showing differences between absolute and relative strength for the man and the woman in the text example. Purple bars represent absolute strength (left *y*-axis); green bars represent strength relative to body weight (right *y*-axis). Notice the significant difference between the man and the woman based on absolute strength (purple bars). However, when body weight is taken into account, overall maximal strength measures are very similar between the man and the woman (green bars). This is a typical response to a training program over time: Although a male's absolute strength will increase more than a female's strength, the relative strength gains between men and women are similar.

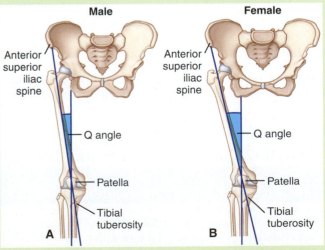

Figure 16-3. Q-angle relationship at the knee in females (A) and males (B).

## Frequency

The intensity and volume of a training program will dictate the frequency with which the program should be performed within a specific period. When the exercise program features a lower volume or lower intensity exercise, less time is required between exercise sessions for adaptation and recovery. When the exercise program features higher intensity loads, or exercises that include more challenging movement patterns or movement velocities, it is these increased demands placed on the neuromuscular system that necessitate longer recovery periods between the workouts to ensure adequate adaptation and recovery.

ACSM guidelines generally recommend a 48-hour recovery before training the same muscle group to ensure adequate time for replenishment of muscle glycogen, synthesis of muscle protein, and recovery of the neuromuscular system (muscle motor units). Although these guidelines provide a general recommendation, more specific recovery periods are recognized according to training **specificity**. Individuals beginning a resistance training program should establish an initial goal of at least two training sessions a week including exercises that address all of the major muscle groups.[1] As the training frequency increases, the exercise sessions can shift to address specific movements or muscle groups within each individual training session. Split routines are workouts where specific muscle groups are targeted within a workout (e.g., chest, shoulders, and biceps on day one; back and biceps on day two) to allow greater volumes and intensities of work for each muscle group or body segment, while allowing appropriate periods of recovery.

An individual with between 2 and 6 months of training experience should have sufficient ability to perform up to four training sessions per week, whereas individuals who have been exercising for at least 1 year should be capable of handling the stress of training up to six times per week, following a split-routine format. Table 16-2 outlines guidelines for resistance training frequency based on training experience.

## Intensity

**Intensity** refers to the specific amount of resistance or the amount of external load applied to the muscles.

Intensity is commonly expressed as a percentage of the **one-repetition maximum** (%1 RM).

This percentage of maximal effort correlates inversely with training volume, implying that, as the intensity increases, the number of repetitions decreases proportionally, as listed in Table 16-3. Higher intensity efforts generally involve lower volumes (i.e., sets and reps) and longer recoveries between the exercise sets and the training sessions. Resistance training programs that utilize lower intensities usually involve larger training volumes or frequency, as long as adequate rest is allowed for a particular muscle group before being exercised again. Using %1 RM allows fitness professionals to assign specific intensities to exercise (e.g., 10 RM or a 10-repetition maximum specifies the maximal amount of load or weight that can be lifted for 10 repetitions in succession before taking a recovery interval).

## Repetitions

**Repetitions** (reps) define the consecutive number of times an exercise movement is performed before taking a rest interval and includes the eccentric (lengthening) and concentric (shortening) phases of the muscle action. The number of reps performed represents a specific quantity of times a complete repetition phase or cycle is completed. As mentioned previously, the intensity of the load determines the number of reps that can be completed as these two variables are inversely related. In a comprehensive review on applying the variables to training for hypertrophy, Schoenfeld[20] identified three specific ranges of repetitions, with each range stimulating different adaptations. Consequently, training objectives or outcomes are influenced by the volume of the training stimulus placed on the muscle, and specific adaptations can be determined by the number of repetitions, as listed in Table 16-4.

## Sets

A set is defined as a group of repetitions completed before taking a rest interval. According to ACSM guidelines, one set of 8–12 repetitions to volitional muscle fatigue provides sufficient overload to stimulate strength improvements in individuals with little-to-no training experience. However, once an individual

**Table 16-2.** Guidelines for Resistance Training Frequency Based on Training Experience

| TRAINING STATUS | TRAINING EXPERIENCE | FREQUENCY GUIDELINES (SESSIONS PER WEEK) | TRAINING INTENSITY |
| --- | --- | --- | --- |
| Beginner | ≤2 months | 2–3 | Low |
| Intermediate | 2–6 months | 3–4 | Medium |
| Advanced | >12 months | 4–7 | High |

## Table 16-3. Relationship Between Intensity (%1 RM) and Repetitions

| NO. OF REPETITIONS | %1 RM |
|---|---|
| 1 | 100 |
| 2 | 95 |
| 3 | 93 |
| 4 | 90 |
| 5 | 87 |
| 6 | 85 |
| 7 | 83 |
| 8 | 80 |
| 9 | 77 |
| 10 | 75 |
| 11 | 70 |
| 12 | 67 |

1 RM, one-repetition maximum.
Data from Baechle T, Earle R. *Essentials of Strength and Conditioning.* 3rd ed. Champaign, IL: Human Kinetics; 2008.

experiences initial strength gains, the number of sets needs to be increased to create the desired overload and training effect. Four sets is generally considered optimal for younger, healthy adults seeking to maximize opportunities for hypertrophy, whereas two to three sets is considered best for older adults seeking similar morphological changes. Increasing the number of sets in a resistance training program requires planning for the additional time to complete those sets. However, sets can be organized in a variety of different ways to increase the training volume of a session without significantly increasing the time needed to complete the allotted exercises. Some examples include:

- **Supersetting**: Traditional supersets involve completing two exercises that target opposing muscle groups that are performed in sequence before taking a rest interval (e.g., one set of seated back rows followed immediately by one set of barbell chest press).
- **Compound sets**: Compound sets involve completion of two exercises that emphasize the same muscle groups before taking a rest interval (e.g., one set of body-weight pull-ups followed immediately by one set of lat

pull-downs for the back). Compound sets can be further subdivided into:
  - √ Tri-sets, when three exercises are performed in a sequence, each targeting the same muscle group.
  - √ Quad sets, where four exercises are performed in a sequence, each targeting the same muscle group.
- **Circuit training**: This form of training, also known as vertical loading, involves organizing multiple exercises into a sequence with shorter or no recovery intervals between each station.
- **Pre-exhaustive sets**: These sets are designed to pre-fatigue assistant muscles (synergists) to place more emphasis on the prime mover (e.g., triceps extensions performed before a barbell bench press fatigue the triceps, shifting more emphasis on the larger pectoralis major muscles).

## Rest and Recovery

Adaptations to the neuromuscular system that create the desired training effects occur primarily during the recovery phase. Adequate recovery between sessions is important to allow trained muscles time to restore glycogen and build or rebuild protein. Insufficient recovery does not allow the body to complete these processes, which may potentially lead to overtraining (Box 16-1), deterioration of muscle function, and injury. All of these conditions compromise an individual's ability to achieve his or her goals. In a review of the literature, Bishop and colleagues[21] identified three types of recovery:

- Immediate recovery, which is the time interval between individual repetitions within one working set
- Short-term recovery, which is the rest interval between sets of the same exercise
- Long-term recovery, which is the period between individual training sessions

Immediate recovery does not generally exert much influence on the exercise outcome until fatigue becomes relevant. Longer recoveries between repetitions may certainly increase the total volume of work performed, but it also decreases the overall amount of muscle overload. It reduces the stimulus for adaptation as less fatigue is imposed on the muscle, and it

## Table 16-4. Relationship Between Training Repetitions and Training Purpose

| REPETITION RANGE | INTENSITY (% 1 RM) | PURPOSE |
|---|---|---|
| High (>12) | <67% | Muscular endurance |
| Medium (6–12) | 67%–85% | Muscular hypertrophy |
| Low (1–5) | 85%–100+ % | Maximum strength |
| | | Maximal effort |

1 RM, one-repetition maximum.

## Box 16-1. Overtraining

The application of physical stress through resistance training stimulates anabolic responses that promote muscle growth. However, various researchers have also found that the accumulation of training stress (volume or load) without sufficient time for recovery and adaptation can trigger a catabolic effect that reduces testosterone levels and produces a concurrent increase in cortisol that promotes muscle breakdown. This response is called *overtraining* (Fig. 16-4) and is characterized by an elevated resting heart rate (RHR) and blood pressure, decreased performance, increased muscle soreness and weakness, general irritability, loss of appetite, and nausea.[21,33–35]

Fitness practitioners and participants should always be aware of overtraining symptoms. Simple strategies one can use to monitor for this potential effect include observing changes in RHRs over time. As one becomes more conditioned, RHR should lower. If RHR is elevated, overtraining may need to be considered. In addition, watch for decrements in exercise performance over a period of 1 to 2 weeks. As an individual improves his or her conditioning status, performance should increase, not decrease, as is often seen with overtraining.

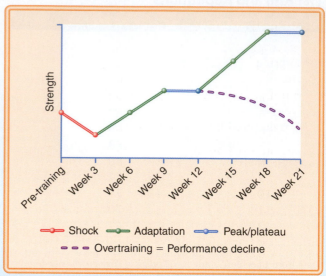

**Figure 16-4.** Potential time course of resistance training adaptations over a period of approximately 5 months. In general, on beginning a new program or experiencing a new overload period, the body may adapt in a manner eliciting a drop in performance (shock phase). Upon reaching the end of this initial phase, the body begins to more positively adapt to the new stress, and training improvements are realized (adaptation phase). At the end of the adaptation phase, the body reaches a plateau or peak phase, where no more improvements in strength occur. At this point, variables within the training program such as intensity, volume, recovery, or type of exercise would need to be changed to begin the next phase of adaptation. If these changes are not planned and administered appropriately, the end result could be overtraining with a resulting decline in performance.

also increases the time required to complete the exercises and sessions.

Short-term recovery is needed to allow adequate muscle (energy pathway) and neural recovery between sets. Heavier intensities require longer recovery periods between sets. Without adequate amounts of short-term recovery, the quality of future sets becomes compromised, decreasing the overall exercise or session efficacy and experience, and increasing the potential for injury. Table 16-5 provides recommended rest interval lengths based on various training goals. Recent research demonstrates that shorter rest intervals do evoke more metabolic stress on the body and may result in higher levels of circulating anabolic hormones.[22]

Long-term recovery between exercise sessions is important to restore muscle glycogen and to promote protein synthesis. Exercise is a catabolic process that often breaks down muscle protein during the actual exercise

session. Following exercise, the body needs time to repair, rebuild, and perhaps add muscle protein (hypertrophy). Muscle hypertrophy refers to an increase in muscle fiber size as a result of resistance training. Hypertrophy can occur by increasing the number and size of the actin and myosin contractile proteins within the myofibrils, increasing the volume of the sarcoplasm and the amount of noncontractile connective tissue within the muscle fiber.[20] Eccentric resistance training, or the lengthening of sarcomeres under tension, creates muscle damage within these contractile proteins. The implication therefore is that metabolic stress (i.e., accumulation of metabolic by-products) and mechanical tension (i.e., load) stimulate this anabolic (building) process.[20] Satellite cells located within the basal lamina of the muscle fiber function to repair damaged muscle tissue and trigger skeletal muscle growth (Fig. 16-5). (See explanatory animation of Mechanisms for Increasing Muscle Size on the Davis*Plus* site at http://davisplus.fadavis.com.)

## Table 16-5. Rest Period as Determined by Training Intensity

| TRAINING GOAL | GENERAL REST INTERVAL | SUGGESTED REST INTERVAL |
|---|---|---|
| Muscular endurance | 0–90 seconds | ≤30 seconds |
| Hypertrophy | 30–90 seconds | 45–60 seconds |
| Strength | 2–5 minutes | 2–3 minutes |
| Power (multiple reps, lower intensities) | | 90–120 seconds |
| Power (single rep, higher intensities) | 2–5 minutes | >3 minutes |

*Source:* Data from Clark MA, Lucett SC, Sutton BG. *NASM's Essentials to Personal Fitness Training.* Philadelphia, PA: Lippincott Williams & Wilkins; 2012; Baechle T, Earle R. *Essentials of Strength and Conditioning.* 3rd ed. Champaign, IL: Human Kinetics; 2008.

When activated by signaling proteins (e.g., myokines and hormones) that increase as a result of mechanical damage and metabolic stress to muscle tissue, satellite cells fuse with the muscle fiber and facilitate the process of hypertrophy by donating their nuclei to that fiber. Muscle fibers are large cells and require many nuclei to function. These signaling proteins and activation of satellite cells initiate muscle hypertrophy and help stop further muscle breakdown. This entire process requires time, and the degree of recovery needed is dependent on the intensity and amount of exercise performed, and the magnitude of muscle damage incurred. Lower intensity training for muscular endurance generally requires only 24 to 36 hours of recovery between sessions that target a specific muscle group, whereas higher intensity hypertrophy and strength training typically require 48 to 72 hours of recovery between sessions that target a specific muscle group. High-intensity power or advanced body-building training may require 72 to 96 hours of recovery between sessions that target a specific muscle group.[23]

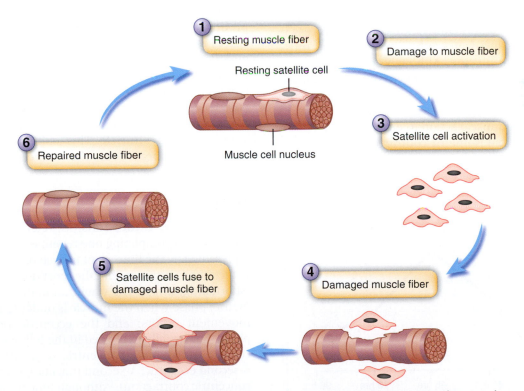

**Figure 16-5.** Overview of the mechanism by which muscle responds to microdamage that occurs from resistance training activities. Step 1 shows the muscle fiber and satellite cell in a resting state. Upon damage to the muscle fiber caused by training (step 2), satellite cells are activated (step 3) by a variety of growth factor signals within the body and migrate to the damaged fiber(s) (step 4). The satellite cells fuse (step 5) to the damaged areas on the muscle fiber and donate their nuclei, which then become muscle cell nuclei. The end result of the process is repair of the damaged muscle fiber, leading to hypertrophy (step 6).

## Delayed Onset of Muscle Soreness

Eccentric training is associated with **delayed-onset muscle soreness (DOMS)**. Individuals who experience DOMS generally notice the onset of muscle pain or discomfort occurring somewhere between 12 and 72 hours after exercise (i.e., during the recovery phase of an exercise program; Fig. 16-6). Mechanical stresses placed on muscle and tissue, especially during eccentric contractions, create disruptions within the microscopic structures of the individual myofilaments, most importantly at the Z-discs.[24] In addition, damage also appears to occur within the muscles' connective tissue. Evidence of this structural damage exists because of the presence of specific muscle enzymes and compounds (e.g., myoglobin) in the blood. Mechanical stress applied to muscle tissue triggers immune responses to repair the damaged tissue that can increase local edema (accumulation of fluid). This tissue damage may also increase the mechanical sensitivity of muscle nociceptors (pain receptors) that are stimulated under muscle lengthening or palpation (touch or pressure). DOMS is a delayed process because this inflammatory response process to sensitize nociceptors takes time. (See explanatory animation of eccentric and concentric muscle action on the Davis*Plus* site at http://davisplus.fadavis.com.)

During this period of muscle damage, however, the muscle demonstrates a reduction in its force-generating capacity as the physical disruption diminishes the capacity for the excitation-contraction coupling process.[24] Impaired muscle glycogen synthesis will also delay muscle recovery and function. Although eccentric training is generally unavoidable during exercise, the magnitude of DOMS can be controlled by implementing specific training strategies, such as the following:

- Limit initial muscle action to emphasize more concentric and isometric contractions.

- Start training at lower intensities and introduce higher levels of intensity gradually.
- Control exercise volume. This is determined by the total amount of time spent performing eccentric contractions. This implies reducing the number of sets and repetitions, as well as the time spent contracting eccentrically.
- Initially limit eccentric muscle lengthening.
- Implement post-exercise stretching and cool-downs.
- Adhere to proper nutrition to manage electrolytes and glycogen before and after exertion.

For example, a new exerciser may find that performing 1 set of 10 repetitions at a light-to-moderate intensity that emphasizes concentric contractions may be more tolerable than a program comprised of multiple sets with slow eccentric contractions.

Muscle does adapt to repeated exposures of this form of training to reduce future damage. Over the duration of a training program, continued application of eccentric loading should result in less soreness, a lower presence of muscle damage indicators (e.g., swelling, reduced strength, and muscle markers in blood), and increased muscle tolerance to eccentric forces.

Last, DOMS should not be confused with acute muscle soreness that is evident during the latter stages of exercise and during immediate recovery period. This is attributed to the accumulation of metabolic by-products within the muscle fibers and interstitial spaces between the muscle fibers. Coupled with the effect of pressure created by exercising muscles collapsing small capillaries in the muscle itself, fluid accumulates within the muscle that may stimulate some pain receptors. This fluid accumulation also helps explain the temporary "muscle pump" often witnessed after exercising a muscle. This acute muscle soreness normally disappears soon after exercise is completed.

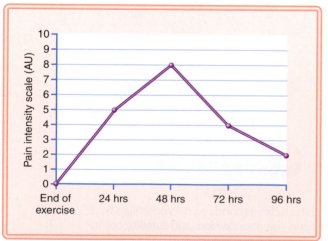

**Figure 16-6.** Time course of delayed-onset muscle soreness (DOMS) as measured by pain intensity (arbitrary units on a scale of 0–10) following resistance training. In general, the most severe pain is experienced within the first 24 to 48 hours after exercise, with the pain subsiding past 72 to 96 hours after exercise training. AU = arbitrary units.

## Tempo

Tempo, or **time under tension**, refers to the speed of movement in completing one repetition and is generally represented by the time spent in each of the three phases of the muscle action within the repetition: the concentric (shortening) phase; the stabilization or transition (isometric) phase when the muscle is under tension, but no movement occurs; and the eccentric (lengthening) phase. It is usually expressed in the following order: eccentric: transitional: concentric (e.g., 4:1:2 implies a 4-second eccentric, 1-second transitional, and 2-second concentric contraction). Although time under tension in the eccentric phase provides a strong stimulus for muscle growth, the training goal and, therefore, exercise intensity should dictate exercise tempo. Heavier loads (strength) require faster tempos, whereas power training requires explosive tempos. Light-to-moderate loads (endurance and hypertrophy training) can be controlled with slower tempos, allowing the muscles to stay under tension for longer periods, providing a strong stimulus for growth. However, DOMS is attributed primarily to extended eccentric phases; thus, longer tempos coupled with increased sets and reps increase the quantity of eccentric work performed. Because muscle soreness can enhance an individual's perception of exercise being painful, it is important to monitor the quantity of muscle soreness and its impact on the overall exercise experience, especially with new exercisers. Table 16-6 presents recommended exercise tempos based on resistance training goals.

## TYPES OF STRENGTH TRAINING

Various modalities of resistance training exist and are organized around volume, load, and power. While volume training manipulates the amount of work performed, load training manipulates the intensity of work performed, and power training manipulates the rate at which work is performed (exercise movements are rapid and explosive). Although they represent three primary methods of applying the variables to resistance training, individuals traditionally use the terms *endurance* (toning and shaping), *hypertrophy, strength* (hypertrophy and strength can both be considered applications of strength training with the focus of hypertrophy being increasing muscle fiber cross-width), and *power* (plyometric) training more frequently. Essentially, endurance training reflects volume, strength training reflects load, and plyometrics reflect power training. These terms are used interchangeably throughout this chapter. Table 16-7 outlines basic differences in intensity and volume (number of sets and repetitions) between these three primary forms of training (volume, load, and power training). Volume training builds both muscular endurance and hypertrophy, whereas load training generally aims to improve muscular strength. Hypertrophy training (discussed later in greater detail) best reflects a blend between moderate levels of volume and load.

## Volume Training

**Volume training** involves the use of submaximal or lighter loads until some defined end point is achieved (e.g., number of repetitions) or until momentary muscle fatigue is achieved. The terms *point of fatigue* or *failure* are often used when training to build muscle size (hypertrophy) or for endurance. Although practitioners and exercisers generally infer the same response with both terms, point of fatigue reflects the initial onset of fatigue (i.e., initial sensation of decreased work capacity), whereas failure represents the point where an additional full repetition cannot be completed without the assistance of other muscles or body segments (i.e., joints). Training to a safe point of muscle failure is important to induce overload and accumulate metabolic by-products (e.g., lactate) within the muscle, which, in turn, lead to improved muscle adaptation. As listed in Table 16-7, moderate volumes are commonly used by bodybuilders and others interested in increasing lean muscle mass, whereas higher volumes are

### Table 16-6. Recommended Exercise Tempos Based on Resistance Training Goals

| TRAINING OUTCOME | ECCENTRIC (SECONDS) | ISOMETRIC (SECONDS) | CONCENTRIC (SECONDS) |
|---|---|---|---|
| Muscular endurance | 2–4 | 1–2 | 1–2 |
| Hypertrophy | 2–4 | 1 | 1–2 |
| Strength | 1–2 | 1 | 1–2 |
| Power | Explosive | n/a | Explosive |

### FROM THEORY TO PRACTICE

Now that you have a general understanding of some of the programming variables that constitute a resistance training program, revisit Marina's goal of toning, losing her added pregnancy weight, and building lean mass while being sensitive to her fear of becoming too muscular. If she commits to training 4 days a week following a split-routine format of two upper and two lower extremity sessions, and decides to target muscular endurance after improving her levels of stability and mobility, how would you organize her programming variables?

Frequency: two upper body sessions; two lower body sessions

**Intensity:** _____ %1 RM

**Sets:** _____

**Reps:** _____

**Rest Interval Between Sets:** _____

**Recovery Interval Between Sessions:** _____

### Table 16-7. Intensity and Repetitions Required for Muscle Force Output

| TYPE OF STRENGTH | DESCRIPTION | INTENSITY | NO. OF REPETITIONS |
|---|---|---|---|
| Load training | The amount of work performed | 85%–100% of maximal effort (1 RM) | 1–5 |
| Volume training | The volume of work performed | Moderate volume: 67%–85% of maximal effort (1 RM) | 6–12 |
| | | High volume: <67% of maximal effort (1 RM) | 13–20 |
| Power training | The rate at which work is performed | Multi-rep events: >30% of maximal effort (1 RM) for repeated efforts | 4–10 (repeated efforts) 1–2 (single-rep efforts) |
| | | Single-rep events: 75%–90% of maximal efforts (1 RM) for single-rep efforts | |

1 RM, one-repetition maximum.

used by individuals who seek to improve muscular endurance without necessarily building more muscle fibers. The differences lie with the primary fibers recruited. More moderate volumes recruit the type II(a) and type II(x) fibers that demonstrate greater capacity for growth, whereas higher volumes primarily recruit the type I fibers that demonstrate smaller potential for growth but greater capacity to resist fatigue.

Volume can be measured several ways. One simple method involves multiplying the number of sets completed by the number of repetitions completed. For example, completing 2 sets of 12 repetitions represents a volume of 24 repetitions. Other methods involve more complicated calculations and include the following:

- Multiply sets × repetitions × tempo (the time interval to complete one repetition). For example, completing 2 sets × 12 repetitions where each repetition is completed in 6 seconds (tempo) represents a volume of 144 (sets × reps × tempo).
- Multiply sets × repetitions × weight lifted. For example, completing 2 sets × 12 repetitions with 135 lb represents a volume of 6,480 lb (2,945 kg). Although this method was more popular 30 to 40 years ago, the complexity of the calculation has made it less popular in present-day training.

It is always important to monitor training volume as it relates to both the quantity and quality of a resistance training program. If the quantity of work is too high, the quality of movements may suffer as fatigue occurs; that is, the risk of injury increases if movement quality decreases. Conversely, if the quantity of work is insufficient, proper motor learning or adaptation may not occur. Total volume of an exercise or workout should be dictated by an individual's training experience and personal goals. During the initial stages of a training program, it is important to keep the volume relatively low to moderate (i.e., one to two sets), where the individual is allowed sufficient repetitions to develop motor skills and experience some adaptation, but also provides positive experiences that promote adherence by controlling the magnitude of DOMS.

### DOING THE MATH

Using the various formulas presented, calculate the total volume of work performed by Kathy and Mike, and answer the question provided. Kathy completes 3 sets × 12 reps using a 25-lb dumbbell at a 4-second tempo, while Mike completes 3 sets of 8 reps using a 40-lb dumbbell at a 6-second tempo. Calculate volume for each using the following formulas:

- Sets × reps
- Sets × reps × tempo

For each formula, who actually performed a higher volume of work?

**Answers:**

- Sets × reps: Kathy = 36 (3 sets × 12 reps); Mike = 24 (3 sets × 8 reps)
- Sets × reps × tempo: Kathy = 144 (3 sets × 12 reps × 4 seconds); Mike = 144 (3 sets × 8 reps × 6 seconds)
- Using the simplest formula, Kathy completed a greater volume, but when including tempo, the volume was equal.

## Load Training

**Load** training emphasizes increased force production by the muscle, requiring greater recruitment of motor units. Discussed previously, a motor unit comprises a motor neuron and the number of skeletal muscle fibers innervated by that neuron. All muscle contractions require groups of motor units to activate and function together, and heavier loads require the activation of more motor units simultaneously to generate greater quantities of force. This entails a progressive recruitment of the larger type II(a) and then even larger type II(x) muscle fibers as additional force is required. This neural recruitment order that engages the larger muscle fibers is important to increasing overall strength. Thus, a primary objective of load training is to improve recruitment of muscle motor units to produce a higher level of force between the involved muscle fibers. As a result of the high levels of stress associated with load training, it is important to use gradual progressions of intensity to appropriately adapt to the heavier loads. This may necessitate monitoring the amount of exposure to heavier loads to reduce the risk for injury or overtraining, and allow maximal recovery and adaptation after training. For example, a coach may progress his athlete's program from 4 sets of 12 reps at 70% of maximal effort to 4 sets of 8 repetitions at 80% of maximal effort, before progressing to 4 sets of 6 repetitions at 85% of maximal effort and monitor for symptoms of overtraining throughout the process.

## Power Training

Power training involves the use of near-maximal or submaximal loads that are moved at the highest attainable velocity. This training mode is the most effective means of increasing the rate of force development and developing the explosive strength required for many sports or dynamic activities. Power training is unique in that it involves a rapid, eccentric lengthening action of the muscle (loading phase), followed by a very brief transition (amortization phase) before executing an explosive, concentric shortening action of the muscle (unloading phase). In practice, this form of training is referred to a plyometrics. A key purpose of this short amortization phase is to harness the elastic energy (recoil) associated with a muscle prestretch or loading, much like when immediately releasing a rubber band after it has been rapidly stretched.

## COMPONENTS AND VARIABLES OF EXERCISE PROGRAM DESIGN

The organization of an exercise program is structured according to specific variables and components. To achieve a specific training outcome, it is necessary to organize the variables and components of exercise program design into structured units of progressively challenging physical work to achieve the specific training outcomes. Understanding how the body adapts to training provides valuable insight to program design. Sex, age, training experience, genetics, rest, nutrition, hydration, and other emotional and physical stressors all affect how human physiological systems adapt to resistance training.

A resistance training program designed to maximize the potential for achieving desired outcomes should include the following components, some of which were described in Chapter 13:

- A thorough health risk and needs assessment to identify the current health status and any special needs of the individual

- Adequate frequency and intensity of exercise consistent with the individual's health status, training experience, current fitness level, and desired goals
- Appropriate exercise selection and sequencing relevant to desired goals
- Appropriate intensity and volume to stimulate desired physiological adaptations
- Sufficient periods of recovery between sets to optimize performance
- Adequate periods of rest between sessions to allow for the necessary adaptation

## EXERCISE SELECTION AND SEQUENCING

Exercise selection should address specific individual needs and personal goals. There is a variety of different resistance exercises to select from, but the challenge lies with how to organize them in a manner that creates an efficient, yet safe method of overload that stimulates adaptation. Identifying and sequencing exercises into a logical order requires prior knowledge of an individual's current strength, training experience, and movement skill. There is no one "right" way to select and organize exercises in a sequential order. It is important for program design to improve stability and mobility at the appropriate joints in order to promote efficient movement and reduce the risk of muscular imbalances. If the program favors certain muscles over others, it may lead to injury.

One method for sequencing exercises is built around the type of exercise performed: Is it machine based or free weight? Machine-based exercises are generally easier to perform and are probably more suitable for new exercisers, whereas free-weight exercises are more challenging and necessitate the need to stabilize the body or specific body segments while performing repetitions. Because resistance training equipment options continue to evolve and expand, and are now available in many shapes and forms (e.g., suspension trainers, kettlebells), the choices and sequences can often be confusing. Figure 13-9 provides a general guideline to follow, illustrating exercise progression over time for novice exercisers, where one would essentially move from exercises that exhibit the trait from the left toward the right. For example, novice individuals should start with exercises that are more machine based (supported), where the machine controls the path of motion and focuses on isolating specific muscle groups, before progressing over time to multijoint or compound movements that require the individual to control multidirectional mobility and stability at every joint. This concept of joint stability and mobility was introduced in Chapter 13.

## Isolation Exercises

Traditional selection and sequencing of exercises focuses on an isolation approach, where programs and sessions are structured around training individual body parts at separate times. These are also known as split routines. Isolation exercises generally focus on specific muscles that work at a particular joint (e.g., biceps curls and lateral raises). This philosophy allows sufficient recovery and adaptation of the exercised muscles or body segment to elicit maximum hypertrophy. For bodybuilders focused on achieving high levels of muscle size and definition, this is still perhaps the most effective and preferred approach to selecting and ordering resistance training exercises. For example, a bodybuilder may favor working his or her arms or biceps and back on one day, while training the chest on another day.

## Compound Exercises

Compound exercises involve exercises or movements where one or more joints and several muscles or muscle groups are trained simultaneously. The barbell squat, for example, is considered a compound exercise because it involves the joints of the ankles, knees, hips, spine, and shoulders, with the muscles responsible for creating movement (mobility) or stability at each joint. Compound movements generally involve a greater degree of difficulty because of the need for multiple muscle actions to move and stabilize joints. Consequently, compound exercises should be performed early in the training session (after a thorough warm-up) when muscles are not fatigued and concentration levels are higher.[20,25–27]

The inclusion of compound-type movements or exercises in resistance training programs has gained popularity given their ability to burn more calories and to better mimic ADLs. Because these movements mimic ADLs more closely than isolation-type training, they provide more effective carryover of any mechanical and biological adaptations into one's daily life. Consequently, these types of exercises are commonly referred to as "functional" exercises. The basic movement patterns that mimic ADLs can be referred to as primary movement patterns and generally include:

- Bend-and-lift patterns that involve lowering the body toward the floor from a standing posture and then rising upward (e.g., deadlifts, squats), flexing and extending the hips and knees as the feet maintain contact with the ground
- Single-leg or lunging patterns that involve raising one foot off the ground to balance or reposition it while moving the entire body (e.g., single-leg balancing, walking, or lunging) in all three planes of motion
- Pushing movement patterns in the upper extremity (e.g., shoulders) that involve movement in all three planes
- Pulling movement patterns in the upper extremity (e.g., shoulders) that involve movement in all three planes
- Rotational movement patterns that integrate the hip complex and trunk

Most of these compound movements connect the lower and upper extremities, creating forces through the lumbo-pelvic hip complex, commonly known as the core region. A strong and stable core is important, not only to protect the low back from injury during these types of exercises or movements, but also to help transfer forces more efficiently between the upper and lower extremities. Research demonstrates how effective core exercises with or without resistance can be to reduce the risk for low-back injuries by conditioning and strengthening the muscles responsible for stabilizing the spine.[28] However, much of this research is relatively recent, and core training has become an integral part of exercise and resistance training programming only over the past few years.

## RESEARCH HIGHLIGHT

### Using Resistance for Core Training

Traditionally, core training is not thought of as a component of a resistance training exercise program. Work done by Canadian researcher Stuart McGill and his colleagues challenges this mind-set by demonstrating that performing core training exercises with resistance can reduce the risk for injury by strengthening the muscles responsible for stabilizing the spine. McGill has identified the inverted or suspended row (body at an incline holding a fixed bar), the bent-over row, and the one-arm cable row as being extremely effective for providing the necessary loading to increase strength in all three planes of motion. The bent-over row placed high loads on the lumbar spine but involved a large amount of muscle responsible for increasing stability. Because of the minimal amount of stress placed on the lumbar spine during the inverted row, which uses primarily the upper back and hip extensor muscles, it is an effective option to enhance stabilization strength for individuals who are experiencing low-back pain. McGill found that the one-arm cable row is an effective exercise for maximizing stability of the spine in the transverse plane of motion. If the purpose of having a client perform core exercises

## RESEARCH HIGHLIGHT—cont'd

is to improve the force production of abdominal and back muscles to enhance the stability of the lumbar spine, then using traditional resistance training exercises can be an effective technique.[28]

Fenwick C, Brown S, McGill S. Comparison of different rowing exercises: Trunk muscle activation and lumbar spine motion, load and stiffness. J Strength Cond Res. 2009;23:350–358.

Although training sessions are often designed around goals (e.g., overall muscle building), available time (e.g., two times a week to train the entire body), or muscle/joint groups (e.g., train pushing muscles—chest, shoulders, and triceps—on Monday; train pulling muscle groups—back and biceps—on Tuesday), functional training is a format of program design that offers an alternative approach by focusing on the type of movement pattern(s) performed. For example, one session may incorporate training bend-and-lift patterns exclusively with squats and deadlifts, whereas another session may target single-leg standing push and pull movements with single-leg cable chests presses, shoulder presses, and high-back rows. Although these sessions may be interpreted as being more functional for improving ADLs, they are not necessarily always better than the isolation approach because it all depends on one's training needs and goals.

Sequencing exercise sessions by muscle group or function continues to remain a popular method for designing resistance training programs (e.g., chest, shoulder, and triceps on Monday; back and biceps on Tuesday). Several reasons are cited for this approach that include time for adequate muscle recovery between sessions (e.g., chest on Monday, with other muscle groups trained on Tuesday and Wednesday, before returning to train the chest on Thursday). Although this method is effective and appropriate for achieving resistance training goals, how the exercises are organized and sequenced within a session is also worthy of consideration. A training session should begin by targeting the larger muscle (primary) groups (e.g., chest) before targeting the smaller muscle (assistant muscles) groups (e.g., triceps). This may enable the exerciser to complete the more challenging exercises with greater effectiveness.

Regardless of preference, selecting appropriate exercises and organizing them into progressively challenging sequences is an important consideration to ensure effective results. Exercise selection should always enhance movement efficiency first to reduce the risk of injury from improper training before increasing the amount of external load to build muscle.

### Assistant Exercises

Assistant exercises are isolation- or single-joint exercises (e.g., biceps curls and triceps extensions) that are often used to complement compound movements in a training session. For example, after completing barbell squats, an individual may complete a leg-extension exercise to increase the total amount of work performed by the quadriceps in a session. Because these exercises are generally less challenging in terms of complexity, they should follow compound movements to ensure that good technique and effectiveness of the movement pattern is maintained. Pre-fatiguing muscles with assistant exercises beforehand may compromise technique and the effectiveness of the compound exercises, potentially increasing the risk for injury.

## FROM THEORY TO PRACTICE

Draw up a short list of two integrated movements that you perform on a regular basis whether they are occupational or recreational. Next, identify two key muscles involved when performing each movement. Last, examine each of these two movements against the list of five movement patterns presented previously to identify the nature of the movement pattern (e.g., bend-and-lift patterns, single-leg patterns, push movements, pull movements, rotational movements, or a combination of any).

- Identify an individual (isolated) exercise to target each of the two muscles of each movement. Complete 1 set × 12 repetitions for each muscle group at a light-to-moderate intensity (volume = 24 for each movement).
- Identify an integrated (compound) exercise you could develop to mimic each movement in an exercise setting using light resistance (e.g., elastic tubing) or just body weight. Complete 2 sets × 12 repetitions of each movement pattern (volume = 24 for each movement).
- Compare the overall perception of effort in completing each task (isolated exercises vs. integrated exercises). Although the overall volume of work performed between the two is equal, did you notice any differences? Do you think there may be a caloric difference between the two modalities?

## Circuit Training

Traditional strength training programs generally include performing one or multiple sets of an exercise before proceeding to the next exercise (also known as a horizontal-loading program in sports conditioning programs). Circuit training is a different modality where the session is organized in such a manner that a set of repetitions for each exercise targeting different muscles groups is completed in succession with little-to-no rest interval between each exercise before completing the second set of a particular exercise (also known as a vertical-loading program in sports conditioning programs). The principles behind this training modality is to create a time-efficient and effective method of targeting multiple muscle groups, increased calorie burn, and muscle conditioning with some simultaneous cardiovascular improvements (achieved as an outcome of potentially maintaining higher heart rates for sustained periods in comparison with traditional resistance training where heart rates fluctuate more significantly between the work and the rest intervals).[29] Although it offers several benefits, this method of training is generally not as effective as a more traditional horizontal-loading format for increasing muscular strength or size.[29]

A circuit can be composed of a variety of different exercises, generally ranging from 4 to 12 movements, each designed to target different muscles. Individuals move from one station to the next with little (15–30 seconds) or no rest, performing a 15- to 45-second work interval that traditionally yields approximately 12 to 20 repetitions at each station (emphasizing primarily endurance). Ideal circuit design alternates between body segments (i.e., lower extremity and upper extremity) and between muscle actions (push-pull) to enable muscle group recovery and greater volumes of work to be completed in shorter periods. Table 16-8 provides an example of a basic circuit training program, listing how exercises alternate between the lower and upper extremities, and between push and pull movements. The traditional circuit format originally created in the 1950s continues to evolve as circuits can now be organized in a multitude of ways, using various integrated exercise sequences, modalities, and work-to-recovery ratios that aim to change or improve many physical parameters that include general physique, fat loss, muscle mass, or strength, or even improve explosiveness (power). Examples of some of these circuit-type programs include CrossFit workouts and many of the commercially available exercise programs sold as DVD compilations to the public (e.g., P90X, Insanity).

Given the minimal frequency recommended by HHS and ACSM for resistance training (targeting a muscle group a minimum of two times a week), circuit training is an appropriate training methodology for individuals who can only afford to train twice or three times a week.[1,12] By comparison, attempting to follow a split-routine–type format where only specific muscle groups are trained once a week (i.e., falling below the minimal guidelines) may minimize some of the benefits of resistance training or lead to some muscle loss because of

### Table 16-8. Sample Circuit Program—Vertical Loading

| | |
|---|---|
| Type of Equipment | Generally machine based for new exercisers |
| No. of circuits | 2 |
| No. of repetitions | 12 repetitions per station |
| Intensity | Feel challenged by the 12th rep on each circuit |
| Recovery between stations | 30 seconds |
| Frequency | 2 times/week |
| Exercise sequence | Leg press |
| | Chest press |
| | Seated row |
| | Hamstrings curl |
| | Front-shoulder press |
| | Leg extensions |
| | Abdominal curls |
| | Low-back extensions |
| | Biceps curl |
| | Triceps pushdowns |
| | Calf raises |

a detraining effect. Circuit training formats are also appropriate for beginning exercisers who are seeking to learn new exercises for multiple muscle groups.

## In Your Own Words

How would you explain the benefits and methodology of circuit training to a friend who is interested in beginning a resistance training program but can only commit to training two times per week?

Many individuals seek opportunities to vary their exercise program by modifying the order of the exercises performed on a frequent basis to keep their program interesting. It is important, however, to consider that while more frequent changes may induce greater levels of both metabolic and mechanical stresses on the body (both are known as effective stimuli for provoking muscle adaptations), more gradual progression and some consistency of exercise selection, especially for new exercisers, allow the individual better opportunities to perfect his or her exercise movement patterns (achieve greater competency and mastery) that may in turn boost self-efficacy and program adherence. Health and fitness professionals should identify the need to start with simpler, supported exercises before advancing the exercise challenge as competency improves.

## EXERCISE PROGRAM DESIGN FOR RESISTANCE TRAINING/PERIODIZATION

Organizing a resistance training program to stimulate the desired adaptations requires planning to vary the training

# VIGNETTE continued

■ After a discussion about Marina's time availability for exercise, she and Geoff decide that a resistance training program consisting of circuit training workouts will benefit her the most. This approach will allow Marina to initially perform whole-body, moderate-intensity workouts and then progress to higher intensity sessions after she masters the movements and develops a certain level of muscular conditioning. When she was doing a split-routine program, Marina was training each muscle group two times per week. Following a program focused on whole-body circuit training will allow Marina to increase the training volume by involving each muscle group three times per week. Furthermore, the variety and efficiency of circuit training appeals to Marina because of her past experience with attending group fitness classes (i.e., she enjoys fast-paced workouts that include elements of muscle conditioning and cardiorespiratory endurance). Lastly, Geoff assures Marina that circuit training workouts are effective at increasing muscular fitness, but they are not designed to promote excessive hypertrophy, or muscle "bulk."

load and volume on a structured basis. Hans Selye's GAS has led to the development of models for periodization, the theory of structuring a training program that is based on the stress–stimulus response. In Matveyev's model of periodization, training intensity and volume vary over the different stages leading up to and following an athletic competition (see Chapter 13).

Training stimuli must progressively challenge the body's physiological systems with overload to trigger biological adaptations. Periodization calls for alternating phases (periods) of training based on volume and intensity, with the goal to create a long-term training plan that controls and manages the application of the training stimuli. The variables gradually increase the intensity of the training to achieve specific training outcomes over a defined period. An individual's specific training goal and needs, competition schedule, and start date determine the length of the plan and the periodization of the training load. For example, when working with a football athlete who has a competitive season spanning September through December, an off-season spanning January through April, and a preseason spanning May through August, his program would be designed around these calendar dates to follow specific training

principles to achieve specific outcomes (e.g., adding 10 lb or 4.5 kg of muscle in the off-season with a generalized, non-football–specific hypertrophy program with greater volume, to a peaking program optimizing the needed skill sets for football performance in the preseason with greater intensity, to a maintenance program implemented during the competitive season with controlled volume and intensity to avoid potential overtraining).

There are two basic methods of organizing the training variables into structured, periodized programs: a linear progression of gradually increasing intensity and volume over time, and a more frequently changing method of alternating volume and intensity in a nonlinear or undulating manner.

## Linear Periodization

Linear periodization involves systematically modifying intensity and volume into distinct training stages where each stage is structured to gradually increase the exercise challenge by increasing load while simultaneously decreasing volume (Fig. 16-7). The overall program, however, should progress through distinct training phases, ultimately peaking performance in preparation for a competition, a competitive season, or a specific goal (e.g., a wedding date). Figure 16-8 provides an example of an 8-month periodization cycle. Furthermore, to accommodate progressive loading with appropriate recoveries, the program should also include timely, short periods of time off or lower intensity and reduced-volume training called *offloading*. An example of linear periodization for a novice individual seeking improvements in strength over a 16-week period is one where an individual may start her resistance training program with a 2-week general conditioning (endurance) phase,

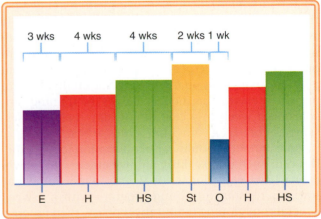

**Figure 16-7.** Example of a linear periodization program. The term *linear* refers to the progression of intensity and volume over weeks until the time of "offloading" when the volume and intensity are greatly reduced. This is a time for the individual to recover from the overall training stress in the program and perform active recovery, cross-training activities. E, endurance; H, hypertrophy; HS, hypertrophy and strength; O, offload; St, strength.

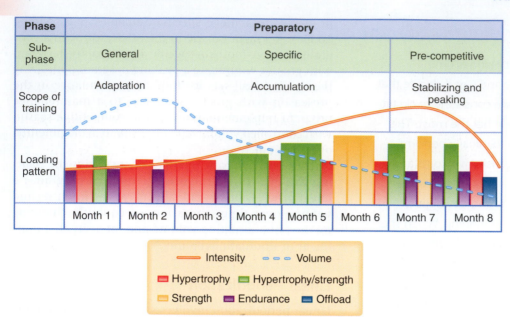

**Figure 16-8.** Eight-month preparatory macrocycle with a linear progression of intensity and volume.

then progress to a 4-week hypertrophy phase, before moving to a 2-week strength training phase. After 8 weeks of training, this individual may take a week off (offload), then return to a 3-week hypertrophy phase, followed by a 4-week strength training phase.

## Nonlinear (Undulating) Periodization

Undulating, or nonlinear, periodization is based on the concept that improved physiological adaptations such as muscle strength can occur as a result of more frequent variations in load (intensity) and volume compared with traditional linear models. As shown in Figure 16-9, this method varies the levels of imposed stress more frequently to stimulate more rapid neuroendocrine responses and adaptations. Support of this method stems from the reduction in accumulated neural and muscular fatigue associated with extended periods of ever-increasing linear stress.[30] Also referred to as "muscle confusion," this method also allows individuals to train and prepare for multiple events throughout a year (multiple peaks), as opposed to the linear program that traditionally prepares an individual for one single event. This model changes the training variables on a week-to-week, day-to-day (between sessions), or between- or within-exercise basis.

An example of nonlinear periodization for an experienced exerciser seeking improvements in power over a 12-week period is one where an individual may start his resistance training program with a 1-week general conditioning (endurance) phase, then progress to a 2-week strength phase, before introducing a 1-week hypertrophy training phase. A 2-week power phase may be introduced next, followed by a planned week off (offload) during week 7, then a return to a 2-week hypertrophy phase, followed by 1-week strength and endurance phases, and culminating in a 2-week power training phase.

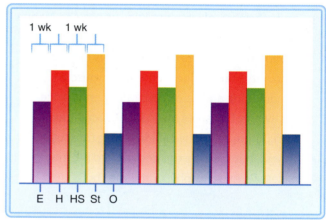

**Figure 16-9.** Example of an undulating progression program. In comparison with the linear progression, this model allows for much greater variation in volume and intensity over the course of a training program. The theoretical advantage of this method over the linear method is that the constant changes in training variables allow for more frequent peaks in preparation for multiple performances or events throughout a season versus building toward one main performance or event. In addition, this method also may hold less of a risk for overtraining because of more frequent adjustments in volume and intensity. E, endurance; H, hypertrophy; HS, hypertrophy and strength; O, offload; St, strength.

Although undulating models have become more popular, the variations between training modalities require greater training experience on the part of the exerciser. Consequently, an individual may need to consider beginning with a linear model initially, then transitioning to nonlinear methods as experience and adaptations occur. In other words, it may not be appropriate to start a novice individual with power and strength training phases until he or she has adapted biologically and mechanically to lower intensity, higher volume (endurance, hypertrophy) training. Keep in mind, however, that too frequent changes that evoke greater levels of stress can also over-tax the body's physiological systems and trigger over-training. There is evidence to suggest that linear and undulating periodization are both effective at producing gains in strength and size. Apel and colleagues[31] discovered that when equating volume and intensity between linear and undulating programs, the linear periodization models produced greater results. Conversely, Prestes and colleagues[30] discovered that undulating models provided greater strength stimuli over linear models. Because both appear to produce similar results, health/fitness practitioners should consider the merits of each and perhaps consider using both when designing a training program.

## VIGNETTE continued

■ Marina has been participating in her exercise program without missing a session, and she is eager to include 1 more day of training in her weekly schedule. After more than a month of circuit training that progressed linearly and became more intense (with respect to increasing load), Geoff asks Marina if she would consider changing her resistance training program to include a day of circuit training, a day of traditional-type load training, and a day of power and agility training. Marina agrees and is excited to start the next phase of her program (i.e., undulating periodization).

## GENERAL CONSIDERATIONS FOR LONG-TERM PROGRAMS

The purpose of planning, organizing, and structuring a resistance training program into separate time units differentiated by intensity, volume, and frequency is to maximize opportunities for adaptation (during recovery), whereas minimizing the accumulation of fatigue or potential for overtraining. This is accomplished with distinct training cycles, each with specific training objectives that progress the training overload, and may also include periods of lighter intensity (offloads) to ensure additional physiological recovery when needed or to accommodate

breaks in the program for other reasons (e.g., vacations or business trips). For the athlete with a specific competition schedule, the program peaks at specifically established times (i.e., competitive events), whereas for individuals with general health/fitness goals (not preparing for events), the program strives to achieve the goal by an established completion date. In Chapter 13, the concept of macrocycles, mesocycles, and microcycles was introduced as the three specific training cycles that are considered when designing a program. These three phases are summarized as follows (see also Table 16-9):

- Macrocycle—represents the overall long-term period of training and can be organized into months, years, or series of years. For an athlete, the macrocycle is typically based on a yearly calendar and organized to achieve and maintain peak strength during his or her competitive season.
- Mesocycle—represents shorter time periods with specific training objectives organized into months or weeks as dictated by the training goals, competition schedule, or work/home-life demands. These represent shorter time periods, each required to achieve a specific training objective. An example of a mesocycle is a 5-week stability training program to prepare the body for strength training.
- Microcycle—represents the shortest period for organizing program variables to help achieve a mesocyle goal and is denoted as daily or weekly training variations in a program. An example of a microcycle is an individual who moves from machine weights to free weights over a microcycle period of 1 week.

## STRENGTH TRAINING EQUIPMENT OPTIONS

The available options of equipment for resistance training are almost endless and appear to be continually evolving, which can prove challenging for both the health/fitness professional and the exerciser. Although each manufacturer may claim to have the latest and best piece of equipment, it is important to recognize that any piece of equipment can be either effective or inappropriate depending on its application. Ultimately, this depends on how the equipment is used to achieve the individual's goal(s). The decisions made regarding which

## FROM THEORY TO PRACTICE

Select a resistance training goal you would like to achieve and identify the timeline in which you desire to achieve this goal. Working with your end goal in mind and using your calendar, develop your macrocycle (timeline to achieve your goal) and three distinct mesocycles you believe you will need to include in your training to achieve the outcome goal. Finally, outline the basic programming variables of a microcycle you would follow in week one or two, and how this would differ from the last 2 weeks of your macrocycle.

### Table 16-9. Phases of Periodization

| CYCLE | TIME AND PURPOSE IN CYCLE | EXAMPLE |
|---|---|---|
| Macrocycle | Months or years<br>Long-term structure of a training plan, aimed at supporting the primary objective(s) of the program | The outline of a program for a woman seeking to tone and shape in time for her wedding 3 months from today |
| Mesocycle | Weeks or months<br>Intermediate period for a training program focused on achieving a specific objective<br>Organizes progressions of training variables into smaller, more manageable periods | Dividing a wrestler's seasonal program into an off-season mesocycle aimed at adding more muscle and a preseason mesocycle aimed at improving explosiveness |
| Microcycle | Days or weeks<br>Shortest periods used when structuring long-term programs<br>Microcycle progresses toward the mesocycle objective or goal | Progressively modifying a deconditioned business executive's program on a weekly basis to progress using selectorized machines to standing and using free weights to improve overall levels of conditioning |

equipment to use therefore should be based on availability; the individual's experience, needs, desires, and goals; and the competency of the health/fitness professional to properly instruct technique with the chosen equipment. An overview of some popular strength training tools that are available on the market is as follows (see also Table 16-10):

- Selectorized weight-stack machines with a fixed path of motion (Fig. 16-10)
- Plate-loaded machines: provide a controlled path of motion; the applied resistance is accomplished through the use of weight plates mounted on a lever system (Fig. 16-11)
- Cable column machines: a cable attached to a weight stack is guided by a pulley system; the actual amount of the applied load is determined by the mass of the weight stack and the leverage of the pulleys (Fig. 16-12)

### Table 16-10. Various Strength Training Options

| EQUIPMENT | FEATURES | BENEFITS | DRAWBACKS |
|---|---|---|---|
| Selectorized machines | • Stacks of weight plates—specific load is selected using a pin<br>• Pulleys and cams to place the highest amount of load on the strongest portion of muscle action<br>• Adjustable for all body types and sizes<br>• The ROM or path of motion of the resistance is dictated and controlled by the design of the machine<br>• Most machines feature bilateral action where both limbs (right and left) are used at the same time to generate force and control motion | • A safe way to apply high amounts of resistance due to controlled ROM of the machine<br>• Easy to learn<br>• Because of the design of the cam or pulley, it can allow a constant resistance or load through the entire ROM | • Require an appropriate amount of space<br>• Difficult to move, not portable<br>• Expensive<br>• Does not train the body how to attenuate the forces created by gravity and ground reaction |
| Plate-loaded machines | • Weight plates are loaded onto a bar, which is attached to a machine with a fulcrum that controls the ROM | • A controlled path of motion that allows emphasis to be on muscle force production | • Require an appropriate amount of space<br>• Difficult to move, not portable |

## Table 16-10. **Various Strength Training Options–cont'd**

| EQUIPMENT | FEATURES | BENEFITS | DRAWBACKS |
|---|---|---|---|
| | • Most are designed to allow unilateral motion where each limb (right and left) can move independent of the other | • Load is adjustable based on the amount of free-weight plates available<br>• A safe way to apply high amounts of resistance due to controlled ROM of the machine | • Expensive<br>• Does not train the body how to attenuate the forces created by gravity and ground reaction<br>• Because of the fulcrum, the load can change based on the position relative to gravity |
| Cable machines | • A weight stack is attached to a handle (or handles) via a pulley system<br>• The action of the pulley can reduce the friction of the load and allow the user to control the specific path of motion<br>• In some machines, the height or position of the pulley can be adjusted to provide for a variety of different movements | • The path of motion is not controlled by the machine and allows an individual to perform a variety of different movements in all planes of motion<br>• Can be used to create loads for specific movement patterns | • Can be difficult to learn proper movement<br>• Because of changing position of the load (based on pivot point of the pulley) could be a higher risk for injury |
| Barbells | • The standard Olympic barbell is 7 feet in length and is designed to accommodate Olympic-style weights<br>• Requires the user to control the entire path of motion<br>• Is adjustable from the weight of the bar to a high amount of load (depending on bar design) | • Allow an individual to control the entire ROM of the exercise<br>• Creates an effective overload on the targeted muscle groups<br>• Uses a higher neuromuscular demand, possibly leading to quicker adaptation to the strength training stimulus<br>• Requires a bilateral application of force from both limbs simultaneously | • Path of motion must be controlled by an individual<br>• An individual without effective movement skill or strength could be at a higher risk for injury<br>• As the joint angle changes, it causes the load to change based on the position relative to gravity |
| Dumbbells | • A handle in the middle of an equally distributed load<br>• Can come in a wide variety of loads and grip styles<br>• Allows the user to train with each arm independently, potentially leading to higher levels of neuromuscular adaptation | • Allows an individual to control the path of motion<br>• Can be used to create specific paths of motion, which could lead to higher levels of specific strength | • As the joint angle changes, it causes the load to change based on the position relative to gravity<br>• Can cause an increased risk for injury because of inherent instability of the load |
| Medicine balls | • A loaded ball that can be lifted or thrown<br>• Available in a variety of styles:<br>  • Sand filled<br>  • Bouncing (live)<br>  • Nonbouncing (dead)<br>  • Rubber coated<br>  • Leather coated | • Allows an individual to control the path of motion<br>• Can be used to create specific paths of motion that could lead to higher levels of specific strength<br>• Can be thrown to generate higher levels of muscle power in the upper body | • As the joint angle changes, it causes the load to change based on the position relative to gravity<br>• Can cause an increased risk for injury because of inherent instability of the load |

*Continued*

**Table 16-10.** Various Strength Training Options—cont'd

| EQUIPMENT | FEATURES | BENEFITS | DRAWBACKS |
|---|---|---|---|
| More common nontraditional strength training | Can refer to a variety of different types of loads that can be used to create a strength training stimulus:<br>• Elastic tubing<br>• Suspension Training–TRX | • Different types of implements can be used to create loads to stimulate specific adaptations required for a training goal<br>• Can elicit higher levels of neuromotor development because of increased challenges<br>• Can create variety for a training program | • As the joint angle changes, it causes the load to change based on the position relative to gravity<br>• Can cause an increased risk for injury because of inherent instability of the load<br>• Can be large and difficult to store |

ROM, range of motion.

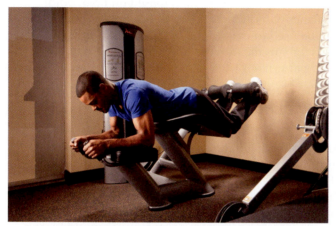

**Figure 16-10.** Prone leg-curl exercise being performed on selectorized equipment. These machines include a weight stack where the resistance is chosen by inserting a metal pin at the level of the weight load. The movement is fixed along a single range of motion.

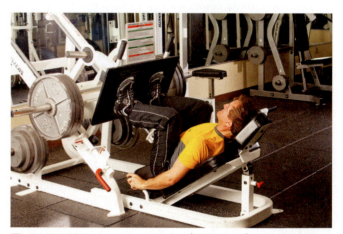

**Figure 16-11.** Leg-press exercise being performed on a plate-loaded machine. This equipment also uses a fixed range of motion, but resistance is adjusted by adding free-weight plates to the machine.

• Barbells: 7-foot (2.1-m) Olympic-style barbells weighing 45 lb (20.5 kg) are the standard piece of strength training equipment used for traditional heavier weight free-weight training (Fig. 16-13); however, shorter, lighter options, commonly used in group exercise or with specific populations (e.g., females, older adults, and youth), are now also available

• Dumbbells: are available in a variety of styles, sizes, and weights; they allow greater freedom of movement when working in all planes of motions to enhance task-specific movements or force outputs (Fig. 16-14)

• Elastic tubing: offers great portability and versatility to resistance training; different densities, thicknesses, and lengths vary the amount of resistance (Fig. 16-15)

• Medicine balls (Fig. 16-16)

• Suspension trainers (Fig. 16-17)

• Body weight (Fig. 16-18)

In addition, a number of other nontraditional forms of resistance training tools have been introduced or re-emerged that can be used effectively to apply external resistance. Many of these have been introduced or developed out of necessity for individuals who are seeking better solutions to their training challenges (e.g., time or cost of equipment). For example, the discovery of training benefits associated with dynamically shifting loads resulted in the creation of slosh pipes—tubes that vary in length and diameter that are filled with water to offer different loads (weights determined by the amount of water in the tube) that can shift as the pipe is moved. This requires greater levels of muscle control and stability. Sand bags allow individuals to quickly and inexpensively fill bags and change the training load anywhere, anytime. Many of these modalities are becoming increasingly popular given their cost, versatility, and portability. A simple Internet search on these tools and more will reveal pictures and videos to help you become more familiar with each piece of equipment.

• Sand bags—durable bags with numerous handles that can be filled to different weights

• Slosh pipes or water-filled equipment—tubes filled with water to offer dynamic resistance or unstable mass caused by constantly shifting center of mass

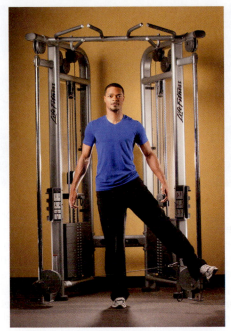

**Figure 16-12.** Standing hip abduction exercise being performed on cable column machines. This equipment uses a weight stack similar to selectorized equipment to apply load for all movements. The advantage of using this type of machine is that the movements are completed in a free range of motion and may be considered more applicable to real-life movement and performance (more functional).

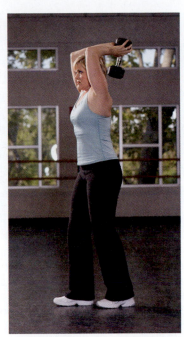

**Figure 16-14.** Example of the standing triceps extension exercise performed with dumbbells. Dumbbells come in a variety of styles, sizes, and weights, and allow for enhanced freedom of movement to improve functional strength and endurance. Creativity in exercise selection and design is much greater with this modality compared with the previous examples of equipment.

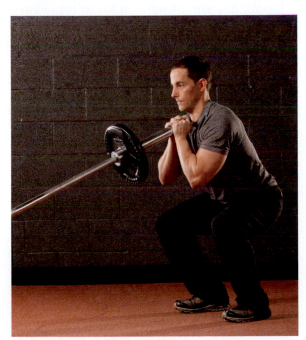

**Figure 16-13.** Barbell jammer exercise. With a free range of motion and required whole-body joint stabilization during movement, these exercises are much more functional compared with fixed range-of-motion and machine-supported exercises.

- Weighted sleds—moveable bases on which resistance can be added that are pulled or pushed
- Kettlebells—cannonball-looking devices with a handle that offers an offset center of mass (because of the position of the handle that requires greater control of the tool during movement)

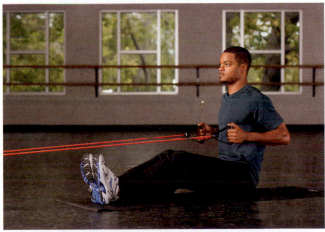

**Figure 16-15.** Seated row exercise performed using elastic tubing. The resistance applied to the working muscles is dependent on the density, thickness, length, and line of force when using resistance bands. Much like cable machines, this modality allows for more freedom in the range of motion per exercise.

- Heavy ropes—industrial-grade ropes that can be pulled, lifted, and shaken at various intensities or speeds to train strength or power
- Chains—heavy chains typically attached to barbells that unravel from the ground as bars are lifted farther from the ground, creating varying levels of resistance throughout the range of motion
- Weighted vests—weighted devices worn during activity to strengthen muscles and increase explosiveness

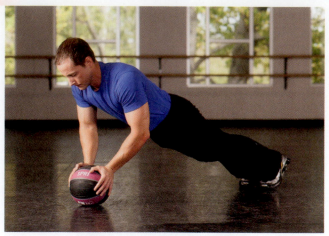

**Figure 16-16.** The use of medicine balls during a push-up exercise. Medicine balls can either be used for resistance purposes or as a means to provide a greater stabilization challenge during training. Medicine balls are also effectively used as resistance when performing power or explosive-type movements for training the upper body and core musculature.

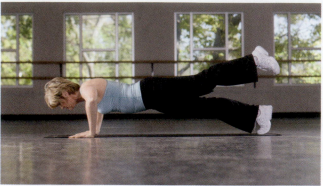

**Figure 16-18.** Push-up with one leg up performed with body weight as the primary resistance. Body weight exercises can be used to supplement a traditional resistance training program or used to create a training specifically utilizing body weight exercises. Body weight programs can be designed to increase intensity through exercise progressions and to enhance range of motion through a wide range of movements.

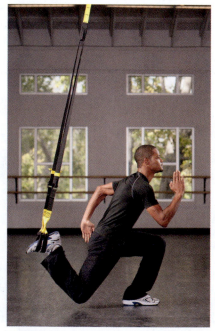

**Figure 16-17.** Single-leg squat exercise being performed using a suspension training system such as TRX. The advantages of using this type of equipment are that it can be performed in a variety of settings, resistance is set using body weight and positioning of the body (i.e., upright vs. prone/supine), resistance can be adjusted quickly based on the abilities of the individual client, and the movements target the core musculature in addition to the prime movers leading to improvements in balance and core stability.

- ViPR—hollow rubber tubes of varying lengths and thicknesses with handles that can be lifted, carried, tilted, thrown, and shifted while moving in all three planes
- Vibration plates—subscribing to Newton's second law (Force = mass × acceleration), these devices

increase muscle force output through acceleration rather than adding load

Regardless of the tools used, it is always important to perform a visual inspection of the equipment before every workout to ensure there is no damage to the equipment. It is not uncommon for bolts to loosen on a dumbbell or the rubber on a piece of resistance tubing to wear away. Taking the time to inspect equipment before its use will ensure the proper operation to achieve the desired training outcome.

## VIGNETTE conclusion

■ After 3 months of training, Marina is very satisfied with her results. She has toned her body, lost weight, and even managed to gain some muscle mass, while overcoming her fear of bulking up too much. She has enjoyed progressing from a linear model, which she followed for the first 6 weeks, to the nonlinear model that she now follows, which appears to keep her more engaged in her workouts. In addition, she has been willing to try a variety of different pieces of equipment and feels this has helped keep her program from becoming stale and "boring." Marina indicates that although she enjoys the convenience of machine-based training, her favorite training tool is the suspension trainer, because it challenges her to control her own body while overcoming the resistance of her own body.

# CRITICAL THINKING QUESTIONS

1. How, if at all, would a resistance training program be different among a teenage boy playing soccer, a middle-aged out-of-shape man, and a 65-year-old woman seeking to improve her overall quality of life? Complete a brief analysis of what resistance training parameters would be important to develop to improve each person's function or performance (i.e., load, volume, and power).

2. What recommendations would you provide to a woman interested in toning her body who had previously tried lifting lighter loads in isolation but failed to achieve any significant improvements? Be sure to consider the most effective and safe methods to incorporate to help her achieve her goals.

3. A person asks for your expertise after seeing a number of advertisements showing athletes pulling sleds, running with parachutes, jumping on and off of boxes, and swinging kettlebells. He asks whether those are appropriate training techniques for his athletic son, a senior and a defensive player on his high-school American football team. He also asks whether that same type of training would be appropriate for him, a 50-year-old deconditioned businessman. What suggestions would you make regarding this man and his son?

## ADDITIONAL RESOURCES

Baechle T, Earle R. *Essentials of Strength and Conditioning*. 3rd ed. Champaign, IL: Human Kinetics; 2008.

Bompa T, Haff G. *Periodization: Theory and Methodology of Training*. 5th ed. Champaign, IL: Human Kinetics; 2009.

Clark MA, Lucett SC, Sutton BG. *NASM's Essentials to Personal Fitness Training*. Philadelphia, PA: Lippincott Williams & Wilkins; 2012.

## REFERENCES

1. American College of Sports Medicine. *ACSM's Guidelines for Exercise Testing and Prescription*. 9th ed. Philadelphia, PA: Lippincott Williams & Wilkins; 2014.

2. Kraemer WJ, Zatsiorsky V. *Science and Practice of Strength Training*. 2nd ed. Champaign, IL: Human Kinetics; 2006.

3. Godfrey R, Blazevich A. Exercise and growth hormone in the aging individual, with special reference to the exercise-induced growth hormone response. *Int Sports Med J* 2004;5:246–261.

4. Ormsbee MJ, Thyfault JP, Johnson EA, Kraus RM, Choi MD, Hickner RC. Fat metabolism and acute resistance exercise in trained men. *J Appl Physiol*. 2007;102:1767–1772.

5. International Health, Racquet and Sportsclub Association/Leisure Trends Group (IHRSA). *The IHRSA Trend Reports*. Boulder, CO: IHRSA; May/August 2012.

6. Hunter RR, Wetzstein CJ, Fields DA, Brown A, Bamman MM. Resistance training increases total energy expenditure and free-living physical activity in older adults. *J Appl Physiol*. 2000;89:977–984.

7. Campbell W, Crim M, Young V, Evans W. Increased energy requirements and changes in body composition with resistance training in older adults. *Am J Clin Nutr*. 1994;60:167–175.

8. Bersheim E, Bahr R. Effect of exercise intensity, duration and mode on post-exercise oxygen consumption. *Sports Med*. 2003;33:1037–1061.

9. Thornton MK, Potteiger JA. Effects of resistance exercise bouts of different intensities but equal work on EPOC. *Med Sci Sports Exerc*. 2002;34:715–722.

10. Willardson JM. A brief review: Factors affecting the length of the rest interval between resistance exercise sets. *J Strength Cond Res*. 2006;20:978–984.

11. Murphy E, Swartzkopf R. Effects of standard set and circuit weight training on excess post-exercise oxygen consumption. *J Appl Sport Sci Res*. 1992;6:88–91.

12. U.S. Department of Health & Human Services. *2008 Physical Activity Guidelines for Americans*. 2008. Available at: www.health.gov/paguidelines/guidelines/default .aspx. Retrieved February 15, 2013.

13. Resnick B, Ory MG. Motivating frail older adults to be physically active. *J Active Aging*. 2006;5:41–50.

14. Ciolac EG, Brech GC, Greve JMD. Age does not affect exercise intensity progression among women. *J Strength Cond Res*. 2010;24:3023–3031.

15. Kerksick C, Wilborn C, Campbell B, et al. Early-phase adaptations to a split-body, linear periodization resistance training program in college-aged and middle-aged men. *J Strength Cond Res*. 2009;23:962–970.

16. Kraemer WJ, Ratamess N. Hormonal responses and adaptations to resistance exercise and training. *Sports Med*. 2005;35:339–361.

17. Kell R. The influence of periodized resistance training on strength changes in men and women. *J Strength Cond Res*. 2011;25:735–744.

18. Huberti HH, Hayes WC. Patellofemoral contact pressures: The influence of Q-angle and tendofemoral contact. *J Bone Joint Surg*. 1984;66A:715–724.

19. Neumann D. *Kinesiology of the Musculoskeletal System*. Philadelphia, PA: Elsevier; 2002.

20. Schoenfeld B. The mechanisms of muscle hypertrophy and their application to resistance training. *J Strength Cond Res*. 2010;24:2857–2872.

21. Bishop PA, Jones E, Woods AK. Recovery from training: A brief review. *J Strength Cond Res*. 2008;22:1015–1024.

22. Rahimi R, Qaderi M, Faraji H, Boroujerdi S. Effects of very short rest periods on hormonal responses to resistance exercise in men. *J Strength Cond Res*. 2010;24: 1851–1859.

23. Bompa T, Haff G. *Periodization: Theory and Methodology of Training*. 5th ed. Champaign, IL: Human Kinetics; 2009.

24. Nosaka K. Muscle soreness and damage and the repeated-bout effect. In: Tiidus PM, ed. *Skeletal Muscle Damage and Repair*. Champaign, IL: Human Kinetics; 2008.

25. Hansen S, Kvorning T, Kjaer M, Sjogaard G. The effect of short-term strength training on human skeletal muscle: The importance of physiologically elevated hormone levels. *Scand J Med Sci Sport*. 2001; 11:347–354.

26. Kraemer WJ, Fry AC, Warren BJ, et al. Acute hormonal responses in elite junior weightlifters. *Int J Sports Med*. 1992;13:103–109.

27. Linnamo V, Pakarinen A, Komi P, Kraemer WJ, Hakkinen K. Acute hormonal responses to submaximal and maximal heavy resistance and explosive exercises in men and women. *J Strength Cond Res*. 2005;19:566–571.

28. Fenwick C, Brown S, McGill S. Comparison of different rowing exercises: Trunk muscle activation and lumbar spine motion, load and stiffness. *J Strength Cond Res*. 2009;23:350–358.

29. Gotshalk LA, Berger RA, Kraemer WJ. Cardiovascular responses to a high-volume continuous circuit resistance training protocol. *J Strength Cond Res*. 2004;18:760–764.

30. Prestest J, Frollini A, De Lima C, et al. Comparison between linear and daily undulating periodized resistance training to increase strength. *J Strength Cond Res*. 2009;22:2437–2442.

31. Apel J, Lacey R, Kell R. A comparison of traditional and weekly undulating periodized strength training programs with total volume and intensity equated. *J Strength Cond Res*. 2011;25:694–703.

32. McGill S. *Low Back Disorders: Evidence Based Prevention and Rehabilitation*. 2nd ed. Champaign, IL: Human Kinetics; 2007.

33. Vingren J, Kraemer W, Ratamess N, Anderson J, Volek J, Maresh C. Testosterone physiology in resistance exercise and training. *Sports Med*. 2010;40:1037–1053.

34. Fry AC, Kraemer WJ, Stone MH, et al. Endocrine responses to overreaching before and after 1 year of weightlifting. *Can J Appl Physiol*. 1994;19:400–410.

35. Raastad T, Glomsheller T, Bjoro T, Hallen J. Changes in human skeletal muscle contractility and hormone status during 2 weeks of heavy strength training. *Eur J Appl Physiol*. 2001;84:54–63.

# *Practice What You Know:* McGill's Torso Muscular Endurance Test Battery

Possessing a strong core is important for the performance of simple ADL, from lifting a heavy laundry basket to swinging a golf club. Core stability involves complex movement patterns that continually change as a function of the three-dimensional torque needed to support the various positions of the body. McGill[32] states that back problems can often be alleviated by improving the motor patterns of the abdominal musculature and then ingraining those new patterns into the neuromuscular system. To determine balanced core strength and stability, it is important to assess all sides of the torso. The benefit of each one of these tests is to assess the inter-relationships among the three torso tests. The tests are evaluated collectively. Poor endurance capacity of the torso muscles or an imbalance among the muscle groups that comprise the trunk flexors, extensors, and lateral flexors is believed to contribute to low-back dysfunction and core instability.

## TRUNK FLEXOR ENDURANCE TEST

The flexor endurance test is the first in the battery of three tests that assesses **muscular endurance** of the deep core muscles (i.e., transverse abdominis, quadratus lumborum, and erector spinae; Fig. 1). It is a timed test that involves a static, isometric contraction of the anterior muscles, stabilizing the spine until the individual exhibits fatigue and can no longer hold the assumed position. As clients move through this battery of tests, make sure they are not holding their breath.

### Contraindications
This test may not be suitable for individuals who suffer from low-back pain, have had recent surgery, or are in the midst of an acute low-back flare-up.

**Equipment**
- Stopwatch
- Board (or step)

**Pretest Procedure**
- After explaining the purpose of the flexor endurance test, describe the proper body position.
  - √ The starting position requires the client to be seated, with the hips and knees bent to 90 degrees, aligning the hips, knees, and second toe.
  - √ Instruct the client to fold his or her arms across the chest, touching each hand to the opposite shoulder, lean against a board positioned at a 60-degree incline, and keep the head in a neutral position (Fig. 1).
  - √ It is important to ask the client to press his or her shoulders into the board and maintain this position throughout the test.
  - √ Instruct the client to engage the abdominals to maintain a flat-to-neutral spine. The back should never be allowed to arch during the test.
  - √ The fitness professional can anchor the toes under a strap or manually stabilize the feet if necessary.
- The goal of the test is to remove the back support and ask the client to hold this 60-degree position for as long as possible.

## *Practice What You Know:* McGill's Torso Muscular Endurance Test Battery

• Encourage the client to practice this position before attempting the test.

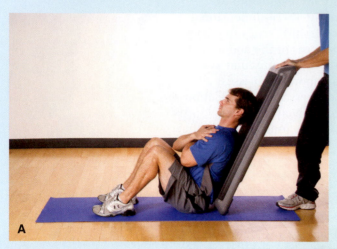

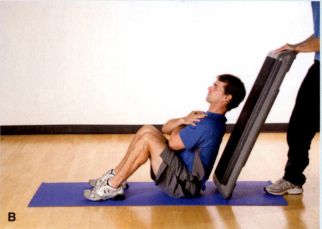

**Figure 1.**

**Test Protocol and Administration**
• The fitness professional starts the stopwatch as he or she moves the board about 4 inches (10 cm) back, while the client maintains the 60-degree, suspended position.
• Terminate the test when there is a noticeable change in the trunk position:
  √ Watch for a deviation from the neutral spine (i.e., the shoulders rounding forward) or an increase in the low-back arch.
  √ No part of the back should touch the backrest.
• Record the client's time on the testing form.

## TRUNK LATERAL ENDURANCE TEST

The trunk lateral endurance test, also called the *side-bridge test*, assesses muscular endurance of the lateral core muscles (i.e., transverse abdominis, obliques, quadratus lumborum, and erector spinae; Fig. 2). Similar to the trunk flexor endurance test, this is a set of timed tests that involve isometric contractions of the lateral muscles on each side of the trunk that stabilize the spine.

### Contraindications
This test may not be suitable for the following individuals:
• Clients with shoulder pain or weakness
• Clients who suffer from low-back pain, have had recent surgery, and/or are in the midst of an acute low-back flare-up

## *Practice What You Know:* McGill's Torso Muscular Endurance Test Battery

**Equipment**
- Stopwatch
- Mat (optional)

**Pretest Procedure**
- After explaining the purpose of this test, describe the proper body position.
  - √ The starting position requires the client to be on his or her side with extended legs, aligning the feet on top of each other or in a tandem position (heel-to-toe).
  - √ Have the client place the lower arm under the body and the upper arm on the side of the body.
  - √ When the client is ready, instruct him or her to assume a full side-bridge position, keeping both legs extended and the sides of the feet on the floor. The elbow of the lower arm should be positioned directly under the shoulder with the forearm facing out (the forearm can be placed palm-down for balance and support), and the upper arm should be resting along the side or across the chest to the opposite shoulder.
  - √ The hips should be elevated off the mat and the body should be in straight alignment (i.e., head, neck, torso, hips, and legs). The torso should be supported only by the client's foot/feet and the forearm (Fig. 2).
- The goal of the test is to hold this position for as long as possible. Once the client breaks the position, the test is terminated.
- Encourage the client to practice this position before attempting the test.

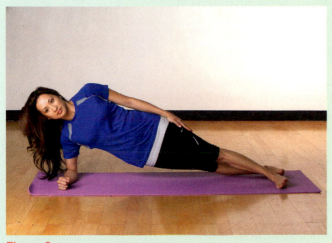

**Figure 2.**

**Test Protocol and Administration**
- The fitness professional starts the stopwatch as the client moves into the side-bridge position.
- Terminate the test when there is a noticeable change in the trunk position.
  - √ A deviation from the neutral spine (e.g., the hips dropping downward)
  - √ The hips shifting forward or backward in an effort to maintain balance and stability
- Record the client's time on the testing form.
- Repeat the test on the opposite side and record this value on the testing form.

### TRUNK EXTENSOR ENDURANCE TEST

The trunk extensor endurance test is generally used to assess muscular endurance of the torso extensor muscles (i.e., erector spinae, longissimus, iliocostalis, and multifidi; Fig. 3). This is a timed test involving an isometric contraction of the trunk extensor muscles that stabilize the spine.

## *Practice What You Know:* McGill's Torso Muscular Endurance Test Battery

### Contraindications

This test may not be suitable for the following individuals:

- A client with major strength deficiencies, where the client cannot even lift the torso for a forward flexed position to a neutral position
- A client with high body mass, in which case it would be difficult for the fitness professional to support the client's suspended upper-body weight
- A client who suffers from low-back pain, has had recent back surgery, and/or is in the midst of an acute low-back flare-up

### Equipment

- Elevated, sturdy examination table
- Nylon strap
- Stopwatch

### Pretest Procedure

- After explaining the purpose of the test, explain the proper body position.
  - √ The starting position requires the client to be prone, positioning the iliac crests at the table edge while supporting the upper body on the arms, which are placed on the floor or on a riser.
  - √ Secure the lower body with the legs supported on a table while the torso, or upper body, is suspended over the ground.
  - √ While the client is supporting the weight of his or her upper body, anchor the client's lower legs to the table using a strap. If a strap is not used, the fitness professional will have to use his or her own body weight to stabilize the client's legs. Client body size in relation to the fitness professional may become a limiting factor in this particular test.
- The goal of the test is to hold this position for as long as possible. Once the client falls below horizontal, the test is terminated.
- Encourage the client to practice this position before attempting the test.

### Test Protocol and Administration

- When ready, the client lifts/extends the torso until it is parallel to the floor with his or her arms crossed over the chest (Fig. 3). This position requires activation of the torso extensor muscles (i.e., erector spinae, longissimus, iliocostalis, and multifidi).
- Start the stopwatch as soon as the client assumes this position.
- Terminate the test when the client can no longer maintain the position.
- Record the client's time on the testing form.

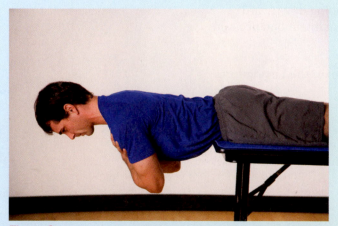

Figure 3.

# *Practice What You Know:* McGill's Torso Muscular Endurance Test Battery

## EVALUATION AND APPLICATION OF PERFORMANCE FOR MCGILL'S TORSO MUSCULAR ENDURANCE TEST BATTERY

Each individual test in this testing battery is not a primary indicator of current or future back problems. McGill[32] has proved that the *relationships* among the tests are important indicators of muscle imbalances that can lead to back pain. In fact, even in a person with little or no back pain, the ratios can still be off, suggesting that low-back pain may eventually occur without diligent attention to a solid core-conditioning program. McGill[32] suggests that the following ratios indicate balanced endurance among the muscle groups:

- Flexion/extension ratio should be less than 1.0.
  - √ For example, a flexion score of 120 seconds and an extension score of 150 seconds generate a ratio score of 0.80.
- Right-side bridge (RSB)/left-side bridge (LSB) scores should be no greater than 0.05 from a balanced score of 1.0.
  - √ For example, an RSB score of 88 seconds and an LSB score of 92 seconds generate a ratio score of 0.96, which is within the 0.05 range from 1.0.
- Side-bridge (either side)/extension ratio should be less than 0.75.
  - √ For example, an RSB score of 88 seconds and an extension score of 150 seconds generate a ratio score of 0.59.

Demonstrated deficiencies in these core functional assessments should be addressed during exercise programming as part of the foundational exercises for a client. The goal is to create ratios consistent with McGill's recommendations. Muscular endurance, more so than muscular strength or even range of motion, has been shown to be an accurate predictor of back health.[32] Low-back stabilization exercises have the most benefit when performed daily. When working with clients with low-back dysfunction, it is prudent to include daily stabilization exercises in their home exercise plans.

## ESTIMATED ONE-REPETITION MAXIMUM TESTS

A 1 RM test is an assessment that attempts to measure a person's strength, which requires an all-out exertion against a heavy load. However, these tests are not appropriate for many individuals.

### Considerations and Contraindications for 1 RM Testing

- Many strength tests are performed using free weights, so proper form and control are necessary elements. Novice exercisers may not have the familiarity or skills to handle the heavier free weights.
- Beginning exercisers are often unsure of their abilities and tend to quit before their true maximum.
- Proper breathing patterns are necessary. Clients should avoid the Valsalva maneuver or any other form of breath-holding.
- Individuals with hypertension and/or a history of vascular disease should avoid a 1 RM testing protocol.

## *Practice What You Know:* McGill's Torso Muscular Endurance Test Battery

When working with inexperienced exercisers or individuals with health considerations that would preclude them from performing a 1 RM test, it is appropriate to assess strength using submaximal efforts. Table 1 provides prediction coefficients of 1 RM for a client completing anywhere between 1 and 10 repetitions at a maximal effort. Submaximal tests that exceed 10 repetitions assess muscular endurance and not muscular strength.

> The following table offers fitness professionals a way to estimate a client's 1 RM without requiring the client to perform an exercise with maximal effort. In fact, the client's 1 RM can be estimated by simply observing a workout and making the appropriate calculation. For example, a client is performing bench presses during his or her workout and the trainer observes that he or she consistently completes 8 repetitions with 160 lb (73 kg). Using the coefficient of 1.255, the client's 1 RM is calculated as follows:
> 1 RM = 160 lb × 1.255 = 201 lb (91 kg)

### Table 1. One-Repetition Maximum Prediction Coefficients

| NUMBER OF REPETITIONS COMPLETED | SQUAT OR LEG-PRESS COEFFICIENT | BENCH- OR CHEST-PRESS COEFFICIENT |
| --- | --- | --- |
| 1 | 1.000 | 1.000 |
| 2 | 1.0475 | 1.035 |
| 3 | 1.13 | 1.08 |
| 4 | 1.1575 | 1.115 |
| 5 | 1.2 | 1.15 |
| 6 | 1.242 | 1.18 |
| 7 | 1.284 | 1.22 |
| 8 | 1.326 | 1.255 |
| 9 | 1.368 | 1.29 |
| 10 | 1.41 | 1.325 |

*Source:* Data from Brzycki M. Strength testing: Predicting a one-rep max from reps-to-fatigue. *J Phys Educ Recreat Dance* 1993;68:88–90.

# *Practice What You Know:* McGill's Torso Muscular Endurance Test Battery

**Testing Protocol**
- Determine the number of repetitions that is appropriate for the client based on his or her current training regimen or experience (e.g., Mary usually performs 3 sets of 8 repetitions at 60 lb [27 kg]).

**Sets**
- Have the client perform one or two warm-up sets at a lower intensity than the target weight and allow 1 to 2 minutes of recovery between the sets.
- Instruct the client to perform the first attempt at a personal best, completing the targeted number of repetitions consistent with his or her current training (e.g., Mary completes 1 set of 8 repetitions at 60 lb [27 kg]).
- If the client is successful, he or she should rest for approximately 2 minutes and repeat the personal-best effort with a heavier load.
- If the client is unsuccessful at achieving the goal repetitions, simply use the actual number completed in the calculation (e.g., Mary completed 3 squat repetitions with 66 lb [30 kg], which equates to a 1 RM equivalent of 71 lb [32 kg]).

## Application

Assessments can also be performed to determine left-to-right muscle balance or appropriate ratios of agonist-to-antagonist muscle strength. Muscle imbalances occur from improper training, overuse of one side of the body (e.g., tennis serves or golf swings), or structural imbalances caused by injury or poor posture or body mechanics. Muscle balance is essential to prevent injury, enhance sports performance, and avoid chronic conditions later in life. Table 2 presents the recommended strength ratios between opposing muscle groups.

**Table 2.** **Appropriate Strength Ratios**

| JOINT | MOVEMENTS | MUSCLES | RATIO |
|---|---|---|---|
| Shoulder | Flexion/Extension | Anterior deltoids/Trapezius, posterior deltoids | 2:3 |
| Shoulder | Internal rotation/ External rotation | Subscapularis/Supraspinatus, infraspinatus, teres minor | 3:2 |
| Elbow | Flexion/Extension | Biceps/Triceps | 1:1 |
| Lumbar spine | Flexion/Extension | Iliopsoas, abdominals/Erector spinae | 1:1 |
| Hip | Flexion/Extension | Iliopsoas, rectus abdominis, tensor fascia latae/Erector spinae, gluteus maximus, hamstrings | 1:1 |
| Knee | Flexion/Extension | Hamstrings/Quadriceps | 2:3 |
| Ankle | Plantarflexion/ Dorsiflexion | Gastrocnemius/Tibialis anterior | 3:1 |
| Ankle | Inversion/Eversion | Tibialis anterior/Peroneals | 1:1 |

*Source:* Heyward VH. *Advanced Fitness Assessment and Exercise Prescription.* 6th ed. Champaign, IL: Human Kinetics; 2010.

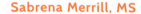

Sabrena Merrill, MS

# CHAPTER 17

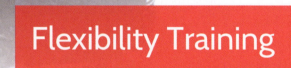

Flexibility Training

## CHAPTER OUTLINE

## CHAPTER OUTLINE–cont'd

## LEARNING OUTCOMES

1. Define *flexibility* and explain its relevance for activities of daily living.
2. Explain the benefits of flexibility training.
3. Identify factors that influence flexibility.
4. Describe mechanical and neurological properties of stretching and how to maximize these properties.
5. Describe the six major stretching modalities.
6. Recommend a flexibility program for an individual based on established stretching guidelines.

## ANCILLARY LINK

Visit Davis*Plus* at http://davisplus.fadavis.com for study and practice resources, including online quizzes, animations that help explain physiological processes, podcasts concerning news and career trends in exercise physiology, and practice references.

## *VIGNETTE*

■ Mike is a competitive cyclist who meets with Noah, his team's athletic trainer, to discuss updating his training goals. Besides increasing fitness, Mike is interested in improving the flexibility in his upper body and relieving intermittent back pain. The inflexibility Mike experiences in his upper extremities is related to years of flexing his spine forward during cycling training and competition. Thus, he exhibits an exaggerated rounded forward position with his spine and shoulders. Mike has received medical clearance from his physician to perform strength and stretching exercises to improve his posture.

How can a program of focused stretching help Mike improve posture and flexibility in his upper extremities?

Flexibility training is an integral part of participation in exercise and sports at all levels, competitive or recreational. It is also an important component in the recommended general guidelines for physical activity for healthy adults.[1,2] Consequently, stretching to improve flexibility is regularly included in warm-up and cooldown exercises. Although stretching before and after participation in physical activity and sport is recommended as a method to enhance performance and prevent injuries, the evidence to support this supposition remains unclear.[3] Nonetheless, having inadequate flexibility that results in stiff or rigid muscles poses a health risk in that the essential activities of daily living, such as bathing, eating, and dressing, in addition to instrumental activities such as cooking and cleaning, become more difficult, especially with increasing age.[4]

The issue of stretching and decreased performance has recently gained attention. It is not clear whether there is an optimal amount of flexibility needed for performance or whether additional flexibility in flexible athletes is needed. Theories that address compromised performance caused by stretching include less efficient movement because of decreased joint stability, injuries resulting from increases in tissue compliance with decreased energy absorption by tendons and muscles, creation of joint positions that could stretch ligaments too far, and increased pain tolerance leading to skeletal and soft-tissue damage. However, research on the adverse effects of stretching and enhanced flexibility is inconsistent, and there is some evidence that increased flexibility may actually enhance performance.[5]

Despite the inconsistency of the evidence supporting or discounting the use of stretching as a means to enhance performance, certain sport-specific tasks seem to be improved when the participant possesses more than average joint extensibility. Athletes such as gymnasts and dancers may prevent muscle strain or joint sprain by maintaining greater than normal joint ranges of motion. This enhanced flexibility allows these athletes to complete the extreme ranges of motion that their sports demand. However, this should not be interpreted to mean that all individuals should strive to achieve maximum joint flexibility to prevent injury.

This chapter describes the many variables that affect flexibility and the acute responses and chronic adaptations to flexibility training. Various stretching modalities and guidelines to maximize performance and function are explored. Understanding the contribution of flexibility to health and physical function helps health and fitness professionals in the promotion and design of safe and effective flexibility training programs for their clients.

## ORIGIN OF FLEXIBILITY TRAINING

Although the origin of training to enhance flexibility is unknown, stretching has been depicted throughout history in paintings, carvings, and literature. Its uses have ranged from constructive (e.g., improving one's well-being and enhancing performance) to destructive (e.g., torture and execution). Thus, when evaluating a client's **range of motion (ROM)** and formulating an exercise program for enhancing flexibility, health and fitness professionals must consider not only the benefits associated with improved flexibility, but also the potential for injury.

Historically, the ancient Greeks used flexibility training to enhance their performances during dancing, acrobatic stunts, and wrestling. Furthermore, it is thought that the Greeks incorporated stretching into their medical and therapeutic programs, military training, and athletic endeavors. In Eastern cultures, stretching postures called **asanas** have been used in yoga practices to develop both a higher state of well-being and improved postural awareness. In addition, Eastern traditions have viewed flexibility as a vital component in developing defensive and offensive skills in various martial arts (e.g., karate and tae kwon do).

In relation to the time stretching has been practiced throughout history, the scientific study of the influence of flexibility on health and performance is still in its infancy. However, the body of research thus far has revealed that flexibility is a significant health-related component of fitness.[1,6]

## FLEXIBILITY AND RANGE OF MOTION

Flexibility is defined as the ROM possessed around a specific joint or series of joints. In biomechanical terms, flexibility refers to changes in the length of a musculotendinous unit as a result of alterations in its viscoelastic properties; that is, the length of a muscle and its attached tendon can be changed given the fact that muscle has some specific mechanical properties, such as elasticity (e.g., rubber band). This viscoelasticity enables the muscle to change length when a load is applied over time (e.g., stretch) and then resume its original size and shape when the force is removed (i.e., when the stretch is removed).

Although there are many explanations of "normal" flexibility, one interpretation is to envision it as the ability to move a joint fluidly through its full ROM without causing undue stress to the musculotendinous unit, and doing so well within the limits of pain or discomfort (i.e., pain free). This ROM must not compromise joint **stability**, which was previously defined as the ability to control the position or movement of a joint. Using the structure of a building as an example, stability is improved by reducing movement at the building joints or within the structure. Although this logic applies in humans, people also need to move, and thus have a need for stability to resist loads (e.g., gravity) while exhibiting necessary amounts of mobility (to move). Joints that are excessively mobile (hypermobile) may compromise stability and increase the potential for injury.

## TYPES OF FLEXIBILITY

There are two basic types of flexibility: static and dynamic. **Static flexibility** refers to the ROM about a joint with no emphasis on the speed of movement. Its limits are defined primarily by the extensibility of the musculotendinous unit. In other words, static flexibility is the ability to assume and maintain an extended position at one end or point in a joint's ROM (e.g., **static stretch**). Examples of static flexibility are holding a modified hurdler hamstrings stretch or maintaining a leg split position on the floor (Fig. 17-1).

**Dynamic flexibility**, in contrast, involves movement and is based on a joint's ability to move through its ROM without resistance. Although a clear-cut definition of dynamic flexibility has yet to be universally accepted, it can be thought of as the ability to move a joint through its ROM while performing a physical task at normal or rapid speeds. Dynamic flexibility represents the resistance encountered within a joint or series of joints to active movement. A movement associated with a high degree of dynamic flexibility is a split leap commonly performed by ballet dancers. A certain degree of functional, dynamic flexibility is required for most athletic endeavors. Figure 17-2 shows an example of dynamic flexibility in the sequence of the inverted flyer exercise.

**Ballistic flexibility**, which is a form of dynamic flexibility, refers to quick bobbing, bouncing, or jerking motions (e.g., **ballistic stretching**). An example of

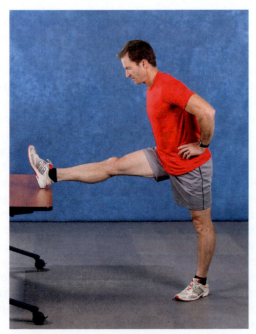

**Figure 17-1.** Example of static stretching with the standing hurdler's stretch.

ballistic stretching is touching the toes repeatedly in rapid succession to stretch the hamstrings.

## BENEFITS OF FLEXIBILITY

There are many purported benefits to good flexibility and participating in a regular program of flexibility training. The potential benefits and common motives for improving ROM include:

- Muscle relaxation and stress reduction
- Decreased risk for low-back pain
- Relief from muscle cramps
- Prevention and/or alleviation of muscle soreness post-activity
- Reduction in the incidence and severity of injury

The results from research regarding both qualitative and quantitative measures of the potential rewards from a regular program of stretching vary, indicating that there is no clear-cut answer to whether regular flexibility training offers the benefits extolled by many.[5,7-9] It is generally accepted that adequate levels of flexibility are required for the maintenance of functional independence and performance of activities of daily living such as stooping down to pick up a pair of shoes or getting out of the back seat of a two-door car. However, compared with research on other components of fitness (i.e., cardiorespiratory endurance, muscle strength, and muscle endurance), studies on flexibility do not substantiate the importance of stretching in health-related fitness.

### Muscle Relaxation and Stress Reduction

Two of the most important benefits of a flexibility program may be to promote muscle relaxation and to reduce stress. Studies have shown that performing stretching exercises reduces mental tension, slows the breathing rate, and reduces blood pressure, which are all important for counteracting the body's physiological response to chronic stress.[10-12] Technically, relaxation is the cessation of muscular tension. Abnormally high levels of muscular tension, whether caused by stress or improper body mechanics, result in several negative side effects. In addition to decreased sensory awareness and increased blood pressure, excessive muscular tension contributes to a waste of energy because a contracted muscle requires more energy to sustain than a relaxed muscle. Furthermore, an undesirable level of muscular tension creates a toxic environment for the affected muscle cells because the resultant decrease in blood circulation to the muscle prevents an optimal amount of oxygen and other essential nutrients from entering the cells. This causes waste products to accumulate in the cells; as a result, fatigue and pain commonly accompany muscular tension.

A contracted and chronically tense muscle is less supple, less strong, and unable to absorb the stress of

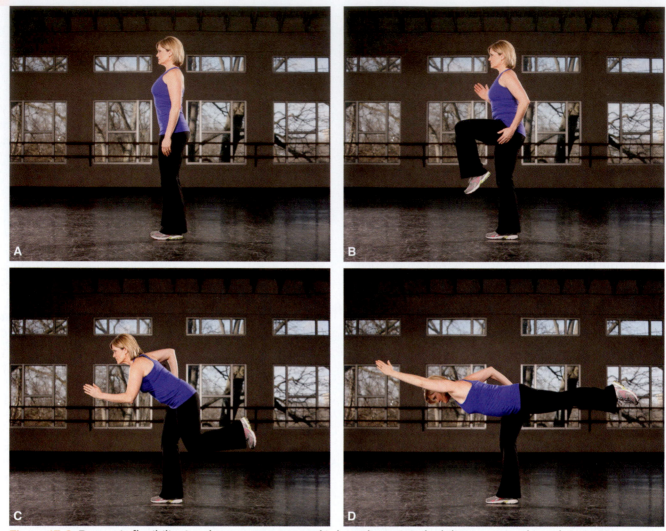

**Figure 17-2.** Dynamic flexibility involves movement and is based on a joint's ability to move through its range of motion without resistance. This sequence shows the inverted flyer exercise.

various types of movement. A stretching program that promotes elongation of tight muscles to facilitate muscular relaxation and to provide relief can help combat this condition. Studies conducted to determine the minimum duration and number of repetitions of stretches required to decrease muscular tension in tight muscles have shown that simple passive stretching techniques can be effective. It appears that passive stretches held for 15 to 60 seconds and repeated up to four times per muscle group can bring about immediate, significant decreases in musculotendinous stiffness.[1,13–17]

## Decreased Low-Back Pain

Low-back pain represents a significant public health problem, as it has become one of the most common ailments in industrialized societies; it can affect up to 80% of the population and is reported to be the most common cause of functional limitation in individuals younger than 45 years.[18] Is flexibility a contributing factor in low-back pain? This remains a controversial topic of study among back pain researchers. Thus, studies investigating the

cause of common low-back pain have been performed to determine the best methods for preventing and rehabilitating the condition.

Results from numerous studies support the theory that adequate flexibility or stretching can help to reduce the risk for or severity of low-back pain.[19–26] However, there is little evidence to support the use of exercises to maintain or increase spinal ROM as a protective measure against back pain.[27] In fact, some exercise programs that include loading of the spine throughout its ranges of motion (i.e., flexion/extension, lateral flexion, and rotation) have produced negative results, and greater spine mobility has been associated with an increase in back problems such that those who have greater spine ROM are at greater risk for future back troubles.[28]

The most successful exercise programs for low-back pain emphasize trunk stabilization through exercises performed with a neutral spine (i.e., maintaining the natural curves of the spine) that emphasize muscles of the trunk (e.g., abdominals) and hip regions (e.g., hamstrings, glutes).[27] In general, for individuals with low-back pain, spine flexibility should be emphasized only after they have undergone a thorough evaluation by a medical professional and then have participated in a program of conditioning of the muscles supporting the spine.

## In Your Own Words

Lisa regularly attends yoga class and is very proficient at mastering the postures. In fact, she is able to flex and extend her joints into extreme ranges as a result of her consistent yoga practice. However, Lisa often suffers from low-back pain, which puzzles her because she is clearly very flexible and had thought that being flexible was the key to a healthy back. How would you explain to Lisa that her hypermobility might be playing a role in her back pain?

## Relief From Muscle Cramps

Stretching has been reported to be effective in reducing the occurrence and severity of muscle cramps.[29] A typical muscle cramp is actually neural in origin and is initiated when a muscle already in its most shortened position involuntarily contracts. Swimmers often experience muscle cramps in their calves, because proper kicking form requires a pointed-toe position with the gastrocnemius in a shortened, contracted state. In addition, most individuals adopt a plantar-flexed ankle position during sleep, which may contribute to nocturnal calf cramps. Studies have shown that muscle cramps cease when the involved muscle group is passively stretched or when there is an active contraction of its **antagonist** (opposite) muscle group.[30–32] Both of these relief-providing actions disrupt the muscle's electrical activity and allow it to relax into a more lengthened state. Other research has supported the use of regular stretching as a preventative measure against painful muscle cramps. In fact, one study found that a group of 44 subjects was cured of nocturnal cramps after 1 week of calf stretches performed three times per day.[33]

## Prevention of Delayed-Onset Muscle Soreness

Overexertion and strenuous muscular exercise often result in muscular pain. One type of post-activity discomfort, **delayed-onset muscular soreness (DOMS)**, involves muscle pain that appears approximately 12 hours after activity and becomes most intense after 24 to 48 hours. Typically, DOMS will gradually subside so that the muscle becomes symptom free after 3 or 4 days. This condition has been described as a syndrome of delayed muscle pain, which leads to increased muscle tension, edema (swelling as a result of a collection of fluid in connective tissue), increased stiffness, and resistance to stretching. Review Chapters 10 and 16 for more information on DOMS.

Muscle soreness may best be prevented by beginning at a moderate level of activity and gradually increasing the intensity of the exercise over time. A popular theory states that the extent of muscular pain, soreness, or stiffness corresponds to the state of training of the structures involved. For example, people with deconditioned, tight muscles usually show a significantly higher DOMS response when subjected to a variety of physical stresses. Thus, fibers and connective tissues are more susceptible to strain and rupture.

In addition to starting an exercise program at a low intensity and gradually building the intensity over time, performing an adequate warm-up before strenuous exercise and stretching may help to prevent DOMS. Without a proper warm-up, cold tendons and muscles have a greater tendency to strain and rupture because of poor blood circulation and resistance to stretch. Currently, there is little experimental evidence with human subjects to support this theory, most likely because researchers are hesitant to conduct experiments in which subjects may be injured. Even so, it is reasonable to assume—based on muscle physiology—that a warm-up is a prudent protective measure.

## Injury Prevention

One of the most debated reasons for participating in a regular stretching program is injury prevention.[3,34] It is commonly believed that individuals who are less flexible are more likely to experience musculoskeletal pain and injury. The resulting presumption is that, in individuals with shortened, tight muscles, stretching increases flexibility by elongating tissues to a more normal range, promoting optimal function and reducing the risk for musculoskeletal injury. However, little evidence exists that documents a relationship between increased flexibility and reduced incidence of injury. Although many studies in sports literature have demonstrated that stretching before or during an athletic activity helps to reduce the incidence of strains and sprains, a roughly equal number of studies have shown that stretching either has no effect on injury rates or may actually increase the risk for musculoskeletal pain or injury in athletes.[5] Furthermore, preparation for athletic activity often includes both stretching and warm-up, making it difficult to assess their independent effects on injury prevention.[3] For example, studies examining stretching combined with warm-up, strength, and balance training suggest that this combination can prevent ankle and knee injuries, but the independent effects of warm-up and stretching were not investigated.[35,36]

Research findings support the hypothesis that more-than-normal joint extensibility is beneficial in some sports (e.g., gymnastics, diving, ice skating, and dance) to prevent injury, but this should not be interpreted to suggest that maximum flexibility will prevent musculoskeletal strain or joint sprain.[3,5] Most studies on flexibility and injury incidence rely on college-age athletes as subjects. It may be erroneous to assume that these athletes behave the same way as the average, nonathletic population. Although research is lacking in support of flexibility training to prevent muscle and connective tissue injuries, conceptually, it is logical to assume that stretching programs for athletes and regular exercisers is advantageous. Refer to Chapter 30 for more information pertaining to common musculoskeletal injuries.

### V I G N E T T E  continued

■ To help Mike achieve his goals of increased health and fitness, together with improved posture and flexibility in his upper extremities, Noah designs a comprehensive program that includes cardiorespiratory endurance exercise, resistance training, and stretching. For his cardiorespiratory endurance exercise, Noah recommends that Mike limit his cycling to team practice time and perform other modalities, such as elliptical training and walking or jogging, as complementary training so that his body can spend time in a more upright position (instead of flexed forward posture on a bike). While whole-body muscular conditioning is implemented, Mike's resistance training has a special focus on exercises that strengthen the posterior trunk and shoulders to help counter the forward (anterior) pull of his imbalanced posture. Mike's stretching program consists of dynamic stretches for the whole body, as well as focused static stretches for the anterior trunk and shoulders.

## CONTRIBUTING FACTORS TO FLEXIBILITY

Effective flexibility training necessitates an understanding of the normal ROM of various movements at the different joints within the body (Table 17-1). An individual who exhibits greater than normal ROM is considered **hypermobile**, whereas an individual demonstrating less than normal ROM is considered **hypomobile**. Familiarity with ROM at these joints allows practitioners and participants of flexibility training to understand which muscle groups appear to have adequate flexibility and which need improvement.

Although Table 17-1 depicts the average ROM for healthy adults, it is important to understand that there are inherent differences between people. Genetic predisposition, age, sex, joint structure, physical activity levels, previous injury, activities of daily living, and body temperature can all influence a person's ROM. Other contributing factors to flexibility include:
- Soft-tissue factors
- Age
- Previous injury
- Tissue temperature

### Soft-Tissue Factors

Muscle and connective tissue are two important determinants of flexibility. The tightness of these soft-tissue structures is a major contributor to both static and dynamic flexibility. Muscle is a complex structure—composed of progressively smaller units—that is very adaptable to the stresses placed on it. Connective tissue structures (i.e., tendons, ligaments, and fascia) contain a wide variety of specialized cells that perform functions including proprioception, protection, storage, binding, connection, and general support and repair. A classic study by Johns and Wright[37] demonstrated the relative contributions of soft tissues to the total resistance encountered by the joint during movement throughout its ROM. The basic types of soft tissue contribute resistance to movement as follows:
- Joint capsule (ligaments)—47%
- Muscle (fascia)—41%
- Tendons—10%
- Skin—2%

### Muscle Tissue

Muscle contraction, relaxation, and elongation are all influenced by the structure of myofibrils discussed previously in Chapter 9. Following is a review of sarcomeres and other specific structures to understand their role in flexibility. A structure called **titin** is a connecting filament thought to be responsible for maintaining myosin's position between the Z lines (even during sarcomere stretching), as well as maintaining some resting tension within the muscle fiber. The titin molecules extend from the Z line to the center of the sarcomere (i.e., M line), where it is firmly bound to the myosin filament. When the sarcomere is stretched, the region of titin attached to myosin behaves as if it were rigidly bound to that thick filament (myosin) and resists elongation. By contrast, the region of titin attached to the Z line acts as an elastic component that allows sarcomere stretching. Thus, when a stretch is applied to a muscle, the segment of titin between the end of the myosin filament and the Z line is the primary contributor that allows sarcomere lengthening.

For a muscle fiber to be lengthened, an external force must act on it. Forces include gravity, momentum, antagonistic muscle contractions (active stretching—e.g., contracting the quadriceps to extend the knee and stretch the hamstrings), and the force provided by another person or one's own body (passive stretch—gently having someone move the knee into an extended position to stretch the hamstrings). To stretch effectively without risking injury, the sarcomere should be elongated to a length at which there is a slight overlap of the filaments, with at least one cross-bridge maintained between the actin and the myosin. This length has been found to be approximately 50% to 67% greater than the sarcomere's resting length, which allows movement through wide ranges of motion.[38]

## Table 17-1. Average Range of Motion for Healthy Adults

| JOINT AND MOVEMENT | ROM* | JOINT AND MOVEMENT | ROM* |
|---|---|---|---|
| **Shoulder/Scapulae** | | **Thoracolumbar Spine** | |
| Flexion | 150–180 | Lumbar flexion | 40–45 |
| Extension | 50–60 | Thoracic flexion | 30–40 |
| Abduction | 180 | Lumbar extension | 30–40 |
| Internal/medial rotation | 70–80 | Thoracic extension | 20–30 |
| External/lateral rotation | 90 | Lumbar rotation | 10–15 |
| Shoulder horizontal adduction | 90* | Thoracic rotation | 35 |
| Shoulder horizontal abduction | 30–40* | Lumbar lateral flexion | 20 |
| **Elbow** | | Thoracic lateral flexion | 20–25 |
| Flexion | 145 | **Hip** | |
| Extension | 0 | Flexion | 100–120 |
| **Radio-ulnar** | | Extension | 10–30 |
| Pronation | 90 | Abduction | 40–45 |
| Supination | 90 | Adduction | 20–30 |
| **Wrist** | | Internal/medial rotation | 35–45 |
| Flexion | 80 | External/lateral rotation | 45–60 |
| Extension | 70 | **Knee** | |
| Radial deviation | 20 | Flexion | 125–145 |
| Ulnar deviation | 45 | Extension | 0–10 |
| **Cervical Spine** | | **Ankle** | |
| Flexion | 45–50 | Dorsiflexion | 20 |
| Extension | 45–75 | Plantarflexion | 45–50 |
| Lateral flexion | 45 | **Subtalar** | |
| Rotation | 65–75 | Inversion | 30–35 |
| | | Eversion | 15–20 |

*Zero point (0 degrees) is with the arms positioned in frontal-plane abduction at shoulder height.
ROM, range of motion.
*Source:* Data from Kendall FP, McCreary, EK, Provance PG, et al. *Muscles Testing and Function with Posture and Pain.*
  5th ed. Baltimore, MD: Lippincott Williams & Wilkins; 2005.

## Connective Tissue

Connective tissue is the material between the cells of the body that gives tissue both form and strength. This "cellular glue" is also involved in delivering nutrients to the tissue. Connective tissue is made up of dozens of proteins, including collagens, proteoglycans, and glycoproteins. Collagen, the most abundant protein in the body, is particularly significant when explaining joint ROM. The two major physical properties of collagen fibers are its tensile strength and relative inextensibility; that is, structures that contain large amounts of collagen tend to limit motion and resist stretch. Thus, collagen fibers are the main constituents of tissues such as ligaments and tendons that are subjected to pulling forces.

One of the mechanisms behind collagen's great tensile strength and relative inextensibility is its banded, or striated, structure (much like the pattern observed in muscle tissue). When viewed under a microscope, collagen in tendons is arranged in wavy bundles called **fascicles**. These fascicles are composed of **fibrils**, which, in turn, consist of bundles of **subfibrils**. Each subfibril is composed of bundles of collagen filaments.

In addition to a striated pattern, connective tissue also contains wavelike folds of collagen fibers known as **crimp**. The mechanical properties of collagen fibers are such that each fibril behaves much like a mechanical spring (each fiber is, therefore, like a collection of springs). When a fiber is pulled, its crimp straightens and its length increases. As in a mechanical spring, energy is stored within the fiber (spring), and it is the release of this energy that returns the fiber to its resting state when the stretch force is removed.

Compared with a sarcomere, a collagenous fiber is relatively inextensible. In a classic study of collagen elasticity, it was demonstrated that the collagen fiber is so inelastic that a weight 10,000 times greater than itself will not stretch it.[39] Other classic research has revealed that collagen fibers may undergo a molecular extension of about 3%, until the slack in their wavy bundles (crimp) is taken up.[40] If the stretch continues, a critical point will be reached where the tissue ruptures.

Elastic fibers, called **elastin** to describe their functional extensibility, also exist. Unlike collagen, these elastic fibers determine the range of extensibility of muscle cells. As their name implies, elastic fibers succumb readily to stretching, and when released, they return to their former length. Only when elastic fibers are stretched to more than 150% of their original length do they reach their rupture point.[41]

A large amount of elastic tissue exists within the connective tissue that surrounds each muscle fiber. They are also found in numerous other organs and structures, where their roles include disseminating mechanical stress, enhancing coordination, maintaining tone during muscular relaxation, defending against excessive forces, and assisting organs in returning to their undeformed state once all forces have been removed.

Elastic fibers are almost always found together with collagen fibers. These two connective tissues work together to support and facilitate joint movement. Elastic fibers are responsible for what is called **reverse elasticity** or temporary deformation (i.e., the ability of a stretched material to return to its original resting state). Collagen, in contrast, provides the rigidity that limits the deformations of the elastic elements and gives tissues their tensile strength and relative inextensibility (sometimes referred to as permanent deformation). In tissues that contain large amounts of collagen, rigidity, stability, tensile strength, and restricted ROM will prevail.

Although connective tissue is found throughout the body, the structures related most to flexibility are tendons, ligaments, and fascia. Tendons are tough, cordlike tissues that connect muscles to bones. Their primary function is to transmit force from muscle to bone, thereby producing motion. Tendons consist of fibrils that are usually oriented toward the direction of normal physiological stress. The amount of deformation (i.e., change in shape) that occurs in a tendon when a stretch load is applied is called a *load-deformation curve* (Fig. 17-3). The wavy bundles of collagen in tendons straighten when a low level of stretch force is applied. Further stretch results in deformation of the tendon that is linearly related to the amount of tension applied. When stretched within a certain range, tendons will return to their original lengths when unloaded. Stretching the tendon beyond its "yield point" results in permanent length changes and microtrauma to the tendon's structural integrity.

Ligaments function primarily to support a joint by attaching bone to bone. Unlike tendons, ligaments take on various shapes, such as cords, bands, or sheets, depending on their location. Ligaments possess a greater mixture of elastic and fine collagenous fibers woven together than their tendinous counterparts. This results in a tissue that is pliant and flexible that allows freedom of movement, but is also strong, tough, and inextensible so as not to yield easily to applied forces. Whereas tendons provide approximately 10% of the resistance experienced during joint movement, the ligaments and joint capsule (a saclike structure that encloses the ends of bones at a joint) contribute about 47% of the total resistance to movement.[37]

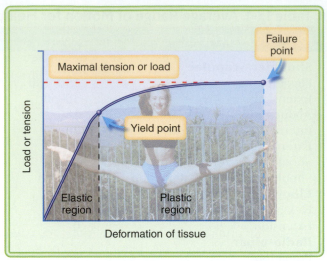

**Figure 17-3.** Relationship between load or tension and the amount of deformation that occurs in the tissue. When stretched up to the yield point, tendinous tissue will not permanently deform because the load or tension provided is not great enough to exceed elastic properties (elastic region). In this case, the tendon would return to its original length following the stretch. However, when the load or tension exceeds this point, microtrauma to the tissue occurs, resulting in permanent length changes and greater extensibility of the tissue.

In gross anatomy, fascia is a term typically used to designate all fibrous connective tissue not otherwise specifically named. Intramuscular fascia (**deep fascia**) is directly related to flexibility and ROM. Its main functions are:

- To provide a framework that ensures proper alignment of muscle fibers, blood vessels, and nerves
- To enable the safe and effective transmission of forces throughout the whole muscle
- To provide the necessary lubricated surfaces between muscle fibers that allow muscles to change shape during contraction and elongation
- To provide proprioceptive support during dynamic movement

During a passive stretching movement, fascia contributes 41% of the total resistance to joint ROM. Thus, fascia is second only to the joint capsule in terms of resistance to movement.[37]

## Mechanical and Dynamic Properties

The soft tissues of the body possess certain mechanical and dynamic properties that allow for performance of necessary functions, as well as protection from forces they may encounter. Whenever a tissue is subjected to a force (e.g., push, pull), a change in the shape of the tissue may occur. These changes are called **deformations**. The extent of deformation depends on variables such as the type of tissue, the amount of force applied, and the temperature of the tissue. When a force is applied to tissue, its length is increased; such lengthening is called **tensile deformation**.

**Elasticity** is the mechanical property that allows a tissue to return to its original shape or size when an applied force is removed. A critical region (**elastic limit** or yield point in Fig. 17-3) is reached when a tissue is stretched beyond the point where it can return back to its normal length after the tensile force is removed. The difference between the original resting length and the new resting length (after being stretched beyond its elastic limit) establishes a new state of permanent elongation called **plastic stretch**.

The mechanical property known as **plasticity** allows a tissue to deform when it is loaded past its elastic limit or yield point. Once a tissue is stretched past this point, it may succumb to considerable amounts of additional deformation with relatively small increases in force (within the plastic region in Fig. 17-3). An example of a substance that demonstrates an extraordinary display of plastic behavior is modeling clay, which exhibits some elasticity when gently stretched very lightly, but then exhibits greater amounts of deformity with additional stretching.

Plasticity of tissues can be observed with long-term, repetitive microtrauma. This type of chronic stress results in tissue that becomes less stable and less efficient, which ultimately contributes to a reduced quality of life. An example of long-term microtrauma is the deformation occurring in postural muscles as a result of poor posture when sitting in a chair. Over time, the body adapts to a faulty sitting posture by increased deformation of the posterior (back) tissue and shortening of the anterior (trunk) tissue. This ultimately leads to reduced ROM and the development of pain. In this example, one would strive to correct the problem by promoting plasticity within the anterior trunk muscles through stretching exercises and developing strength in the posterior back muscles using some muscle conditioning.

**Viscosity** is the property of tissues to resist loads and, unlike elasticity and plasticity, is dependent on time and temperature. An example of a viscous substance dependent on time and temperature is honey. Imagine squeezing honey out of its container when it has been chilled in the refrigerator. The flow of the honey is slow, and the harder you squeeze the container, the more resistance you will experience. Now imagine squeezing honey from its container after it has been heated. The honey is thinner and quickly flows out of the small opening in the container with little or no squeezing force. Tissue viscosity is an important principle for exercisers and athletes. Properly warming up the body's tissues and fluids reduces viscosity and allows adequate extensibility.

As the name implies, **viscoelasticity** is the property that allows tissues to exhibit both plastic and elastic behaviors. Most structures in the body are neither completely elastic nor completely plastic. Instead, they exhibit a combination of both properties. When subjected to low loads, most tissues exhibit elastic behavior. Conversely, when subjected to higher loads, tissues exhibit a plastic response. Furthermore, when loads are repeated over time, tissues exhibit viscous deformation.

## Age

Children are generally considered to be quite supple. Flexibility decreases slowly until puberty and then increases throughout adolescence. After adolescence, flexibility levels off and then begins to decrease as people age.[38,42] Although flexibility has been shown to decrease with age, the loss seems to be minimized in those who remain physically active.

Decades of research on flexibility in growing children reveal potential explanations for the variability in muscular tightness as the body matures. One hypothesis for the decline in flexibility seen in children growing into adolescence is that during periods of rapid growth, bones grow much faster than the muscles stretch.[43–46] Consequently, there is an increase in musculotendinous tightness at the joints. Another theory is that the decrease in flexibility, specifically in the hamstrings, is a direct result of prolonged sitting in school.[28,47] Most individuals sit with the pelvis in a posteriorly tilted position. Initially, this causes the hamstrings to become slack. Over time, sitting in this position causes the hamstrings to adaptively shorten to take up the slack. An extension of this hypothesis that applies to all age groups is that decreases in flexibility and increased tightness could be the result of a less physically active population as a whole.

The aging process inevitably brings about a decrease in normal muscle function including strength, endurance, flexibility, and agility. These functions are even more adversely affected when inactivity, disease, and injury (which are commonly associated with aging) are present. Part of the decline in age-related muscle function is due to the progressive atrophy, or wasting away, of muscle tissue. This loss is due to the reduction in both size and number of the muscle fibers. As muscle fibers undergo atrophy, they are replaced by collagen, the fatty and fibrous inelastic tissue described earlier in this chapter. Collagen contributes to the stiffening

### FROM THEORY TO PRACTICE

Think of any repetitive postures or habits that you have maintained for an extended period (e.g., months or years). For example, sitting at desk, working at a computer, or driving—when performed for prolonged periods without breaks—can produce positions that over time cause tissues on one side of the joint to lengthen (i.e., plastic deformation), whereas the tissues on the opposite side of the joint become tight (i.e., hypertonicity). How would you approach evening out these imbalances in your body?

and decreased mobility of aging muscle. With aging, collagen fibers lose water, gradually increasing their density and stiffness, which decreases tissue flexibility. However, an effective stretching program can help slow this process and help maintain pliability and mobility within the collagen fibers.[48]

Similar to collagen, the elastic fibers also deteriorate with age. Studies have shown that elastic fibers experience fragmentation, fraying, and calcification caused by the aging process. These alterations may be partly responsible for the loss of resiliency and increased joint rigidity experienced by older individuals. Furthermore, Buckwalter[49] demonstrated that cell function deteriorates in cartilage, ligaments, tendons, and muscles with aging, thus compromising flexibility.

Physical activity can improve flexibility through mechanisms such as increasing collagen turnover in ligaments and building muscle mass (which decreases the likelihood that muscle tissue will be replaced with inelastic collagen and fatty tissue, as is commonly seen in sedentary older adults),[50] enhancing collagen fiber cross-linkage formation, and increasing the viscosity of joint synovial fluid.[51] Thus, a physically active lifestyle is associated with less functional impairment, even in already frail older individuals.[52] In addition, resistance training together with stretching exercises may contribute to an increase in flexibility because its action is through a full ROM that is similar to the natural movement of a joint. Importantly, when combined with gains in strength, increased flexibility provides for greater bodily control and stability in everyday functional activities.[51]

## Injury

With advancing age, certain levels of trauma may be endured by the body. There are many levels of injury, or trauma, from acute injury to repetitive motion or sustained awkward positions. The effect of these traumatic events can alter joint function, muscular efficiency, and neural pathways. Repetitive microtrauma can lead to chronic injuries that inhibit muscular patterns, and acute trauma can lead to more severe injuries. These injuries can be more destructive and alter the structural properties of the bones and connective tissue permanently.

Bony structures can restrict the endpoint in a joint's ROM. In many instances, joints rely on bony prominences to stop movements at normal endpoints in the range. However, an elbow that has been fractured through the joint might lay down excess calcium in the joint space, causing the joint to lose its ability to fully extend. In addition, skin might be a contributor to limited movement. For example, an individual who has had some type of injury or surgery involving a tearing, incision, or laceration of the skin, particularly over a joint, will have inelastic scar tissue formed at that site. This scar tissue is incapable of stretching with joint movement. Over time, however, the elasticity of skin

contractures caused by scarring of ligaments, joint capsules, and musculotendinous units can be improved through stretching.

## Tissue Temperature

Effectively warming up the body for activity is imperative in preparing the muscles and connective tissue for activity. This also holds true for any liquid mediums present within the body (e.g., blood and synovial fluid). An effective warm-up provides optimal extensibility that helps minimize the potential for injury. In colder climates, an increased time allotment for a warm-up is recommended.

## Warming Up

Intramuscular temperature should be increased before any stretching activities are performed (e.g., warm-up or exercise) to most effectively stretch a muscle. Warming up before exercise or activity provides a period of adjustment from rest to exercise to improve performance and decrease the chance of injury by preparing the individual mentally and physically for activity. Increasing core temperature enhances the ability of collagen and elastin components within the musculotendinous unit to deform and the ability of the Golgi tendon organ (GTO) to reflexively relax through autogenic inhibition. Classic studies on the optimal temperature of muscle and connective tissue to achieve these benefits appears to be 103°F to 104°F (39°–40°C).[44,53,54]

The most common method of elevating body temperature and reducing tissue viscosity is performing several minutes of self-initiated active movement. This may include activities such as light calisthenics, walking, jogging, or stationary bicycling. The warm-up activities should be intense enough to increase the body's core temperature and cause some sweating, but not so intense as to cause fatigue.

## In Your Own Words

Clients often perform static stretches before engaging in physical activity with the goal of "warming up." How would you explain to a client that stretching before exercise is not the same as actually warming up?

## Cooling Down

Cooling down provides a period of adjustment returning from exercise back to rest, and it may include a group of low-intensity activities or exercises performed immediately after a workout. The main objectives of a cooldown are to facilitate muscular relaxation, promote the removal of muscular waste products by the blood, reduce muscular soreness, and allow the cardiovascular system to adjust to lowered demand. The general consensus from fitness organizations and the research on flexibility generally agree that some form of static stretching should be incorporated as part of this cooldown period when tissue temperatures are highest.

## SEX DIFFERENCES

### ANATOMY AND PHYSIOLOGY AFFECT FLEXIBILITY

In general, females usually exhibit consistently greater flexibility than their male counterparts of the same age.[42,55,56] Several factors, including anatomical and physiological differences, may account for the disparity in flexibility between the sexes. A key explanation for this difference is related to skeletal structure and specific differences in soft-tissue structures and hormone receptors throughout the body.[38] Specifically, the pelvic regions of males and females are shaped differently. When compared with a female's pelvis, a male's pelvis is generally larger, heavier, and rougher; the cavity between the bones is not as spacious; the sacrosciatic notch, pubic arch, and sacrum are narrower; and the acetabulae are closer together than a female's. Females tend to have broader and shallower hips than males. Collectively, these anatomical differences allow for a greater potential for ROM in the pelvic region for childbirth and movement. Furthermore, females usually have a greater range of extension in the elbow because of having a shorter upper curve of the olecranon process of the elbow than males. It has also been suggested that girls have greater potential for flexibility after puberty because of their lower center of gravity and shorter leg length compared with boys. Because female hormones such as relaxin (the hormone involved with preparing the pelvis for childbirth and the letdown response of breast milk) generally improve tissue compliancy, females in the latter trimesters of pregnancy and those who are lactating possess increased levels of this hormone. Consequently, they demonstrate further increases in flexibility through the lumbar, pelvic, and hip region.

## VIGNETTE *continued*

Mike has been enjoying his conditioning program for several weeks and, although his posture is still noticeably rounded forward at rest, he claims that he feels like it is easier for him to adopt and maintain an ideal posture during his training activities. In addition to progressing the posture-enhancement exercises (i.e., posterior trunk and shoulder exercises) that Noah gave Mike to help strengthen areas of his body that are lengthened and weak, Noah introduced more focused dynamic stretching movements into the warm-up before each of Mike's workout sessions. Teaching Mike how to safely and effectively take his shoulders and spine through their intended ROM using rhythmic movements, such as neck rotations, spine extensions, side bends, and arm circles, helps him incorporate even more flexibility work into his exercise sessions without spending more time to accomplish it.

## STRETCHING MODALITIES

Stretching with a goal of improving flexibility has been performed throughout history. In a fundamental sense, stretching involves moving the origin and insertion points of a muscle away from each other following the muscle's fiber arrangement and direction. Stretching may be performed as a dynamic activity, or it may be accomplished as a static hold near the joint's end ROM.

Various methods of stretching exist and each aims to achieve specific outcomes:

- **Static stretching** involves stretching a muscle to the point of mild tension or discomfort and then holding it at that point for an extended period. This method aims to elongate resting lengths of the sarcomeres by manipulating its viscoelastic properties and involves the neurological principle of autogenic inhibition discussed in Chapter 10.
- **Proprioceptive neuromuscular facilitation (PNF)** stretching techniques are more advanced forms of static stretching that achieve similar outcomes but involve the application of specific methodologies (e.g., specific isometric holds, alternating contractions and stretches) that are typically applied by a skilled partner.
- **Active isolated stretching (AIS)** is a technique that incorporates short-duration static stretches in combination with active muscle contractions between muscles at or around the joint (agonists, synergists, antagonists) to improve joint mobility and movement efficiency.
- **Myofascial release**, although not quite considered stretching, is a newer method of tissue manipulation of the fascia to improve mobility. Myofascial release will be discussed in greater detail later in this chapter. Because fascia forms complex webbing in and through all muscles to create one interconnected network, this method focuses on mobilizing larger sections of the body in an integrated manner rather than the practice of isolated lengthening of one single muscle.
- **Dynamic stretching**, or dynamic range of motion (DROM), generally involves integrated movements that rely on force production and momentum to move joints through functional ranges. The coordinated action of agonists and

antagonists produces movements that function primarily under the neurological principle of reciprocal inhibition.

- *Ballistic stretching* is an advanced form of dynamic movement that makes use of repetitive, but more explosive or bouncing movements as a method to enhance sport-specific mobility. It demonstrates a higher potential for injury; thus, it is generally advised for only well-conditioned athletes and is sometimes featured as a component of certain activity-specific conditioning programs.

These methods are performed either actively or passively, or in some cases both can be used. An **active** process requires the participant to provide the force to the stretch by voluntarily contracting his or her own muscles to perform the movement without the aid of an external force (Fig. 17-4). As illustrated in Figure 17-4, the participant voluntarily moves his body into the crossover lunge position with a trunk rotation via coordinated muscle actions. A **passive** process, in contrast, requires little-to-no effort by the participant to generate the stretch force. Instead, the stretch movement is performed with the assistance of an external agent such as a partner, piece of stretching equipment, or sturdy object (Fig. 17-5). As illustrated in Figure 17-5, the participant is using the table edge as a prop to help hold the hamstring muscle group in an extended position.

## Static Stretching

Perhaps because of its simplicity, the most widely used form of flexibility exercise is static stretching. This technique involves passively stretching a muscle by placing it in a maximal or near-maximal stretch position and then holding it there for an extended period (e.g., 15–60 seconds). This stretch should be performed at least

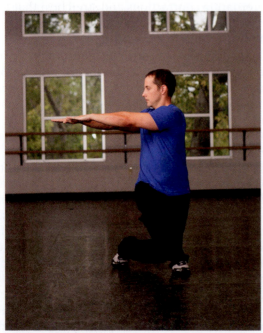

**Figure 17-4.** A crossover lunge exercise combined with trunk rotation, demonstrating an active flexibility exercise.

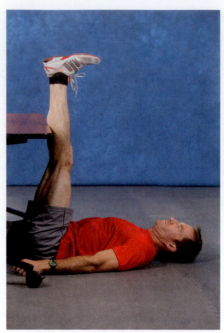

**Figure 17-5.** A static stretch activity for the hamstrings, demonstrating a passive flexibility exercise.

four times on the same muscle group.[1] Table 17-2 provides general instructions on performing static stretching. The key qualities to static stretching are the ability to control the range of movement using points of tension and use of simple methods. Consequently, these types of stretches may be preferred over more complex dynamic movements for deconditioned or novice population groups. Furthermore, it can be performed anywhere and within the constraints of limited time and space. Static stretching is also preferable to ballistic stretching because it requires less energy, results in less muscle soreness, and provides more qualitative relief from muscular distress.

Static stretching can also be boring and it is not specific to the types of dynamic movements commonly associated with exercise and sports activities. For these individuals, a blend of both static and dynamic techniques may solve their problem. Nonetheless, much research has been done comparing dynamic with static stretching techniques for the improvement of flexibility, and they appear to be equally effective in increasing ROM.[38] However, it is reasonable to conclude that with static stretching there is less danger of exceeding the extensibility limits of the involved joints because the stretch is more controlled.

## In Your Own Words

Explain to a peer why you might favor static stretching over more ballistic-type stretching with a deconditioned individual.

## Proprioceptive Neuromuscular Facilitation Techniques

Commonly used in rehabilitation and athletic training, proprioceptive neuromuscular facilitation (PNF) is a specialized stretching technique that involves various

## Table 17-2. General Overview of Various Stretching Methods

| METHOD | STATIC | PROPRIOCEPTIVE NEUROMUSCULAR FACILITATION | ACTIVE ISOLATED STRETCHING |
|---|---|---|---|
| Neurological principle | Autogenic inhibition | Variety of techniques (contraction and stretching)<br>• Autogenic inhibition<br>• Reciprocal inhibition | Reciprocal inhibition |
| Variables | ≥4 reps × 15–60 sec each | 1–3 reps with:<br>• 6–15 sec contraction<br>• 20–30 sec stretch | • 1–2 sets × 5–10 reps, holding end ROM for no longer than 2 sec |

| METHOD | MYOFASCIAL RELEASE | DYNAMIC MOVEMENT | BALLISTIC MOVEMENT |
|---|---|---|---|
| Neurological principle | Autogenic inhibition | Reciprocal inhibition<br>• Begin with basic movements in sagittal plane<br>• Gradually introduce frontal and transverse plane | Reciprocal inhibition |
| Variables | • Apply constant pressure back and forth rolling 2–6 inches for 30–60 sec (>30 reps)<br>• Continue until noticeable decrease in tenderness/tension | • 1 set × 10 reps at a controlled tempo<br>• Progressively increase movement complexity, mimicking forthcoming activities | **Zachazewski model:**<br>• Start with static stretches<br>• Progress to slow, short, end-range ballistic stretches<br>• Progress to slow, full-range ballistic stretches<br>• Progress to fast, short, end-range ballistic stretches<br>• Progress to fast, full-range ballistic stretches |

combinations of muscle contractions coupled with stretching to improve flexibility. Various forms of PNF stretching exist that range from the simple (e.g., "hold-relax") to the complex (e.g., "contract-relax-antagonist-contract"). The three main PNF techniques will be introduced along with instructions on performing each modality.

PNF techniques are based on several vital neurophysiological mechanisms that stimulate the musculotendinous proprioceptors (i.e., muscle spindles and GTO) to facilitate or inhibit muscle action, thereby incorporating autogenic or reciprocal inhibition, or both. **Facilitation** is the process of increasing motor nerve excitability, whereas **inhibition** is designed to decrease excitability, or promote relaxation. These two mechanisms are essentially inseparable from one another, implying that any technique that promotes facilitation of an agonist will simultaneously promote inhibition of the antagonist. For example, implementing any strategy to help activate the quadriceps (agonist in this example) will inhibit the hamstrings (antagonist in this example). The underlying assumption is that through inhibition, the antagonistic muscles relax and therefore will provide less resistance to

either movement of the agonist or lengthening of the antagonist. This is primarily achieved through specific strategies that involve isometric contractions with no change in muscle length (known as "hold") or isotonic contractions with changes in muscle length (known as "contract") that are performed in alternating manners between muscles or coupled with muscle relaxation. The three main PNF techniques commonly used to enhance ROM are:

- Hold-relax
- Contract-relax
- Contract-relax-agonist-contraction, also known as **slow reversal-hold-relax**

### Hold-Relax Technique

The following sequence outlines the hold-relax technique:

- The stretch begins with the partner gently moving the participant's body part passively to an end position that stretches the antagonist (i.e., moving in the direction of the agonist). This end position is where the participant experiences resistance or limitations to further stretching. For example, as illustrated in Figure 17-6, when

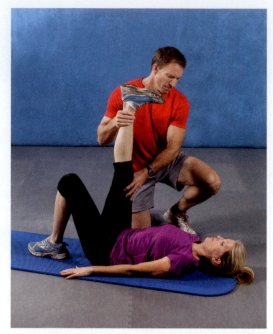

**Figure 17-6.** Example of the hold-relax hamstrings stretch. Following a passive stretch to the endpoint in the range of motion, the participant gently contracts (isometric) the targeted muscle and holds this position for a short period. Once this period is complete, the partner moves the body part deeper into the stretch.

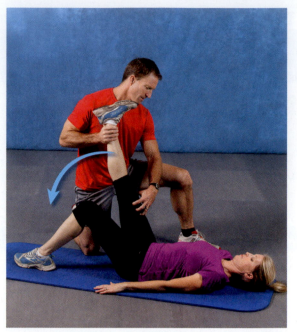

**Figure 17-7.** Example of the contract-relax hamstrings stretch technique. Following a passive stretch up to end-point resistance, the participant performs a light concentric contraction of the targeted muscle for a short period. Afterward, the partner moves the body part farther into the stretch to the new point of resistance.

the hamstrings are being targeted, the partner moves the extended leg into hip flexion.

- The participant is then instructed to contract or push lightly against the partner with an isometric contraction of the antagonist (e.g., hamstrings) for 6 to 15 seconds (performing a "hold" contraction with no movement).[1]
- The participant then relaxes that antagonist (e.g., hamstrings) for 2 to 3 seconds before the partner passively moves the body part deeper into the stretch, achieving as much extension as possible to a new point of resistance.
- This new end position is held approximately 20 to 30 seconds.[1]
- Additional repetitions can be performed.

### Contract–Relax Technique

The following sequence outlines the contract-relax technique:

- Similar to the hold-relax technique, the stretch begins with the partner gently moving the participant's body part passively to an end position that stretches the antagonist (i.e., moving in the direction of the agonist). This end position is where the participant experiences resistance or limitations to further stretching (Fig. 17-7).
- Again, the participant is instructed to contract or push against the partner, but this time the action involves a light concentric contraction of the antagonist (e.g., hamstrings) for 6 to 15 seconds that moves the limb back toward its starting position (e.g., contracting the hamstrings to move the elevated leg back toward the floor).[1]

- The participant then relaxes the antagonist (e.g., hamstrings) for 2 to 3 seconds before the partner passively moves the body part deeper into the stretch, achieving as much extension as possible to a new point of resistance.
- This new end position is held approximately 20 to 30 seconds.[1]
- Additional repetitions can be performed.

### Contract-Relax-Agonist-Contraction Technique

The following sequence outlines the contract-relax-agonist-contraction technique:

- Similar to the contract-relax technique, the stretch begins with the partner gently moving the participant's body part passively to an end position that stretches the antagonist (i.e., moving in the direction of the agonist). This end position is where the participant experiences resistance or limitations to further stretching (Fig. 17-8).
- The individual now initiates a brief isotonic contraction (<5 seconds) of the agonist (e.g., quadriceps) attempting to move the limb deeper into the stretch.
- This is followed by a light isometric contraction of the antagonist (e.g., hamstrings) for 6 to 15 seconds and then relaxation as the partner now moves the limb deeper into the stretch and repeats the sequence of agonistic and antagonistic actions. This can be repeated two to three times.

### Active Isolated Stretching

Active isolated stretching (AIS) is a technique that blends portions of active and passive stretching and was

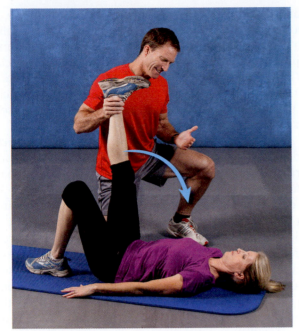

**Figure 17-8.** Example of the contract-relax-agonist-contraction stretch technique for the hamstrings. This technique begins similarly to the hold-relax and contract-relax exercises. However, in this exercise, the participant contracts the opposite muscle (quadriceps), followed by a brief contraction of the targeted muscles and then relaxation to allow for a deeper passive stretch.

originally used during rehabilitation for surgery patients. As the name indicates, this is an active technique that requires muscle activity on the part of the participant.

- The participant actively moves the body part to a desired end position where resistance to movement is encountered (Fig. 17-9A), but instead of holding a lengthened position for longer durations (e.g., 30 seconds), this lengthened position is never held for more than 2 seconds.[57]
- The stretch is then released, returning the body segment to the starting position (Fig. 17-9B); the

stretch is repeated for several repetitions, with each subsequent movement exceeding the resistance point by a few degrees (Fig. 17-9C). Increasing the stretch by a few degrees at a time allows the muscle to adjust more gradually to the stretch.

- The stretches are typically performed in sets of 5 to 10 repetitions with a goal of isolating an individual muscle in each set.
- Proponents of AIS claim that this technique targets specific muscles and prepares the body for physical activity better than static stretching can, while also protecting the joint attachments that static stretching can sometimes weaken.[57]

As Figure 17-9 illustrates, the quadriceps muscles are contracted to extend the knee, stretching the hamstrings while using an external device to hold that end position briefly. While the quadriceps reciprocally inhibit the hamstrings, it is also believed that this external device allows the hamstrings to relax more completely and receive full benefit from the stretch. However, some experts believe that holding a stretch for only 2 seconds is not adequate to have an effect on the connective tissue that surrounds and runs through muscles.[1,13–17] Table 17-2 provides general instructions on performing AIS stretching.

## Myofascial Release

Myofascial release or self-myofascial release (self-administered) is a technique that applies pressure to tight, restricted areas of fascia and underlying muscle in an attempt to relieve tension and improve flexibility. It is thought that applying sustained pressure to a tight area can inhibit the tension in a muscle by stimulating the GTO to bring about autogenic inhibition.[58] Perhaps the most common technique used is one where the participant positions his or her body on a foam roller and allows the combination of gravity and body weight to control the amount of pressure. Tender areas of soft

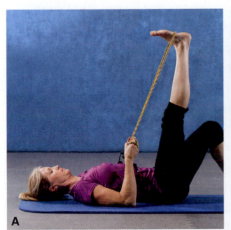
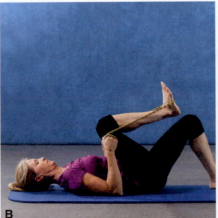
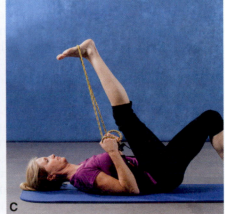

**Figure 17-9.** Active isolated stretching (AIS) technique. This technique involves short bouts (<2 seconds) of both active and passive stretching to improve range of motion. First, the participant moves the body part to a point where resistance to stretch is encountered (A). After ≥2 seconds in this position, the participant returns back to the unstretched position (B) and then back to the stretched position (C). This cycle is repeated 5 to 10 times with a greater stretch being applied from repetition to repetition.

tissue (also called *trigger points*) can be diminished through the application of pressure (myofascial release) followed by static stretching of the tight area. The benefits of this method include a reduction in soft-tissue tension (which may also reduce discomfort associated with this muscle tightness), restoration of normal muscle length–tension relationships, and an improvement in muscle function.

Understanding the concept behind myofascial release requires an understanding of the fascial system itself. As described previously, fascia is a densely woven, specialized system of connective tissue that covers and unites all of the body's compartments. The result is a system in which each part is connected to the other parts through this web of tissue. In this web-like structure, fascia interacts differently at multiple levels in the body, from the superficial layers to the deep layers. As the research of fascia's function continues to evolve, we do know it plays an essential role in providing the following[59]:

- **Proprioception**: Fascia is considered the largest and richest sensory organ in the body with nine times more sensory nerve endings than muscles. Myers[59] estimates that for every muscle spindle, there are 10 GTOs and sensory receptors relaying information on any mechanical forces to tissue (e.g., loading and tension).
- **Protective**: Fascia is considered a tension distributor that allows the body the opportunity to dissipate and/or distribute forces to minimize localized trauma to muscle. Many injuries previously diagnosed as muscle injuries are, in fact, fascial injuries.
- **Mobility**: Fascia has attachments with muscles and other connective tissue (e.g., tendons and ligaments), and when it is unable to move efficiently (called adhesions or knots in the fascial tissue) it limits mobility of the underlying tissue (e.g., muscles) by compressing that tissue.
- **Stabilizer**: The fascial web is designed in such a manner to provide integrity by balancing and distributing tension forces (called *tensegrity*), which provides greater amounts of strength and resiliency. Because fascia is more plastic in nature, this property allows it to hold positions and provide stability.
- **Force transmission**: Like muscle, fascia is also capable of creating tension and producing motion. Its structure creates a weave of tissue capable of producing both force and power.
- **Adaptability**: When placed under strain, fascia changes its architecture. Following Davis's law, this tissue models itself along the demands imposed on itself, which can be both good (good movement, good posture, and proper technique) or bad (poor movement, poor posture, and improper technique).

In a normal, healthy state, fascia has a relaxed and wavy configuration. It has the ability to stretch and move without restriction. However, with physical trauma, scarring, or inflammation, fascia loses its pliability. It becomes tight, restricted, and a potential source of pain. An acute injury, habitual poor posture over time, and repetitive stress injuries can be damaging to the fascia. As a result, the damaged fascia can exert excessive pressure, producing pain or restriction of motion, which, in turn, may induce adaptive shortening of the muscle tissue associated with the fascia.

As mentioned previously, one technique instructs individuals to perform small, continuous, back-and-forth movements on a foam roller, covering an area of 2 to 6 inches (5–15 cm) over the tender region for 30 to 60 seconds (Fig. 17-10). Because exerting pressure on an already tender area requires a certain level of pain tolerance, the intensity of the application of pressure determines the duration in which the individual can withstand the discomfort. For example, a person with a high pain tolerance can position his or her body on the foam roller *directly over a tender area* and hold the applied pressure for 30 seconds. In contrast, an individual with low pain tolerance can position his or her body *near the focal point of the tender area* and hold the applied pressure for 60 seconds. Table 17-2 provides general instructions on performing myofascial release.

Ultimately, myofascial release realigns the elastic muscle and connective tissue fibers from a bundled position (called a knot or adhesion) into a straighter arrangement and resets the proprioceptive mechanisms of the soft tissue, thus reducing hypertonicity within the underlying muscles.

## VIGNETTE *continued*

■ After 6 months of his new training regimen, Mike has progressed nicely in his program for increased fitness and improved posture and upper body flexibility. He is satisfied with his ability to realign his spine and upper extremity into a more ideal postural position during his exercise training. Specifically, he reports that he can maintain an upright, stable posture longer without becoming fatigued and reverting back to his rounded forward posture that was so prevalent before starting his training with Noah. To help Mike continue on his path to improved posture and flexibility, Noah introduces Mike to self-myofascial release (especially of the pectorals and latissimus dorsi muscle groups) and teaches him how to use a foam roller to help release any fascial restrictions that might contribute to poor posture. Noah encourages Mike to use the foam roller daily, if possible, and to perform self-myofascial release before and after his workout sessions to promote enhanced ROM.

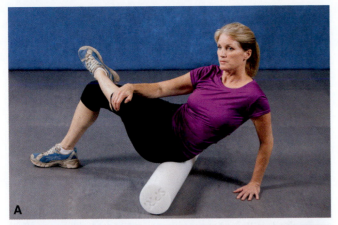

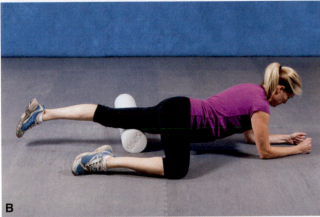

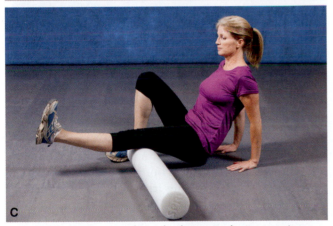

**Figure 17-10.** The myofascial release technique, using a foam roller to apply pressure massage. The exercises shown in the three images involve the glutes (A), quadriceps (B), and hamstrings (C). The technique works by targeting trigger points through pressure to release tension in the fascia and improve flexibility.

## Dynamic Stretching or Dynamic Range of Motion Movements

Stretching that is dynamic in nature implies that instead of remaining still and holding a stretch, the participant keeps the body parts involved in the stretch moving continuously. This type of flexibility training is common among athletes who use stretching as a pre-event warm-up strategy. A dynamic stretch uses controlled speed of movement as a component of the exercise. The participant moves his or her joints through the ROM at a speed that is slower than what is experienced during competition. Gradually the athlete increases the speed of the dynamic stretch to mimic the speed of movement required during the sport-related activity. For example, a track sprinter preparing for an event would perform long strides, which emphasize hip mobility, while maintaining a posterior pelvic tilt. This dynamically stretches the hip flexors, which are used vigorously during competition, providing flexibility about the hip joints.

Dynamic stretching is popular among athletes primarily because of the specificity of the activity. That is, most sports require athletes to move rapidly through different planes of movement, and stretching activities that mimic these dynamic sport demands have more carryover to the sport than do slow, static stretches. Also, by performing dynamic stretches before a competitive event, athletes recruit the same muscles used in competition, thereby using a "rehearsal effect" that prepares the neuromuscular system for higher levels of performance. Table 17-2 provides general instructions on performing dynamic ROM movements.

## Ballistic Stretching

Ballistic stretching is a controversial topic in sports medicine. The technique involves repetitively contracting an agonist muscle to produce quick stretches of the antagonist muscle.[60] The controversy is complicated further by the lack of available research on ballistic flexibility because of the difficulty of assessing it in individuals.[61] Proponents of ballistic stretching tout its ability to enhance dynamic flexibility, its effectiveness as a means of increasing ROM, and its role in improving adherence in a stretching program.[60] Perhaps most important, ballistic stretching helps to develop dynamic flexibility. Because most activities are dynamic in nature, ballistic stretching allows for specificity in both training and the warm-up. Lastly, supporters of ballistic stretching cite that, because it involves rapid movement, it is less boring than static stretching and individual compliance is therefore higher.[60]

Arguments against ballistic stretching are based on the following factors:

- Inadequate tissue adaptation
- Soreness resulting from injury
- Initiation of the stretch reflex
- Inadequate neurological adaptation

The rapid motion involved in ballistic stretching does not allow the muscle and its supporting connective tissues adequate time to adapt. If tissues are stretched too rapidly, lasting flexibility cannot be achieved. Permanent increases in flexibility have been shown to occur most effectively when tissues are stretched by lower force for longer duration at an elevated temperature. Also, rapid bouncing movements that take the limbs to their end ranges of motion often exceed the tensile absorbing capacity of the tissues being stretched and may cause injury.

Ballistic stretching may cause soreness or injury. When a tissue is stretched too fast, it can be strained or ruptured, which results in pain and a decrease in ROM.

Ballistic stretching also raises concerns about the stretch reflex. If a sudden stretch is applied to a muscle, a reflexive action brought on by the muscle spindle causes the muscle to contract. The resultant increase in muscular tension makes it difficult to stretch the connective tissue and defeats the original purpose of the stretch, as well as increases the likelihood of soft-tissue injury.

Last, the argument that ballistic stretching does not allow adequate neurological adaptation is based on classic studies that found that the amount of tension for a given amount of stretch is more than doubled by a quick stretch as compared with a slow stretch.[62,63] The slower stretch reduced the frequency of motor neuron firing and subsequently reduced tension in the muscle.

In general, experts recommend that sedentary individuals, laypeople, and athletes who have sustained musculoskeletal injuries avoid ballistic stretching. However, there is no evidence that, if performed properly, ballistic stretching results in injury.[61] In fact, ballistic stretching may be an important program component for individuals whose sports and activities involve ballistic movements.[1]

Proponents of ballistic stretching maintain that it has benefits if implemented correctly for the right population. The Zachazewski model, developed and named after James Zachazewski, incorporates a ballistic stretching method that is progressive in nature and allows the body to adapt to the increasing demands of the functional movement patterns (Fig. 17-11). Zachazewski[64] briefly describes the model as follows:

> The athlete progresses from an environment of control to activity simulation, from a slow-velocity methodical activity to high-velocity functional activity. After static stretching, slow short end range (SSER) ballistic stretching is initiated.

The athlete then progresses to slow full range stretching (SFR), fast short end range (FSER) and fast full range (FFR) stretching. Control and range of motion are the responsibility of the athlete. No outside force is exerted by anyone else.

Zachazewski and Reischl[60] state, "Ballistic activities may play a vital role in the conditioning and training of the athlete. If ballistics are utilized, they should be preceded by static stretching and confined to a small range of motion, perhaps no more than 10% beyond the static range of motion." After consistently practicing the Zachazewski model, the athlete goes through "a series of stretching exercises in which the velocity and range of lengthening are combined and controlled on a progressive basis."[64] This gradual program permits the muscle and its associated tendon to adapt progressively to functional ballistic movements, thus reducing the risk for injury.

## FLEXIBILITY PROGRAMMING FOR GENERAL HEALTH AND FITNESS

To ensure a safe and effective approach to developing flexibility, the simplest tactic is to perform a moderate, activity-specific warm-up for the muscle groups involved in the upcoming activity. For example, runners can begin a long-distance run with a slow 10-minute jog before they pick up the pace. Gentle static stretching after an adequate warm-up appears to do no harm, but many exercisers will find it cumbersome to perform a warm-up, stop and stretch, and then continue on with their workout.

Guidelines for static stretching are presented in Table 17-2, but dynamic or ballistic, PNF, AIS, and self-myofascial release techniques can also be used to effectively improve joint ROM and enhance flexibility. Recommendations for the optimal time for holding a static stretch vary, ranging from as little as 2 seconds to as much as 60 seconds.[1,57] Stretches that last longer

### FROM THEORY TO PRACTICE

Flexibility programs may be corrective, active, or functional in nature. Corrective stretching programs aim to improve muscle imbalances, altered joint kinematics, and postural dysfunction. Active flexibility training aims to improve soft-tissue extensibility and neuromuscular control. Stretching that focuses on functional significance uses dynamic, integrated, multiplanar movement patterns to improve performance.

The design of a stretching program varies within a workout session. Pre-workout stretches to correct muscle imbalance include myofascial or self-myofascial release to inhibit tight muscles, followed by static stretches to improve tissue extensibility. Throughout the workout, dynamic stretching can be used between sets to offset the concentric contractions during a weight-lifting set that tend to increase muscle tonicity. This facilitates tissue extensibility while maintaining neuromuscular efficiency. Post-exercise stretching most likely provides the greatest potential for ROM improvements because of the increased muscle temperature gained during the workout. Flexibility training performed after a workout can help reduce muscle tonicity through myofascial release followed by static or PNF stretches. As a result, the reduction in hypertonicity can improve overall flexibility.

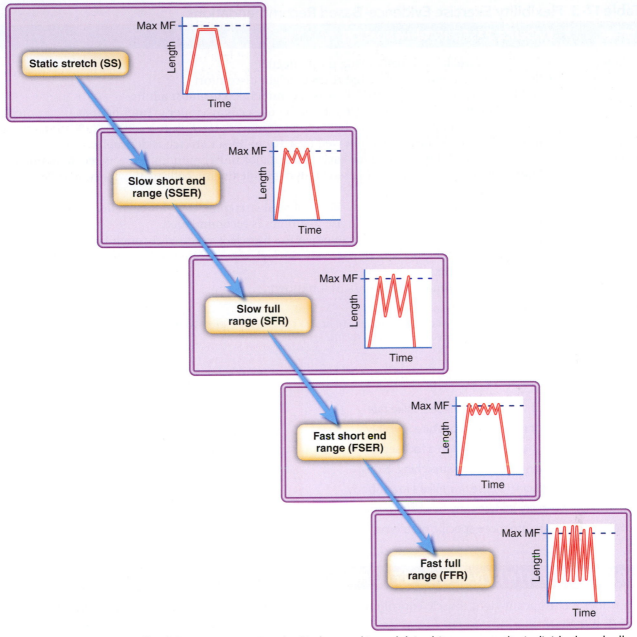

**Figure 17-11.** Progressive flexibility program using the Zachazewski model. In this program, the individual gradually progresses from controlled static stretching to more active, high-velocity functional movement. Proponents of this model contend that this is more specific and beneficial to improve athletic activities. MF, maximal force.

than 30 seconds may seem to be uncomfortable for participants, especially when they exhibit muscular tightness. Static stretches should be performed for all the major muscle groups in the body and repeated three or four times after the muscle group is warm. Thus, whole-body static stretching can be conveniently performed at the conclusion of each workout. Guidelines on the frequency for participating in stretching exercises suggest a minimum of 2 days per week, but may be increased to 5 or even 7 days per week depending on the frequency of exercise sessions.[1] Table 17-3 lists the programming guidelines for safe and effective stretching.

From the volumes of available research,[3,5] it is clear that sufficient and conclusive evidence is lacking

from which evidence-based recommendations can be made about the role of stretching in injury prevention. Although the evidence is insufficient to endorse pre- or post-exercise stretching, research does support that stretching improves flexibility, posture, and body awareness, and helps to relieve stress.[38] In addition, lack of flexibility resulting in limited joint ROM predisposes individuals to injuries. Essentially, flexibility is an important component of fitness that must not be ignored. The inconclusive results of a limited amount of research should not be the basis for deeming flexibility any less important for overall health. Clearly, there is a need for more research in this area before any evidence-based recommendations can be made.

## Table 17-3. Flexibility Exercise Evidence-Based Recommendations

| FITT-VP | EVIDENCE-BASED RECOMMENDATION |
|---|---|
| Frequency | • ≥2–3 days/week, with daily being most effective |
| Intensity | • Stretch to the point of feeling tightness or slight discomfort |
| Time | • Holding a static stretch for 10–30 sec is recommended for most adults. |
| | • In older individuals, holding a stretch for 30–60 sec may confer greater benefit. |
| | • For PNF stretching, a 3- to 6-sec light-to-moderate contraction (e.g., 20%–75% of maximum voluntary contraction) followed by a 10- to 30-sec stretch is desirable. |
| Type | • A series of flexibility exercise for each of the major muscle-tendon units is recommended. |
| | • Static flexibility (i.e., active or passive), dynamic flexibility, ballistic flexibility, and PNF are each effective. |
| Volume | • A reasonable target is to perform 60 sec of total stretching time for each flexibility exercise. |
| Pattern | • Repetition of each flexibility exercise 2–4 times is recommended. |
| | • Flexibility exercise is most effective when the muscle is warmed through light-to-moderate aerobic activity or passively through external methods such as moist heat packs or hot baths. |
| Progression | • Methods for optimal progression are unknown. |

PNF, proprioceptive neuromuscular facilitation.
Data from American College of Sports Medicine (ACSM) (2014). *ACSM's Guidelines for Exercise Testing and Prescription* (9th ed.). Philadelphia, PA: Wolters Kluwer/Lippincott Williams & Wilkins.

## V I G N E T T E  conclusion

■ After 1 year of working with Noah, Mike rarely experiences back pain and his posture is visibly improved. Together, they develop a focused program of dynamic and static stretching, along with self-myofascial release, for Mike's lower body that will potentially address any flexibility problems before they turn into more specific problems involving pain or loss of ROM. Mike's case illustrates the concept that repetitive activities can cause the soft tissues to deform or become hypertonic, thereby resulting in loss of function or development pain. His case also demonstrates that flexibility is joint specific, and that to promote appropriate ROM in all joints requires a thoughtful approach to stretching that considers a person's physical activity habits and daily repetitive patterns.

## CRITICAL THINKING QUESTIONS

1. How does a chronically tight muscle contribute to loss of function?

2. What is likely the most effective approach to prevent DOMS (besides avoiding eccentric contractions)?

3. If a muscle is stretched and relaxed, then why is it that tension within that muscle can be felt (i.e., touching a person's arm that is relaxed, yet "muscle tone" can still be felt)?

4. Using the neurological principle behind static stretching (i.e., autogenic inhibition) and the neurological principle behind dynamic ROM movements (e.g., reciprocal inhibition), explain why dynamic movement would be more effective before exercise, whereas static stretching would be more effective after exercise.

## ADDITIONAL RESOURCES

American Council on Exercise (ACE). *ACE Personal Trainer Manual*. 5th ed. San Diego, CA: American Council on Exercise; 2014.

American Council on Exercise (ACE). *ACE's Essentials of Exercise Science for Fitness Professionals*. San Diego, CA: American Council on Exercise; 2010.

McAtee RE. *Facilitated Stretching*. 3rd ed. Champaign, IL: Human Kinetics; 2007.

# REFERENCES

1. American College of Sports Medicine (ACSM). *ACSM's Guidelines for Exercise Testing and Prescription.* 9th ed. Philadelphia, PA: Wolters Kluwer/Lippincott Williams & Wilkins; 2014.

2. U.S. Department of Health and Human Services. Office of Disease Prevention and Health Promotion. *2008 Physical Activity Guidelines for Americans.* 2008. www.health.gov/PAGuidelines/pdf/paguide.pdf. Accessed 04/07/14.

3. Gremion G. The effect of stretching on sports performance and the risk of sports injury: A review of the literature. *Sportmedizin Sporttraumatol.* 2005;53:6–10.

4. Lees FD, Clark PG, Nigg CR, Newman P. Barriers to exercise behavior among older adults: A focus-group study. *J Aging Phys Act.* 2005;13:23–33.

5. Thacker SB, Gilchrist J, Stroup DF, Kimsey CD. The impact of stretching on sports injury risk: A systematic review of the literature. *Med Sci Sports Exerc.* 2004;36:371–378.

6. Caspersen CJ, Powell KE, Christenson GM. Physical activity, exercise, and physical fitness: Definitions and distinctions for health-related research. *Public Health Rep.* 1985;100:126–131.

7. Herbert RD, Gabriel M. Effects of stretching before and after exercising on muscle soreness and risk of injury: Systematic review. *Br Med J.* 2002;325:468.

8. Hess JA, Hecker S. Stretching at work for injury prevention: Issues, evidence, and recommendations. *Appl Occup Environ Hyg.* 2003;18:331–338.

9. Weldon SM, Hill RH. The efficacy of stretching for prevention of exercise-related injury: A systematic review of the literature. *Man Ther.* 2003;8:141–150.

10. De Vries HA, Wiswell RA, Bullbulion R, Moritani T. Tranquilizer effect of exercise. *Am. J Phys. Med.* 1981;60:57–66.

11. Entyre B, Abraham L. Effects of three stretching techniques on the motor pool excitability of the human soleus muscle. *Absracts of Research Papers 1984.* Reston, VA: American Alliance for Health, Physical Education, and Recreation; 1984:90.

12. Thigpen LK. Neuromuscular variation in association with static stretching. *Abstracts of Research Papers 1984.* Washington, DC: American Alliance for Health, Physical Education, and Recreation; 1984:28.

13. Boyce D, Brosky JA. Determining the minimal number of cyclic passive stretch repetitions recommended for an acute increase in an indirect measure of hamstring length. *Physiother Theory Pract.* 2008;24:113–120.

14. Magnusson SP, Simonsen EB, Aagaard P, Kjaer M. Biomechanical responses to repeated stretches in human hamstring muscle in vivo. *Am J Sports Med.* 1996;24:622–628.

15. McNair PJ, Dombroski EW, Hewson DJ, Stanley SN. Stretching at the ankle joint: Viscoelastic responses to holds and continuous passive motion. *Med Sci Sports Exerc.* 2001;33:354–358.

16. Ryan ED, Herda TJ, Costa PB, et al. Determining the minimum number of passive stretches necessary to alter musculotendinous stiffness. *J Sports Sci.* 2009;27:957–961.

17. Yeh CY, Chen JJ, Tsai KH. Quantifying the effectiveness of the sustained muscle stretching treatments in stroke patients with ankle hypertonia. *J Electromyogr Kinesiol.* 2007;17:453–461.

18. Van der Wees PJ, Jamtvedt G, Rebbeck T, de Bie RA, Dekker J, Hendriks EJ. Multifaceted strategies may increase implementation of physiotherapy clinical guidelines: A systematic review. *Aust J Physiother.* 2008;54:233–241.

19. Cailliet R. *Low Back Pain Syndrome.* 4th ed. Philadelphia: F.A. Davis; 1988.

20. Carey TS. Comparative effectiveness studies in chronic low back pain: Comment on 'A randomized trial comparing yoga, stretching, and a self-care book for chronic low back pain.' *Arch Intern Med.* 2011;171:2019–2026.

21. Deyo RA, Walsh NE, Martin DC, Schoenfield LS, Ramamurthy S. A controlled trial of transcutaneous electrical nerve stimulation (TENS) and exercise for chronic low back pain. *New Engl J Med.* 1990;322:1627–1634.

22. Khalil TM, Asfour SS, Martinez LM, Waly SM, Rosomoff RS, Rosomoff HL. Stretching in rehabilitation of low back pain patients. *Spine.* 1992;17:311–317.

23. Locke JC. Stretching away from back pain injury. *Occup Health Saf.* 1983;52:8–13.

24. Rasch PJ, Burke J. *Kinesiology and Applied Anatomy.* 7th ed. Philadelphia, PA: Lea & Febiger; 1989.

25. Russell GS, Highland TR. Care of the Low Back. Columbia, MO: *Spine;* 1990.

26. Sherman KJ, Cherkin DC, Wellman RD, et al. A randomized trial comparing yoga, stretching, and a self-care book for chronic low back pain. *Arch Intern Med.* 2011;171:2019–2026.

27. McGill S. *Ultimate Back Fitness and Performance.* 2nd ed. Waterloo, Ontario, Canada: Wabuno Publishers, Backfitpro; 2004.

28. Pheasant S. *Bodyspace—Anthropometry, Ergonomics and Design.* London: Taylor and Francis; 1986.

29. Stone MB, Edwards JE, Stemmans CL, Ingersoll CD, Palmieri RM, Krause BA. Certified athletic trainers' perceptions of exercise-associated muscle cramps. *Sport Rehabil.* 2003;12:333–342.

30. Bertolasi L, De Grandis D, Bongiovanni LG, Zanette GP, Gasperini M. The influence of muscular lengthening on cramps. *Ann Neurol.* 1993;33:176–180.

31. Fowler AW. Relief of cramp. *Lancet.* 1973;1(7794):99.

32. Graham G. Cramp. *Lancet.* 1965;2:537.

33. Weiner IH, Weiner HL. Nocturnal leg muscle cramps. *J Am Med Assoc.* 1980;244:2332–2333.

34. Hume PA, Cheung K, Maxwell L, Weerapong P. DOMS: An overview of treatment strategies. *Int Sportmed J.* 2004;5:98–118.

35. Ekstrand J, Gillquist J, Liljedahl S. Prevention of soccer injuries: Supervision by doctor and physiotherapist. *Am J Sports Med.* 1986;11:116–120.

36. Hewitt TE, Lidenfeld TN, Riccobene JV, Noyes FR. The effects of neuromuscular training on the incidence of knee injury in female athletes. *Am J Sports Med.* 1999;27:699–704.

37. Johns RJ, Wright V. Relative importance of various tissues in joint stiffness. *J Appl Physiol.* 1962;17:824–828.

38. Alter MJ. *Science of Flexibility.* 3rd ed. Champaign, IL: Human Kinetics; 2004.

39. Verzar F. Aging of collagen fiber. In: Hall DA, ed. *International Review of Connective Tissue Research.* New York: Academic Press; 1964:244–300.

40. Ramachandran GW. Structure of collagen at the molecular level. In: Ramachandran GW, ed. *Treatise of Collagen.* Vol. 1. New York, NY: Academic Press; 1967:103–179.

41. Bloom W, Fawcett DW. *A Textbook of Histology.* 11th ed. Philadelphia, PA: WB Saunders; 1986.

42. Youdas JW, Krause DA, Hollman JH, Harmsen WS, Laskowski E. The influence of gender and age on hamstring muscle length in healthy adults. *J Orthop Sports Phys Ther.* 2005;35:246–252.

43. Kendall HO, Kendall FP. Normal flexibility according to age groups. *J Bone Joint Surg.* 1948;30:690–694.

44. Laban MM. Collagen tissue: Implications of its response to stress in vitro. *Arch Phys Med Rehabil.* 1962;43:461–465.

45. Leard JS. Flexibility and conditioning in the young athlete. In: Micheli LJ, ed. *Pediatr Adolesc Sports Med.* Boston, MA: Little, Brown; 1984:194–210.

46. Sutro CJ. Hypermobility of bones due to "overlengthened" capsular and ligamentous tissues. *Surgery.* 1947;21:67–76.

47. Pheasant S. *Ergonomics, Work and Health.* Gaithersburg, MD: Aspen; 1991.

48. Bassey EJ, Morgan K, Dallosso HM, Ebrahim SB. Flexibility of the shoulder joint measured as range of abduction in a large representative sample of men and women over 65 years of age. *Eur J Appl Physiol Occup Physiol* 1989;58:353–360.

49. Buckwalter JA. Maintaining and restoring mobility in middle and old age: The importance of the soft tissues. *Instruct Course Lect.* 1997;46:459–469.

50. Goldspink G. Cellular and molecular aspects of adaptation skeletal muscle. In Komi PV, ed. *Strength and Power in Sport.* London, U.K.: Blackwell Science; 1992:231–251.

51. Billson JJ, Cilliers JF, Pieterse JJ, Shaw BS, Shaw I, Toriola AL. Comparison of home-based and gymnasium-based resistance training on flexibility in the elderly. *South Afr J Res Sport Phys Educ Recreat.* 2011; 33:1–9.

52. Fiatarone MA. Physical activity and functional independence in aging. *Res Q Exerc Sport.* 1996;67:S70–S71.

53. Lehmann JF, Masock AJ, Warren CG, Koblanski JN. Effect of therapeutic temperature on tendon extensibility. *Arch Phys Med Rehabil.* 1970;51:481–487.

54. Mason T, Rigby BJ. Thermal transition in collagen. *Biomech Biophys Acta.* 1963;79:448–450.

55. Allander E, Bjornsson OJ, Olafsson O, Sigfusson N, Thorsteinsson J. Normal range of joint movements in shoulder, hip, wrist and thumb with special reference to side: A comparison between two populations. *Int J Epidemiol.* 1974;3:253–261.

56. Bell RD, Hoshizaki TB. Relationships of age and sex with range of motion of seventeen joint actions in humans. *Can J Appl Sport Sci.* 1981;6:202–206.

57. Mattes AL. *Active Isolated Stretching: The Mattes Method.* Sarasota, FL: Aaron Mattes Therapy; 2000.

58. Clark MA, Lucett SC, eds. *NASM Essentials of Corrective Exercise Training.* Baltimore, MD: Lippincott Williams & Wilkins; 2011.

59. Myers T. *Anatomy Trains: Myofascial Meridians for Manual and Movement Therapists.* 2nd ed. Philadelphia, PA: Churchill Livingstone; 2008.

60. Zachazewski JE, Reischl SR. Flexibility for the runner: Specific program considerations. *Top Acute Care Trauma Rehabil.* 1986;1:9–27.

61. Ratamess NA, Alvar BA, Evetoch TK, et al. ACSM Position Stand: Progression models in resistance training for healthy adults. *Med Sci Sports Exerc.* 2009;34:364–380.

62. Granit R. Muscle tone and postural regulation. In: Rodahl K, Hovrath SM, eds. *Muscle as Tissue.* New York, NY: McGraw-Hill; 1962:190.

63. Walker SM. Delay of twitch relaxation induced by stress and stress-relaxation. *J Appl Physiol.* 1961;16: 801–806.

64. Zachazewski JE. Flexibility in sports. In: Sanders B, ed. *Sports Physical Therapy.* Norwalk, CT: Appleton & Lange; 1990.

## *Practice What You Know:* Flexibility Assessments

A health and fitness professional may opt to assess a client's flexibility within specific areas of the body that demonstrate tightness or limitations to movement. The following flexibility assessments can be used to measure ROM at specific joints.

### PASSIVE STRAIGHT-LEG RAISE

**Objective**
The objective of the passive straight-leg raise is to assess the length of the hamstrings.

**Equipment**
• Stable table or exercise mat

**Instructions**
• Explain the objective of the test and allow a warm-up if necessary.
• Instruct the client to lie supine on a mat or table with the legs extended and the low back and sacrum flat against the surface.
• Place one hand under the calf of the leg that will be raised while instructing the client to keep the opposite leg extended on the mat or table. Restrain that leg from moving or rising during the test.
• Slide the other hand under the lumbar spine into the space between the client's back and the mat or table (Figure 1).

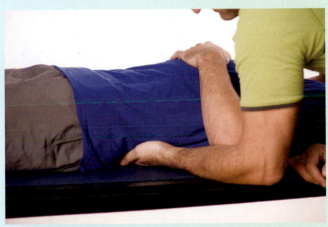

**Figure 1.** Passive straight-leg raise: tester's hand position.

• Advise the client to gently plantar-flex his or her ankles to point the toes away from the body. This position avoids a test limitation because of a tight gastrocnemius muscle (which would limit knee extension with the ankle in dorsiflexion). In addition, a straight-leg raise with dorsiflexion may increase tension within the sciatic nerve and create some discomfort.
• Slowly raise the one leg, asking the client to keep that knee loosely extended throughout the movement.
• Continue to raise the leg until firm pressure can be felt from the low back pressing down against the hand (Figure 2).

## *Practice What You Know:* Flexibility Assessments–cont'd

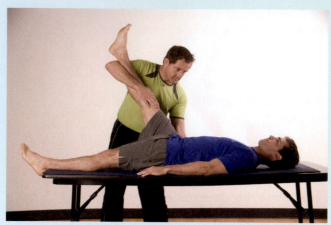

**Figure 2.** Passive straight-leg raise: test position.

- This indicates an end ROM of the hamstrings with movement now occurring as the pelvis rotates posteriorly.
- Throughout the movement, the client needs to maintain extension in the opposite leg and keep the sacrum and low back flat against the mat or table.
- If the test is performed with the opposite hip in slight flexion, this allows the pelvis more freedom to move into a posterior tilt, allowing a greater ROM and falsely increasing the length of the hamstrings.

### Observation
- Note the degree of movement attained from the table or mat that is achieved before the spine compresses the hand under the low back or the opposite leg begins to show visible signs of lifting off the table or mat.
  - The mat or table represents 0 degrees.
  - The leg perpendicular to the mat or table represents 90 degrees.

### General Interpretation
Use the information provided in Table 1 to determine the limitation(s).

### Table 1. Interpretation of the Passive Straight-leg Raise

| MOVEMENT/LIMITATION | HAMSTRINGS LENGTH |
| --- | --- |
| The raised leg achieves ≥80 degrees of movement before the pelvis rotates posteriorly. | Normal hamstrings length |
| The raised leg achieves <80 degrees of movement before the pelvis rotates posteriorly or there are any visible signs in the opposite leg lifting off the mat or table. | Tight hamstrings |

Data from Kendall FP, McCreary, EK, Provance PG, et al. *Muscles Testing and Function with Posture and Pain.* 5th ed. Baltimore, MD: Lippincott Williams & Wilkins; 2005.

## THOMAS TEST FOR HIP FLEXION/QUADRICEPS LENGTH

### Objective
- The objective of the Thomas test is to assess the length of the muscles involved in hip flexion. This test can actually assess the length of the primary hip flexors:
  - Hip flexors or iliopsoas
  - Rectus femoris (one of the four quadriceps muscles)
- This test should not be conducted on clients suffering from low-back pain, unless cleared by their physician.

## Practice What You Know: Flexibility Assessments—cont'd

**Equipment**
• Stable table

**Instructions**
• Given the nature of the movement associated with this test, trainers may want to consider draping a towel over the client's groin area.
• Explain the objective of the test and allow a warm-up if necessary.
• Instruct the client to sit at the end of a table with the mid-thigh aligned with the table edge. Place one hand behind the client's back and the other under his or her thighs (Figure 3).

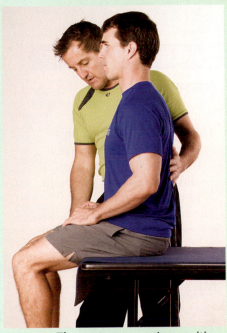

**Figure 3.** Thomas test: starting position.

• While supporting the client, instruct him or her to gently flex both thighs toward the chest, and gradually assist as the client rolls back onto the table to touch the back and shoulders to the tabletop.
  • Instruct the client to slowly pull one thigh (hip) toward the chest, reaching with both hands to grasp the thigh or the area behind the knee without raising or moving the torso.
  • Ask the client to slowly relax the opposite leg, allowing the knee to slowly fall toward the table and the lower leg to hang freely off the table edge (a 1-inch [2.5-cm] spacing between the back of the knee and the table edge is adequate) (Figure 4).

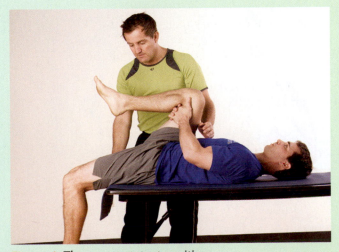

**Figure 4.** Thomas test: test position.

## *Practice What You Know:* Flexibility Assessments–cont'd

### Observations

- Observe whether the back of the lowered thigh touches the table (hips positioned in 10 degrees of extension).
- Observe whether the knee of the lowered leg achieves 80 degrees of flexion.
- Observe whether the knee remains aligned straight or falls into internal or external rotation.

### General Interpretations

Use the information provided in Table 2 to determine the location and identity of the tight or limiting muscles.

### Table 2. Interpretation of the Thomas Test

| MOVEMENT/LIMITATION | SUSPECTED MUSCLE TIGHTNESS |
| --- | --- |
| With the back and sacrum flat, the back of the lowered thigh does not touch the table and the knee cannot flex to 80 degrees. | Primary hip flexor muscles |
| With the back and sacrum flat, the back of the lowered thigh does not touch the table, but the knee does flex to 80 degrees. | The iliopsoas, which is preventing the hip from rotating posteriorly (this would allow the back of the thigh to touch the table) |
| With the back and sacrum flat, the back of the lowered thigh does touch the table, but the knee does not flex to 80 degrees. | The rectus femoris, which does not allow the knee to bend |

Data from Kendall FP, McCreary, EK, Provance PG, et al. *Muscles Testing and Function with Posture and Pain.* 5th ed. Baltimore, MD: Lippincott Williams & Wilkins; 2005.

### APLEY'S SCRATCH TEST FOR SHOULDER MOBILITY

#### Objective

The objective of Apley's scratch test is to assess simultaneous movements of the shoulder girdle (primarily the scapulothoracic and glenohumeral joints). *Note:* There are no quantitative measurements for this assessment—only a visual inspection to see how close the fingers get to the landmark on the scapula.

#### Movements

Movements include:

- Shoulder extension and flexion
- Internal and external rotation of the humerus at the shoulder
- Scapular abduction and adduction

#### Instructions

- Explain the purpose of the test and allow a warm-up if necessary (e.g., forward and rearward arm circles).
- From a sitting or standing position, the client raises one arm overhead, bending the elbow and rotating the arm outward while reaching behind the head with the palm facing inward to touch the medial border of the contralateral scapula or to reach down the spine (touching vertebrae) as far as possible (Figure 5).

## *Practice What You Know:* Flexibility Assessments–cont'd

- The client should avoid any excessive arching in the low back or rotation of the torso during the movement.
- Have the client repeat the test with the opposite arm.

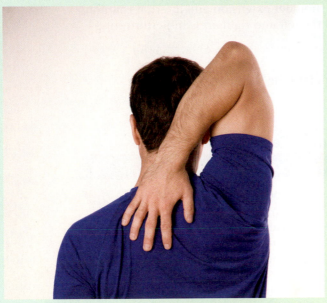

**Figure 5.** Apley's scratch test: shoulder flexion, external rotation, and scapular abduction.

- From a sitting or standing position, ask the client to reach one arm behind the back, bending the elbow and rotating the arm inward with the palm facing outward to touch the inferior angle of the contralateral scapula, or to reach up the spine (touching vertebrae) as far as possible (Figure 6).
- The client should avoid any excessive arching in the low back or rotation of the torso during the movement.
- Have the client repeat the test with the opposite arm.

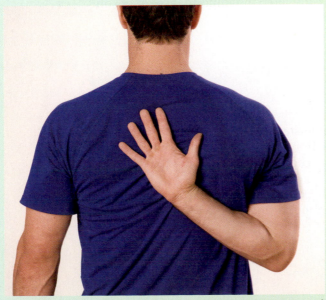

**Figure 6.** Apley's scratch test: shoulder extension, internal rotation, and scapular adduction.

## *Practice What You Know:* Flexibility Assessments–cont'd

### Observations
• Note the client's ability to touch the medial border of the contralateral scapula or how far down the spine he or she can reach with shoulder flexion and external rotation.
• Note the client's ability to touch the opposite inferior angle of the scapula or how far up the spine he or she can reach with shoulder extension and internal rotation.
• Observe any bilateral differences between the left and right arms in performing both movements.

### General Interpretations
Use the information provided in Table 3 to determine the limitation(s) in this flexibility test.

### Table 3. Interpretation of Apley's Scratch Test

| MOVEMENT/LIMITATION | SHOULDER MOBILITY* |
|---|---|
| Ability to touch specific landmarks | Good shoulder mobility |
| Inability to reach or touch the specific landmarks or discrepancies between the limbs | Requires further evaluation to determine the source of the limitation (i.e., which of the movements is problematic)<br>• Shoulder flexion and extension<br>• Internal and external rotation of the humerus<br>• Scapula abduction and adduction |

*Tightness of the joint capsules and ligaments may also contribute to limitations. It is common to see greater restriction on the dominant side because of increased muscle mass.

Data from Kendall FP, McCreary, EK, Provance PG, et al. *Muscles Testing and Function with Posture and Pain*. 5th ed. Baltimore, MD: Lippincott Williams & Wilkins; 2005.

## THORACIC SPINE MOBILITY SCREEN

### Objective
The objective of the thoracic spine mobility screen is to examine bilateral mobility of the thoracic spine. Lumbar spine rotation is considered insignificant, as it offers only approximately 15 degrees of rotation.

### Equipment
• Chair
• Squeezable ball or block
• 48-inch (1.2-m) dowel

### Instructions
• Briefly discuss the protocol so the client understands what is required.
• Instruct the client to sit upright toward the front edge of the seat with the feet together and firmly placed on the floor. The client's back should not touch the backrest.
• Place a squeezable ball or block between the knees and a dowel across the front of the shoulders, instructing the client to hold the bar in his or her hands (i.e., front barbell squat grip) (Figure 7).

# *Practice What You Know:* Flexibility Assessments–cont'd

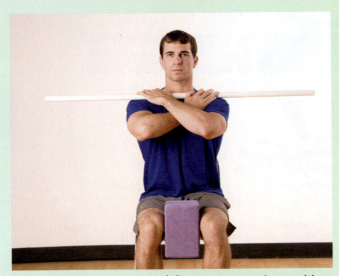

**Figure 7.** Thoracic spine mobility screen: starting position.

- While maintaining an upright and straight posture, the client squeezes the ball to immobilize the hips and gently rotates left and right to an end ROM without any bouncing (Figure 8).

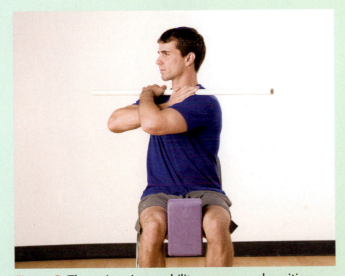

**Figure 8.** Thoracic spine mobility screen: end position.

- Do not cue the client to use good technique, but instead observe his or her natural movement.
- Ask the client to perform a few repetitions in each direction, slowly and with control.

## Observation
Observe any bilateral discrepancies between the rotations in each direction (see Table 4).

*Practice What You Know:* Flexibility Assessments—cont'd

### Table 4. Thoracic Spine Mobility Screen

| VIEW | JOINT LOCATION | COMPENSATION | POSSIBLE BIOMECHANICAL PROBLEMS |
|------|----------------|--------------|-------------------------------|
| Transverse | Trunk | None if trunk rotation achieves 45 degrees in each direction | |
| Transverse | Trunk | Bilateral discrepancy (assuming no existing congenital issues in the spine) | Side dominance<br>Differences in paraspinal development<br>Torso rotation, perhaps associated with some hip rotation<br>*Note:* Lack of thoracic mobility will negatively impact glenohumeral mobility |

Data from Sahrmann, S.A. (2002). *Diagnosis and Treatment of Movement Impairment Syndromes.* St. Louis, MO: Mosby.

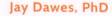

**CHAPTER 18**

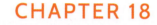

# Skill-Related Training

## CHAPTER OUTLINE

## CHAPTER OUTLINE–cont'd

*Training for Power*
   PHASES OF PLYOMETRIC EXERCISES
   GUIDELINES
   PROGRAM DESIGN
*Training for Speed, Agility, and Quickness*
   GUIDELINES
   PROGRAM DESIGN
**Vignette Conclusion**
**Critical Thinking Questions**
**Additional Resources**
**References**
**Practice What You Know**

## LEARNING OUTCOMES

1. Define the following skill-related components of fitness: *balance, coordination, power, speed, agility,* and *reaction time*.

2. Explain the five basic concepts and principles associated with skill-related training.

3. Describe the components of a sports conditioning training program.

4. List the components of a comprehensive training program that integrates the skill-related components of fitness with other modalities of training.

5. Describe key techniques to proper form for a variety of drills that improve balance, power, speed, agility, and quickness.

## ANCILLARY LINK

Visit Davis*Plus* at http://davisplus.fadavis.com for study and practice resources, including online quizzes, animations that help explain physiological processes, podcasts concerning news and career trends in exercise physiology, and practice references.

## VIGNETTE

■ Ben is a strength and conditioning coach for a Division III football team in a small college town. He holds a certification from the National Strength and Conditioning Association and has been working toward his master's degree. His goal is to start his own business providing sport-specific training to athletes and fitness enthusiasts in the community.

After earning his degree, Ben retains his job with the football team and begins offering small-group training sessions in the evenings. Among his first clients are Ryan, Parker, and Antonio, three friends who are in excellent physical condition and who play together in a recreational soccer league.

What aspects of athletic performance should Ben focus on when training his new clients?

Skill-related training, a long-standing training modality for improving sports performance, has recently emerged as a popular modality of training within health and fitness, and it will likely continue to increase in popularity in the future. Although many exercise enthusiasts have traditionally viewed skill-related training as a modality reserved primarily for improving performance, it has become apparent that the benefits of training these parameters has relevancy to all exercisers, whether seeking to improve health, fitness, or performance. In this chapter, however, the terms *skill-related* and *sports conditioning* are used interchangeably.

The skill-related components of fitness include balance, coordination, power, speed, agility, and reaction time. Although commonly associated with athletic performance, these skills can be equally important for the nonathlete, because they have a positive impact on an individual's overall quality of life. The relevance and importance of each of these components depends on the needs of the individual in the following areas:

- Joint angles and ranges of motion needed
- Forces and torques that must be incurred
- Speeds that must be achieved
- Distances that must be traveled

These same biomechanical and physiological factors apply to nonathletes. For example, the basic fundamental movement skills required by a running back on the playing field may be remarkably similar to the movement patterns performed by a father playing with his children on the playground. Furthermore, the need to produce force rapidly, or rate of force development, is important for the sprinter to best an opponent, but may be equally as important for a police officer rushing to the aid of a victim of crime. Therefore, each of these components should be considered when developing a training program either for athletes or for the general population. However, priority and time commitments to developing these attributes should be based on an individual's specific needs and goals.

When incorporating specific skills training into a client's general training programs, however, health and fitness professionals should develop an appropriate training base or foundation to accommodate the stress that this form of training places on the body. For this reason, the higher the level of skill-related component required, the more important a solid base of the requisite health-related components of fitness becomes to support these movements and minimize injury risk. This chapter explores each of these components in detail and discusses their relevance to human performance in a variety of settings. Specific training considerations are also described in detail.

## SKILL-RELATED COMPONENTS OF FITNESS

This section describes in detail the following skill-related components of fitness: balance, coordination, power, speed, agility, and reaction time.

## Balance

The ability to maintain one's **balance**, or **center of gravity (COG)**, over a fixed and changing **base of support (BOS)** is critical for movement efficiency (Fig. 18-1). COG is the point at which the distribution of body weight would be considered equal in all directions and is generally located slightly anterior to the S1-S2 joint at the sacrum. This point is usually higher in men than in women because of body mass distribution (i.e., men demonstrate increased amounts of upper-extremity mass), but this location varies within individuals according to differences in body shape.

COG differs slightly in definition from **center of mass (COM)**, which defines the location in which the majority of a person's weight is concentrated. BOS, in contrast, is generally defined as the space under and between a person's feet. BOS plays an important role in maintaining balance; a wider BOS is established by moving the feet farther apart to increase stability, whereas moving the feet closer or standing on one foot reduces the BOS and decreases stability. Given the importance of balance to good posture and all movement, and considering how balance serves as the foundation to essentially all forms of training, this topic will be discussed in more detail in the next section.

Balance is typically categorized as either static or dynamic.[1,2] **Static balance** requires an individual to shift or alter his or her COM over an unchanging, or fixed, BOS. For example, static balance is required when an individual initially stands from a seated position before attempting to move. **Dynamic balance**, or the ability

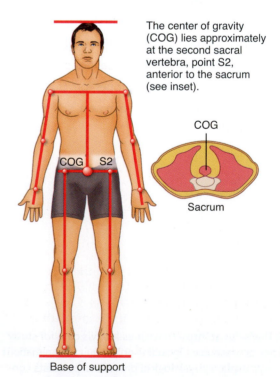

The center of gravity (COG) lies approximately at the second sacral vertebra, point S2, anterior to the sacrum (see inset).

COG

S2

COG

Sacrum

Base of support

**Figure 18-1.** Center of gravity is the point at which the distribution of body weight would be considered equal in all directions.

to maintain balance while moving, requires an individual to lose, manipulate, and regain control of his or her COM over a changing BOS, such as when walking, marching, running, skipping, and jumping.[2]

Without the ability to maintain balance, most movements that are influenced by gravity, momentum, inertia, and ground reaction forces (GRFs) would be too difficult, if not impossible, to perform safely. The reality is that many sports and recreational activities require rapid multidirectional movements ranging from brief bursts of activity to statically controlled positions in which the COG is pushed toward the edge of the BOS.[3] For example, an athlete attempting to keep a basketball in play at the sideline may need to turn to run toward the sideline, decelerate rapidly while keeping both feet in-bounds, then reach his upper extremity over the line toward the ball to put it back into play. For this reason and many others, balance could be considered the underlying component of most functional human movements.[4,5]

Although balance appears to be a relatively simple concept, it is actually a very complex process that is dependent on the successful interaction and coordination of several systems and subsystems in the body, such as the visual, vestibular, and somatosensory systems.[1] Each of these systems provides individuals with visual, tactile, and perceptual feedback about their environment, the body's location, and the direction and speed of movements to aid in maintaining both static and dynamic postural equilibrium. When the functional abilities of these systems are reduced, the ability to balance may be compromised. For example, vertigo is a condition that affects the vestibular system; individuals with vertigo perceive the body is in motion while it is actually stationary (e.g., standing). For this reason, people who suffer from vertigo are unable to orient themselves in their environment and often experience sensations of dizziness and nausea, and have difficulty ambulating.

In recent years, the use of balance training has gained popularity among fitness and rehabilitation professionals as a method for improving performance and reducing risks of injuries, especially in older adults who exhibit greater propensities for falls.[3,6,7] This form of training is commonly used in conjunction with traditional strength and conditioning exercises as a method to enhance balance, dynamic joint stabilization, and neural efficiency with **perturbation training** (Fig. 18-2)[1,7-9] For example, nontraditional training implements, such as chains, sandbags, and slosh pipes (pipes filled partially with water), are commonly used forms of perturbation training because they provide a predictable, yet slightly varying movement path when performing an exercise.[10] Practitioners may also create these small multidirectional forces by using resistance tubing. For instance, as an athlete attempts to perform a squat while using his or her own body weight, the trainer uses a resistance tube positioned around the athlete's waist to add consistent, yet unpredictable balance disturbances. This forces the

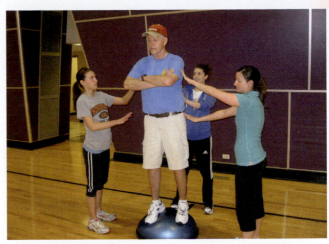

**Figure 18-2.** Perturbation training is the use of randomized and unpredictable, yet controlled, multidirectional forces to create subtle disturbances in an individual's balance. *(Photo courtesy of Lance Dalleck)*

athlete to adjust his or her body position in relation to these forces to maintain balance.

Although numerous research studies discuss the benefits of balance training as a method for fall or injury prevention or rehabilitation, this form of training has also been shown to negatively impact force and power production.[11] For this reason, this form of training may have a limited application when developing training programs for apparently healthy or athletic populations.[6] Therefore, the amount of time and emphasis placed on this type of unstable training must be considered in terms of the individual's strengths, weaknesses, and goals.

Most balance training programs progress from exercises performed on stable surfaces (e.g., the ground) to more unstable surfaces (e.g., balance/rocker boards, domed training devices, and pads). This progressively increases the proprioceptive demands of the exercise (Box 18-1). However, in recent years, some professionals have questioned whether a more sport-specific method of balance training should be used for athletes.[6,12]

## Coordination

**Coordination** means that the muscles of the body are working in an organized and synergistic fashion to produce both simple and complex movement patterns.[13,14] Physiologically speaking, coordination is typically considered in terms of intramuscular (within muscles) and intermuscular (between or within a group of muscles) coordination.

- **Intramuscular coordination** refers to the number of motor units an individual is able to simultaneously activate.[15,16]
- **Intermuscular coordination** refers to an individual's ability to activate certain muscles, or muscle groups, in a specific order to perform skilled movements or actions.[15]

Both the number of motor units and the order in which they are stimulated can have a profound impact

## FROM THEORY TO PRACTICE

Balance is influenced by the visual, vestibular, and somatosensory systems. To illustrate this point, stand on a single leg with your hands outstretched to assist you in maintaining your balance. Perform the following actions:

- To challenge the somatosensory system, place your hands on your hips and extend your leg in front of you.
   √ How did you have to adjust your body to maintain equilibrium?
- To challenge the vestibular system, slowly turn your head to the right and then the left. Look upward and then downward. Slightly speed up this movement.
   √ How was your balance influenced by changing your head position and speed of movement?
- While looking straight ahead, close one eye and then the other eye.
   √ What systems do you feel working harder to help you stay oriented?

### Box 18-1. Active Resistance

*Active resistance* is a term coined by Hedrick[6] to describe a method of training that uses "active" resistance (e.g., water-filled devices, sandbags, and kettlebells to a lesser degree where the mass of the device shifts with movement). It is considered an advanced form of balance training that places additional demands on the body that may need to constantly adapt with movement. This type of training is different from more traditional forms of static resistance (e.g., barbell, dumbbells), where the mass of the device does not shift. Because athletes must often control, redirect, or overcome active resistance for effective movement while shifting their BOS on a stable surface (e.g., trying to hold on to a ball as an opponent attempts to strip it away, or redirecting an opponent's body weight to avoid being tackled), this form of training may add an advanced but appropriate level of training to an athlete's conditioning program.[12] Although a greater emphasis is being placed on this method of training, research is still needed to validate its effectiveness.

on human movement. An increase in the rate or frequency of neural firing also occurs with the increased intensity of a stimulus. This increase in neural transmission rate, also known as rate coding, can increase force production in a given motor unit.[17] Individuals with higher levels of intermuscular coordination are able to move more efficiently and, therefore, may be able to perform movements with a higher level of proficiency in the skill than their less coordinated counterparts. Consequently, individuals with greater coordination are able to execute both basic and complex movements with greater movement economy.

Although coordination may be driven to a large extent by genetics, it is a trainable skill. Evidence indicates that certain stages of growth and development may be ideal for optimizing coordination.[18] This may be accomplished by emphasizing the fundamental movement skills within an individual's training program.[4,5,19,20,20a] For example, when an adolescent is undergoing a growth spurt, the rapid changes in limb lengths may decrease coordination as the body grows; therefore, the opportunity to reinforce balance and coordination skills during this growth phase may prove valuable in maintaining some athletic competency.

### Power

In mechanical terms, **power** is defined as the rate of doing work[21] and can be calculated as work divided by the time in which the work is done (Power = work ÷ time).[22] Power can also be described as the combination of force (strength) and velocity (speed).[23,24] Some power movements favor strength (i.e., require lower velocities with heavier loads), such as power lifting, whereas other movements favor speed (i.e., high velocities with light loads), such as punching, kicking, and swinging a tennis racket. In essence, all movements exist along a power continuum of strength and speed.[24] Therefore, when designing a power training program, the fitness professional should determine where a particular skill exists on this continuum and then select exercises with similar speed and load requirements to the target activity in which power improvements are being sought.

Numerous factors influence one's ability to produce power, including the elastic and proprioceptive properties of a muscle, neuromuscular efficiency, body composition, and functional strength levels.[1] In many sports where explosive movements are needed, power may contribute to athletic success.[21] Thus, training programs should include strategies to improve power that ideally transfer to sports performance.

In addition, power training should be specific to the plane of movement in which the skill is performed to provide the greatest carryover effect to the target activity. For example, if a coach or fitness professional is seeking to improve rotational power for a golfer, power training in the transverse plane, such as a medicine ball rotational throw, would likely translate better to performance than a vertical jump, because of the greater biomechanical similarities between these movements. In addition, for athletes who need to produce power in more horizontal rather than vertical directions (e.g., accelerating into a sprint, blocking a defensive lineman in American football, or throwing the shot put), training in these planes and replicating these specific propulsive forces should be emphasized in their training program.

## Speed

**Speed** is defined as the ability to cover a given distance in a certain amount of time.[25] **Linear speed**, or straight-line speed, is determined by the combination of **stride frequency** (the number of strides per unit of time) and **stride length** (the distance covered in a single stride). Linear speed can be improved by enhancing either or both of these elements.[26] The importance of linear speed is imperative in most track and field events. However, for many athletes, such as field sport athletes, linear speed is likely to be less important than good multidirectional speed (i.e., quickness in changing direction as in a basketball game).[27]

The ability to improve speed is of great importance to many athletes. However, speed is composed of several subqualities, including acceleration, maximal velocity, and speed-endurance.[28]

- **Acceleration** is the rate of change in velocity. In sports, acceleration typically refers to the speed generated in the first 5 to 10 m from a stationary or moving start.[29,30]
- **Maximal velocity** can be defined as the highest speed attained during an event or performance. For field sports, an athlete's maximum velocity is usually attained within 30 to 40 m (33–44 yards),[31] and for track athletes, maximum velocity likely occurs between 40 and 50 m (44 and 55 yards).[31]

- **Speed-endurance** is the ability to maintain top or near-top speed performance. This includes the ability to withstand fatigue and sustain high intensities without significant reductions in speed (e.g., 400-m run). Speed-endurance may also refer to the ability to perform repeated sprints in intermittent sports, such as soccer, lacrosse, and ice hockey.

## Agility

**Agility** is most often defined as the ability to start, stop, and change directions rapidly and efficiently either in response to a stimulus or while performing a preprogrammed movement pattern.[28,32] Plisk[33] defines agility as an athlete's collective coordinative abilities. Agility performance is influenced by numerous physical and cognitive factors. Young, Jones, and Montgomery[34] separated these factors into two broad categories: perceptual/decision-making factors and change of direction speed (Fig. 18-3).

The first category addresses the cognitive/mental aspects of agility performance, or perceptual and decision-making factors. This category addresses how an individual gains awareness and processes sensory information from the environment to select an appropriate response movement. For example, as a tennis player waits for a serve from the opponent, he or she processes information in relation to the speed and position of the server's arm and racket to get an anticipatory clue as to where the ball will land. This assists the athlete in making a mental plan for how he or she will need to be positioned in relation to the serve to be in the best position to return the ball over the net.

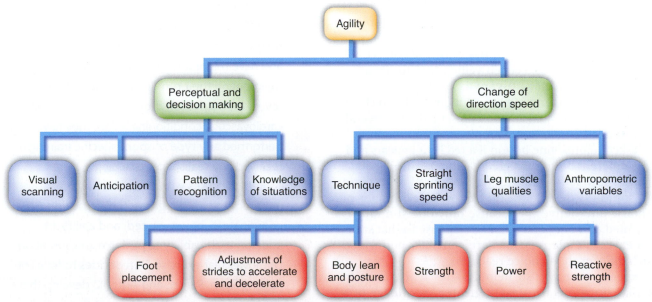

**Figure 18-3.** Agility performance is influenced by numerous physical and cognitive factors that can be divided into two categories: perceptual/decision-making factors and change of direction speed. *(Adapted from Young WB, James R, Montgomery I. (2002). Is muscle power related to running speed with changes of direction? J Sports Med Phys Fitness, 2002;43:282–288, by permission.)*

Often this form of agility is referred to as **reactive agility**.[35]

The second category addresses those factors related to the physical attributes that allow individuals to change direction rapidly. In this category, factors such as technique, linear speed, leg muscle qualities, and anthropometric variables are considered.

## Reaction Time

**Reaction time** is defined as the time elapsed from a stimulus to the initiation of a movement or the production of force.[36] Reaction time is highly dependent on perceptual and decision-making skills. To react appropriately to stimuli, individuals must collect information from their environment via the visual, auditory, and somatosensory systems.[37] Once sensory input is collected, the individual must then make a decision regarding whether to react. If the decision to react is made, then the decision must be made to determine how to react to successfully perform the skill or task required. Therefore, by enhancing an individual's speed of recognition, the ability to make quick and accurate decisions regarding the requisite movement skills to successfully execute a task may also be improved.[38] The ability to recognize these stimuli are heavily dependent on the type of stimuli (visual, auditory, or tactile), the number of stimuli, and one's experience.

The type of stimuli received has a profound impact on the speed the stimulus is received and processed. According to Vickers,[39] the time required to respond to a visual stimuli is approximately 180 to 200 milliseconds, to an auditory stimuli is about 140 to 160 milliseconds, and to a kinesthetic stimuli is approximately 120 to 140 milliseconds.

The number of stimuli in the environment also impacts reaction time. According to Schmidt and Lee,[40-42] reactions can be categorized as either simple or choice.

- **Simple reaction** can be defined as the display of a single stimulus that has only one correct response, such as a coach yelling "go" to signal an athlete to run a 40-yard dash.
- **Choice reactions** require an individual to pick an appropriate response when presented with several possible stimuli. For example, a person might be asked to press one button if a red light appears and a different button if a green light appears.

Hick's law states that the time required to respond to a stimuli is dependent on the possible number of response alternatives.[43] Because only one stimulus is presented and only one possible response to that stimulus exists, simple reactions are generally performed much quicker than choice reactions.[40-42]

Experience may also help athletes react faster in familiar situations because of greater knowledge of a situation. For example, experienced athletes typically have a better working knowledge of offensive and defensive strategies used in specific game situations and the tendencies of certain players/teams. Thus, they use different visual search patterns to find relevant anticipatory cues than an inexperienced individual.[43] For example, during a baseball game, a third baseman realizes that, based on the situation, the batter may try to lay down a bunt. The fielder would look for visual cues, such as the batter pivoting in the batter's box, to gain a signal that she may need to charge a bunted ball. This would be very different from responding to a generic stimulus, such as a flashing light positioned on a speed training device that signals an athlete to react in a certain way. Although this form of training may improve reaction time in a specific drill, it does not necessarily help the athlete learn how to read and react to the ball coming off the bat. Thus, the transfer of such a stimulus to an actual game situation may be irrelevant because the context of the drill is not similar to a real game situation.[44] An agility training drill in which the athlete is required to react to a coach either bunting or rolling a baseball would be more contextually appropriate and may transfer better to on-field performance because it more closely relates to what the athlete would experience in a real game scenario.

By creating appropriate training drills similar to real game situations, the coach/trainer may be able to enhance an athlete's ability to identify task-relevant cues and improve the synaptic linkages required to retrieve specific motor patterns and movements in competitive or real-world situations.[45] This presents a strong rationale for progressing or incorporating sport-specific agility training drills into an athlete's training program.

## VIGNETTE *continued*

■ During his first sessions with Ryan, Parker, and Antonio, Ben learns that they met while competing on the cross-country running team in high school and have maintained their high level of fitness by maintaining their running program. They also reveal that, although they clearly have excellent cardiovascular conditioning levels, they have never performed any type of sport-specific training or received any real soccer coaching.

Ben discusses with them the physical requirements of the game, which include coordination, power, speed, and agility, in addition to the ability to perform long-duration cardiovascular exercise. Ben decides to focus on helping Ryan, Parker, and Antonio develop these skills, while allowing them to continue with their running program on their own.

## FROM THEORY TO PRACTICE

Think of three different sports: soccer (or football as it is called internationally), volleyball, and the shot put in track and field events. Given your understanding of the six skill-related parameters of fitness, identify how each, if applicable, would be critical to success in each sport. A collaborative effort with peers may help to better understand the needs of each sport.

## BASIC TRAINING CONCEPTS AND PRINCIPLES

When performing any activity that requires powerful, swift, and efficient movements, several basic concepts and principles should be considered. Having a base level of understanding about how each of these concepts applies to performance will greatly enhance the fitness professional's understanding of how to teach and correct movement mechanics, and how to optimize performance for the athlete-client. Specific movement mechanics are addressed later in this chapter; however, a global understanding of movement is essential before progressing forward. The basic training concepts and principles include:

- The kinetic chain concept
- COG and COM
- BOS and stability
- The force/velocity continuum

### Kinetic Chain Concept

The term **kinetic chain** was coined by Steindler,[45] who used an engineering model to describe human movement. This concept is used to illustrate the dynamic and integrated fashion in which the human body functions. It consists primarily of the body's segments (i.e., body and extremities—legs, arms) that are linked together via joints (articular systems) to create movement and includes all of the muscles, ligaments, tendons, fascia, and neural systems.[1] Each of these systems works in concert with one another to create efficient movement. This is outlined in more detail in Chapter 14. Consequently, the position and function of each of these links affects each subsequent link in the chain. For example, during foot-strike, if the foot overly pronates (collapses inward) the knee will adduct (collapse inward) toward the midline of the body. This leads to a condition known as **valgus collapse**, which makes an individual more prone to injury.

Furthermore, when the joints are not in proper biomechanical alignment, forces cannot be effectively transferred from the ground up through the entire kinetic chain. Therefore, good movement mechanics are highly dependent on the body's ability to transfer forces produced at foot-strike from the foot, up through the legs, trunk, and extremities. During movement, it is critical that the hip, knee, and ankle extend simultaneously with as much force as possible to maximize force production. This concept directly relates to Newton's third law of motion, which addresses action-reaction. When a person exerts force into the ground, the ground will exert an equal and opposite force on that person's body. The forces the ground exerts on the body are known as **ground reaction forces (GRFs)**. The better able a person is harnessing the GRFs and transfering them through the kinetic chain, the greater the opportunity for powerful, explosive, and efficient movements. For example, when running or jumping, a person must first flex at the ankle, knee, and hip (i.e., **triple flexion**) to then push off the ground, increasing GRFs to forcefully extend these joints (i.e., **triple extension**) and transfer these forces up the kinetic chain for explosive athletic-type movements.[46]

### Center of Gravity and Center of Mass

As a person shifts his COM, his COG is altered, which causes him to move. Thus, to create efficient movement, it is important that the body is positioned in a way that allows a person to control his COG. If an individual is unable to control movement as this shifting occurs, the by-product will be awkward, inefficient movement patterns. If an individual shifts her COM too far outside the limits of stability, the COG may be significantly altered to the point at which the individual can no longer maintain her balance and may even fall[32] (Fig. 18-4). This is one of the reasons balance, especially dynamic balance, is so critical to movements that require speed and power.

For example, when accelerating to a sprint, an individual must create a **positive shin angle (PSA)**, or an angle in which the shin is pointed in the intended direction of movement, the individual must have a slight forward lean at the torso, and the foot must be behind the COG. If the foot is in front of the COG, the GRFs created at foot-strike will transfer in a more vertical fashion, creating more of a braking force than one optimal for horizontal propulsion.[29] Figure 18-5 shows the proper acceleration technique for a nontrack athlete. Notice the PSA created by the athlete's front leg, the neutral posture of the torso, and the triple extension of the rear leg to generate explosive GRFs. This position will allow the athlete to maximize the transfer of energy throughout the kinetic chain to propel the individual in the intended direction.

### Base of Support and Stability

The *BOS* is defined as the space that exists between and under the feet, and changes as a person moves foot position.[22] For example, when standing with a

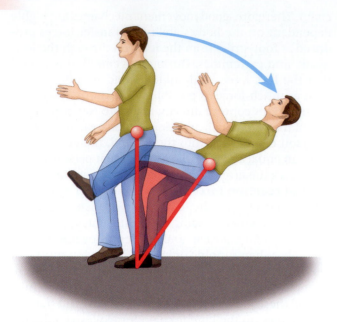

**Figure 18-4.** If an individual shifts his or her center of mass too far outside the limits of stability, the center of gravity may be significantly altered to the point at which the individual can no longer maintain balance and may even fall.

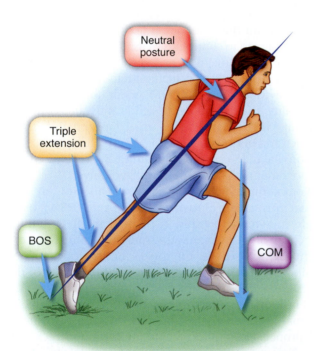

**Figure 18-5.** Efficient acceleration technique. Notice the positive shin angle created by the athlete's front leg, the neutral posture of the torso, and the triple extension of the rear leg to generate explosive ground reaction forces. BOS, base of support; COM, center of mass.

wide stance, the BOS represents the space between and under the feet. Moving the feet closer together reduces the BOS, and moving onto one foot represents a further reduction in the BOS. BOS is an important concept when seeking to improve stability. **Stability** is the ease or difficulty with which balance can be disturbed.

A common stance used by athletes to optimize stability is the **universal athletic position (UAP)**, shown in Figure 18-6. This position provides an individual with good stability, especially in the frontal plane.[15] Manipulating the BOS has a profound impact on a person's stability. For example, by bringing the feet closer together, the COM rises while the BOS becomes narrower. Consequently, a person is less stable in this position than in the UAP, in which the COM is lower and the BOS is wider. For example, a linebacker in football or rugby player preparing to make a tackle would want to increase his BOS to enhance stability in preparation to make his tackle in comparison to standing with a narrow BOS (more upright) where he may be pushed over by the ball carrier.

However, it is important to understand that during movement, the BOS is constantly changing. For instance, when running at maximal velocity, BOS would be greatest in the split-stance position; although this position may be ideal for linear sprinting performance and generating maximal velocity, it is a poor position for directional changes because stability in the frontal plane is reduced. Therefore, if an individual performed an agility movement requiring a directional change, widening the BOS and lowering the COM can significantly improve balance and body control without too much loss of speed. Consider this concept in terms of automobile performance: A Formula One car has a wide BOS and a low COM to enhance its ability to make quick directional changes and turns. A drag racing car is narrow

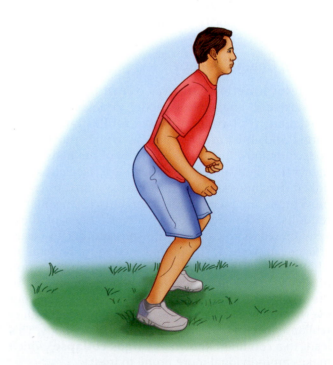

**Figure 18-6.** The universal athletic position (UAP), often referred to as neutral stance (feet placed at shoulder-width position), provides an individual with good stability, especially in the frontal plane.

because lateral stability is less of a factor for this vehicle, as it is designed to go as fast as possible in a straight line.

## Force/Velocity Continuum

Power exists on a continuum, and the power demands required to perform successfully vary widely between activities and sports. The force-velocity continuum, illustrated in Figure 18-7, shows that maximal speed and maximal force exist at different ends of a scale. An example of maximal force is a one-repetition maximum squat performed at a moderate pace, whereas maximal speed is swinging a golf club at faster speeds and less force. Optimal amounts of speed and force needed for all activities fall somewhere along this curve. Maximal force cannot be produced during high-speed activities, such as sprinting, because the foot is not in contact with the ground long enough to allow the muscles adequate time to generate forces at this pace (the foot is only in contact with the ground for fractions of a second). For this reason, in many sports and even activities of daily living, the rate at which the body can generate force is as important as the ability to produce maximal force. The goal, therefore, of many training programs seeking to improve performance is to improve the amount of force over the time interval during which the force acts (known as **impulse**). Many sports require explosive-type movements (e.g., volleyball, tennis), and thus exist more toward the maximal velocity end of the continuum, rather than toward maximal force.

## SPORTS CONDITIONING TRAINING PROGRAM COMPONENTS

Constructing a sports conditioning program can initially be very challenging because of the wide array of training options and programs that are available.

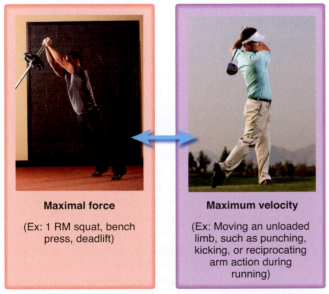

**Maximal force**

(Ex: 1 RM squat, bench press, deadlift)

**Maximum velocity**

(Ex: Moving an unloaded limb, such as punching, kicking, or reciprocating arm action during running)

**Figure 18-7.** Force/velocity continuum. Note that maximal speed and maximal force exist at different ends of the continuum.

However, regardless of the approach, several training variables can be manipulated to elicit the desired training adaptation. These variables include frequency of training, intensity of the training drill(s), volume of work performed, periodization, and drill selection and progression. Each of these variables is described in this section and then applied to specific training methods later in this chapter.

Programming variables such as frequency and intensity contribute to successful sports conditioning program design. They are discussed in detail in Chapters 13 and 15. Within a sports conditioning program, however, volume, previously defined as the amount of work performed in a session, may be described as the total amount of distance traveled in a session, or the amount of time spent performing drills. For plyometric (explosive training) drills, the volume of training is often based on the number of foot contacts (either double or single legged) performed during a training session. Table 18-1 presents a progressive model for selecting plyometric training volumes based on the intensity of the drills selected and the conditioning levels of the individual. Foot contact is not universal to all plyometric drills, because volume for some horizontal plyometrics drills, such as bounding, may use distance to calculate volume.

## Periodization

The concept of **periodization**, which was introduced in Chapter 13, is essentially a systematic planning method used to maximize performance while managing fatigue, resulting in strategically achieving predetermined periods of peak performance. Chapter 13 also introduced the concept of specific time periods known as a **macrocyle**, **mesocycle(s)**, and **microcycle(s)**. The following is a brief review:

- Macrocycles comprise the entire training period.
- Mesocycles represent blocks of training that last several weeks to months.
- Microcycles range between a few sessions and 1 to 4 weeks in duration.

Transition periods (offloading) are used between training cycles as a method of recovery. In traditional resistance training programs, these cycles are generally used to delineate a change from high-volume training to high-intensity training.[47]

For the general population, periodization cycles that include speed, agility, and power training are usually less structured, because many recreational enthusiasts really have no need to peak for a specific event. For athletes, however, it is important to plan these cycles in the context of the sports season. According to Wathen, Baechle, and Earle,[47] the sport season can be broken down into four periods:

- Off-season
- Preseason
- In season
- Postseason

**Table 18-1. Guidelines for Plyometric Training Volumes (Foot Contacts) and Intensities**

| ATHLETIC LEVEL | LOW-INTENSITY DRILLS | MODERATE-INTENSITY DRILLS | HIGH-INTENSITY DRILLS |
|---|---|---|---|
| Beginner | 80–100 | 60 (100–120 total*) | 40 (100–120 total*) |
| Intermediate | 100–150 | 80–100 (150–200 total*) | 60–80 (150–200 total*) |
| Advanced | 140–200 | 100–120 (180–220 total*) | 80–100 (180–220 total*) |

*Includes some low-intensity drills as movement preparation for the more advanced drills.

## Off-season Period

**Off-season** is the period between the postseason and approximately 6 weeks (although this may vary) before the first contest or competition of the following year's season. During the first portion of this preparatory phase, the main emphasis is on general conditioning to build a solid foundation of fitness for the intense training the individual will be expected to perform in future training cycles. During this phase, there should be no competitions and minimal sport-specific skills practices. Conditioning activities during this phase focus on higher training volumes and use lower-intensity training drills that emphasize developing fundamental movements. As this preparatory period progresses, there will be a gradual shift from higher to lower training volumes and from lower to higher intensities to help improve sport-specific strength and fitness, and allow adequate recovery for the athlete as more attention is placed on the development of sport-specific skills.

## Preseason Period

The **preseason** period immediately follows the off-season training program and lasts approximately 2 to 4 months for most sports. Between these periods it is beneficial to add a transition phase of 1 to 2 weeks to transition from higher-volume/lower-intensity training to higher-intensity/lower-volume training. During this period, a greater emphasis is placed on skill-related training practices, and the conditioning drills selected should become increasingly more sport specific in nature.

## In-Season Period

The **in-season** period is the time frame in which the athletes are actually competing in their sport. During this time frame, the major emphasis of the training program should be to maintain the strength and power gained in the offseason so the athletes do not experience performance decrements as the season progresses.

When working with a multisport high school athlete or an athlete who plays sports year-round, the volume and intensity of the training program may need to be periodically adjusted (lowered) to ensure recovery between sessions and competitions. For these athletes, the trainer or coach can prioritize their training cycle based on the most important competition or sport that takes priority for the athlete. Another alternative would be to divide the training week up into heavy, moderate, and light training days.

## Postseason Period

The **postseason** commences after the completion of the in-season period and is generally devoted to recovery, allowing athletes much needed time to recover from the stress of competition (offloading). Light-active recoveries often are implemented at this time, during which athletes may select or participate in general, non–sport-specific activities that minimize the stresses placed on their bodies or that they enjoy doing (e.g., cross-training).

## Drill Selection and Progression

When selecting drills and exercises for sports conditioning programs, a motor development approach should be followed. This approach emphasizes a logical progression from simple, preprogrammed drills with a high degree of focus on skill acquisition to drills that require greater mental and cognitive demands in a more contextually appropriate environment. The long-term goal of this approach is to assist individuals in learning specific movement patterns and reinforce faster, more precise motor recruitment patterns to enhance movement quality and control.[48] The following subsections describe closed versus open drills and blocked versus random practice.

## Closed Versus Open Drills

Drills for improving speed, agility, and power are generally classified as closed or open.

- **Closed drills** are preprogrammed training drills that are performed in a predictable and unchanging environment. These types of drills require the individual to perform a preset movement pattern that minimizes the amount of environmental feedback required to perform the drill. For example, a closed training drill may require an individual to stand on a starting line, run in a straight line to a cone, and then backpedal until returning to the starting line.
- **Open drills** require athletes to accurately respond to a variety of environmental stimuli to select an appropriate movement pattern based on the context of the situation. For example, a game such as tag is considered an open drill because there are no set patterns, and individuals must read the body movements and actions of their competitors to determine the appropriate movement pattern to tag an opponent or avoid a tag.

For beginners, closed training drills should be emphasized to help maximize learning and master the fundamental movement skills. To determine which drills should be priority, the fitness professional should perform a basic movement needs analysis of an activity or sport and break down the tasks into specific movements, or discrete tasks.[49]

A **discrete task** is one with a clear beginning and end, and should be the focus of drill selection at this stage. An example of a discrete task would be a forward run, backpedal, or lateral shuffle. These drills are typified by an emphasis on motor learning and skill development, rather than decision making. Once each of these skills has been mastered, the fitness professional may now combine these movements to create a **serial task**, which is a combination of discrete tasks. For example, running forward to a cone, shuffling sideways to another, and sprinting back to the starting line would be a serial task. This type of programming is also referred to as part-to-whole learning.

Once clients or athletes become proficient in their movement abilities, a greater emphasis can be placed on the use of open drills. This requires the individual to adapt these skills learned in a closed environment to real-life situations, rather than performing them as a preprogrammed pattern or drill.[40-42] This type of training places a greater emphasis on an athlete's perceptual and decision-making skills. During this stage, there is a certain amount of automaticity that should occur when executing a specific movement pattern. In other words, movement skills have been mastered so that the athlete no longer has to consciously think about the skill.

### Blocked Versus Random Practice

When designing a practice session, the fitness professional can use blocked or random practice sessions.

- **Blocked practice sessions**: These sessions primarily focus on closed drills and are performed repeatedly to improve movement mechanics and efficiency. All of the sets and repetitions for each drill are completed before moving on to the next drill. The goal of this training is to make a movement pattern automatic. When first learning to perform drills, a block-type practice setting using closed drills may be most beneficial.[20,48,49]
- **Random practice sessions**: Once the athlete refines his or her technique and skills, random practice sessions may be used to further challenge the athlete's cognitive abilities. During these sessions, rather than following a repetitive drill format, drills are performed in random (e.g., switching the nature of an agility drill with each repetition).[49]

Blocked training may be most effective for developing closed skills and to promote rapid short-term learning, and therefore may be beneficial for novice athletes who are learning new skills.[49] For example, for an athlete learning to perform a specific sequence of movements

in a play, the coach may break the movement sequence into segments, teaching each in segments with multiple repetitions until mastered before joining the individual segments together. Although effective for learning, random practices may yield the greatest long-term learning effect on motor performance and should be used when athletes have the requisite fundamental movement skills to perform each drill with precision.[49]

### VIGNETTE continued

■ Ben uses a variety of training modalities and tools, ranging from agility ladders and wobble boards to balance and power training, to address the various needs of his new clients. The program also addresses reaction time and the ability to quickly change directions and accelerate and decelerate safely and effectively. Ryan, Parker, and Antonio were initially surprised to learn how many aspects of physical fitness were involved with playing soccer, as they had thought their endurance would be enough to allow them to excel at the game. That said, the three friends soon see dramatic improvements in their performance during games and refer some of their teammates to Ben's business.

## PROGRAMMING GUIDELINES AND CONSIDERATIONS

Although fitness professionals may find it valuable to incorporate many specific skills into their clients' general training programs, it is important that they have developed an appropriate training base or foundation to accommodate the stressors this form of training may place on the body. For this reason, the higher the level of skill-related component required, the more important a solid base of the requisite health-related components of fitness becomes to support these movements and minimize injury risk. When designing training programs aimed at improving the skill-related components of fitness, the fitness professional must consider several factors to ensure optimal development of these skills and to minimize injury risk:

- Fitness level
- Age (chronological vs. physiological)
- Sport and activity assessment
- Training for balance
- Training for power
- Training for speed, agility, and quickness (SAQ)

### Fitness Level

Before conducting skill-related fitness training, it is critical to determine the current health status of the client.

This can be accomplished with a basic physical activity readiness questionnaire or a more detailed medical questionnaire. During the collection of this information, any health issues or previous injuries that may be exacerbated by this type of training should be discussed. This will allow the fitness professional to determine what assessment tests can be performed safely and serve as an opportunity to identify an individual's current strengths, weaknesses, and opportunities for improvement.

Because of the intense nature required to improve many of these components, such as speed, power, and agility, individuals at increased risk for adverse effects should not participate in these activities until they have been released to do so by a medical doctor and have achieved the necessary level of health and fitness to perform these activities safely. For example, individuals with orthopedic injuries or limitations, or who have any known cardiovascular diseases or disorders (e.g., high blood pressure or heart disease) should refrain from these types of activities because of the increased physiological and musculoskeletal stresses placed on the body.

## Age: Chronological Versus Physiological

Chronological age is the number of years a person has lived, whereas physiological aging is determined by the physical maturation and aging process of the body and its various systems. For older individuals this term is often used to describe the age of an individual based on his or her health or life expectancy. For example, with aging, various systems age at different rates that impact a person's functional capabilities (e.g., muscular power may deteriorate faster than strength, thus compromising balance and reactivity to a greater extent than an individual's ability to rise out of a chair).[9] By contrast, in young athletes or children, physiological aging focuses on their level of physical maturation, or growth and development. For this reason, when introducing training methods to improve muscular power in youth and adolescent athletes, one of the most important periods of motor development is between the ages of approximately 6 and 9 years. Therefore, at this stage, the coach or trainer should focus on developing fundamental movement skills.

In regard to speed training, a window for accelerated adaptation in the development of these skills generally occurs somewhere between the ages of 6 and 8 years for girls and 7 and 9 years for boys once their neuromuscular systems develop. Thus, during these stages, sport-specific movements such as linear and lateral change of direction, and agility movements should be developed through games and fun activities to maintain their interest and attention. Speed/agility bouts within the training session should last no more than 5 seconds. Suslov[18] states that improvements in basic reaction speed can be observed as early as 7 years of age, with significant increases in reactivity to more complex movements occurring between the ages of 11 and 16 years. Suslov[18] also states that the most advantageous time for the development of coordination occurs between the ages of 12 and 18 years. Therefore, failing to take full advantage of these stages may compromise athletic development, reducing the chances of the child reaching his or her full athletic potential.

Although a full discussion of these critical windows of adaptation is beyond the scope of this chapter, this information provides an overview of the importance of training young athletes based on periods of accelerated adaptations to maximize their long-term athletic potential. For more detailed discussion of training based on stages of development and long-term athletic development, refer to the works of Dr. Istvan Balyi (see Additional Resources).

## Conducting Needs Assessments for Sport

The training program should be individualized to reflect the specific needs of the sport to ensure optimal transfer of skills acquired during training to a sport. Therefore, an important step in program design is to conduct a detailed needs analysis that considers the biomechanical factors (e.g., movements), physiological demands (e.g., energy systems), and primary injuries associated with the particular sport or activity.[50] The following are examples of questions fitness professionals should consider to develop a comprehensive training program to improve performance and reduce injury risk:

1. What are the primary muscles used to perform the target activities?
2. What types of muscle actions are used (concentric, eccentric, or isometric), and in what context (agonists, antagonists, or synergists)?
3. What joint angles/velocities are common during performance of the sport/activity?
4. What factors are inherent in the operational environment (gravity, inertia, momentum, GRF, etc.) and how must the body respond to these forces (force production, reduction, and stabilization)?
5. What energy systems (ATP-PC, glycolytic, aerobic) are used and in what ratios?
6. What are common injuries, or injury sites, related to the sport/activity?

Once these questions have been answered, the fitness professional can develop a testing battery to assess the athlete/client's current strengths, weakness, and opportunities to impact performance via safe and effective training strategies. Other training considerations include:

- How much time can the individual commit to training?
- What types of equipment/facilities are available?
- What part of the season is the athlete in (off-season, preseason, or in season)?

Once this needs analysis has been completed, the fitness professional can begin developing a training program to address the specific needs, goals, strengths, and weaknesses of the client.

## Training for Balance

Balance serves as the foundation to all movement, and many of the drills and exercises individuals perform probably contain some element of balance. However, fitness professionals should intentionally include specific balance training exercises and appropriate progressions to improve balance within the individual. This is perhaps most relevant with older population groups who are faced with balance challenges and anxieties over the fear of falling.

The physiological limitations imposed by loss of balance can have significant negative effects on an individual's cognitive and affective (emotional) states. For older adults faced with the fear of falling, reassurances from health and fitness professionals that their program will incorporate balance training in a safe, effective, and progressive manner is important to emphasize. Developing self-efficacy to improve one's confidence levels to function more autonomously (independently) should always be a consideration with balance training. Additional information on exercise training for balance and fall prevention in older adults is included in Chapter 26.

## Guidelines

When designing a balance training program, a wide array of drills can be selected. The following guidelines will assist the practitioner in making the most appropriate initial balance exercise selections. In addition, these guidelines will provide the practitioner with a basic framework for progressing the physiological and proprioceptive demands of these drills.

1. *Progress from static balance drills to more dynamic drills:* Individuals must be stable before they can be mobile. Therefore, balance training drills should emphasize maintaining postural equilibrium from a stationary position before incorporating any dynamic movements. An example is progressing an exercise position where the individual starts by standing stationary with both feet together on the ground (static) to positions that include taking half steps or full steps forward (dynamic).
2. *Range of motion:* Balance training programs should be progressed from using small ranges of joint movement to larger ranges. For example, progress exercises from a basic forward arm reach to a full overhead arm reach.
3. *BOS:* Altering one's BOS from a bilateral (e.g., training on both feet or with extremities in unison), to staggered (e.g., walking position), split (e.g., feet aligned in sagittal plane), or tandem (e.g., heel-to-toe) positions, to single-leg stance (e.g., unilateral) positions reduces the amount of surface area in contact with the ground and makes maintaining balance more challenging because an individual is less stable.

For example, progress exercises from standing on both feet to single-leg stands.
4. *Unstable surface:* Unstable training devices can also be used to increase the proprioceptive and neural challenges of the training drill and are an excellent tool for prehabilitative and rehabilitative purposes. For example, progress exercises from the ground to standing on foam or air-filled devices. Unstable training surfaces, however, should be used sparingly because of their lack of specificity and poor carryover to performance-related activities.
5. *Speed of movement:* As neuromuscular efficiency improves, an individual may increase the speed of dynamic balance drills to add increasingly greater neuromuscular and stabilization challenges. For example, use progressive exercises that incorporate slow rhythmic movements to moving more explosively.
6. *Static to active resistance:* Progressing from static resistance to active resistance may increase the sport/activity specificity of many balance training activities and add a reactive component to these drills. This can be accomplished via the use of perturbation training. For example, progress exercises from holding a medicine ball in both hands to performing trunk rotations with offset or asymmetrical resistance (load is not held in front of body, but offset to one side).
7. *Plane of movement:* Initially, single planes of movement should be emphasized; but once an individual is able to demonstrate proficiency in a single plane, introduce multiplanar drills to increase movement specificity and increase the kinesthetic and proprioceptive demands. An example is progressing drills that train in the sagittal plane (e.g., single-leg forward reaches) to multidirectional reaches (e.g., single-leg squats with trunk rotations and reaches).

## Program Design

The inclusion of balance training as a component of a total fitness program has generally focused on older adults and is not usually emphasized to the same degree as strength, flexibility, or aerobic fitness in younger adults. Thus, much of the recommendations for younger adults are based on a fitness professional's judgment and experience. In general terms, the amount of time and emphasis spent working on balance drills for individuals who are apparently healthy or athletic is relatively low in comparison with other training modalities. However, when working with populations who experience more balance challenges, such as older adults, balance training may be the main focus of their training program. Balance training drills tend to work well during a dynamic warm-up routine, between exercises in a circuit, or as a form of active recovery from more intense working sets during a resistance training program. Box 18-2 includes sample balance exercises that can be incorporated into a client's overall conditioning program.

## Box 18-2. Balance Drills

- Stork stand drill (see Practice What You Know at the end of this chapter)
- Leaning towers
  - While standing on a single leg, extend both arms overhead, aligning the arms with the ears. While keeping the foot flat on the ground and a rigid torso, push the hips forward while reaching back as far as possible without losing balance. Continue pushing the hips forward until the knee is over the toes (not in front of them) or until balance can no longer be maintained. This movement should be initiated from the hips and not from the knee of the stance (support) leg (i.e., flexing the knee to drive the body forward).
- Star excursions
  - Position a cone on the floor, then set up five cones in the shape of a star around that central cone (arrange cones 2 feet from the central cone). Standing at the central cone, assume a single-leg stance position, with the support foot in full contact with the ground. While controlling your balance, slowly reach the foot of the raised leg out as far as possible toward the first cone in the configuration without letting it make contact with the floor. This movement should be initiated from the hips and not by flexing the knee of the stance (support) leg knee. Hold this end position for 5 seconds, then return to your starting position. Repeat this movement to the remaining four cones, and repeat with the opposite leg.
- Multiplanar reaches
  - Using the same configuration as described for the star excursion, assume a single-leg stance with the support foot making full contact with the ground. While maintaining a neutral spine, slowly bend at the waist to reach the opposite hand to touch the cone in front of the body. Return to the starting position, then repeat this drill touching the opposite hand to each cone and repeat with the opposite leg.
- Body-weight squat with band perturbations
  - Begin in the UAP described earlier, keeping both feet flat on the floor. The health/fitness professional should wrap an elastic resistance band around the participant's waist and then apply pulls to the band in multiple directions while the participant attempts to resist these forces and maintain a stable body position.
- Multidirectional jumps-to-stick
  - From a UAP, jump up and forward land approximately 2 to 3 feet from your original starting position. Land in a UAP with the feet approximately shoulder width apart, chest up, and shoulders back. Allow the knees, hips, and ankles to bend slightly to absorb the force and "stick" the landing position. Jump back to the starting position, stick the landing, and repeat this movement pattern jumping laterally to the left, right, and at a 45-degree angle.

*Note:* It is helpful to instruct the client to visualize the face of a clock on the ground. The instructor can then cue the participant to jump to various positions, or numbers, based on this visual.

## Training for Power

There are numerous ways to improve power. Some of these methods include traditional heavy resistance training, ballistic and explosive resistance training, and plyometrics.[24] This section focuses primarily on plyometric training, which is derived from its Latin origins, where the terms *plio* and *metric* literally mean "measurable increases."[51,52] Although legendary track and field coach Fred Wilt introduced the term *plyometrics* in the United States in 1975, this form of training was used by Russian athletes as early as the mid-1960s.[52] Considering how many studies have demonstrated the effectiveness of plyometric training for improving power[53] and the similarity of many plyometric activities to actual sporting and recreational activities, the inclusion of some plyometric training as a portion of a power training program is logical.

### Phases of Plyometric Exercises

Plyometric training relies heavily on the utilization of the **stretch-shortening cycle** to produce powerful and explosive movements.[53] An example of a plyometric exercise is the squat jump (Table 18-2). When performing this exercise, the individual begins by dropping his or her COG into a squat position (eccentric phase) in a rapid, but controlled manner, which signals the muscle spindles. While the muscle spindles trigger sensory transmission (via afferent pathways) to the spine to elicit a reflexive action via the alpha motor neuron in the ventral root of the spinal cord, there is a very slight delay (less than 50 milliseconds) during the

### FROM THEORY TO PRACTICE

Take a moment to perform and experience each of the balance drills. Using the knowledge acquired in the earlier Training for Balance section, order the exercise sequentially for an individual interested in improving his skiing ability. Plan to progress your choices from simple to more advanced following the balance training variables provided.

## Table 18-2. Distinct Phases of Plyometric Exercises

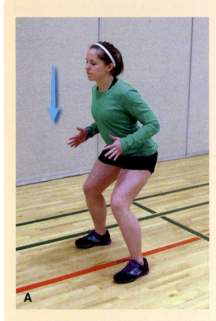

**A. Eccentric phase**: During this phase, the muscles are rapidly stretched (loaded). This rapid eccentric movement stimulates the muscle spindles located within the muscle tissue. These proprioceptors are sensitive to the amount and rate of stretch in a muscle,[50] and stimulation activates the stretch reflex, facilitating a powerful concentric action of the agonist muscle group to protect the muscle from overstretching.

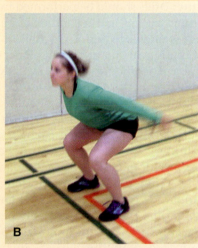

**B. Amortization phase**: This transitional phase between loading and unloading is critical in plyometrics in that it needs to remain short to avoid losses of stored elastic energy created by the stretch-shortening cycle in the musculotendinous unit. This will reduce the transfer of stored elastic energy into the concentric contraction and force output as more energy is dissipated as heat.[50]

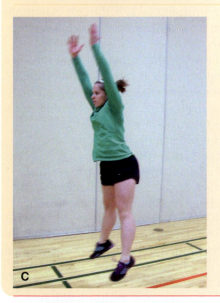

**C. Concentric phase**: During this phase, the muscles contract to shorten powerfully (unload). The muscles harness the energy of the stretch-shortening cycle and stored elastic energy gained from the eccentric and amortization phases to generate a rapid, forceful contraction.

A squat jump is shown as an example.
Source: Photos are courtesy of Lance Dalleck.

amortization phase.[32] The alpha motor neurons transmit an impulse to the agonist muscle group to contract (concentric phase), allowing the individual to produce an explosive upward movement.[51,52]

## Guidelines

Before participating in most plyometric training programs, several safety issues and guidelines should be considered:

- **Perform a warm-up.** To warm up, perform 3 to 5 minutes of a general warm-up, consisting of walking, jogging, or cycling. Immediately after, perform activity-specific movements and/or drills, such as dynamic balance drills shuffling, backpedaling, or sprinting 5 to 10 yards for 5 to 10 minutes.

- **Age:** Prepubescent athletes should not perform high-intensity plyometric drills such as depth or drop jumps because of the increased stress that may be placed on the epiphyseal (growth) plates. An example of a depth or drop jump is one in which the individual starts on an elevated platform (e.g., 18- to 24-inch riser), drops to the floor, landing, and then explosively jumps upward. Plyometrics for children should initially focus on low-intensity drills used to develop neuromuscular control and be progressed to moderate-intensity drills as the athlete matures and gains more strength and training experience.[9,51] Examples of low-intensity drills include jumping jacks, alternating toe taps to a low riser (e.g., less than 6 inches), a standing vertical jump, or a partner-assisted medicine ball chest toss for the upper extremity. Examples of moderate-intensity drills include multiple forward linear jumps (leap frogging), multidirectional jumps around cones, or medicine ball overhead slams for the upper extremity. Furthermore, high-intensity plyometrics should also be avoided in middle-aged or older adults who may be more prone to injury because of the natural aging process. Generally, low- to moderate-level plyometric exercises tend to be most appropriate and beneficial for improving power for athletes of all ages.[9,51]

- **Body weight:** Larger athletes (more than 220 lb) should avoid performing depth jumps from a drop greater than 18 inches because of greater amounts of stress being placed on the joints.[54,55]

- **Strength requirements for lower-body plyometrics:** For high-intensity lower-body plyometrics, the traditional recommendation has been that an athlete be capable of squatting at least 11/2 times his or her body weight before performing any drills.[54,55] Given how strength (force production) differs slightly from power (rate of force production), Wathen[53] provided another criteria whereby the individual should be able to perform five squats in 5 seconds or less with 60% of his or her total body weight. For

example, if an athlete weights 180 lb (81.8 kg), he or she should be able to squat 96 lb (49 kg) five times in no more than 5 seconds. According to McNeely,[56] for athletes performing low- to moderate-level plyometrics, as long as they land with proper form, they should be able to safely perform any drills at these levels.

- **Strength requirements for upper-body plyometrics:** Athletes should be able to bench-press at least their body weight before performing upper-body plyometric exercises. Another recommendation suggested is that individuals perform an explosive bench-press movement using 60% of total body weight, completing five repetitions in 5 seconds or less.[51]

- **Experience:** Athletes should have a good base of strength before incorporating these drills into their training sessions. Therefore, it is recommended that athletes engage in a structured resistance training program for a minimum of 8 to 12 weeks before performing moderate- to higher-intensity drills.

- **Proper technique:** Drills should be performed in a controlled manner with proper technique at all times. If an athlete is unable to perform a drill correctly, a basic strength assessment should be performed to determine if additional strength training may be required before performing plyometric work. Remember, it is essential that an individual know how to land before they learn how to jump.

  As the demands of the environment change, so too do the amplitudes, torques, and forces that these movements produce and they vary dramatically. For example, a jumping jack is performed at a much lower amplitude (height or intensity) and requires much less time on the ground between eccentric and concentric movements (amortization time) when compared with the vertical jump. Therefore, the jumping jack, although essentially using the same basic technique, is much less stressful on the body than a vertical jump.

- **Footwear:** Footwear that provides good foot and ankle support, such as cross-training shoes, are essential for safety when performing plyometric training drills. Running shoes would not be appropriate because they typically have a narrow sole and offer poor ankle support.[51]

- **Training surface and equipment:** All plyometric drills should be performed on a nonslip, shock-absorbing surface. Grass fields, suspended wood flooring, or rubberized mats are all acceptable surfaces for plyometric training.[51,54,55] Plyo boxes used for box and depth jumps should also have a nonslip surface on the top.[51] However, the trainer or coach may also have to consider the real surface on which an individual competes if it lacks shock-absorbing properties. Training will need to ultimately mimic the true surface, without being excessive where it can result in injury.

- **Single-response versus multiple-response drills:** Progress training drills that require only one explosive jump or throw whereas multiple-response drills require several repetitions in a row while attempting to minimize the transition time between each repetition.
- **Fatigue:** Because of the high neural demands associated with plyometric training, these drills should be performed earlier in a training session if performed with other forms of training within the same session (e.g., cardio and resistance training), or by themselves, to allow adequate recovery to ensure best efforts during each repetition and reduction of injury risks.
- **Weight selection for medicine ball drills:** Currently, there are no standardized recommendations on what training load should be used for medicine ball throws and tosses. However, beginning with a ball that is approximately 4% to 5% of total body weight is a good place to start. For example, a 220-lb (100-kg) athlete would use an 8- to 11-lb (3.5- to 5-kg) ball, whereas a 120-lb (54.5-kg) individual would start with a ball between 5 and 6 lb (approximately 2.5 kg).

## Program Design

Plyometric training sessions typically are performed between 1 and 4 days per week. However, this largely depends on the clients/athlete's training goals and status, ability to recover, time of year (off-season, pre-season, in season), other activities, and sports participation.[9,51,54,55]

The intensity of plyometric drills can vary tremendously. According to Ratamess,[9] the intensity of plyometric exercises is based on the drill complexity, loading, speed, and height and distances of boxes and barriers. However, with the exception of high-intensity plyometric drills sometimes referred to as "shock drills," there appears to be a great deal of controversy regarding the intensity level of many plyometric drills. The term *shock* originated from Dr. Yuri Verkoshanski, who used a specific method of applying mechanical shock to force the muscles to produce as much force as possible.[57] This method involved drills using a relaxed drop from a predetermined height, an impact force as the feet hit the

ground, and then an explosive rebound afterword. Allerheiligen and Rogers[54,55] state that the intensity of a drill is dependent on the rate of the stretch-shortening cycle, and this rate is, in turn, dependent on several variables that include height of the COG (amount of the drop), horizontal speed, body weight, effort of the individual, and ability of the muscles to overcome load. Drill intensity, however, should ultimately be based on the client's/athlete's current training status and experience, strength and technique level, physiological age, injury profile, and specific needs and goals.

As discussed previously in this chapter, plyometric training volume is typically measured by foot or hand contacts and/or by distance traveled.[9,51,54,55] Some authors count a foot contact as each time a foot or feet contact a surface.[9,51,54,55] For example, performing the tuck jump, where the jumper drives her knees to her chest during each jump, for 3 sets × 10 repetitions would equate to a total volume of 30. Other authors, however, count foot contacts as each time each foot hits the ground.[56,58,58a] Thus, using the same example, performing tuck jumps for 3 sets × 10 repetitions would equate to a total volume of 60. Although this may appear to be semantics, it does have practical implications when programming exercise volume based on current recommendations. If the first definition were used, the individual would perform twice the volume of work to achieve a desired number of contacts. This text defines a foot contact as each time a single foot hits the ground on a single-leg drill or every time the feet land together. Earlier in the chapter, Table 18-1 provided some basic guidelines for volume based on the individual's experience level and the time of year (e.g., pre-season, in-season, post-season). These are simply guidelines and special modifications may be necessary based on the athlete's ability to recover and the time allotted to this and other methods of training. In addition, much like with resistance training, there is an inverse relation between volume and intensity that should be considered when designing plyometric training sessions.

Rest interval lengths for plyometric drills are intensity and goal specific. Longer rest periods will be required between more intense drills than lower-intensity drills.[9,51] For example, because a set of jumping jacks is less intense than a set of cone hops, more rest would be required between the cone hops (e.g., 2–3 minutes) versus the jumping jacks (e.g., 30 seconds to 1 minute). Depletion of the anaerobic energy systems and quality of repetitions are critical considerations:

- Higher-intensity, yet submaximal plyometric exercises (e.g., submaximal depth jumps) may require 5- to 10-second rest periods between each repetition within the set and 2- to 3-minute rest periods between sets.
- For maximal, high-intensity exercises (e.g., maximal effort depth jumps), longer rest periods, perhaps as long as 5 to 10 minutes, may be needed between sets to allow for optimal ATP-PC system recovery for 100% effort.

### FROM THEORY TO PRACTICE

To get a real feel for the prerequisite requirement for higher-intensity plyometric programs, attempt to complete the five repetitions in 5 seconds test with 60% of your body weight. Use a stopwatch, count, or metronome to monitor your cadence and always consider safety. Learn how to properly squat first and include a warm-up before attempting this activity.

**DOING THE MATH**

Using this text's definition of foot contacts and the information presented in Table 18-1, calculate Joe's volume for his preseason plyometric workouts, and assess what changes you might suggest for his training volume if he is an experienced basketball player who plays for his university.

**Low-Intensity Drills (warm-up)**
- Jumping jacks (2 sets × 30 repetitions)
- Plyo box jumps—12-inch (30 cm) box (2 sets × 20 repetitions)
- Lateral cone jumps (2 sets × 15 repetitions in each direction)
- Multidirectional cone jumps (2 sets × 10 repetitions)

**Answers:** Jumping jacks = 60; 12-inch box jumps = 40; lateral cone jumps = 60; multidirectional jumps = 20

**Moderate-Intensity Drills**
- Knee tucks (4 sets × 10 repetitions)
- Plyo box jumps—24-inch (60 cm) box (4 sets × 10 reps)
- Leap frog jumps (4 sets × 10 reps)
- Multiple vertical jumps (4 sets × 10)
- 180-degree multiple vertical jumps (4 × 10 repetitions)

**Answers:** Knee tucks = 40; 24-inch box jumps = 40; leap frogs = 40; multi-vertical jumps = 40; 180-degree jumps = 40

**High-Intensity Drills**
- Depth (drop) jumps (20 repetitions)
- Single-leg vertical hops (2 sets × 10 repetitions per leg)
- Single-leg lateral hops (2 sets × 10 repetitions per leg)

**Answers:** Depth = 20; single-leg hops = 40, single-leg lateral hops = 40

Although it is common practice to see plyometric drills conducted with little-to-no rest intervals in fitness and with various commercial exercise programs, for the purposes of burning more calories per session or for aerobic conditioning, this practice should be avoided because it may increase an individual's risk for injury and hinder power development.

Box 18-3 includes sample plyometric drills ranging from low to high intensity. Each drill should be progressed from single-response (one jump with a rest) jumps for beginners to multiple-response jumps (several repetitions performed with little amortization time between repetitions). Technique is paramount to maximize the benefit of plyometric training. Thus, if the individual is unable to maintain good form and technique during any of the exercise movements, the intensity or volume of training should be altered accordingly.

## Box 18-3. Sample Plyometric Drills

**Low-Intensity Drills**
- Jumping jacks—The progressive sequence of exercise form for this drill is shown in Figure 18-8.
- Alternating toe taps—The progressive sequence of exercise form for this drill is shown in Figure 18-9.
- Plyo box jumps—The progressive sequence of exercise form for this drill is shown in Figure 18-10. Performing the plyo box jumps to a higher box ( ≥24 inches or 60 cm) or for multiple repetitions while attempting to minimize the amortization phase between sets would be classified as a moderate-intensity drill.
- Lateral cone jumps—The progressive sequence of exercise form for this drill is shown in Figure 18-11.
- Multidirectional jumps—The progressive sequence of exercise form for this drill is shown in Figure 18-12. *Note:* The athlete should perform this drill with his or her COG shifted toward the center to move as quickly as possible.
- Seated chest pass—The progressive sequence of exercise form for this drill is illustrated in Figure 18-13.
- Front toss—The progressive sequence of exercise form for this drill is shown in Figure 18-14.

## Box 18-3. **Sample Plyometric Drills—cont'd**

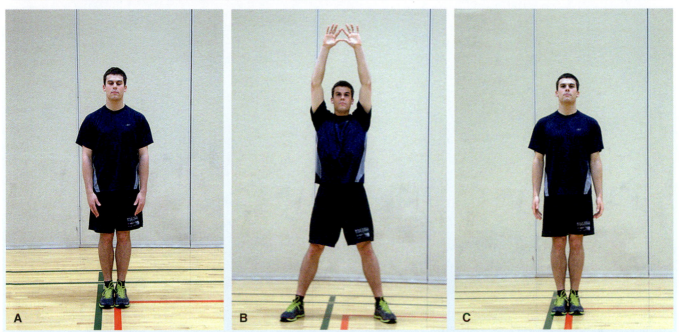

**Figure 18-8.** Jumping jacks. A, Begin with the feet together and arms down to the sides. B, Jump upward (not shown in photos), abducting the arms and legs until the feet are slightly wider than shoulder width apart and the hands touch over the head. C, Quickly jump back to the starting position while simultaneously adducting the arms and legs.

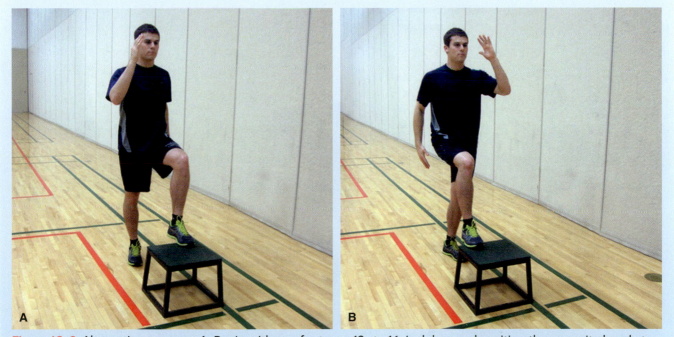

**Figure 18-9.** Alternating toe taps. A, Begin with one foot on a 12- to 16-inch box and position the opposite hand at chin level, with the same-side hand on the hip pocket. B, Rapidly switch the feet in a scissoring-type action and move the arms in a reciprocating fashion similar to a running motion. The foot on the box will not be load bearing, but rather simply tap the top of the box. Repeat this action for the desired number of repetitions.

*Continued*

**Box 18-3. Sample Plyometric Drills—cont'd**

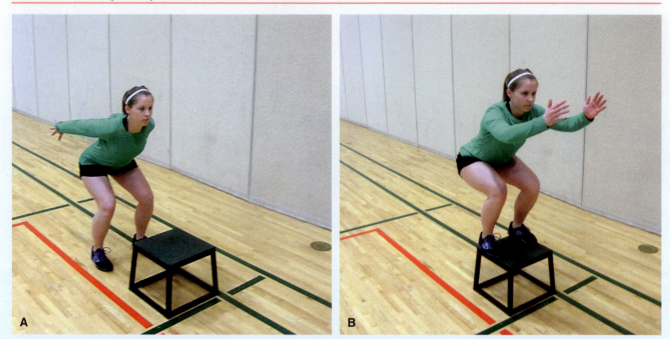

**Figure 18-10.** Plyo box jump. A, Stand in the universal athletic position facing a plyo box. Perform a rapid counter-movement arm swing while simultaneously performing a three-quarter squat to eccentrically load the muscles of the shoulders and lower body. B, Quickly swing the arms forward and at the same time extend the ankles, knees, and hips to jump up and forward. Land on top of the box in an athletic position.

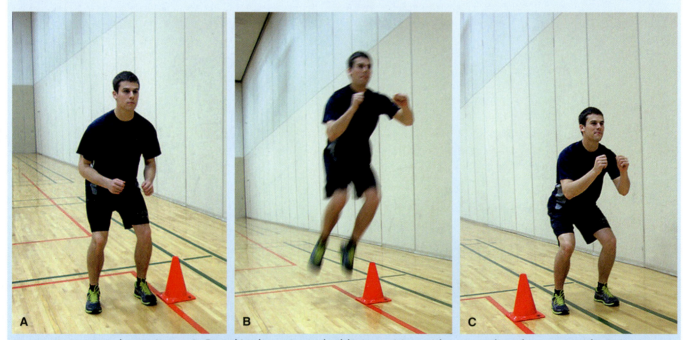

**Figure 18-11.** Lateral cone jump. A, Stand in the universal athletic position with a cone directly to your side. B, Jump up and laterally over the cone. C, Land in an athletic position with the feet approximately shoulder width apart, chest up, and shoulders back. Allow the knees, hips, and ankles to bend just slightly to prepare the body for the next jump. Upon landing, spring back over the cone as quickly as possible (e.g., similar to a ball bouncing off the ground).

## Box 18-3. Sample Plyometric Drills—cont'd

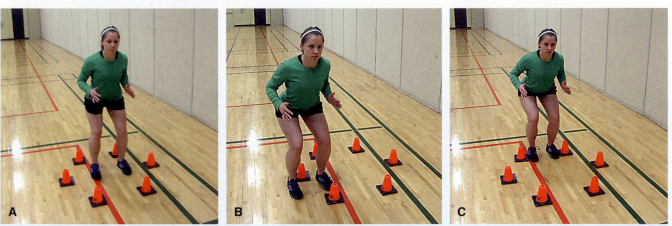

**Figure 18-12.** Multidirectional jump. A, Begin by positioning six small cones in a hexagon pattern. Stand in the center of the hexagon in the universal athletic position directly facing the first cone. B, Jump forward over the first cone and immediately upon landing jump backward to return to the center. C, Repeat this pattern jumping forward, backward, laterally, and diagonally over each cone. The athlete can perform this drill by jumping over the cones in a clockwise, counterclockwise, or randomized fashion.

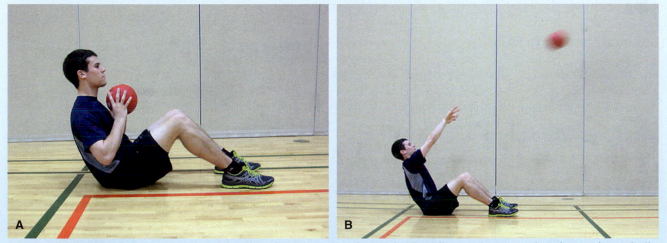

**Figure 18-13.** Seated chest pass. A, While seated on the ground with the feet flat on the ground and a medicine ball in hand, lean back slightly at the torso while maintaining a neutral spine position and braced core. B, Bring the medicine ball to the chest and explosively pass the ball forward as far as possible.

*Continued*

**Box 18-3. Sample Plyometric Drills—cont'd**

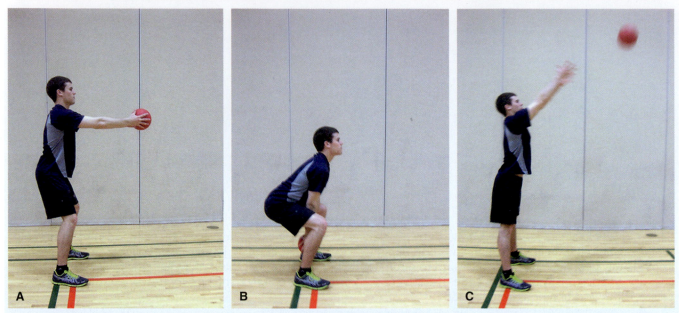

**Figure 18-14.** Front toss. A, Hold a medicine ball in both hands. B, Rapidly bend at the hips and swing the ball down and back between the legs. C, Throw the ball forward and up as far as possible.

**Moderate-Intensity Drills**

- Knee tucks—The progressive sequence of exercise form for this drill is shown in Figure 18-15.
- Leap frog jumps—The progressive sequence of exercise form for this drill is shown in Figure 18-16.
- Standing chest pass—The progressive sequence of exercise form for this drill is illustrated in Figure 18-17.
- Slams—The progressive sequence of exercise form for this drill is shown in Figure 18-18.
- Medicine ball side toss—The progressive sequence of exercise form for this drill is shown in Figure 18-19.

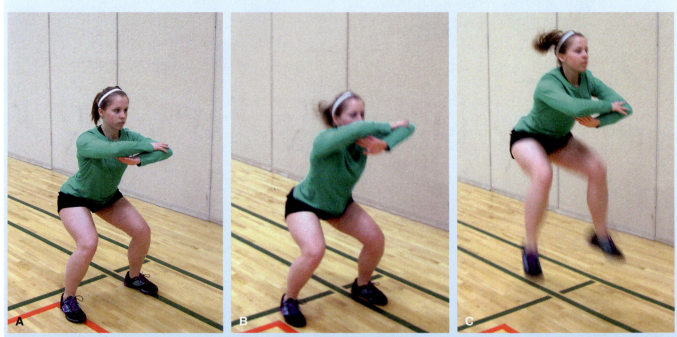

**Figure 18-15.** Knee tucks. A, Begin by standing in the universal athletic position with the feet approximately hip width apart. B, Fold the arms and raise them so the upper arms are approximately parallel to the ground. C, Rapidly sit the hips back and then jump vertically, pulling the knees up toward the chest. Land on the balls of the feet and with "soft knees" to absorb the shock of the landing.

## Box 18-3. Sample Plyometric Drills—cont'd

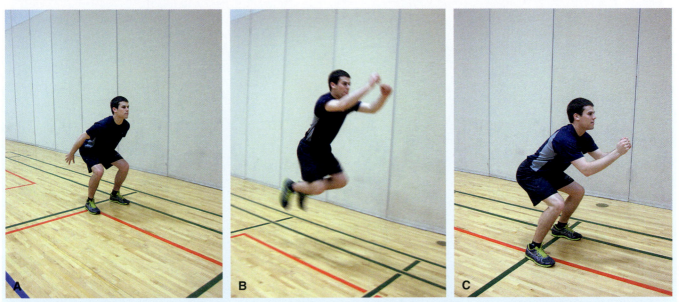

**Figure 18-16.** Leap frog jumps. A, Begin by standing in the universal athletic position. B, Sit the hips backward and perform a rapid countermovement arm swing, bringing the arms back toward the hip pocket. C, Swing the arms outward and extend at the hip, knee, and ankle, projecting the body horizontally as far as possible.

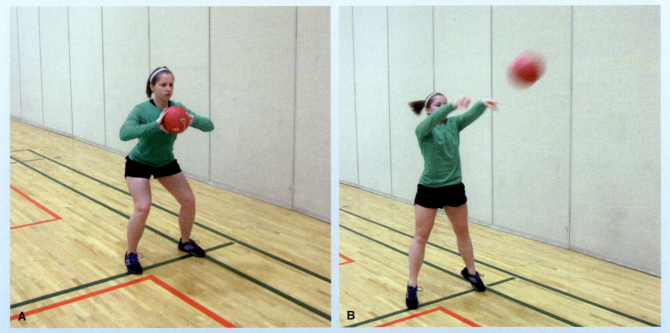

**Figure 18-17.** Standing chest pass. A, Stand in the universal athletic position with a medicine ball in hand. B, Bring the medicine ball to the chest and explosively pass the ball forward as far as possible or to a partner.

*Continued*

**Box 18-3. Sample Plyometric Drills—cont'd**

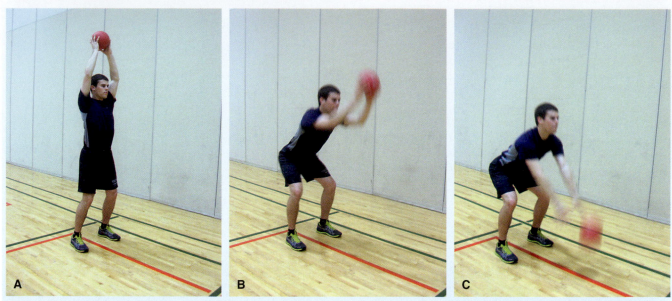

**Figure 18-18.** Slam. A, Hold a medicine ball with both hands above the head and position the upper arms beside the ears, eccentrically loading the abdominal muscles. B, Quickly contract the abdominals. C, Slam the medicine ball to the ground directly in front of you.

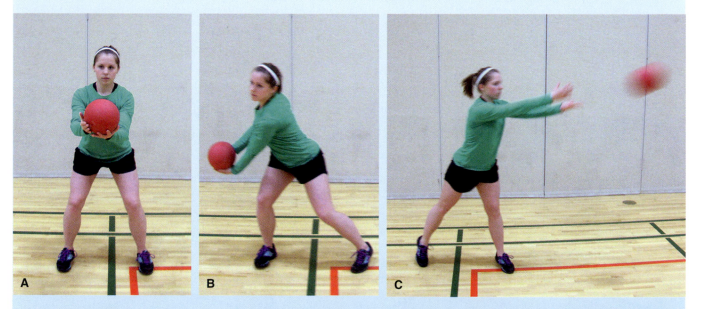

**Figure 18-19.** Medicine ball side toss. A, Stand laterally and hold a medicine ball in front of the body with both hands at navel height. B, Twist and bring the ball to the back hip, then quickly change directions. C, Throw the ball to a partner or to the wall. Repeat for the desired number of repetitions, then repeat on the opposite side.

## Box 18-3. Sample Plyometric Drills—cont'd

**High-Intensity Drills**
- Depth (drop) jumps—The progressive sequence of exercise form for this drill is shown in Figure 18-20.
- Single-leg vertical hops—The progressive sequence of exercise form for this drill is shown in Figure 18-21.
- Single-leg lateral hops—The progressive sequence of exercise form for this drill is shown in Figure 18-22.
- Drop push-up progression—The progressive sequence of exercise form for this drill is shown in Figure 18-23.

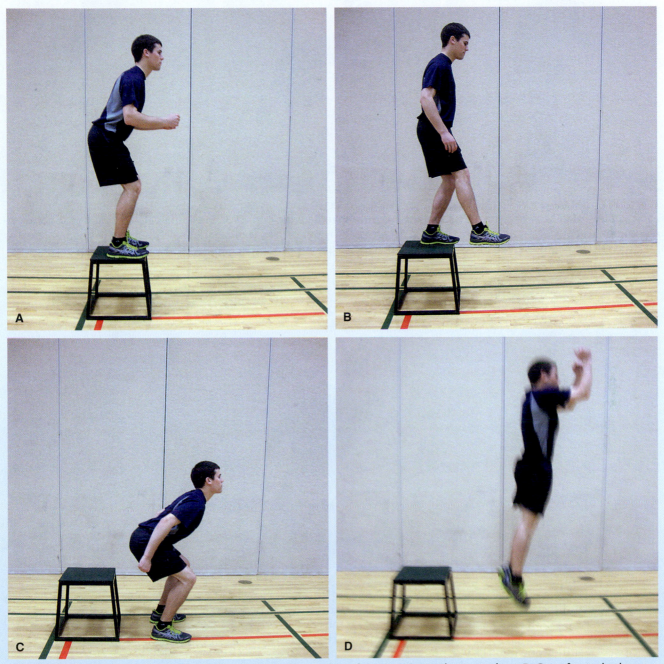

**Figure 18-20.** Depth (drop) jump. A, Stand on the front edge of a 12- to 24-inch riser or box. B, Step from the box. C, Drop and land on both feet with the ankles, knees, and hips slightly flexed to absorb the landing and preload the body for the next movement. D, Immediately on contact with the ground, rebound up as quickly as possible into a vertical jump.

*Continued*

## Box 18-3. Sample Plyometric Drills—cont'd

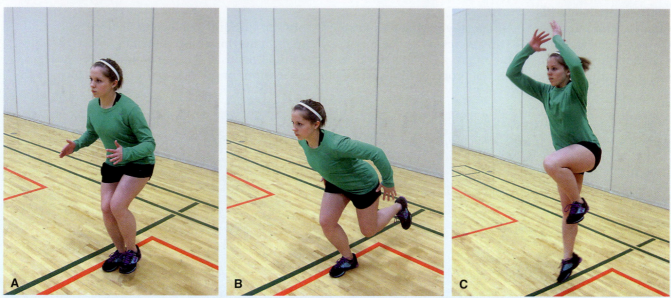

**Figure 18-21.** Single-leg vertical hop. A, Stand on a single leg and hop up as high as possible, then stick the landing. B, Allow the knees, hips, and ankles to bend just slightly to reduce the impact of the landing. C, Repeat this action hopping laterally over the line. This exercise can be progressed by performing multiple hops without rest (e.g., upon landing the individual would minimize the amortization phase and attempt to spring back over the line as quickly as possible).

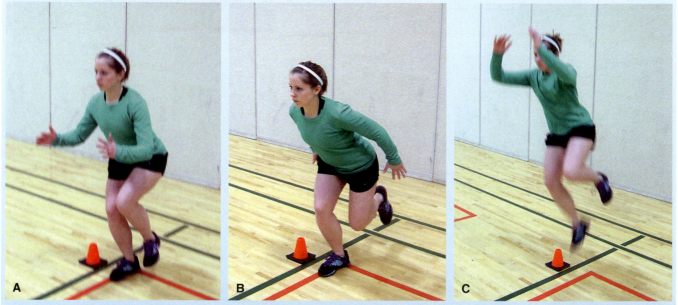

**Figure 18-22.** Single-leg lateral hop. A, Stand on a single leg with a cone directly to your side. B–D, Hop up and laterally over the cone and stick the landing. Allow the knees, hips, and ankles to bend just slightly to reduce the impact of the landing. E, Repeat this action, hopping laterally back over the cone. This exercise can be progressed by performing multiple hops without rest (e.g., upon landing the individual would minimize the amortization phase and attempt to spring back over the cone as quickly as possible).

## Box 18-3. Sample Plyometric Drills—cont'd

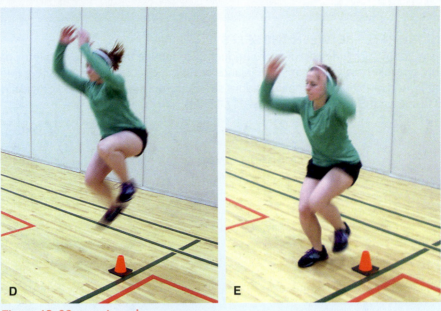

D          E

Figure 18-22—continued

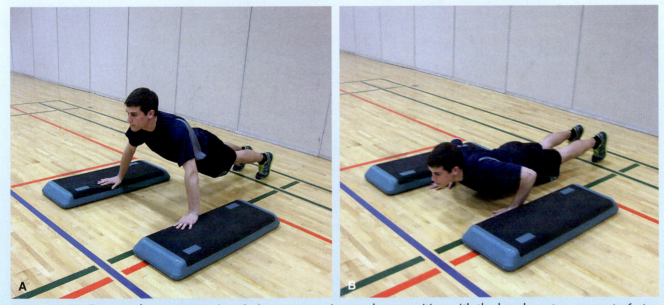

A          B

Figure 18-23. Drop push-up progression. A, Assume a supine, push-up position with the hands on two separate 6- to 12-inch risers or boxes. Ensure there is enough space between the risers/boxes to perform a push-up. B, Simultaneously lift both hands and drop to the ground. Land with the hands flat on the ground and allow the elbow and shoulder to flex, to absorb the shock of the landing, and preload the muscles to return to the box. The torso should remain rigid throughout the entire drill and you should be able to visualize a straight line extending from the torso down through the hips, knees, and ankles. Forcefully extend the elbows and shoulders and explode upward, returning back to the starting position with the hands back on top of the box.

## SEX DIFFERENCES

### ■ INJURY RATES BETWEEN THE SEXES

Anterior cruciate ligament (ACL) injuries occur more frequently in female than in male athletes participating in the same sports. Notably, approximately 70% of these injuries occur in noncontact activities (e.g., jumping, landing, quick stopping, cutting, and directional changes). Various structural, hormonal, and neurological differences help explain differences in injury rates between the sexes (Fig. 18-24).

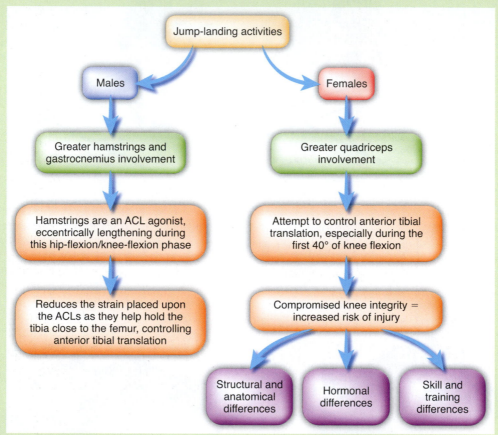

**Figure 18-24.** Structural, hormonal, and neurological differences that help explain differences in injury rates between the sexes.

- Structurally, females have a wider pelvis, which, when coupled with shorter bones, increases the Q-angle between the quadriceps muscle on the front of the thigh and the patellar tendon (female angle averages 18 degrees vs. approximately 13 degrees in males). The Q-angle represents the deviation in alignment of the long axis of the tibia versus that of the femur, and the larger the deviation, the greater the degree of instability at the knee. In addition, females exhibit a narrower intercondylar notch in the femur (space between the two epicondyles at the distal or lower end of the femur) that may cause a "shearing" effect (fraying and weakening) on the ACL ligament by bone during ballistic or rotational movement. The intercondylar notch represents the grove between the two condyles of the femur through which the ACL and posterior cruciate ligaments pass. Furthermore, females have smaller ligaments and bone surfaces for ligament attachment, thus weakening the knee.
- Hormonally, females have greater levels of hormones (estrogen, progesterone, relaxin) that increase joint laxity (looseness), but this may increase the potential for injury.
- Skill and training differences also increase the potential for injury. Boys often begin involvement in organized sports at a younger age and this may facilitate earlier development of footwork, eye–hand coordination, and catching and throwing skills, all of which develop the neuromuscular system. Thus, it is assumed that females generally exhibit lower neuromuscular coordination levels, which may help explain the greater incidence of female knee injuries in high school sports. It is believed that because girls may often miss early exposure to motor learning, it creates motor skill disadvantages when they become involved in high school

## SEX DIFFERENCES—cont'd

sports. Consequently, as they demonstrate lower abilities and skills and potentially inferior technique from a lack of organized coaching, they may exhibit greater propensity for knee injury. However, considering how greater quantities of younger females are now participating in organized sports at an earlier age, this sex difference may be insignificant.

Considering these differences that may place females at a disadvantage for a knee injury, any health/fitness practitioner who works with females should devote adequate time to:

- Improve lower extremity mechanics in all three planes of movement.
- Increase knee stability and strength.
- Teach proper technique for jumping, landing, turning, and so on.
- Develop necessary levels of neuromuscular coordination for sport-type movement patterns.

## Training for Speed, Agility, and Quickness

Speed is a function of stride length × stride frequency (number of strides). Although we all differ in terms of our anatomical design, the goal of improving SAQ in general is to positively impact one or both variables in such a manner that it results in an increased rate at which we move. When developing SAQ, it is imperative to follow a systematic approach to maximize the benefits experienced from this form of training. This section discusses basic guidelines for coaching and technique in addition to program design recommendations.

### Guidelines

- **Experience:** Similar to plyometric exercises, athletes should have a good base of strength before incorporating these drills into their training sessions. Therefore, it is recommended that athletes participate in a structured resistance training program for a minimum of 8 to 12 weeks before performing moderate- to higher-intensity drills. However, lower-level drills, such as ladder drills and A-Marches (high-knees, power skipping), may be incorporated into a dynamic warm-up routine within the first few training sessions. Many of these drills are detailed in the following sections.
- **Proper technique:** Drills should be performed in a controlled manner with proper technique at all times. Individuals should be encouraged to "Go as fast as they can, not as fast as they can't." To be fast, you must train fast. However, when an individual is unable to control his movements, he is more prone to injury. If drills are not performed at high speeds, muscle activation patterns may be altered and speed development may be hindered.[59] However, fast movement with poor technique may engrain poor motor programs and patterns. Therefore, individuals should be encouraged to perform drills as fast as possible with good technique and form.
  - When teaching technique, it is helpful to use the PAL approach—posture, arm action, and leg

action.[49] This concept is outlined in Table 18-3. Depending on what type of speed individuals are training, postures may be quite different. For example, sprinters will adopt a more upright stance with a higher COM after they have finished accelerating. This is quite different from field sport athletes. Typically, these athletes will tend to maintain a lower COM to prepare for multidirectional changes over relatively short distances, often within 5 to 15 yards. This lowered COM provides a means to prepare the body for quick accelerations and decelerations.[29] Therefore, running posture will vary slightly depending on the demands of the sport and is contextually specific to the athlete's goal (e.g., whether it be straight line, maximal velocity, or quick changes in direction). The upper body contributes to total speed by improving leg turnover.[60] In fact, many believe that arm speed governs leg speed. For this reason, good arm mechanics are just as important for speed development as leg movement. When performing activities that require the legs and arms to work in a reciprocating fashion, such as walking, marching, skipping, jogging, and running, the arms should swing forward and backward in a reciprocating manner (e.g., when the right leg is in front of the body, the left arm should also be in front). This helps create counterbalance between both sides of the body, and allows sufficient transverse-plane rotation that will use the stored elastic energy without any loss of energy. The amplitude, range of motion, direction of motion, and length of the lever arm must all be evaluated for each drill to ensure that GRFs that push back into the body, propelling us forward, and leg speed (turnover) are maximized.[60]

- Leg actions include foot placements, stride adjustments, and alignment. Speaking in general terms, individuals should aim to run more on the ball of the foot and not on the heel or toe. When turning the legs over, the ankle of the swing leg should be dorsiflexed while the knee and hip are flexed. This allows the rear foot to pass directly under the buttocks, which is important for accelerating turnover at the hip and stride rate.[33]

Furthermore, PSAs, as discussed previously, are critical for maximizing force reduction and reducing injury potential. Thus, creating PSAs should be a primary focus for the coach/instructor to maximize force in the intended direction of movement.

- **Footwear:** Footwear that provides good foot and ankle supports, such as cross-training shoes, are essential for safety when performing agility drills. Running shoes would not be appropriate because they typically have less lateral support.[51]
- **Training area:** Agility and speed training should ideally be performed in a large, open area, free of sharp objects and clutter, and with plenty of room outside of the drill area to decelerate without risk for injury.
- **Fatigue:** Because of the high neural demands associated with speed and agility training, these drills should be performed early in a training session if performing other forms of training on the same day, or by themselves, to allow adequate recovery to ensure best efforts during each repetition and reduction of injury risks.

### Program Design

The frequency of SAQ training will vary dramatically based on the needs and demands of a sport. In general,

### FROM THEORY TO PRACTICE

As stated earlier, arm swing governs leg speed. For this reason, proper arm mechanics is critical to generating the necessary propulsive forces to run fast. To illustrate this point, perform the arm swing drill at half, three-quarters, and full speed. As the speed of your arms increases you will notice your lower body will start to move back and forth more rapidly. Now stand up and grab your shirt at about chest height. Run as fast as possible. Now perform the same task with the hands moving freely and using proper arm mechanics. You should notice a measurable increase in speed.

it is recommended for most athletes to perform 1 to 4 days of speed and agility training per week. However, this will depend on how well they are able to recover from previous training sessions and other demands that are placed on the athletes, such as other methods of training (e.g., plyometric and resistance), practice and competition schedules, and time available for training.[9] According to Vescovi,[59] when developing a training program, if maximal linear speed development is the goal, then 3 to 4 days per week may be devoted to developing this skill with occasional agility training for variety. If both speed and agility are desired, they

### Table 18-3. Posture, Arm, and Leg Action During Acceleration

| POSTURE | ARMS | LEGS |
|---|---|---|
| • The jaw should be relaxed, eyes should be gazing forward, and the trainer should be able to see a straight line from the top of the head, through the torso, hip, and knee of the drive leg. The foot (BOS) of the drive leg should be behind the COM. <br> • A pronounced forward lean should be observed as a result of the COM's displacement outside of the BOS, the pelvis should be neutral, and the trunk should be braced. <br> *Note:* The extent of the forward lean needed will depend on the distance to be travelled. | • Arm swing should originate at the shoulder with the elbows flexed at approximately 90 degrees. <br> • Keep the hands relaxed and attempt to swing the arms aggressively, yet controlled, from the cheeks to the back hip pocket. *Note:* If greater changes of direction are required and more frequent stride adjustments are required, the hands may not reach either the cheek or back hip pocket. However, this movement path should still be followed to minimize rotational forces that may pull the runner out of proper alignment. | • Extend the hip, knee, and ankle of the support foot and exert force against the ground, as if "trying to push the ground away." <br> • Keep the ankles in a dorsiflexed position throughout the running cycle. <br> • At foot-strike, the weight should be on the ball of the foot, directly under the athlete to minimize braking forces and maximize propulsive force. <br> • The shin angle should be sharp (less than 90 degrees) initially and increase slightly with each successive stride. |

BOS, base of support.

Adapted from description provided by Dawes, J. & Lentz, D. (2012) Methods of Improving Power for Acceleration for the Non-track Athlete. *Strength and Conditioning Journal.* 34(6):44-S1; and Brewer C. *Strength and Conditioning for Sport: A Practical Guide for Coaches.* The National Coaching Foundation. Leeds, United Kingdom. 2008:54–58.

suggest dedicating 1 to 2 days per week to linear speed and 1 to 2 days per week to agility training.

The intensity of speed and agility drills will depend on a variety of factors as well, such as the movement velocities, effort, sharpness of angles, and number of directional changes.[59] Although maximal sprinting efforts are highly demanding, submaximal efforts can be used to refine movement technique and reduce the overall intensity of a drill or workout. Agility drills that require rapid deceleration and multiple changes of direction are generally more intense than drills that involve fewer changes of direction. Open or reactive drills for agility are generally more stressful than closed drills because of the increased forces and torques placed on the joints during this unplanned movement. Intensity can be increased with **resisted** or **assisted** running.

- Resisted running techniques, including running with a harness attached to sleds or parachutes, are generally used to help improve acceleration and stride length.
- Assisted running or overspeed training techniques, including running while being towed or running downhill, are used to help improve leg turnover (increase number of steps per minute).

Although both are effective methods to improve speed, these techniques are quite advanced and probably better suited to more experienced athletes. For more novice individuals, a more appropriate approach may be to work on simple running techniques that improve movement efficiency for speed.

The volumes and specific type of speed training will also vary dramatically based on the athlete's sport. For track and field athletes, the majority of their time will be spent developing linear speed, especially maximal velocity training and linear acceleration. However, for the field or court sport athlete, such as soccer, hockey, or baseball, more time will be spent working on acceleration over short distances and for quick changes of direction. This places less emphasis on developing linear speed that traditionally involves distances greater than 30 m (33 yards). Volume can be quantified by distances traveled or by the time spent performing each drill.[48,59] As with plyometric training, there is an inverse relation between volume and intensity; therefore, both must be balanced. This can create great challenges for fitness professionals because there is little guidance in the literature on balancing volume and intensity with speed and agility drills. For this reason, a qualitative assessment may also be necessary to determine appropriate workloads. If the coach or instructor notices a significant breakdown in running mechanics, or noticeably slower running speed as drills progress (around a 10% drop-off from maximal movement velocities), the training session should be stopped and future sessions should be adjusted accordingly. In Table 18-4, Raether and Sandler[48] provide some general guidelines regarding

### Table 18-4. Agility Training Volume Based on Experience Level

| EXPERIENCE LEVEL | WORK VOLUME PER SESSION TRAINING | REST BETWEEN DRILLS* |
|---|---|---|
| Beginner | 2 minutes | 30 seconds |
| Intermediate | 3 minutes | 30–40 seconds |
| Advanced | 4 minutes | 30–50 seconds |

*As the number of drills increases, rest time should also increase if maximal speed is desired. The cumulative effect of fatigue will play a role in both technique and speed breakdown.
*Source:* Reprinted from Raether J, Sandler DJ. Agility and quickness program design. In: Dawes JJ, Roozen M, eds. In: *Developing Agility and Quickness.* Champaign, IL: Human Kinetics; 2011.

the appropriate volume of training for speed and agility work. This primarily applies to multidirectional speed development; thus, track athletes may need a greater volume of training depending on their event and whether speed-endurance versus maximal speed is of greater importance.

Ratamess[9] recommends performing:
- One to three sets of technique or form drills and dynamic exercises, then performing three to five sets for sprint and agility drills
- Limiting acceleration and maximum speed drills to no more than 20 to 80 yards
- Limiting training volume within a workout to a range between 300 and 500 yards for acceleration and 300 and 800 yards for maximum speed in college-level athletes; for younger or older athletes, these guidelines require some adjustment to accommodate their current training status and account for other age-related factors

Rest periods are critical for maximizing speed and agility. To maximize speed development, it is recommended that 1 to 3 minutes be provided between sets to allow for recovery of the phosphagen system, and that 1:5 to 1:20 work-to-recovery ratios are used between repetitions. For example, if an agility drill takes 5 seconds to perform and a 1:10 work-to-recovery ratio is used, the rest period would be 50 seconds. These work-to-recovery ratios will be highly dependent on the intensity of the training drill. For instance, a ladder training drill that is performed at a relatively low intensity may require only a 1:7 work-to-recovery ratio, whereas a more intense agility drill involving multiple changes of direction may require a 1:10 work-to-recovery ratio. If work periods are extended beyond this point or the recovery periods are reduced excessively, then these drills become focused on conditioning and contribute less to improving SAQ. However, it is also important to remember that recovery rates may also need to mimic true time intervals reflected within the sport. For example, in

American football, a single play may take 5 seconds to complete and although the athlete physiologically needs 30 to 100 seconds, this may not be possible given the rules of the game, which involve a play clock in which the next play must be initiated to avoid a delay-of-game penalty. Consequently, the coach or trainer may need to train his or her athletes using work-to-recovery ratios used during the sport.

Box 18-4 outlines sample SAQ drills ranging from low to high intensity.

Table 18-5 provides a sample plyometric, speed, and agility training program for a moderately conditioned recreational athlete. This program will use a nonlinear periodization design, as it is assumed that the athletes participate in their sport year-round and are not required to peak for a specific competition.

---

### Box 18-4. Sample Speed, Agility, and Quickness Drills

**Low-Intensity Drills**
- Arm-swing drill
  - Sit on the ground with the knees slightly bent, heels on the ground, and the arms bent at 90-degree angles. Place one hand at eye level and the other at the back hip pocket. Swing the arms from the shoulder, moving the front arm to the back as the back arm simultaneously moves to the front, while maintaining a 90-degree bend in the elbow.
- A-March and skip
  - With the arms bent at 90-degree angles, march forward driving or "punching" the knee up and forward until the foot is just higher than the support leg knee while using a good reciprocating arm action. Focus on keeping the ankle dorsiflexed, the eyes and chest up, and the torso in a neutral and upright position. As soon as peak knee height is reached, drive the foot downward as if trying to push the ground away. The mid-foot should strike the ground first, directly beneath the hips. This action should then be repeated driving with the opposite leg. Once this movement pattern is mastered, complexity can be added to this drill by performing an A-skip, which can be cued as a simple step-hop pattern.
- Icky shuffle
  - Begin standing on the end of the ladder and to the side of the first square. Facing the ladder, step laterally into the first square of the ladder with the foot closest to the ladder, followed by the trailing foot. Immediately step out with the lead foot and place the foot still in the square forward into the next square in the ladder. Then step with the outside foot into the second square. Continue this pattern, moving as quickly as possible through the ladder while maintaining good body control.

**Medium-Intensity Drills**
- Ball drops
  - Assume an athletic stance (two- or three-point stance) approximately 10 yards away from the trainer who should be holding a racquet ball directly out to his side at shoulder height. When the trainer drops the ball, immediately sprint toward the ball and attempt to catch it in as few bounces as possible.
- 20-yard shuttle (pro agility)
  - Start in the UAP, straddling the center line. Turn to the right and sprint 5 yards touching the line with the right hand. Turn to the left and sprint 10 yards touching the line with the left hand. Turn to the right and sprint 5 yards to the center starting line.
- L-run
  - Begin by setting up four cones in the shape of an L. Begin at the first cone and sprint forward 5 yards to cone 2; turn right as soon as you pass the cone and sprint 10 yards to cone 3. Round cone 3 and sprint back to cone 2. Round cone 2 and return to cone 1.

**High-Intensity Drills**
- Four corners drill
  - Begin by setting up four cones, 10 yards apart, in the shape of a square. Starting at cone 1, assume an athletic stance (two- or three-point stance). Sprint 10 yards forward to cone 2, shuffle laterally to cone 3, backpedal to cone 4, then shuffle returning back to cone 1.
- Reactive cone drills
  - The following are examples of ways to progress a closed agility drill to a reactive agility drill using both auditory and visual cues. Begin by positioning three cones approximately 10 yards apart on two separate lines. Stand behind cone 1 and assume an athletic stance (two- or three-point stance). The trainer will call out a specific number (1, 2, or 3). Then sprint to the corresponding number on the opposite row of cones, and stand behind the cone and wait on the next directional cue. Two to four changes of direction should be used for this drill.

**Table 18-5. Sample Nonlinear Plyometric, Speed, and Agility Program**

| MONDAY | | |
|---|---|---|
| **DRILL** | **SETS** | **REPS/TIME** |
| Star excursions | 2 (1 per r/l leg) | 30 seconds |
| Multiplanar reaches | 2 ( 1 per r/l leg) | 30 seconds |
| Jumping jacks | 2 | 20 reps |
| Knee tucks | 3 | 10 reps |
| Leap frog jumps | 3 | 5 reps |
| Box jumps (24 in.) | 3 | 10 reps |
| Pro agility | 3 | 5 reps |
| Ball drops | 10 | 1 reps |

| WEDNESDAY | | |
|---|---|---|
| **DRILL** | **SETS** | **REPS/TIME** |
| Leaning towers | 2 (1 per r/l leg) | 15 seconds |
| Body-weight squats with band | 2 | 20 seconds |
|    perturbations | 3 | 10 seconds |
| Arm-swing drill | 3 | 15 seconds |
| A- March | 3 | 20 reps |
| Alternating toe taps | 3 | 10 reps |
| Chest pass | 3 | 6 reps |
| Multidirectional jump to stick | 3 | 5 reps |
| Front toss | | |

| FRIDAY | | |
|---|---|---|
| **DRILL** | **SETS** | **REPS/TIME** |
| Multiplanar reaches | 2 (1 per r/l leg) | 30 seconds |
| Jumping jacks | 2 | 20 reps |
| Alternating toe taps | 2 | 20 reps |
| Vertical jumps | 3 | 5 reps |
| Lateral cone jumps | 3 | 10 reps |
| Slams | 3 | 10 reps |
| Four corners | 4 | |
| Reactive cone drill | 4 | 3 Cycles per set (2–4 sec/sprint) |

l, left; r, right.

## VIGNETTE conclusion

■ Six months after opening his business, Ben has seen a major shift in his career. Based almost exclusively on word of mouth, his training business has expanded considerably. His clients run the gamut from recent graduates of the university who are working to maintain their elite athletic abilities to weekend golfers looking to improve their swing. Ben enjoys the challenge of evaluating each client's specific needs, as well as the unique movements and the muscles used in each sport, and then turning that knowledge into effective training programs.

As for Ryan, Parker, and Antonio, they have progressed enough to incorporate plyometric movements into their training sessions once each week. Ben is even working with them to develop an off-season periodization program that will allow their fitness and skill levels to peak in time for the beginning of next year's soccer season.

## CRITICAL THINKING QUESTIONS

1. Sarah is a high school volleyball player and would be considered a novice regarding her level of strength and conditioning experience. She would like to start a plyometric training program to improve her vertical jump. However, when conducting an initial athletic testing battery with her, you notice that when she performs the vertical jump she experiences fairly significant valgus collapse upon landing. What actions would you recommend Sarah take before engaging in a plyometric training program?

2. How might a non-athletic client benefit from training more like an athlete?

3. You volunteer to take on the role of conditioning coach for a youth soccer program that fields two teams: boys aged 13 to 15 years and girls aged 13 to 15 years. Your primary responsibility is to help make them more explosive. Briefly outline your needs assessment process, identifying the needs of the sport, the prevalent injuries, and the key anatomical/structural differences between both sexes that should be considered during program design.

4. As a conditioning coach aiming to develop SAQ, you plan to use various tools including cones and agility ladders to improve these skills over a 6-week time frame. Select one drill that will improve multidirectional SAQ and outline your idea on how it will progress over a period from a simple, sagittal-motion foot drill (i.e., stepping sequence moving forward in a straight line) to a complex multidirectional drill involving eye–hand coordination (i.e., stop-and-start motion, moving in multiple directions while catching and passing a ball).

## ADDITIONAL RESOURCES

Baechle TR, Earle RW, eds. *Essentials of Strength Training and Conditioning.* 3rd ed. Champaign, IL: Human Kinetics; 2008.

Balyi I, Hamilton A. Long-Term Athlete Development: Trainability in Childhood and Adolescence. Windows of Opportunity. Optimal Trainability. Victoria, BC: National Coaching Institute British Columbia & Advanced Training and Performance Ltd.; 2004.

Dawes J. Agility training for general populations. *ACSM Certified News.* 2010;20:5–6.

Dawes J. Learning to react. *Prof Strength Cond.* 2008; 9:25–27.

## REFERENCES

1. Clark MA. Integrated Training for the New Millennium. Chandler, AZ: National Academy of Sports Medicine; 2001.
2. Roetert EP. 3-D balance and core stability. In: Foran B, ed. *High Performance Sports Conditioning: Optimum Training for Ultimate Athletic Development.* Champaign, IL: Human Kinetics; 2001.
3. Yagee JA, Campbell BM. Effects of balance training on selected skills. *J Strength Cond Res.* 2006;20:422–428.
4. Gambetta V. Everything in balance. In: Gambette V, ed. *The Gambetta Method.* Sarasota, FL: Gambetta Sports Training Systems, Inc.; 1998.
5. Gambetta V. Fundamental fun. In: Gambette V, ed. *The Gambetta Method.* Sarasota, FL: Gambetta Sports Training Systems, Inc.; 1998.
6. Hedrick A. Implement Training. NSCA Hot Topics. 2008. http://www.nsca.com. Accessed October 10, 2012.
7. Taylor JB. Lower-extremity perturbation training. *Strength Cond J.* 2011;33:76–83.
8. Myer GD, Ford KR, Brent JL, Hewett TE. The effects of plyometrics vs. dynamic stabilization and balance training on power, balance, and landing force in female athletes. *J Strength Cond Res.* 2006;20:345–353.
9. Ratamess N. *ACSM's Foundations of Strength Training and Conditioning.* Philadelphia, PA: Lippincott Williams & Wilkins; 2012;pp.238–243.
10. McMasters DT, Cronin J, McGuigan M. Forms of variable resistance. *Strength Cond J.* 2009;31:27–30.
11. Cressey EM, West CA, Tiberio DP, Kraemer WJ, Maresh CM. The effects of ten weeks of lower-body unstable surface training on markers of athletic performance. *J Strength Cond Res.* 2007;21:561–567.
12. Dawes J, Vives D. Active resistance as a dynamic warm-up modality. *J Austral Strength Cond.* 2009;17:35–36.
13. Coker CA. *Motor Learning and Control for Practitioners.* 2nd ed. Scottsdale, AZ: Holcomb and Hathaway Publishers; 2009.
14. Turvey MT. Coordination. *Am Psychol.* 1991;45:938–953.
15. Klavora P. *Foundations of Kinesiology: Studying Human Movement and Health.* 2nd ed. Toronto, ON: Sports Book Publishers; 2010.
16. Stanganelli LC, Duardo AC, Oncken P, Mancan S, da Costa SC. Adaptations on jump capacity in Brazilian volleyball players prior to the under-19 world championship. *J Strength Cond Res.* 2008;22:741–749.
17. Kenney, WL, Wilmore, JH, & Kenney, DL. *Physiology of Sport and Exercise,* 5th edition. Champaign, IL: Human Kinetics. 2012.
18. Suslov F. About the sensitive age periods in the development of physical capacities. *Modern Athlete and Coach.* 2002;40:31–33.
19. Balyi I, Hamilton A. (2004). Long-Term Athlete Development: Trainability in Childhood and Adolescence. Windows of Opportunity. Optimal Trainability. Victoria: National Coaching Institute British Columbia & Advanced Training and Performance Ltd.
20. Dawes, J & Lentz, D. (2012). Methods of improving power for acceleration for the non-track athlete. *Strength and Conditioning Journal.* 34(6):44-51.
20a. Dawes J. Learning to react. *Prof Strength Cond.* 2008;9:25–27.
21. Knudson D. Correcting the use of the term "Power" in the strength and conditioning literature. *J Strength Cond Res.* 2009;23:1902–1908.
22. Newton RU. Biomechanics of Conditioning Exercises. In: Chandler TJ, Brown LE, eds. *Conditioning for Strength and Human Performance.* Philadelphia, PA: Lippincott Williams & Wilkins; 2008.

23. O'Shea P. Toward an understanding of power. *Strength Cond J.* 1999;21:34–35.

24. Cavanaugh B. Specificity of power training for sports performance: A review of the literature. *J Austral Strength Cond.* 2010;18:25–29.

25. Harmon EA, Pandorf C. Principles of test selection and administration. In: Baechle TR, Earle RW, eds. *Essentials of Strength Training and Conditioning.* 2nd ed. Champaign, IL: Human Kinetics; 2000.

26. American Council on Exercise (ACE). *Sports Conditioning Workshop Manual.* San Diego, CA: ACE; 2011.

27. Sayers M. Running techniques for field sport players. *Sports Coach* 2000;23:26–27.

28. Sheppard JM, Young WB. Agility literature review: Classifications, training and testing. *J Sport Sci.* 2006;24:919–993.

29. Benton D. Sprint running needs of field sport athletes: A new perspective. *Sports Coach.* 2001;24:2–14.

30. Ebben W, Davies J, Clewien R. Effect of the degree of hill slope on acute downhill running velocity and acceleration. *J Strength Cond Res.* 2008;22:898–902.

31. Australian Strength and Conditioning Association (ASCA). Module 4 – Speed and Agility – Elite Training Theory and Current Practices. ASCA Level 3 Coaches Course, Queensland, Australia, November 9, 2011.

32. Roozen M, Suprak D. Change of direction factors. In: Dawes JJ, Roozen M, eds. *Developing Agility and Quickness.* Champaign, IL: Human Kinetics; 2011.

33. Plisk SS. Speed, agility, and speed-endurance development. In: Baechle TR, Earle RW, eds. *Essentials of Strength Training and Conditioning.* 3rd ed. Champaign, IL: Human Kinetics; 2008:458–485.

34. Young WB, James R, Montgomery I. Is muscle power related to running speed with changes of direction? *J Sports Med Phys Fitness.* 2002;43:282–288.

35. Sheppard JM, Young WB, Doyle TLA, Sheppard TA, Newton RU. An evaluation of a new test of reactive agility and its relationship to sprint speed and change of direction speed. *J Sci Med Sports.* 2006;9: 342–349.

36. Kovacs MS. Movement for tennis: The importance of lateral training. *Strength Cond J.* 2009;31:77–85.

37. Schmidt &Wrisberg, 2007. *Motor Learning and Performance* (4th ed). Champaign, Ill. Human Kinetics, p.51.

38. Serpell BG, Young WB, Ford M. Are the perceptual and decision-making components of agility trainable? A preliminary investigation. *J Strength Cond Res.* 2011;25:1240–1248.

39. Vickers JN. *Perception, Cognition, and Decision Training: The Quiet Eye in Action.* Champaign, IL: Human Kinetics; 2007:30–31, 48.

40. Schmidt RA, Lee TD. *Motor Control and Learning: A Behavioral Emphasis.* 4th ed. Champaign, IL: Human Kinetics; 2005:91–101.

41. Schmidt RA, Lee TD. *Motor Control and Learning: A Behavioral Emphasis.* 4th ed. Champaign, IL: Human Kinetics; 2005; 280–285.

42. Schmidt RA, Lee TD. *Motor Control and Learning: A Behavioral Emphasis.* 4th ed. Champaign, IL: Human Kinetics; 2005; 401–431.

43. Abernethy B, Russell DG. Expert-novice difference in an applied selective attention task. *J Sport Psychol.* 1987;9:326–345.

44. Jeffreys I. A task-based approach to developing context-specific agility. *Strength Cond J.* 2011;33:52–59.

45. Steindler A. *Kinesiology of the Human Body: Under Normal and Pathological Conditions.* Springfield, IL: Charles C Thomas; 1955.

46. Viitasalo JT, Komi PV. Effects of fatigue on isometric force- and relaxation-time characteristics in human muscle. *Acta Physiol Scand.* 1981;111:87–95.

47. Wathen D, Baechle TR, Earle RW. Periodization. In: Baechle TR, Earle RW, eds. *Essentials of Strength and Conditioning.* 3rd ed. Champaign, IL: Human Kinetics; 2008:507–522.

48. Raether J, Sandler DJ. Agility and quickness program design. In: Dawes JJ, Roozen M, eds. In: *Developing Agility and Quickness.* Champaign, IL: Human Kinetics; 2011.

49. Jeffreys I. *Total Soccer Fitness.* Monterey, CA: Coaches Choice; 2007.

50. Reiman MP, Lorenz DS. Integration of strength and conditioning principles into a rehabilitation program. *Int J Sports Phys Ther.* 2011;6:241–253.

51. Potach DH, Chu DA. Plyometric training. In: Baechle TR, Earle RW, eds. *Essentials of Strength and Conditioning.* 3rd ed. Champaign, IL: Human Kinetics; 2008:507–522.

52. Fowler K, Kravitz L. Explosive power. *IDEA Fitness J.* 2011;8:38–45.

53. Wathen D. Literature review explosive/plyometric exercises. *Natl Strength Cond Assoc J.* 1993;15:46–48.

54. Allerheiligen B, Rogers R. Plyometrics program design. *Strength Cond.* 1995;17:26–31.

55. Allerheiligen B, Rogers R. Plyometrics program design, part 2. *Strength Cond.* 1995;17:33–39.

56. McNeely E. Introduction to plyometrics: Converting strength to power. *NSCA's Perform Train J.* 2005;6:19–22.

57. Siff MC. *Facts and Fallacies of Fitness.* 5th ed. Denver, CO: Mel Siff; 2002.

58. Sandler DJ. *Sports Power.* Champaign, IL: Human Kinetics; 2005.

58a. Schmidt R, Wrisberg CA. *Motor Learning and Performance.* 4th ed. Champaign, IL: Human Kinetics; 2008. P.51.

59. Vescovi JD. Plyometric, speed and agility prescription. In: Chandler TJ, Brown LE, eds. *Conditioning for Strength and Human Performance.* Baltimore, MD: Lippincott Williams & Wilkins; 2008.

60. Jeffreys I. *Gamespeed: Movement Training for Superior Sports Performance.* Monterey, CA: Coaches Choice; 2010.

# *Practice What You Know:* Skill-Related Assessments

Given the increased popularity of sports conditioning, some clients may desire or need assessments of the skill- or performance-related parameters of fitness, which include:

• Balance
• Power (anaerobic power and anaerobic capacity)
• Speed
• Agility
• Reactivity
• Coordination

The following assessments can be used to measure the skill-related components of fitness.

## BALANCE ASSESSMENTS

Baseline assessments of balance are important to evaluate the need for comprehensive balance training and core conditioning during the early stages of an exercise program. The following two tests measure a client's basic level of static balance.

### Stork-Stand Balance Test

**Objective**

The objective of the stork-stand balance test is to assess static balance by standing on one foot in a modified stork-stand position.

**Equipment**
• Firm, nonslip surface
• Stopwatch

**Test Protocol and Administration**
• Explain the purpose of the test.
• Ask the client to remove his or her shoes and stand with feet together and hands on the hips.
• Instruct the client to raise one foot off the ground and bring that foot to lightly touch the inside of the stance leg, just below the knee (Figure 1).

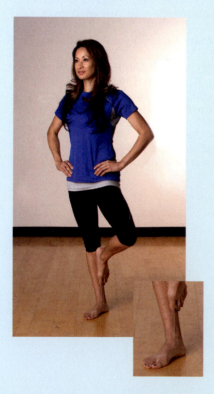

**Figure 1.** Stork-stand balance test: starting position.

- The client must raise the heel of the stance foot off the floor and balance on the ball of the foot (Figure 2).

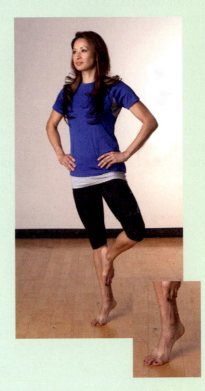

**Figure 2.** Stork-stand balance test: test position.

- Stand behind the client for support if needed.
- Allow 1 minute of practice trials.
- After the practice trial, perform the test, starting the stopwatch as the heel lifts off the floor.
- Repeat with the opposite leg.
- Allow up to three trials per leg position and record the best performance on each side.

### Observations

Timing stops when any of the following occurs:

- The hand(s) come off the hips
- The stance or supporting foot inverts, everts, or moves in any direction
- Any part of the elevated foot loses contact with the stance leg
- The heel of the stance leg touches the floor
- The client loses balance

### General Interpretation

Use the information provided in Table 1 to categorize the client's performance.

### Table 1. The Stork-Stand Balance Test

| | RATING | | | | |
|---|---|---|---|---|---|
| SEX | EXCELLENT | GOOD | AVERAGE | FAIR | POOR |
| Male | >50 seconds | 41–50 seconds | 31–40 seconds | 20–30 seconds | <20 seconds |
| Female | >30 seconds | 25–30 seconds | 16–24 seconds | 10–15 seconds | <10 seconds |

Data from Johnson BL, Nelson JK. *Practical Measurements for Evaluation in Physical Education*. 4th ed. Minneapolis, MN: Burgess; 1986.

## *Practice What You Know:* Skill-Related Assessments—cont'd

### Sharpened Romberg Test

#### Objective
The objective of the sharpened Romberg test is to assess static balance and postural control while standing on a reduced BOS while removing visual sensory perception.

#### Equipment
- Firm, flat, nonslip surface
- Stopwatch

#### Test Protocol and Administration
- Explain the purpose of the test.
- Instruct the client to remove his or her shoes and stand with one foot directly in front of the other (tandem or heel-to-toe position) with the eyes open.
- Ask the client to fold his or her arms across the chest, touching each hand to the opposite shoulder (Figure 3).

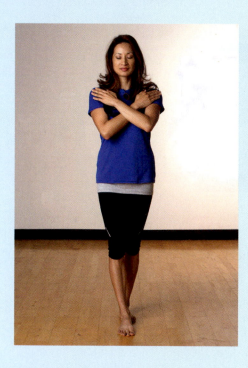

**Figure 3.** Sharpened Romberg test.

- Allow sufficient practice trials. Once the client feels stable, instruct the client to close his or her eyes. Start the stopwatch to begin the test.
- Always stand in close proximity as a precaution to prevent falling.
- Continue the test for 60 seconds or until the client exhibits any test-termination cue, as listed in the following Observations section.
- Allow up to two trials per leg position and record the best performance on each side.

#### Observations
Continue to time the client's performance until one of the following occurs:

- The client loses postural control and balance
- The client's feet move on the floor
- The client's eyes open
- The client's arms move from the folded position
- The client exceeds 60 seconds with good postural control

#### General Interpretations
- The client needs to maintain his or her balance with good postural control (without excessive swaying) and not exhibit any of the test-termination criteria for ≥30 seconds.
- The inability to reach 30 seconds is indicative of inadequate static balance and postural control.

## ANAEROBIC POWER ASSESSMENTS

Human power is the rate at which mechanical work is performed under a defined set of conditions. Power correlates to the immediate energy available through the anaerobic energy system, specifically the phosphagen energy system. Anaerobic power involves a single repetition or event and represents the maximal amount of power the body can generate, whereas anaerobic capacity represents the sustainability of power output for brief periods.

Strength and power are closely related, but for assessment purposes, they should be evaluated independently. Power is also sport or activity specific. Evaluation and subsequent correction of athletic performance is closely related to body mechanics and movement. Evaluation of fluid movements like a golf swing or a swimming stroke requires digital movement analysis or other technology. The power assessments covered in this section are also related to skills and performance in a variety of sports and are significant indicators of sports success.

### CONSIDERATIONS AND CONTRAINDICATIONS FOR FIELD TESTS OF POWER, SPEED, AGILITY, AND QUICKNESS

Because these tests are intended for athletes and those interested in advanced forms of training, individuals in "special populations" are not likely candidates. When working with a client who is still recovering from an injury, it is wise to omit these tests.

Fitness professionals must keep in mind that power tests are designed for clients interested in training at very intense levels, or for high-level athletic performance. Therefore, the majority of normative data presented with these tests have been obtained from studies involving college and professional athletes. Little, if any, data exist for middle-aged or older adults. The results of these tests are perhaps best used as baseline data against which to measure a client's future performance.

### Vertical Jump Test

The vertical jump test is a simple way to measure anaerobic power and is quick to administer. It is especially valuable when assessing the vertical jump height in athletes who participate in sports that require skill and power in jumping (e.g., basketball, volleyball, and swimming).

#### Equipment
- A smooth wall with a relatively high ceiling
- A flat, stable floor that provides good traction
- Chalk (different color than the wall)
- Measuring tape or stick
- Stepstool or small ladder
- Vertical jump tester (e.g., Vertec) (optional)

#### Pretest Procedure
- After explaining the purpose of the vertical jump test, describe and demonstrate the procedure. Allow the client to perform a few practice trials before administering the test.
- Instruct the client to stand adjacent to a wall, with the inside shoulder of the dominant arm approximately 6 inches (15 cm) from the wall. Measure the client's standing height by marking the fingers with chalk, extending the inside arm overhead, and marking the wall (Figure 4A).

## *Practice What You Know:* Skill-Related Assessments—cont'd

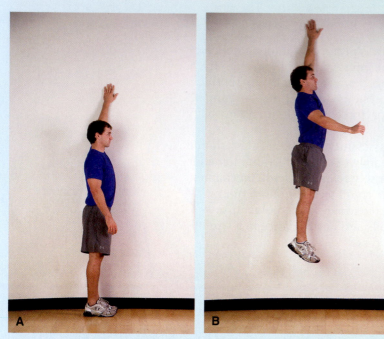

**Figure 4.** Vertical jump test.

   This mark will then be compared with the maximum height achieved on a vertical jump.

- The goal of this test is to jump as high as possible from a standing position.
- Because proper technique plays a role in achieving maximum jump height, encourage the client to use the arms and legs for propulsion.

### Test Protocol and Administration
- The client stands adjacent to the wall, 6 inches (15 cm) away from the wall, with both arms extended overhead and feet flat on the floor.
- The client then lowers the arms and, without any pause or step, drops into a squat movement before exploding upward into a vertical jump.
- At the highest point the athlete touches the wall, marking it with chalk (Figure 4B).
- The vertical jump measurement is determined by the vertical distance between the new chalk mark and the starting height.
- Allow three repetitions and record the maximum height achieved on the testing form.

### General Interpretation
Use Table 2 to rank the client's performance.

### Table 2. Vertical Jump Descriptive Data* for Various Groups

| GROUP, SPORT, OR POSITION | VERTICAL JUMP (IN.) |
|---|---|
| NCAA Division I college football split ends, strong safeties, offensive and defensive backs | 31.5 |
| NCAA Division I college football wide receivers and outside linebackers | 31 |
| NCAA Division I football linebackers, tight ends, and safeties | 29.5 |
| College basketball players (men) | 27–29 |
| NCAA Division I college football quarterbacks | 28.5 |
| NCAA Division I college football defensive tackles | 28 |
| NCAA Division I college basketball players (men) | 28 |
| NCAA Division I college football offensive guards | 27 |

## Vertical Jump Descriptive Data* for Various Groups–cont'd

| GROUP, SPORT, OR POSITION | VERTICAL JUMP (IN.) |
| --- | --- |
| Competitive college athletes (men) | 25–25.5 |
| NCAA Division I college football offensive tackles | 25–26 |
| Recreational college athletes (men) | 24 |
| High school football backs and receivers | 24 |
| College baseball players (men) | 23 |
| College tennis players (men) | 23 |
| High school football linebackers and tight ends | 22 |
| College football players | 21 |
| College basketball players (women) | 21 |
| 17-year-old boys | 20 |
| High school football lineman | 20 |
| NCAA Division II college basketball guards (women) | 19 |
| NCAA Division II college basketball forwards (women) | 18 |
| NCAA Division II college basketball centers (women) | 17.5 |
| Sedentary college students (men) | 16–20.5 |
| 18- to 34-year-old men | 16 |
| Competitive college athletes (women) | 16–18.5 |
| College tennis players (women) | 15 |
| Recreational college athletes (women) | 15–15.5 |
| Sedentary college students (women) | 8–14 |
| 17-year-old girls | 13 |
| 18- to 34-year-old sedentary women | 8 |

*The values listed are either means or 50th percentiles (medians). There was considerable variation in sample size among the groups tested. Thus, the data should be regarded as only descriptive, not normative.

Reprinted with permission from Baechle, T.R. & Earlie, R.W. (2008). *NSCA's Essentials of Strength Training and Conditioning* (3rd ed.). Champaign, Ill.: Human Kinetics, p. 278.

## Anaerobic Capacity Step Test

The anaerobic capacity step test is considered "long" for an anaerobic test because its duration is 60 seconds, whereas shorter anaerobic capacity tests range from 10 to 30 seconds (e.g., the Wingate test is 30 seconds). In this procedure, one foot remains on the step for the duration of the test. Thus, it is essentially a one-legged step test. The performance of the anaerobic capacity step test is fueled primarily by the glycolytic pathway (lactate system) of metabolism and secondarily by the phosphagen system.

### Objective
The objective of the anaerobic capacity step test is to perform as many step-ups as possible on leg with all-out effort for 60 seconds.

### Equipment
- Bench (40 cm or 15.75 inches in height)
- Stopwatch
- Calculator
- Body-weight scale

### Pretest Procedure
- Measure the participant's body weight in the same shoes and clothes that are worn during the test.
- Because of the intensity of this test, it is recommended that the participant perform a 5- to 7-minute warm-up that includes walking with high knees; stretching of the hips, quadriceps, and calves; and low-intensity stepping on a bench (approximately 20 steps/min). However, the client should avoid becoming fatigued at any time during the warm-up.
- The client should become familiar with the stepping technique before the test, because it is different from typical stepping procedures.

## *Practice What You Know:* Skill-Related Assessments—cont'd

- Have the client stand alongside the bench, not in front of it. The test leg (preferred, dominant, or support leg) rests on top of the bench in preparation for the start of the test (Figure 5A).
- The other leg, called the "free" leg, need not touch the bench when the test leg lifts the body (Figure 5B).

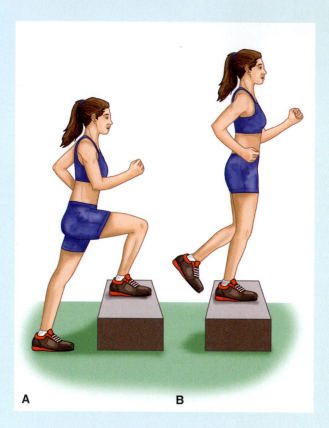

A                           B

**Figure 5.** Positions for the anaerobic capacity step test.

The free leg dangles in a straight position during the ascent and then supports and pushes off when the foot contacts the floor.
- The legs and the back should straighten with each step. In fact, the back should start in a straight position and never be changed throughout the test.
- The arms may be used for balance but cannot be pumped vigorously during the test.
- The cadence for the test is a 1–2 count (i.e., 1 is up and 2 is down), which is different than the typical 4-count cadence of aerobic step tests.
- The participant should be instructed to go all out without pacing for the duration of the test. Thus, the participant should be exhausted, or nearly so, by the end of the test. Exhaustion is defined in this case as the inability to take another step.

### Test Protocol and Administration
- A step is counted for each time the participant's support leg is straightened and then returned to the starting position. Steps are not counted if the participant does not straighten the support leg or if the participant's back is not straight.
- Count aloud for the participant as follows: "Up-1, up-2, up-3," and so on. Thus, a full step is considered to be a return to the starting (down) position after the ascent.
- Record the number of steps at the 60th second. The 60th-second score is used to calculate anaerobic capacity.
- The duration of the test is 60 seconds. The time begins with the first upward movement of the participant. The technician should call out the time to the participant every 15 seconds.
- Mild walking or walking in place is recommended immediately after the test.

General Interpretation

Calculate anaerobic capacity using the following equations:

**Anaerobic capacity**

Body weight (kg) × (0.40 m × number of steps in 60 seconds) × 1.33

To compare scores based on standardized norms (see Tables 3 and 4), convert anaerobic capacity from kg/sec to watts. Divide anaerobic capacity by the conversion factor (1 W = 6.12 kg/min = 9.81 W).

## Table 3. Comparative Scores (Anaerobic Capacity) for the Anaerobic Power Step Test

| | ANAEROBIC CAPACITY | | | |
| | MEAN | | HIGHEST | |
| GROUP | KG/MIN | W | KG/MIN | W |
| --- | --- | --- | --- | --- |
| **Active college students** **(repeat trial)** | | | | |
| Men (n = 14) | 2,778 | 454 | 3,571 | 583 |
| Women (n = 11) | 2,068 | 338 | 2,794 | 457 |
| **Pro football players** | 3,381 | 626 | 4,957 | 810 |
| **(n = 15; offseason)** | | (SD 108) | | |
| **Active adults** | | | | |
| Men (n = 130; 17–30 yr old) | 2,815 | 460 | (SD 90) | |
| Women (n = 70; 18–30 yr old) | 1,879 | 307 | (SD 61) | |

Data from Adams, G.M. (1990). *Exercise Physiology Laboratory Manual*. Dubuque, IA: Wm. C. Brown Publishers

## Table 4. Norms for Anaerobic Power Step Test for Active Men (n = 130) and Women (n = 70) Between 18 and 30 Years Old

| PERCENTILE | MEN POWER (W) | FEMALE POWER (W) |
| --- | --- | --- |
| 99 | 730 | 490 |
| 95 | 608 | 407 |
| 90 | 584 | 391 |
| 85 | 554 | 370 |
| 80 | 536 | 358 |
| 75 | 520 | 348 |
| 70 | 507 | 339 |
| 65 | 495 | 331 |
| 60 | 483 | 322 |
| 55 | 472 | 315 |
| 50 | 460 | 307 |
| 45 | 448 | 299 |
| 40 | 438 | 292 |
| 35 | 425 | 283 |
| 30 | 413 | 275 |
| 25 | 400 | 266 |
| 20 | 384 | 258 |
| 15 | 366 | 244 |
| 10 | 336 | 223 |
| 5 | 312 | 207 |

Data from Adams, G.M. (1990). *Exercise Physiology Laboratory Manual*. Dubuque, IA: Wm. C. Brown Publishers.

*Practice What You Know:* Skill-Related Assessments–cont'd

**Example:**
A 68-kg client completes 50 steps in the 60-second period.
Anaerobic capacity: 68 kg × (0.40 m × 50) × 1.33 = 1,809 kg/min
Watt conversion: 1,809 kg/min ÷ 6.12 kg/min = 302 W

## SPEED, QUICKNESS, AND AGILITY ASSESSMENTS

### 40-Yard Dash

**Objective**
- The purpose of the 40-yard dash is to determine acceleration and speed. This test is simple to administer and does not require much time or equipment. The 40-yard dash or variations on the test that use other distances are performed extensively in football and other sports that require quick bouts of speed.
- Weather conditions and running surface can greatly affect the speed of the client. On follow-up assessments, it is important to test on the same running surface and in the same conditions as in the initial test.

**Equipment**
- Running track, marked field, or measuring tape and unobstructed surface (of at least 60 yards)
- Stopwatch
- Cones
- Timing gates (optional)

**Pretest Procedure**
- After explaining the purpose of the 40-yard dash, describe the test to the client. The client should warm up before the actual test and even perform some practice starts to work on acceleration techniques.
- The goal of the test is to run as quickly as possible. The client begins in a four-point (track start) or three-point stance if that is more comfortable (Figure 6) and runs past the 40-yard (37-m) mark.

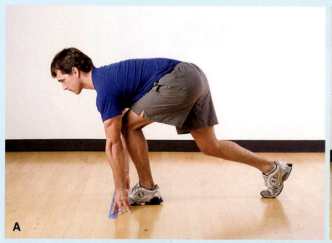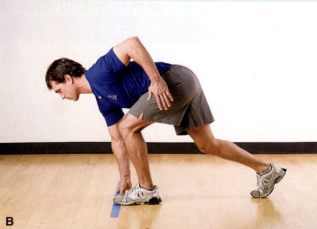

**Figure 6.** Forty–yard dash starting positions. A, Four-point stance (track start). B, Three-point stance.

**Test Protocol and Administration**
- The client starts in a four-point (track start) or three-point stance with the front foot positioned on or behind the starting line. He or she should place the hands and feet on the line, but not beyond it. The client can lean across the line but is not permitted to rock. This position must be held for at least 3 seconds before starting.
- Start the stopwatch at the first movement and stop it when the client's chest crosses the finish line.

- The time is measured to one hundredth (0.00) of a second.
- Have the client perform two trials with appropriate recovery (at least 2 minutes) between the trials and record the average of the two trials on the testing form.

### General Interpretation

Refer to Table 5 for descriptive data that can be used to show clients where their performance might rank among various groups of athletes.

#### Table 5. 40-Yard Dash–Descriptive Data

| GROUP, SPORT, OR POSITION | 40-YARD (37-M) SPRINT (SEC) |
| --- | --- |
| **NCAA Division I college American football players** | |
| Split ends, wide receivers, strong safeties, outside linebackers, and offensive and defensive backs | 4.6–4.7 |
| Linebackers, tight ends, safeties, and quarterbacks | 4.8–4.9 |
| Defensive tackles | 4.9–5.1 |
| Defensive guards | 5.1 |
| Offensive tackles | 5.4 |
| College American football players | 5.35 |
| **Competitive college athletes** | |
| Men | 5.0 |
| Women | 5.5–5.96 |
| **Recreational college athletes** | |
| Men | 5.0 |
| Women | 5.8 |
| **Sedentary college students** | |
| Men | 5.0 |
| Women | 6.4 |
| **High school American football players** | |
| Backs and receivers | 5.2 |
| Linebackers and tight ends | 5.4 |
| Linemen | 4.9–5.6 |

Data listed are either means or 50th percentiles (medians). There was considerable variation in sample size among the groups tested. Thus, the data should be regarded as only descriptive, not normative.
Data from Baechle TR, Earle RW. *Essentials of Strength Training and Conditioning*. 3rd ed. Champaign, IL: Human Kinetics; 2008.

## Pro Agility Test

The pro agility test is sometimes called the 20-yard agility test or the 5-10-5 shuttle run. The National Football League and USA Women's Soccer Team use this assessment as part of their battery of tests.

### Objective

This test quickly and simply measures an individual's ability to accelerate, decelerate, change direction, and then accelerate again.

### Equipment

- A marked football field, but the test can be conducted on any hard, flat surface that offers good traction
- Measuring tape
- Cones or tape
- Stopwatch
- Timing gates (optional)

*Practice What You Know:* Skill-Related Assessments—cont'd

**Pre-test Procedure**
• Set up the cones as shown in Figure 7.

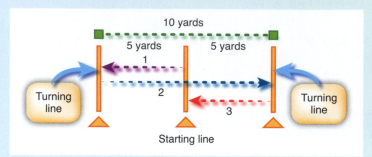

**Figure 7.** The Pro Agility test.

• After explaining the purpose of the test, describe and demonstrate the proper route and technique. Allow the client to warm up and perform a few practice trials before administering the test.
• The goal of the test is to complete the course as quickly as possible.
• The client does not need to touch the cone with his or her hand, but must touch the line with either foot. Proper technique must be followed or the test run will not count.

**Test Protocol and Administration**
• The trainer is positioned as the timer/judge at the center cone or line marker.
• Ask the client to straddle the middle cone or line marker facing the trainer and assume a three-point stance (see the figure above for the 40-yd dash).
• On the trainer's command, the client turns and sprints to the cone or line marker to the left, making foot contact with the marker before changing direction and sprinting 10 yards across the center marker to make foot contact with the cone or line marker on the right, then changes direction once again and sprints back through the center line.

- Record the time needed to complete the test to the nearest one-hundredth of a second.
  - The pro agility test is then repeated two more times. The client can take a few minutes to recover between tests.
- The fastest of the three trials is noted as the final test score on the testing form.

**General Interpretation**

Use Table 6 to rank the client's performance. *Note:* The test can be run in either or both directions.

**Table 6. Percentile Ranks for the Pro Agility Test for NCAA Division I Athletes (time in seconds)**

| PERCENTILE RANK | MEN'S BASKETBALL | MEN'S BASEBALL | MEN'S FOOTBALL | WOMEN'S VOLLEYBALL | WOMEN'S BASKETBALL | WOMEN'S SOFTBALL |
|---|---|---|---|---|---|---|
| 90th | 4.22 | 4.25 | 4.21 | 4.75 | 4.65 | 4.88 |
| 80th | 4.29 | 4.36 | 4.31 | 4.84 | 4.82 | 4.96 |
| 70th | 4.35 | 4.41 | 4.38 | 4.91 | 4.86 | 5.03 |
| 60th | 4.39 | 4.46 | 4.44 | 4.98 | 4.94 | 5.10 |
| 50th | 4.41 | 4.50 | 4.52 | 5.01 | 5.06 | 5.17 |
| 40th | 4.44 | 4.55 | 4.59 | 5.08 | 5.10 | 5.24 |
| 30th | 4.48 | 4.61 | 4.66 | 5.17 | 5.14 | 5.33 |
| 20th | 4.51 | 4.69 | 4.76 | 5.23 | 5.23 | 5.40 |
| 10th | 4.61 | 4.76 | 4.89 | 5.32 | 5.36 | 5.55 |

Adapted with permission from Hoffman J. *Norms for Fitness, Performance, and Health.* Champaign, IL: Human Kinetics; 2006.

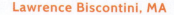

Lawrence Biscontini, MA

## CHAPTER 19

# Mind–Body Exercise and Fitness

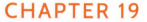

## CHAPTER OUTLINE

## LEARNING OUTCOMES

1. Define the concepts of *mindfulness* and *mind-body fitness.*

2. Describe the most common mind-body fitness disciplines, including their country of origin; age; approach to and methods of training the body in terms of cardiovascular strength, flexibility, and balance; and how they incorporate equipment, if at all.

3. Describe breathing techniques from the most common mind-body disciplines, including their purpose, technique, and applicability to improving overall wellness.

4. Explain how to introduce components of mind-body exercise into traditional fitness training regimens by manipulating a mental, breathing, and speed focus.

5. Define some aspects of mind-body training that can be implemented within traditional group fitness and personal training settings.

## ANCILLARY LINK

Visit Davis*Plus* at http://davisplus.fadavis.com for study and practice resources, including online quizzes, animations that help explain physiological processes, podcasts concerning news and career trends in exercise physiology, and practice references.

## VIGNETTE

■ Tanya, a young mother of three small boys, has been working with Dennis, a personal trainer at a local fitness studio, since the birth of her first son 7 years ago. During this time, Dennis has helped Tanya manage her weight and regain her fitness level after each of her three pregnancies, and the two of them have developed a tremendous amount of rapport over the years. Her current regimen consists of 2 days of resistance training with Dennis, as well as three or four evening walks each week. She is getting bored with her walking routine and asks Dennis for some ideas for incorporating mind-body exercise into her program because she has read many good things about yoga in various parenting magazines.

Dennis encourages the idea of adding variety and mindfulness to Tanya's exercise program and asks if she is willing to replace two of her weekly walks with mind-body workouts under the supervision of Elijah, a yoga instructor who works at the studio. Dennis suggests that she continue walking at least two nights a week, as the cardiorespiratory benefits of moderate-intensity walking will not be derived from the yoga program. In addition, Dennis tells Tanya that he will also add some mindful elements to her two resistance training sessions each week.

What is the best way for Dennis to incorporate those elements into Tanya's workouts, and what benefits can she expect from participating in the yoga sessions?

According to a recent report of the Sports & Fitness Industry Association (formerly the Sporting Goods Manufacturers Association), mind–body fitness activities (namely, yoga and Pilates) are fast-growing and popular forms of physical activity in the United States, boasting approximately a combined 31 million participants.[1] To be sure, other types of classes appear on class schedules across the globe on a daily basis, but the fact remains that mind–body classes, such as Pilates, are gaining more and more acceptance among gym-goers. What is special about the disciplines called *mind–body*? What is the benefit of slowing down and adding an inward focus on training? Most importantly, why is this type of training among the fastest-growing trends in the fitness industry?[2]

Pilates, like other mind–body disciplines, offers its participants the ability to train more than the body's muscles and bones. Mind–body disciplines include a keen attention to training speeds that are slower than traditional approaches, an emphasis on breath work that proves crucial to the execution of the exercises, and a strong, inward mental focus. Furthermore, research reveals that mind–body fitness definitely increases the body's ability to recruit more muscle fibers than when the body alone works without a strong component of mindfulness, which includes a strong emphasis on concentration.[3] Ultimately, mind–body fitness trains more than just the physical body; it trains the breath and brain as well, resulting in a more complete experience involving the whole person.

## THE FITNESS BODY AS A TRILOGY: MIND, BODY, AND SPIRIT

Traditional fitness modalities address the body and, collectively, these forms have long focused on the physical parameters of health (Fig. 19-1), with little consideration given to the **mind–body connection**. Occasionally, exercise and fitness professionals reference breathing in a general sense, but they rarely go beyond the two most common recommendations: avoiding the **Valsalva maneuver** (or holding one's breath) and exhaling on exertion.[2,4]

Using a driving analogy, mind–body fitness includes more than just putting gas in the car; it encompasses attentional focus at the wheel, adjustment of mirrors for greater depth perception and peripheral vision, and even seat adjustment to enhance efficiency of posture.

The **mind–body concept** considers each individual as a trilogy of not only the traditional body, but also of brain and breath. Consequently, mind–body fitness includes a strong training component that addresses each of those aspects of the person—a triangular fitness vision, as illustrated in Figure 19-2.

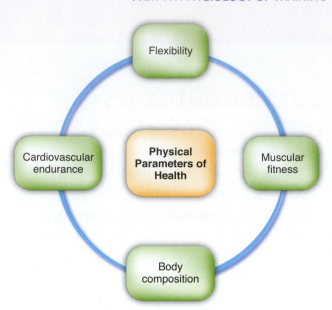

**Figure 19-1.** The four main factors that comprise the basic physical parameters of health.

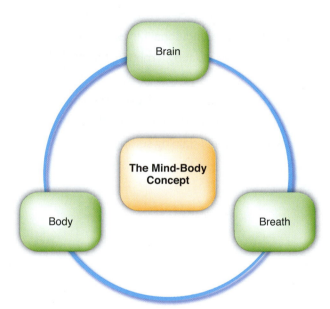

**Figure 19-2.** The three main factors that comprise the mind–body concept.

## COMMON MISCONCEPTIONS

The traditional words used to describe the fitness approach explained in this chapter are *mind, body,* and *spirit,* but these words can sometimes be disconcerting to some individuals and cultures because of preconceptions, misinformation, and stereotypes. Common misconceptions for "mind" include thinking that mind–body fitness includes a component of mind-altering techniques, influencing communication, or religious practices, when, in fact, it really refers to a strong mental component that involves keen concentration on, and co-ordination of, the other two points of the triangle. Many practitioners replace "mind" with "brain" to make the concept seem more related to traditional fitness because "brain" denotes a more tangible, anatomical reality that proves less threatening to some.

Common misconceptions for "spirit" include references to a particular cult, sect, or religious organization or affiliation. In mind–body fitness, however, "spirit" refers to the sharp focus on breathing in conjunction with the other components of the trilogy; the etymology of the word derives from the Greco-Latin word *spiritos,* meaning both "breath" and "energy." The breath, therefore, is a common thread woven among most of the mind–body disciplines discussed in this chapter. Where the word *spirit* may alienate some individuals from the real intent behind mind–body–spirit fitness, some professionals adopt the term *brain–body–breath* fitness to convey the emphasis of this discipline.

## STABILITY–MOBILITY CIRCLE

Practitioners of mind–body fitness recognize that each person needs to train to enhance cardiovascular fitness, strength, and flexibility on all or most days of the week.[5] A mind–body approach can be viewed as an essential component to each of these health-related parameters. Considering the conceptualization of *who* humans are, represented by the trilogy, and *what* humans need,

represented by the health-related parameters of fitness, mind–body fitness proposes a game plan for *how* humans achieve it in training. More specifically, the concepts of stability and mobility unite all mind–body disciplines, because these two concepts convey the framework under which all the disciplines operate.

Figure 19-3 demonstrates this attention to the fundamental principles of stability and mobility with the ancient Chinese yin-yang. Notice how the concepts are related to each in the formation of the circle: Each has a specific role within the framework of the other. In other words, part of the concept of "stability" lies within the concept of "mobility" and vice versa. Together, these individual concepts form a complete circle explaining movement, but the two concepts themselves are both independent and interdependent to each other.

As discussed in Chapter 13, **stability**, in the realm of programming, is generally defined as the ability to control the position or movement of a joint and involves **proprioception**, muscular balance, and isometric muscular strength, but can be also expanded within the mind–body concept to include nutritional balance. Conversely, **"mobility"** within the realm of programming is defined as the ability to move a joint through a functional range of motion and involves flexibility, muscular coordination and sensory–motor integration, movement patterns, and isotonic muscular strength. Collectively, these two properties summarize human movement.[6]

All mind–body disciplines, regardless of country of origin or age, share a commonality of addressing the brain–body–breath (mind–body–spirit) trilogy. This chapter addresses the important comparisons and contrasts (summarized in Table 19-1) among some of the most popular mind–body disciplines of yoga, T'ai chi, qigong, Pilates, and Feldenkrais, and how each discipline addresses the trilogies and stability–mobility circle.

### FROM THEORY TO PRACTICE

#### ■ MINDFUL REVERSE BREATHING

Read this paragraph once before beginning the exercise. Sit comfortably in a chair as you read, then, using a clock or watch, set aside this text and *inhale* through the mouth and *exhale* through the nose for 3 full minutes. Gently inhale through the mouth and then close the lips as you gently exhale through the nose. As you do so, notice how mindful you need to be to accomplish this unique breathing technique. When the 3 full minutes are up, return to the text.

Did you notice how mindful you needed to be to accomplish this task? The first objective was to make the body acutely aware of breathing, because this is not normally a conscious process. The second objective of this exercise is to introduce a new breathing technique. If "reverse breathing" seemed completely foreign to you, remember that there are times when this type of breathing would be appropriate (e.g., when performing high-intensity cardiovascular routines).

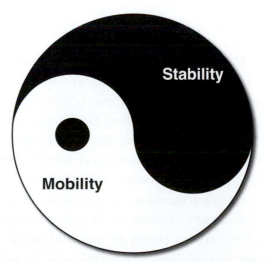

**Figure 19-3.** Relationship between stability and mobility illustrated by the concept of the Chinese yin and yang model.

## Table 19-1. Comparison of Common Mind–Body Disciplines

| DISCIPLINE | METHOD | BREATHING | SPEED | EQUIPMENT |
|---|---|---|---|---|
| Yoga | Primarily isometric | Nose | Slow moving with an emphasis on holding postures | Sticky mat, optional straps and blocks |
| Pilates | Isotonic | Nasal inhalation and mouth exhalation | Usually slow with exceptions | Mat class requires mat, optional rings and balls |
| Qigong | Isotonic | Nose and pursed lips | Variable; individual's choice | None |
| T'ai Chi | Isotonic | Nose and pursed lips | Super slow | None |
| Feldenkrais | Isotonic | Individual choice | Slow at individual's choice | None required |

| DISCIPLINE | FOCUS | ORIENTATION | FLEXIBILITY | EMPHASIS |
|---|---|---|---|---|
| Yoga | Holding a posture | Standing and floor | Static and active | Individual movement |
| Pilates | Isotonic arms and legs challenge isometric core | Mostly floor | Mostly active | Individual movement |
| Qigong | Waking energy through the body based on individual need | Standing | Active | Individual movement |
| T'ai Chi | Slow synchronization with others based on group choreography | Standing | Active | Group movement |
| Feldenkrais | Slow, repeated patterns to increase efficiency | Mostly floor | Mostly active | Individual movement |

## VIGNETTE continued

■ When Dennis and Tanya meet the following week, Dennis asks her if she enjoyed her first beginner's yoga class, and Tanya tells him that she loved it. While discussing Tanya's experience, Dennis finds that she particularly enjoyed the meditative and breathing-focused elements of the class, as well as the mental challenge involved in achieving and maintaining certain poses. To draw some of that experience into Tanya's resistance training sessions, Dennis decides to add some yogic breathing exercises into the warm-up and cool-down portions of their sessions together, and

to end each session with a few minutes of meditative visualization that will help Tanya cope with the stresses of her daily life. Dennis makes a note to ask Elijah about some poses that he may be able to incorporate into future workouts. Before Tanya leaves, Dennis obtains her written permission to discuss her routine with Elijah.

## YOGA

It is important for health and fitness professionals to know the difference between "yoga" and what much of the fitness industry refers to as yoga exercise or hatha yoga. According to Patañjali's philosophical analyses contained in the *Yoga Sutra*, yoga historically refers to the complex system of physical and spiritual disciplines that are fundamental to Buddhist, Jain, and Hindu religious practice throughout Asia. It is important to differentiate a "yogic lifestyle" from participation in hatha yoga classes, such as those offered in yoga studios and fitness centers in the United States (e.g., Iyengar yoga and power yoga classes). Individuals who live yogic lifestyles, although perhaps not in full compliance with the teachings of the *Yoga Sutra*, generally embark upon daily dietary, meditation, and spiritual centering and regular hatha yoga exercise, whereas the routine practice of hatha yoga poses may or may not include dietary or other lifestyle changes. This is an important point because some yoga research outcomes are based on following yogic lifestyle principles that clearly transcend the mere practice of yoga exercise.

Hatha yoga is the physical aspect of yogic disciplines and includes a vast repertoire of physical postures, or asanas, done seated, standing, or lying prone or supine on the floor, and, in some instances, inverted positions. Several basic movement patterns are involved in most asanas: backbends, twists, and forward bends.

The principal challenge of hatha yoga is to become proficient at handling increasingly greater amounts of "resistance" (i.e., complexity and the degree of difficulty) in the various postures and breathing patterns while maintaining a steady and comfortable equilibrium of mind and body. As a general rule, hatha yoga sessions start and end with a relaxation pose (a savasana, or corpse pose) and include a variety of asanas focusing on spinal, postural, and limb muscle groups so that the exerciser spends 30 seconds to 1 minute with each pose before transitioning to the next. In virtually all forms of hatha yoga, it is paramount that yogic breathing be executed in synchrony with each pose. As a general rule, yogic breathing is combined with yoga exercise in a very logical way. Whenever a yoga movement or pose expands the chest or abdomen, the participant inhales. Conversely, when a movement contracts or compresses the chest or abdomen, the participant exhales.

## General Precautions With Hatha Yoga Programs

Because many styles of hatha yoga involve acute dynamic changes in body position, it is important to understand the **hemodynamic** and cardiovascular responses to such exercise and how these may alter cardiac function in people diagnosed with cardiovascular disease, including hypertension or diabetes. Inverted poses in which the head is below the heart (e.g., downward facing dog, headstands) and sequences in which a head-down position is alternated with a head-up pose should be avoided, at least in the early stages of a yoga program. In most cases, those who are initially deconditioned or have a chronic disease should: (1) minimize acute rapid changes in body position (e.g., changes in the limbs and trunk in relation to the heart) in early stages of hatha yoga training, and/or (2) use slower transitions from one yoga pose to the next.

Some yoga asanas and sequences require considerable muscular strength and mental concentration. Therefore, they may be more appropriate for higher-functioning individuals (i.e., those with >11–12 metabolic equivalents **[MET]** exercise capacity). Some may cause significant and rapid changes in blood pressure and may be inappropriate for those with stage 2 or higher hypertension (i.e., those with blood pressures ≥160/100 mm Hg). DiCarlo and colleagues[7] demonstrated significantly greater **systolic blood pressure**

## RESEARCH HIGHLIGHT

### Yoga, Relaxation, and Stress Reduction

Researchers compared yoga with relaxation techniques as treatment approaches to reduce stress, anxiety, and blood pressure, and promote overall improvement in health. The study recruited 131 subjects with mild-to-moderate levels of stress who were randomly assigned to either group and participated in 10 weekly, 60-minute sessions of relaxation or hatha yoga. Following the 10-week intervention, yoga was found to be equally effective as relaxation techniques in reducing stress, anxiety, and improving health status, but was more effective than relaxation in improving mental health. At the end of a 6-week follow-up period, no differences were observed between the groups for stress, anxiety, and several health domains, although vitality, social function, and mental health scores became higher in the relaxation group during this period. Based on these findings, the researchers concluded that yoga appears to provide comparable improvements in stress, anxiety, and health status when compared with relaxation techniques.

Smith C, Hancock H, Blake-Mortimer J, Eckert K. A randomized comparative trial of yoga and relaxation to reduce stress and anxiety. *Complement Ther Med.* 2007;15:77–83.

and **diastolic blood pressure** in yoga practitioners practicing Iyengar-style yoga when compared with moderate treadmill walking (~4 miles/hr).

Because some yoga programs involve advanced breathing techniques (e.g., breath retentions and breath suspensions), caution must be used with those who have cardiovascular or pulmonary disease. Breath retentions are brief pauses (2 to 4 seconds) taken at the end of a controlled inspiration. Breath suspensions are similar pauses taken at the end of controlled expirations. Although very brief pauses appear to be relatively safe, individuals with cardiovascular disease, hypertension, obstructive pulmonary disease, or asthma should avoid retentions or suspensions of longer than 4 to 5 seconds and focus on the standard breathwork taught in most yoga programs.

## Equipment

Yoga does not require equipment; in fact, it requires little more than an open mind and heart. However, many practitioners find that a nonstick yoga mat assists with comfort for asana on the floor (Fig. 19-4). Many yoga mats are biodegradable, recyclable, and offer "sticky" surfacing to prevent accidental slips when perspiration hits the mat. In addition, a sticky mat will offer "mat memory," illustrating where bony landmarks (e.g., elbows, knees, and feet) have left imprints as participants flow through asanas more than once.

Other yoga props include straps, blocks, blankets, and bolsters. Straps allow for an extension of arms and legs where flexibility falls short. Blocks (originally made of hard wood and now usually made of more "giving" foamlike material) generally exist in three heights and serve to raise the floor or contact points toward the upper extremity when flexibility is limited. Blankets allow for bundling under different body parts to act as bolsters and support mechanisms, and cover the body for temperature management. Finally, bolsters provide more support to hips and legs in certain positions like sitting. Restorative yoga involves gentle yoga postures done on the floor with equipment to help facilitate the attainment of the poses. Instead of "doing asana," in restorative yoga,

props are used to "let the asana do you." Overall, equipment can enable participants to access asana that they otherwise may not be able to do.

## Applications

Hatha yoga is appropriate for anyone willing to focus on a well-being program to increase their overall quality of life. Many insurance companies offer health insurance premium discounts to individuals as an incentive to practice hatha yoga regularly.[8] Yoga has been associated with increases in muscular endurance and strength, flexibility, stamina, kinesthetic awareness, balance, and overall well-being.[9] Exercise professionals who wish to incorporate yoga practices should take yoga classes and seek out specialty certificates.

A common perception is that fitness involves active, isotonic movements, which is contrary to the principles of yoga, which address the concepts of stability, isometric work, breathing techniques, and an inward focus. Whereas some traditional Western practices traditionally begin with a large-to-small muscle group progression and an outward focus, the Eastern discipline of yoga brings into play an opposing view that commences with the smallest core muscles first (pelvic floor, called "mula bandha" or "root lock of the body") and works outward with a completely introspective and inward focus. In essence, yoga may offer the traditional exercise and fitness professional a new way to view training to enhance mindfulness by working from the center outward.

### FROM THEORY TO PRACTICE

#### ■ YOGA CHAIR POSE

The chair pose is also known as the power pose, squatting pose, and lightning bolt pose, or *utkasana* in Sanskrit (Fig. 19-5). While barefoot, stand comfortably and perform the breathing technique from the previous exercise. Relax your eyes and face, but stand tall with feet together and activate your pelvic floor and transverse abdominis. Adduct your femurs (i.e., bring the knees together) and imagine holding a piece of paper between the knees. Slowly squat down to a depth that is challenging, while keeping your knees behind your toes. If possible, raise your arms overhead with elbows extended, and bring your upper arms to align with your ears, framing the sides of the head with palms facing each other. If possible, raise the heels to balance on the forefeet. After attaining this position, concentrate on prolonging the inhalation and exhalation for five breath cycles, or about 30 seconds.

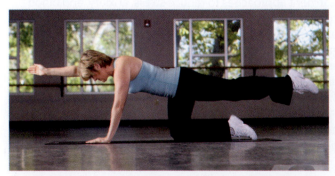

**Figure 19-4.** A basic yoga pose, called the bird-dog or sunbird, using minimal equipment such as a soft yoga mat.

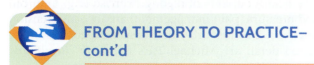

## FROM THEORY TO PRACTICE– cont'd

This pose strengthens the front, inner, and outer sides and the back of the legs and glutes, engages the core muscles, and stretches the latissimus dorsi muscles. If you choose to raise one or both heels, then you are also training the calves and proprioceptors of the feet and ankles.

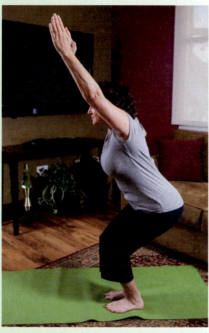

**Figure 19-5.** Another basic yoga pose, the chair pose, can be safely performed by older or deconditioned individuals.

## Common Misconceptions

Contrary to many popular beliefs, the practice of asana, pranayama, and dharana do not involve any particular religious beliefs or aspirations. No deities are associated with this type of physical yoga; anyone of any faith or lack thereof can practice yoga. Some yoga classes include chanting as a method of centering the body and mind, and of bringing healing to the world through vibration and sound therapy. Although no religious connotation is associated with chanting in most yoga classes throughout the world, any particular student who may be uncomfortable can sit quietly and refrain from vocalizing. Furthermore, in classes involving chanting in other languages, such as common Sanskrit chants, most instructors explain the meanings behind the chants before inviting everyone to participate.

## In Your Own Words

A colleague who has poor kinesthetic awareness asks you what possible benefits he could achieve from starting to practice yoga. He also asks you which "type" of yoga he should investigate first as a novice. How would you respond?

## VIGNETTE continued

■ Two weeks later, with Tanya still enjoying her yoga classes, Dennis decides to incorporate some additional mind–body elements into her resistance training sessions. Elijah recommended that Tanya perform certain exercises with a deeper internal awareness, meaning that she should prioritize her mental focus on the kinesthesis of each muscle contraction, as well as her breath. This will enable Tanya to think about the movements themselves, as opposed to thinking about the physical effort involved, which can sometimes act as a deterrent to optimal exercise performance. Dennis tells Tanya that she can use this same technique during her evening walks by focusing on the joy of movement as opposed to any difficulty getting motivated or the distance still left to complete her walking workout. Tanya agrees to try it the following evening.

## T'AI CHI AND QIGONG

Although yoga may be the oldest individual mind–body discipline in which *individuals* practice postures of stability and mobility with a strong, individual, inner focus, the oldest *group* mind–body discipline are **T'ai chi** and one of its building blocks, **qigong**. Both forms evolved from China, and whereas T'ai chi is a form of martial art practiced for both its defense training and health benefits, qigong is a practice of aligning breath, movement, and awareness for exercise, healing, and meditation.

### T'ai Chi

T'ai chi (shorthand for t'ai chi chuan or taijiquan) is only one form of the more ancient practice of qigong. T'ai chi chuan is a complex martial arts choreography of 108 flowing graceful movements that can be practiced for health, meditation, and self-defense. In t'ai chi, students are taught to allow the practice to evolve into a free-flow exercise such that the movements and breathing become one unified energy flow (Fig. 19-6). As with hatha yoga, it is important that the movements and breathing are coordinated so that the student may derive the energy-centric benefits (i.e., unobstructed flow of perceived positive energy).

There are numerous forms or styles of t'ai chi chuan, including the original Chen, and the relatively more recent Yang, Chang, and Wu styles. It is commonly accepted that all t'ai chi styles follow similar essential principles: deep synchronous breathing, profound mental concentration, and perceptive and intentional movement of chi. The Yang form is the most widely practiced form in the West today. Originated by Yang Lu-chan in the 1800s, the original Yang form consists of 108 movements (Yang Long Form); however, the Yang 24–Short Form is a popular modification practiced today. As with all styles of t'ai chi, Yang-style movements reflect the principle of opposites commonly called *yin* and *yang*, in which offensive and defensive movements unite to form a graceful flow of martial arts choreography and, more importantly, chi.

## Qigong Exercise

Qigong is a system of self-healing exercise and meditation that is executed at very low metabolic levels, usually between 2 and 4 METs. Exercises include standing, seated, and supine positions with the ultimate goal to improve the balance of the functions of the body. There are perhaps many thousands of qigong exercise styles all based on balance, relaxation, breathing, and good posture.

One simple qigong series is Taiji qigong, which consists of only 18 movements taken from the t'ai chi and qigong forms.[10] Figure 19-7 shows the four-movement Taiji qigong sequence called Pushing the Wave. Taiji qigong is ideal as a preparation for higher-intensity conditioning exercise or as a cooldown. Numerous published studies, mostly with small subject numbers, have demonstrated

many health benefits of qigong exercise (e.g., reduced blood pressure, pain management, anxiety, and tension reduction). Two resources that describe qigong exercise in good detail are Michael Tse's *Qigong for Health and Vitality* and Kenneth Cohen's *The Way of Qigong*.

## Breathing

The most popular qigong and t'ai chi breathing technique is "pursed lip breathing." This technique involves inhaling through the nose and exhaling through the mouth without any sound, and the lips are pursed (i.e., about to kiss or drink through a large straw). This breathing technique helps regulate strength and control the flow of body movements without going too fast. Breathing should be mindful and slow, and should flow freely with emphasis on when to inhale and exhale. Finally, the tongue is placed on the palate (just behind the top teeth) with slight pressure and remains there throughout the practice. This tongue position stimulates the neck flexor muscles to stabilize the head and contributes to proper upper-neck and head alignment posture, which also improves balance and concentration. Anchoring the tongue against the palate also joins the many meridians of energy in the body into one central place, called the "bye way."

## Equipment

Because qigong and t'ai chi emphasize functional, standing stability and mobility work, there is no required equipment. To be sure, participants with special needs can practice next to a wall, ballet barre, or chair for

### FROM THEORY TO PRACTICE

■ **T'AI CHI BREATHING**

Stand comfortably with the feet hip-width apart, called the "closed door stance." Rest your arms at your sides in a relaxed position and place the tongue behind the top row of teeth and then draw it back to your palate (until you cannot feel your teeth with your tongue). This is the contact point where the tip of the tongue should remain. The tongue actively touches the palate during the inhalation and exhalation phase, with sufficient and constant pressure that it can remain in this position for the entire practice of t'ai chi or qigong without fatiguing, whether it be 15, 30, 45, or 60 minutes. Inhale through your nose and, when exhaling, form pursed lips and exhale around your tongue. Continue breathing this way for 3 minutes while attempting to perceive any different sensations within your body (i.e., the energy, or chi, in comparison with what you felt before this breathing exercise).

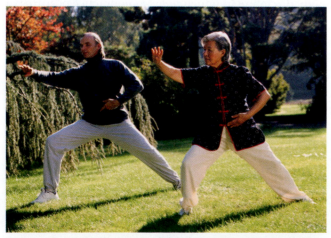

**Figure 19-6.** The practice of t'ai chi can be done individually or in a group setting. This activity has been shown to improve balance, posture, and flexibility in a wide range of individuals. *(Courtesy of Duncan Smith.)*

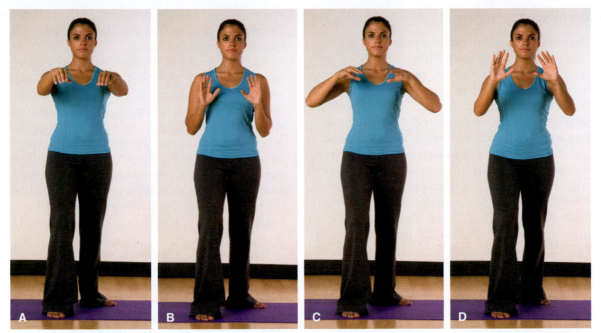

**Figure 19-7.** (A–D) Example of a qigong exercise series called Pushing the Wave. When done properly, qigong can influence the body's health by improving blood pressure and posture, and reducing stress and anxiety.

additional security, but, unlike yoga, equipment is not common in these Chinese disciplines.

## Applications

Participants do not need to practice hours of qigong and t'ai chi to reap the benefits. Just 5 minutes in the morning demonstrates increased synovial fluid and improved circulation to prepare the body for its required **activities of daily living (ADL)**.[11] Participants in other mind–body disciplines such as yoga have found that fusing qigong and t'ai chi into their warm-ups can increase their heart rate and joint range of motion before deepening their practice of asana.[12] Group exercise managers find that classes with these disciplines attract a large number of first-timers or novice exercisers, because they do not feature complicated choreography,

equipment, or muscle soreness. Health and fitness professionals implementing mindful techniques into their exercise training programs with clients often incorporate some of the limbering movements and active stretches as part of the warm-up and cooldown periods.

Qigong and t'ai chi are practiced differently from other mind–body forms of fitness. Whereas some practices, like yoga, make use of the floor and require closed eyes while working in a relatively confined space, these disciplines (qigong and t'ai chi) require awareness of the environment as an exerciser moves as one with those around him or her. During qigong, individuals practice exercises as a group while accounting for individual differences, whereas in t'ai chi, movements are synchronized. This stems from the Asian tradition of recognizing the importance of the group over the individual, where conformity is a key principle.

## FROM THEORY TO PRACTICE

### ■ FLYING ROOSTER

Stand in the "closed door" position described previously with your arms at your sides and slightly behind you; abduct your shoulders until the humerus bones are parallel to the floor, but with your wrists below shoulder level and palms facing down. Maintain a relaxed sensation in the wrists and elbows without hyperextending these joints. Return the arms to the sides and repeat, slowly. Notice how this rhythmic movement generates a stretch for the pectoralis major and some intercostal muscles between the ribs. Also, notice how your supraspinatus and medial deltoids begin to tire as you continue to perform repetitions. Shift into a single-leg stance as your arms float upward, raising the elevated leg by flexing at the hip until the knee aligns with the belly button (a key body landmark in qigong). When the arms float downward, return the lifted foot to its starting position and repeat on the other side. This adds an element of balance and strength for the lower body, making the "flying rooster" an ideal exercise for fusing bilateral upper-body mobility with unilateral lower-body stability.

## Common Misconceptions

The most common misconceptions regarding qigong and t'ai chi are that these disciplines are appropriate only for seniors. The slow speeds, easier movements, and ability to perform arm movements while seated all appeal to older adults with health issues. However, both qigong and t'ai chi are appropriate for other populations as well. Children and teens cultivate discipline while learning movements performed at slower speeds. Athletes may learn to harness their ability to recruit muscular efficiency at their regular movement speeds when incorporating super-slow eccentric training into their workouts. In addition, qigong and t'ai chi also are appropriate for conditioned individuals who seek a less intense workout on a recovery day from the gym. Individuals with vertigo, Parkinson's disease, fibromyalgia, and muscular dystrophy have all demonstrated benefits from practicing qigong and t'ai chi.[11]

## In Your Own Words

Explain to another student how incorporating the super-slow speed of T'ai chi with individuals during muscular contractions can serve as an effective training variable. Also, describe how standing, slow muscular work can be valuable for different populations as a component of fitness.

## VIGNETTE continued

■ During the warm-up phase of a workout a few weeks later, Dennis notices how excited Tanya is to talk about how much she is enjoying the new mindful approach she has taken not only in her workouts, but also in the rest of her life. She has been enjoying the yoga sessions with Elijah and has seen some real improvements in her performance. In addition, she has been pleased with the new meditative approach she has been using during her walks. Impressed by Tanya's rediscovered enthusiasm for exercise, Dennis tells her how wonderful it is that she is now seeing exercise as its own reward, instead of dwelling on losing baby weight or regaining a certain level of fitness.

## PILATES

Joseph Pilates was born in 1883 in Mönchengladbach, Germany, and immigrated to the United States in 1926. Since his youth, Pilates had endured poor health and took it upon himself to develop exercises to stay strong even when confined to home and, later, to a hospital-like bed when incarcerated during World War I. Some of his exercise inventions have come to be known as

Pilates today. The term *Pilates*, therefore, describes a German discipline that was both practiced and perfected in the United States.

Pilates referred to his own work as "Contrology" to signify the use of the mind to control the muscles in a variety of positions, mostly on, but not limited to, the floor. He invoked twisting, stretching, pushing, pulling, and rolling movements, both on mats and when using other various forms of equipment, all drawn from his experiences in other disciplines. His familiarity with yoga, rehabilitation, and dance therapy helped him examine isometric, stabilizing postures of the body, while his military callisthenic training helped him add isotonic (dynamic), mobilizing sequences to traditional fitness postures.

Because its founder emphasized mindful movement that commenced with the mind first, the Western world viewed Pilates as one of the original true mind–body disciplines originating in the Western world. Most of his clients were performers, dancers, and female socialites of New York City, including high-profile individuals who popularized his practice, like George Balanchine and Martha Graham.[13] He trained these individuals based on what they needed, never taking the one-size-fits-all approach that t'ai chi features, although he taught key exercises he believed most people should use.[14] Similar to yoga's eightfold path and the eight historical moves of qigong, Pilates developed eight principles to enhance mind–body movement:

1. Concentration
2. Control
3. Interdependence/dynamic stabilization
4. Alignment/centering
5. Endurance/stamina
6. Balance
7. Breath
8. Purpose

## Training Methods

Pilates began training the body using postures and positions similar to yoga, but added movement emphasizing the mobility, stamina, and endurance for performing ADL. In most of his exercises, he emphasized keeping the core isometrically braced while isotonically mobilizing the distal body parts. In most supine Pilates exercises, for example, the spine maintains a flexed position, called a "C curve," while the arms and legs move isotonically away from the core and then back to it.

## Breathing

Pilates emphasized a breathing technique called "complete forced exhalation."[13] He created movements that actually work better when accompanied by his breathing techniques. There are different interpretations of the Pilates breathing technique in today's evolutions of the discipline. The exercise shown in Figure 19-8 illustrates one of the interpretations of his breathing technique.

## FROM THEORY TO PRACTICE

### ■ THREE-PART DEEP DIAPHRAGMATIC BREATHING: "COMPLETE EXHALATION" BREATHING

Lay supine on a comfortable surface with your legs fully extended and heels hip-width apart. Place your right hand, fingers spread open, over your chest so that the thumb points toward your throat and your smallest finger is touching your belly button. Place your left hand just below this area with fingers spread open, placing your left thumb on your navel, touching the smallest finger of the right hand. Inhale through the nose and exhale through the mouth as it opens naturally, without trying to make any particular sound, but try to hear your exhalation. For some, emphasizing a sound like a prolonged *shhhh, ahhhh,* or *chhhh* on the exhalation helps coordinate breathing with concentration. Without forcing the breath into any unnatural movement, inhale and exhale more slowly. Notice the movements and feelings under the right and left hands. Now, as you inhale, try to connect with the diaphragm by feeling the left hand raise. Toward the second half of your inhalation, notice how the breathing moves upward toward the thorax as the lungs expand, and raise the right hand. Reverse this process as you exhale through the mouth. As you start to exhale, notice how the right hand over the lungs starts to lower first as the lungs begin to empty, followed by the left hand returning to its original, lowered position. Laying supine enhances this breathing technique because it facilitates the diaphragmatic movement that flexed hips (i.e., sitting) can inhibit.[15]

## Equipment

Other than a mat to make being on the floor comfortable, no other equipment is required for most of the original exercises of Pilates. Joseph Pilates, however, did infuse his creativity into the training of his clients by developing several pieces of equipment, some of which are still used to this day. Some of this equipment is used during mat exercises including rings, small balls, and towels.

Other, more complex pieces of equipment that Pilates developed evolved into what is now called a *reformer* (Fig. 19-9). These larger pieces of equipment are commonly used for personal and small-group Pilates training today. Some instructors fuse concepts and exercises of Pilates with newer equipment that was not available in the previous century. For example, some instructors teach Pilates-based exercises with evolved rings called "magic circles," foam rollers, small inflated balls, small weighted balls, the BOSU Balance Trainer, elastic tubing and bands, stability balls, and other apparatuses.

## Applications

The applications of Pilates to the fitness industry today are vast. Some instructors choose to follow exercises and methodology much in the same way Joseph Pilates did.[13] Alternatively, recent trends have updated Pilates's methodology from the 1950s with a more sophisticated understanding of human biomechanics, special populations, and spinal deviations. For example, whereas Pilates emphasized flattening or "imprinting" the lumbar area of the spine into the mat when in a supine position, practitioners now emphasize a more neutral spinal posture whenever possible. Regardless of whether instructors choose a classical or evolved approach, they still hold firm attention to the principles of Pilates. Many

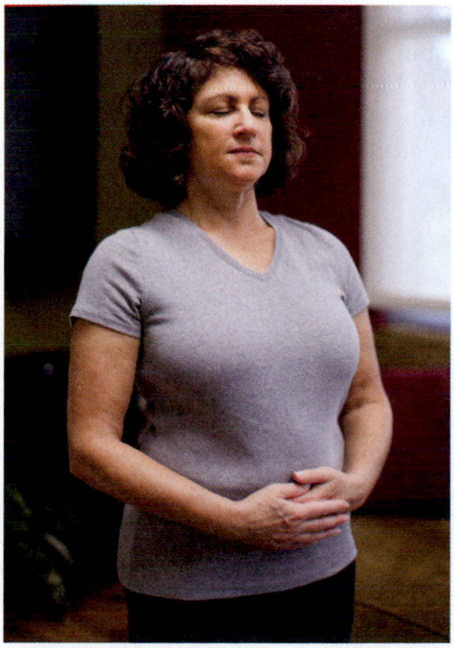

**Figure 19-8.** Example of posture and hand placement when engaging in deep diaphragmatic breathing exercises.

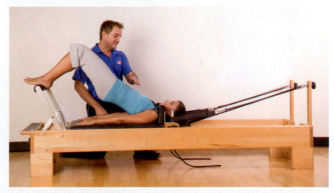

**Figure 19-9.** The reformer is a piece of equipment used during modern Pilates training.

health and fitness professionals incorporate some Pilates exercises (especially mat-based exercises) into training regimens with their clients. Unlike the discipline of yoga that sometimes proves challenging to incorporate into one-on-one training, the discipline of Pilates easily adds exercises into the health and fitness professional's toolbox.

## Common Misconceptions

Common misconceptions about Pilates include misunderstanding its place in the mind–body genre. Pilates does require a crucial mind–body connection to execute the principles of *concentration, control,* and *centering.* The strong emphasis on technique and timing of breathing also enhances the mind–body connection. Unlike yoga, however, which typically ends with a supine meditation that emphasizes stillness, or qigong and t'ai chi, which also can include moments of stillness at the end of classes, Pilates classes traditionally do not involve movement until the very end of class. Pilates can be used to complement other systems for training core strength, muscular endurance, and flexibility. Whereas most practitioners believe that the purpose of Pilates is to develop an increased sense of flexibility, the constant isotonic, dynamic nature of Pilates can improve muscular strength and endurance for some individuals.[14]

Finally, some critics of Pilates say that method does not feature enough prone and rotational work. While the majority of Pilates work does occur in the supine position and sagittal plane, Joseph Pilates did create exercises in the prone position (such as "swimming" and "starfish"), as well as transverse-plane movement (rotation) in a variety of body positions.

## In Your Own Words

Explain to a fellow student why core stability is important before adding distal mobility. Be sure to describe how "bracing" the transverse abdominis both protects from injury and prepares the body for further movement.

---

## FROM THEORY TO PRACTICE

### ■ NEUTRAL "DEAD BUG" CORE BRACING

Lay supine on a comfortable, padded surface. Flex your shoulders and hips, moving both your arms and femurs perpendicular to the floor with your fingers pointing toward the sky. Flex your knees to 90 degrees, positioning your tibia and fibula parallel to the floor (Fig. 19-10). Make a conscious connection to the pelvic floor muscles and try to tighten this area (i.e., perform a Kegel squeeze). Next, contract your rectus abdominis muscle (this will also engage transversus abdominis) without drawing your belly button in toward your spine (called "abdominal bracing"; Fig. 19-10). Abdominal bracing promotes enhanced spinal stability. Perform this bracing maneuver without any movement of rib cage or hips and keeping the lumbar spine in a neutral (curved) position. Try to keep the proximal core stable while adding the challenge of distal mobility. While keeping your arms shoulder-distance apart, slowly move one arm overhead toward the floor until the thumb touches the floor, and return to the starting point. Repeat with the other arm before progressing to moving both arms simultaneously. The goal is to maintain proximal spinal stability (i.e., no movement of your lumbar spine) while challenging the core with distal mobility. When you are comfortable with the movement, try incorporating Pilates breathing, which involves maintaining this "bracing" position, inhaling to prepare for movement, and exhaling slowly through the lips as you lower and return the arm to the starting point.

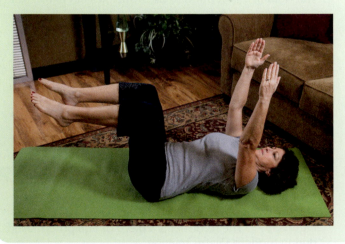

**Figure 19-10.** The "dead bug" is a basic floor-based Pilates exercise that emphasizes neutral lumbar spine position while challenging the core musculature through movements of the legs and arms.

## FELDENKRAIS

Moshé Feldenkrais (1904–1984) was born in the Ukraine. As a gifted athlete in his youth, he suffered a debilitating knee injury. Like Joseph Pilates, he guided himself to recovery through rehabilitation derived from his own research, both in Israel, where he lived until the age of 13, and then in Paris. In France, he diligently studied mental and physical disciplines, and was the first Western man to receive a black belt in Judo.

Drawing from his own method of self-discovery and from an intense observation of the movement of babies, he dedicated himself to helping others become aware of their movement patterns and to reprogramming their bodies to become more functional and efficient. He emphasized the power of the body and the influence of the mind, and constantly questioned his students in his Awareness Through Movement (ATM) sessions. "I'm not interested in flexible bodies," he was famous for saying, "because, first, I am interested in flexible minds."

### Training Methods

Unlike some of the aforementioned mind–body disciplines, the Feldenkrais technique does not contain specific exercises always done in a sequential order. Dr. Feldenkrais looked at individuals and devised movements to enhance their awareness based on his observations. Although an oversimplification of his technique, Feldenkrais classes generally place students in a variety of positions, then implements super-slow movements using one or two body parts like the eyes, lower body, upper body, head, fingers, and feet. Feldenkrais encouraged originating all movements in the imagination and mind first, then followed with body movements, performed repeatedly to induce a sense of awareness about total-body integration. No ATM exercise particularly addresses strength or flexibility, but instead the quality of overall movement.

### Breathing

Feldenkrais would devote entire lessons to the importance of breathing and the awareness of its place of origin in the body and its ability to assist or resist our movements. In some lessons, teachers address the breath to show the difference in how movements feel when breathing in assistive and resistive ways. For instance, a lesson can involve supine spinal flexion, and practicing inhalation and exhalation on the exertion to

---

## FROM THEORY TO PRACTICE

### ■ FELDENKRAIS EXPLORATORY BREATHING

The purpose of this lesson is to explore different breathing techniques for self-discovery. Lay supine with your legs extended and place your hands at your sides, palms facing down. Gently perform an abdominal curl, flexing your spine to move your rib cage toward your hips (Fig. 19-11). Inhale through your nose on the way up and exhale through the nose on the way down. Notice how this feels? Change your breathing to inhale through the nose on the way up and exhale through the mouth on the way down. Change your breathing once again to inhale through the mouth on the way up and down, exhaling between repetitions. Repeat all three breathing techniques, but perform your exhalations on the way up and your inhalation on the way down. After completing all six techniques, pause and notice which breathing technique most facilitated breathing for you. The goal is not to judge or to compare, but to be aware and decide for yourself which breathing technique best facilities your movements. The point of breathing in Feldenkrais is not only to explore breathing, but to discover for yourself which particular breathing technique works best.

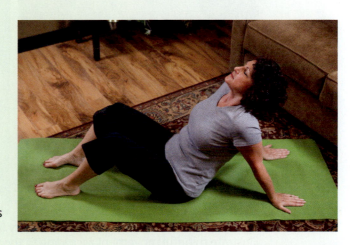

Figure 19-11. Proper positioning during a Feldenkrais exploratory breathing exercise.

enable participants to make their own decisions about what breathing format best facilitates movement. Feldenkrais did not mention specific techniques for breathing, such as through the nose or mouth.

## Equipment

Feldenkrais did not depend on particular pieces of equipment. While he would place foam pads under participants lying supine, he was adamant that awareness of movement could occur without any props. Popular equipment pieces used by instructors today include towels, pillows, hard and soft foam rollers of various sizes, and pads similar to those used for kneeling by gardeners.

## Applications

As demonstrated in the previous exercise, Feldenkrais lessons aim to teach choices, not standards. There are no correct or incorrect choices made by students, but a Feldenkrais instructor's goal is to teach anyone, from athletes to the sedentary, how to become more efficient at movement through their own increased awareness.

Individuals who aim to extrapolate Feldenkrais principles can begin by creating movement with a super-slow

## FROM THEORY TO PRACTICE

### ■ NECK TURNS

Sit comfortably upright in a chair and breathe normally. Keeping your chin level and cervical vertebrae in a neutral extended position, slowly turn your head to the left (Fig. 19-12A). Find your point of tightness. Maintain this position for a few breaths, noticing what it feels like to be at your point of tightness, then slowly return to your starting position. Now, imagine turning your head to the right. Imagine feeling the same point of tightness, but being able to turn the head even farther to the right while maintaining an even breathing pattern. After visualizing turning to the right side, slowly close your eyes and begin turning the head to the right side (Fig. 19-12B). When you find your point of tightness, maintain that position with even breathing. Slowly open your eyes and see if you have gone past your range of motion on this right side compared with the original left side.

Return to your starting position. To re-pattern movement, slowly repeat this pattern of closed-eye, conscious movement five times to the left side. When finished, repeat to the right side five times. Constantly ask yourself throughout the cervical rotations what you are feeling in terms of breathing, tightness, and overall body compensation. Do you feel that at the end of the exercise there is less restriction in your movement on one or both sides? Do you notice that adding an inhalation or an exhalation furthers your range of motion? Do you notice that parts of your body compensate for neck tightness such as observing a muscle tightening in shoulders, abdominals, or even knees, hips, and ankles?

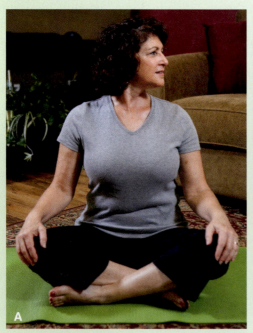
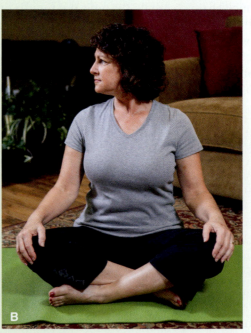

**Figure 19-12.** Example of a neck turn activity (A) to the left and (B) to the right to illustrate mindful movement according to the Feldenkrais technique.

approach, with eyes closed to induce a deeper sense of mindfulness, and by imagining how the body recruits muscles before actually initiating the movement. Whereas today's fitness professionals subscribe to the learning approach of "tell, show, do," the Feldenkrais practitioner advocates a "tell, show, imagine, explore, and repeat" approach to encourage self-discovery through quality repetitions to re-pattern the neuromuscular pathways of less efficient movement.

## Common Misconceptions

Because Feldenkrais exercises are lesser known worldwide than the other disciplines outlined in this chapter, few misconceptions exist other than the common thought that Feldenkrais is highly esoteric, difficult to find, and expensive. Feldenkrais group and individual lessons are not as common or popular as yoga and Pilates, but they are becoming increasingly available. Others believe that Feldenkrais is the mind–body practice performed when one cannot do anything else, but the opposite is true. A true Feldenkrais lesson enhances one's movement at any level, from novice to elite athlete, by educating the participant how to refine movement through the use of eyes, visualization, and breathing exploration.

## OTHER MIND–BODY DISCIPLINES

Over the past century, various other mind–body practices have been introduced, either as derivatives of existing classical practices (e.g., yoga, qigong, t'ai chi) or as more contemporary practices derived from emerging science and applications (e.g., neuromuscular integrative approach [NIA] or Alexander technique).

To deepen an understanding of yoga, for example, prospective students should use the Internet to find local facilities that offer different styles of hatha yoga. Once they find both an instructor and a format that feels comfortable, challenging, and enjoyable, students should try to attend practice a minimum of three times per week and monitor their feelings after a period of 2 weeks.

If you are interested in learning more about these disciplines or expanding your knowledge of the more traditional practices, visit any of the websites presented later in the Additional Resources section.

## VIGNETTE conclusion

■ Dennis decides to review some of the benefits of mind–body exercise with Tanya so that she can see how much value her new program truly has. He tells her that in addition to the more obvious benefits that she has been able to see in her own life–reduced stress, decreased fatigue, and improved psychological well-being–yoga has many other research-supported benefits. These include decreased blood pressure, improved cardiovascular disease risk profile, improved posture, and increased balance control. He tells her that these and other benefits only become more pronounced and valuable as people age.

Like many exercisers, Tanya is not so inspired by the listing of benefits. Recognizing this, Dennis reminds her of her renewed interest in exercising and the resultant improvement in program adherence. Tanya agrees that she looks forward to all of her workouts, not just the yoga sessions, more than she did in the past. That, Dennis tells her, is one of the greatest benefits that mind–body exercise has provided in her life.

## CRITICAL THINKING QUESTIONS

1. An individual asks what the purpose of moving so slowly is in yoga. She says she is "type A" and has to move quickly and aggressively to get the intensity she needs to achieve her fitness goals. "All of that slow moving seems boring to me," she claims, "so what's the point?" How do you respond as a fitness consultant?

2. How could a personal trainer incorporate the Eastern, yogic philosophy of training from the inside out into the regimen of a fitness client without totally changing the client's approach?

3. How can a basic qigong and T'ai chi movement that involves slowly transferring one's weight from one leg to the other be a functional exercise that complements ADL? (*Hint:* Think of getting in and out of a car or shower and stepping over curbs in the street).

4. How could a fitness enthusiast incorporate T'ai chi breathing at certain times during a workout to induce mindfulness and balance?

5. How can the concept of proximal stability and distal mobility apply to anyone's fitness regimen? Think of common ADL and how exercises to enhance them could train both stability and mobility simultaneously. Consider picking up objects, bending over, sitting and twisting as in a car, and gardening.

6. What would be the value in asking exercisers to verbalize their own thoughts regarding breathing as they perform movements? Could this experimentation further one's kinesthetic awareness of the body?

## ADDITIONAL RESOURCES

Finding qigong and t'ai chi classes in local areas is becoming less difficult as more options surface, especially in larger cities. As with all mind–body classes, searching an online search engine for "qigong" and a local zip code or city name usually reveals enough local options to serve as a starting point to find classes. Two principal website sources for more information are http://qi.org and http://drtaichi.com.

The Pilates Method Alliance (http://pilatesmethodalliance .org) is an organization dedicated to standards and testing of Pilates instructors.

The Feldenkrais Institute (http://feldenkraisinstitute.com) offers in-depth information on the Feldenkrais method.
For further information on the Alexander technique, visit http://alexandertechnique.com.
Balanced Body: http://pilates.com
Mad Dogg Athletics (Peak Pilates): http://spinning.com
NIA: http://nianow.com
Stott Pilates: http://stottpilates.com
Yoga Alliance: https://www.yogaalliance.org/
YogaFit: http://yogafit.com

## REFERENCES

1. Sporting Goods Manufacturers Association. *2012 Tracking the Fitness Movement: The Annual Review of Fitness Participation in America*. Juniper, FL: SGMA Research/Sports Marketing Surveys USA; 2013.
2. Austin JA, Shapiro SL, Eisenberg DM, Forys KL. Mind–body medicine: State of the science, implications for practice. *J Am Board Fam Pract*. 2003;16:131–147.
3. Goleman D, Gurin J. What is mind/body medicine? In Goleman D, Gurin J, eds. *Mind/Body Medicine: How to Use Your Mind for Better Health*. Yonkers, NY: Consumer Reports Books; 1993:3–18.
4. Benson H, Klipper MZ. *The Relaxation Response* (updated and expanded edition). New York, NY: HarperTorch; 2000.
5. American College of Sports Medicine. *ACSM's Guidelines for Exercise Testing and Prescription*. 9th ed. Philadelphia, PA: Lippincott Williams & Wilkins; 2014.
6. Houglum PA. *Therapeutic Exercise for Musculoskeletal Injuries*. 2nd ed. Champaign, IL: Human Kinetics; 2005.
7. Basmajian J, DeLuca, C. *Muscles Alive—Their Functions Revealed By Electromyography*. 4th ed. Baltimore, MD: Williams and Wilkins; 1979.
8. Ornish D, Scherwitz LW, Billings JH, et al. Intensive lifestyle changes for the reversal of coronary heart disease. *JAMA*. 1998;280:2001–2007.
9. Hagins M, Moore W, Ruddle A. Does practicing hatha yoga satisfy recommendations for intensity of physical activity which improves and maintains health and cardiovascular fitness? *BMC Complement Altern Med*. 2007;7:40–49.
10. Tse YK, Guo X, Quin I, Lam TP, Ng BK, Cheng JC. Association of osteopenia with curve severity in adolescent idiopathic scoliosis: A study of 919 girls. *Osteopor Intern* 2005;16(12):1924–1932. The Upledger Institute Inc., Eastland Press.
11. Xin L, Miller YD, Burton NW, Brown WJ. A preliminary study of the effects of Tai chi and Qigong medical exercise on indicators of the metabolic syndrome, glycaemic control, health related quality of life, and psychological health in adults with elevated blood glucose. *Br J Sports Med*. 2010;44(10):704–709.
12. Kabat-Zinn J. Mindfulness meditation: Health benefits of an ancient Buddhist practice. In Goleman D, Gurin J, eds. *Mind/Body Medicine: How to Use Your Mind for Better Health*. Yonkers, NY: Consumer Reports Books; 1993:259–275.
13. Breibart J. *The Body Biz: The Pilates Story*. New York, NY: PMI Publishers; 2006.
14. Curnow D, Cobbin D, Wyndham J, Boris Choy ST. Altered motor control, posture and the Pilates method of exercise prescription. *J Bodyw Mov Ther*. 2009;13:104–111.
15. Farhi D. *The Breathing Book*. New York, NY: Henry Holt and Company; 1996.

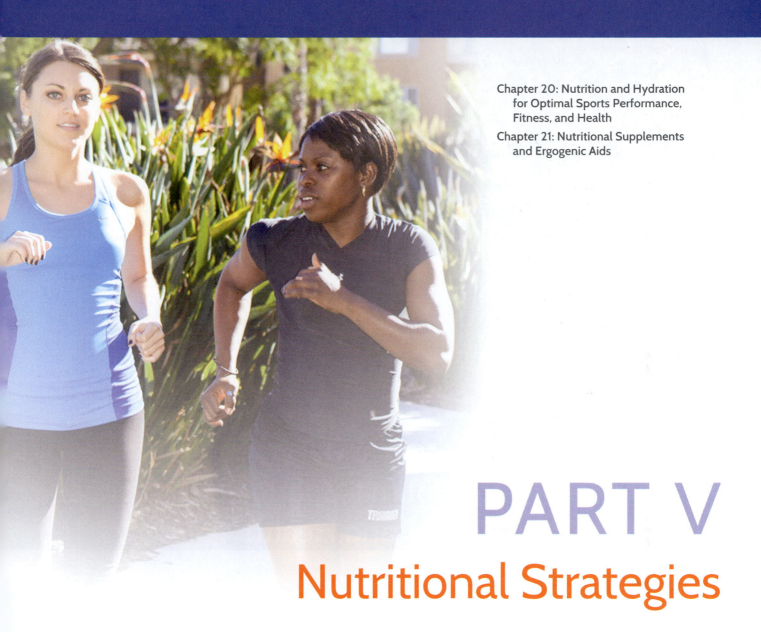

# PART V
# Nutritional Strategies

This part of the book provides the latest information relative to nutrition, hydration, and ergogenic aids for exercise and sports. Chapter 20 focuses on nutritional and hydration strategies that can be followed before, during, and after exercise to optimize exercise performance. Chapter 21 provides a solid overview of the regulation of nutritional supplements. In addition, the rationale and efficacy of the most common nutritional supplements and ergogenic aids on the market are described.

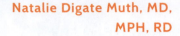

Natalie Digate Muth, MD,
MPH, RD

CHAPTER 20

# Nutrition and Hydration for Optimal Sports Performance, Fitness, and Health

## CHAPTER OUTLINE

## CHAPTER OUTLINE–cont'd

## LEARNING OUTCOMES

1. List the major goals of pre-exercise, during-exercise, and post-exercise nutritional strategies.

2. Describe several strategies to optimize pre-exercise, during-exercise, and post-exercise nutrition.

3. List ways in which hydration status affects athletic performance.

4. Apply the current, research-based hydration recommendations for before, during, and after exercise.

5. Calculate sweat rate using the protocol provided by the USA Track & Field Association.

6. Explain how to identify and respond to a client with an eating disorder.

7. Explain how gluten sensitivity and a vegetarian diet can affect athletic performance.

8. List three ways in which sports nutrition for children is different than for adults.

## ANCILLARY LINK

Visit Davis*Plus* at http://davisplus.fadavis.com for study and practice resources, including online quizzes, animations that help explain physiological processes, podcasts concerning news and career trends in exercise physiology, and practice references.

## VIGNETTE

■ Layla is a 23-year-old recreational athlete who stands 5'9'' (1.75 m) and weighs 135 pounds (61.4 kg). She is intensifying her training in hopes of qualifying for the Boston Marathon. Layla has finished three marathons, but despite her best efforts, she has yet to run the 26.2 miles in the qualifying time of 3 hours 40 minutes (her personal record is 4 hours). During her prior training, she focused exclusively on physical training and made no changes to her diet or eating habits. She is convinced that if she optimizes her nutrition, she will easily be able to shave the needed 20 minutes off of her run time, so she enlists the help of Enrique, a Certified Specialist in Sports Dietetics.

How might the application of basic sports nutrition principles help Layla run faster and give her the energy she needs to train for peak performance?

Today, it's not just elite athletes who triumphantly finish 26.2-mile runs and other physically strenuous ventures. Recreational athletes from teenagers to the elderly repeatedly accomplish these feats. Some strive for peak performance, whereas others participate for the sense of satisfaction and accomplishment of finishing. In any case, with the right preparations, including a sound training regimen and a little bit of sports nutrition know-how, the body can be trained to perform at high levels under stressful conditions with minimal discomfort and risk for injury. Regardless of whether clients are preparing for a 10K run, a century bike ride, an Ironman triathlon, or something in between, what they eat and drink before, during, and after exercise plays an important role in determining exercise comfort and athletic performance.

This chapter introduces key fundamentals of sports nutrition, discusses nutritional needs for active individuals and how energy intake and hydration affect athletic performance, explains how to effectively implement appropriate pre-exercise and post-exercise refueling strategies, and prepares you to recognize eating disorders and other nutrition issues relevant to active individuals today.

## FUNDAMENTALS OF SPORTS NUTRITION

Some of the most common questions active individuals ask relate to sports nutrition. These questions can range from an avid early-morning indoor cycling class attendee who wants to know what to eat, if anything, before heading to the gym, to a distance runner who is prone to stomach cramping during long, strenuous runs who wants some recommendations for less cramp-provoking snacks, to a triathlete who struggles to excel during his evening swims on days when he did morning cycling rides who asks for help with his post-ride recovery snack. For each of these athletes, the answers include consuming the right foods and drinks in the right combinations and quantities to meet nutritional needs.

This starts with determining caloric needs (see Chapter 24), followed by ensuring an appropriate breakdown of carbohydrates, protein, fat, micronutrients, and fluids. From there, athletes need to consider the best timing of their food and fluid intake.

### Macronutrient, Micronutrient, and Fluid Needs

The Institute of Medicine's (IOM's) **Dietary Reference Intakes (DRI)** recommend that approximately 45% to 65% of calories come from carbohydrates, 10% to 35% from protein, and 20% to 35% from fats.[1] Although active individuals require ample carbohydrates to maintain blood glucose during exercise and to replace muscle glycogen expended during exercise, as well as increased protein for muscle repair, research

suggests that active individuals do not need a greater *percentage* of calories from carbohydrate or protein than the average population.[1] Therefore, active individuals are able to meet increased demands through a greater overall caloric intake.

The Academy of Nutrition and Dietetics (formerly known as the American Dietetic Association) and the American College of Sports Medicine (ACSM) suggest that active individuals consume between 6 and 10 g carbohydrate per kilogram of body weight per day (2.7–4.5 g/lb) depending on their total daily energy expenditure, type of exercise done, sex, and environmental conditions.[2] Generally, inactive adults require 3 to 5 g carbohydrate per kilogram of body weight per day (1.4–2.3 g/lb), whereas moderately active individuals require 5 to 7 g carbohydrate per kilogram body weight each day (2.3–3.2 g/lb). Very active individuals and athletes may require in excess of 10 g carbohydrate per kilogram body weight (>4.5 g/lb), depending on the volume and intensity of work performed.[2]

As discussed in Chapter 3, an important role of proteins is in the growth, maintenance, and synthesis of muscle tissue. The Recommended Daily Allowance (RDA) for the general population is 0.8 g protein per kilogram of body weight (g/kg), or 0.36 g/lb, although the average adult in the United States consumes well in excess of that recommendation. The average American man consumes 1.15 g protein per kilogram of body weight (approximately 44% higher than the RDA), whereas the average woman consumes approximately 0.95 g protein per kilogram of body weight (up to 20% higher than the RDA).[3] Both Academy of Nutrition and Dietetics and ACSM suggest that athletes have higher protein needs than the general population. They advise endurance athletes to consume 1.2 to 1.4 g protein per kilogram of body weight and resistance trained athletes to consume up to 1.8 g protein per kilogram body weight (0.55–0.82 g/lb).[2] These recommendations can usually be met through diet alone, without the need for protein supplementation.[2]

Athletes generally do not have increased fat needs compared with their inactive counterparts, but they may need to monitor fat intake to ensure adequate intake of essential fats.

Active individuals who eat a well-balanced diet are not at increased risk for micronutrient deficiencies compared with their sedentary counterparts. However, athletes who restrict caloric intake, eliminate one or more food groups from their diets, or consume diets low in micronutrients are at risk for micronutrient deficiencies. Overall, to avoid deficiency, athletes should consume at least the RDA for each of the micronutrients. DRI tables that include RDAs for each of the micronutrients are available at the Food and Nutrition Center web page of the U.S. Department of Agriculture (USDA): http://fnic.nal.usda.gov. Typically, no vitamin and mineral supplements are necessary beyond those recommended for the average population and for reasons unrelated to exercise, such as folic acid in women of childbearing age.

How to determine an individual's fluid needs is discussed later in this chapter.

## VIGNETTE *continued*

■ Layla entered her age, sex, height (5'9"), weight (135 pounds), and physical activity level (greater than 60 min/day) into the ChooseMyPlate (http://choosemyplate.gov) food tracker (Supertracker), which calculated her total daily energy expenditure at approximately 2,400 calories/day. She asks Enrique to help her optimize her nutritional intake while staying at or below this threshold.

## Nutrient Timing

Specific timing of nutrient and fluid intake, composition of both nutrients and fluids, and the quantities ingested greatly impact athletic performance. Nutrient timing is a deliberate approach to consuming foods and beverages in relation to the planned exercise that will help the individual achieve the following benefits[4]:

- Increase levels of available fuel to provide energy for the training session.
- Establish total body water and fluid balance to optimize thermoregulatory mechanisms.
- Optimize recovery and the process of repair, replenishment, and muscle synthesis to prepare the body again for subsequent events.
- Enhance immune function, especially after strenuous activity that compromises overall immune function.
- Reduce potential for injury considering how poor nutritional and hydration levels negatively impact mental concentration, physical skills, and fatigue.

## ENERGY INTAKE AND ATHLETIC PERFORMANCE

An optimal eating plan combined with well-planned physical training and rest sets the stage for peak athletic performance. An ideal eating plan contains the right mix of foods and drinks to ensure adequate carbohydrates, protein, fat, and micronutrients to support the specific exercise demands on the body.

The body uses the macronutrients to meet its energy needs, using a greater percentage of fats at lower intensities and carbohydrates at higher intensities. If needed, the body can also use proteins to supply needed energy; this is discussed in detail in Chapter 4. Proteins generally contribute 2% to 5% of the body's

total daily energy needs in the average adult, but this amount can easily increase to approximately 10% in athletes.

## Carbohydrates

Carbohydrates play a critical role in athletic performance and exercise. They serve as a primary and preferred fuel for muscle activity, and for optimal brain and central nervous system function. Carbohydrates also are a source of quick energy given their rapid transit time through the gastrointestinal (GI) tract and rapid utilization rates within the body. It typically takes carbohydrates less than 4 hours to be digested, absorbed, and broken down to supply energy to fuel activity, or to be stored as glycogen in the muscles or liver.

In addition to the energy available from foods consumed before and during exercise (**exogenous sources**), the body also relies on its stored energy reserves to help fuel exercise (**endogenous sources**). When metabolic demands increase, glucose-releasing enzymes free stored glycogen within the muscles. In addition, the liver's unique ability to release glucose into circulation allows it to combine exogenous and endogenous sources, and maintain circulatory levels needed to fuel organs and to contribute to exercising muscles.

Carbohydrate availability is important for endurance performance, especially during higher-intensity exercise or when individuals begin training with lower levels of muscle glycogen (e.g., not carbohydrate loaded or have not consumed pre-exercise meals or snacks).[5] Interestingly, it appears that carbohydrates can even improve performance without the body actually absorbing the nutrients. In one study, researchers investigated the role that carbohydrate receptors located within the mouth play on influencing exercise performance (Fig. 20-1).[6] At timed intervals during an intense 60-minute exercise bout, subjects rinsed with either water or a 6.4% maltodextrin (MT) solution (Box 20-1) for 5 seconds before spitting. Results demonstrated improved average power output with the carbohydrate rinse, supporting the notion that a central drive or internal motivation can improve performance rather than only a metabolic drive (i.e., the perception of consuming carbohydrates without actually absorbing them improves performance).

Supplying the exercising body with carbohydrates is important before, during, and after exercise. For most individuals, a small snack or meal consumed a few hours before exercise is usually adequate to supply and/or top off their fuel reserves for their training or event. However, for more serious endurance athletes, the practice of carbohydrate loading is oftentimes followed. More information on carbohydrate loading is presented in Box 20-2. Also, see Chapter 3 for more information on the various forms and qualities of carbohydrates, glycemic index, and glycemic load, and the basic role of carbohydrates during exercise.

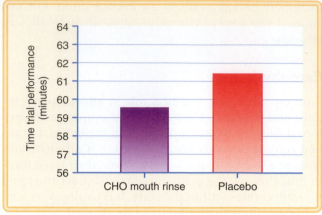

**Figure 20-1.** Mean cycle trial performance time for the carbohydrate (CHO) mouth rinse and placebo experimental conditions. Participants completed two performance trials under each experimental condition (CHO mouth rinse and placebo), during which they were required to finish a designated amount of work (914 kJ) as rapidly as possible. At timed intervals during each exercise bout, the participants either rinsed with water or a 6.4% maltodextrin solution for 5 seconds before spitting. Results showed an average improvement of 2.9% in the CHO mouth rinse experimental condition.

## Box 20-1. Maltodextrin

MT is an easily digestible carbohydrate commonly made from rice, corn, or potato starch that is used as a food additive, filler, or even sweetener. It is manufactured by first cooking the starch and then chemically or enzymatically breaking it down into smaller chains that vary in length between 3 and 20 glucose units. Being somewhat short in length and composed of glucose units, they are digested and absorbed quickly. The shorter MT chains are sweeter, have a higher glycemic index score, and can provide a rapid source of energy, but like glucose, they can increase blood glucose levels.

## Protein

Protein plays an important role in both endurance and muscle-strengthening exercise. Both modes of exercise stimulate muscle protein synthesis,[7] which is further enhanced with consumption of protein around the time of exercise.[8]

## Box 20-2. Carbohydrate Loading

Individuals training for long-distance endurance events lasting more than 90 minutes, such as a marathon or triathlon, may benefit from **carbohydrate loading** in the days or weeks before competition. The practice of carbohydrate loading has demonstrated various levels of improvement in endurance-type events as the body adapts by storing more glycogen within liver and muscle cells. For many endurance athletes, this is critical to athletic success for the following reasons:

- Carbohydrate stores in tissues are limited and generally insufficient to fuel many endurance events. Expanding one's glycogen tank can avoid potentially "hitting the wall" or "bonking" that sometimes happens when athletes run out of available glycogen.
- Higher intensities of exercise rely more on carbohydrates as a fuel; thus, expanding the quantities available can help an athlete sustain higher intensities.

A Position Statement by the American Dietetic Association (now known as the Academy of Nutrition and Dietetics) and ACSM[2] reviewed 23 studies that have examined rates and amounts of macronutrient consumption during the training period before an athletic competition. Although different study designs revealed different results, the general consensus appears to be that carbohydrate loading increases muscle glycogen concentrations and can contribute to improved performance. However, it appears that there is a threshold limit to the amount of carbohydrates consumed (e.g., 6 g carbohydrates per kilogram of body weight) and a sex difference whereby women may be less able to increase their muscle glycogen concentrations than men.

The primary goal behind carbohydrate loading is to increase the muscle's glycogen-storage capacity. This is accomplished by increasing carbohydrate intake and exercising at an intensity that is capable of depleting the body's stored glycogen. Various carbohydrate loading regimens exist, including 7-, 6-, 3-, and 1-day protocols, but they typically involve two stages:

- **Glycogen-depletion stage**: moderate- to high-intensity exercise to deplete glycogen stores, coupled with low-to-moderate carbohydrate intakes (<55% of total kilocalories)
- **Glycogen-loading stage**: tapered exercise (low intensity, short duration), coupled with high carbohydrate intakes (>70% of total kilocalories)

Carbohydrate loading may contribute to water-based weight gain because carbohydrates require sizeable amounts of water for storage (1 g glycogen pulls approximately 2.4–2.7 g water into storage).

The following is a sample 1-week plan:

- Days 1–3: Moderate-carbohydrate diet (50% of calories): this is coupled with intense exercise to intentionally deplete glycogen stores

## Box 20-2. Carbohydrate Loading—cont'd

- Days 4–6: High-carbohydrate diet (up to 80% of calories): this is coupled with exercise that tapers down to no exercise to optimally expand glycogen stores
- Day 7: Competitive event: pre-event meal (typically dinner the night before the event) with more than 80% of calories from carbohydrates

Although carbohydrate loading may benefit athletic performance during a prolonged endurance session, it is not without drawbacks. Mental and physical fatigue, irritability, mood disturbances, poor recovery, and increased risk for injury can occur during the glycogen-depletion stage. Bloating, GI distress, weight gain, lethargy, and frustration associated with altered training schedules frequently occur during carbohydrate loading stages.[50] Also, it is notable that carbohydrate loading may not always contribute to increased athletic performance. Multiple variables, including the loading strategy, type of carbohydrate consumed (low vs. high glycemic), timing, sex, and exercise characteristics (e.g., endurance or sprint) affect performance.[50] Individuals seeking full-menu plans to carbohydrate load should consider consulting with a qualified sports nutritionist.

Although the amount of protein that should be consumed by athletic individuals continues to remain hotly debated, the general consensus is that athletic individuals require greater quantities of protein in their diets than their sedentary counterparts to support protein synthesis.[2,9] To help provide evidence-based recommendations, in 2009, the American Dietetic Association (currently known as the Academy of Nutrition and Dietetics), Joint Dietitians of Canada, and ACSM[2] released a joint position statement on protein intake for endurance (defined as ≥10 hr/week of training) and strength-training athletes (aiming to build muscular mass, strength, and power). They recommended intakes between 1.2 and 1.7 g/kg body weight (0.55–0.77 g/lb) and suggested that this intake could be met through diet alone (i.e., without the use of protein or amino acid supplements) as long as the individual's total energy intake was adequate to maintain body weight for optimal protein use and performance. This was further subdivided into:

- 1.2 to 1.4 g protein per kilogram of body weight (0.55–0.64 g/lb) for endurance-trained individuals
- 1.4 to 1.7 g protein per kilogram of body weight (0.64–0.77 g/lb) for strength-trained individuals
- 1.3 to 1.8 g protein per kilogram of body weight (0.59–0.82 g/lb) for vegetarian athletes, given the fact that protein quality of nonanimal and nondairy source is lower

Campbell and Spano[10] examined current research and suggested that there is growing evidence to support strength athletes ingesting protein and amino acid quantities at the upper end of the range of 1.5 to 2.0 g protein per kilogram of body weight per day (0.68–0.91 g/lb) before, during, and/or after exercise to optimize training adaptations. Regardless, there appears to be an upper limit, after which additional protein no longer provides significant benefits and may actually begin to induce more harm than good.[2]

Although these position statements differ slightly, the apparent consensus and a practical guideline to follow is one where aerobic endurance athletes should aim to consume between 1.2 and 1.4 g protein per kilogram of body weight per day (0.55–0.64 g/lb), whereas anaerobic athletes (e.g., strength and power lifters) should aim to consume between 1.4 and 2.0 g protein per kilogram of body weight per day (0.64–0.91 g/lb). For example, a 185-lb (84.1-kg) endurance athlete should consume between 101 and 118 g protein daily, whereas a similar 185-lb (84.1-kg) strength-trained athlete should consume between 118 and 168 g protein daily (Table 20-1).

Consumption of protein immediately post-exercise helps in the repair and synthesis of muscle proteins.[11] Although some research does support protein consumption before exercise, protein intake during exercise probably does not offer any additional performance benefit if sufficient amounts of carbohydrate—the body's preferred energy source—are consumed (0.7 g/kg body weight/hr).[11] However, for endurance athletes who may struggle to consume adequate calories to fuel extended training sessions, or for the average exerciser striving to lose weight, research suggests that protein helps to preserve lean muscle mass and assure that the majority of weight lost comes from fat rather than lean tissue.[7] Although protein typically is used to build muscle, tissue, and other compounds, in times of short carbohydrate supply, the carbon skeleton of some amino acids can be converted to glucose through **gluconeogenesis**

## Table 20-1. Examples of Suggested Protein Intakes for 145-and 185-Pound Individuals

| TYPE OF INDIVIDUAL | 145 LB (65.9 KG) | 185 LB (84.1 KG) |
|---|---|---|
| Average adult | 53 g | 67 g |
| Endurance athlete | 79–92 g | 101–118 g |
| Resistance-trained athlete | 92–32 g | 118–168 g |
| Upper tolerance | <131 g | <168 g |

through pathways such as the glucose-alanine pathway discussed in Chapter 4.

Although these may seem like great reasons to boost protein intake, it is worth noting that many people habitually consume more than even the most liberal protein intake recommendations. Protein consumption beyond recommended amounts is unlikely to result in further muscle gains because the body has a limited capacity to use amino acids to build muscle.[7]

## Fat

The effectiveness of various dietary strategies to use fat as an ergogenic aid are inconclusive. According to a Position Statement of the Academy of Nutrition and Dietetics and ACSM, to date there is no evidence for performance benefit from a very low-fat diet (<15% of total calories) or from a high-fat diet.[2] However, there has been interest in **fat loading**, a dietary approach in which an athlete increases consumption of fat in an effort to provide a ready supply of fat as an energy source. Fat loading can be done immediately before exercise or long term by adopting a high-fat, low-carbohydrate diet. The theory is that if a progressively greater percentage of fat is consumed in the diet, fat oxidation will be increased during exercise. Energy can be produced from fat; therefore, carbohydrate stores can be spared. Typically, carbohydrate stores can only fuel about 3 hours of endurance activity. By using more fat for fuel, the belief is that it will take longer to deplete muscle glycogen stores and the athlete will be able to maintain long-distance activities for a longer period at a higher intensity. However, studies examining the short-term and long-term effects of fat loading on endurance performance have not demonstrated consistent benefits.

## NUTRITIONAL STRATEGIES FOR OPTIMAL PERFORMANCE

Whether training for endurance activities or trying to maximize power and strength, athletes need the right types and amounts of food before, during, and after exercise to maximize the amount of energy available to fuel optimal performance and minimize the amount of GI distress. Sports nutrition strategies should address three exercise stages: pre-exercise, exercise, and post-exercise (Fig. 20-2).

## Pre-exercise Fueling

The primary goals associated with pre-exercise fueling are: (1) to optimize glucose availability and glycogen stores, and (2) to provide the fuel needed for exercise performance.[4] Keeping this in mind, in the hours, days, and sometimes even up to a week before a strenuous endurance effort, an athlete should consider what nutritional strategies might best facilitate optimal performance.

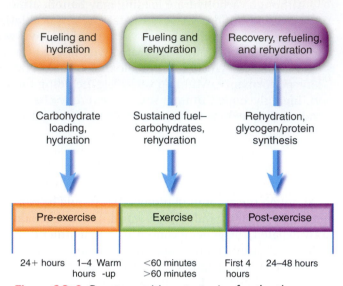

**Sports nutritional strategies should address three exercise stages:**

1. *Pre-exercise:* Beginning 1 week prior to the event through warm-up
2. *During exercise*
3. *Post-exercise:* Up to 48 hours post-exercise

**Figure 20-2.** Sports nutrition strategies for the three exercise stages.

For the most part, carbohydrate consumption is the most critical component of a pre-exercise fueling regimen, and some research supports protein consumption before exercise.

An athlete who is preparing for a long endurance event might consider the pros and cons of carbohydrate loading in the week before the event to help increase glycogen stores. All athletes should aim to begin their pre-exercise fueling regimen at least within the 4 to 6 hours before the event to minimize GI distress and optimize performance. Four hours after eating, the food will already have been digested and absorbed; now liver and muscle glycogen levels are at their highest. Thus, eating a carbohydrate-rich snack 4 to 6 hours before an event allows for peak liver and muscle glycogen levels at the onset of exercise. Athletes who work out in the early afternoon will benefit most from a wholesome carbohydrate-rich breakfast. Athletes who exercise in the early morning may benefit from a carbohydrate-rich snack before going to bed.

Some research also suggests that eating a relatively small carbohydrate- and protein-containing snack (e.g., 50 g carbohydrate and 5–10 g protein) 60 to 120 minutes before exercise helps increase glucose availability near the end of the workout and helps to decrease exercise-induced protein catabolism.[12] Athletes who are preparing for high-performance endurance activities may benefit from a regimented carbohydrate feeding plan. Research supports that competitive endurance athletes should consume pre-exercise snacks or meals containing between 1 and 4 g carbohydrate per kilogram of body weight (0.45–1.8 g/lb).[13,14]

To avoid potential GI distress when blood is diverted from the gut to exercising muscles, the carbohydrate and calorie content of snacks and meals should be reduced as one gets closer to the start of exercise. For example, a carbohydrate feeding of 1 g/kg body weight (0.45 g/lb) is more appropriate an hour before exercise, whereas an individual can consume 4.0 g/kg body weight (1.8 g/lb) 4 hours before exercise.[14] Table 20-2 presents a simplistic guide to follow for pre-exercise carbohydrate regimens.[14,15]

Health and fitness professionals can implement the following strategies when planning pre-exercise strategies for carbohydrates[8,16,17]:

- *Pre-exercise meal:* Aim to consume 2 to 4 g/kg body weight (0.91–1.8 g/lb) of moderate glycemic carbohydrates a minimum of 2 to 3 hours before exercise to allow sufficient time for gastric emptying, digestion, and absorption.
  - *Example:* Feed a 175-lb (79.5-kg) athlete 159 to 318 g (636–1,272 kcal) of more moderate glycemic carbohydrates 3 to 4 hours before his or her 4-hour training session.
- *Pre-exercise snack:* Aim to consume 1.0 to 1.5 g/kg body weight (0.45–0.68 g/lb) 60 to 90 minutes before exercise to allow sufficient time for gastric emptying, digestion, and absorption.
  - *Example:* A 145-lb (65.9-kg) athlete eats 66 to 99 g (264–396 kcal) low-glycemic carbohydrates 90 minutes before a 2-hour training session.

*Note: When training a regular client who expends 300 to 450 kcal in a session, there is probably no need for either strategy. A 50- to 150-kcal snack consumed within 60 to 90 minutes of the exercise session may be more appropriate, especially if the client is in a fasted state (e.g., has not eaten in the past 4–5 hours). For example, an average client who ate lunch at 12 p.m., but plans to exercise at 5 p.m. performing 45 to 60 minutes of moderate-intensity exercise, would be advised to consume a small snack up to 150 calories 60 to 90 minutes before working out. Good examples of carbohydrate-rich foods for pre-exercise meals include fruit, cereal, bread products (adding jam or jelly increases the carbohydrate content), and low-fat or nonfat yogurt. Ultimately, the exact timing and size of the snack for peak performance will vary by athlete.*

Historically, endurance athletes had been advised to avoid carbohydrates in the hour before exercise—the most convenient time for many athletes to consume a pre-exercise snack—because of concern for rebound or reactive hypoglycemia (a drop in blood sugar because of a surge in insulin) and diminished performance. However, evidence suggests that carbohydrate consumption in the hour before exercise provides more benefit than potential harm, although it probably does not provide the same performance boost as carbohydrates consumed at least 2 hours before the onset of exercise.[2]

Ultimately, carbohydrate consumption before training should be based on training session goals, as well as the exercise demands for each individual. For instance, athletes in sports involving running (e.g., basketball and soccer) and contact (e.g., boxing and wrestling) may only tolerate small volumes of liquid fuel before training that empty from the stomach quickly and limit potential GI distress (e.g., stomach distension) caused by up-and-down movements. By contrast, cyclists and golfers, who demonstrate less dynamic trunk displacement, may tolerate larger, more solid carbohydrate sources that empty more slowly before training.

Despite the performance benefits from carbohydrates, some athletes may hesitate to consume recommended amounts because of concerns of GI distress. If carbohydrates are not rapidly digested and absorbed, it can contribute to performance-limiting cramps, dizziness, nausea, vomiting, and diarrhea. The likelihood of GI problems increases with consumption of fiber, fat, protein, and concentrated carbohydrate-containing foods and drinks. A pre-exercise meal or snack should have the following characteristics to minimize GI discomfort:

- Relatively high in carbohydrates to maximize blood glucose availability
- Relatively low in fat and fiber to minimize GI distress and facilitate gastric emptying
- Moderate in protein
- Well tolerated by the individual

## Fueling During Exercise

The goal of during-exercise fueling is to provide the body with the essential nutrients needed by muscle cells and to maintain optimal blood glucose levels. When exercise lasts longer than 60 minutes, blood glucose levels may begin to decrease. After 1 to 3 hours of continuous moderate-intensity exercise , muscle glycogen stores may become depleted. If no glucose is consumed, the blood glucose levels decline, resulting in further depletion of muscle glycogen. When this happens, regardless of the athlete's internal toughness or desire to maintain intensity, performance falters. During a prolonged endurance effort, such as a marathon, an athlete is at risk for "hitting the wall"—a phenomena that can occur around or after mile 20 when glycogen stores become depleted. This is when extreme fatigue

## Table 20-2. Pre-exercise Carbohydrate Feeding Guidelines

| TIMING BEFORE EXERCISE | CARBOHYDRATE QUANTITY | CARBOHYDRATE TYPE |
|---|---|---|
| 1 hour | 1.0 g/kg body weight (0.45 g/lb) | Low glycemic preferred |
| 2 hours | 2.0 g/kg body weight (0.91 g/lb) | Lower-to-moderate glycemic |
| 3 hours | 3.0 g/kg body weight (1.4 g/lb) | Moderate glycemic preferred |
| 4 hours | 4.0 g/kg body weight (1.8 g/lb) | Any |

tends to set in because of drained fuel stores, although there are gradations on the physical demands of exercise based on the duration of the exercise session. Exercise lasting less than 1 hour can be adequately fueled with existing glucose and glycogen stores. No additional carbohydrate-containing drinks or foods are necessary.

## Recommendations

To maintain a ready energy supply during prolonged exercise sessions (>60 minutes), athletes should consider consuming glucose-containing beverages and snacks. The Academy of Nutrition and Dietetics, Dietitians of Canada, and ACSM recommend that athletes consume 30 to 60 g carbohydrate per hour of training,[2] or 0.7 g/kg body weight/hr of exercise. This is especially important for athletes who: (1) engage in prolonged exercise and exercise in extreme heat, cold, or high altitude; (2) did not consume adequate amounts of food or drink before the training session; and (3) did not carbohydrate load, who restrict energy intake for weight loss, or who participate in more vigorous intensities of exercise. In general, for most individuals participating in moderate-to-vigorous levels of recreational exercise, the recommendations provided in Figure 20-3 can be followed.

Carbohydrate consumption during prolonged exercise should begin shortly after the initiation of the workout. The carbohydrate will be more effective if the 30 to 60 g/hr (0.7 g/kg body weight/hr) are consumed in small amounts every 15 to 20 minutes rather than as a large bolus after 2 hours of exercise.[2] Some experts believe that adding protein to carbohydrate during exercise will help to improve performance, but to date this evidence is inconclusive.[18]

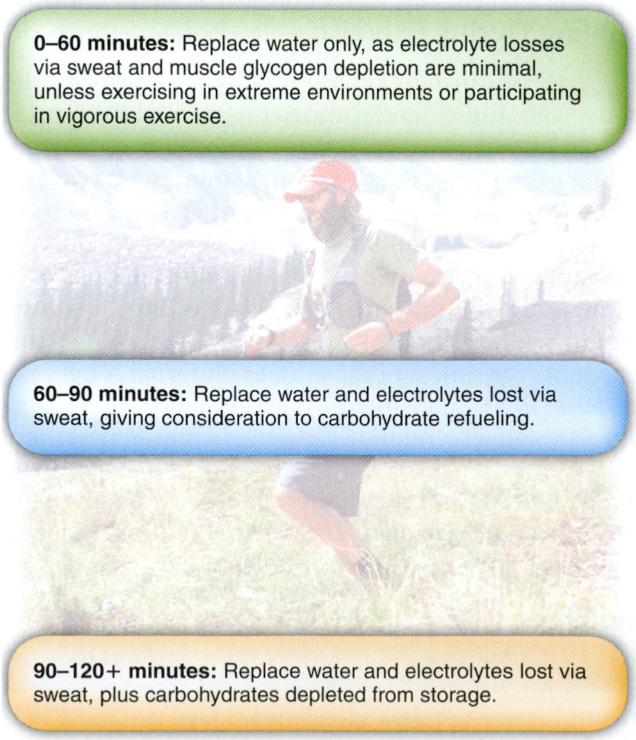

Many athletes choose to meet carbohydrate needs during exercise with consumption of sports drinks. Most sports drinks are made with a combination of the sugars glucose and fructose. As discussed in Chapter 3, glucose sources are absorbed more rapidly than fructose sources, and thus are considered a better carbohydrate source for fueling the muscles. In addition, whereas glucose is used directly by muscle cells, fructose is generally transported to the liver first, for conversion to glucose, and thus delays delivery of fuel to muscle cells. Furthermore, given the delayed passage of fructose through the GI, high fructose concentrations in beverages may increase the likelihood of GI distress, such as diarrhea.[19]

Whereas ideal total carbohydrate concentrations should be no higher than 8%, fructose concentrations exceeding 4% can increase the risk for GI distress. To calculate total carbohydrate concentration, for example, if a sports drink contains 14 g carbohydrates per 8 oz (approximately 240 mL) serving (listed on the label), the carbohydrate concentration can be calculated as follows:

- Concentration = 14 g ÷ 240 mL
- = 0.058 × 100
- = 5.8% solution

Unfortunately, labels do not separate glucose from fructose; therefore, the health and fitness professional needs to read the list of ingredients to identify whether the primary carbohydrate sugars are derived from glucose or fructose.

**0–60 minutes:** Replace water only, as electrolyte losses via sweat and muscle glycogen depletion are minimal, unless exercising in extreme environments or participating in vigorous exercise.

**60–90 minutes:** Replace water and electrolytes lost via sweat, giving consideration to carbohydrate refueling.

**90–120+ minutes:** Replace water and electrolytes lost via sweat, plus carbohydrates depleted from storage.

**Figure 20-3.** Recommendations for the ingestion of water and glucose-containing beverages/snacks during prolonged exercise in recreational exercisers.

### DOING THE MATH

- Calculate the carbohydrate concentration in a beverage containing 22 g sugar per 8 oz serving.
- Calculate the carbohydrate concentration in a beverage containing 32 g sugar per 8 oz serving.

**Answers:**
9.2%; 13.3%

## The Gut and Gastric Emptying

To supply the body with sufficient energy to fuel exercise, athletes often must consume foods during exercise. The GI system must then rapidly digest and absorb fluids and nutrients that fuel exercise. Although this is in many cases essential for optimal performance, many athletes can experience GI distress, including cramping, reflux, heartburn, bloating, side-stitch, gas, nausea, vomiting, the urge to defecate, loose stool, bloody stool, and diarrhea during intense activity. These GI ailments occur in response to: (1) reduced gastric emptying,

(2) delayed transit time, or (3) decreased blood flow. Knowledge of factors that affect the GI system's ability to adapt to exercise-induced stresses can help to prevent GI upset and optimize athletic performance.

**Gastric emptying** refers to the passage of food and fluid from the stomach to the small intestines for further digestion and absorption. When gastric emptying is reduced, food remaining in the stomach for a longer period can cause stomach distension, movement, and distress. High-intensity exercise, dehydration, hyperthermia, and consumption of more concentrated (**hypertonic**) drinks with carbohydrate concentrations exceeding 8% slow gastric emptying. A hypertonic solution is defined as one having concentrations of substrate (e.g., sodium, glucose, and amino acids) that are greater than their concentration in human blood. For example, many sports drinks, energy drinks, and juices all are more concentrated than blood (i.e., hypertonic), whereas water is less concentrated than blood (i.e., hypotonic).

In contrast, low- to moderate-intensity exercise helps to speed digestion by stimulating intestinal muscles to contract and push more food waste through the digestive system. Endurance-trained athletes enjoy faster gastric emptying than their untrained counterparts, as the body adapts to larger and more frequent meals. This translates into quicker energy availability and decreased GI discomfort following fueling.[17]

Exercise-induced sympathetic stimulation diverts blood flow from the GI system to the heart, lungs, and working muscles. The higher the exercise intensity, the more blood flow and **colonic tone** (the functionality of the colon in absorbing and moving food along its length) decrease, causing waste to accumulate in the colon and rectum. The high amount of waste at the end of the GI tract may signal the stomach to slow down, leading to reduced gastric emptying and prolonged transit time. A bulky high-fiber snack increases intestinal distension and water content, contributing to decreased gastric emptying, as well as discomforts such as loose stool and an urge to defecate. Box 20-3 lists practical suggestions on how to prepare the gut for an athletic competition.

## Post-exercise Refueling

The main goal of post-exercise fueling is to replenish glycogen stores and facilitate muscle repair. The average client training at moderate intensity and duration (~45–60 minutes) every few days does not need any aggressive post-exercise replenishment. Normal dietary practices following exercise will facilitate recovery within 20 to 48 hours. But athletes following vigorous training regimens, especially those who will participate in multiple training sessions in a single day (like a triathlete), benefit from strategic refueling.

Studies show that the best post-workout meals include mostly carbohydrates accompanied with some protein.[12] Box 20-4 outlines post-workout snack and meal ideas. Refueling should begin within 30 minutes

### Box 20-3. Practical Tips to Prepare the Gut for Competition

1. Familiarize your body with drinking practices during training before attempting strategies on race days.
2. Drink frequently to maintain some stomach volume (7–10 oz or 200–300 mL every 15 minutes), but avoid overdrinking at one time that distends the stomach (i.e., beyond 23 oz or 700 mL).
3. Get fit and acclimatized to heat; allow 9 to 14 days to properly acclimatize to hot and/or humid environments.
4. Avoid overeating too soon before and during exercise; as GI function slows down during exercise, food takes longer to digest and may cause GI distress.
5. Avoid high-energy, hypertonic food and drinks (greater than 8% concentrations) within 30 to 60 minutes of exercise; this slows absorption and may interfere with fuel utilization. Limit fat and excessive amounts of protein intake before exercise and opt for more carbohydrate-based snack and meals, but avoid high-fiber foods.
6. After exercise, plan to refuel and rehydrate as soon as possible, but monitor for any GI distress with food or beverages consumed too soon after exercise.
7. Limit nonsteroidal anti-inflammatory drugs, alcohol, caffeine, antibiotics, and nutritional supplements before and during exercise. Rather, try to experiment with those products during training to identify which are triggers to potential adverse effects.
8. Aim to void (urinate and defecate) before exercise to avoid GI or bladder discomfort.
9. If GI distress exists and persists with training (especially abdominal pain, diarrhea, or bloody stool), consult with a physician.

### Box 20-4. Post-workout Snack and Meal Ideas

In the several hours following a prolonged and strenuous workout, consuming snacks and meals high in carbohydrate with some protein can set the stage for optimal glycogen replenishment and subsequent performance. Here are a few snack and meal ideas that fit the bill:

- Snack 1: In the first several minutes after exercise, consume 16 oz Gatorade™ or other sports drink, a power gel such as a Clif Shot™ or Goo™, and a medium banana. This quickly begins to replenish muscle carbohydrate stores. *Carbohydrates: 73 g; Protein: 1 g; Calories: 288*

*Continued*

## Box 20-4. Post-workout Snack and Meal Ideas–cont'd

- Snack 2: After cooling down and showering, grab another quick snack such as 12 oz orange juice and 1/4 cup of raisins. *Carbohydrates: 70 g; Protein: 3 g; Calories: 295*
- Small meal appetizer: Enjoy a spinach salad with tomatoes, chickpeas, green beans, and tuna and a whole-grain baguette. *Carbohydrates: 70 g; Protein: 37 g; Calories: 489*
- Small meal main course: Replenish with whole-grain pasta with diced tomatoes. *Carbohydrates: 67 g; Protein: 2 g; Calories: 292*
- Dessert: After allowing ample time for the day's snacks and meals to digest, finish your refueling program with 1 cup of frozen yogurt and berries. *Carbohydrates: 61 g; Protein: 8 g; Calories: 280*

after exercise and be followed by a high-carbohydrate meal within 2 hours.[12] The carbohydrates replenish the used-up energy that is normally stored as glycogen in muscle and liver. The protein helps to rebuild the muscles that were fatigued with exercise. The Academy of Nutrition and Dietetics and other leading organizations recommend carbohydrate intakes between 1.0 and 1.5g/kg body weight within the first 30 minutes after exercise, then repeating this amount within the first 2 hours, and then every 2 hours for a total of 4 to 6 hours.[2] After that, the athlete can resume his or her typical, balanced diet. Of course, the amount of refueling necessary depends on the intensity and duration of the training session. A long-duration, low-intensity workout may not require such vigorous replenishment.

### DOING THE MATH

If John weighs 176 lb (80 kg) and follows the recommendation presented in this chapter, how many grams of carbohydrates and calories (from carbohydrates) would he actually consume within the first hour? If he repeated this amount two more times, for how many minutes would he need to run to match the total number of calories if his running pace of 8 miles/hr consumed 18.6 cal/min?

- First, calculate the number of grams of carbohydrate:
  - 1.0–1.5 g/kg body weight × 80 kg = 80–120 g
- Next, calculate the number of calories of carbohydrate:
  - 80–120 g × 4 kcal/g = 320–480 kcal
- Total calories consumed over the three meals = 320–480 kcal × 3 = 960–1,440 kcal
- At 1.0 g/kg body weight: 960 kcal ÷ 18.6 kcal/min = 51. 6 minutes
- At 1.5 g/kg body weight: 1,440 kcal ÷ 18.6 kcal/min = 77.4 minutes

## HYDRATION FOR OPTIMAL PERFORMANCE

Although some individuals may still subscribe to the practice of replacing lost fluids and electrolytes only after they start sweating, effective hydration strategies should include all three stages (pre-, during, and

---

### RESEARCH HIGHLIGHT

### Chocolate Milk and Recovery

In recent years, researchers have examined the efficacy of low-fat or nonfat chocolate milk as a recovery beverage given its blend of whey and casein, coupled with its 4:1 carbohydrate/protein ratio (1 serving generally contains 28 g carbohydrates and 7 g protein). In one study, researchers examined nine endurance-trained cyclists who performed an interval workout, followed by 4 hours of recovery, and a subsequent workout to exhaustion at 70% $\dot{V}O_2$max.[20] On testing days, subjects ingested an isovolumic (same volume) amount of chocolate milk, fluid replacement drink, or a carbohydrate-replacement drink immediately after the first workout and then again 2 hours into recovery. Results measuring time to exhaustion, heart rate response, and ratings of perceived exertion demonstrated that chocolate milk was an effective recovery aid (Figure 20-4).

Overall consuming about 1.0-1.5g/kg/h of chocolate milk immediately after exercise and at 2 hours post-exercise may be optimal for exercise recovery and minimizing muscle damage in endurance athletes.[21]

Karp JR, Johnston JD, Tecklenburg S, Mickleboroughm TD, Fly AD, Stager JM. Chocolate milk as a post-exercise recovery aid. *Int J Sports Nutr Exerc Metab.* 2006;16:78–91.

Ferguson-Stegall L, McCleave E, Ding Z, et al. Aerobic exercise training adaptations are increased by post-exercise carbohydrate-protein supplementation. *J Nutr Metab.* 2011. doi: 10.1155/2011/623182

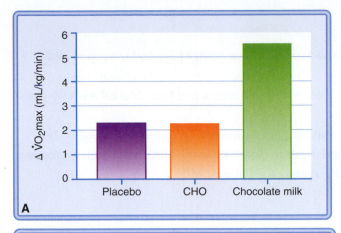

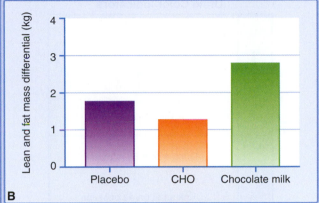

Figure 20-4. Greater improvements in maximal oxygen uptake (VO$_2$max) and body composition (calculated by lean and fat mass differential) were found following 4.5 weeks of aerobic training in a group who consumed chocolate milk post-exercise when compared with groups who consumed carbohydrate (CHO) or placebo post-exercise, respectively.

post-exercise) to promote optimal performance. Figure 20-5 shows the overall timeframes to achieve effective hydration and rehydration.

Much has been studied and written about euhydration (maintaining normal total body water content), hyperhydration (excessive fluid intake or leading to excessive total body water content), hyponatremia (condition marked by low blood sodium levels), and dehydration (condition marked by excessive fluid loss; usually accompanied by, or attributed to, electrolyte losses).

## Euhydration and Estimating Fluid Needs

Various methods exist to determine the body's fluid needs for euhydration, including[4,22–24]

1. Body weight measurement:
   - Establishing baseline body weight using several days of first morning body weight (after voiding), following conscientious hydration the preceding evening
2. Consistent urine color and volume:
   - Consistent, larger volumes excreted during the first morning void with a lemonade color usually indicate euhydration (Fig. 20-6)
   - Consistent, smaller volumes excreted during the first morning void with an apple juice to iced tea color usually indicate dehydration
   - Exceptions:
     - B vitamins, betacyanins (pigments in dark red vegetables—beets), and artificial food color can discolor urine. If an individual follows a 7-day washout period where he or

## VIGNETTE continued

The following table presents Layla's planned workout program for the next week:

| MONDAY | TUESDAY | WEDNESDAY | THURSDAY | FRIDAY | SATURDAY | SUNDAY |
|--------|---------|-----------|----------|--------|----------|--------|
| 5-mile recovery jog | 6 × 400-meter sprints, weight lifting | 6-mile jog | 6 × 400-meter sprints, weight lifting | Marathon pace 10-mile run | Rest | 20-mile run (long, slow distance) |

Layla and Enrique are preparing a pre-, during, and post-exercise fueling plan for her 20-mile run on Sunday. Because Layla plans to wake up early to begin the run, she will have little opportunity for pre-fueling before the workout. To address this, she plans to consume a high-carbohydrate dinner and ample fluids on Saturday evening. During the Sunday run, Layla will carry some sports gels, gummies, and jelly beans in her fuel belt to supply about 11 g carbohydrate every 15 minutes. On Enrique's recommendation, within 30 minutes of finishing the run Layla will begin a several-hour refueling plan to help replenish her glycogen stores at a rate of 1.0 to 1.5 g/kg body weight, as follows:

- Snack 1: In the first several minutes after exercise, she will consume a 16 oz (~0.5 L) sports drink, a power gel, and a medium banana. This will quickly begin to replenish muscle carbohydrate stores. *Carbohydrates: 73 g; Protein: 1 g; Calories: 288*

*Continued*

## VIGNETTE *continued*

- Snack 2: Ninety minutes later, she will eat another quick snack, such as 12 oz orange juice and 1/4 cup of raisins. *Carbohydrates: 70 g; Protein: 3 g; Calories: 295*
- Lunch: Layla will prepare a salad with spinach, tomatoes, chickpeas, green beans, and tuna, and eat a whole-grain baguette. *Carbohydrates: 69 g; Protein: 37 g; Calories: 489*
- Small dinner: 1.5 cups of whole-grain pasta with diced tomatoes. *Carbohydrates: 67 g; Protein: 2 g; Calories: 292*
- Dessert: After allowing ample time for the day's snacks and meals to digest, Layla will finish her refueling program with 1 cup of frozen yogurt and berries. *Carbohydrates: 61 g; Protein: 8 g; Calories: 280*

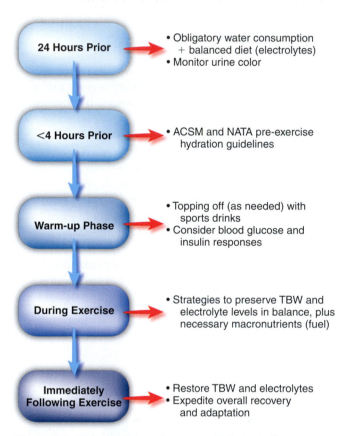

**Figure 20-5.** Overall time frames to achieve effective hydration and rehydration. ACSM, American College of Sports Medicine; NATA, National Athletic Trainers' Association; TBW, total body water.

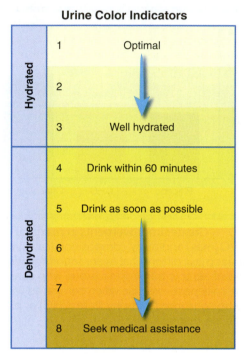

**Figure 20-6.** Urine color comparison chart. Urine color is a marker of hydration.

she stops taking multivitamins, continues drinking fluids as usual, and observes urine color, this may provide insight into his or her level of euhydration.

- Some medications (e.g., diuretics) will consistently increase urine volume and potentially lighten urine color.
- Protein supplements can consistently discolor urine. If an individual follows a 7-day washout period from protein supplements, continue drinking fluids as usual and observe urine color; this may provide insight into the level of euhydration.

  - Urine volumes and color can be misleading during rehydration stages. For example, a dehydrated individual who is consuming a large amount of hypotonic fluids will produce large volumes of clear urine, creating the perception of euhydration, even though the individual may still be dehydrated.

3. Pre-and post-exercise weight differences:
   - Comparing pre-exercise weight (voided), either naked or in light clothing, and post-exercise weight can help to determine fluid needs, provided that the individual is euhydrated before exercise.

   Fluid requirement = pre-exercise weight – post-exercise weight

   *Note: There are approximately 16 oz or 480 mL in 1 lb.*
   - *Example:* If Janelle weighed 145 lb (65.9 kg) before exercise (voided, dry) and then weighed 142 lb (64.5 kg) following exercise,

she needs to replace 3 lb (3 lb × 480 mL = 1.44 L) of fluid lost during the exercise session.
- 1–2: Well hydrated—equivalent to less than 1% loss in body weight
- 3–4: Minimal dehydration—equivalent to 1% to 3% loss in body weight
- 5–6: Significant dehydration—equivalent to 3% to 5% loss in body weight
- >6: Severe dehydration—equivalent to more than 5% loss in body weight

## Estimating Fluid Needs

Using an individual's body weight is a method by which we can estimate daily fluid needs following some simple guidelines.[25] However, these guidelines provide estimates of fluids needed to maintain total body water and do not include additional fluids needed to replace that lost to sweat.

1. Consume 30 to 40 mL/kg body weight (convert pounds to kilograms by dividing by 2.2).
   - For example, if an individual weighs 150 lb (68.2 kg), he or she will need 2,046 to 2,728 mL or 69.2 to 92.3 oz of fluid daily.
2. Fluid needs (in ounces) equals body weight divided by two.
   - For example, for that same 150-lb individual, he or she would need to consume 75 oz (2,218 mL) of fluid daily.

In 2004, the IOM set a general fluid intake recommendation (adequate intake) for women at approximately 2.7 L (91 oz) of total water from beverages and food, and for men at approximately 3.7 L (125 oz daily) of total water from beverages and food.[26] U.S. data collected from the most recent National Health and Nutrition Examination Survey demonstrate that beverages provide approximately 81% of total daily water intake, whereas foods contribute the remaining 19%.[27] Given this information, the average woman should consume 2.2 L (approximately 74 oz or 9 cups, 81% of 2.7 L) each day, whereas the average man should consume 3.0 L (approximately 101 oz or 12.5 cups, 81% of 3.7 L) each day. The IOM also set adequate intakes for children and adolescents[26]:

- Boys
  - 4–8 years old: Total fluid = 1.7 L (57.5 oz); 1.2 L (40.5 oz) from fluids
  - 9–13 years old: Total fluid = 2.4 L (81 oz); 1.8 L (61 oz) from fluids
  - 14–18 years old: Total fluid = 3.3 L (112 oz); 2.6 L (88 oz) from fluids
- Girls
  - 4–8 years old: Total fluid = 1.7 L (57.5 oz); 1.2 L (40.5 oz) from fluids
  - 9–13 years old: Total fluid = 2.1 L (71 oz); 1.6 L (54 oz) from fluids
  - 14–18 years old: Total fluid = 2.3 L (78 oz); 1.8 L (61 oz) from fluids

As mentioned previously, these guidelines provide estimates of fluids needed to maintain total body water and do not include additional fluids needed to replace water lost to sweat. Although the panel did not make recommendations for athletic individuals, they did suggest that these individuals consume fluids in quantities larger than the guidelines.

### DOING THE MATH

Various methodologies were presented to determine minimal water intake for euhydration. Using an example of a 34-year-old, 165-lb (75-kg) man who consumes 2,400 calories daily, estimate his minimal water requirements for euhydration using each of the methodologies presented.

**Answers:**
- 30–40 mL/kg: 2.25 L (76 oz) to 3.0 L (101.5 oz)
- ½ body weight (in ounces): 75 oz (2.2 L)
- IOM method: 3.7 L × 81% (fluid intake) = 3.0 L (101 oz)
- Consensus of all these methods ranges between 2.2 and 3.0 L (76 and 101.5 oz) daily

## Hyperhydration and Hyponatremia

Athletes who are prone to dehydration during intensive training may benefit from **hyperhydration**. By consuming large amounts of fluids before exercise, the athlete increases fluid reserves and delays the onset of dehydration. The excess fluid also helps to offset increases in body heat (an especially serious concern when exercising in the heat) and maintain a high volume status for optimal cardiac output. Excess fluid intake also leads to increased urination, which can offset the benefits of hyperhydration. To limit urination, some athletes incorporate **glycerol**-containing beverages into their hyperhydration regimen. Glycerol creates an osmotic gradient in the circulation favoring fluid retention, which subsequently reduces fluid excretion from the kidneys and decreases urination (see Fig. 20-7).[28] Glycerol supplementation is banned by the World Anti-Doping Agency.

Any athlete who drinks more fluid than what is lost from sweat is at increased risk for hyponatremia, or low blood sodium levels (<135 mEq/L); however, slower athletes are at highest risk because they are more likely to consume large amounts of **isotonic fluids** that far exceed the rate of fluid lost from sweat.[29] Hyponatremia can also be caused by excessive loss of sodium because of vomiting, diarrhea, or even sweating.[9,22,25,30] Sodium losses typically reduce fluid volume as the body loses its primary solute, and thus loses its ability to retain fluid. This signals the release of antidiuretic hormone that stimulates water retention, diluting blood sodium and increasing the risk for hyponatremia.

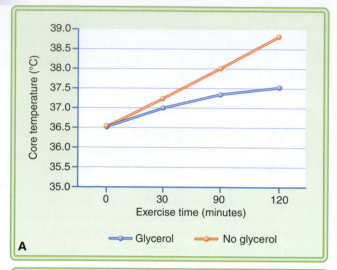

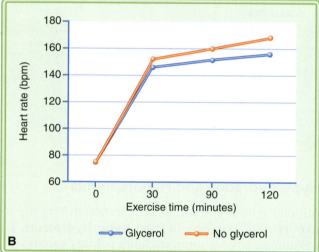

**Figure 20-7.** Physiological benefits of glycerol ingestion for prolonged exercise performance in (A) core temperature and (B) heart rate. The capacity to hyperhydrate with ingestion of glycerol-containing beverages specifically benefits individuals by prevention of excessive body core temperatures and reduced cardiovascular strain (i.e., lower heart rate) during prolonged exercise. A practical recommendation based on research findings is that ingestion of a 1.0 g/kg glycerol dosage mixed with approximately 20 mL/kg water 60 to 120 minutes pre-exercise accomplishes hyperhydration.[51]

When sodium levels within blood and the extracellular fluid compartments become low, water is pulled inside cells as the body attempts to restore normal intracellular/extracellular sodium concentrations. This shift of body water can trigger a variety of symptoms that include mild GI distress, confusion, fatigue, nausea, vomiting, headache, and some swelling within the extremities (edema). More advanced stages of this condition may be life-threatening. For example, as water passes into the brain, it causes swelling within brain tissue (encephalopathy), and because the brain is encased within the skull, this swelling causes excessive pressure on the brain, resulting in seizures and death. Within the lungs, water can accumulate and cause pulmonary edema, increasing the difficulty of breathing.

One of the factors that makes hyponatremia difficult to diagnose is that some of the initial symptoms of hyponatremia (e.g., confusion, fatigue, headache, muscle cramps, nausea, and vomiting) are similar to those of dehydration and heat illness (discussed in the next section), but this condition is distinguished from heat illnesses by the presence of weight gain and swelling.

## Dehydration and Caffeine

The sensation of thirst in adults younger than 50 years is generally initiated at about 1% dehydration or loss of body weight. At 2% dehydration, performance is compromised. Performance diminishes and symptoms become more severe with increased levels of dehydration until around 8% loss of body weight when the risk for development of severe heat illnesses like exertional heat stroke becomes significant.[9]

Prolonged exposure to hot environments or excessive metabolic heat production can lead to heat-related illnesses (hyperthermia) that vary in symptomology and severity. Heat illness is discussed in detail in Chapter 12.

Contrary to popular belief, research now demonstrates that coffee, tea, and other caffeine-containing beverages do not increase urine output significantly, nor do they negatively impact hydration status in individuals who are desensitized to the potential diuretic effects of caffeine (i.e., in habitual caffeine users).[31] Even in nonhabitual caffeine drinkers, although caffeine may have a diuretic effect, the fluid consumption rate versus fluid loss rate favors fluid uptake into the body (i.e., the net difference between volume ingested and volume lost to diuresis will favor fluid intake). Some individuals (e.g., nonhabitual caffeine users) lose 1 mL of fluid for every milligram of caffeine consumed.[26] Thus, while one 8-oz cup (240 mL) of drip-brewed coffee may contain somewhere between 60 and 120 mg caffeine, which can lead to 60 to 120 mL of water loss, the net intake is still positive because the cup contained 240 mL water (i.e., net gain of 120–180 mL). Given this evidence, the 2004 IOM report suggests that caffeinated beverages appear to contribute to the daily total water intake similar to that contributed by noncaffeinated beverages.[26] Although coffee is the chief source of caffeine in the United States, many other sources of caffeine exist that are consumed on a regular basis (Table 20-3). It is estimated that the average daily caffeine intake of a U.S. adult is between 120 and 200 mg/day.[26,32]

The ergogenic properties of caffeine ingestion are multifactorial (Fig. 20-8). Of recent interest is the finding that combined caffeine plus carbohydrate intake post-exercise contributes to increased muscle glycogen synthesis. In the first study, researchers reported that co-ingestion of 2 mg/kg/hr caffeine with 1.0 g/kg/hr carbohydrate resulted in a 66% greater increase in muscle-glycogen synthesis rates over 4 hours of post-exercise recovery.[33] More recently, a separate study[34] showed combined CHO + caffeine intake resulted in improved high-intensity interval-running capacity (Fig. 20-9).

### Table 20-3. Caffeine Content in Various Foods and Beverages

| SOURCE | SERVING SIZE | CAFFEINE QUANTITY |
| --- | --- | --- |
| Coffee (plain, drip method) | 8 oz (240 mL) | 60–120 mg |
| Espresso | 1 oz (30 mL) | 30–50 mg |
| Black/Oolong tea | 8 oz (240 mL) | 40–70 mg |
| Green tea | 8 oz (240 mL) | 25–40 mg |
| Colas | 12 oz (355 mL) | 45–45 mg |
| Energy drinks | 8–16 oz (240–480 mL) | 80–200 mg |
| Chocolate bar | 2 oz (57 g) | 10–25 mg |
| Painkillers (with caffeine) | Per tablet | 65–100 mg |
| Stimulant tablets | Per tablet | 35–200 mg |

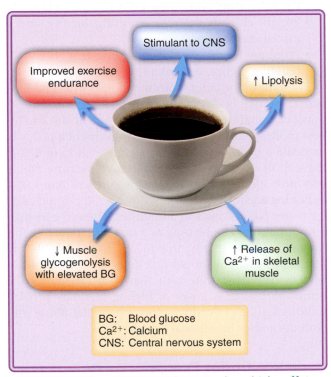

BG: Blood glucose
Ca²⁺: Calcium
CNS: Central nervous system

**Figure 20-8.** The various mechanisms by which caffeine ingestion may provide an ergogenic benefit.

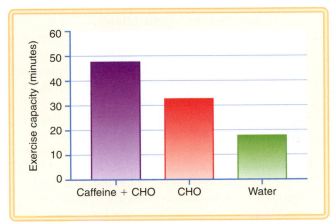

**Figure 20-9.** Combined caffeine + carbohydrate (CHO) intake has been shown to improve high-intensity interval-running capacity. Participants initially completed a maximal exercise test to exhaustion. Throughout a 4-hour recovery period, participants ingested 8 mg/kg/hr caffeine combined with 1.2 g/kg/hr CHO. Subsequent high-intensity interval-running performance was enhanced with this nutritional intake strategy compared with a condition where a similar CHO intake (i.e., 1.2 g/kg/hr) was combined with water.

## Fluid Balance and Hydration Before Exercise

A primary goal of prehydration is to ensure the individual begins activity in an euhydrated state with normal plasma electrolyte levels. In particular, this is an important consideration for early-morning exercisers who may find it challenging to implement any strategies when exercising so early. For them, a viable solution may lie with drinking appropriate amounts the night before.

### General Guidelines

The following fluid intake guidelines serve as a starting point in developing an athlete's hydration plan:

1. Because some individuals may only think consciously about drinking when thirsty (i.e., 1% dehydrated state), aim to implement a strategy that helps promote conscious and obligatory (required) fluid consumption beginning 24 hours before the event. This does not imply excessive water intake, but simply the practice of increasing their normal fluid intake slightly. For most, water is preferred over sports drinks because their balanced diet should provide adequate electrolytes to establish normal plasma levels and they may not need the additional calories. However, preferences and palatability should always be considered. Fluid temperatures influence the amount consumed; thus, temperatures between 10°C and 15°C (50°F and 59°F) are considered optimal.[30]

- Monitor consistent urine color: scores between 1 and 2 indicate well-hydrated states (see Fig. 20-6), equivalent to less than 1% loss in baseline body weight.
- Use body weight fluctuations by first establishing baseline body weight following several days of first morning body weights (after

voiding) coupled with sound hydration practices the prior evening.

2. ACSM recommendations[22]: Consume approximately 5 to 7 mL/kg (0.37–0.52 oz/lb) at least 4 hours before activity. This allows ample time for urine output before exercise. If the individual does not produce urine colors scoring between 1 and 2 over the next 2 hours, consume an additional 3 to 5 mL/kg (0.22–0.37 oz/lb) about 2 hours before activity. This still allows sufficient time for urine output. Although water is emphasized, ingesting sports drinks with some sodium (20–50 mEq/L or approximately 110–270 mg per 8-oz [240-mL] serving) or consuming some sodium-containing foods may help stimulate thirst and preserve ingested fluids.

- For example, a 100-lb (45.5-kg) gymnast may need to consume 225 to 320 mL (7.5–10.5 oz) 4 hours before her workout, plus an additional 135 to 225 (4.5–7.5 oz) 2 hours later if her urine color is still too dark.

3. National Athletic Trainers' Association (NATA) Recommendation[30]: Consume 500 to 600 mL (17–20 oz) of fluid 2 to 3 hours before exercise.

4. Although pre-exercise snacks and meals do provide some fluid, this amount is marginal and probably inadequate to properly hydrate an individual.

5. Should the event include a warm-up phase, a pre-event "topping off" is suggested to replace any potentially lost fuel, and fluids and electrolytes lost to sweat. Consume 200 to 300 mL (7–10 oz) water or sports drink 10 to 20 minutes before exercise.

- When ingesting fluids before exercise (inside of 45–60 minutes from the start), sports drinks with high glycemic loads may prove detrimental to performance because they stimulate the release of insulin, an anabolic hormone that inhibits the normal catabolic processes associated with exercise (e.g., mobilization of fat stores and breakdown of glycogen in liver tissue). However, once the individual falls under the influence of his or her sympathetic nervous system or flight-or-fight response (i.e., during warm-up, building anxiety before the event), this naturally inhibits insulin release and thus will not interfere with many catabolic processes that occur during exercise. Consequently, some athletes prefer sports drinks over water at this point to help "top off" carbohydrates, electrolytes, and fluids.
- If sports drinks are being consumed, they should not be more concentrated than an 8% carbohydrate solution.

6. Provide adequate education on the effects of dehydration and performance, and instruct athletes or parents how to effectively monitor hydration status outside of the exercise session. Implement a policy of collecting pre-exercise (voided) body weight measurements.

Although hydration protocols should always consider the unique features of a sport, the fact that the primary goal of pre-exercise hydration is to establish euhydration, these guidelines apply to all sports, including:

- Middle-distance, long-distance, and ultra-endurance training
- Field and court-based sports (e.g., soccer, rugby, tennis, volleyball, and basketball)
- Power-based sports (e.g., football, ice hockey, and field events in track)
- Artistic and extreme sports (e.g., gymnastics, figure skating, and many X-Game type events)
- Weight-class sports (e.g., wrestling, boxing, and mixed martial arts)
- Physique training and competition (e.g., body building, figure, and bikini)

For some of the latter sports mentioned where athletes perform in weight classes, abuse with diuretics and intentional dehydration occurs frequently. As a health and fitness professional, it is advisable to implement a policy to mandate a hydration status check at weigh-in or before the start of exercise. The most effective measure would be a urine specific gravity test with a score less than 1.020, indicating adequate hydration. However, it is impractical for many professionals to administer. Therefore, consistent urine color can be used as a measure for acceptable hydration.[30] Essentially, this means that a health and fitness professional should first determine the athlete's baseline consistent urine color; then if on a weigh day the urine color score is lower or higher, this may provide some indication of overhydration or potential abuse with diuretics and/or intentional dehydration.

## Hydration During Exercise

The primary goal of drinking fluids during exercise is to avoid dehydrated states where body weight loss exceeds ≥2% and to avoid excessive losses of electrolytes, both of which will compromise performance. Ideally,

### FROM THEORY TO PRACTICE

Map out the pre-exercise hydration strategies using ACSM guidelines for a 175-lb (79.5-kg) tennis player who, after his 4-hour hydration practice, still shows discolored urine (color score = 5). What is the total volume of fluid consumed before exercise? How much sodium should he consume in this same time frame if you aimed for 180 mg/240 mL?

*Hint:* Use 5 to 7 mL/kg four hours before activity and an additional 3 to 5 mL/kg two hours before activity.

the amount and rate of fluid replacement should match the rate of fluid lost from the body, but unfortunately, this is difficult to accurately quantify and to accomplish. Because sweat rates are influenced by multiple variables (e.g., body size, environmental conditions, and intensity) and opportunities to drink during exercise can prove to be equally challenging, determining this amount is no easy task. Furthermore, during exercise, blood flow to the GI tract decreases; therefore, our ability to digest and absorb fluids, even if we were able to successfully determine fluid needs, may not enable us to match our rate of fluid loss. What is recommended is the calculation of sweat rates described previously to determine individual fluids needs during exercise and the implementation of proper pre-exercise hydration strategies to complement what may need to be an aggressive during-exercise protocol to preserve total body water and electrolytes.[30]

### General Guidelines[22,30,31]

Although individual determination of sweat rates is the most effective method to determine exercise fluid needs, several organizations have provided general guidelines based on the duration of the event that can help preserve total body water (Table 20-4). The main highlights of these recommendations include:

- The IOM provides a general guideline for fluid intakes during prolonged activity in hot weather.[26] Neither duration of exercise nor a definition of what constitutes hot weather is provided, but IOM recommends that fluids contain approximately 20 to 30 mEq/L (460–690 mg/L) or 110 to 165 mg sodium in an 8-oz serving (240 mL), and contain approximately 2 to 5 mEq/L (75–195 mg/L) or 18 to 46 mg potassium in an 8-oz serving (240 mL).

- When exercising, athletes are advised to consume 200 to 300 mL (7–10 oz) every 10 to 20 minutes. This is similar to the research presented earlier that indicated that consuming approximately 150 to 200 mL (5.1–6.7 oz) of fluid every 10 to 15 minutes maintains stomach distension and accelerates gastric emptying rates. If hydration opportunities are frequent (e.g., football and baseball), individuals can consume smaller volumes at a more convenient pace. If hydration opportunities occur at specific times (e.g., half time of soccer match or marathon hydration stations), then athletes may need to consume larger quantities, monitor gastric emptying rates, and be cautious of any GI distress associated with larger volumes.

- Fluid replacement beverages should be palatable and meet individual preferences. Beverage temperatures not only influence consumption amounts, but also can help cool the body while stimulating gastric emptying. Ideal fluid temperatures are between 10°C and 15°C (50°F and 59°F).

- Fluids should be accessible and served in clearly marked containers (e.g., every 100 mL) to consciously remind individuals to drink appropriate amounts. Furthermore, this facilitates measurement of fluids consumed during exercise.

- Finally, if sports drinks are consumed, then they should not exceed 8% carbohydrate concentrations (Table 20-5).

### Post-exercise Rehydration

Following exercise the athlete should aim to correct any fluid and electrolyte imbalances that occurred during the exercise session. This includes consuming water to restore hydration, carbohydrates to replenish glycogen stores, and electrolytes to speed rehydration. If the

### Table 20-4. General Fluid and Electrolyte Recommendations for Events of Differing Durations

| EXERCISE DURATION | HYDRATION STRATEGY |
|---|---|
| Events ≤60 minutes | Generally, water is *all* that is needed (assuming a balanced diet and pre-exercise euhydration) unless: <br> • Performing high-intensity exercise (high sweat rates): may require electrolyte replacement <br> • Exercising in extreme environments (high sweat rates): may require electrolyte replacement <br> • Dehydrated and fasted (improper preparation): may require fluid, electrolytes, and carbohydrates |
| Events lasting 60–90 minutes | Fluid and electrolyte replacement are most important, with carbohydrate replacement needed to a lesser extent |
| Events lasting 90–120 minutes | Generally require fluid, electrolyte, and carbohydrate replacement |
| Events ≥120 minutes | Require fluid, electrolyte, more complex-carbohydrate replacement <br> Merits consideration for the inclusion of amino acids (e.g., branched chain amino acids) as glycogen stores become depleted |

## Table 20-5. Evaluating Sports Drinks, 8-oz Serving Size

| DRINK | CALORIES (KCAL) | SODIUM (MG) | CARBOHYDRATE (G) | CARBOHYDRATE CONCENTRATION (%) |
|---|---|---|---|---|
| Gatorade | 50 | 110 | 14 | 6 |
| Gatorade Endurance Formula | 50 | 200 | 14 | 6 |
| Powerade | 70 | 55 | 19 | 8 |
| Ultima | 12.5 | 37 | 3 | 1 |
| Power Bar Endurance | 70 | 160 | 17 | 7 |
| Propel Zero | 0 | 75 | 2 | <1 |
| Zico coconut water | 34 | 91 | 7.4 | 3 |

*Source:* Data from sports drink websites including http://gatorade.com, http://powerade.com, http://ultimareplenisher.com, http://powerbar.com, http://propelzero.com, and http://zico.com.

### FROM THEORY TO PRACTICE

Map out a hydration strategy for a 200-lb (70.9-kg) boxer who usually trains for 60 minutes in the boxing ring, then proceeds to run (steady-state continuous) for an additional 30 minutes following his boxing workout. How often would you ideally like to have him drinking fluids during his training session? What volume of fluid should he consume each time for both modalities? How much sodium would you want him to consume during his entire workout?

*Hint:* Remember to consider stomach volume, fluid temperature, hydration opportunities (i.e., frequency), and the relationship between sport modality and GI distress (e.g., body orientation, sport demands, and stomach volume).

athlete will have at least 12 hours to recover before the next strenuous workout, then rehydration with the usual meals, snacks, and plain water is adequate. The sodium in the foods will help retain fluids and stimulate the sensation of thirst.

If rehydration needs to occur more rapidly, then the individual should consume more fluid than was lost during exercise to restore lost fluid and compensate for increased urine output that occurs with rapid consumption of large amounts of fluid. A severely dehydrated athlete can lose upward of 6% body water during training or competition, which may increase the likelihood for development of heat illness and a variety of symptoms. These individuals will obviously need to implement aggressive rehydration strategies that may also include intravenous fluid replacement by a medical professional if necessary.

### General Guidelines

Recommendations for post-exercise fluid replacement suggest drinking up to 1.5 L (51 oz) of fluid for each kilogram (or 681 mL or 23 oz of fluid for each pound) of body weight lost.[22] While the consumption of water (as opposed to a sports drink) creates greater urine losses because of the dilutional effect of water on the blood, slower rates of rehydration, and a potential need for food to replace carbohydrates, sodium, and potassium, it is calorie free. Sports drinks, in contrast, result in faster rehydration rates and less fluid lost to urine, but they do include additional calories. The choice of water versus a sports drink should be determined by caloric need, palatability, and the rate at which rehydration is required.

Although individuals should always strive to hydrate and rehydrate (during and following exercise), it is important to replace both fluids and electrolytes in proportion. Because it is challenging to accurately determine the amounts of electrolytes needed, some simple guidelines can be followed to establish total body water in a balanced ratio with electrolytes:

1. Outside of exercise, drink when thirsty and try to drink smaller volumes when not thirsty. Avoid drinking excessive amounts of water when not feeling thirsty (i.e., forcing large volumes of water).
2. Monitor water needs during exercise. Although many variables influence this amount, determining your water needs via pre- and post-body weight differences is a useful tool. Aim to drink to replace fluid the body loses to sweat and not more (i.e., not gaining weight during the exercise bout).
3. During exercise, make a conscious effort to consume products (food or liquid) that contain sodium; many commercially available sports drinks provide appropriate quantities of sodium. For any event lasting longer than 60 minutes, especially if significant sweat rates are evident (e.g., high-intensity exercise, extremely hot/humid environments), individuals should consume a sports drink that contains electrolytes.

## VIGNETTE *continued*

■ On the morning of her 20-mile training run, Layla recorded her body weight at 135 lb (61.4 kg). During the workout, Layla ran 20 miles over the course of 3 hours, during which she consumed 64 ounces (1.9 L) of water. Enrique recorded her post-workout weight to be 132 lb (60 kg). She lost 2.2% of her body weight during the run, which qualifies as mild dehydration, and her total fluid loss over the 3 hours was 3,300 mL (111.6 oz). Enrique calculated Layla's sweat to be 1,100 mL/hr, or 37.2 oz/hr. Enrique tells Layla that she needs to consume about 37.2 oz of fluid per hour (9.3 oz every 15 minutes) to maintain euhydration during her long training runs and on the day of the marathon.

## ATHLETES AND EATING DISORDERS

Participation in ample physical activity and consumption of a nutrient-dense and healthful diet are defining features of a healthy lifestyle. Oftentimes, athletes are the model citizens of excellent health and nutrition. However, a sizeable number of athletes have taken healthful habits to an extreme such that their behaviors become pathologic and detrimental to overall health and well-being. An **eating disorder** is a severe alteration in eating patterns linked to psychological or emotional factors. Eating disorders are usually more evident in young female athletes, but can affect any segment of the population.

### Anorexia Nervosa

The most well-known of the eating disorders is **anorexia nervosa**. Anorexia nervosa must be diagnosed by a physician using *Diagnostic and Statistics Manual,* 5th ed. (DSM-5). The diagnostic criteria include[35]:

1. Restriction of energy intake leading to a significantly low body weight for age, sex, developmental trajectory, and physical health.
2. Intense fear of gaining weight or becoming fat, or persistent behavior that interferes with weight gain, even though at a significantly low weight.
3. Disturbance in the way in which one's body weight or shape is experienced, undue influence of body weight or shape on self-evaluation, or persistent lack of recognition of the seriousness of the current low body weight.

Anorexia nervosa is further classified into two subtypes:

**Restricting type**: During the past 3 months, the individual has not engaged in recurrent episodes of binge eating or purging behavior (i.e., self-induced vomiting or the misuse of **laxatives**, **diuretics**, or **enemas**).

**Binge-eating/purging type**: During the last 3 months, the individual has engaged in recurrent episodes of binge eating or purging behavior (i.e., self-induced vomiting or the misuse of laxatives, diuretics, or enemas).

This definition is updated from the previous diagnostic criteria that required four strict criteria: refusal to maintain body weight of at least 85% of expected weight, intense fear of gaining weight or becoming fat, body image disturbances including a disproportionate influence of body weight on self-evaluation, and the absence of at least three consecutive menstrual periods (**amenorrhea**).[36]

The causes of anorexia are multifactorial and not fully understood. A combination of genetic predisposition; personality traits of perfectionism and compulsiveness; anxiety; family history of depression and obesity; and peer, cultural, and familial ideals of beauty interact to trigger anorexia in some individuals. The most severe potential consequences of the disorder include osteoporosis, miscarriage, low infant birth weights, abnormalities in cognitive functioning, suicide, and death from starvation or heart arrhythmias.[2,37,38] Although many people with anorexia nervosa are resistant to change and may need inpatient treatment in a psychiatric hospital, full recovery of body weight, growth, menstruation, and normal eating behavior and attitudes regarding food and body shape occurs in 50% to ≥70% of treated adolescents.[37] Only 25% to 50% of adults with anorexia severe enough to require hospitalization fully recover.[37]

### Bulimia Nervosa

Bulimia nervosa is more difficult to identify than anorexia because people with bulimia nervosa are often normal weight or sometimes overweight. Bulimia nervosa is diagnosed when the following criteria are met[35]:

1. Individual has recurrent episodes of **binge eating**. An episode of binge eating is characterized by:
   - Eating, in a discrete period (e.g., within any 2-hour period), an amount of food that is definitely larger than most people would eat during a similar period under similar circumstances; AND
   - A sense of lack of control over eating during the episode (e.g., a feeling that one cannot stop eating or control what or how much one is eating)
2. Recurrent inappropriate compensatory behaviors to prevent weight gain, such as self-induced vomiting; misuse of laxatives, diuretics, or other medications; fasting; or excessive exercise
3. The binge eating and inappropriate compensatory behaviors both occur, on average, at least once per week for 3 months
4. Self-evaluation is unduly influenced by body shape and weight

## Binge Eating Disorder

**Binge eating disorder** falls along the continuum of **disordered eating** with anorexia and bulimia. Binge eating disorder is characterized by repeated overconsumption of large amounts of food in a short period. The condition frequently co-occurs with mental health disorders such as anxiety and depression, and it is highly associated with obesity.[35,39] Some people associate binge eating disorder with **food addiction**, although the physiological basis for each is a source of ongoing research.[2,40]

For the diagnosis of binge eating disorder, the person must meet the following characteristics:

1. Recurrent episodes of binge eating
2. The binge-eating episodes are associated with three (or more) of the following:
   - Eating much more rapidly than normal
   - Eating until feeling uncomfortably full
   - Eating large amounts of food when not feeling physically hungry
   - Eating alone because of feeling embarrassed by how much one is eating
   - Feeling disgusted with oneself, depressed, or very guilty after overeating
3. Marked distress regarding binge eating is present
4. The binge eating occurs, on average, at least once a week for 3 months
5. The binge eating is not associated with the recurrent use of inappropriate compensatory behavior and does not occur exclusively during the course of bulimia nervosa or anorexia nervosa

## V I G N E T T E  continued

■ Layla complains that she has experienced lower energy and decreased performance during her long runs. After further questioning and evaluation, Enrique notes that while Layla began her intensive marathon training program 2 months ago at a weight of 135 lb, at a more recent pre-exercise weight check before a long run, she only weighed 120 lb. Layla reveals that she has not had a menstrual period since she began to intensify her training. While she denies trying to lose weight, Layla is at high risk for the **female athlete triad**.

## Female Athlete Triad

Whether done inadvertently or purposefully, somewhere around 25% of elite female athletes in endurance sports, aesthetic sports, and weight-class sports suffer from disordered eating and some variation of the female athlete triad.[41]

The **female athlete triad** is characterized by **amenorrhea** (at least 3 months without a menstrual period), **osteoporosis** (weakened bones and increased risk for fracture), and disordered eating. The path from optimal health to full manifestation of the triad exists along a continuum; that is, an athlete's eating and activity habits can range from optimal health to severe anorexia nervosa. Her bones can be incredibly strong to extremely frail and fracture prone. She may have regular, monthly menstrual periods or prolonged amenorrhea.

The triad results when an athlete burns more calories than she consumes, creating a state of decreased energy availability. This can happen when an athlete increases her physical activity without appropriately increasing caloric intake or restricting her caloric intake. When this happens, the body attempts to restore energy balance by using less energy for growth, reproduction, and various other important bodily functions. Menstruation halts and hormonal imbalance ensues, which often leads to decreased bone strength and increased risk for fracture.

Athletes at highest risk for low energy availability and manifestation of the triad are those who restrict caloric intake, exercise for prolonged periods, are vegetarian, and limit the types of foods that they will eat. Other risk factors include sport-specific training at an early age, dieting, sports injury, and sudden increase in training volume[41] (also see Chapter 23).

## Preventing Eating Disorders in High-Risk Populations

Health and fitness professionals who work with young people and others at risk for eating disorders play a critically important role in helping to prevent the onset of an obsession with weight, body image, and exercise. The National Eating Disorders Association (http://nationaleatingdisorders.org) offers the following tips for health and fitness professionals to help prevent eating disorders:

- Take warning signs seriously. Box 20-5 lists the signs and symptoms of an eating disorder. If you believe someone may have an eating disorder, share your concerns in an open, direct, and sensitive manner.
- De-emphasize weight. Eliminate comments about weight, especially with those individuals you believe may be at risk for an eating disorder.
- Do not assume that reducing body fat or weight will improve performance.
- Help other health and fitness professionals recognize the signs of eating disorders and be prepared to address them.
- Provide accurate information about weight, weight loss, body composition, nutrition, and sports performance. Have a broad network of referrals (such as physicians, clinical psychologists, and registered dietitians) that may also be able to help your clients when appropriate.

## Box 20-5. Signs and Symptoms of an Eating Disorder

*Anorexia nervosa:* extreme thinness; excessive exercise; fine, soft hair that covers the body; easily broken bones; obsessive behavior; cognitive impairment; depression; low self-esteem; extreme perfectionism; self-consciousness; self-absorption; and ritualistic behavior

*Bulimia nervosa:* "Chubby cheeks" from swollen parotid glands; eroded dental enamel; scars on back of hands from repeated self-induced vomiting; irregular menstruation; loss of normal bowel function; acid reflux; depressed mood; anxiety; alcohol and drug use; low self-esteem; irritability; impulsive spending; shoplifting; sexual impulsivity; and concentration and memory impairments

*Binge eating disorder:* No definitive physical cues; repeated overconsumption of large amounts of food in a short period; mental health disorders such as anxiety and depression; eating when full or not hungry; eating until uncomfortably full; feeling ashamed or guilty about eating habits; feeling isolated; and losing and gaining weight repeatedly (i.e., yo-yo dieting)

Reprinted with permission from Muth, N.D. (2013). *ACE Fitness Nutrition Manual.* San Diego, CA: American Council on Exercise.

---

- Emphasize the health risks of low weight, especially for female athletes with menstrual irregularities (in which case, referral to a physician, preferably one who specializes in eating disorders, is warranted).
- Avoid making any derogatory comments about weight or body composition to or about anyone.
- Do not curtail athletic performance and gym privileges to an athlete or client who is found to have eating problems unless medically necessary. Consider the athlete's physical and emotional health and self-image when deciding how to modify exercise participation level.
- Strive to promote a positive self-image and self-esteem in clients and athletes. Carefully assess your own assumptions and beliefs.

## SPECIAL POPULATIONS, SPORTS NUTRITION, AND PERFORMANCE

Health and fitness professionals work with individual who have different nutritional preferences, restrictions, and limitations. Being familiar with the basics of the most common alternative eating patterns will help these professionals provide the best nutritional guidance, information, and understanding for these clients.

**VIGNETTE** *continued*

■ Layla tells Enrique that she has adopted a vegetarian diet in hopes of leading an overall healthier lifestyle and increasing her vegetable and fruit intake. After inadvertently losing 15 pounds during her training, she makes a conscious effort to consume adequate calories and iron from a varied meat-free diet. With this renewed attention to her eating and focused effort to consume adequate nutrients, her performance and energy level improve.

## Vegetarian Athletes

From the millions of readers buying best-selling books proclaiming the animal-friendly, nutrient-dense, energy-lite plan for weight loss to world-class athletes breaking world records, an increasing number of Americans have adopted vegetarian diets. Elite athletes, including Olympic track star Carl Lewis, tennis champ Martina Navratilova, power lifter Pat Reeves, and ultramarathoner Scott Jurek, have opted to buy in to the vegetarian fanfare. Although in the past it was thought that vegetarian diets might impair athletic performance, scientists, coaches, and athletes alike now agree that with proper planning, the diet can effectively fuel peak performance.

Vegetarian diets come in several forms, all of which are healthful, nutritionally adequate, and effective in disease prevention if carefully planned. A **lacto-ovo-vegetarian** does not eat meat, fish, or poultry, but does consume dairy products and eggs. A **lacto-vegetarian** does not eat eggs, meat, fish, or poultry, but does consume dairy products. A **vegan**, in contrast, does not consume any animal products.

Vegetarian diets provide several health advantages. To start, they are low in saturated fat, cholesterol, and animal protein, and high in fiber, folate, vitamins C and E, carotenoids, and some phytochemicals. Compared with nonvegetarians, vegetarians have lower rates of obesity, death from cardiovascular disease (Fig. 20-10), hypertension, type 2 diabetes, and prostate and colon cancer.[42,43] However, if poorly planned, vegetarian diets may include insufficient amounts of protein, iron, vitamin $B_{12}$, vitamin D, calcium, and other nutrients.[42] These diets also include a variety of mild negative side effects that include increased flatulence because of the increased bean content in the diet and more frequent bowel movements because of the high fiber content.

Although vegetarian diets are capable of providing sufficient energy, some vegetarian athletes may be challenged to eat enough calories to fuel their exercise. Some suggestions to increase caloric intake include eating more frequent meals and snacks, including meat alternatives,

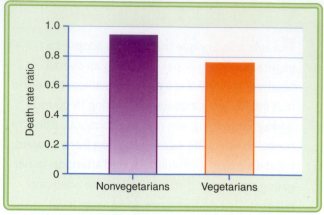

**Figure 20-10.** Mortality from ischemic heart disease has been reported to be 24% lower in vegetarians compared with nonvegetarians (death rate ratio: 0.76 vs. 0.94). Moreover, the lower mortality rates were more pronounced at younger ages and were exclusive to those individuals who maintained their current diet for more than 5 years.

and adding dried fruit, seeds, nuts, and other healthful calorie-dense foods. Although vegetarians do not consume complete proteins unless they eat a lot of soy, flax, chia, and other complete plant-based proteins, vegetarians can assure adequate protein intake if they choose a variety of foods throughout the day.

People are drawn to vegetarian diets for various reasons including weight control (these diets tend to be lower in calories than other eating plans), health benefits (research has shown that vegetarians have reduced risk for diabetes, obesity, hypertension, cardiovascular disease, and some cancers), perceived performance benefits (because of the high carbohydrate content of vegetarian diets), and ethical or philosophical beliefs.[44] Yet, because vegetarian diets are restrictive, people who adhere to these eating plans face potential nutrient deficits including creatine, iron, zinc, vitamin $B_{12}$, calcium, riboflavin, and vitamin D.[44] Some of these deficits can be detrimental to athletic performance. However, with appropriate planning, vegetarian athletes can consume a balanced and complete diet that prepares them for peak performance.

A registered dietitian with a focus on sports nutrition can help clients adopt a well-designed and individualized vegetarian eating plan to fuel optimal health and athletic performance. For reference, following are a few general nutrition guidelines for vegetarian athletes:

- *Ensure adequate carbohydrate and high-quality protein intake.* Because carbohydrates are the preferred energy source during exercise, and vegetarian diets typically contain higher amounts of carbohydrates than omnivorous diets, a vegetarian diet may be an optimal diet for athletes. Most endurance athletes, in particular those who train more than 60 to 90 min/day, are advised to consume a diet that is 60% to 70% carbohydrate to optimize glycogen synthesis. A typical vegetarian

diet parallels that goal with 50% to 65% of calories from carbohydrates.[44] The typical vegetarian diet contains about 10% to 12% of calories from protein, compared with 14% to 18% in omnivorous diets,[44] causing some to worry that vegetarians may be unable to consume adequate amounts of protein to repair damaged muscle and facilitate muscle hypertrophy. Legumes, dried beans, peas, nuts, soy, and meat alternatives provide ample protein, although few vegetarian foods provide all of the essential amino acids, making it necessary for vegetarians to consume a variety of protein-rich plant foods throughout the day to meet protein requirements. Because plant proteins are not as readily digested as animal proteins, vegetarians should consume about 10% more grams of protein than the standard recommendations.[42] That is, if an athlete consumes a 3,000-calorie diet with 10% from protein, approximately 300 calories (75g) are from protein. A vegetarian should consume about 30 extra protein calories (7–8 g), for a total of 330 calories from protein.

- *Consume enough calories.* Athletes have increased energy needs because of the demands of physical activity. Depending on the duration and intensity of exercise, body composition, sex, and training regimen, a typical athlete needs from 2,000 to 6,000 cal/day or more.[44] Although a vegetarian diet can provide sufficient energy to meet these needs, vegetarians need to make special efforts to get enough calories to support optimal performance, maintain lean tissue, and support immune and reproductive functions.[42] Vegetarian athletes can optimize caloric intake if they eat more frequent meals and snacks, include meat alternatives such as tofu and textured vegetable protein, and opt for healthy, calorie-dense snacks such as dried fruit or fruit juice, jams, avocados, nuts, and seeds.

- *Consider creatine supplementation, if peak performance is essential.* Research suggests that those who consume a vegan or other vegetarian diet have decreased total muscle creatine concentration.[44] Muscle creatine stores are important for energy metabolism, in particular for exercises that are short term and high intensity. Vegetarian athletes may be more responsive to creatine supplementation–related improvements in sports performance compared with their meat-eating counterparts.[44] However, remember that a registered dietitian, preferably one with a focus on sports nutrition, or a licensed physician is best equipped to discuss supplementation with an individual.

- *Prevent iron-deficiency anemia.* Iron is a critical nutrient for optimal athletic performance because it is necessary for the synthesis of hemoglobin and myoglobin, iron–protein complexes that deliver oxygen from the lungs to the working muscles. Athletic training combined with low dietary intake can lead to a depletion of iron stores and subsequently hampered athletic performance, although iron-deficiency anemia is rare among vegetarian athletes, affecting only about 10% of them.[44] Vegetarian athletes can prevent anemia by consuming a diet rich in fortified breakfast cereals, bread, textured vegetable protein, legumes, dried beans, soy foods and meat alternatives, nuts, dried fruits, and green leafy vegetables. Vegetarian iron sources are not as well absorbed as their animal counterparts, but absorption can be enhanced with a diet rich in vitamin C.

- *Get enough zinc.* Zinc is important for immune function, protein synthesis, and blood formation. It is readily lost from the body following strenuous exercise, especially in hot, humid environments. Although animal sources provide the most bioavailable zinc, legumes, whole grains, cereals, nuts, and seeds are good sources. Consuming foods rich in vitamin C and soaking beans, grains, and seeds enhances absorption.

- *Eat fortified foods to optimize vitamin B$_{12}$, riboflavin, vitamin D, and calcium intake.* The best sources of each of these nutrients are derived from animal products, dairy products, and eggs. However, vegans can assure adequate amounts from fortified soy products, cereals, and, in the case of calcium, from low-oxalate green vegetables like broccoli, bok choy, and kale. Along with folic acid, vitamin B$_{12}$ is important for the normal metabolism of nerve tissue, protein, fat, and carbohydrate. It is especially important for women of childbearing age to consume enough of the vitamin to prevent neural tube defects in a developing fetus. Riboflavin is an essential nutrient for energy production; the nutrient is stored in muscles and used most in times of muscular fatigue. Vitamin D is necessary for calcium absorption, bone growth, and mineralization. Although necessary for maintaining bone structure and vitamin D metabolism, calcium is also important for blood clotting, nerve transmission, and muscle stimulation.[44] Each of these nutrients makes an important contribution to optimal athletic performance.

## Gluten Sensitivity

A strenuous endurance workout demands careful nutrition planning to optimize athletic performance and minimize the GI distress—cramps, bloating, abdominal pain, and generalized fatigue—that plagues many recreational and elite athletes. In an effort to avoid these unpleasant GI symptoms, many athletes have experimented with adopting a gluten-free diet. **Gluten** is a protein compound made up of two proteins called gliadin and glutenin that are found joined with starch in the grains wheat, rye, and barley. With scientific evidence lacking, the success (or lack of success) of a gluten-free diet in improving athletic performance is theoretical and anecdotal.

Historically (and scientifically), a gluten-free diet only has been considered necessary for people with celiac disease. Celiac disease affects almost 1% of the population and is characterized by an allergic response to gluten-containing foods. Exposure to gliadin—the "toxic" component of gluten for people with celiac disease—causes the body to go into immunological overdrive. One of the consequences is decreased nutrient absorption. When the gut is unable to absorb nutrients, anemia, weight loss, abdominal pain, bloating, diarrhea, and vitamin deficiencies may occur. The only definitive treatment for celiac disease is strict avoidance of gluten-containing foods.

Over the past several years, a growing number of people without diagnosed celiac disease have experimented with gluten-free diets. In some cases, people have adopted the diet in simple protest against the current American culture of overconsumption of heavily processed, nutritionally poor foods, as many fresh, wholesome foods like fruits and vegetables are gluten free. Other people report that symptoms like tiredness, abdominal pain, and diarrhea or constipation are decreased after adopting a gluten-free diet. These people are said to have "gluten sensitivity." Gluten sensitivity is much more common and less understood than celiac disease. It occurs when the body has a pronounced response to gluten-containing foods; it is not clear what causes the symptoms or the body's actual response to the gluten. Anyone with gluten sensitivity should be tested for celiac disease before adopting a gluten-free diet, as tests done after gluten has already been eliminated from the diet are unreliable.[45]

Whether adopting a gluten-free diet affects athletic performance has not been adequately studied to draw any concrete conclusions. Each athlete must weigh what is known about eating for optimal athletic performance with his or her individual experiences and discomforts during strenuous training. For example, many of the best sources of carbohydrate, the body's preferred energy source during intense exercise, contain gluten. Thus, anyone who adopts a gluten-free diet needs to be especially careful to eat enough gluten-free carbohydrates to fuel the exercise session. Fortunately, there are many high-carbohydrate, gluten-free foods to choose from, including rice, corn, soy, potato, tapioca, beans, quinoa, millet, buckwheat, flax, nut flours, and uncontaminated oats. Other inherently gluten-free products include milk, butter, cheese, fruits and vegetables, meat, fish, poultry, eggs, beans, and seeds.

If an athlete experiences GI symptoms during an endurance session, it is important to investigate other potential culprits in addition to (or instead of) gluten. For example, many high-carbohydrate products have large amounts of fiber. Although fiber is a nutrient that most people do not consume in high enough quantities for optimal health, it is also a source of GI discomfort when consumed with or soon before strenuous exercise.

Ultimately, a conscientious and nutrition-savvy athlete could successfully adopt a gluten-free eating plan to meet nutritional needs. It may be helpful to think of a gluten-free diet in the same way as a vegan diet—because the diet is restrictive, people who adhere to the eating plan face potential nutrient deficits that could be detrimental to athletic performance. However, with appropriate planning, both vegan and gluten-free athletes can consume a balanced and complete diet that prepares them for peak performance. A registered dietitian with a focus on sports nutrition can help design an individualized gluten-free eating plan to fuel optimal health and athletic performance.

## Youth Sports Nutrition

A lot of attention has focused on the problem of childhood obesity and inactivity, but there has been little mention of the growing number of highly active children engaged in competitive sports. These youth athletes push themselves physically and mentally to achieve impressive levels of athletic performance. The high training loads create unique nutritional demands. Children are not just "little adults," and the rules of adult sports nutrition do not necessarily apply.

A highly active youth athlete requires first and foremost an adequate number of calories to fuel not only the strenuous exercise regimen but also optimal growth and development. Individuals involved in endurance sports, aesthetic sports like gymnastics and cheerleading, and weight-class sports are at highest risk for not consuming adequate calories. Young athletes can get a general idea of how many calories they need per day based on their age, weight, height, and activity level by referring to the USDA's Supertracker website (http://www.supertracker.usda.gov). The website provides users with an individualized eating plan that can help athletes consume an optimally healthy diet including all of the essential nutrients they need, like iron and calcium, which are deficient in a lot of preteens and teens. This individualized plan will work for most children, although athletes should be sure to let hunger be their guide and choose nutrient-dense meals and snacks to fuel their activity.

Adults are advised to consume a carbohydrate-rich food within 30 minutes of finishing exercise for optimal recovery and then to have an overall increased protein intake to help rebuild muscles, but nutrient recommendations for children are a little less clear. The Recommended Dietary Allowance of carbohydrate for most children is 130 g/day regardless of body weight, totaling 520 calories.[46] Ideally, athletes will get this from a diet rich in whole grains like cereals, rice, and pasta; fruits and vegetables; and limited in simple sugars. This recommended amount is based on the body's need to provide glucose for brain development and does not include the needs for active children to replenish glucose stores. But children metabolize sugars differently than adults, and it is not entirely clear whether and

how much more carbohydrate youth athletes need for optimal performance. Likewise, it is not clear whether children involved in long-distance endurance events benefit from carbohydrate loading the same way adults do. Generally, most young athletes will do well eating a healthy, nutrient-dense diet that contains at least 50% of calories from carbohydrate. As far as protein intake goes, most young athletes will meet their protein needs with the standard recommendation of 0.8 to 1.2 g protein/kg/day. Some athletes may have higher needs, but most will spontaneously increase their caloric and protein intake.[46] Any protein consumed in excess of what the body needs will likely be used as energy or stored as fat.

Driven to excel, many young athletes push through sports practices and games to the point of exhaustion. Although this physical exertion can benefit cardiovascular fitness, a developing competitive spirit, and a child's enjoyment of the game, without appropriate attention to hydration, young athletes can suffer serious consequences, especially when exercising in the heat.

It is commonly taught that children have a more difficult time regulating body temperature than adults, especially in extreme environments like a hot and humid summer day. Consequently, children are taught to pay careful attention to consuming sufficient fluids. Frequently, sports drinks, energy drinks, and other flavored beverages are the young athlete's drink of choice. In one study, more than 50% of adolescents used sports drinks and 42% used sports drinks in the 2 weeks preceding the survey.[47] Although in some cases sports drinks (but not energy drinks) may provide benefits to young athletes, in other cases the reliance on sweetened beverages does little more than negate the health benefits of exercise and contribute to the worldwide problem of childhood obesity.

In an effort to avoid confusion and guide pediatricians, coaches, parents, and young fitness professionals, the American Academy of Pediatrics has published two important articles related to optimal hydration for young athletes: a policy statement on heat stress and exercise[48] and a clinical report on sports drinks and energy drinks for children and adolescents.[49] Following is a brief recap of the major conclusions and recommendations from these reports:

1. Contrary to previous thinking, children do *not* have less effective ability to regulate body temperature and tolerate high levels of physical exertion when exercising in the heat compared with their adult counterparts *as long as they maintain appropriate hydration*. This conclusion is a major departure from the previous caution that children innately have a poor ability to regulate body temperature.

2. Proper hydration is essential for optimal health and athletic performance. Thirst is generally a good guide in determining intake. A more precise method of monitoring hydration status is to weigh the child before and after exercise. The

goal is to avoid weight loss. If weighing is not possible, the AAP suggests that consumption of 100 to 250 mL (approximately 3–8 oz) every 20 minutes for 9- to 12-year-olds and up to 1.0 to 1.5 L (approximately 34–50 oz) per hour for adolescents is sufficient to avoid dehydration, as long as the athlete's prehydration status is good. Fluid needs may differ based on heat and humidity, diet, medications, and illness or chronic health conditions.

3. Most children and adolescents can safely participate in outdoor sports and other physically challenging endeavors in a variety of climates, including warm to hot conditions. However, in addition to ensuring adequate hydration, coaches, parents, and other supervising adults need to ensure the children are allowed sufficient recovery between workouts, same-day training sessions, or rounds of sports competition; that they wear appropriate clothing, uniforms, and protective equipment (when necessary) to not retain excessive heat; and that the adults consider the child's fitness level and gradually (rather than abruptly) increase exercise exertion.

4. Sports drinks play a role in ensuring appropriate hydration and nutrition for optimal performance in combination with water during intense and prolonged exercise lasting more than 1 hour or multiple strenuous workouts in a single day. However, consumption of sports drinks for the average child engaged in routine physical activity or in place of water in the lunchroom or at home can lead to excessive calorie intake and increased risk for overweight and dental problems. This has become an especially widespread problem as sports drinks have replaced soda in school vending machines and cafeterias.

5. Energy drinks—that is, beverages containing caffeine or other supplements in addition to carbohydrate—should be avoided. Although caffeine may provide performance benefits for adults, its effects have not been well studied in children. Furthermore, it is difficult to know the true caffeine content for many drinks. Some may contain as much as 500 mg of caffeine, which is equivalent to about 14 cans of soda. A lethal dose of caffeine is somewhere around 100 to 200 mg/lb body weight (thus the impact of caffeine is most significant for younger and lighter children), but caffeine toxicity can occur at much smaller doses. The guidelines suggest that parents, coaches, and schools should not offer or allow children to drink energy drinks. Energy drinks pose potential health risks mostly because of their stimulant (caffeine) content and are never safe for children.

How can a parent or coach put all of this into action? They can start with a sample meal plan from ChooseMyPlate.gov and divide the recommended types of food into a daily plan based on the athlete's exercise schedule. Pregame meals should be eaten about 1.5 to 3 hours before the event. Easily digestible snacks that are high in carbohydrate and moderate in protein are ideal, such as pasta with ground turkey. A glass of low-fat chocolate milk or a granola bar and an orange are good snacks following a moderately strenuous practice or game. If an all-day tournament is under way, snacks like these, which contain about 200 to 300 calories, spaced throughout the day will help to sustain energy. Fluids should be emphasized throughout the game or practice, and sports drinks might be a good idea for events in warm temperatures that last longer than about an hour. A post-game dinner of pizza loaded with veggies on a whole-grain crust would give an athlete a sufficient number of calories and nutrients to get him or her ready for the next day.

Ultimately, when it comes to youth sports nutrition, the goal is for the athlete to consume enough calories and fluids to fuel the exercise and enough nutrients to meet the body's demands for growth and strength. Additional topics related to exercise in children and adolescents are addressed in Chapter 25.

## VIGNETTE conclusion

■ After 18 weeks of intensive physical training and a concerted effort to optimize nutrition in preparation for a 26.2-mile run, Layla was able to complete the marathon in 3:39:30, achieving her goal. Through the process of working with Enrique, she learned about major sports nutrition principles and carefully planned her pre-, during-, and post-exercise nutrition and hydration. Although she adopted vegetarianism and for a short period consumed inadequate calories to maintain a healthy weight during her strenuous training program, Enrique helped her find the right balance to not only achieve her performance goal, but also improve her overall energy level and health status.

## CRITICAL THINKING QUESTIONS

1. What advice would you give an athletic individual to help minimize the likelihood that she will have GI distress on race day?

2. An endurance cyclist asks you about the benefits and risks of carbohydrate loading. What do you tell him? He also asks you to help him develop a carbohydrate-loading regimen. How do you respond?

3. A client tells you that she read in a magazine that protein supplements help to build increased muscle mass. She asks you if that is true, and if so what supplements you recommend. How do you respond?

4. Your friend recently learned that Scott Jurek, a record-setting ultramarathoner, follows a strictly vegan diet. She tells you that she would like to try a vegetarian diet in hopes of improving her athletic performance and overall health. What are some considerations she should keep in mind?

5. You notice that a client has lost a lot of weight since she has intensified her marathon training program. How might you go about assessing whether she is at risk for the female athlete triad? How might you go about sharing any concerns with this client?

## ADDITIONAL RESOURCES

Casa DJ, Armstrong LE, Hillman SK, et al. National Athletic Trainers' Association (NATA) position statement: Fluid replacement for athletes. *J Athl Train.* 2000;35:212–224.

Clark N. *Nancy Clark's Sports Nutrition Guidebook.* 5th ed. Champaign, IL: Human Kinetics; 2013.

Kerksick C, Harvey H, Stoutm J, et al. International Society of Sports Nutrition position stand: Nutrient timing. *J Int Soc Sports Nutr.* 2008;5:17.

Nattiv A, Loucks AB, Manore MM, Sanborn CF, Sundgot-Borgen J, Warren MP. American College of Sports Medicine position stand. The female athlete triad. *Med Sci Sports Exerc.* 2007;39:1867–1882.

Rodriguez NR, Di Marco NM, Langley S. American College of Sports Medicine position stand. Nutrition and athletic performance. *Med Sci Sports Exerc.* 2009;41:709–731.

Sawka MN, Burke LM, Eichner ER, Maughan RJ, Montain SJ, Stachenfeld NS. American College of Sports Medicine position stand. Exercise and fluid replacement. *Med Sci Sports Exerc.* 2007;39:377–390.

Skolnik H, Chernus A. *Nutrient Timing for Peak Performance.* Champaign, IL: Human Kinetics; 2010.

**Websites**

ChooseMyPlate.gov: http://choosemyplate.gov

Food and Nutrition Center, USDA: http://fnic.nal.usda.gov

National Eating Disorders Association: http://nationaleatingdisorders.org

USDA: http://usda.gov

## REFERENCES

1. Institute of Medicine, National Academy of Sciences, Food and Nutrition Board. *Dietary Reference Intakes.* Washington, DC: The National Academies Press, 2005.

2. Rodriguez NR, DiMarco NM, Langley S; American Dietetic Association; Dietitians of Canada; American College of Sports Medicine: Nutrition and Athletic Performance. Position of the American Dietetic Association, Dietitians of Canada, and the American College of Sports Medicine: Nutrition and athletic performance. *J Am Diet Assoc.* 2009;109:509–527.

3. Katch VL, McArdle WD, Katch FL. *Essentials of Exercise Physiology.* 4th ed. Baltimore, MD: Lippincott Williams & Wilkins; 2011.

4. Skolnik H, Chernus A. *Nutrient Timing for Peak Performance.* Champaign, IL: Human Kinetics; 2010.

5. Widrick JJ, Costill DL, Fink WJ, Hickey MS, McConell GK, Tanaka H. Carbohydrate feedings and exercise performance: Effect of initial muscle glycogen concentration. *J Appl Physiol.* 1993;58:2998–3005.

6. Carter JM, Jeukendrup AE, Jones DA. The effect of carbohydrate mouth rinse on 1-hour cycle time trial performance. *Med Sci Sports Exerc.* 2004;36:2107–2111.

7. Phillips SM. Dietary protein for athletes: From requirements to metabolic advantage. *Appl Physiol Nutr Metab.* 2006;31:647–654.

8. Hayes A, Cribb PJ. Effect of whey protein isolate on strength, body composition and muscle hypertrophy during resistance training. *Curr Opin Clin Nutr Metab Care.* 2008;11:40–44.

9. Gisolfi CV, Wenger CB. Temperature regulation during exercise: Old concepts, new ideas. *Exerc Sport Sci Rev.* 1984;12:339–372.

10. Campbell BI, Spano MA. *NSCA's Guide to Sport and Exercise Nutrition.* Champaign, IL: Human Kinetics; 2011.

11. Gibala MJ. Protein metabolism and endurance exercise. *Sports Med.* 2007;37(4-5):337–340.

12. Kreider RB, Wilborn CD, Taylor L, et al. ISSN exercise & sport nutrition review: Research & recommendations. *J Int Soc Sports Nutr.* 2010;7:7.

13. Nutrition Working Group. Nutrition for athletes: A practical guide for eating for health and performance. Medical Commission of the International Olympic Committee, International Consensus Conference; Lausanne, Switzerland; 2003.

14. Burke LM, Hawley JA, Wong S, Jeukendrup AE. Carbohydrates for training and competition. *J Sports Sci.* 2011; 8:1–11.

15. Thomas DE, Brotherhood JR, Brand JC. Carbohydrate feeding before exercise: Effect of Glycemic Index. *Int J Sports Med.* 1991;12:180–186.

16. Hoek HW, van Hoeken D. Review of the prevalence and incidence of eating disorders. *Int J Eat Disord.* 2003;34:383–396.

17. Murray R. Training the gut for competition. *Curr Sports Med Rep.* 2006;5:161–164.

18. Kerksick C, Harvey H, Stoutm J, et al. International Society of Sports Nutrition position stand: Nutrient timing. *J Int Soc Sports Nutr.* 2008;5:17.

19. Hoswill CA. Effective fluid replacement. *Int J Sports Nutr.* 1998;8:175–195.

20. Karp JR, Johnston JD, Tecklenburg S, Mickleboroughm TD, Fly AD, Stager JM. Chocolate milk as a post-exercise recovery aid. *Int J Sports Nutr Exerc Metab.* 2006;16:78–91.

21. Pritchett, K., Pritchett, R. Chocolate milk: a post-exercise recovery beverage for endurance sports. *Med Sci,* 2012, 59: 127–134.

22. Sawka MN, Burke LM, Eichner ER, Maughan RJ, Montain SJ, Stachenfeld NS. American College of Sports Medicine position stand. Exercise and fluid replacement. *Med Sci Sports Exerc.* 2007;39:377–390.

23. Fink HH, Mikesky AE, Burgoon LA. *Practical Applications in Sports Nutrition.* 3rd ed. Burlington, MA: Jones & Bartlett Learning; 2012.

24. Morimoto T, Miki K, Nose H, Yamada S, Hirakawa K, Matsubara C. Changes in body fluid volumes and its composition during heavy sweating and the effect on fluid and electrolyte replacement. *Jpn J Biometeorol.* 1981;18:31–39.

25. Berardi J, Andrews R. *The Essentials of Sport and Exercise Nutrition.* 2nd ed. Toronto, ON: Precision Nutrition; 2012.

26. Institute of Medicine. *Dietary Reference Intakes: Water, Potassium, Sodium, Chloride, and Sulfate.* Washington, DC: National Academies Press; 2004.

27. National Center for Health Statistics. *National Health and Nutrition Examination Survey.* Atlanta, GA: Centers for Diseases Control and Prevention; 2008.

28. van Rosendal SP, Osborne MA, Fassett RG, Coombes JS. Guidelines for glycerol use in hyperhydration and rehydration associated with exercise. *Sports Med.* 2010;40:113–129.

29. Almond CS, Shin AY, Fortescue EB, et al. Hyponatremia among runners in the Boston Marathon. *New Engl J Med.* 2005;352:1550–1556.

30. Casa DJ, Armstrong LE, Hillman SK, et al. National Athletic Trainers' Association (NATA) position statement: Fluid replacement for athletes. *J Athl Train.* 2000;35:212–224.

31. Grandjean AC, Reimers KJ, Bannick KE, Haven MC. The effect of caffeinated, non-caffeinated, caloric and non-caloric beverages on hydration. *J Am Coll Nutr.* 2000;19:591–600.

32. National Center for Health Statistics. *National Health and Nutrition Examination Survey.* Atlanta, GA: Centers for Diseases Control and Prevention; 2008.

33. Pedersen DJ, Lessard SJ, Coffey VG, et al. High rates of muscle glycogen resynthesis after exhaustive exercise when carbohydrate is coingested with caffeine. *J Appl Physiol.* 2008;105:7–13.

34. Taylor C, Higham D, Close GL, Morton JP. The effect of adding caffeine to postexercise carbohydrate feeding on subsequent high-intensity interval-running capacity compared with carbohydrate alone. *Int J Sport Nutr Exerc Metab.* 2011;21:410–416.

35. American Psychiatric Association. *Diagnostic and Statistical Manual of Mental Disorders.* 5th ed. Washington, DC: American Psychiatric Association; 2013.

36. American Psychiatric Association. *Diagnostic and Statistical Manual of Mental Disorders.* 4th ed. Washington, DC: American Psychiatric Association; 2000.

37. Yager J, Andersen AE. Clinical practice. Anorexia nervosa. *N Engl J Med.* 2005;353:1481–1488.

38. Arcelus J, Mitchell AJ, Wales J, Nielsen S. Mortality rates in patients with anorexia nervosa and other eating disorders. A meta-analysis of 36 studies. *Arch Gen Psychiatry.* 2011;68:724–731.

39. Wonderlich SA, Gordon KH, Mitchell JE, Crosby RD, Engel SG. The validity and clinical utility of binge eating disorder. *Int J Eat Disord.* 2009;42:687–705.

40. Corsica JA, Pelchat ML. Food addiction: True or false? *Curr Opin Gastroenterol.* 2010;26:165–169.

41. Nattiv A, Loucks AB, Manore MM, Sanborn CF, Sundgot-Borgen J, Warren MP. American College of Sports Medicine position stand. The female athlete triad. *Med Sci Sports Exerc.* 2007;39:1867–1882.

42. Craig WJ, Mangels AR. Position of the American Dietetic Association: Vegetarian diets. *J Am Diet Assoc.* 2009;109:1266–1282.

43. Key TJ, Fraser GE, Thorogood M, et al. Mortality in vegetarians and nonvegetarians: Detailed findings from a collaborative analysis of 5 prospective studies. *Am J Clin Nutr.* 1999;70(3 Suppl):516S–524S.

44. Venderley AM, Campbell WW. Vegetarian diets: Nutritional considerations for athletes. *Sports Med.* 2006; 36:293–305.

45. Niewinski MM. Advances in celiac disease and gluten-free diet. *J Am Diet Assoc.* 2008;108:661–672.

46. Nemet D, Eliakim A. Pediatric sports nutrition: An update. *Curr Opin Clin Nutr Metab Care.* 2009;12:304–309.

47. O'Dea JA. Consumption of nutritional supplements among adolescents: Usage and perceived benefits. *Health Educ Res.* 2003;18:98–107.

48. Bergeron MF, Devore C, Rice SG. Policy statement: Climatic heat stress and exercising children and adolescents. *Pediatrics.* 2011;128:e741–e747.

49. American Academy of Pediatrics Committee on Nutrition and the Council on Sports Medicine and Fitness. Sports drinks and energy drinks for children and adolescents: Are they appropriate? *Pediatrics.* 2011;127: 1182–1189.

50. Sedlock DA. The latest on carbohydrate loading: A practical approach. *Curr Sports Med Rep.* 2008;7: 209–213.

51. Nelson JL, Robergs RA. Exploring the potential ergogenic effects of glycerol hyperhydration. *Sports Med.* 2007;37:981–1000.

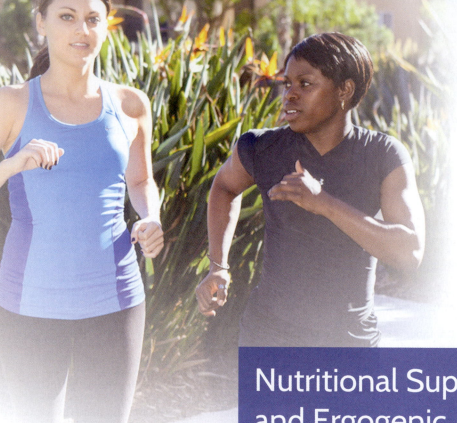

Natalie Digate Muth, MD,
MPH, RD

CHAPTER 21

## Nutritional Supplements and Ergogenic Aids

## CHAPTER OUTLINE

## CHAPTER OUTLINE–cont'd

Scope of Practice
  *Practical Guidelines for Health and Fitness Professionals*
Vignette Conclusion
Critical Thinking Questions
Additional Resources
References

## LEARNING OUTCOMES

1. Define a dietary supplement and what substances are considered dietary supplements.
2. Explain the limitations of dietary supplement regulation in the United States.
3. Describe the product claims, efficacy, and safety of popular, commonly used dietary supplements for weight loss, health, and performance.
4. List the potential harmful effects associated with key dietary supplements.
5. Define the scope of practice for health professionals with regard to the recommendation and sale of dietary supplements.

## ANCILLARY LINK

Visit Davis*Plus* at http://davisplus.fadavis.com for study and practice resources, including online quizzes, animations that help explain physiological processes, podcasts concerning news and career trends in exercise physiology, and practice references.

## VIGNETTE

■ Anne Marie is a 37-year-old advertising executive who is very motivated to continue improving her overall fitness. During the time Anne Marie has worked with her personal trainer (more than one year), she has exceeded her initial fitness goals. Outside of an existing diagnosis of mild hypertension, she is otherwise very healthy but wants to accomplish more–push herself harder, lose weight, and get stronger. In an effort to continue her progress, she asks her personal trainer for advice on nutritional supplements. Given Anne Marie's desire to boost her fitness and performance, her personal trainer suggests a combination of different supplements that he believes will help her achieve her goals. They include:

- Thermadrene, a thermogenic stimulant containing ephedrine
- Yohimbe, an extract of a tree bark that is thought to increase athletic performance
- Whey protein to improve muscle strength
- Essential fatty acids (Omega-3 fatty acids) that can benefit heart health
- Lean-mass enhancement shakes (high-protein meal replacement) consumed twice a day

Anne Marie decides to purchase each of the recommended supplements and begins using them as a complement to her training program.

As a health/fitness professional, do you see any potential concerns regarding the actions of the trainer, that is, when he makes supplement recommendations to his client?

The use of dietary supplements is widespread as individuals at all levels of athleticism strive to improve their overall health, fitness outcomes, and performance. Individuals frequently ask health and fitness professionals for information, guidance and advice on various products. These professionals therefore need to be well informed on dietary supplements and regulations surrounding these products, and be prepared to answer questions or refer clients to qualified professionals when necessary.

## OVERVIEW OF DIETARY SUPPLEMENTS

From multivitamins and herbal supplements to weight-loss pills and muscle boosters, **dietary supplements** comprise a multibillion-dollar industry playing to people's desire to quickly and easily get or stay healthy, lose weight, gain muscle, improve memory, enhance sexual function, and achieve various other desires. This interest has translated into robust retail sales of sports nutrition supplements that have increased at an annual compounded growth rate of approximately 10% since 2005.[1] It is estimated that more than 50% of the adult U.S. population uses some kind of dietary supplement, a figure that has increased from a little more than 40% between 1988 and 1994.[2] However, the use of dietary supplements, in particular, those intended to improve fitness and performance, is more specific to more athletic populations. A study of Finnish Olympic athletes found that 73% of the athletes used some form of a dietary supplement.[3] However, this widespread use is not only limited to the realm of sports, because 84% of all individuals who attend health clubs consider themselves users of some kind of supplements for health, fitness, or performance.[4]

Yet, despite the rising popularity, supplements are not regulated by the U.S. Food and Drug Administration (FDA) like foods and drugs, and therefore are not subject to the same degree of thorough examination. This essentially means there is no guarantee that they are safe, effective, or free of contaminants that may cause potential harm or trouble. It is estimated that approximately 25% of supplements are contaminated with harmful substances such as heavy metals, with the most common contaminate being anabolic steroids.[5] For athletes, taking such products could unknowingly lead to positive drug testing and subsequent disqualification or bans from competition.

## SUPPLEMENT REGULATION

Supplement regulation continues to be an ongoing source of controversy and debate. Whereas foods and drugs are tightly regulated by the FDA, manufacturers of dietary supplements are not required to prove their products are safe, or effective. In fact, they only need to provide reasonable evidence of product safety before bringing new products to market. Unlike new drugs that undergo extensive testing for safety and efficacy before the FDA approves their use, supplement manufacturers have to notify the FDA only 75 days before marketing a new product to the public. Manufacturers are asked to include, with the notification, a statement that the product is thought to be generally safe to the consumer. Beyond that, the FDA does not play a major role in preventing the distribution of fraudulent supplements in the marketplace. It does, however, monitor those supplements that are available to the consumer and investigate those with high suspicion for health or safety threats.

### Dietary Supplement and Health Education Act

In 1994, the **Dietary Supplement Health and Education Act (DSHEA)** was signed into law.[61] In the DSHEA, a dietary supplement was defined as any product other than tobacco that is taken by mouth that contains a dietary ingredient intended to supplement the diet. This may include vitamins, minerals, herbs and other botanicals, amino acids, enzymes, organ tissues, metabolites, extracts, constituents, concentrates, any dietary substance that increases total daily intake, or some combination of the above ingredients.[6] Under DSHEA, dietary supplements in the United States became regulated, in part, as a subset of food by the FDA, which outlined guidelines for product manufacture, claims, and labeling.

The DSHEA does include regulation against the nature of claims on supplement products made by manufacturers where they cannot claim that a supplement can cure, treat, or mitigate symptoms of a disease. For example, a claim that "glucosamine may support joint health" is legal, whereas a therapeutic claim such as "glucosamine cures osteoarthritis" is not.

Certain types of claims are permissible on supplements. These include:
- Nutrient content claim (e.g., this supplement contains as much calcium as a glass of milk)
- Structural claim (e.g., calcium builds strong bones)
- Functional claim (e.g., calcium can help reduce losses in bone strength and reduce the risk for fractures)

Alongside any claim, though, the manufacturer must also include a disclaimer that "This statement has not been evaluated by the Food and Drug Administration. This product is not intended to diagnose, treat, cure, or prevent any disease."[7] Box 21-1 differentiates between structure/function and disease claims.

Nonetheless, false claims and misleading advertising remain rampant. Supplement manufacturers often flood the market, making assertions without proof that their products work as claimed. In the United States, the Federal Trade Commission works in collaboration with the FDA to identify false advertising and hold companies accountable for deceptive advertising of dietary supplements. To date, the Federal Trade Commission has filed numerous complaints against companies regarding their supplement claims.[6]

## Box 21-1. Examples of Structure/Function Versus Disease Claims

**FDA Approval Not Needed (Structure/Function Claim)**

- Enhances muscle tone or size.
- Improves memory.
- Supports the immune system.
- Arouses sexual desire.
- Boosts stamina.
- Promotes relaxation.
- Calcium builds strong bones.
- Fiber maintains bowel regularity.
- Antioxidants maintain cell integrity.

**FDA Approval Needed (Disease Health Claim)**

- Lowers cholesterol.
- Suppresses appetite to treat overweight or obesity.
- Provides relief of chronic constipation.
- Helps relieve persistent heartburn or acid indigestion.
- Retains healthy lung function in smokers.
- Diets low in sodium may reduce the risk for high blood pressure, a disease that is associated with many factors.
- Diets low in saturated fat and cholesterol that include 25 g/day soy protein may reduce the risk for heart disease.

*Source:* U.S. Food and Drug Administration.[8,9]

The DSHEA also requires supplements to contain an ingredient label including the name and quantity of each dietary ingredient (Fig. 21-1) and requires that such products be identified as "dietary supplements."

Safety standards provide that the Secretary of the Department of Health and Human Services may declare that a supplement poses imminent risk or hazard to public safety. A supplement is considered *adulterated* if it or one of its ingredients presents a "significant or unreasonable risk of illness or injury" when used as directed, or under normal conditions. It may also be considered adulterated if too little information is known about the risk of an unstudied ingredient. The FDA does have the authority to remove a product from the market if the product presents an unreasonable risk for causing illness or injury when used as directed, but the FDA holds the burden of proof for doing so. Frequent reports of adverse events trigger investigation by the FDA, as was the case when the sale of ephedrine (also ephedra and ma huang) was banned in 2004.[10] Portions of the ban were struck down by a federal court, and the law currently allows ephedrine supplements containing less than 10 mg to be sold in the United States. However, individual states including New York and California still prohibit the sale of this supplement.

Overall, although the DSHEA was intended to help protect consumers, the safety and legitimacy of any supplement cannot be assumed. With little federal accountability or oversight, many savvy product manufacturers and marketing experts have found ingenious ways to get around many of the rules. Box 21-2 offers a strategy to help protect consumers from experiencing harm from supplements.

## Current Good Manufacturing Practices

In June 2007, the FDA issued regulations that require **Current Good Manufacturing Practices (CGMPs)** for dietary supplements.[6] CGMPs ensure that dietary supplements made in the United States and abroad are consistently produced and of acceptable quality. The CGMPs apply to all companies that test, produce, package, label, and distribute supplements in the United States. The CGMPs include regulations related to the following:

- Design and construction of physical plants that facilitate maintenance
- Cleaning

## RESEARCH HIGHLIGHT

### Advertising Claims on Sports Performance Supplements

Researchers analyzed print advertisements in 92 health, fitness, and sports-related consumer magazines and 1,035 web pages making claims on sports performance supplements. Of the 431 performance-enhancing claims made for 104 different products, 52.8% of the web pages provided no references. Furthermore, researchers identified only 146 references cited that appeared to support the claims but could critically review only 74 of these references as they were published. Based on the quality of the research (i.e., methodology—sample size, randomized protocol, human vs. animal studies), the researchers concluded that only 3 of the 74 studies (2.7%) were judged to be of high quality. The takeaway message was that the evidence used to support supplement claims is often poor at best, and improvements are needed in the quality and reporting of research.

Heneghan C, Howick J, O'Neil B, et al. The evidence underpinning sports performance products: a systematic assessment. *BMJ Open.* 2012:2:e001702.

Dietary supplement of amino acids:

# Supplement Facts

Serving Size 1 Tablet

Amount Per Tablet

| | |
|---|---|
| Calories | 15 |
| Isoleucine (as L-isoleucine hydrochloride) | 450 mg* |
| Leucine (as L-leucine hydrochloride) | 620 mg* |
| Lysine (as L-lysine hydrochloride) | 500 mg* |
| Methionine (as L-methionine hydrochloride) | 350 mg* |
| Cystine (as L-cystine hydrochloride) | 200 mg* |
| Phenylalanine (as L-phenylalanine hydrochloride) | 220 mg* |
| Tyrosine (as L-tyrosine hydrochloride) | 900 mg* |
| Threonine (as L-threonine hydrochloride) | 300 mg* |
| Valine (as L-valine hydrochloride) | 650 mg* |

*Daily Value not established

Other ingredients: Cellulose, lactose, and magnesium stearate.

### What must be included in a supplement label?

**General information**
- Name of product (including the word "supplement" or a statement that the product is a supplement)
- Amount of contents
- Name and place of business of manufacturer, packer, or distributor
- Directions for use

**Supplement facts panel**
- Serving size, list of dietary ingredients, amount per serving size (by weight), percent of Daily Value (%DV), if established
- If the dietary ingredient is a botanical, the scientific name of the plant or the common or usual name
- If the dietary ingredient is a proprietary blend (a blend exclusive to the manufacturer), the total weight of the blend in order of predominance by weight

**Other ingredients**
- Non-dietary ingredients such as fillers, artificial colors, sweeteners, flavors, or binders; listed by weight in descending order of predominance and by common name or proprietary blend

**Figure 21-1.** The Dietary Supplement Health and Education Act (DSHEA) requires supplements to contain an ingredient label.

- Proper manufacturing operations
- Quality-control procedures
  - Testing final products or testing incoming materials
  - Handling consumer complaints
  - Maintaining records

All companies were required to be in compliance with the CGMPs by mid-year 2010. The benefits to the consumer include assurance that supplements are of acceptable quality and accurately labeled, and are of consistent identity, purity, strength, and composition. The CGMPs do not address supplement safety or their effect on health. The major goals of the CGMPs are to prevent:
- Imprecise dosages of ingredients
- Wrong ingredients

## Box 21-2. Key Points to Ponder When Considering Supplement Use

- **Think twice about chasing the latest headline.** Sound health advice is generally based on research over time, not a single study. Be wary of results that claim a "quick fix" that depart from scientific research and established dietary guidance. Keep in mind that science does not generally proceed by dramatic breakthroughs, but rather by taking many small steps, slowly building toward scientific agreement.
- **We may think,** *Even if a product may not help me, at least it won't hurt me.* **It is best not to assume that this will always be true.** Some product ingredients, including nutrients and plant components, can be toxic based on their activity in your body. Some products may become harmful when consumed in high enough amounts, for a long enough time, or in combination with certain other substances.
- **The term *natural* does not always mean safe.** Do not assume this term assures wholesomeness or that these products have milder effects, making them safer to use than prescribed drugs. For example, many weight-loss products claim to be "natural" or "herbal," but this does not necessarily make them safe. The product's ingredients may interact with drugs or may be dangerous for people with certain medical conditions.
- **Spend your money wisely.** Some supplement products may be expensive and may not work, given your specific condition. Be wary of substituting a product or therapy for prescription medicines. Be sure to talk with your health-care team to help you determine what is best for your overall health.
- **Remember: safety first.** Resist the pressure to decide "on the spot" about trying an untested product or treatment. Ask for more information and consult your doctor, nurse, registered dietitian, pharmacist, and/or caregiver about whether the product is right for you and safe for you to use.

*Source:* U.S. Food and Drug Administration.[11]

- Contaminants (e.g., bacteria, pesticide, glass, lead)
- Foreign material in a dietary supplement container
- Improper packaging
- Mislabeling[12]

## Monitoring Systems

Several nongovernmental organizations implement monitoring systems to help ensure compliance with FDA regulations. The U.S. Pharmacopeia (USP) is a nonprofit organization that offers a set of guidelines for the quality, purity, strength, manufacturing practices, and ingredients in dietary supplement products. Dietary supplement manufacturers can choose to voluntarily subject their products to USP testing. If the supplement passes the testing, the manufacturer is authorized to display the USP symbol on its labels. ConsumerLab.com also offers supplement testing and is a ready source of supplement information for subscribers.

For athletes, taking such products could unknowingly lead to positive drug testing and subsequent disqualification or bans from competition. Fortunately, institutions such as the National Sanitation Foundation (NSF), which was originally founded to standardize sanitation and food safety, has expanded into the supplement industry. NSF provides independent screening of supplements for banned substances (steroids, stimulants, hormones, etc.) for consumer assurance and monitors manufacturing facilities for compliance with the FDA's Good Manufacturing Practices (GMPs). NSF's certification service includes product testing, GMPs inspections, and ongoing monitoring. Supplements that pass NSF testing may be eligible for NSF certification, a recognizable "seal of approval" (access the NSF website for more information: www.nsf.org). Therefore, an individual purchasing a supplement that contains the NSF mark can be assured that a standard of quality has been met and that the product is free of potential contaminants that might be of concern. Sports organizations such as Major League Baseball (MLB), the National Football League (NFL), the National Collegiate Athletic Association (NCAA), and their players associations have partnered with companies like the nonprofit NSF International that test and certify dietary supplements.

## VIGNETTE *continued*

■ After taking the recommended supplements for about 3 months, Anne Marie collapses during an early-morning workout. She is rushed to the hospital, but by late evening she is pronounced dead from a massive brain hemorrhage. After investigation, the ephedra-containing Thermadrene is believed to be the most likely culprit. The Chinese botanical ma huang, also known as ephedra, reduces appetite, but also is associated with significant life-threatening adverse effects, including dangerously increased blood pressure, heart attacks, seizure, stroke, and serious psychiatric illness.[13] Anne Marie's pre-existing hypertension combined with physical exertion and ephedra use presumably predisposed her to the massive brain hemorrhage that ultimately took her life.[14]

## In Your Own Words

Given what you have just read about supplement regulation and considering the popularity of supplements, how would you respond to a friend who asked your opinion on taking supplements?

## WEIGHT-LOSS SUPPLEMENTS

With millions of Americans following some form of a diet at any given time, it is not surprising that weight-loss supplements are so popular. Supplement marketers skillfully depict these products as a "quick fix" and a surefire way to lose unwanted weight. Manufacturers claim their supplements help the body lose fat, enhance metabolism, suppress appetite, and promote weight loss, sometimes without any need to significantly change physical activity or dietary intake. A popular group of weight-loss supplements is termed "thermogenic," implying *increased production of heat in the body*. The claim is that thermogenic products alter metabolism in a way that causes the body to use more energy. The reality is that these claims are largely unsubstantiated, and these supplements are poorly regulated and potentially harmful. Most weight-loss supplements contain several ingredients including herbs and botanicals, vitamins, minerals, and sometimes caffeine or laxatives. These chemicals can interact with other medication and/or supplements, causing harmful consequences. The reality is that anyone considering using a weight-loss supplement should discuss this first with his or her physician, especially if the person is taking prescription or over-the-counter medications or other supplements.

Table 21-1 highlights the characteristics of some of the most commonly used weight-loss substances, although the list is far from exhaustive. Health and fitness professionals should feel confident in sharing this information with individuals, but should also direct clients to their primary care physician for further discussion of whether it is safe for a client to consume any of these supplements.

## DIETARY SUPPLEMENTS FOR HEALTH

From vitamins and minerals to proteins, essential fatty acids, and various herbs, many supplements make health-related claims that are unsubstantiated. Although some actually provide some health benefits, supplements should not be considered a substitute for a healthy diet. Whole foods offer many important health and nutritional benefits that are not offered by dietary supplements, such as providing rich sources of a variety of important nutrients (rather than just one) like health-promoting fiber and **phytochemicals** (naturally occurring protective substances that may help protect against myriad diseases and conditions). Whereas a healthy, balanced diet rarely results in individuals over- or under-consuming important vitamins

## Table 21-1. Weight-Loss Supplements

| PRODUCT | CLAIM | EFFECTIVENESS | SAFETY |
|---|---|---|---|
| Alli, over-the-counter version of prescription drug orlistat (Xenical) | Decreases fat absorption | Effective, though weight-loss usually less for OTC versus prescription | FDA is investigating reports of liver injury |
| Bitter orange | Weight loss, among other health claims | Insufficient evidence to confirm health benefit | Similar to ephedra, and insufficient information to confirm if safer |
| Conjugated linoleic acid (CLA) | Reduces body fat and builds muscle | Possibly effective | Possibly safe |
| Ephedra | Decreases appetite | Possibly effective | Likely unsafe and is banned by FDA |
| Green tea extract | Increases calorie and fat metabolism, and decreases appetite | Insufficient reliable evidence to rate | Possibly safe |
| Human chorionic gonadotropin (HCG) | "Reset metabolism" and change "abnormal eating patterns" | No evidence that increases weight loss beyond caloric restriction (which pill manufacturers typically advise in conjunction with pill) | Sold illegally with unsubstantiated claims, target of FDA investigation |
| Hoodia | Decreases appetite | Insufficient reliable evidence to rate | Insufficient information |

FDA, U.S. Food and Drug Administration; OTC, over-the-counter.
*Source:* National Center for Complementary and Alternative Medicine website: http://nccam.nih.gov/health

and minerals, this is more likely with a supplement that sometimes includes megadoses of one or various nutrients that may prove harmful. Thus, although some supplements may benefit overall health, others may do harm in some way that is not yet fully understood.

The exotic fruit juice industry is one example where the supplement industry is experiencing a boom with a growing list of hard-to-pronounce, antioxidant-rich, high-priced "super-fruit" juices lining health food shelves and popping up in Internet ads. These exotic juices proclaim promises of improved health, but the reality is that little human research has been done to support or reject these claims. Some of the most phytochemical-rich fruits are outlined in Table 21-2.

## Vitamin and Mineral Supplements for Health

Clients who have been paying attention to the latest research on vitamins may be wondering whether these nutritional supplements are worthwhile and may find the information confusing. Physicians, scientists, dietitians, and other health professionals have long touted

## Table 21-2. Supplement-Inspiring Fruits

| FRUIT | ORIGIN | NUTRIENTS | CLAIMS | EVIDENCE FROM HUMAN STUDIES |
|---|---|---|---|---|
| Pomegranate | Mediterranean, India, Israel, China, Japan, Russia, Afghanistan, United States (California and Arizona) | Highest concentration of antioxidants, specifically ellagitannins and anthocyanins | Decreased risk for cardiovascular disease, decreased periodontal disease, decreased erectile dysfunction | All from small studies: improved blood flow in men with cardiovascular disease,[15] reduced atherosclerosis and blood pressure,[16] improved cholesterol,[17] no effect on erectile dysfunction |

## Table 21-2. Supplement-Inspiring Fruits–cont'd

| FRUIT | ORIGIN | NUTRIENTS | CLAIMS | EVIDENCE FROM HUMAN STUDIES |
|---|---|---|---|---|
| Acai (ah-SIGH-ee) | Brazil | Antioxidants, monounsaturated fat, 19 amino acids, dietary fiber, phytosterols, many vitamins and minerals | Removes wrinkles, cleanses body of toxins, quickens weight loss | Two small studies showed increased serum antioxidant capacity after consumption of acai juice[18,19] |
| Goji berries (Go-jee) | China | Antioxidants beta-carotene and lycopene, 19 amino acids, 21 trace minerals, protein, high vitamin C, vitamin E, essential fatty acids (in seeds) | Varied including: anti-aging; prevention and treatment of cancer, diabetes, arthritis, and digestive problems; and weight loss | One small study paid for and conducted by a company that sells goji juice reported increased feelings of well-being, reduced fatigue and stress, and improved regularity of gastrointestinal function after 15 days of 4 oz. goji juice daily[20] |
| Mangosteen | Southeast Asia/ India | Xanthone antioxidant, otherwise lacking in vitamin and mineral content | Maintain intestinal health, neutralize free radicals, support cartilage and joint function, promote healthy seasonal respiratory system, and myriad traditional medicinal properties | One human study in 1932 showed benefit in treating dysentery in Singapore[21] |
| Noni (NO-knee) | Tropical Asia, Pacific islands | "Mystery ingredients"; a small amount of vitamins and minerals, moderate antioxidant potency | Boosts your immune system, delivers superior antioxidants, increases energy and physical performance, and many users believe it helps to cure cancer | None found |

the importance of getting enough of these nutrient powerhouses, and for many this came in the form of a daily tablet or two. However, the latest research, which has mostly been done to evaluate whether megadoses of vitamins offer additional benefits, has largely been disappointing.

A study of 15,000 physicians from the Physician's Health Study found no difference in heart disease in men taking vitamins E and C compared with those taking placebo[22] (Fig. 21-2). Another study failed to show that vitamin E and selenium supplements change the risk for development of prostate cancer in older men,[23] and other research has shown that mega-doses of vitamins may actually be harmful.[24,25] An analysis of randomized

controlled trials (the gold standard in research design) studying the role of **antioxidants** in disease found that people who take antioxidant supplements, especially vitamin A, beta carotene, and vitamin E, had higher mortality rates, whereas vitamin C and selenium supplements seemed to provide no benefit or harm.[26]

Contemporary research now shows exercise-induced reactive oxygen species (ROS) mediates a number of the key health benefits accrued from exercise training. For example, it has been shown that exercise-induced ROS production decreases insulin resistance and causes a beneficial adaptive response promoting natural antioxidant defense capacity.[27] However, blocking exercise-dependent formation of ROS with the

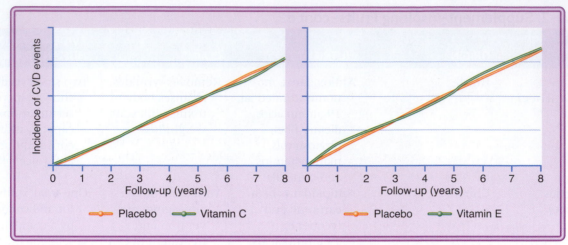

**Figure 21-2.** During a mean follow-up of 8 years, neither vitamin C nor vitamin E supplementation was reported to reduce the incidence of cardiovascular events in a long-term trial of male physicians. Accordingly, it was concluded that there was no evidence to support the use of supplements for cardiovascular disease prevention in men.

ingestion of antioxidant supplements abolishes the health-promoting effects of exercise (Fig. 21-3).

Overall, most studies have shown no significant association between vitamin supplements and improved health, with few exceptions including folic acid supplementation in pregnant women and calcium in the prevention of recurrent precancerous colon polyps. In addition, researchers are continuing to investigate whether vitamin D supplementation might help ward off a variety of health conditions, but thus far, conclusive research is lacking.[28]

Many athletes suffer from iron deficiency because of inadequate intake or excessive iron losses that can occur with exercise. Iron is necessary for optimal oxygen delivery to working cells. When iron levels decrease, aerobic athletic performance falters. Some athletes may require iron supplementation to restore normal levels. However, this should be discussed with a registered dietitian or physician.

Ultimately, if individuals consume a balanced enough diet, it is safe to assume that they are ingesting adequate vitamins and minerals to prevent any nutritional deficiency, and thus do not need vitamin or mineral supplementation (Tables 21-3 and 21-4 outline the recommended amounts and best food sources of vitamins and minerals, respectively). Clients who suspect that they may suffer from a nutritional deficiency should discuss this matter with a qualified professional to determine whether supplementation beyond a multivitamin is advantageous.

## Macronutrient Supplements for Health

Generally, individuals consume macronutrient supplementations such as whey protein or essential fatty acids to improve performance, but some are consumed to improve overall health.

### Protein Supplements

The most common reason cited for protein supplementation is to enhance muscular growth and strength. The rationale for taking protein supplements to gain a

## RESEARCH HIGHLIGHT

### Multivitamins, Disease, and Mortality

In a study from the Women's Health Initiative clinical trials, 161,808 participants were followed for approximately 8 years. The investigation examined individuals on hormone therapy, dietary modification, and calcium and vitamin D supplements. The study documented the incidence of cancers of the breast, colon/rectum, endometrium, kidney, bladder, stomach, ovary, and lung; cardiovascular diseases (CVDs) such as myocardial infarction, stroke, and venous thromboembolism; and total mortality. Results reported that 41.5% of the participants used multivitamins. When rates of cancers, CVD, and overall mortality were analyzed statistically, the study provided convincing evidence that multivitamin use had little or no influence on reducing the risk for common cancers, CVD, or total mortality in postmenopausal women.

Neuhouser ML, Wassertheil-Smoller S, Thomson C, et al. Multivitamin use and risk of cancer and cardiovascular disease in the Women's Health Initiative cohorts. *Arch Intern Med.* 2009;169:294–304.

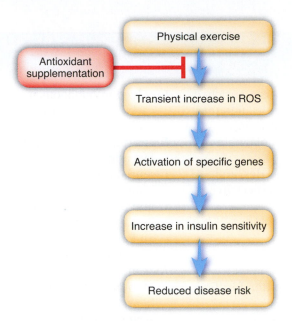

**Figure 21-3.** Exercise-induced reactive oxygen species (ROS) mediates a number of the key health benefits accrued from exercise training.

competitive edge is discussed in the Performance-Enhancing Supplements section later in this chapter.

Individuals may also take protein supplements to improve general health. For example, many people consume soy protein supplements because they believe this protein form to be good for their health. Soy isolates are 90% protein and contain some isoflavones (phytoestrogens that mimic estrogen function), albeit less than in regular soy. They are highly digestible and easily added to sports drinks, health beverages, and infant formulas.[29] Early studies suggested that isolated soy protein might reduce low-density lipoprotein cholesterol and blood pressure, potentially protect against breast cancer, maintain bone density, and decrease menopausal symptoms.[30] Given what seemed to be compelling evidence of benefit, the FDA approved labeling for food containing soy protein as protective against heart disease in 1999. Shortly thereafter, the American Heart Association (AHA) released a statement concluding that "it is prudent to recommend including soy protein foods in a diet low in saturated fat and cholesterol."[30] Food manufacturers and grocery

## Table 21-3. Vitamin Facts

| VITAMIN | RDI/AI* | | BEST SOURCES | FUNCTIONS |
|---|---|---|---|---|
| | MEN[†] | WOMEN[†] | | |
| A (carotene) | 900 mcg | 700 mcg | Yellow or orange fruits and vegetables, green leafy vegetables, fortified oatmeal, liver, dairy products | Formation and maintenance of skin, hair, and mucous membranes; helps people see in dim light; bone and tooth growth |
| B$_1$ (thiamine) | 1.2 mg | 1.1 mg | Fortified cereals and oatmeal, meats, rice and pasta, whole grains, liver | Helps the body release energy from carbohydrates during metabolism; growth and muscle tone |
| B$_2$ (riboflavin) | 1.3 mg | 1.1 mg | Whole grains, green leafy vegetables, organ meats, milk, eggs | Helps the body release energy from protein, fat, and carbohydrates during metabolism |
| B$_5$ (pyridoxine) | 1.3 mg | 1.3 mg | Fish, poultry, lean meats, bananas, prunes, dried beans, whole grains, avocados | Helps build body tissue and aids in metabolism of protein |
| B$_{12}$ (cobalamin) | 2.4 mcg | 2.4 mcg | Meats, milk products, seafood | Aids cell development, functioning of the nervous system, and the metabolism of protein and fat |
| Biotin | 30 mcg | 30 mcg | Cereal/grain products, yeast, legumes, liver | Involved in metabolism of protein, fats, and carbohydrates |
| Choline | 550 mg | 425 mg | Milk, liver, eggs, peanuts | A precursor of acetylcholine; essential for liver function |
| Folate (folacin, folic acid) | **400 mcg** | **400 mcg‡** | Green leafy vegetables, organ meats, dried peas, beans, lentils | Aids in genetic material development; involved in red blood cell production |

*Continued*

## Table 21-3. Vitamin Facts–cont'd

| VITAMIN | RDI/AI* | | BEST SOURCES | FUNCTIONS |
| | MEN† | WOMEN† | | |
| --- | --- | --- | --- | --- |
| Niacin | **16 mg** | **14 mg** | Meat, poultry, fish, enriched cereals, peanuts, potatoes, dairy products, eggs | Involved in metabolism of carbohydrates, protein, and fat |
| Pantothenic acid | 5 mg | 5 mg | Lean meats, whole grains, legumes | Helps release energy from fats and vegetables |
| C (ascorbic acid) | **90 mg** | **75 mg** | Citrus fruits, berries, and vegetables—especially peppers | Essential for structure of bones, cartilage, muscle, and blood vessels; helps maintain capillaries and gums and aids in absorption of iron |
| D | 5 mcg | 5 mcg | Fortified milk, sunlight, fish, eggs, butter, fortified margarine | Aids in bone and tooth formation; helps maintain heart action and nervous system function |
| E | **15 mg** | **15 mg** | Fortified and multigrain cereals, nuts, wheat germ, vegetable oils, green leafy vegetables | Protects blood cells, body tissue, and essential fatty acids from harmful destruction in the body |
| K | 120 mcg | 90 mcg | Green leafy vegetables, fruit, dairy, grain products | Essential for blood-clotting functions |

*Recommended Daily Allowances (RDAs) are presented in boldface; adequate intakes (AIs) are not in boldface.
†RDAs and AIs given are for men aged 31–50 years and nonpregnant, nonlactating women aged 31–50 years.
‡This is the amount women of childbearing age should obtain from supplements or fortified foods.
*Source:* Reprinted with permission from Dietary Reference Intakes (various volumes). Copyright 1997, 1998, 2000, 2001 by the National Academy of Sciences. Courtesy of the National Academies Press, Washington, DC.

## Table 21-4. Mineral Facts

| MINERAL | RDI/AI* | | BEST SOURCES | FUNCTIONS |
| | MEN† | WOMEN† | | |
| --- | --- | --- | --- | --- |
| Calcium | 1,000 mg | 1,000 mg | Milk and milk products | Strong bones, teeth, muscle tissue; regulates heartbeat, muscle action, and nerve function; blood clotting |
| Chromium | 35 mcg | 25 mcg | Corn oil, clams, whole-grain cereals, brewer's yeast | Glucose metabolism (energy); increases effectiveness of insulin |
| Copper | 900 mcg | 900 mcg | Oysters, nuts, organ meats, legumes | Formation of red blood cells; bone growth and health; works with vitamin C to form elastin |
| Fluoride | 4 mg | 3 mg | Fluorinated water, teas, marine fish | Stimulates bone formation; inhibits or even reverses dental caries |
| Iodine | 150 mcg | 150 mcg | Seafood, iodized salt | Component of hormone thyroxine, which controls metabolism |
| Iron | 8 mg | 18 mg | Meats, especially organ meats, legumes | Hemoglobin formation; improved blood quality; increases resistance to stress and disease |

## Table 21-4. Mineral Facts—cont'd

| MINERAL | RDI/AI*  MEN[†] | WOMEN[†] | BEST SOURCES | FUNCTIONS |
|---------|------|--------|--------------|-----------|
| Magnesium | 420 mg | 320 mg | Nuts, green vegetables, whole grains | Acid–alkaline balance; important in metabolism of carbohydrates, minerals, and sugar (glucose) |
| Manganese | 2.3 mg | 1.8 mg | Nuts, whole grains, vegetables, fruits | Enzyme activation; carbohydrate and fat production; sex hormone production; skeletal development |
| Molybdenum | 45 mcg | 45 mcg | Legumes, grain products, nuts | Functions as a cofactor for a limited number of enzymes in humans |
| Phosphorus | 700 mg | 700 mg | Fish, meat, poultry, eggs, grains | Bone development; important in protein, fat, and carbohydrate utilization |
| Potassium | 4,700 mg | 4,700 mg | Lean meat, vegetables, fruits | Fluid balance; controls activity of heart muscle, nervous system, and kidneys |
| Selenium | 55 mcg | 55 mcg | Seafood, organ meats, lean meats, grains | Protects body tissues against oxidative damage from radiation, pollution, and normal metabolic processing |
| Zinc | 11 mg | 8 mg | Lean meats, liver, eggs, seafood, whole grains | Involved in digestion and metabolism; important in development of reproductive system; aids in healing |

*Recommended Daily Allowances are presented in boldface; adequate intakes (AIs) are not presented in boldface.
†RDAs and AIs given are for men aged 31–50 years and nonpregnant, nonlactating women aged 31–50 years.
*Source:* Reprinted with permission from Dietary Reference Intakes (various volumes). Copyright 1997, 1998, 2000, 2001 by the National Academy of Sciences. Courtesy of the National Academies Press, Washington, DC.

stores eagerly diversified soy product offerings (including various forms of soy supplements and additives), and consumers readily boosted their soy consumption. Shortly thereafter, following a comprehensive review of current scientific research, the Nutrition Committee of the AHA released an updated statement in 2006, concluding that "the direct cardiovascular benefit of soy protein or isoflavone supplements is minimal at best."[31] The authors of this statement recommended against use of soy protein isolates (with isoflavones) in foods or pills, but did continue to encourage consumption of *whole* soy products such as tofu, soy burgers, and soy nuts, which contain high levels of nonprotein nutrients including heart-healthy polyunsaturated fats, fiber, vitamins, and minerals, and low levels of saturated fat.[31]

The scientific research on soy protein and isoflavones continues to evolve, with mostly conflicting findings. Once again, American consumers are left in the familiar situation of not knowing what evidence to believe.

### Essential Fatty Acids

Although omega-3 and omega-6 fatty acids and healthy ratios of each are discussed in detail in Chapter 3, this section also addresses these fatty acids because of their relevance as a health supplement. The numerous health benefits of omega-3 essential fatty acids have gained popularity recently among consumers. Savvy food manufacturers and marketers have managed to add these fatty acids to a variety of foods and offer a variety of omega-3 supplements. The reasons driving consumer interest may be associated with a growing body of research[32] and media attention suggesting that omega-3 and healthy omega-6 fatty acids offer numerous health benefits, including decreased risk for heart disease by reducing cholesterol and triglyceride levels, while reducing blood clotting and dilating blood vessels (Fig. 21-4). They are also known to reduce inflammation associated with many autoimmune inflammatory diseases such as colitis. Furthermore, they are important for healthy eye and brain development (especially important for a growing fetus in the late stages of pregnancy and in young children), and can reduce disabilities related to mental illnesses.[32]

Notably, most Americans do not consume enough omega-3 fatty acids in their diets. Although natural food sources such as egg yolk and cold-water fish like

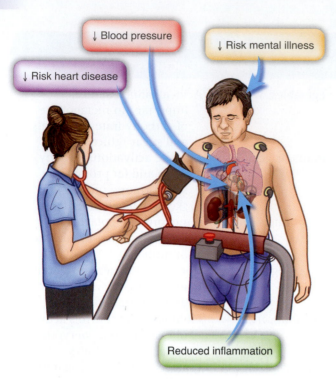

↓ Blood pressure

↓ Risk mental illness

↓ Risk heart disease

Reduced inflammation

**Figure 21-4.** Various health benefits have been linked to omega-3 fatty acid intake, including decreased risk for heart disease, reduced inflammation, healthy eye and brain development, and reduced disabilities related to mental illnesses.

tuna, salmon, mackerel, cod, crab, shrimp, and oyster are all rich sources of these fatty acids, some evidence suggests that people who do not eat sufficient omega-3 may benefit from supplementation or from fortified foods. In fact, many cardiologists recommend that their patients take "fish oils" to supplement the low quantities normally consumed through their diets.

Although there is no established Dietary Reference Intake (DRI) that is considered optimal for omega-3,

some expert panels have recommended an intake between 250 and 500 mg/day.[33] This dosage is likely safe and effective to achieve the benefits of omega-3 without increased risk for complications such as bleeding caused by increased clotting times. Individuals who are considering fish oil supplementation should talk with their physician and pay close attention to the dosage of omega-3 in the supplement.

## Herbal Supplements

**Herbal supplements**, or **botanicals**, are plant-derived substances used for medicinal purposes. Plants have been used as medicine for thousands of years, long before Westernized medicine evolved. Community healers throughout the world continue to prescribe plant extracts to fend off physical and mental ailments. Many Westerners have now turned to herbal supplements for more "natural" ways to heal. Two key concerns associated with this practice include: (1) herbal supplements have not been as thoroughly studied and evaluated as medications to understand their effects on health, and (2) herbal supplements are not as closely regulated as medications. As a result, consumers have no guarantee that the supplement they consume is not adulterated, contaminated, or otherwise different from the supplement they believed they purchased.

The most commonly used herbal supplements that health and fitness professionals will probably encounter include gingko biloba, an herb thought to improve memory; Saint-John's-wort, given to help with depression; echinacea, to fight off cold symptoms and boost the immune system; and flaxseed/flaxseed oil, which provides the essential fatty acids (omega-3 and omega-6) to improve cardiovascular health. The characteristics of each of these and other popular herbal supplements are highlighted in Table 21-5. For information on herbal supplements not specifically described in Table 21-5, health and

## Table 21-5. Commonly Used Herbal Supplements

| HERB | SOURCE | CLAIM | EFFECTIVENESS | SAFETY |
|---|---|---|---|---|
| Arnica | Flowering head of the plant | Anti-inflammatory and antimicrobial activity; used as a remedy for sports injuries and to reduce delayed-onset muscle soreness | Topical herbal cream widely used and minimally studied Homeopathic oral preparation, with unproven effectiveness | Topical herbal cream—Safety unknown Homeopathic oral supplement, highly diluted and safe for oral use |
| Bee pollen | Pollen granules from stamens of flowers and flower nectar collected by bees | "Super-food" that boosts athletic performance | Minimal effect | Generally safe but may cause anaphylaxis on those with bee allergy |
| Echinacea | Coneflower found in the United States and southern Canada | Treatment and prevention of colds, flu, and other infections | May possibly be beneficial in treating upper respiratory infections, but study results are mixed | Usually no adverse effects if taken by mouth, although some people experience allergic reactions |

## Table 21-5. Commonly Used Herbal Supplements–cont'd

| HERB | SOURCE | CLAIM | EFFECTIVENESS | SAFETY |
|---|---|---|---|---|
| Flaxseed and flaxseed oil | Oil of the flaxseed that is the seed of the flax plant | Laxative effects, arthritis relief, treatment of hot flashes and breast pain, treatment of high cholesterol, cancer prevention | Study results are mixed whether flaxseed claims are accurate; probably does have a laxative effect because of fiber content | Generally well tolerated with few adverse effects |
| Ginseng | Chinese herb | Improve cardiorespiratory function, increase aerobic and anaerobic performance, improve mental acuity | Claims have not been substantiated | Easily contaminated, little standardization of ingredients |
| Gingko biloba | Eastern Asia Maidenhair tree | Aid memory, improve circulation, prevent altitude sickness | Research is ongoing; large study showed no improvement in memory, Alzheimer's disease risk, cognitive function, blood pressure, or hypertension | Adverse effects include headache, nausea, gastrointestinal upset, dizziness, and allergic reactions; may increase bleeding risk |
| Garlic powder | Herb grown in many countries | Prevents fatigue | May improve circulation and slightly lower blood pressure; could help prevent colorectal and stomach cancer | Safe for most adults; may thin blood; adverse effects include breath and body odor, stomach upset, and allergic reactions |
| Guarana | Climbing plant in Amazon basin | Reduced fatigue, increased alertness, ergogenic aid | Stimulant with twice the amount of caffeine as the coffee bean | Generally safe, but lethal overdose possible |
| Saint-John's-wort | Yellow flowering plant, medicinal use first recorded in ancient Greece | Treatment of depression, anxiety, and sleep disorders; balm for wounds, burns, and insect bites | Mixed results in treatment of depression | Interacts with many medications that could lead to serious adverse effects |

*Source:* Data from Stear S, Burke L, Castell LM. BJSM reviews: A-Z of nutritional supplements: Dietary supplements, sports nutrition foods and ergogenic aids for health and performance part 3. *Br J Sports Med.* 2009;43:890–892; Burke L, Castell LM, Stear S, et al. BJSM reviews: A-Z of nutritional supplements: Dietary supplements, sports nutrition foods and ergogenic aids for health and performance part 4. *Br J Sports Med.* 2009;43:1088–1090; National Center for Complementary and Alternative Medicine website. http://nccam.nih.gov.

fitness professionals (and their clients) should refer to the Office of Dietary Supplements of the National Institutes of Health (http://ods.od.nih.gov) or National Center for Complementary Medicine of the National Institutes of Health websites (http://nccam.nih.gov).

## PERFORMANCE-ENHANCING SUPPLEMENTS

Numerous supplements claim to provide **ergogenic** effects or promises of increased athletic performance. This obviously holds appeal to athletes, whether recreational,

professional, or Olympian, who are constantly striving for that edge to beat their personal record and achieve athletic success. Ergogenic aids are generally defined as substances or devices intended to enhance physical development or performance above normal expectations. It is a broad definition with various categories that include mechanical devices (e.g., belts or shoes), psychological strategies (mental skills training like imagery), pharmacological substances (e.g., caffeine or steroids), physiological practices/substances (e.g., blood doping), and nutritional practices/substances (macronutrients, cellular components like carnitine and coenzyme Q10, and anabolic substances such as creatine).

## Banned Substances and Doping

Given the uncertain safety, yet potential efficacy, of some supplements (and the well-known risks and hazards of a few), plus the unfair advantage they could provide, the International Olympic Committee (IOC), NCAA, and other organizations have published position statements describing the risks and restrictions of supplement use for athletes. The World Anti-Doping Agency (WADA) code explicitly describes those supplements that are banned from use given their ergogenic effect. (Access the report online at www.wada-ama.org for a complete listing of prohibited or banned substances.) Despite the ban, athletes frequently get caught with various levels of banned substances in their blood and urine during random testing.

One form of **doping** is the practice of ingesting a banned substance in an effort to improve athletic performance. It is relatively common among elite athletes and has especially plagued the Tour de France; only three winners between 1998 and 2012 have not tested positive or been involved in controversies surrounding performance-enhancing drugs. In the most widely publicized downfall of a world-class athlete, seven-time Tour de France winner Lance Armstrong was stripped of his medals after he was exposed for what the United States Anti-Doping Agency (USADA) called "the most sophisticated, professionalized and successful doping program that sport has ever seen." Armstrong ultimately admitted to using blood doping and a cocktail of banned substances including erythropoietin (EPO), testosterone, cortisone, and human growth hormone.[62] Another disgraced Tour de France "winner," Alberto Contador, was stripped of his 2010 victory after he screened positive for the performance-enhancing and illegal drug clenbuterol.

However, Contador maintained his innocence, claiming it was a contaminant in a cut of steak he ate. (Sometimes cattle are given the drug to improve their value, but investigators found no evidence that the meat was tainted.) For Armstrong, Contador, and other athletes found guilty of doping, a lifetime of intense physical training, competition, and success is nullified by cheating.

Because supplements are not closely regulated and rates of **contamination** are high, some athletes test positive for banned substances without even being aware of their ingestion, which is referred to as **inadvertent doping**. For example, former U.S. track and field athlete Carl Lewis tested positive at the 1988 Olympic Trials for small amounts of several banned substances. After being nearly disqualified from the Seoul Olympics, the United States Olympic Committee accepted his claim that an allowable herbal supplement he was taking was contaminated with the banned substances, unbeknownst to Lewis.[63]

Although anabolic steroids represent the banned substance that most frequently contaminates products, the rates of inadvertent doping are highest with the banned stimulants ephedrine, sibutramine, and methylhexaneamine.[34] Products that contain ephedrine often are labeled with the herbal names *ma huang* or *ephedra sinica* and not by the more easily identifiable names of ephedrine, pseudoephedrine, or methylephedrine. The unclear labeling poses a trap for less sophisticated athletes. Because of its potent potential adverse effects, such as stroke or heart attack in certain individuals, sibutramine is approved only as a prescription medication for weight loss. When sibutramine is present in a supplement, the consumer may only know that the product they are ingesting has "pure herbal ingredients" and that it is advertised to induce weight loss. The supplement name and ingredient list may not include the word *sibutramine* anywhere, leaving it up to the individual to recognize that this banned substance may be a hidden ingredient.

Methylhexaneamine is also frequently inadvertently ingested because of confusing labeling. This substance can be found on supplements labels as dimethylamylamine, dimethylpentylamine, pentylamine, geranamine, and Forthane, among others. On WADA's 2013 prohibited list, only methylhexaneamine (dimethylpentylamine) is mentioned.[35]

## Steroids

**Anabolic steroids** are strictly prohibited by the WADA code. There is irrefutable evidence that the use of steroids increases muscle mass and strength, thus giving users an unfair competitive advantage. However, their use is also accompanied by serious adverse effects including high blood pressure, rage, gynecomastia (enlarged breast size), decreased testicle size in men, and increased testosterone, facial hair growth, and deepening of the voice in women. Although most elite and recreational athletes know to avoid these substance, many supplements on the market may contain anabolic steroid contaminants, sometimes intentionally, of which the consumer may not be aware.[34] Consumers should proceed with caution when considering trying any product that boasts of its ability to quickly boost muscle mass.

Androstenedione, a precursor to testosterone, is commonly referred to as a "natural alternative" to anabolic steroids. Androstenedione supplements claim to increase testosterone levels and promote muscle size and strength. Research in men does not support these claims, and the effect of androstenedione intake in women has not been studied.[36] Repeated use of androstenedione supplements poses significant health risks, including decreased high-density lipoprotein (the "healthy" cholesterol) levels and increased CVD risk, increased risk for prostate cancer and pancreatic cancer, baldness, and gynecomastia (development of breast tissue) in men.[36] Although androstenedione is not banned by MLB, it is banned by WADA and the IOC, the NCAA, the NFL, the National Basketball Association (NBA), and the National Hockey League (NHL).

The FDA has also banned the sale of androstenedione in the United States.

Similar to androstenedione, dehydroepiandrosterone (DHEA) is a precursor to testosterone and is also banned by WADA and various other organizations. Despite claims of promoting youthfulness, virility, and enhanced strength, research consistently shows that it does not affect strength, lean body mass, or athletic performance.[37]

## Hormones

Some athletes turn to **hormones** to gain an unfair athletic advantage. From erythropoiesis-stimulating hormones, which lead to increased red blood cell production and consequently increased oxygen-carrying capacity, to human growth hormone (HGH) and androgenic (sex) hormones that boost testosterone levels, most hormone supplements are strictly banned and should be avoided by all athletes.

### Human Growth Hormone

HGH is a peptide hormone that has gained notoriety in recent years in light of its abuse by various professional athletes in sports such as baseball and football. HGH is naturally produced by the pituitary gland and stimulates growth, cell reproduction, and regeneration of tissue, particularly in children and adolescents, for whom HGH helps all internal tissue (except the brain) grow, including the skeleton. However, HGH also helps to regulate body composition and metabolism of fats and carbohydrates, stimulating fat oxidation to fuel growth and repair. Given its ability to stimulate muscle growth, promote fat metabolism, and therefore alter body composition, it should come as no surprise to learn that HGH is abused by athletes and bodybuilders. However, HGH is on the WADA prohibited substances list and is also banned by many professional organizations and the FDA, which has not approved it as an ergogenic aid.

HGH levels naturally decrease with age. Therefore, for adults who have very small levels of this hormone, HGH is also promoted as an antiaging compound to reverse age-related bodily deterioration, although these claims are unsubstantiated. Likewise, its use to slow aging is not approved by the FDA.

Increased levels of HGH in adults may promote increased muscle synthesis, greater fat oxidation, and overall growth. However, HGH is also associated with numerous adverse effects, including[38]:

- Neural, muscle, and joint pain
- Increased retention of water in body tissue (edema)
- Soft-tissue complication at joints (e.g., carpal tunnel syndrome)
- Increased lipid (e.g., cholesterol) levels
- Increased risk for diabetes
- Potential increase in risk for growth of cancerous tumors

### Erythropoietin

Erythropoietin (EPO) is a hormone that is naturally found within the body and that regulates erythropoiesis, or red blood cell production within bone marrow. Exogenous EPO (administered into the body) is classified as an erythropoiesis-stimulating agent and is used as a performance-enhancing drug that has been widely abused by many athletes in endurance sports, in particular, in cycling.

Doping with EPO improves overall oxygen delivery by increasing normal red blood cell levels that subsequently also increase blood volume (to accommodate additional cells), stroke volume, and overall blood oxygen levels, which all improve overall endurance performance. However, EPO also is a banned substance by most organizations and can be detected in blood by more modern tests that can identify the slight differences between the body's natural endogenous proteins that comprise this hormone and those created in a laboratory.[39]

## Diuretics

A **diuretic** is any substance that promotes the production of urine by removing sodium from the body, resulting in increased water loss. Oftentimes, athletes who are attempting to "make weight" in various weight-categorized sports (e.g., boxing, wrestling, and Mixed Martial Arts [MMA]) will abuse diuretics. Although diuretics can stimulate some rapid weight loss, and thus are banned by WADA and other professional organizations, they can also be dangerous to human health. Known adverse effects of abuse by diuretics include[40]:

- Hypovolemia or decreased blood volume
- Hyponatremia or reduced serum sodium concentration (<135 mEq/L) if only water and not the lost sodium is replaced; this can trigger organ failure (e.g., kidneys), heart failure, and swelling within brain cells
- Potassium alterations in the body (e.g., hypokalemia and hyperkalemia)
- Metabolic changes (e.g., alkalosis and acidosis) that alter blood and tissue pH that can negatively impact structure and function of many protein compounds within the body

## Stimulants

A **stimulant** is a substance that activates the central nervous system and may be found in various forms, with perhaps the most commonly abused stimulant being caffeine. Stimulants increase heart rate, cardiac output, and glucose availability, and may even suppress appetite. In addition to their potential performance-enhancing attributes, stimulants can also have serious and significant adverse effects. A telling example of this is ephedra—a supplement that was once widely used in the bodybuilding arena to increase metabolism and burn fat. Ephedra has since been banned and removed from the market because of multiple cases of life-threatening side effects and death associated with its use. WADA prohibits stimulant use during competition, with the exception of caffeine.

Given the popularity of caffeine and its widespread use (habitual) and abuse (by athletes or individuals seeking increased mental alertness or enhanced fat oxidation), it merits further discussion as a stimulant. Caffeine is found in multiple forms, including traditional products like coffee, tea, chocolate, and 60+ foods and drinks, and in various nontraditional sources such as soaps, lip balm, and chewing gum. Individuals do not need to look far to get their daily fix. In addition, countless cleverly disguised caffeine-loaded products also exist—all promising a performance-enhancing, metabolism-boosting jolt—such as guarana and kola nut. The stimulant's potent ability to ward off sleep, improve athletic performance, decrease pain and fatigue, boost memory, and enhance mood[41] make it America's drug of choice, with more than 90% of Americans admitting to regular caffeine use.[42] About 20% to 30% of Americans consume a whopping 600 mg (equivalent to about 6 cups of coffee) or more each day.[41]

Caffeine rapidly enters the bloodstream and within a short 40 to 60 minutes reaches all organs of the body, causing physiological changes that last for up to 6 hours in most people.[43] Some of these positive or ergogenic effects increase metabolism and fat oxidation, increase mental alertness, and decrease perceived exertion, thereby allowing individuals to train longer with greater intensity.[44] The following section provides more detailed explanations of these effects and of performance. However, caffeine can also produce some adverse effects, especially in nondesensitized individuals, that include increased heart rate and blood pressure, gastrointestinal distress and anxiety, and sleep disturbances (by temporarily binding with adenosine receptors in the brain and preventing adenosine, a natural sedative, from making a person feel drowsy). To nerve cells in the brain, caffeine resembles adenosine, a molecule that normally slows nervous system transmission, helps dilate blood vessels, and allows sleep. Because the nerve's adenosine receptor cannot differentiate between the two molecules, they essentially compete for receptor binding. When caffeine is consumed and crosses into the brain, it wins. An exaggerated stress response takes hold where nerve cell activity accelerates (i.e., mental alertness), brain blood vessels constrict (reducing headaches), and neuron firing rates increase. Because of caffeine's lipophilic or "fat-loving" chemical structure, it crosses the blood–brain barrier easily to enter the brain and it affects brain function as mentioned earlier. The blood–brain barrier is essentially the brain's security system that prevents many water-soluble compounds from potentially altering brain function or, worse, damaging itself. For example, too much tryptophan, an essential amino acid, crossing into the brain may increase levels of serotonin, a sedative neurotransmitter that produces states of relaxation.

In response to this increase in neural activity in the brain, the pituitary gland responds to the increased activity by sending a message to the adrenal glands to produce catecholamines, our primary fight-or-flight hormones. This activates many sympathomimetic responses that include dilation of the pupils and breathing tubes, increases in heart rate and blood pressure, increased blood flow shunts to muscles, mobilized fat stores, and increased glycogenolysis or glucose release from the liver, thus sparing muscle glycogen stores.[14] During exercise, caffeine prolongs time to fatigue, increases high-intensity performance (maximizing effort at 85% $\dot{V}O_2$max in cyclists and increasing speed in endurance events[43]), and decreases perceived exertion, making high-intensity efforts seem less taxing.[41]

Given all these physiological responses to caffeine, it should come as no surprise that the research findings on caffeine are consistent and clear: Caffeine enhances athletic performance, especially in nondesensitized individuals. Also, contrary to popular opinion, research suggests that caffeine during exercise does not cause the generally believed negative effects such as dehydration, water-electrolyte imbalances, hyperthermia, or reduced exercise-heat tolerance.[41] It appears, therefore, that although caffeine improves performance, it does so without causing much harm. Although most research studying caffeine's ergogenic potential has used doses around 400 to 600 mg in capsule form, benefits are evident at doses as low as 250 mg.[43] There is a catch, however. Caffeine's performance-enhancing benefits are stronger in nonhabitual users (<50 mg/day) than in regular users (>300 mg/day),[45] because the brain adapts to chronic caffeine use by producing more adenosine receptors for adenosine binding. Thus, caffeine's effects are lessened and the same dose produces fewer desirable physiological changes. Consequently, in a chronically sleep-deprived, high-achieving culture, a common response to increased caffeine tolerance is consumption of more caffeine. While extra caffeine binds up the newly created adenosine receptors, the brain also adapts by further increasing receptor production. As dosages continue to increase in pursuit of the invigorating caffeine jolt, risk for severe consequences multiply. In addition to its toxicity at high doses, when combined with other substances such as alcohol, ephedrine, or anti-inflammatory medications, even moderate caffeine use can be dangerous. The NCAA and IOC consider intakes up to approximately 800 mg or less than 9 mg/kg body weight to be habitual and acceptable doses (cutoffs are based on caffeine amounts in urine testing).

## Proteins and Amino Acids

Proteins and amino acids are among the most popular and commonly used supplements by competitive athletes, particularly recreational and competitive bodybuilders, as well as the general population of gym-goers and weekend athletes.

## Whey and Casein

Two of the most common forms of supplemented proteins are the milk proteins whey and casein. Whey, given its high degree of solubility, is quickly assimilated into the body. It is often described as a "fast" protein among practitioners, because it is ideally suited for ingestion before and immediately after exercise. Casein, by comparison, is insoluble, forming a gel or clot in the stomach, which delays gastric emptying, digestion, and absorption. This protein is described as a "slow" protein. It is ideally suited for sustaining protein delivery into the body and positive nitrogen balance hours after exercise when the body generally reverts back to a state of muscle degradation. These two proteins and their structure and benefits are described in detail in Chapter 20.

## Amino Acids

Branched-chain amino acids (BCAAs) comprise leucine, isoleucine, and valine, and they play an important role in muscle building. Although results are inconsistent, some research has found that following exercise, the administration of BCAAs, especially leucine, increases the rate of protein synthesis and decreases the rate of protein catabolism.[46] Given these findings, the supplement industry has made numerous BCAA and leucine supplement products widely available to consumers. However, because these research findings are inconsistent and little is known about the safety of these products, the Academy of Nutrition and Dietetics advises against individual amino acid supplementation and protein supplementation overall.[47] Arginine and aspartate/aspartic acid are additional frequently supplemented amino acids, but supplementation is likely unnecessary to achieve the purported benefits. It may be that food sources of these proteins and amino acids provide the same effect for a small fraction of the cost. Table 21-6 highlights readily available amino acid supplements.

## Table 21-6. Readily Available Amino Acid Supplements

| AMINO ACID | CLASSIFICATION | ERGOGENIC FUNCTION | DESCRIPTION | EFFICACY OF SUPPLEMENTATION |
|---|---|---|---|---|
| Alanine (and dipeptide carnosine) | Nonessential | Combines with histidine to form carnosine; synthesis of carnosine dependent on availability of alanine; increases muscle buffering capacity | Buffer | Attenuates decline in blood pH during high-intensity exercise, leading to increased capability to perform strenuous exercise |
| Valine | Essential | Stimulates protein synthesis in muscle | BCAA | |
| Leucine | Essential | Stimulates protein synthesis in muscle | BCAA | |
| Isoleucine | Essential | Stimulates protein synthesis in muscle | BCAA | |
| Arginine | Nonessential | Facilitates vasodilation as a nitrous oxide precursor and improves muscle strength as substrate for creatine formation | Formed in urea cycle, essential for nitric oxide signaling pathway; necessary for creatine formation; may stimulate growth hormone and recovery of muscle after exercise | Could enhance muscle gain from resistance training, but effect may be minimal in athletes who already eat enough protein; supplementation is unnecessary for most; research supporting nitrous oxide and improved performance is weak |
| Aspartic acid/ aspartate | Nonessential | Glucose and energy production | Easily converted to oxaloacetate, an intermediary of the Krebs (citric acid) cycle | Supplementation increases time to exhaustion when combined with asparagine in rat studies, but results are not confirmed in human study of triathletes |

*Continued*

## Table 21-6. Readily Available Amino Acid Supplements—cont'd

| AMINO ACID | CLASSIFICATION | ERGOGENIC FUNCTION | DESCRIPTION | EFFICACY OF SUPPLEMENTATION |
|---|---|---|---|---|
| Glutamic acid/ glutamine | Nonessential | Increases athletic performance—preferred fuel of immune cells during periods of stress; aids in recovery and supports post-exercise adaptive responses (e.g., muscle synthesis) | Many metabolic roles; excitatory neurotransmitter; food flavoring "umami" | Mixed evidence of efficacy when used alone, but significant improvements when combined with carbohydrate or other amino acids (BCAA) |
| Cysteine | Essential (in infants and those with chronic disease) | Increases exercise performance | Essential for glutathione synthesis (important antioxidant in cellular signaling) | May be beneficial because of its ability to increase levels of glutathione |

BCAA, branched-chain amino acid.

*Source:* Data from Burke LM, Castell LM, Stear SJ. BJSM reviews: A-Z of supplements: Dietary supplements, sports nutrition foods and ergogenic aids for health and performance—part 1. *Br J Sports Med.* 2009;43:728–729; Castell LM, Burke L, Stear S, McNaughton LR, Harris RC. BJSM reviews: A-Z of nutritional supplements: Dietary supplements, sports nutrition foods and ergogenic aids for health and performance—part 5. *Br J Sports Med.* 2010;44:77–78; and Newsholme P, Krause M, Newsholme EA, Stear S, Burke L, Castell LM. BJSM reviews: A to Z of nutritional supplements: Dietary supplements, sports nutrition foods and ergogenic aids for health and performance—part 18. *Br J Sports Med.* 2011;45:230–232.

## Creatine

Creatine is a compound that is derived from the amino acids glycine, arginine, and methionine. It is synthesized within the body (approximately 1 g/day), ingested through foods (approximately 1 g/day), and primarily stored within skeletal muscle. It functions as the primary source of energy for the phosphagen energy system, fueling short bouts of high-intensity activity lasting less than 10 seconds, such as sprinting, weight lifting, and other sports involving repeated explosive movements such as tennis, football, basketball, and soccer. Creatine's involvement within the phosphagen energy system is discussed in greater detail in Chapter 4.

Raising muscle stores of creatine is believed to provide additional fuel for explosive activities, which allows athletes to perform more repetitions, which, in turn, leads to greater strength and size gains. The other theory supporting creatine's ergogenic effect involves cell volumizing, whereby creatine pulls additional water into the muscle cell, increasing sarcoplasmic volume within the muscle cell, thereby increasing muscle mass.

Creatine is perhaps one of the most researched supplements on the market. It is most commonly sold as creatine monohydrate, a more efficiently digested and absorbed form than other creatine compounds such as creatine citrate or creatine malate.

Multiple studies have demonstrated that many individuals who consume creatine supplements during training gain an average of 1 to 2 kg (2.2–4.5 lb) of additional muscle mass over periods of 4 to 12 weeks compared with those taking placebos.[48–50] In fact, several hundred peer-reviewed research studies have validated creatine as an effective dietary supplement for increasing high-intensity exercise capacity and lean body mass in conjunction with resistance training.[51] Approximately two thirds of these studies have demonstrated significant improvement in performance with creatine supplementation, while the remaining third reported performance improvements that were statistically insignificant.

Studies support that ingestion of a variety of creatine dosages (up to 20–30 g/day for up to 2 weeks) can increase muscle creatine stores by 10% to 30% and can boost muscle strength by about 10% when compared with resistance training alone (Fig. 21-5).[52,53] Muscle stores can be elevated by adopting a loading phase consisting of 0.3 g/kg (0.14 g/lb) of body weight per day (~20 g) for 3 to 5 days, followed by a maintenance phase of 3 to 5 g/day for 4 to 12 weeks to keep muscle stores elevated.[54] However, loading phases are generally not considered necessary anymore because muscle can essentially achieve the same creatine levels through maintenance dosing, albeit more slowly.

Because creatine is a natural substance produced by the body, it is not included on any doping lists, but it is prohibited by the NCAA, on the basis that it is thought to provide athletes with an unfair advantage. Overall, creatine is generally considered safe in healthy adults and there are limited known adverse effects. Some anecdotal reports include muscle cramping and heat intolerance, although the research has not confirmed these findings.[53] People with potential risk for renal dysfunction, such as those with diabetes, hypertension, and

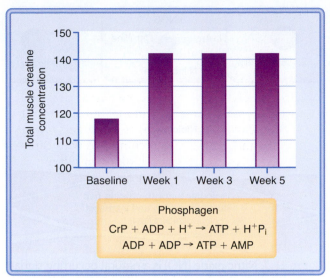

**Figure 21-5.** Creatine monohydrate ingestion has been reported to increase total concentration of muscle phosphocreatine (CrP), which is a required substrate for short-term intense exercise. Supplementation with creatine monohydrate has been linked to an improved ability to maintain force production and power output. Initially, a dosage of 20 g/day creatine monohydrate is required to increase muscle creatine levels. Subsequently, a dosage of 2 g/day has been shown to maintain increased muscle creatine levels for more than a month.

decreased kidney function, should not use creatine unless its use has been advised or cleared by a physician. Anyone who uses creatine on a long-term basis should undergo routine monitoring by a physician. Because creatine holds water and triggers a cell-volumizing effect, this may prove undesirable for athletes who participate in sports where performance may be impaired by additional weight; however, this is likely a nonissue for athletes seeking to increase lean body mass.

## Other Popular Ergogenic Aids

Other ergogenic aids show promise in their ability to boost athletic performance, although the short- and long-term effects are not known for some. Examples include sodium bicarbonate (Fig. 21-6) and sodium citrate to effectively buffer metabolic acidosis that occurs during intense physical activity that accumulates hydrogen ions. Chapter 4 presents a Research Highlight feature that demonstrates the ergogenic effect of supplementing with sodium bicarbonate, although this practice is not common among athletes given its negative side effects.

### Beta-hydroxy-beta-methylbutyrate

Beta-hydroxy-beta-methylbutyrate (HMB) is another popular supplement used by individuals seeking increases in muscle size and strength. It is formed in the body as a by-product of leucine breakdown. HMB reduces muscle damage after exercise in trained and untrained individuals by inhibiting protein breakdown

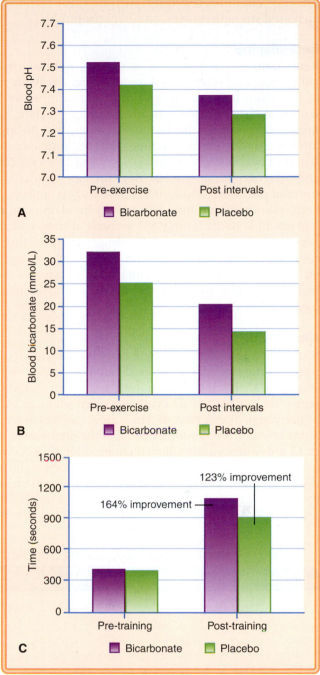

**Figure 21-6.** Muscle buffering capacity can be augmented by various nutritional strategies. Alkalizing agents have been studied extensively for their potential to enhance performance by attenuating the extent to which metabolic acidosis contributes to fatigue during high-intensity exercise performance. One such alkalizing substance that has been found to improve recovery by increasing the muscle buffering capacity is sodium bicarbonate. One study[55] found that chronic sodium bicarbonate ingestion increased blood pH (A) and blood bicarbonate (B) levels during interval training when compared with a placebo. This strategy resulted in greater improvements in time to fatigue (C) following 8 weeks of training.

and increasing protein synthesis, thereby enhancing the recovery process.[56] With appropriate exercise protocols (i.e., hypertrophy, strength, and power workouts), dosages of 38 mg/kg (17.3 g/lb) of body weight per day administered over two to three servings increased strength, power, and hypertrophy.[57]

## Beta-alanine

Beta-alanine is a naturally occurring nonessential amino acid that is converted to carnosine, a scavenger of hydrogen ions that helps buffer lactate produced within skeletal muscle. Accumulation of lactate in muscle tissue results in the burning sensation during intense exercise and subsequent fatigue. Supplementation of beta-alanine in dosages varying between 2.4 and 6.4 g/day for at least 21 days increases muscular stores of carnosine. Also, studies have shown improved performance of high-intensity activity involving single and multiple bouts lasting ≥60 seconds, during which muscle pH declines because of hydrogen accumulation resulting from lactate production.[58] Although research on this supplement is limited, no significant adverse effects have been noted when consumed at recommended doses.

## Nitric Oxide

Nitric oxide (NO) in the human body is a natural neurotransmitter that promotes vasodilation of blood vessels (Fig. 21-7). NO supplements often contain arginine (converted to NO by NO synthase) or citrulline as the primary ingredients, both of which are converted to NO. Some research has demonstrated that the ingestion of 4 to 12 g/day of arginine supplementation for 8 weeks in healthy men increased plasma arginine levels significantly and improved one-repetition maximum bench press scores, but other studies have reported no effects on muscle endurance in trained men.[59,60] Citrulline is

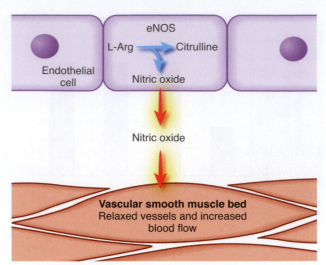

**Figure 21-7.** Nitric oxide (NO) is a natural occurring signaling molecule that promotes relaxation of the smooth muscle–its production in endothelial cells is facilitated by the enzyme nitric oxide synthase (eNOS). Increased production of NO is believed to enhance blood flow, increase cellular uptake of energy and nutrients, and facilitate the removal of waste products.

also used in NO supplements because it is converted in the body to arginine (the precursor to NO) and is not subject to breakdown during digestion or to breakdown by the enzyme arginase in the body. Because the research is conflicting, no definitive answers have been formulated regarding this supplement's efficacy and safety. Information on other potential performance-enhancing supplements is outlined in Table 21-7.

## Table 21-7. Performance-Enhancing Supplements

| SUPPLEMENT | CLAIM | EFFECTIVENESS | SAFETY |
|---|---|---|---|
| Androstenedione | Promotes muscle size and strength | No more effective than resistance training alone | May increase risk for cardiovascular disease, cancer, baldness, and gynecomastia (development of breast tissue) |
| Sodium bicarbonate and sodium citrate | By buffering metabolic acidosis, reduces or delays onset of fatigue during strenuous exercise | Effective, especially at optimal amounts of 0.3 g/kg body weight | May contribute to GI upset |
| Caffeine | Improves athletic capacity and performance | Effective | May develop dependency, toxic at very high doses |
| Bovine colostrum | Contains growth factors that mediate protein synthesis | Limited studies, but may provide ergogenic benefits | No safety information |
| Creatine | Improves athletic performance for high-intensity exercise, especially when combined with resistance training | Consistently provides benefit | Appears safe |
| Dehydroepiandrosterone (DHEA) | Enhances muscle strength and lean body mass | Consistently provides NO benefit | Possibly safe for short-term use and possibly unsafe for long-term use |

## Table 21-7. Performance-Enhancing Supplements–cont'd

| SUPPLEMENT | CLAIM | EFFECTIVENESS | SAFETY |
|---|---|---|---|
| Pyruvate | No plausible ergogenic mechanism, but marketed to improve athletic performance and enhance weight loss | No scientific basis as ergogenic aid | Appears safe |
| Hydroxymethyl butyrate | Increases muscle size and strength, and decreases muscle damage and soreness associated with resistance training | May enhance strength training adaptations slightly in untrained athletes and negligibly in trained athletes | Short-term supplementation appears safe |
| Ribose | Increases the rate of ATP resynthesis and the speed of recovery following high-intensity exercise | Little published evidence to suggest benefit | Appears safe, even at high doses |
| Nitrates | Reduces oxygen cost of activity and could improve exercise performance | Studies to date confirm claims | Nitric oxide–induced vasodilation could lead to a decline in blood pressure |

ATP, adenosine triphosphate; GI, gastrointestinal.

*Source:* Data from Castell LM, Burke L, Stear S, McNaughton LR, Harris RC. BJSM reviews: A-Z of nutritional supplements: Dietary supplements, sports nutrition foods and ergogenic aids for health and performance—part 5. *Br J Sports Med.* 2010;44:77–78; Castell LM, Burke L, Stear S. BJSM reviews: A-Z of supplements: Dietary supplements, sports nutrition foods and ergogenic aids for health and performance—part 2. *Br J Sports Med.* 2009;43:807–810; and Stear S, Castell LM, Burke L, et al. BJSM reviews: A-Z of nutritional supplements: Dietary supplements, sports nutrition foods and ergogenic aids for health and performance—part 10. *Br J Sports Med.* 2010;44:688–690.

## VIGNETTE continued

■ The story of Anne Marie's death played out in the media in the case of *Capati v Crunch Fitness*, in which Anne Marie's personal trainer and fitness center were sued for $320 million. Ultimately, the case was settled before going to trial, with the gym and the trainer liable for $1,750,000.

## SCOPE OF PRACTICE

Although it is outside the scope of practice of health and fitness professionals to provide specific and individualized nutrition eating plans, they can use well-established guidelines to help clients adopt healthful and appropriate nutrition habits. Many clients may have medical diagnoses that require special nutrition recommendations beyond those discussed in the government guidelines. In these cases, it is advisable that the client work closely with his or her physician and a registered dietitian to develop an individualized eating plan. Often the health and fitness professional's role will be to provide support and encouragement for the client to follow the recommended plan. This is especially important when working with individuals with complex medical histories and special nutritional requirements and needs.

Health and fitness professionals' competencies include *knowledge* of basic nutrition and weight-management information; they are not expected to—and should not—*calculate, outline, counsel,* or *prescribe* individual nutrition or weight-management plans. As several lawsuits have demonstrated, health and fitness professionals tread especially treacherous waters if they recommend supplements or other risky substances.[61]

Although each state has different laws and regulations regarding who can practice dietetics, the standard in Ohio serves as a useful example to describe scope of practice for health and fitness professionals. Ohio legislators passed a statute in 2006 titled "Unauthorized Practice of Dietetics" that may help clarify scope of practice for "nonlicensed individuals"—that is, individuals with occasion to discuss nutrition but without the registered dietitian credential and state license, where necessary (more than 30 states require licensing). Nonlicensed individuals can provide only "general nonmedical nutrition information" such as a cooking demonstration; endorsement of government recommendation guidelines and programs such as the *Dietary Guidelines* and MyPlate; discussion of macronutrients and micronutrients, and how requirements vary by life stage; information about statistics relating to nutrition and chronic disease; and education about nutrients contained in particular foods or substances.[61] Health and fitness professionals should consult their state laws and statutes that delineate the scope of practice of a licensed dietitian versus a nonlicensed individual.

When asked to advise on supplements, the health and fitness professional should inform individuals that supplements are not regulated by the FDA and, therefore, not thoroughly examined. Not only does this not guarantee efficacy, but supplements may also increase potential risks for harm. Health and fitness professionals should always try to redirect individuals toward sensible eating plans with common foods that meet individual needs. Encourage individuals to look beyond product labels and be skeptical of claims that sound too good to be true, and become familiar with state laws on standards and respect scope of practice for dispensing nutritional information. Health and fitness professionals should be educated on supplement claims, efficacy, and potential harmful effects, so that they can provide credible information and allow individuals to make their own informed decisions or guide them to talk to their physician.

## Practical Guidelines for Health and Fitness Professionals

To summarize and provide practical guidelines, it is important for health and fitness professionals to subscribe to a code of conduct that covers both legal and ethical behavior. For some, there is the option of some financial gain through the sale and distribution of supplements that may come at the expense of doing harm. Although it is important to adhere to this code of conduct to protect clients and athletes, it is equally important to protect yourself from potential liability.

Because the FDA loosely regulates supplements through the DSHEA, it is important for health and fitness professionals to understand scope of practice with regard to supplements. The following points are practical guidelines to follow when working with individuals and supplements:

1. Inform individuals that supplements are not regulated by the FDA and, therefore, are not thoroughly examined in the same manner as food and drugs. This means there is no guarantee that they safe, effective, or free of contaminants that may cause potential harm or trouble.
2. Always try to direct individuals toward strategic and sensible eating plans that include the consumption of common foods and beverages that meet individual needs.
3. Encourage individuals to look beyond product labels and claims, and be skeptical of claims that sound too good to be true.
4. Be familiar with your own state or nation's laws on standards and scope of practice for recommending nutritional information.
5. Develop credibility by providing evidence-based facts and information on supplements via reputable scientific research and allow individuals to make their own informed decisions.

6. The following resources provide credible information on supplements and should be used to develop your credibility:
   - National Institutes of Health database: Office of Dietary Supplements
     - International Bibliographic Information on Dietary Supplements (IBIDS): http://ods.od.nih.gov/Health_Information/IBIDS.aspx
     - Computer Access to Research on Dietary Supplements Database (CARDS): http://dietary-supplements.info.nih.gov
   - FDA (www.fda.gov)—provides supplement warnings
   - Center for Food Safety & Applied Nutrition (FDA): http://www.fda.gov/AboutFDA/CentersOffices/OfficeofFoods/CFSAN/default.htm
   - Institute of Medicine (IOM) Food and Nutrition Board: www.iom.edu
   - Credible independent organizations providing independent research:
     - ConsumerLab.com: www.consumerlab.com
     - Quackwatch: www.quackwatch.com
     - www.supplementwatch.com

## In Your Own Words

Health and fitness professionals are often asked many questions about nutrition and dietary supplements by clients who want to lose weight or enhance their performance. Although it may seem pretty obvious that psychologists should not be treating a toothache, the line separating the practice of health and fitness professionals and registered dietitians can be much less clear. Where does one draw the line when it comes to nutrition advice?

Following are examples of appropriate and inappropriate remarks in a theoretical conversation between a personal trainer and client:
- Acceptable: "Fish is a good source of healthy fats."
- Not acceptable: "You should take fish oil supplements to get more healthy fats."

The first remark is merely a statement of fact. The second is a *recommendation*, which is much different. Until supplements are regulated by the FDA, with guidelines from the U.S. Department of Agriculture (USDA), it will be very difficult for the health and fitness professional to recommend them without stepping outside their scope of practice.
- Acceptable: "According to the USDA *Dietary Guidelines*, you should try to consume 2 to 3 servings of meat to help meet your daily

protein needs. Examples of a serving include an egg, 1/4 cup beans, 1 tbsp. peanut butter, or 1/2 oz. nuts or seeds."
- Not acceptable: "I recommend that you eat one egg for breakfast, a turkey sandwich for lunch, and a 3-oz. portion of salmon for dinner to meet your protein needs."

The difference here involves citing published guidelines rather than your own personal recommendations, and health and fitness professionals should never provide a meal plan.

When discussing sports nutrition, do the same with the delivery of educational information:
- Acceptable: "According to the American College of Sports Medicine, you should consume 7 to 10 oz. of fluids every 15 minutes during exercise."
- Not acceptable: "I recommend that you drink 8 oz. of PowerAde and take a protein supplement."

The difference again is citing published guidelines rather than your own personal recommendations.

## VIGNETTE Conclusion

■ The tragic loss of Anne Marie's life was caused, in part, by an overzealous fitness professional who stepped outside the scope of practice of the profession. Unless a personal trainer is qualified to do so (e.g., the trainer is also a medical doctor), he or she should never recommend nutritional supplements, because a personal trainer is not qualified to analyze a client's health history and medication use, and then "prescribe" a supplement. Had Anne Marie been referred to her personal physician at the outset, this entire tragedy would likely have been avoided. The bottom line is: *No matter how harmless a supplement seems, health and fitness professionals should never recommend supplements to clients. Not only is it outside the scope of practice, but recommending supplements without a full medical history and physical examination is dangerous.*

## CRITICAL THINKING QUESTIONS

1. How would you respond to an individual who states the following reasons for taking a particular supplement? What factors will you consider in determining your response?
   a. Prevent or treat nutritional deficiency
   b. Provide a more convenient form of nutrients
   c. Performance-enhancing effect
   d. Everyone else is doing it

2. As a group, identify two supplements that are not discussed in detail in this chapter but appear to be popular among athletes or exercisers at the local fitness clubs or centers. Take time to research these supplements using the resources provided and share your discoveries with your peers.

3. An individual informs you that he is planning to try an ergogenic supplement, but before he takes it he wants to be certain that this supplement is safe and effective. What process might you recommend that he undertake to get a better idea of the safety and efficacy of the supplement? How is this process different from the process he might take to understand the safety and efficacy of a medication prescribed by his physician?

Now, choose a supplement of interest and find out for yourself whether it is considered to be safe and effective. (Go through the process you would recommend to this client.) What did you find? After this research, would you consider taking this supplement? Why or why not?

4. Describe the current state of supplement regulation and oversight in the United States (note that you may need to look up the latest laws and regulations as changes may have occurred since publication of this textbook, and in fact, some new regulations were under consideration at the time of printing).

5. Health and fitness professionals are often asked to comment on the usefulness of taking various supplements. What is the scope of practice related to nutrition advice in your state? Describe several ways you may talk about supplements with your clients while staying within your scope of practice. Refer to the Commission on Dietetic Registration website (http://www.cdrnet.org/certifications/licensure/index.cfm) to get started.

## ADDITIONAL RESOURCES

**Dietary Supplements Labels Database**
(http://dsld.nlm.nih.gov/dsld/):The database has information on the ingredients for thousands of dietary supplements sold in the United States. Look up products by brand name, uses, active ingredient, or manufacturer.

**Office of Dietary Supplements** of the National Institutes of Health (http://ods.od.nih.gov): Aims to strengthen knowledge and understanding of dietary supplements by evaluating scientific information, stimulating and supporting research, disseminating research results, and educating the public to foster an enhanced quality of life and health for the U.S. population.

**National Center for Complementary and Alternative Medicine** (NCCAM) of the National Institutes of Health (http://nccam.nih.gov): The NCCAM maintains a list of supplements that are under regulatory review or that have been reported to cause adverse effects in addition to a general listing of dietary and herbal supplements.

**Food and Drug Administration (FDA) Dietary Supplements Alerts and Safety Information:**
http://www.fda.gov/Food/RecallsOutbreaksEmergencies/ SafetyAlertsAdvisories/ The FDA website provides information and updates regarding supplement regulations and safety issues.

The following three organizations provide supplement testing and assurances of compliance with FDA regulations:
• **U.S. Pharmacopeia** (www.usp.org)
• **ConsumerLab.com** (www.consumerlab.com)
• **NSF International** (www.nsf.org)

**PubMed Dietary Supplement Subset**
(http://ods.od.nih.gov/Research/PubMed_Dietary_ Supplement_Subset.aspx): PubMed provides an easy-to-use search engine to identify published scientific literature of interest. The subset is designed to limit search results to citations from a broad spectrum of dietary supplement literature including vitamin, mineral, phytochemical, ergogenic, botanical, and herbal supplements in human nutrition and animal models.

**IOC/WADA—Prohibited List of Substances and Methods:** http://www.wada-ama.org/en/World-Anti-Doping-Program/Sports-and-Anti-Doping-Organizations/ International-Standards/Prohibited-List/

**NCAA Banned Drug List:** http://www.ncaa.org/ health-and-safety/policy/2013-14-ncaa-banned-drugs

## REFERENCES

1. National Business Journal. *Sports Nutrition & Weight Loss Report.* New York, NY: Penton Media, Inc.; 2012.
2. Gahche J, Bailey R, Burt V, et al. *Dietary Supplement Use Among U.S. Adults Has Increased Since NHANES III (1988–1994). National Center for Health Statistics, HCHS Data Brief Number 61, April 2011.* Atlanta, GA: Centers for Diseases Control and Prevention; 2011.
3. Heikkinen, A., Alaranta, A, Helenius, I, & Vasankari, T. Use of dietary supplements in Olympic athletes is decreasing: a follow-up study between 2002 and 2009. *Journal of the International Society of Sports Nutrition.* 2011: 8:1. http://www.jissn.com/content/8/1/1
4. Anni Heikkinen A, Alaranta A, Helenius I, Vasankari T. Use of dietary supplements in Olympic athletes is decreasing: A follow-up study between 2002 and 2009. *J Int Soc Sports Nutr.* 2011;8:1.
5. Watson E. *Bodybuilding.com steroid spiking guilty plea is a wake-up call for industry.* 2012. http://www.nutraingredients-usa.com/Regulation/Bodybuilding.com-steroids-spiking-guilty-plea-is-a-wake-up-call-for-industry-says-lab-director. Retrieved May 12, 2013.
6. Food and Drug Administration. *Q&A on Dietary Supplements.* 2013. http://www.fda.gov/Food/ DietarySupplements/QADietarySupplements/ default.htm#what_is. Retrieved May 13, 2013.
7. Dietary Supplement Health and Education Act of 1994.
8. U.S. Food and Drug Administration. Structure/ function claims. http://www.fda.gov/Food/ IngredientsPackagingLabeling/LabelingNutrition/ ucm2006881.htm
9. U.S. Food and Drug Administration. Guidance for industry: FDA's implementation of "qualified health claims": Questions and answers; final guidance. May 12, 2006. http://www.fda.gov/Food/GuidanceRegulation/ GuidanceDocumentsRegulatoryInformation/ LabelingNutrition/ucm053843.htm
10. Food and Drug Administration. *FDA Issues Regulation Prohibiting Sale of Dietary Supplements Containing Ephedrine Alkaloids and Reiterates Its Advice That Consumers Stop Using These Products.* 2004. http://www.fda.gov/NewsEvents/ Newsroom/PressAnnouncements/2004/ucm108242. htm. Retrieved May 13, 2013.
11. U.S. Food and Drug Administration. Tips for dietary supplement users: Making informed decisions and evaluating information. January 2002. http://www.fda.gov/ Food/DietarySupplements/UsingDietarySupplements/ ucm110567.htm
12. Food and Drug Administration. *Dietary Supplement Current Good Manufacturing Practices (CGMPs) and Interim Final Rule (IFR) Facts;* 2007.
13. Jenkinson DM, Harbert AJ. Supplements and sports. *Am Fam Physician.* 2008;78:1039–1046.
14. O'Neill A. Fatal choice. *People Magazine* 1999. Vol 52, 4, 105-109. Available at http://www.people.com/people/ archive/article/0,,20128865,00.html; Accessed 5/10/2014.
15. Sumner MD, Elliott-Eller M, Weidner G, et al. Effects of pomegranate juice consumption on myocardial perfusion in patients with coronary heart disease. *Am J Cardiol.* 2005;96:810–814.
16. Aviram M, Rosenblat M, Gaitini D, et al. Pomegranate juice consumption for 3 years by patients with carotid artery stenosis reduces common carotid intima-media thickness, blood pressure and LDL oxidation. *Clin Nutr.* 2004;23:423–433.
17. Rosenblat M, Hayek T, Aviram M. Anti-oxidative effects of pomegranate juice (PJ) consumption by diabetic patients on serum and on macrophages. *Atherosclerosis.* 2006;187:363–371.
18. Mertens-Talcott SU, Rios J, Jilma-Stohlawetz P, et al. Pharmacokinetics of anthocyanins and antioxidant effects after the consumption of anthocyanin-rich acai juice and pulp (Euterpe oleracea Mart.) in human healthy volunteers. *J Agric Food Chem.* 2008;56:7796–7802.
19. Jensen GS, Wu X, Patterson KM, et al. In vitro and in vivo antioxidant and anti-inflammatory capacities of an antioxidant-rich fruit and berry juice blend. Results of a pilot and randomized, double-blinded, placebo-controlled, crossover study. *J Agric Food Chem.* 2008;56:8326–8333.
20. Amagase H, Nance DM. A randomized, double-blind, placebo-controlled, clinical study of the general effects of a standardized Lycium barbarum (Goji) Juice, GoChi. *J Altern Complement Med.* 2008;14:403–412.

21. Pedraza-Chaverri J, Cardenas-Rodriguez N, Orozco-Ibarra M, Perez-Rojas JM. Medicinal properties of mangosteen (Garcinia mangostana). *Food Chem Toxicol.* 2008;46:3227–3239.

22. Sesso HD, Buring JE, Christen WG, et al. Vitamins E and C in the prevention of cardiovascular disease in men: The Physicians' Health Study II randomized controlled trial. *Jama.* 2008;300:2123–2133.

23. Gaziano JM, Glynn RJ, Christen WG, et al. Vitamins E and C in the prevention of prostate and total cancer in men: The Physicians' Health Study II randomized controlled trial. *Jama.* 2009;301:52–62.

24. Mursu J, Robien K, Harnack LJ, Park K, Jacobs DR Jr. Dietary supplements and mortality rate in older women: The Iowa Women's Health Study. *Arch Intern Med.* 2011;171:1625–1633.

25. Klein EA, Thompson IM Jr, Tangen CM, et al. Vitamin E and the risk of prostate cancer: The Selenium and Vitamin E Cancer Prevention Trial (SELECT). *Jama.* 2011;306:1549–1556.

26. Bjelakovic G, Nikolova D, Gluud LL, Simonetti RG, Gluud C. Mortality in randomized trials of antioxidant supplements for primary and secondary prevention: Systematic review and meta-analysis. *Jama.* 2007;297:842–857.

27. Ristow M, Zarse K, Oberbach A, et al. Antioxidants prevent health-promoting effects of physical exercise in humans. *Proc Natl Acad Sci USA.* 2009;106:8665–8670.

28. Slomski A. IOM endorses vitamin D, calcium only for bone health, dispels deficiency claims. *Jama.* 2011;305:453–454, 456.

29. Hoffman JR, Falvo MJ. Protein: Which is best? *J Sports Sci Med.* 2004;3:118–130.

30. Erdman JW Jr. AHA Science Advisory: Soy protein and cardiovascular disease: A statement for healthcare professionals from the Nutrition Committee of the AHA. *Circulation.* 2000;102:2555–2559.

31. Sacks FM, Lichtenstein A, Van Horn L, Harris W, Kris-Etherton P, Winston M. Soy protein, isoflavones, and cardiovascular health: An American Heart Association Science Advisory for professionals from the Nutrition Committee. *Circulation.* 2006;113:1034–1044.

32. Riediger ND, Othman RA, Suh M, Moghadasian MH. A systemic review of the roles of n-3 fatty acids in health and disease. *J Am Dietet Assoc.* 2009;109:668–679.

33. Kris-Etherton PM, Grieger JA, Etherton TD. Dietary reference intakes for DHA and EPA. *Prostaglandins Leukot Essent Fatty Acids.* 2009;81:99–104.

34. Geyer H, Braun H, Burke L, Stear S, Castell LM. A-Z of nutritional supplements: Dietary supplements, sports nutrition foods and ergogenic aids for health and performance - part 22. *Br J Sports Med.* 2011;45:752–754.

35. *The World Anti-Doping Code: The 2013 Prohibited List: International Standard.* World Anti-Doping Agency, Montreal (Quebec), Canada; 2013.

36. Burke LM, Castell LM, Stear SJ. BJSM reviews: A-Z of supplements: Dietary supplements, sports nutrition foods and ergogenic aids for health and performance Part 1. *Br J Sports Med.* 2009;43:728–729.

37. Currell K, Syed A, Dziedzic CE, et al. BJSM reviews: A-Z of nutritional supplements: Dietary supplements, sports nutrition foods and ergogenic aids for health and performance part 12. *Br J Sports Med.* 2010;44:905–907.

38. Houglum J, Harrelson GL. *Principles of Pharmacology for Athletic Trainers.* 2nd ed. Thorofare, NJ: Slack Incorporated; 2011.

39. Lasne F, Martin L, Crepin N, de Ceaurriz J. Detection of isoelectric profiles of erythropoietin in urine: Differentiation of natural and administered recombinant hormones. *Anal Biochem.* 2002;311:119–126.

40. Boron WF, Boulpaep EL. *Medical Physiology: A Cellular and Molecular Approach.* Philadelphia, PA: Elsevier/Saunders; 2012.

41. Armstrong LE, Casa DJ, Maresh CM, Ganio MS. Caffeine, fluid-electrolyte balance, temperature regulation, and exercise-heat tolerance. *Exerc Sport Sci Rev.* 2007;35:135–140.

42. Frary CD, Johnson RK, Wang MQ. Food sources and intakes of caffeine in the diets of persons in the United States. *J Am Dietet Assoc.* 2005;105:110–113.

43. Keisler BD, Armsey TD 2nd. Caffeine as an ergogenic aid. *Curr Sports Med Rep.* 2006;5:215–219.

44. Diepvens K, Westerterp KR, Westerterp-Plantenga MS. Obesity and thermogenesis related to the consumption of caffeine, ephedrine, capsaicin, and green tea. *Am J Physiol.* 2007;292:R77–R85.

45. Bell DG, McLellan TM, Sabiston CM. Effect of ingesting caffeine and ephedrine on 10-km run performance. *Med Sci Sports Exerc.* 2002;34:344–349.

46. Blomstrand E. A role for branched-chain amino acids in reducing central fatigue. *J Nutr.* 2006;136:544S–547S.

47. Rodriguez NR, Di Marco NM, Langley S. American College of Sports Medicine position stand. Nutrition and athletic performance. *Med Sci Sports Exerc.* 2009;41:709–731.

48. Beque MD, Lochmann JD, Melrose DR. Effects of oral creatine supplementation on muscular strength and body composition. *Med Sci Sports Exerc.* 2000;32:654–658.

49. Brose A, Parise G, Tarnopolsky MA. Creatine supplementation enhances isometric strength and body composition improvements following strength exercise training in older adults. *J Gerontol A Biol Sci Med Sci.* 2003;58:11–19.

50. Volek JS, Rawson ES. Scientific basis and practical aspects of creatine supplementation for athletes. Review. *Nutrition.* 2004;20:609–614.

51. Cooper R, Naclerio F, Allgrove J, Jimenez A. Creatine supplementation with specific view to exercise/sports performance: An update. Review. *J Int Soc Sports Nutr.* 2012;9:33.

52. Rawson ES, Volek JS. Effects of creatine supplementation and resistance training on muscle strength and weightlifting performance. *J Strength Cond Res.* 2003;17:822–831.

53. Poortmans JR, Rawson ES, Burke LM, Stear SJ, Castell LM. A-Z of nutritional supplements: Dietary supplements, sports nutrition foods and ergogenic aids for health and performance Part 11. *Br J Sports Med.* 2010;44:765–766.

54. Buford TW, Kreider RB, Stout JR, et al. International Society of Sports Nutrition position stand: Creatine supplementation and exercise. *J Int Soc Sports Nutr.* 2007;4:6.

55. Edge J, Bishop D, Goodman C. Effects of chronic $NaHCO_3$ ingestion during interval training on changes to muscle buffer capacity, metabolism, and short-term endurance performance. *J Appl Physiol.* 2006;101:918–925.

56. Nissen S, Sharp R, Ray M. Effect of leucine metabolite beta-hydroxy-beta-methylbutyrate on muscle metabolism during resistance-exercise training. *J Appl Physiol.* 1996;81:2095–2104.

57. Ahtiainen JP, Pakarinen A, Alen M, Kraemer WJ, Hakkinen K. Muscle hypertrophy, hormonal adaptations and strength development during strength training in strength-trained and untrained men. *Eur J Appl Physiol.* 2003;89:555–563.

58. Baguet A, Reyngoudt H, Pottier A, et al. Carnosine loading and washout in human skeletal muscles. *J Appl Physiol.* 2009;106:837–842.

59. Campbell B, Roberts M, Kerksick C, et al. Pharmacokinetics, safety, and effects on exercise performance of L-arginine alpha-ketoglutarate in trained adult men. *Nutrition.* 2006;22:872–881.

60. Greek BK, Jones BT. Acute arginine supplementation fails to improve muscle endurance or affect blood pressure responses to resistance training. *J Strength Cond Res.* 2011;25:1789–1794.

61. Sass C, Eickhoff-Shemek JM, Manore MM, Kruskall LJ. Crossing the line: Understanding the scope of practice between registered dietitians and health/fitness professionals. *ACSM Health Fitness J.* 2007;11:12–19.

62. USADA. Statement from USADA CEO Travis T. Tygart regarding the U.S. postal service pro cycling team doping conspiracy. Statement released 10-10-12. http://cyclinginvestigation.usada.org/. Accessed May 10, 2014.

63. BBC Sport. *Lewis escapes doping punishment.* April 30, 2003. http://news.bbc.co.uk/sport2/hi/athletics/2989361.stm. Retrieved May 10, 2014.

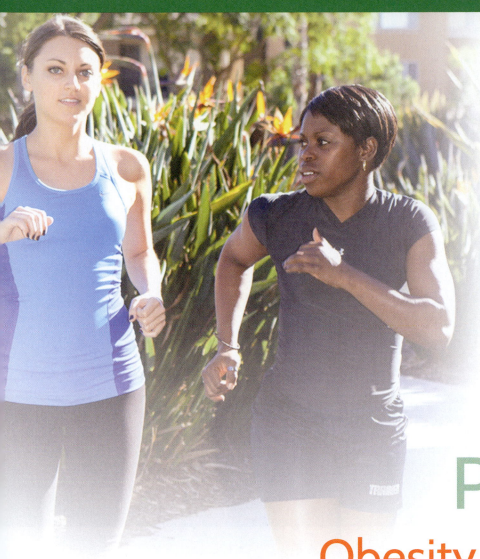

# PART VI

# Obesity and Weight Management

Part VI of this book covers a topic that is of major concern for many of the clients with whom health and fitness professionals work on a daily basis. The latest information on the science of obesity is covered in Chapter 22, with a focus on the adverse health consequences of this condition. Chapter 23 provides current information on body composition assessment techniques and focuses on the accuracy and limitations of each technique. Chapter 24, the final chapter in this section, provides information on the components of a successful weight-management program. Understanding behavior change is a major focus of Chapter 24 because it plays such a critical role in helping people adopt effective weight-management strategies. The synergistic role of sound exercise and nutritional programming is also highlighted, as are practical suggestions for relapse prevention.

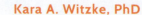

Kara A. Witzke, PhD

CHAPTER 22

# Physiology of Obesity

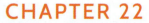

## CHAPTER OUTLINE

## LEARNING OUTCOMES

1. Describe factors related to the increase in the prevalence of overweight and obesity among adults and children in the United States.

2. Explain the differences between overweight, overfat, and obesity.

3. Describe the use of body mass index (BMI) for population studies and its limitations for use with individuals.

4. Describe several health consequences of overweight and obesity.

5. Define the components of energy balance and describe the relationship of dietary intake and physical activity to each component.

6. Identify the hormones responsible for short- and long-term regulation of energy intake.

7. Describe the environmental and genetic factors that regulate body weight.

## ANCILLARY LINK

Visit Davis*Plus* at http://davisplus.fadavis.com for study and practice resources, including online quizzes, animations that help explain physiological processes, podcasts concerning news and career trends in exercise physiology, and practice references.

## VIGNETTE

■ Lucinda is a 45-year-old working mother of two daughters, ages 7 and 10. Like many women her age, she has experienced gradual weight gain since the birth of her children. Standing 5'2" (1.6 m) tall and now weighing 160 pounds (73 kg), she is experiencing difficulty performing the everyday tasks associated with her busy lifestyle. Lucinda also was recently told by her physician that, in addition to being obese, she is starting to display other characteristics of metabolic syndrome, including hypertension and glucose intolerance.

Lucinda has "yo-yo dieted" in the past, usually resorting to very low-calorie diets, and does not exercise. She is convinced that her weight problem is genetic, because she and her mother look very similar despite their desire to be thinner. She is getting concerned that her daughters will also someday look just like her and does not want to live the rest of her life with health problems. Lucinda tries to "eat healthy," but resorts to eating at fast-food restaurants most days for the sake of convenience. This lifestyle has reduced her lean body mass over the years, and a recent body composition test conducted using a BOD POD revealed that she has 47% body fat.

How can a basic understanding of the physiology of obesity and the relationship between genetics and environment help Lucinda turn things around for herself, and also help her two young daughters avoid going down the same road as Lucinda and her mother?

**Obesity** is defined as having an excessive amount of **body fat**. This excess is associated with many adverse health outcomes, such as cardiovascular disease, metabolic disease, and cancer. Despite an increased awareness of these negative health risks, the prevalence of **overweight** (a higher weight than recommended) and obesity is on the rise in the United States. In fact, the rise in childhood obesity has never been more rapid, and a clear understanding of this complex disease is imperative.

This chapter describes the prevalence and consequences of the obesity epidemic, as well as prevailing theories about its cause. Information about the interaction of genetic and environmental factors on the development of obesity is also presented.

## PREVALENCE OF OVERWEIGHT AND OBESITY

According to the Centers for Disease Control and Prevention (CDC),[1] American society has become "**obesogenic**," meaning that it is an environment that tends to generate or create a state of obesity. An increasingly convenient lifestyle, characterized by environments that promote unhealthy food intake and physical inactivity, has contributed to an increase in the percentage of *obese* adults from just 13.3% in 1960 to 33.9% in 2008.[2] The number of adults categorized as *overweight* or *obese* has increased from 44.8% in 1960 to 68.0% in 2008 (Table 22-1).[3] It is estimated that by 2015, more than 40% of U.S. adults will be obese.[4] Key facts about obesity are presented in Box 22-1.[5]

Unfortunately, the unhealthy habits of American adults have been passed down to their children. Results from the 2007–2008 National Health and Nutrition Examination Survey (NHANES)[3] using measures of body mass index (BMI) indicate that 16.9% of all children and adolescents ages 2 to 19 years are now obese (Fig. 22-1). In the 1960s, this number was only 4.4%. The chance of having a BMI greater than 25 starts to rise around age 35 years and declines around age 75 years in both men and women. However, women are still more likely to be obese at all ages. Not surprisingly, these trends are similar for other countries throughout the world.

There are differences in overweight and obesity prevalence by racial/ethnic group (see Table 22-1). It is estimated that 54% of non-Hispanic black women are considered obese compared with 32% of Mexican American and 30% of non-Hispanic white women of the same age. Among men, 34% of black men compared with 31% of white and 32% of Mexican American men are obese.[6] Among children of color, these estimates are also alarming, with 24.5% of non-Hispanic black children and 22.1% of Mexican American children now meeting the criteria for obesity.[7]

These racial differences may be explained by a combination of genetics, food, and exercise habits, as well as cultural attitudes toward body weight. On average, non-Hispanic black women burn about 100 fewer calories each day during rest than white women, which translates into nearly 1 lb (0.5 kg) of body fat gained each month.[8] Non-Hispanic black women also tend to experience a more dramatic lowering of their **resting metabolic rate (RMR)** during dieting than white women, which may also help to explain why they tend to have greater difficulty in achieving a goal body weight than overweight white women.[9] However, the trend toward increasing overweight and obesity continues to increase among all racial/ethnic and socioeconomic groups.

## Overweight Versus Obesity

Some confusion exists regarding the precise meaning of the terms *overweight*, *overfat*, and *obesity* as they pertain to **body composition** and an individual's risk for health problems. In proper context, the term *overweight* simply refers to a body weight that exceeds some predetermined average for height. A person who is overweight has usually experienced an increase in body fat, but not always, as in the case of muscular athletes.

*Overfat* is a term used to describe the condition of having more than a healthy amount of body fat. This is determined by measuring a person's percent body fat. Men with 25% or more body fat and women with 32% or more body fat are considered to be overfat (as well as obese).

The term *obesity* refers to the overfat condition that accompanies a host of comorbidities, including **glucose** intolerance, insulin resistance, dyslipidemia, type 2 diabetes, **hypertension**, elevated plasma leptin concentrations, increased visceral fat tissue, and increased risk for coronary heart disease and cancer. Research indicates a much clearer relation between these conditions and increased body fat, rather than merely an increase in body weight. It is certainly possible for an individual to be overweight or overfat but not exhibit these comorbidities.

In most medical literature, the term *overweight* is used to describe an *overfat* condition, even in the absence of accompanying body-fat measures. In this context, obesity then refers to individuals at the extreme end of the overweight continuum. This is the framework used to determine body fatness using BMI.

## Estimation of Body Fatness Using Body Mass Index

BMI, the most common technique for estimating fatness, is calculated as the ratio of one's weight to height:

$$BMI = weight\ (kg)/height^2\ (m^2)$$

*Example:*
Male: 5'9", 214 lb
5'9" = 69 in. 69 in. × 0.0254 m/in. = 1.753 m
214 lb = 214 lb ÷ 2.2 kg/lb = 97.3 kg
BMI = 97.3 ÷ (1.753)² = 31.7 kg/m²

## Table 22-1. Prevalence of Obesity and Overweight for Adults Aged 20 Years and Older

| CATEGORIES BY AGE | ADULTS (%) (95% CI) | | |
| --- | --- | --- | --- |
| | ALL ADULTS* | NON-HISPANIC WHITE | NON-HISPANIC BLACK |
| **BMI ≥ 30** | | | |
| All, age (y) | | | |
| ≥20 | 33.9 (31.7–36.1) | 32.8 (29.4–36.1) | 44.1 (39.9–48.3) |
| ≥20‡ | 33.8 (31.6–36.0) | 32.4 (28.9–35.9) | 44.1 (40.0–48.2) |
| Men, age (y) | | | |
| ≥20‡ | 32.2 (29.5–35.0) | 31.9 (28.1–35.7) | 37.3 (32.3–42.4) |
| 20–39 | 27.5 (23.8–31.2) | 26.3 (20.9–31.7) | 34.7 (28.5–40.9) |
| 40–59 | 34.3 (29.8–38.8) | 34.0 (28.1–39.8) | 39.7 (30.0–49.5) |
| ≥60 | 37.1 (33.1–41.0) | 38.4 (34.1–42.6) | 38.0 (31.3–44.7) |
| Women, age (y) | | | |
| ≥20‡ | 35.5 (33.2–37.7) | 33.0 (29.3–36.6) | 49.6 (45.5–53.7) |
| 20–39 | 34.0 (29.0–39.1) | 31.3 (23.3–39.3) | 47.2 (41.3–53.1) |
| 40–59 | 38.2 (33.8–42.6) | 35.7 (29.7–41.7) | 51.7 (47.2–56.1) |
| ≥60 | 33.6 (30.2–36.9) | 31.4 (27.3–35.5) | 50.5 (40.5–60.5) |
| **BMI ≥ 25** | | | |
| All, age (y) | | | |
| ≥20 | 68.3 (66.6–70.0) | 67.5 (65.0–70.1) | 73.7 (71.2–76.2) |
| ≥20‡ | 68.0 (66.3–69.8) | 66.7 (64.1–69.3) | 73.8 (71.3–76.3) |
| Men, age (y) | | | |
| ≥20‡ | 72.3 (70.4–74.1) | 72.6 (69.9–75.3) | 68.5 (65.2–71.8) |
| 20–39 | 63.5 (60.8–66.2) | 62.6 (58.0–67.2) | 61.5 (54.6–68.5) |
| 40–59 | 77.8 (74.0–81.7) | 77.7 (72.8–82.6) | 73.5 (65.9–81.2) |
| ≥60 | 78.4 (74.8–81.9) | 81.4 (77.9–84.9) | 72.5 (65.2–79.8) |
| Women, age (y) | | | |
| ≥20‡ | 64.1 (61.3–66.9) | 61.2 (56.7–65.7) | 78.2 (74.5–81.9) |
| 20–39 | 59.5 (54.5–64.5) | 54.9 (46.3–63.6) | 78.0 (71.8–84.2) |
| 40–59 | 66.3 (63.3–69.3) | 63.8 (59.8–67.8) | 78.4 (74.1–82.6) |
| ≥60 | 68.6 (64.4–72.7) | 67.6 (62.2–73.1) | 78.2 (70.7–85.8) |

| CATEGORIES BY AGE | ADULTS (%) (95% CI) | | |
| --- | --- | --- | --- |
| | ALL ADULTS* | HISPANIC ADULTS | MEXICAN AMERICAN |
| **BMI ≥ 30** | | | |
| All, age (y) | | | |
| ≥20 | 33.9 (31.7–36.1) | 37.9 (32.3–43.4) | 39.3 (32.0–46.6) |
| ≥20‡ | 33.8 (31.6–36.0) | 38.7 (33.5–43.9) | 40.4 (34.2–46.6) |
| Men, age (y) | | | |
| ≥20‡ | 32.2 (29.5–35.0) | 34.3 (28.2–40.3) | 35.9 (26.3–44.4) |
| 20–39 | 27.5 (23.8–31.2) | 32.3 (23.9–40.7) | 33.8 (22.7–44.9) |
| 40–59 | 34.3 (29.8–38.8) | 37.4 (29.0–45.8) | 38.2 (26.3–50.1) |
| ≥60 | 37.1 (33.1–41.0) | 32.6 (23.5–41.7) | 35.8 (21.9–49.8) |
| Women, age (y) | | | |
| ≥20‡ | 35.5 (33.2–37.7) | 43.0 (37.9–48.2) | 45.1 (28.9–51.2) |
| 20–39 | 34.0 (29.0–39.1) | 37.6 (32.3–42.8) | 39.6 (33.7–45.5) |
| 40–59 | 38.2 (33.8–42.6) | 46.6 (37.3–55.9) | 48.9 (38.0–59.8) |
| ≥60 | 33.6 (30.2–36.9) | 46.7 (41.0–52.3) | 48.1 (43.0–53.3) |
| **BMI ≥ 25** | | | |
| All, age (y) | | | |
| ≥20 | 68.3 (66.6–70.0) | 76.9 (72.9–80.8) | 77.5 (73.4–81.6) |
| ≥20‡ | 68.0 (66.3–69.8) | 77.9 (74.5–81.4) | 78.8 (75.2–82.4) |
| Men, age (y) | | | |
| ≥20‡ | 72.3 (70.4–74.1) | 79.3 (74.7–83.9) | 80.0 (75.5–84.5) |
| 20–39 | 63.5 (60.8–66.2) | 74.2 (66.8–81.5) | 75.0 (67.4–82.7) |
| 40–59 | 77.8 (74.0–81.7) | 87.2 (81.4–93.0) | 88.0 (80.8–95.1) |
| ≥60 | 78.4 (74.8–81.9) | 75.4 (70.2–80.7) | 75.8 (68.4–83.1) |
| Women, age (y) | | | |
| ≥20‡ | 64.1 (61.3–66.9) | 76.1 (72.0–80.1) | 76.9 (71.8–81.9) |
| 20–39 | 59.5 (54.5–64.5) | 68.5 (61.4–75.7) | 70.3 (62.7–77.9) |
| 40–59 | 66.3 (63.3–69.3) | 81.2 (77.3–85.1) | 80.3 (73.6–87.0) |
| ≥60 | 68.6 (64.4–72.7) | 80.7 (77.3–84.1) | 82.6 (77.2–88.0) |

*Includes racial and ethnic groups not shown separately.

†Includes Mexican Americans.

‡Age adjusted by the direct method to the year 2000 U.S. Census population using the age groups 20–39, 40–59, and ≥60 years.

BMI, body mass index (calculated as weight in kilograms divided by height in meters squared); CI, confidence interval.

*Source:* Based on data from the National Health and Nutrition Examination Survey (NHANES) 2007–2008. Reprinted from Flegal KM, Carroll MD, Ogden CL, Curtin LR. Prevalence and trends in obesity among US adults, 1999-2008. *JAMA.* 2010;303:235–241.

## Box 22-1. Key Facts About Obesity

- Worldwide obesity has nearly doubled since 1980.
- In 2008, 1.4 billion adults aged 20 years and older were overweight. Of these, more than 200 million men and nearly 300 million women were obese.
- Thirty-five percent of adults aged 20 and older were overweight in 2008, and 11% were obese.
- 65% of the world's population lives in countries where overweight and obesity kill more people than underweight.
- More than 40 million children younger than age 5 years were overweight in 2011.
- Obesity is preventable.

Data from the World Health Organization. (2013, March). *Obesity and Overweight.* www.who.int/mediacentre/factsheets/fs311/en/ Accessed April 30, 2014.

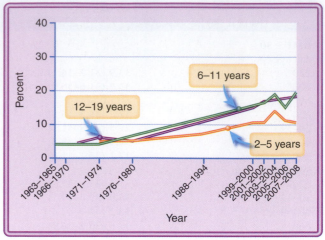

**Figure 22-1.** Trends in obesity among children and adolescents: United States (1963–2008). Note: Obesity is defined as body mass index (BMI) greater than or equal to sex- and age-specific 95th percentile from the 2000 U.S. Centers for Disease Control and Prevention (CDC) Growth Charts. (Data from CDC/NCHS, National Health Examination Surveys II [ages 6–11 years], III [ages 12–17 years], and the National Health and Nutrition Examination Surveys [NHANES] I–III, and NHANES 1999–2000, 2001–2002, 2003–2004, 2005–2006, and 2007–2008.)

Table 22-2 provides a simple way to determine BMI by intersecting an individual's height and weight in standard units. An easy-to-use BMI calculator is available at the American Council on Exercise website (www.acefitness.org/calculators/default.aspx).

In 1997, the World Health Organization developed guidelines that classified people with BMIs greater than 25 as overweight, and those with BMIs greater than or equal to 30 as obese.[10] Individuals with BMIs greater than or equal to 40 are considered morbidly, or extremely, obese (Table 22-3). These individuals clearly have a higher risk for death and disability because of their weight. These standards place 97 million Americans in the overweight and obese categories, up from 72 million people when using previously accepted standards.

## Use of Body Mass Index in the Clinical Setting

Although BMI does not measure body fat, it is considered one of the best ways to quickly approximate an individual's degree of body fatness, as opposed to looking at weight alone. It not only provides a simple baseline measure against which progress can be compared, but it also provides useful information about an individual's potential health risk factors. For example, if an individual is classified as being overweight or obese using BMI, it would be a good idea for the fitness or health professional to inquire about the client's health history related to blood pressure, cholesterol, and heart health. At the very least, it does provide a platform from which to discuss the relationship between body fatness and chronic disease, and provides both the individual and the professional with a starting point for more in-depth discussion.

## Limitations of Body Mass Index

Despite its convenience and popularity, some researchers still consider BMI a relatively crude index of body composition, because BMI fails to consider the body's proportional distribution of body fat and the lean tissue. Healthy adults can be misdiagnosed by BMI as overweight or obese, when body composition mass is verified by a criterion method such as dual-energy x-ray absorptiometry (DEXA) or hydrostatic weighing. For instance, BMI may overestimate "fatness" in athletes and others who have a muscular build (false positive), and it may underestimate fatness in older persons and others who have lost muscle (false negative). The possibility of misclassifying someone as overweight using BMI standards applies particularly to large-size field athletes, bodybuilders, heavier wrestlers, and football players who tend to have large amounts of muscle mass, which *weighs* more than fat *per unit volume* (i.e., muscle is more dense than fat), but does not contribute to a higher percentage of body fat (Fig. 22-2).

Although there are inherent problems with assessing fatness of an individual using the BMI method, it remains the method of choice for large-scale epidemiological studies because of the ease of obtaining the two measurements required for BMI calculation and its acceptable correlation with more technical measures (e.g., DEXA, hydrostatic weighing, and skinfold measurements). Notably, however, the number obtained using BMI is *not* a measure of body composition (i.e., percent body fat) per se, but merely a calculated *ratio* using height and weight.

The measurement of body composition—whether using sophisticated methods such as hydrostatic weighing, DEXA, or air displacement plethysmography (e.g., BOD POD) or less-sophisticated methods such as bioelectrical impedance, skinfold measurements, or near-infrared interactance—produces *estimates* of the percentage of the body composed of fat versus fat-free mass. When working with *individuals*, body composition measurement is considered a much better method of assessing overall fatness and risk for disease than BMI. Chapter 23 provides a more detailed discussion of these methods.

## In Your Own Words

How would you respond to someone who says, "I know that body composition is more important than body weight, and I'd like to be able to measure my progress, but getting my body composition measured is just too complicated and too expensive."

## Fat Cell Size and Number: Hypertrophy Versus Hyperplasia

Obesity can also be classified by fat cell size and number:
- Fat cell **hypertrophy**: an increase in fat cell size
- Fat cell **hyperplasia**: an increase in total fat cell number

The development of obesity involves an intricate process and is dependent on the interplay between adipocyte hypertrophy and adipocyte hyperplasia (Fig. 22-3). Adipocyte hyperplasia represents a complex process by which new fat cells are developed from adipocyte precursor fat cells called **preadipocytes**.[11] This process of **adipogenesis** involves two major events: the recruitment and proliferation of preadipocytes followed by their subsequent differentiation into mature fat cells containing stored **triglyceride** (the major form of fat stored in the body). The recruitment and proliferation phase represents hyperplasia (Fig. 22-3, obesity example 1), and the differentiation phase reflects hypertrophy (Fig. 22-3, obesity example 2). Although evidence from cell line studies suggests that the proliferation of preadipocytes occurs before differentiation,[12] human preadipocyte studies indicate that partially differentiated cells can also replicate.[13]

Most cases of adult obesity previously were attributed solely to adipocyte hypertrophy, where existing adipocytes hypertrophy because of an excessive accumulation of lipids from excessive energy intake versus energy expenditure (positive energy balance). However, evidence suggests that adipogenesis occurs throughout the lifetime of an individual, both in response to normal cell turnover and the need for additional fat mass stores when caloric intake exceeds the body's requirements.[13–15] Studies in the 1970s showed that in adults who achieved body weights of 170% of ideal (moderately severe obesity), adipocytes reached a maximum size with roughly 1.0 μg lipid per cell, which was about twice their normal size. Over this level of obesity, the degree of hyperplasia, not hypertrophy, correlated well with the severity of obesity. This concept is reflected in Figure 22-3

when comparing fat cell number with fat cell volume changes from the lean to severely obese categories. Note that transitioning from lean to overweight mostly involves an increase is cell volume (hypertrophy) with a relatively stable fat cell number (hyperplasia). However, on reaching the category of obesity, fat cell volume begins to plateau as fat cell number begins to increase. This pattern holds through increasing severity of obesity. Whereas hyperplasia was previously shown to occur in those with early-onset obesity, this work showed significant hyperplasia even in individuals with a later onset of obesity.[15]

Animal studies have corroborated the notion that adipocytes have a "critical size" at which cellular hyperplasia is triggered.[16] Rats force-fed up to 200% of their usual caloric intake showed an increase in fat cell number in all fat pads in a two-step manner as the overfeeding progressed. First, there was an initial increase in fat cell number, believed to be due to lipid filling of existing cells to a measurable cell size, which was followed several weeks later by a second increase in cell number thought to be due to true cellular hyperplasia.[17] Human studies show similar results, whereby preadipocytes extracted from the adipose tissue of both young and old individuals can be induced to differentiate in vitro, thereby providing additional evidence for the continued adipogenic capacity of fat cells throughout life.[18] In normal human growth and development, however, the differentiation of preadipocytes to mature fat cells is a process that begins during embryonic development and continues until shortly after birth, during which time the majority of differentiation-related events occur.[19]

Obesity that occurs during the first year of life or during the adolescent growth spurt (ages 9–13 years) with a BMI greater than 40 can induce adipocyte hyperplasia and predispose an individual to hyperplastic obesity into adulthood. In fact, children who are obese between the ages of 6 and 9 years have a 55% chance of becoming obese adults, which is 10 times the risk of children of normal weight. These children do not generally "outgrow" obesity. In fact, once established, the number of fat cells remains relatively constant in spite of weight gain or loss. Reducing body fatness is especially difficult, although not impossible, for individuals with a high number of fat cells. Individuals with hyperplastic obesity are not easily treated with ordinary dietary and exercise regimens. When treated with a conventional low-energy diet, they seem to fail to lose weight after reaching a certain fat-cell size. Obese people who have lost weight by restricting energy intake are very prone to weight regain. Unfortunately for these individuals, no amount of dietary restriction or exercise can reduce fat-cell number.[20] Therefore, lifestyle-modification plans that strive to reduce overall body fat will only function to reduce the amount of fat in each existing cell, which may still translate into a higher body-fat percentage merely because of the higher number of fat depots.

## Table 22-2. Determination of Body Mass Index

| | BMI | | | | | | | | | | | | | | | | |
|---|---|---|---|---|---|---|---|---|---|---|---|---|---|---|---|---|---|
| | NORMAL | | | | | | OVERWEIGHT | | | | | OBESE | | | | | |
| HEIGHT (IN.) | 19 | 20 | 21 | 22 | 23 | 24 | 25 | 26 | 27 | 28 | 29 | 30 | 31 | 32 | 33 | 34 | 35 |
| | BODY WEIGHT IN POUNDS | | | | | | | | | | | | | | | | |
| 58 | 91 | 96 | 100 | 105 | 110 | 115 | 119 | 124 | 129 | 134 | 138 | 143 | 148 | 153 | 158 | 162 | 167 |
| 59 | 94 | 99 | 104 | 109 | 114 | 119 | 124 | 128 | 133 | 138 | 143 | 148 | 153 | 158 | 163 | 168 | 173 |
| 60 | 97 | 102 | 107 | 112 | 118 | 123 | 128 | 133 | 138 | 143 | 148 | 153 | 158 | 163 | 168 | 174 | 179 |
| 61 | 100 | 106 | 111 | 116 | 122 | 127 | 132 | 137 | 143 | 148 | 153 | 158 | 164 | 169 | 174 | 180 | 185 |
| 62 | 104 | 109 | 115 | 120 | 126 | 131 | 136 | 142 | 147 | 153 | 158 | 164 | 169 | 175 | 180 | 186 | 191 |
| 63 | 107 | 113 | 118 | 124 | 130 | 135 | 141 | 146 | 152 | 158 | 163 | 169 | 175 | 180 | 186 | 191 | 197 |
| 64 | 110 | 116 | 122 | 128 | 134 | 140 | 145 | 151 | 157 | 163 | 169 | 174 | 180 | 186 | 192 | 197 | 204 |
| 65 | 114 | 120 | 126 | 132 | 138 | 144 | 150 | 156 | 162 | 168 | 174 | 180 | 186 | 192 | 198 | 204 | 210 |
| 66 | 118 | 124 | 130 | 136 | 142 | 148 | 155 | 161 | 167 | 173 | 179 | 186 | 192 | 196 | 204 | 210 | 216 |
| 67 | 121 | 127 | 134 | 140 | 146 | 153 | 159 | 166 | 172 | 178 | 185 | 191 | 198 | 204 | 211 | 217 | 223 |
| 68 | 125 | 131 | 138 | 144 | 151 | 158 | 164 | 171 | 177 | 184 | 190 | 197 | 203 | 210 | 216 | 223 | 230 |
| 69 | 128 | 135 | 142 | 149 | 155 | 162 | 169 | 176 | 182 | 189 | 196 | 203 | 209 | 216 | 223 | 230 | 236 |
| 70 | 132 | 139 | 146 | 153 | 160 | 167 | 174 | 181 | 188 | 195 | 202 | 209 | 216 | 222 | 229 | 236 | 243 |
| 71 | 136 | 143 | 150 | 157 | 165 | 172 | 179 | 186 | 193 | 200 | 208 | 215 | 222 | 229 | 236 | 243 | 250 |
| 72 | 140 | 147 | 154 | 162 | 169 | 177 | 184 | 191 | 199 | 206 | 213 | 221 | 228 | 235 | 242 | 250 | 258 |
| 73 | 144 | 151 | 159 | 166 | 174 | 182 | 189 | 197 | 204 | 212 | 219 | 227 | 235 | 242 | 250 | 257 | 265 |
| 74 | 148 | 155 | 163 | 171 | 179 | 186 | 194 | 202 | 210 | 218 | 225 | 233 | 241 | 249 | 256 | 264 | 272 |
| 75 | 152 | 160 | 168 | 176 | 184 | 192 | 200 | 208 | 216 | 224 | 232 | 240 | 248 | 256 | 264 | 272 | 279 |
| 76 | 156 | 164 | 172 | 180 | 189 | 197 | 205 | 213 | 221 | 230 | 238 | 246 | 254 | 263 | 271 | 279 | 287 |

*Source:* Adapted from National Heart, Lung, and Blood Institute. Clinical Guidelines on the Identification, Evaluation, and Treatment of Overweight and Obesity in Adult: The Evidence Report. http://www.nhlbi.nih.gov/guidelines/obesity/bmi_tbl.htm

| | | | | BMI | | | | | | | | | | | | | | |
|---|---|---|---|---|---|---|---|---|---|---|---|---|---|---|---|---|---|---|
| | | | | **EXTREME OBESITY** | | | | | | | | | | | | | | |
| 36 | 37 | 38 | 39 | 40 | 41 | 42 | 43 | 44 | 45 | 46 | 47 | 48 | 49 | 50 | 51 | 52 | 53 | 54 |
| | | | | **BODY WEIGHT IN POUNDS** | | | | | | | | | | | | | | |
| 172 | 177 | 181 | 186 | 191 | 196 | 201 | 205 | 210 | 215 | 220 | 224 | 229 | 234 | 239 | 244 | 248 | 253 | 258 |
| 178 | 183 | 188 | 193 | 198 | 203 | 208 | 212 | 217 | 222 | 227 | 232 | 237 | 242 | 247 | 252 | 257 | 262 | 267 |
| 184 | 189 | 194 | 199 | 204 | 209 | 215 | 220 | 225 | 230 | 235 | 240 | 245 | 250 | 255 | 261 | 266 | 271 | 276 |
| 190 | 195 | 201 | 206 | 211 | 217 | 222 | 227 | 232 | 238 | 243 | 248 | 254 | 259 | 264 | 269 | 275 | 280 | 285 |
| 196 | 202 | 207 | 213 | 218 | 224 | 229 | 235 | 240 | 246 | 251 | 256 | 262 | 267 | 273 | 278 | 284 | 289 | 295 |
| 203 | 208 | 214 | 220 | 225 | 231 | 237 | 242 | 248 | 254 | 259 | 265 | 270 | 278 | 282 | 287 | 293 | 299 | 304 |
| 209 | 215 | 221 | 227 | 232 | 238 | 244 | 250 | 256 | 262 | 267 | 273 | 279 | 285 | 291 | 296 | 302 | 308 | 314 |
| 216 | 222 | 228 | 234 | 240 | 246 | 252 | 258 | 264 | 270 | 276 | 282 | 288 | 294 | 300 | 306 | 312 | 318 | 324 |
| 223 | 229 | 235 | 241 | 247 | 253 | 260 | 266 | 272 | 278 | 284 | 291 | 297 | 303 | 309 | 315 | 322 | 328 | 334 |
| 230 | 236 | 242 | 249 | 255 | 261 | 268 | 274 | 280 | 287 | 293 | 299 | 306 | 312 | 319 | 325 | 331 | 338 | 344 |
| 236 | 243 | 249 | 256 | 262 | 269 | 276 | 282 | 289 | 295 | 302 | 308 | 315 | 322 | 328 | 335 | 341 | 348 | 354 |
| 243 | 250 | 257 | 263 | 270 | 277 | 284 | 291 | 297 | 304 | 311 | 318 | 324 | 331 | 338 | 345 | 351 | 358 | 365 |
| 250 | 257 | 264 | 271 | 278 | 285 | 292 | 299 | 306 | 313 | 320 | 327 | 334 | 341 | 348 | 355 | 362 | 369 | 376 |
| 257 | 265 | 272 | 279 | 286 | 293 | 301 | 308 | 315 | 322 | 329 | 338 | 343 | 351 | 358 | 365 | 372 | 379 | 386 |
| 265 | 272 | 279 | 287 | 294 | 302 | 309 | 316 | 324 | 331 | 338 | 346 | 353 | 361 | 368 | 375 | 383 | 390 | 397 |
| 272 | 280 | 288 | 295 | 302 | 310 | 318 | 325 | 333 | 340 | 348 | 355 | 363 | 371 | 378 | 386 | 393 | 401 | 408 |
| 280 | 287 | 295 | 303 | 311 | 319 | 326 | 334 | 342 | 350 | 358 | 365 | 373 | 381 | 389 | 396 | 404 | 412 | 420 |
| 287 | 295 | 303 | 311 | 319 | 327 | 335 | 343 | 351 | 359 | 367 | 375 | 383 | 391 | 399 | 407 | 415 | 423 | 431 |
| 295 | 304 | 312 | 320 | 328 | 336 | 344 | 353 | 361 | 369 | 377 | 385 | 394 | 402 | 410 | 418 | 426 | 435 | 443 |

## Table 22-3. Interpretation of Body Mass Index Scores

| BMI SCORE | INTERPRETATION |
|---|---|
| 18 | Underweight |
| 18–24.9 | Normal weight |
| 25–29.9 | Overweight |
| 30–39.9 | Obese |
| ≥40 | Morbidly obese |

Body mass index (BMI) = weight (kg)/height (m²).
*Source:* Adapted from National Heart, Lung, and Blood Institute. Clinical Guidelines on the Identification, Evaluation, and Treatment of Overweight and Obesity in Adult: The Evidence Report. http://www.nhlbi.nih.gov/guidelines/obesity/bmi_tbl.htm

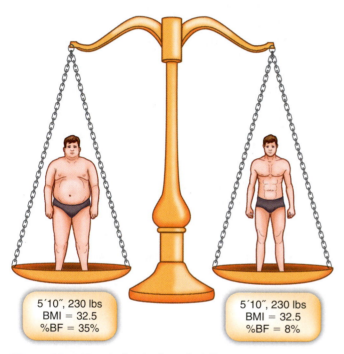

**5´10˝, 230 lbs**
**BMI = 32.5**
**%BF = 35%**

**5´10˝, 230 lbs**
**BMI = 32.5**
**%BF = 8%**

**Figure 22-2.** Two individuals with differing percent body fat values but similar body mass index (BMI) values. In this example, BMI does not distinguish between individuals who are lean and muscular and individuals who are obese. Thus, on an individual level, BMI is limited in determining the composition of fat and lean tissue that make up the total body weight. However, at the larger population level, BMI is much more effective at determining the rates of obesity.

## HEALTH CONSEQUENCES OF OBESITY

Obesity is considered the third leading cause of preventable death in the United States, with smoking and hypertension being first and second, respectively.[21] In two longitudinal analyses adjusted for smoking status, annual death risk among nonsmokers was 12% to 40% higher among overweight individuals and 50% to 150% higher among obese individuals.[22,23] Other studies have

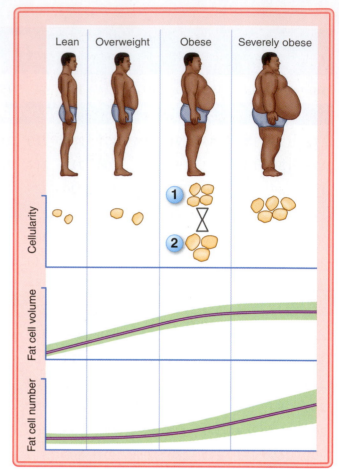

**Figure 22-3.** The state of fat cells (adipocytes) and adipogenesis in lean and obese individuals. Fat mass in humans is the product of two factors: adipocyte size or volume and total number of cells. Overweight individuals usually will have larger adipocytes than lean individuals without significant changes in the total number. A greater number of and larger adipocytes will accompany obese individuals compared with their leaner counterparts. These two factors are used to characterize the two main types of obesity: hyperplastic (obese example 1) and hypertrophic (obese example 2). As shown at the bottom of the figure, when the individual moves further into the range of severe obesity, hyperplasia (cell number) becomes the greater contributing factor to the increase in fat mass compared with cell volume. Cell volume at this point demonstrates a plateau response with no further increase in the severely obese range.

## VIGNETTE continued

■ The good news for Lucinda is that, because she was not an overweight child and is not above 170% of ideal body weight, it is unlikely that her obesity as an adult is due to adipocyte hyperplasia. The hypertrophic obesity that she has experienced is more likely due to poor dietary choices and being sedentary that have created years of positive energy balance, leading to excess calories that have been stored as triglyceride. The bad news is that years of poor dietary choices and lack of exercise have now led to adverse health conditions that will only get worse if she does nothing to change her lifestyle.

Lucinda reaches out to Destiny, a life coach whom one of her friends recommended. In addition to teaching Lucinda about physical activity, Destiny recommends a series of behavioral change techniques that Lucinda can incorporate into her lifestyle. Lucinda can then choose the ones that work best for her. For example, Lucinda begins waking up about 20 minutes earlier each morning so she has time for food preparation so that she can prepare a healthy dinner when she gets home from work. She also packs a few healthy snacks to eat throughout the day. With Destiny's help, Lucinda begins to embrace the long-term changes necessary to improve her health, as opposed to going to bed each night feeling like she "blew her diet."

concluded that obesity is an independent risk factor for coronary heart disease, even when adjusted for the influences of other risk factors such as age, cholesterol, systolic blood pressure, smoking, left ventricular hypertrophy, and glucose intolerance.[24] It has been estimated that obesity directly or indirectly results in 188,000 to 237,000 premature deaths in the United States each year,[25] at a cost of more than $147 billion annually.

## Specific Health Risks of Excessive Body Fat

According to the National Institutes of Health, obesity represents a chronic, degenerative disease, even at low levels of excessive body fat. A moderate 4% to 10% increase in body weight after the age of 20 years correlates with a 50% greater risk for death from coronary artery disease and nonfatal heart attack.[26] Of particular importance is the strong association between excess body fat and diabetes mellitus. Not surprisingly, overweight children are more prone to becoming overweight adults, especially if they have an obese parent or have higher BMIs.[27,28] Obesity during adolescence is associated with many adverse health consequences in adulthood, even if the obesity does not persist.[29]

Excessive body fat is closely related to the explosion of type 2 diabetes diagnosed in children. Even long-term body weight at the high end of the normal range increases heart disease and cancer risk.[30] In the Nurses' Health Study, nurses of average weight experienced 30% more heart attacks compared with their thinnest counterparts, and the risk for a moderately overweight nurse was 80% higher.[30] This means that a woman

who gains only 20 pounds (9 kg) from her late teens to middle age doubles her risk for having a heart attack. Research now identifies obesity as an independent heart disease risk, similar in nature to cigarette smoking, high cholesterol, and hypertension. It also appears to correspond to higher levels of arterial inflammation that slowly and progressively increases heart attack and stroke risk over many years.

Specific health risks of excessive body fat include (Fig. 22-4):

- Impaired cardiac function
- Hypertension
- Stroke
- Deep-vein thrombosis
- Increased insulin resistance
- Renal disease
- Sleep apnea and pulmonary disease
- Problems receiving anesthesia during surgery
- Osteoarthritis, degenerative joint disease, and gout
- Endometrial, breast, prostate, and colon cancers
- Abnormal plasma lipid and cholesterol levels
- Menstrual irregularities
- Gallbladder disease
- Psychological distress

## Importance of Body-Fat Distribution Pattern

Where on the body a person tends to store body fat is also an important determinant of future health. Studies suggest that weight gain in the abdominal area, or **android**

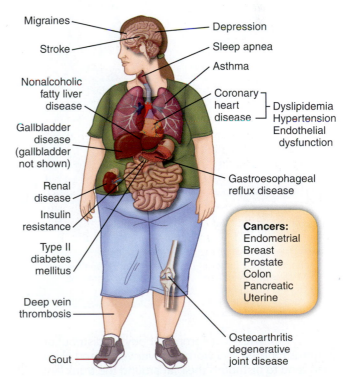

**Figure 22-4.** Specific health consequences of excessive body fat. Note that these health outcomes are systemic, affecting tissues such as the brain, heart, blood vessels, liver, and bone.

obesity, doubles the risk for coronary heart disease, high blood pressure, diabetes, and stroke compared with individuals of the same overall body fat who tend to store fat in the **gynoid** pattern, that is, in the hip, buttocks, and thighs (see Fig. 22-5). The reason for this difference appears to be that fat in the abdomen is more easily mobilized into the bloodstream, increasing the disease-related blood-fat levels. In general, men tend to gain weight in the android pattern, whereas women tend to store fat in the gynoid pattern, although any person with android obesity carries increased health risks.

To determine body-fat distribution pattern, a simple waist-to-hip ratio can be performed, whereby the girth of the waist at the smallest point at or near the navel is divided by the girth of the hip at the largest point around the buttocks (see Chapter 23 for a more detailed discussion of waist-to-hip ratio). If the ratio exceeds 0.80 for women and 0.95 for men, this is indicative of a central body-fat distribution pattern (android). Therefore, it is associated with higher blood cholesterol, triglycerides, insulin levels, and blood pressure, and lower high-density lipoprotein cholesterol, in addition to increased left ventricular wall thickness.[31]

Some clinicians use waist girth as a simple gauge of abdominal obesity and to complement measures of body fat for normal-weight individuals. Waist girth alone has been shown to correlate more strongly to direct measures of abdominal visceral fat accumulation and other heart disease risks than even waist-to-hip ratio.[32] Men with waist circumferences larger than 40 inches (102 cm) and women with waist circumferences larger than 35 inches (88 cm) have increased cardiovascular risk profiles.[33]

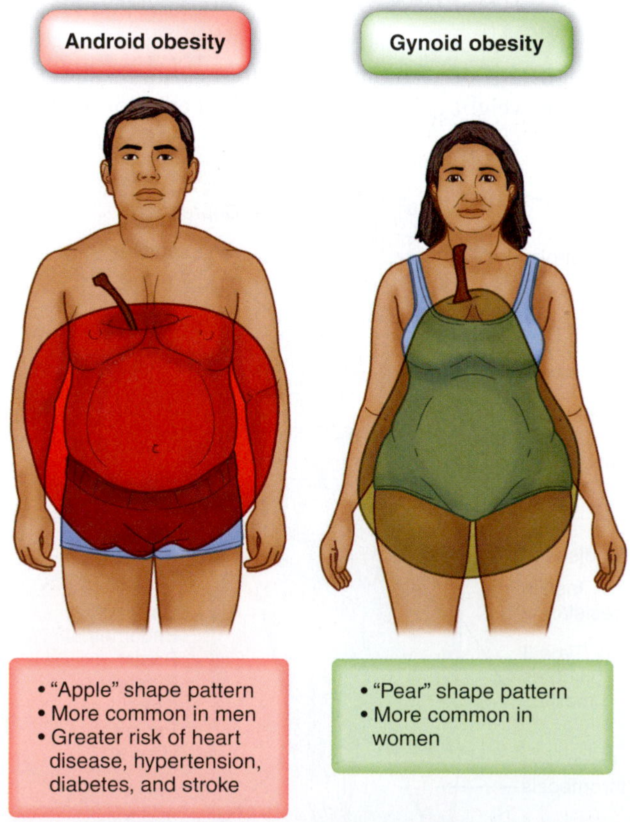

## Impact of Obesity Across Race and Sex

Because being overweight or obese increases risk for cardiovascular disease, diabetes, and some types of cancer, it follows that overweight individuals would also be at a greater risk for hospitalization than normal-weight individuals. In a study examining the association between weight status and all-cause and cause-specific hospitalizations between white and black men and women, researchers reported the average number of all-cause hospitalization per 1,000 adults to be 1,316 for normal-weight individuals versus 1,543 for overweight adults and 2,025 for obese adults.[34] Normal-weight women had fewer hospitalizations overall than normal-weight men, but the increase associated with obesity on all-cause hospitalizations was greater in women than in men. The differences between the number of hospitalizations for either normal-weight white and black adults and overweight/obese white and black adults were not significant.

Other research, however, has shown that obese individuals in general have longer hospital stays, and that obese black adults have longer hospital stays than obese white adults.[35] This work clearly demonstrates the cumulative burden of overweight and obesity on hospitalizations, including the myriad of comorbidities that underlie these conditions. Given the high prevalence of obesity in these population groups, obesity-prevention programs that target ethnic minorities in particular have a high potential to reduce health-care costs associated with obesity-related hospital admissions.

## CAUSE OF OBESITY

The exact cause of obesity remains a mystery. If obesity was a simple disorder caused by overindulgence, then reducing food intake should cause permanent weight loss and improved health. Unfortunately, obesity involves a complex interaction of many factors with psychological, environmental, evolutionary, biologic, and genetic causes. In its simplest context, the maintenance of body weight can be seen as involving three main factors: metabolic utilization of nutrients, dietary habits, and physical activity. In turn, these factors are affected by susceptibility genes, which may influence energy expenditure, fuel metabolism, muscle fiber function, and appetite or food choices. Certainly, the increasing rates of obesity cannot be explained solely by changes in the gene pool, but it is possible that genetic variants

**Android obesity**

**Gynoid obesity**

- "Apple" shape pattern
- More common in men
- Greater risk of heart disease, hypertension, diabetes, and stroke

- "Pear" shape pattern
- More common in women

**Figure 22-5.** The most common body fat distribution patterns for men and women. Overweight and obese men tend to distribute their fat around the trunk (android obesity) and women around the hips and thighs (gynoid obesity). The android obesity pattern is associated more often with a greater risk of cardiovascular disease and type 2 diabetes compared with gynoid obesity.

are more often triggered now by an "obesogenic" environment that includes high availability of energy- and fat-dense foods and by society's increasingly sedentary lifestyles (Fig. 22-6). The following sections review how excess energy intake, sedentary lifestyle, and genetics influence the presence of obesity.

## Energy Intake

Probably the most obvious, but most misunderstood, theory of why individuals become obese is because they simply consume too many calories. Short-term overeating (e.g., eating too much over the holidays) is a common habit that does little to adversely affect health, whereas overeating over long periods can create a health risk.

Overeating can be either active or passive and can be induced by a number of conditions (Box 22-2). **Active overeating** can be caused by a cognitive drive to consume too many calories (driven by internal or external cues), a physical defect in appetite and/or satiety regulation, or an inappropriate psychological response to stress. **Passive overeating** is a different phenomenon, in which the consumption of what would otherwise be a "normal" amount of food becomes excessive because of a sedentary, inactive lifestyle.

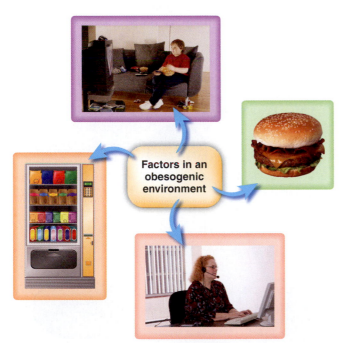

**Figure 22-6.** Factors that may play a role in creating an "obesogenic environment" in the United States: increased sedentary behaviors in children and adults; continued development and overuse of technology that reduces energy expenditure; high-fat, calorically dense convenience food sources (e.g., fast-food outlets, convenience stores); and readily available snack food options (i.e., public vending machines). Other factors may include an expanded food supply, food advertising strategies, increased alcohol consumption, and sociocultural issues related to food and eating. *(Boy on sofa from Digital Vision; bacon cheeseburger from Brand X Pictures.)*

## Box 22-2. Active and Passive Overeating

Overeating can be either active or passive and can be induced by a number of conditions.

### Active Overeating

One of the clearest examples of active overeating is illustrated by what happens to laboratory rats when their normal, bland food is replaced by chocolate-chip cookies and other high-calorie foods. This substitution disrupts energy balance, which normally defends the body's set-point weight, and replaces it with a fourfold fat gain in these animals.[85]

Active overeating in humans can occur because of cultural norms that favor fatness and regard high body weight (in women in particular) as a symbol of affluence and attractiveness. In Western society, however, active overeating is mostly driven by marketing. Huge portion sizes and fast-food "combo" meals that are less expensive than the à la carte option and generally more convenient to order provide an excessive amount of calories that bear no relationship to the single-meal energy requirement of most individuals. Dr. Barbara Rolls calls this phenomenon "volumetrics."[86]

In 1 study, 23 normal-weight men and women were presented standard-portion meals for 11 consecutive days and large-portion meals (additional 50%) for 11 days. When larger meals were an option, subjects consumed approximately 423 additional calories per day. Therefore, it appears that the availability of larger portions contributed to energy overconsumption and excess body-weight gain.[86] However, evidence suggests that active overeating contributes to the obesity epidemic to a lesser degree in the general population than does passive overeating.[73]

### Passive Overeating

It is easy to demonstrate how increases in energy intake lead to positive energy balance and weight gain. In contrast, there is strong evidence to suggest that the modern sedentary lifestyle, and resultant low levels of energy expenditure, is the driving force behind the obesity epidemic. In fact, there is evidence to suggest that reduced energy expenditure increases a person's vulnerability to overeating, primarily because of the fat content of foods that provide excessive amounts of calories even though overall "portions" of these high-fat foods may be quite normal.

In an interesting study of this phenomenon, men were allowed to eat freely from seemingly identical diets that had been secretly manipulated to contain 20%, 40%, or 60% energy from fat. Regardless of the fat content of their diets, each group of men ate the same bulk of food. Therefore, the energy overload provided in the 60% fat

*Continued*

## Box 22-2. Active and Passive Overeating–cont'd

diet was an "accidental" phenomenon (thus the term *passive overeating*).[87] The results showed a significantly higher fat balance in men consuming the highest fat diet.[88]

Independent of fat content, low-energy–dense diets generate greater satiety than high-energy–dense diets, suggesting that an important regulatory signal may be the weight or volume of food consumed rather than the actual caloric content of the food.[89] Therefore, high-fat foods do not decrease consumption, but rather only serve as a source of unnecessary excessive calories.

Whether overconsumption is accomplished through active or passive overeating, the result is the same: The excessive intake of energy will be stored and can increase the size and/or number of adipocytes depending on the person's age and the size of existing adipocytes, as described earlier. Although it is a common belief that "a calorie is a calorie" regardless of its nutrient composition, and a diet in which energy intake matches energy expenditure has no impact on weight gain or loss, research indicates that not all of the macronutrients contribute to obesity equally. For instance, Flatt et al.[36] and Schutz et al.[37] demonstrated that a high-fat meal that provides more calories than are immediately necessary stimulates fat storage without a similar increase in fat utilization.

A positive energy balance because of an increase in carbohydrate ingestion, however, stimulates a rapid increase in carbohydrate oxidation, which spares fat utilization. This seems to suggest that a positive energy balance caused by excess fat intake will promote more fat storage than if the excess calories come from carbohydrate sources. Furthermore, the storage of dietary fat into adipose tissue is associated with a very low metabolic cost (0%–2%)[38] compared with the thermic effect for carbohydrate (6%–8%) and protein (25%–30%).[39] Therefore, of the three macronutrients, it is more metabolically costly to convert and store dietary protein as fat than it is for either dietary carbohydrate or fat.

Many studies have also examined the effects on weight loss of varying macronutrient compositions in diets with identical caloric content. In a study evaluating weight loss in participants consuming a hypocaloric diet with high-protein versus high-carbohydrate content, researchers concluded that the replacement of some dietary carbohydrate with protein improves weight and fat loss, and spares protein loss by promoting lipid oxidation in the fasting state.[40] Randomized, controlled trials continue to show comparable or superior effects of high-protein diets on weight loss, preservation of **lean body mass**, and improvement in several cardiovascular risk factors for up to 12 months.[41] Evidence that chronic high-protein intake affects glucose metabolism, however, is inconclusive.

Despite their appeal for weight loss, high-protein diets remain controversial because of questions about their safety, especially if consumed long term. Animal studies confirm that long-term intake of very high-protein diets (35% of calories from protein) promotes kidney damage in animals.[42] Diets with moderately increased protein and modestly restricted carbohydrate and fat contents (especially saturated fat) can have beneficial effects on body weight, body composition, and metabolic parameters. Key issues regarding their safety over the long term, however, warrant further study.

## Energy Expenditure

In the classic sense, there are three components of human daily energy expenditure: basal metabolic rate, thermic effect of food, and thermic effect of physical activity (see Fig. 22-7). **Basal metabolic rate** is the amount of energy required to maintain bodily functions at rest; it accounts for approximately 60% to 75% of daily energy expenditure in a sedentary person. Most of the variability across individuals is accounted for by differences in lean body mass, which is more metabolically active than fat mass.

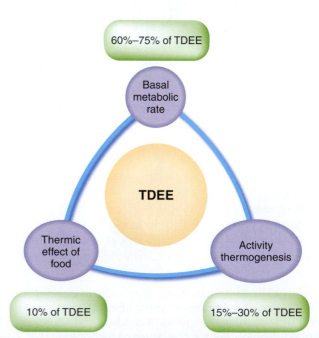

**Figure 22-7.** Factors that contribute to total daily energy expenditure (TDEE). Basal metabolic rate determines approximately 60% to 75% of TDEE and remains relatively stable on a day-to-day basis. The thermic effect of food (up to 10% of TDEE depending on diet) is composed of the digestion and assimilation of food stuffs within the body. The last factor, activity thermogenesis, presents the most variability (15%–30%) in determining TDEE.

The **thermic effect of food** is the energy required to digest, absorb, and store ingested food energy, and accounts for about 10% of daily energy expenditure in most people. The remaining component, activity thermogenesis, represents between 15% and 30% of daily energy expenditure and can be further subdivided into exercise and **nonexercise activity thermogenesis (NEAT)**. In contrast with the other two components of energy expenditure, activity thermogenesis is highly variable across individuals and can easily vary by as much as 2,000 kcal/day between individuals.[43] The majority of individuals in the world do not participate in purposeful exercise for the sake of fitness, so for them, exercise thermogenesis is negligible. In those who do exercise, expenditure can be quite small, accounting for less than 200 kcal/day of energy expenditure. Therefore, it stands to reason that the variability between individuals for activity thermogenesis is largely accounted for by NEAT associated with occupation and leisure (e.g., going to work or school, performing household tasks, and ambulation). It also stands to reason that increasing energy expenditure by increasing NEAT may hold significant promise in combating the obesity epidemic.

The notion that obesity may be more related to energy expenditure related to NEAT than to energy expenditure related to exercise is supported by the literature. When positive energy balance is imposed through overfeeding, Levine and colleagues[44] demonstrated that obese subjects sat 2.5 hours per day more than lean subjects. The lean sedentary volunteers stood and walked for more than 2 hours per day longer than obese sedentary subjects, even though all subjects lived and worked in similar environments. Therefore, those who voluntarily increase their NEAT the most (primarily through walking) gain the least fat, and those who consume excess calories but do not increase their NEAT gain the most fat.[44]

These researchers also calculated that, if the obese subjects were to adopt the same activity patterns as the lean subjects, they could expend an additional 350 kcal/day because of their larger size. Thus, NEAT and specifically walking are of substantial energetic importance in obesity. It might seem obvious that because people with obesity are heavier, they sit more than lean people. However, these differences are not due to greater body weight alone, because when lean subjects gained weight through overfeeding, their tendency to stand/ambulate persisted, and when obese subjects became lighter, their tendency to sit did not change.[45]

Research in this area supports the notion that perhaps peoples' environments need to be re-engineered to promote NEAT (see Figs. 22-8 and 22-9). This argument makes sense, especially given the fact that, despite the best efforts nationally, participation in physical activity is at an all-time low and obesity rates are at an all-time high.

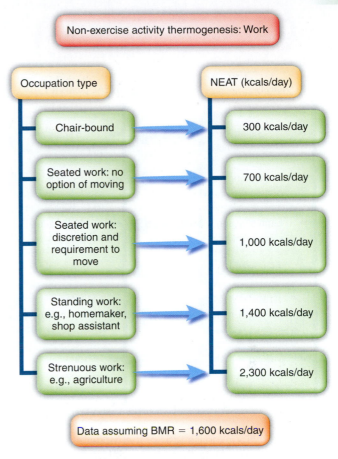

**Figure 22-8.** Nonexercise activity thermogenesis (NEAT) in the working environment. Data show the variability in NEAT (kcal/day) in occupations with significantly differing requirements of activity. The greatest difference (2000 kcal/day) in NEAT occurs between those whose work requires prolonged sitting and work that requires strenuous activity. By introducing some movement requirement on the job, one can increase NEAT up to 700 kcal/day or more, which can be a significant addition to total daily energy expenditure (TDEE). *(Data based on Black AE, Coward WA, Cole TJ, Prentice AM. Human energy expenditure in affluent societies: An analysis of 574 doubly-labelled water measurements. Eur J Clin Nutr. 1996;50:72–92.)*

## Possible Mechanisms of Obesity

In addition to the contributors to obesity mentioned previously, several hormones, genetic components, and secreted substances have been implicated in the cause of obesity. Some of these have an effect on long-term control of energy intake (e.g., insulin and leptin). Signals that provide short-term information about hunger and satiety include gut hormones, such as cholecystokinin, ghrelin, and peptide YY (PYY), and signals from vagal afferent neurons within the gastrointestinal tract that respond to fullness, macronutrients, pH, tonicity, and hormones. Neural and humoral signals are then integrated in the arcuate nucleus, a group of cells in the hypothalamus, and are mediated by two types of neurons: the appetite-inhibiting proopiomelanocortin

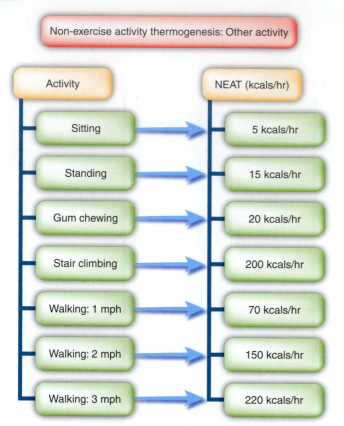

Non-exercise activity thermogenesis: Other activity

| Activity | NEAT (kcals/hr) |
|---|---|
| Sitting | 5 kcals/hr |
| Standing | 15 kcals/hr |
| Gum chewing | 20 kcals/hr |
| Stair climbing | 200 kcals/hr |
| Walking: 1 mph | 70 kcals/hr |
| Walking: 2 mph | 150 kcals/hr |
| Walking: 3 mph | 220 kcals/hr |

**Figure 22-9.** Nonexercise activity thermogenesis (NEAT) for other activities. Data illustrate the differences between common activities individuals may perform on a daily basis. By limiting time while sitting, individuals can significantly increase energy expenditure throughout the day. *(Data based on Levine JA. Nonexercise activity thermogenesis (NEAT): environment and biology. Am J Physiol Endocrinol Metab. 2004;286:E675–E685.)*

### FROM THEORY TO PRACTICE

Do the research findings related to NEAT mean that people do not need to exercise? Not at all. What this research does indicate, however, is that *in addition to* purposeful physical activity and exercise routines, people need to make a conscious effort to "undo" their technologically geared lifestyles. Although all of the modern conveniences people enjoy make working "easier," they have also successfully engineered physical activity right out of most people's lives. Putting it back *in* now requires behavior change.

The best advice is to sit less. Many activities that involve sitting can be done while standing, pacing, or walking instead. The additional calories expended by doing these activities while *not* seated add up and contribute to an overall healthier lifestyle, not only because of the calories being expended, but also because of the thought process that people engage in when they make the choice to be active continuously throughout the day.

## *In Your Own Words*

Your best friend, who has always struggled with her weight, tells you, "There is just no way I can lose weight. I sit all day in an office and have to care for my family when I get home. When do I have time to exercise?" What quick tips could you give your friend to change her thinking about her opportunities for physical activity?

(POMC) and the appetite-stimulating neuropeptide Y (NPY). These neurons relay feedback signals to the hypothalamus via the central nervous system, digestive tract, thyroid gland, adrenal glands, and pancreas to signal the individual to either start or stop eating (Fig. 22-10). The following section discusses the role that several key hormones, neuropeptides, and other factors may play in the development of obesity.

### Long-Term Control of Energy Intake

Insulin and leptin have an effect on long-term control of energy intake.

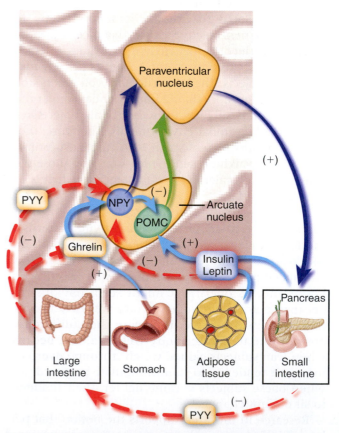

**Figure 22-10.** Interactions among hormonal and neural pathways that regulate food intake and body fat mass. Dashed lines indicate inhibitory effects; solid lines indicate stimulatory effects. The paraventricular and arcuate nuclei each contain neurons that are capable of stimulating or inhibiting food intake. NPY, neuropeptide Y; POMC, proopiomelanocortin; PYY, peptide YY.

## RESEARCH HIGHLIGHT

### Chronic Inflammation and Obesity

Research has shown that chronic inflammation is a risk factor for chronic diseases including diabetes mellitus, heart disease, osteoporosis, Alzheimer's disease, cancer, rheumatoid arthritis, and others.[46-49] In addition, it appears that obesity, especially abdominal obesity, increases this risk because of elevated concentrations of inflammatory cytokines, released from the adipocytes themselves.[48,50] Although inflammation is an important part of the body's normal immune response, chronic upregulation of the innate immune system's inflammatory cytokines such as interleukin (IL)-6, IL-1, and tumor necrosis factor-$\alpha$ can have negative effects on the body. Specifically, these molecules increase systemic inflammation by stimulating proinflammatory molecules in other tissues such as C-reactive protein secretion from the liver.[51]

It has also been observed that oxygen levels in adipose tissue are reduced in obese individuals, accompanied by local vasoconstriction in those tissues. This hypoxic state, possibly because of a reduction in the formation of new blood vessels (angiogenesis), may contribute to further inflammation.[52] In addition, many obese individuals also display significant damage to endothelial cells that line the arteries presumably caused by increased activity of macrophages that release additional inflammatory cytokines into the bloodstream.[51]

Therefore, in obese individuals, enlarged adipose cells not only cause an increase in local inflammation in and around the adipose tissue itself, but also cause systemic inflammation associated with the innate immune response that damages vessels everywhere in the body. Because obesity damages blood vessels, at least indirectly, thereby interfering with nutrient delivery to all tissues, it is easy to see how obesity is related to the development of many other diseases.

Support is mounting for a relation between physical activity and chronic inflammation levels, and strategies to reduce obesity have been shown to reduce a person's likelihood of development of comorbid secondary diseases.[53,54] Exercise has been shown to have a very positive effect on circulating levels of inflammatory cytokines. The positive influence of exercise is best when weight loss occurs, but the reduction in adipose hypoxia that occurs with exercise training appears to occur independent of weight loss.[51] The bottom line is that excess body fat predisposes an individual to a host of otherwise preventable chronic diseases, and that weight loss reverses this risk. Exercise, in and of itself, however, counteracts many of the devastating effects of obesity, even in the absence of weight loss.

*Please see reference list at the end of the chapter.*

## Insulin

**Insulin** is a peptide hormone produced by the pancreatic beta cells and secreted in response to increased blood glucose levels. Insulin is an anabolic hormone for both muscle and fat cells, and it plays an important role in the storage and utilization of energy in the adipocytes. Circulating levels of insulin are directly proportional to adipose level and increase rapidly after eating. Similar to leptin, insulin suppresses NPY and stimulates POMC to regulate feeding in response to the amount of stored calories. Through coordinated action on hypothalamic neurons that stimulate or inhibit feeding behavior, insulin and leptin function centrally as satiety signals to decrease food intake when energy levels are met and adipose tissue has been restored.

## Leptin

Leptin is a cytokine hormone produced by the *ob* gene and secreted by adipose tissue in direct proportion to the total amount of body fat. Leptin has been called a regulator of appetite, but more specifically, it is a hormone that acts on the hypothalamus in the brain via a negative feedback loop to regulate energy intake.[55] Animal studies indicate that it may also increase energy expenditure by increasing the activity of the sympathetic nervous system.[56] In a normal situation, increases in triglyceride deposits into the adipocyte cause a release of leptin from the adipocyte, which, in turn, triggers the hypothalamus to reduce appetite and the drive to eat. Fasting induces a decrease in leptin produced in adipose tissue and a subsequent decrease in serum leptin levels, which stimulates hunger.[55]

Although it was initially hypothesized in 1994 when leptin was discovered that obese individuals must have low leptin levels, research has now shown that most obese individuals actually have increased plasma leptin levels.[55] In obese children and adults, plasma leptin circulates in direct proportion to adipose tissue mass when weight is stable, in amounts four times higher than in lean individuals.[57] Analogous to insulin resistance in obese individuals with moderate type 2 diabetes, it is now thought that perhaps obese individuals are "leptin resistant." This theory is supported by the observation that leptin transport across the blood–brain barrier is impaired in obese individuals. It cannot be shown, however, that the hypothalamic response of obese and lean individuals is any different from similar levels of circulating leptin. It is possible that increased leptin levels may reflect increased adiposity, just as insulin is elevated in response to increased blood glucose after a meal. Another explanation is that leptin cannot counteract overfeeding behaviors (hedonistic eating) that are not regulated by feelings of satiety, but rather by the pleasure one receives from the act of eating.

Weight loss reduces serum leptin levels, and weight gain increases circulating levels. Even without significant weight loss, a prolonged state of negative caloric balance or fasting decreases circulating leptin concentrations and increases hunger sensations.[58] Interestingly, neither short- nor long-term exercise significantly affects leptin independently of the effects of exercise on total body-fat loss. Injections of leptin in obese subjects who produce adequate amounts of leptin, but are resistant to it, do not stimulate an increase in fat loss. This may indicate that physiologically, leptin may be more important as an indicator of energy deficiency and may be a possible mediator of an adaptation to starvation.[59]

Leptin alone does not determine whether a person becomes obese, nor does it explain why some people can eat without restriction and maintain a stable body weight, whereas others become overfat with the same caloric intake. It may, however, be a very important regulatory component of the obesity puzzle. For instance, leptin administration may have a clinical application in the treatment of weight-loss maintenance. Weight loss reduces leptin concentrations, which may activate neuroendocrine mechanisms that stimulate hunger and decrease energy expenditure by decreasing thyroid hormone levels, which slows metabolism.[60] Thus, replacing leptin may restore these neuroendocrine abnormalities and prevent the adverse effects of "yo-yo" dieting.

## Short-Term Control of Energy Intake

Signals that provide short-term information about hunger and satiety include gut hormones, such as cholecystokinin, ghrelin, and PYY.

### Cholecystokinin

Cholecystokinin (CCK) is a peptide hormone secreted in the duodenum and jejunum of the small intestine in response to digestive enzymes. It slows emptying of the stomach and sends satiety signals to the hypothalamus, which should inhibit food consumption. CCK administration reduces food intake, meal size, and meal duration when given to rodents and humans, but rodents compensate for the reduction in meal size by eating more frequently with no effect on overall body weight.[61] Although its role in obesity is not known, drugs called CCK-A promoters that enhance the effects of CCK-A, an intestinal hormone that may inhibit appetite, are currently in development.[62]

### Ghrelin

Ghrelin, a hormone discovered in 1999, is produced mainly in the stomach. It is responsible for stimulating appetite via stimulation of the NPY receptors and by stimulating growth hormone release from the pituitary gland. Ghrelin concentrations in the blood vary widely throughout the day, with higher levels during sleep and before meals and lower levels after meals. For this reason, ghrelin was thought to be a "hunger hormone" responsible

for meal initiation, but it is more likely that ghrelin functions to prepare the body for an influx of food.[63] Ghrelin levels in the blood are inversely correlated with weight, meaning that high ghrelin levels are associated with low body weight. Research using ghrelin administration in **anorexia nervosa** and obesity suggest a potential for future use of ghrelin antagonists and agonists in the treatment of anorexia, as well as in the prevention of weight recovery in obesity.[62]

### Peptide YY

Peptide YY (PYY) is a hormone that is rapidly released from the descending colon and rectum in proportion to the number of calories consumed. PYY acts on the hypothalamus to suppress appetite, especially 2 to 6 hours after a meal, on the pancreas to increase its exocrine secretion of digestive juices, and on the gallbladder to stimulate the release of bile. The appetite suppression mediated by PYY works more slowly than that of cholecystokinin and more rapidly than that of leptin. Subjects given PYY were less hungry and ate less food over the next 12 hours than those who received a placebo.[64] In obese individuals, circulating levels of PYY are decreased and release of PYY following a meal is lower than in normal-weight individuals.[65] In addition, PYY also reduces ghrelin secretion, which may be an additional effect that promotes weight loss.

## INFLUENCE OF GENETICS VERSUS ENVIRONMENT

Genetic and environmental factors affect metabolism and appetite, with a larger percentage explained by environmental influences. The epidemic of obesity, begun decades ago, has occurred within a gene pool that has not changed in 100 years or more. Nonetheless, it is clear that genetic factors play an important role in a person's susceptibility to becoming obese in an obesogenic environment, rich with sedentary and stressful activities and ready access to inexpensive, large-portion, high-calorie, good-tasting food. Researchers have established that genetics contributes to the development of obesity in two ways:

- Single, rare mutations in certain genes that wholly explain the development of obesity (monogenic obesity): There are now at least 20 single-gene disorders that result in an autosomal form of obesity, but these forms are rare, very severe, and generally begin in childhood (e.g., lacking the gene that produces leptin).[66]
- Several genetic variants that interact with an "at-risk" environment (polygenic obesity): In this case, each gene, taken individually, would only contribute to body weight in a small way, and the cumulative effect of these genes would only become significant when there is an interaction with environmental factors that cause their expression (e.g., overeating and sedentary lifestyle).

The unique interaction between an individual's genetic composition and the environment in which his or her genes have an opportunity to express themselves makes it difficult to quantify the role of each in the development of obesity. Although an individual's genes do not necessarily cause obesity, they may lower the threshold for its expression. Researchers are just now starting to identify key genes and specific deoxyribonucleic acid (DNA) sequences that relate to the causes of appetite regulation and predispose a person to obesity. To date, more than 50 genes and **polymorphisms** (natural variations in a gene, DNA sequence, or chromosome) have been tested and implicated in controlling food intake, energy expenditure, and fat and carbohydrate metabolism. Although no conclusive role in obesity development has been established for these genes, certain variants are associated with different types of obesity (child vs. adult onset), metabolic and cardiovascular complications, appetite, and the interaction between excess body weight and physical activity.[67] This area of research, however, is extremely complex, and progress in the knowledge of the human genome and the development of computing tools and new analysis strategies that can handle several hundreds of items of genetic and environmental information at once will be necessary to tackle these questions.[67]

## Genetic Factors

The first significant advances in the discovery of obesity susceptibility gene loci were made in 2007 through genome-wide association studies.[68] Many genes that are being targeted for their possible role in obesity development fall within two broad categories: genes that affect the central nervous system and those that operate peripherally via adipose tissue. Insightful information about the causes of obesity has come from the cloning of obesity genes in animals. Molecular and reverse genetic studies (using mouse **"knockouts"** [mice that have all or part of a gene eliminated or inactivated by genetic engineering]) have also helped to establish important pathways that regulate body fat and food intake. Leptin deficiency, produced by a single gene mutation, as described earlier in this chapter, has shown that true metabolic-gene pathways do exist.[66] Similar deficiencies in genes that regulate food intake have been found, such as fat mass and obesity associated (FTO) and melanocortin-4 receptor (MC4R), where changes to the amino acid sequence of a key regulator of food intake causes uncontrolled appetite similar to that seen in leptin deficiency. These insights into biology have shown that body-fat regulation may be independent of willpower.

In a landmark study by Bouchard et al.,[69] the importance of genetics in body-weight regulation was clearly shown. Researchers intentionally overfed 12 pairs of male identical twins for 100 days (total overfeeding of 84,000 kcal) to observe differences within and between twin pairs. What they found was a striking similarity in the amount of weight gain, skinfold changes, and changes in BMI *within* the twin pairs, but three times more variance *between* twin pairs for these same variables. The within-pair similarity was particularly evident with respect to the changes in regional fat distribution and amount of abdominal visceral fat, with about six times as much variance between pairs as within pairs. They concluded that the most likely explanation for the similarity within pairs of twins in the adaptation to long-term overfeeding and for the large variations in weight changes and body-fat distribution between pairs of twins is that genetic factors were involved. These genetic factors may regulate a person's tendency to store extra calories as either fat or lean tissue and alter resting metabolism accordingly.

## Environmental Factors

There has been increasing interest in the role of the environment in the determination of dietary behavior among individuals. This "social ecological" view of health takes into account the fact that individuals interact with their environments, which ultimately influence their health behaviors.[70] Higher rates of obesity are found in individuals with the lowest incomes and the least education, especially among women and certain ethnic groups. This association may be partially explained by the relatively low cost of energy-dense, high-fat food, and the association of lower incomes and unavailability of fresh fruits and vegetables.[71] Observational studies in many different countries confirm that dietary patterns and obesity rates vary among neighborhoods, where living in a low-income neighborhood is independently associated with obesity and a poor diet.[72] These environmental influences on diet involve two pathways: access to foods for home consumption from supermarkets and grocery stores, and access to ready-made food from fast-food restaurants and convenience stores.

Studies on the built environment (the human-made space in which people live, work, and recreate on a day-to-day basis) consistently show that the presence of supermarkets is associated with a lower prevalence of obesity. In the United States and Canada, "healthier" and more expensive foods are less available in poorer communities, and access to supermarkets is more difficult in low-income neighborhoods, where independent stores dominate and tend to charge higher prices. Foods purchased from fast-food and other restaurants are becoming an increasingly important part of people's diets, especially in the United States (Fig. 22-11). These foods, which can be up to 65% more energy dense than the average diet, provide fewer nutrients and higher amounts of fat, and tend to be larger in portion size than foods consumed at home.[73,74] Current statistics show that 11.3% of calories consumed in the United States by adults older than 20 years comes from fast food.[68] These data also show that non-Hispanic black individuals between the ages of 20 and 39 years consume 21.1% of their total calories from fast food.

Several components of the food supply and food "environment" may be important determinants of obesity. Research on portion sizes or packages and servings clearly indicates that when more food is provided, more food is eaten.[75] Portion sizes have increased dramatically over the past decades, and although containers do state that a particular package may contain more than one serving, it is common to consume food by the package and not by the serving size (Fig. 22-12).

The creation of built environments that encourage people to adopt, or further increase levels of, physical activity is another strategy that is becoming increasingly popular. A focus on modifying residential neighborhoods to support physical activity is especially important,

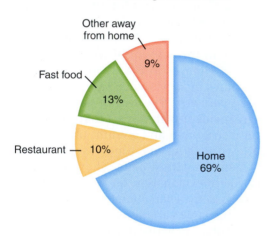

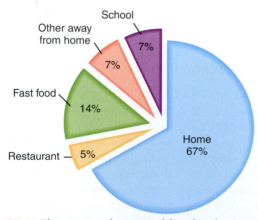

**Figure 22-11.** The preponderance of fast food as a relative percentage of the diet outside the home for adults 20 years and older and children between the ages of 2 and 19 years. In children, the percentage of food in the diet coming from fast and convenient sources is double or more of that coming from school or other restaurants. *(Befort, CA, Nazir, N, & Perri, MG. (2012). Prevalence of Obesity Among Adults From Rural and Urban Areas of the United States: Findings From NHANES (2005-2008). J Rural Health. Fall; 28(4): 392-397. doi: 10.1111/j.1748-0361.2012.00411.x)*

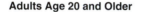

### FROM THEORY TO PRACTICE

Overweight and obesity are largely preventable. Individual choices are influenced by supportive communities and environments. Making the healthy choices easier to select will go a long way in preventing obesity. Individuals can reduce their obesity risk by:
- Engaging in daily physical activity according to the Surgeon General's guidelines
- Limiting sedentary/inactive time
- Increasing consumption of fruits, vegetables, legumes, whole grains, and nuts
- Limiting sugar intake
- Achieving a healthy weight and maintaining energy balance

Society can help prevent obesity in individuals by:
- Supporting healthy decision-making through collaboration of public and private stakeholders
- Making regular physical activity and healthy diets affordable and accessible to all individuals, especially to members of groups with the largest health disparities

The food industry can promote healthy diets by:
- Reducing the fat, sugar, and salt content in processed foods
- Ensuring that nutritious food options are accessible to all
- Practicing responsible marketing

*Source:* World Health Organization. Obesity and overweight. Fact sheet No 311. March 2011. Retrieved from http://www.who.int/mediacentre/factsheets/fs311/en/

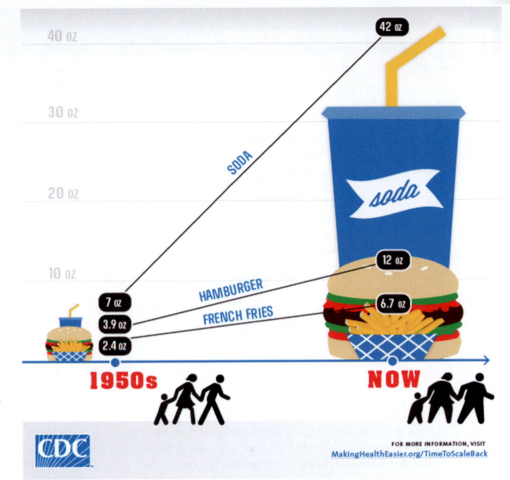

**Figure 22-12.** Large portion sizes served at home and in restaurants can contribute to the overconsumption of food. The relative increase in fast-food portion sizes from the 1950s to the present day. It is clear that the larger portion sizes seen in restaurants today are the new norm. *(From Making Health Easier, the Centers for Disease Control's Division of Community Health (DCH). The New (Ab)normal. http://makinghealtheasier.org/newabnormal.)*

because that is where the majority of physical activity, including walking, is undertaken. Positive associations between walking for transport and access to and quality of pedestrian infrastructure such as maintained sidewalks, pedestrian-level lighting and shade, and street furniture have been reported.[76] Ongoing research in this area continues to examine the potential short- and long-term effects of built environment interventions on physical-activity behavior, as well as the cost-effectiveness of creating walkable neighborhoods.

## RESEARCH HIGHLIGHT

### The Set-Point Theory of Obesity

The concept of a "set point" for body weight has been debated for many decades. Initially, this theory proposed that adult body weight is regulated at some predetermined or "preferred" level by a simple feedback control system regulated by the hypothalamus[77] (see Fig. 22-13). This was based on studies of rats[78] and humans[79] that showed that weight gained or lost by overfeeding or underfeeding was restored to the original control weight once feeding returned to normal. The homeostatic control mechanisms involved in this process were argued to include an adaptation in the energy economy of metabolic processes, whereby they became more or less wasteful to maintain fixed fat stores and body weight.[80] A low RMR is most often blamed for this phenomenon, but the simple notion that RMR is downregulated during weight loss, and therefore responsible for weight regain, remains controversial.[81]

Roland Weinsier, a prominent obesity researcher, sought to answer the question, "Do adaptations in energy economy explain the weight-gain tendency of obesity-prone persons?" To fully answer this question, he and his colleagues designed a series of experiments that addressed five important research questions:

1. Is RMR reduced after weight loss to a post-obese state? To address this question, 70 obese women were recruited. Through dietary restriction, they lost approximately 16% to 17% of their body weight so that each woman had a BMI less than 25 kg/m². Although RMR *did* decline after losing weight, RMR was *normal* when adjusting for changes in body composition. The researchers concluded that women are not more energy conservative and do not have a lower body composition–adjusted RMR after losing weight.[82]

*Continued*

# RESEARCH HIGHLIGHT–cont'd

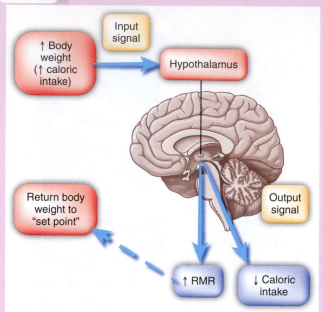

**Figure 22-13.** Physiological set-point theory. Regulation of the hypothalamus over the maintenance of body weight at a level specific to the individual is shown. In this model, the hypothalamus receives peripheral input regarding changes in body weight caused by increased caloric intake. The hypothalamus sends out information to suppress appetite and increase metabolic rate to compensate for the increased body weight. The outcome of these physiological adjustments is a return of body weight to the "normal" or preferred level specific to the individual.

2. Is RMR low in post-obese versus never-obese women? To address this question, the RMR of the post-obese group was compared with a group of matched never-obese women. The RMRs between the two groups were actually within 1% to 4% of each other and not statistically different, even after adjusting for small differences in body composition. The researchers concluded that RMRs are *comparable* between obesity-prone, weight-reduced women and obesity-resistant women.[82]

3. Does low RMR predict weight regain in post-obese women? In the same study, women were followed for 4 years to observe their weight-gain patterns. The never-obese women had a mean BMI increase from 21.3 to 21.8, whereas the previously obese women went from an initial BMI of 28 to 23 during weight loss, and then regained to a BMI of 27 after 4 years. More importantly, body composition–adjusted RMR in the weight-reduced state did not correlate with the weight-regain patterns, nor was there a tendency for those with a lower RMR to regain more weight than those with a higher RMR. Therefore, the researchers concluded that factors other than variation in RMR were responsible for the weight gain of the obesity-prone women.[82]

4. Are black women more energetically economical than white women? To address this question, Byrne et al.[83] studied 18 white and 22 matched black women in the overweight state, after weight reduction to normal weight (with diet only, no exercise), and after 1 year without intervention. What they found was that white and black women did not differ in their weight loss and subsequent regain, but RMR was higher in white women than in black women. They attributed this, however, to differences in trunk lean body mass, possibly attributable to lower organ mass in the black women. Because organ tissue is more metabolically active than skeletal muscle tissue during rest, this could explain some of the variation in RMR.

5. Do differences in energy economy favor greater weight gain in black versus white women? In a study of 23 obese white and 23 matched obese black women and 38 never-obese control subjects, weight loss through diet alone was induced in the obese subjects. A host of metabolic measures were tracked, including activity energy expenditure, sleeping energy expenditure, free-living energy expenditure, body composition, and aerobic fitness. What they found was that weight-reduced white women increased their activity energy expenditure and consequently their aerobic fitness, while the black women appeared to produce a more obesity-prone sedentary state that favored weight relapse.[84] Their earlier findings confirmed that after 1 year, black women tended to regain more weight than their weight-reduced white counterparts.[81]

What this elegant series of studies underscores is that the maintenance of a healthy body weight is achieved through a complex interaction among physical activity, food choice, and individual metabolism, and is influenced by hormonal, environmental, and genetic factors. One is not necessarily "programmed" to be a certain body weight, but someone who has lost weight will naturally tend to return to his or her pre-weight-loss state if the **behaviors** that led to the overweight state are not properly addressed.

*Please see reference list at the end of the chapter.*

## In Your Own Words

An African-American colleague asks, "My whole family is overweight, including my parents, siblings, and children. Isn't it true that African Americans are just genetically programmed to be heavy?" How would you respond to this question?

## VIGNETTE conclusion

Lucinda's choice to opt for convenience over planned, healthy food choices had been compromising her health, setting a poor example for her daughters, and contributing to an unhealthy environment for her family. The fast food that she chose to consume was calorically dense and nutrient sparse. In addition, her omission of physical activity in her daily routine had reduced her lean body mass, which reduces metabolically active tissue and favors weight gain. Lucinda's assumption that she is "destined to be overweight" because her mother is overweight is probably better explained by their common tendency to actively and passively consume too many calories (environment) rather than to a shared family predisposition to obesity (genetics). In her effort to help her new client turn things around, Destiny educates Lucinda about the composition and quantity of her current diet, and the effect of these choices and her lack of physical activity on her increasing weight and declining health status.

Destiny is glad that Lucinda has been taking steps to improve her nutritional intake, although consistency is still an issue. As it appears that Lucinda is receptive to learning new techniques to change her behavior, Destiny introduces the idea of packing workout clothes the night before and taking the bag with her into the office, where Lucinda can place it by the door of her office as a reminder to go to the gym on the way home.

Lucinda is still in the early stages of behavioral change and has a long way to go before achieving a healthy weight, but by combining knowledge of physiology, physical activity, nutrition, and behavioral change, Destiny has enabled Lucinda to start making better choices over the long haul.

## CRITICAL THINKING QUESTIONS

1. Many overweight individuals are convinced that to lose weight by exercising, they would have to perform hours of structured exercise every day. How would you explain to an overweight individual that this may not be the case, paying particular attention to the components of activity thermogenesis?

2. Many people have heard that it is better to consume a meal slowly to allow time for "the stomach to communicate with the brain" that it is full. Explain how this is indeed true, with respect to the hormones involved in the short-term regulation of energy intake.

3. Individuals are bombarded with environmental barriers to maintaining a normal, healthy weight. Explain how the environment is increasingly "obesogenic" and how this relates to the skyrocketing obesity rates in the United States.

## ADDITIONAL RESOURCES

American Heart Association: http://www.heart.org

American Diabetes Association: http://www.diabetes.org

Centers for Disease Control. Obesity: Halting the Epidemic by Making Health Easier at a Glance 2011. http://www.cdc.gov/chronicdisease/resources/publications/AAG/obesity.htm

Donnelly JE, Blair SN, Jakicic JM, Manore MM, Rankin JW, Smith BK. Appropriate physical activity intervention strategies for weight loss and prevention of weight regain for adults. *Med. Sci. Sports Exerc.* 2009;41:459–471.

Expert Panel on the Identification, Evaluation, and Treatment of Overweight and Obesity in Adults. Executive summary of the clinical guidelines on the identification, evaluation, and treatment of overweight and obesity in adults. *Arch Intern Med.* 1998;158:1855–1867.

National Institutes of Health, National Center for Biotechnology Information, U.S. National Library of Medicine. Obesity. http://www.ncbi.nlm.nih.gov/pubmedhealth/PMH0004552/

Obesity Society: www.obesity.org

A BMI calculator is available on the American Council on Exercise website: www.acefitness.org/calculators/default.aspx.

# REFERENCES

1. Centers for Disease Control and Prevention. What are the health consequences of living in an 'obesogenic' society? Retrieved November 22, 2010, from http://www.cdc.gov/speakers/subtopic/speechTopics.html
2. Ogden CL, Lamb MM, Carroll MD, Flegal KM. Obesity and socioeconomic status in adults: United States, 2005–2008. *NCHS Data Brief.* 2010:1–8.
3. Flegal KM, Carroll MD, Ogden CL, Curtin LR. Prevalence and trends in obesity among US adults, 1999–2008. *JAMA.* 2010;303:235–241.
4. Wang Y, Beydoun MA. The obesity epidemic in the United States—gender, age, socioeconomic, racial/ethnic, and geographic characteristics: A systematic review and meta-regression analysis. *Epidemiol Rev.* 2007;29:6–28.
5. Obesity and overweight. Fact sheet No 311. Retrieved March 2011, from http://www.who.int/mediacentre/factsheets/fs311/en/
6. Ogden CL, Carroll MD, Curtin LR, McDowell MA, Tabak CJ, Flegal KM. Prevalence of overweight and obesity in the United States, 1999–2004. *JAMA.* 2006;295:1549–1555.
7. Ogden CL, Lamb MM, Carroll MD, Flegal KM. Obesity and socioeconomic status in children and adolescents: United States, 2005–2008. *NCHS Data Brief.* 2010:1–8.
8. Carpenter WH, Fonong T, Toth MJ, et al. Total daily energy expenditure in free-living older African-Americans and Caucasians. *Am J Physiol.* 1998;274:E96–E101.
9. Foster GD, Wadden TA, Swain RM, Anderson DA, Vogt RA. Changes in resting energy expenditure after weight loss in obese African American and white women. *Am J Clin Nutr.* 1999;69:13–17.
10. Obesity: Preventing and managing the global epidemic. Report of a WHO consultation. *World Health Organ Tech Rep Ser.* 2000;894:i–xii, 1–253.
11. Hausman DB, DiGirolamo M, Bartness TJ, Hausman GJ, Martin RJ. The biology of white adipocyte proliferation. *Obes Rev.* 2001;2:239–254.
12. Cornelius P, MacDougald OA, Lane MD. Regulation of adipocyte development. *Ann Rev Nutr.* 1994;14:99–129.
13. Prins JB, O'Rahilly S. Regulation of adipose cell number in man. *Clin Sci.* 1997;92:3–11.
14. Crandall DL, DiGirolamo M. Hemodynamic and metabolic correlates in adipose tissue: Pathophysiologic considerations. *FASEB J.* 1990;4:141–147.
15. Hirsch J, Batchelor B. Adipose tissue cellularity in human obesity. *Clin Endocrinol Metab.* 1976;5:299–311.
16. Faust IM, Johnson PR, Stern JS, Hirsch J. Diet-induced adipocyte number increase in adult rats: A new model of obesity. *Am J Physiol.* 1978;235:E279–E286.
17. Harris RB, Ramsay TG, Smith SR, Bruch RC. Early and late stimulation of ob mRNA expression in meal-fed and overfed rats. *J Clin Invest.* 1996;97:2020–2026.
18. Entenmann G, Hauner H. Relationship between replication and differentiation in cultured human adipocyte precursor cells. *Am J Physiol.* 1996;270:C1011–C1016.
19. Burdi AR, et al. Adipose tissue growth patterns during human gestation: A histometric comparison of buccal and gluteal fat depots. *Int J Obes.* 1985;9:247–256.
20. Vinten J, Galbo H. Effect of physical training on transport and metabolism of glucose in adipocytes. *Am J Physiol.* 1983;244:E129–E134.
21. Danaei G, Ding EL, Mozaffarian D, et al. The preventable causes of death in the United States: Comparative risk assessment of dietary, lifestyle, and metabolic risk factors. *PLoS Med.* 2009;6:e1000058.
22. Adams KF, Schatzkin A, Harris TB, et al. Overweight, obesity, and mortality in a large prospective cohort of persons 50 to 71 years old. *N Engl J Med.* 2006;355:763–778.
23. Lawlor DA, Hart CL, Hole DJ, Davey Smith G. Reverse causality and confounding and the associations of overweight and obesity with mortality. *Obesity.* 2006;14:2294–2304.
24. Hubert HB, Feinleib M, McNamara PM, Castelli WP. Obesity as an independent risk factor for cardiovascular disease: A 26-year follow-up of participants in the Framingham Heart Study. *Circulation.* 1983;67:968–977.
25. Allison DB, Fontaine KR, Manson JE, Stevens J, VanItallie TB. Annual deaths attributable to obesity in the United States. *JAMA.* 1999;282:1530–1538.
26. Rosengren A, Hagman M, Wedel H, Wilhelmsen L. Serum cholesterol and long-term prognosis in middle-aged men with myocardial infarction and angina pectoris. A 16-year follow-up of the Primary Prevention Study in Goteborg, Sweden. *Eur Heart J.* 1997;18:754–761.
27. Guo SS, Chumlea WC. Tracking of body mass index in children in relation to overweight in adulthood. *Am J Clin Nutr.* 1999;70:145S–148S.
28. Whitaker RC, Wright JA, Pepe MS, Seidel KD, Dietz WH. Predicting obesity in young adulthood from childhood and parental obesity. *N Engl J Med.* 1997;337:869–873.
29. Must A, Jacques PF, Dallal GE, Bajema CJ, Dietz WH. Long-term morbidity and mortality of overweight adolescents. A follow-up of the Harvard Growth Study of 1922 to 1935. *N Engl J Med.* 1992;327:1350–1355.
30. Manson JE, Willett WC, Stampfer MJ, et al. Body weight and mortality among women. *N Engl J Med.* 1995;333:677–685.
31. Freedman DS, Dietz WH, Srinivasan SR, Berenson GS. The relation of overweight to cardiovascular risk factors among children and adolescents: The Bogalusa Heart Study. *Pediatrics.* 1999;103:1175–1182.
32. Despres JP. Health consequences of visceral obesity. *Ann Med.* 2001;33:534–541.
33. Executive summary of the clinical guidelines on the identification, evaluation, and treatment of overweight and obesity in adults. *Arch Intern Med.* 1998;158:1855–1867.
34. Han E, Truesdale KP, Taber DR, Cai J, Juhaeri J, Stevens J. Impact of overweight and obesity on hospitalization: Race and gender differences. *Int J Obes.* 2009;33:249–256.
35. Ferraro KF, Shippee TP. Black and white chains of risk for hospitalization over 20 years. *J Health Soc Behav.* 2008;49:193–207.
36. Flatt JP, Ravussin E, Acheson KJ, Jéquier E. Effects of dietary fat on postprandial substrate oxidation and on carbohydrate and fat balances. *J Clin Invest.* 1985;76:1019–1024.
37. Schutz Y, Flatt JP, Jéquier E. Failure of dietary fat intake to promote fat oxidation: A factor favoring the development of obesity. *Am J Clin Nutr.* 1989;50:307–314.
38. Jequier E, Tappy L. Regulation of body weight in humans. *Physiol Rev.* 1999;79:451–480.
39. Jequier E. Nutrient effects: Post-absorptive interactions. *Proc Nutr Soc.* 1995;54:253–265.
40. Labayen I, Díez N, González A, Parra D, Martínez JA. Effects of protein vs. carbohydrate-rich diets on fuel utilisation in obese women during weight loss. *Forum Nutr.* 2003;56:168–170.
41. Brehm BJ, D'Alessio DA. Benefits of high-protein weight loss diets: enough evidence for practice? *Curr Opin Endocrinol Diabetes Obes.* 2008;15:416–421.

42. Wakefield AP, House JD, Ogborn MR, Weiler HA, Aukema HM. A diet with 35% of energy from protein leads to kidney damage in female Sprague-Dawley rats. *Br J Nutr.* 2011;106:656–663.

43. Levine JA. Nonexercise activity thermogenesis—liberating the life-force. *J Intern Med.* 2007;262:273–287.

44. Levine JA, Eberhardt NL, Jensen MD. Role of nonexercise activity thermogenesis in resistance to fat gain in humans. *Science.* 1999;283:212–214.

45. Levine JA, Lanningham-Foster LM, McCrady SK, et al. Interindividual variation in posture allocation: Possible role in human obesity. *Science.* 2005;307:584–586.

46. Ridker PM, Hennekens CH, Buring JE, et al. C-reactive protein and other markers of inflammation in the prediction of cardiovascular disease in women. *N Engl J Med.* 2000; 342:836–843.

47. Wilson PW, Nam BH, Pencina M, et al. C-reactive protein and risk of cardiovascular disease in men and women from the Framingham Heart Study. *Arch Intern Med.* 2005;165:2473–2478.

48. Patel PS, Buras ED, Balasubramanyam A. The role of the immune system in obesity and insulin resistance. *J Obes.* 2013;2013:616193.

49. Derdemezis CS, Voulgari PV, Drosos AA, Kiortsis DN. Obesity, adipose tissue and rheumatoid arthritis: Coincidence or more complex relationship? *Clin Exp Rheumatol.* 2011;29:712–727.

50. Visser M, Bouter LM, McQullan GM, et al. Elevated C-reactive protein levels in overweight and obese adults. *JAMA.* 1999;282:2131–2135.

51. You T, Arsenis NC, Disanzo BL, LaMonte MJ. Effects of exercise training on chronic inflammation: Current evidence and potential mechanisms. *Sports Med.* 2013;43:243–256.

52. Pasarica M, Sereda OR, Redman LM, et al. Reduced adipose tissue oxygenation in human obesity: Evidence for rarefaction, macrophage chemotaxis, and inflammation without an angiogenic response. *Diabetes.* 2009;58:718–725.

53. Balducci S, Zanuso S, Cardelli P, et al. Changes in physical fitness predict improvements in modifiable cardiovascular risk factors independently of body weight loss in subjects with type 2 diabetes participating in the Italian diabetes and exercise study (IDES). *Diabetes Care.* 2012;35:1347–1354.

54. Balducci S, Zanuso S, Cardelli P, et al. Supervised exercise training counterbalances the adverse effects of insulin therapy in overweight/obese subjects with type 2 diabetes. *Diabetes Care.* 2012;35:39–41.

55. Arch JR. Central regulation of energy balance: inputs, outputs and leptin resistance. *Proc Nutr Soc.* 2005;64:39–46.

56. Seals DR, Bell C. Chronic sympathetic activation: Consequence and cause of age-associated obesity? *Diabetes.* 2004;53:276–284.

57. Gutin B, Ramsey L, Barbeau P, et al. Plasma leptin concentrations in obese children: Changes during 4-mo periods with and without physical training. *Am J Clin Nutr.* 1999;69:388–394.

58. Boden G, Chen X, Mozzoli M, Ryan I. Effect of fasting on serum leptin in normal human subjects. *J Clin Endocrinol Metab.* 1996;81:3419–3423.

59. Kelesidis T, Kelesidis I, Chou S, Mantzoros CS. Narrative review: The role of leptin in human physiology: Emerging clinical applications. *Ann Intern Med.* 2010;152:93–100.

60. Rosenbaum M, Goldsmith R, Bloomfield D, et al. Low-dose leptin reverses skeletal muscle, autonomic, and neuroendocrine adaptations to maintenance of reduced weight. *J Clin Invest.* 2005;115:3579–3586.

61. Moran TH, Dailey MJ. Minireview: Gut peptides: Targets for antiobesity drug development? *Endocrinology.* 2009;150:2526–2530.

62. Boguszewski CL, Paz-Filho G, Velloso LA. Neuroendocrine body weight regulation: integration between fat tissue, gastrointestinal tract, and the brain. *Endokrynol Pol.* 2010;61:194–206.

63. Drazen DL, Vahl TP, D'Alessio DA, Seeley RJ, Woods SC. Effects of a fixed meal pattern on ghrelin secretion: Evidence for a learned response independent of nutrient status. *Endocrinology.* 2006;147:23–30.

64. Batterham RL, Cohen MA, Ellis SM, et al. Inhibition of food intake in obese subjects by peptide YY3-36. *N Engl J Med.* 2003;349:941–948.

65. Daniels J. Obesity: America's epidemic. *Am J Nurs.* 2006;106:40–49, quiz 49–50.

66. O'Rahilly S. Human genetics illuminates the paths to metabolic disease. *Nature.* 2009;462:307–314.

67. Clement K. Genetics of human obesity. *Proc Nutr Soc.* 2005;64:133–142.

68. Frayling TM, Timpson NJ, Weedon MN, et al. A common variant in the FTO gene is associated with body mass index and predisposes to childhood and adult obesity. *Science.* 2007;316:889–894.

69. Bouchard C, Tremblay A, Després JP, et al. The response to long-term overfeeding in identical twins. *N Engl J Med.* 1990;322:1477–1482.

70. Giskes K, Kamphuis CB, van Lenthe FJ, Kremers S, Droomers M, Brug J. A systematic review of associations between environmental factors, energy and fat intakes among adults: Is there evidence for environments that encourage obesogenic dietary intakes? *Public Health Nutr.* 2007;10:1005–1017.

71. Turrell G, Hewitt B, Patterson C, Oldenburg B, Gould T. Socioeconomic differences in food purchasing behaviour and suggested implications for diet-related health promotion. *J Hum Nutr Diet.* 2002;15:355–364.

72. Cummins S, Macintyre S. Food environments and obesity—neighbourhood or nation? *Int J Epidemiol.* 2006;35:100–104.

73. Prentice AM, Jebb SA. Fast foods, energy density and obesity: A possible mechanistic link. *Obes Rev.* 2003;4:187–194.

74. Rolls BJ. The supersizing of America: Portion size and the obesity epidemic. *Nutr Today.* 2003;38:42–53.

75. Diliberti N, Bordi PL, Conklin MT, Roe LS, Rolls BJ. Increased portion size leads to increased energy intake in a restaurant meal. *Obes Res.* 2004;12:562–568.

76. McCormack GR, Shiell A. In search of causality: A systematic review of the relationship between the built environment and physical activity among adults. *Int J Behav Nutr Phys Act.* 2011;8:125.

77. Mrosovsky N, Powley TL. Set points for body weight and fat. *Behav Biol.* 1977;20:205–223.

78. Cohn C, Joseph D. Influence of body weight and body fat on appetite of "normal" lean and obese rats. *Yale J Biol Med.* 1962;34:598–607.

79. Sims EA, Horton ES. Endocrine and metabolic adaptation to obesity and starvation. *Am J Clin Nutr.* 1968;21:1455–1470.

80. Bennett WI. Beyond overeating. *N Engl J Med.* 1995;332:673–674.

81. Weinsier RL. Etiology of obesity: Methodological examination of the set-point theory. *JPEN J Parenter Enteral Nutr.* 2001;25:103–110.

82. Weinsier RL, Nagy TR, Hunter GR, Darnell BE, Hensrud DD, Weiss HL. Do adaptive changes in metabolic rate favor weight regain in weight-reduced individuals? An examination of the set-point theory. *Am J Clin Nutr.* 2000;72:1088–1094.

83. Byrne NM, Weinsier RL, Hunter GR, et al. Influence of distribution of lean body mass on resting metabolic rate after weight loss and weight regain: Comparison of responses in white and black women. *Am J Clin Nutr.* 2003;77:1368–1373.

84. Weinsier RL, Hunter GR, Schutz Y, Zuckerman PA, Darnell BE. Physical activity in free-living, overweight white and black women: Divergent responses by race to diet-induced weight loss. *Am J Clin Nutr.* 2002;76:736–742.

85. Jequier E. Pathways to obesity. *Int J Obes Relat Metab Disord.* 2002;26(Suppl. 2):S12–S17.

86. Rolls BJ, Roe LS, Meengs JS. The effect of large portion sizes on energy intake is sustained for 11 days. *Obesity.* 2007;15:1535–1543.

87. Prentice AM. Overeating: The health risks. *Obes Res.* 2001;9(Suppl. 4):234S–238S.

88. Lissner L, Levitsky DA, Strupp BJ, Kalkwarf HJ, Roe DA. Dietary fat and the regulation of energy intake in human subjects. *Am J Clin Nutr.* 1987;46:886–892.

89. Poppitt, S. D., & Prentice, A. M. (1996). Energy density and its role in the control of food intake: evidence from metabolic and community studies. *Appetite.* 26(2): 153–174.

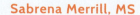

Sabrena Merrill, MS

**CHAPTER 23**

# Body Composition

## CHAPTER OUTLINE

## LEARNING OUTCOMES

1. Describe the various models of body composition, including how they are applied in body composition assessment.

2. List the determinants of body composition and describe how they affect the accuracy of body composition assessment across different populations.

3. Identify the health risks of having too much or too little body fat.

4. Explain the difference between assessments that measure body weight and those that assess body composition.

5. Calculate ideal body weight based on percent body fat.

6. Calculate body mass index.

7. Describe commonly used techniques for body composition assessment and explain appropriate uses for each.

8. Give general guidelines for follow-up body composition assessment measures.

## ANCILLARY LINK

Visit Davis*Plus* at http://davisplus.fadavis.com for study and practice resources, including online quizzes, animations that help explain physiological processes, podcasts concerning news and career trends in exercise physiology, and practice references.

## VIGNETTE

■ Suzanne is a 60-year-old woman who was recently diagnosed with type 2 diabetes. At her last doctor's visit, Suzanne expressed concern about the accuracy of the diagnosis because she had always heard that type 2 diabetes is associated with obesity, and she is not obese. In fact, although she is not physically active, Suzanne has a slender build and has never had a weight problem. Over the past 15 years, Suzanne has gained about 7 pounds, but even with added weight, she wears the same size clothing she has always worn throughout her adulthood. Suzanne's physician assures her that his diagnosis is correct and, in addition to prescribing her oral diabetes medication and referring her to a registered dietitian, he encourages her to start a regular exercise program that focuses on improving her body composition.

How is it possible that a slender person, like Suzanne, would need to take actions to improve his or her body composition?

The interest in studying human body composition stems from the intention to determine the absolute and relative (%) contributions of water, protein, minerals, and fat in the human body, and to describe either deficiencies or excesses of a bodily component that is related to health risk, performance, or both. For example, bone mineral density (BMD) is monitored in individuals with osteoporosis (a disease related to deficient bone mass), and body-fat percentage is often assessed in individuals who are obese (a condition of excess adipose tissue, or body fat). Height and weight are measured in children to monitor growth and maturation changes across the early life span. In fitness and sports, understanding an individual's body composition provides useful information for predicting athletic performance, because a high level of **fat mass (FM)** is generally detrimental to performance.

The available measurement methods for assessing body composition range from simple to complex, with all methods having limitations and some degree of measurement error. Choosing the most appropriate assessment method—whether evaluating an individual's health risk or performance potential—reduces the margin of measurement error and leads to a more effective tracking of body-fat percentage as the client progresses toward his or her body composition goals. This chapter presents the science and application of body composition assessment, as well as the rationale behind various techniques for measuring body composition.

## BODY COMPOSITION AND HEALTH RISKS

Overweight refers to a total body weight above the recommended range for good health [or a body mass index (BMI) between 25 and 29.9], whereas obesity refers to severe overweight and a high body-fat percentage. Both overweight and obesity increase the risk for certain chronic health conditions (Table 23-1). When reviewing an individual's health-assessment data, it is important to consider what proportion of a person's total body weight is fat (i.e., body fat percentage [%BF]).

At its most practical level, body composition refers to the proportion of lean tissue (also called fat-free mass [FFM]) to body-fat tissue. FFM is composed of muscles, connective tissue, bones, blood, nervous tissue, skin, and organs. For the most part, FFM is metabolically active tissue that allows the body to perform work. A certain amount of body fat, called **essential fat**, is necessary for hormone production, cushioning of vital organs, and maintenance of certain body functions. The remainder of body fat is stored throughout the body in adipose tissue, either subcutaneously or viscerally; it acts as a readily available source of energy, protects vital organs, and assists in insulation and thermoregulation.

A certain amount of body fat is necessary for overall health and well-being, although too much body fat can be detrimental to health and increases the risk for many diseases, ranging from cardiovascular disease to osteoarthritis. A person's health can also be compromised if his or her body-fat percentage decreases to less than recommended levels. Table 23-2 presents the general body-fat percentage categories for men and women.

## BODY COMPOSITION MODELS

To study body composition, it is necessary to break the body down into its component parts so that researchers can compare the components with reference models. There are various models for studying body composition, ranging from two-component up to six-component models (Fig. 23-1). Multicomponent models divide the body into compartments consisting of minerals, chemicals, soft tissues, and fluids. As physics and chemistry technology continues to advance, the biological complexity of the models also increases, showing subdivisions from atoms and molecules to cells and tissue systems.

The most widely used model in body composition research is the two-component, whole-body model, which divides the body into FM and FFM compartments, where FM consists of all extractable lipids, and

## Table 23-1. Increased Risk for Obesity-Related Diseases With Higher Body Mass Index

| DISEASE | BMI (kg/m²) | | | |
|---------|-------------|---------|---------|-------|
|         | <25         | 25–<30  | 30–35   | >35   |
| Arthritis | 1.00 | 1.56 | 1.87 | 2.39 |
| Heart disease | 1.00 | 1.39 | 1.86 | 1.67 |
| Diabetes (type 2) | 1.00 | 2.42 | 3.35 | 6.16 |
| Gallstones | 1.00 | 1.97 | 3.30 | 5.48 |
| Hypertension | 1.00 | 1.92 | 2.82 | 3.77 |
| Stroke | 1.00 | 1.53 | 1.59 | 1.75 |

A value of 1.00 equals a standard level of risk, whereas values exceeding 1.00 represent increased risk. For example, a value of 1.87 means that the individual is at an 87% greater level of risk.

*Source:* Centers for Disease Control and Prevention. Third National Health and Nutrition Examination Survey. Analysis by The Levin Group; 1999. http://www.cdc.gov/nchs/nhanes.htm

## Table 23-2. General Body-Fat Percentage Categories

| CLASSIFICATION | FAT (%) WOMEN | FAT (%) MEN |
|---|---|---|
| Essential fat | 10–13 | 2–5 |
| Athletes | 14–20 | 6–13 |
| Fitness | 21–24 | 14–17 |
| Average | 25–31 | 18–24 |
| Obese | ≥32 | ≥25 |

FFM components include water, proteins, and minerals.[1] The classic research that originated the two-component model was conducted in the early 1960s based on dissection data collected from three white male cadavers aged 25, 35, and 46 years.[2] The densities of the fat and FFM components of these cadavers were used to develop a "reference body" with which other methods of body composition assessment were developed. The FFM components of the reference body are assumed to be 73.8% water, 19.4% protein, and 6.8% mineral.[2]

When researchers apply the classic two-component model in their investigations, the following assumptions are made[1,2]:

- Fat density is 0.901 g/cubic centimeter (cc).
- FFM density is 1.10 g/cc.
- The density of fat and FFM components are the same for all individuals.
- The FFM tissue components are constant throughout an individual (73.8% water, 19.4% protein, and 6.8% mineral), and their proportional contribution to the lean component remains constant.

The assumptions associated with the classic two-component model served as the cornerstone on which

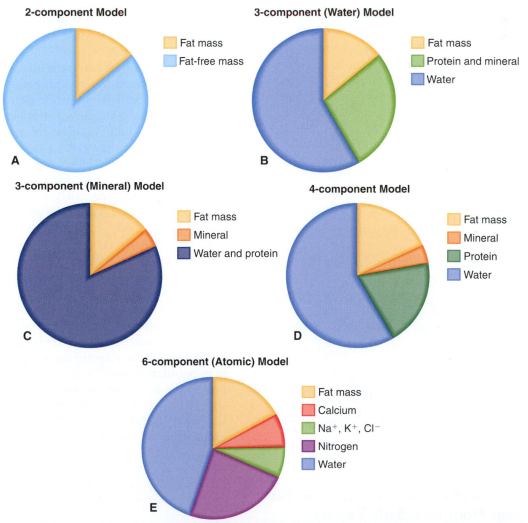

Figure 23-1. The variety of body composition models that can be applied to understand the individual constituents that make up the human body. These models can range from (A) the simple two-component model that divides the body into fat mass and fat-free mass (FFM); (B) the three-component (water) model; (C) the three-component (mineral) model; (D) the four-component model, which best demonstrates the individual contributions of bone mineral (6.8%), protein (19.4%), and water (73.8%) in determining the FFM of the body; and (E) the complex six-component model that shows the body at the atomic level.

the **hydrostatic weighing** (i.e., underwater weighing) method was developed. Using this method, the assumed proportions and their respective densities, listed in Table 23-3, can be used to convert an individual's **total body density** into his or her relative %BF. Two classic formulas used for this process are the Siri[1] and Brozek et al.[2] equations (Table 23-4).

### DOING THE MATH
### Calculating Total Body Density

Using the Siri[1] equation for a person with a measured body density of 1.0500 g/cc yields a %BF estimate of 21.4%. For the same person, the Brozek et al.[2] equation produces a %BF estimate of 21.0%. See the following calculations:

- Siri[1] equation: $([4.95 \div 1.0500 \text{ g/cc}] - 4.50) \times 100 = 21.4\%$
- Brozek et al.[2] equation: $([4.57 \div 1.0500 \text{ g/cc}] - 4.142) \times 100 = 21.0\%$

The two equations yield very similar results. However, the two-component model equations provide accurate estimates of %BF only as long as the basic assumptions of the model are met. Ensuring that all assumptions are met is problematic because there is no guarantee that the FFM composition of the person being assessed exactly matches the values assumed for the reference body.

### Table 23-3. Assumed Values for Fat Mass and Fat-Free Mass Components

| COMPONENT | DENSITY (g/cc) | PROPORTION OF BODY WEIGHT (%) |
|---|---|---|
| Fat mass | 0.9007 | 15.3 |
| Fat-free mass | | |
| Water | 0.9937 | 73.8 |
| Protein | 1.34 | 19.4 |
| Mineral | 3.038 | 6.8 |

Data from Brozek et al.[2]

### Table 23-4. Formulas for Deriving Body Fat Percentage From Total Body Density

| EQUATION | FORMULA |
|---|---|
| Siri[1] | %BF = $([4.95/Db] - 4.50) \times 100$ |
| Brozek et al.[2] | %BF = $([4.57/Db] - 4.142) \times 100$ |

%BF, percentage of body fat; Db, total body density.
*Sources:* Siri[1] and Brozek et al.[2]

The two-component model based on the Siri[1] and Brozek et al.[2] equations can be used to accurately estimate %BF in white male individuals aged 19 to 55 years, but for other populations—such as individuals in various age and ethnic groups—there can be a high degree of individual variation.[3,4] In addition, researchers have reported that the density of FFM composition varies with age, ethnicity, level of body fatness, and physical-activity level.[5–7] For example, it was found that the densities of FFM components of black men and women are higher than the original reference body because of their higher mineral content and bone density.[8–10] As such, the %BF of black individuals will be consistently underestimated when two-component model equations are used. Children possess a relatively high body-water content and low mineral density compared with the reference body.[11] Older adults also exhibit less mineral density than the reference body.[12] Thus, the relative %BF of children and older adults will be systematically overestimated using the Siri[1] and Brozek et al.[2] equations.

As a health and fitness professional, the choice of which %BF prediction equation to use with a client will ultimately determine the accuracy of the assessment. Prediction equations are either population specific or generalized. Population-specific equations are intended for use for the body composition estimation of only the individuals who belong to one homogenous group. For example, a skinfold equation has been developed for prepubescent black boys and a separate one for prepubescent white boys.[13] Thus, if population-specific equations are applied to individuals who are not in the specified subgroup, the %BF estimations will be either too high or too low, depending on the individual being assessed.

Generalized equations are developed from diverse, heterogeneous samples and can be applied to individuals who differ greatly in physical characteristics. For example, a commonly used generalized skinfold equation[14] takes into account age and sex so that it can be applied to men and women between the ages of 18 and 55 years to determine body density.

It is beyond the scope of this chapter to detail the various population-specific equations that are available. For example, there are more than 100 population-specific equations for the skinfold method alone.[15] However, useful generalized equations that apply to a broad range of individuals will be presented in subsequent sections. See also the Additional Resources list at the end of this chapter for more information on population-specific prediction equations for the estimation of body composition.

## DETERMINANTS OF BODY COMPOSITION

To a large extent, a person's individual characteristics influence his or her body composition. Genetics, heredity, bone structure, and body type explain most of the

## VIGNETTE *continued*

■ Suzanne has several individual characteristics that put her at increased risk for an unfavorable body composition. Her age, sex, and physical-activity status set the stage for loss of FFM, and hence higher FM. To address Suzanne's concerns about her type 2 diabetes diagnosis, her doctor refers her to the hospital wellness center to undergo a body composition assessment. There she meets Alonzo, a laboratory technician who performs a dual-energy x-ray absorptiometry (DEXA) scan, which will provide a clearer picture of Suzanne's body composition.

variation in body weight and body composition among people. Energy balance (caloric intake vs. caloric expenditure) plays a significant role in regulating body composition. A healthy diet and daily exercise are the two most important factors that affect the ability to reach and sustain an ideal body weight and %BF. Genetics, however, plays the most significant role in the extent to which body composition can be changed.[16] The main determinants of body composition are age, sex, ethnicity, and physical-activity participation.

### Age

As described earlier, children and older adults tend to have less FFM than young and middle-aged adults. From birth to 22 years of age, FFM steadily increases in humans[17,18] (with the exception of water content, which decreases slightly—about 5%—until age 20 years).[19] This increase indicates that for the first two decades of life, children and adolescents have less FFM than that of adults. From ages 25 to 65 years, decreases in bone mass, skeletal muscle, and **total body water (TBW)** result in a significant reduction in FFM (10%–16%) by the time a person reaches the seventh decade of life.[12,20]

In addition, with aging, adipose tissue is redistributed with relatively more subcutaneous and internal fat deposited in the trunk than the extremities,[21,22] and an infiltration of fat into skeletal muscle tissue.[22,23] Fatty-tissue infiltration of muscle and decreases in muscle mass result in reduced function, which contribute to physical inactivity. These factors play a major role in the tendency for older adults to experience an increase in body fat as they continue to age.

### Sex

Men tend to be taller, have a more dense skeleton, and possess more muscle mass and a lower body-fat content than women.[24–27] It is likely that hormonal differences (specifically, variations in testosterone) play a major role in the body composition differences between men and women.

### Ethnicity

Individuals of particular ethnicities—Native Americans, African Americans, and Hispanics—have a relatively greater risk than other ethnic groups for obesity and its associated comorbidities (e.g., cardiovascular disease, hypertension, type 2 diabetes, certain cancers, and osteoarthritis).[28,29] Asian populations, especially Asian women, tend to have less BMD than other ethnicities, placing them at increased risk for osteoporosis.[30–32]

Compared with white men and women, black men and women tend to have relatively greater muscle mass, bone mineral mass, and BMD,[9,10,33,34] which can serve as a protective factor against the risk for osteoporosis. Lastly, although the prevalence is not as high as in minority populations, excess body fat is also a problem for white individuals, with more than 25% of white men and women being overweight or obese.[29,35,36]

### Physical-Activity Participation

In general, for both men and women, athletes and physically active individuals are leaner than sedentary individuals.[37–39] Regular physical activity and exercise training typically result in decreased FM and increased FFM. Researchers have reported that physically active individuals and athletes have greater BMD and skeletal muscle mass than their inactive counterparts.[40–46] The exception to these findings is female athletes with amenorrhea who may actually have less FFM than sedentary women because of significant loss of BMD as a result of intense physical training and lack of adequate nutrition.[47,48]

## DESIRABLE BODY FAT PERCENTAGE

A person's %BF will vary depending on his or her sex, age, race, and physical-activity level. In addition, hormonal changes in women because of pregnancy, menopause, and menstruation can cause water retention that can account for variations in outcomes between tests.

Whether someone's %BF is too high for good health depends on a number of variables. For example, some people may fall into the high range of acceptability for %BF, but otherwise be healthy and physically active. Others may have acceptable %BF levels but have an elevated risk for chronic illness and disease because of poor lifestyle choices. A person's overall health and lifestyle choices should be taken into account before making a decision about whether their %BF is acceptable or unacceptable. A large and convincing body of literature confirms an increased risk for chronic illness and disease with high %BF levels of more than 32% in women and more than 25% in men.[49]

For both men and women, there exists a lower body-fat limit at which reducing levels of body fat beyond this value ultimately impairs health status or alters normal physiological function. For men, the average lower limit appears to be 3%; for women, it is approximately 12%.[45] These lower body-fat limits are often observed in athletes who participate in sports that require competition in certain weight classes, such as bodybuilding and wrestling, or that focus on aesthetics, such as gymnastics or dance. Some athletes get close to or below minimal ranges for %BF for brief periods because of their training and higher-than-average FFM. Low %BF levels may be appropriate for some athletes, as long as they are otherwise in good health and are getting all of their daily nutritional requirements.

However, a low %BF alone is not a guarantee of athletic success.

An example of disrupted physiological function in women with extremely low body fat is **amenorrhea** (absence of menstruation). In competitive athletic women, a condition called the **female athlete triad** has been observed in those who engage in intense training and dietary restriction. The female athlete triad is a collection of three conditions: (1) disordered eating, (2) amenorrhea or menstrual irregularities, and (3) osteoporosis. Although the research on the amount of body fat that triggers a woman to stop menstruating is inconclusive, investigators have reported that a range of 12% to 17% body fat is necessary for normal menstrual function.[50–52]

## RESEARCH HIGHLIGHT

### The Female Athlete Triad

Low caloric intake (with or without eating disorders), amenorrhea, and osteoporosis, alone or in combination, pose significant health risks to physically active girls and women. The female athlete triad refers to the interrelationships among energy availability, menstrual function, and BMD, which, if left untreated, may develop into clinical conditions including eating disorders, amenorrhea, and osteoporosis (see Fig. 23-2). The potentially irreversible consequences of these clinical manifestations have prompted the medical community to emphasize efforts for prevention, early diagnosis, and treatment. The following sections highlight the findings from the 2007 American College of Medicine "Position Stand: The Female Athlete Triad."[53]

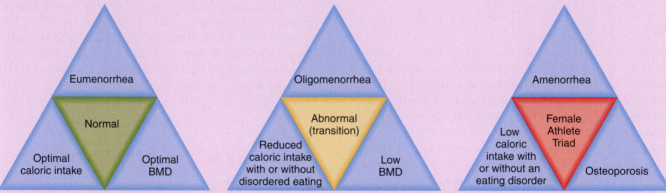

**Figure 23-2.** The development of characteristics associated with the female athlete triad—amenorrhea or menstrual irregularies, low caloric intake with or without an eating disorder, and osteoporosis—occur across a continuum from normal function (green) to altered physiological changes and caloric intake (yellow) to significant clinical signs of this disorder (red). Changes that occur along this continuum may or may not be reversible depending on the severity of the condition at that point in time. Eumenorrhea is normal or regular menstrual periods; oligomenorrhea is very light or infrequent menstrual periods.

### ■ ENERGY INTAKE

Deficient energy intake reduces the amount of energy available for cellular maintenance, thermoregulation, growth, and reproduction, which ultimately leads to impaired health. Low energy availability can result from athletes increasing energy expenditure more than energy intake, or from reducing energy intake more than exercise energy expenditure. Others practice abnormal eating behaviors such as fasting, binge eating and purging, or use diet pills, laxatives, diuretics, and enemas. Some athletes also suffer from eating disorders, such as anorexia nervosa and bulimia nervosa, which are clinical mental disorders that result in disruption of normal daily caloric intake. Notably, however, low energy availability may occur inadvertently without clinical eating disorders or even dietary restriction, but as a result of dramatically increased energy expenditure during physical training without the biological drive to match the expenditure through diet. Athletes at highest risk for low energy availability and manifestation of the triad are those who restrict caloric

## RESEARCH HIGHLIGHT–cont'd

intake, exercise for prolonged periods, are vegetarian, and limit the types of foods that they will eat. Other risk factors include sport-specific training at an early age, dieting, sports injury, and sudden increase in training volume.

### ■ MENSTRUAL FUNCTION

A disruption in an athlete's normal menstrual cycle of 3 or more months is called *secondary amenorrhea*. Primary amenorrhea occurs when the age of menarche (the first menstrual period) is delayed (i.e., ≥15 years). Regardless of the type of amenorrhea, serious medical complications are associated with amenorrheic menstrual dysfunction including infertility, decreased BMD, and increased risk for stress fractures.

### ■ BONE MINERAL DENSITY

Osteoporosis is a skeletal disorder characterized by compromised bone strength, which predisposes a person to an increased risk for fracture. One factor in bone strength is BMD. In female athletes, BMD declines as the number of missed menstrual cycles accumulates, resulting in a loss of BMD that may not be fully reversible. As such, stress fractures are more common in physically active women with menstrual irregularities and/or low BMD, with a relative risk for stress fracture two to four times greater in athletes with amenorrhea than in those with eumenorrhea.

### ■ RECOMMENDATIONS

The American College of Sports Medicine recommends a multidisciplinary approach to dealing with the female athlete triad. Typically, sport participation requires a preparticipation physical examination. During this examination, the physician should ask the appropriate questions to elicit whether the athlete has any signs of the female athlete triad. If she does, a multidisciplinary team including a physician, a registered dietitian, and, if the athlete is thought to have an eating disorder such as anorexia or bulimia, a mental health professional, will work together to help the athlete regain her health. The athlete's coach, an exercise physiologist, a certified athletic trainer, parents, and other family members also play an important role in her recovery.

American College of Sports Medicine. Position Stand: The female athlete triad. *Med Sci Sports Exerc.* 2007;39:1867–1882.

## BODY COMPOSITION ASSESSMENT TECHNIQUES

Assessment of body composition is often of great interest to a client. In fact, many clients are compelled to enroll in a fitness-training program for the sole purpose of changing their body composition. Accordingly, it is important to be able to accurately assess a person's body composition to determine a reasonable body-weight goal and to develop a safe and effective exercise program to reach it. Depending on the test, the assessment of body composition can be quite invasive. It is important for allied health and fitness professionals to conduct these assessments in a private area to put the client at ease.

An accurate body-composition assessment measures the relative percentages of FFM and FM within a particular individual. Routine assessment of body composition is an effective way to show clients how successful their weight-management efforts have been (Box 23-1).

Furthermore, it is not uncommon for an exerciser to lose fat weight and gain muscle weight without any change in total body weight. In reality, such a transformation would be very favorable from an overall health and functional performance perspective. However, without an accurate assessment of a person's level of body composition, this positive change could go undetected and possibly lead to frustration on the part of the exerciser.

A number of body composition assessment techniques are available, including:

- Height and weight tables
- Body mass index (BMI)

### Box 23-1. Purpose of Body Composition Assessment

- To get baseline information
- To document for program assessment
- To use as a motivational tool
- To monitor development- and age-related changes in body composition
- To help formulate dietary recommendations
- To monitor changes in body composition that are associated with certain diseases
- To identify a client's health risk for excessively high or low levels of body fat
- To promote a client's understanding of body fat
- To monitor changes in body composition
- To assess the effectiveness of nutrition and exercise choices
- To help estimate healthy body weight for clients and athletes
- To assist in exercise programming

- Anthropometric measurements
- **Bioelectrical impedance analysis (BIA)**
- Hydrostatic weighing
- Other methods

The assessments presented in Table 23-5 are used to assess body composition. Because of the cost and limited availability of the equipment needed, not all assessments are practical in a fitness setting.

## Table 23-5. Body Composition Assessments

| METHOD | SETTING | DESCRIPTION |
|---|---|---|
| BIA* | Whole-body BIA machines are found primarily in laboratory settings <br> Less sophisticated BIA devices are found in fitness settings | BIA measures electrical signals as they pass through fat, lean mass, and water in the body. In essence, this method assesses leanness, but calculations can be made based on this information. BIA accuracy is based primarily on the sophistication of the machine and consistency of measurement procedures. <br> Many fitness centers use BIA because of the simplicity of use. Optimal hydration is necessary for accurate results. |
| ADP (e.g., BOD POD [PEA POD for children]) | Marketed for the fitness setting, but it is cost-prohibitive for most facilities | The BOD POD is an egg-shaped chamber that measures the amount of air that is displaced when a person sits in the machine. Two values are needed to determine body fat: air displacement and body weight. ADP has a high accuracy rate, but the equipment is expensive. |
| DEXA* | May be found in exercise physiology departments at colleges and universities | DEXA ranks among the most accurate and precise methods. DEXA is a whole-body scanning system that delivers a low-dose x-ray that reads body and soft-tissue mass. DEXA has the ability to identify regional body-fat distribution. |
| Hydrostatic weighing† (underwater weighing) | May be found in exercise physiology departments at colleges and universities | This method measures the amount of water a person displaces when completely submerged, thereby indirectly measuring body fat. It is not practical in a fitness center setting because of the size of the apparatus and the complexity of the technique required for accurate measurements, which involves the individual going down to the bottom of a tank, exhaling all air from the lungs (expiratory quotient), and then holding his or her breath until the scale settles and records an accurate weight. The assessment must then be repeated to ensure accuracy. |
| NIR* (e.g., Futurex) | Marketed for the fitness setting, tends to not be as accurate as other methods | NIR uses a fiber-optic probe connected to a digital analyzer that indirectly measure tissue composition (fat and water). Typically, the biceps are the assessment site. Calculations then are plugged into an equation that includes height, weight, frame size, and level of activity. This method is relatively inexpensive and fast, but not as accurate as most assessments. |
| Skinfold measurement | Commonly used in fitness settings | Skinfold calipers are used to "pinch" a fold of skin and fat. Several sites of the body are typically measured. The measurements are plugged into an equation that calculates body-fat percentage. Accuracy highly dependent on the experience of the technician. |

*These body composition assessment techniques are not accurate when used with obese clients.
†The gold standard: many later methods of body-fat assessment are based on calculations derived from hydrostatic weighing.
ADP, air displacement plethysmography; BIA, bioelectrical impedance analysis; DEXA, dual energy x-ray absorptiometry; NIR, near-infrared resistance.

## In Your Own Words

### Discussing Body-Composition Assessment Results With Clients

Body composition results can be used to help motivate clients and help them set realistic body-weight or fat-loss goals. They should never be used to humiliate, degrade, or categorize people. In addition, fitness and health professionals should be mindful to use positive and encouraging language. For example, avoid saying, "Mr. Jones, your body composition results indicate that your %BF is high, which means that you fall into the obese category. Boy, we sure have a lot of work ahead of us, don't we?" Although this statement may be true, health and fitness professionals would be wise to be more encouraging. For example, you could say, "Mr. Jones, your body composition results indicate that you are above the range for good health, so I'm glad you made this appointment and I'm excited to be working with you. The diet and exercise goals we agreed on will help bring your percent body fat down into a healthier range."

How would you deliver body composition assessment results to your clients? Practice delivering results statements so that the language you use is positive and encouraging.

## Height and Weight Tables

The usual way that weight-conscious people track their body weight (not body composition) is to step on the bathroom scale. Periodically weighing oneself on a scale can help track weight gain or loss over time, but doing so provides no information about FM or FFM changes over time.

In 1943, the Metropolitan Life Insurance Company gave scale weight more meaning when they published desirable weight tables for men and women.[54] The tables, which are based on people who applied for life insurance policies, identify desirable weights based on height and frame size. For the Metropolitan Life Insurance Company, the tables determined the policy applicants with the lowest mortality rates. The tables became known as height–weight tables, and eventually became a universal standard for deciding desirable weight for anyone, not just life insurance applicants. When the tables were revised in 1983, all of the weight ranges increased.[55] The term *ideal weight* gradually became associated with these tables, although the word *ideal* was never specifically published in this context.

## Body Mass Index

More useful estimates of body composition can be obtained by adjusting weight for height or stature and calculating a height-normalized index. The most commonly used index is BMI.

Table 22-2 can be used to determine BMI. People in a normal weight range usually have a BMI between 18.5 and 24.9 kg/m². According to National Health and Nutrition Examination Survey 2003–2004 data, approximately two-thirds of U.S. adults aged 20 years and older are either overweight or obese: 34.1% are overweight, defined as having a BMI of 25.0 to 29.9 kg/m²; and 32.2% are obese, with a BMI ≥30 kg/m².

BMI can also be used to predict body-fat percentages, although the method is still in its initial stages of development and can have a high degree of variability (Table 23-6).

Similar to height–weight tables, BMI also fails to consider the body's proportional distribution of body fat and the composition of overall body weight. Because BMI uses total body weight (i.e., not estimates of FM and FFM separately) in the calculation, it does not discriminate between the overfat and the athletic or more muscular body type. The possibility of misclassifying someone as overweight using BMI standards applies particularly to shot-putters, bodybuilders, heavier wrestlers, and football players. Although there are inherent problems with assessing fatness of an individual using this method, it remains the method of choice for large-scale epidemiological studies because of the ease of obtaining the two measurements required and its acceptable correlation with more technical measures (e.g., hydrostatic weighing and skinfolds). It should be emphasized, however, that the number obtained using BMI is not a measure of body composition per se, but merely a calculated ratio using height and weight. Therefore, BMI ideally should be used in conjunction with other body composition assessments.

### DOING THE MATH
#### Calculating Body Mass Index

BMI (kg/m²) = weight (in kg)/height² (in meters)

Example:
- *Convert weight from pounds to kilograms by dividing by 2.2:*

Weight = 209 lb

209 lb/2.2 = 95 kg

- *Convert height from inches to centimeters, and then to meters, by multiplying by 2.54 and then dividing by 100:*

Height = 68 in.

68 in. × 2.54 = 173 cm

173 cm/100 = 1.73 m

**BMI = 95/(1.73)² = 95/2.99 = 31.8 kg/m²**

**Table 23-6. Body Fat Percentage Based on Body Mass Index for African American and White Adults**

| BMI (kg/m²) | HEALTH RISK | BODY FAT (%) BY AGE (YR) | | |
| | | 20–39 | 40–59 | 60–79 |
| --- | --- | --- | --- | --- |
| **Men** | | | | |
| ≤18.5 | Elevated | <8 | <11 | <13 |
| 18.6–24.9 | Average | 8–19 | 11–21 | 13–24 |
| 25.0–29.9 | Elevated | 20–24 | 22–27 | 25–29 |
| ≥30 | High | ≥25 | ≥28 | ≥30 |
| **Women** | | | | |
| ≤18.5 | Elevated | <21 | <23 | <24 |
| 18.6–24.9 | Average | 21–32 | 23–33 | 24–35 |
| 25.0–29.9 | Elevated | 33–38 | 34–39 | 36–41 |
| ≥30 | High | ≥39 | ≥40 | ≥42 |

Standard error estimate is ±5% for predicting body fat from body mass index (BMI; based on a four-compartment estimate of body fat percentage).

*Source:* Data from Gallagher D, Heymsfield SB, Heo M, Jebb SA, Murgatroyd PR, Sakamoto Y. Healthy percentage body fat ranges: An approach for developing guidelines based on body mass index. *Am J Clin Nutr.* 2000;72:694–701.

## VIGNETTE continued

■ Before her body composition assessment, Alonzo helps Suzanne calculate her BMI. She is 5'4" and weighs 115 lb, which places her toward the low end of the normal weight category, with a BMI of 18.9 kg/m². This further confuses Suzanne, particularly because her doctor told her to work on improving her body composition and her BMI confirms that she does not have a "weight problem."

## In Your Own Words

An active, well-muscled client has recently visited his physician for an annual medical evaluation. He reports to you that, after taking his weight and height measurements, his physician placed him in the overweight category. However, according to the body composition assessment you have conducted with him, he is considered healthy and not in danger of being overweight. How would you explain this discrepancy to your client?

## Anthropometric Measurements

Anthropometric assessments of body composition are perhaps the easiest and least expensive methods for assessing body composition. These include circumference and skinfold measures, which are readily used in the field. Anthropometric measures also can be used to estimate body fat and its distribution (i.e., central vs. peripheral or upper body vs. lower body).

## Circumference Measurements

Circumference, or girth, measures can easily be used to assess body composition, even with significantly overweight clients (see Figs. 23-3, 23-4, and 23-5 for examples of these measures). These measurements are not only good predictors of health problems (e.g., waist circumference as it correlates to cardiometabolic disease), but an overall body assessment will also provide

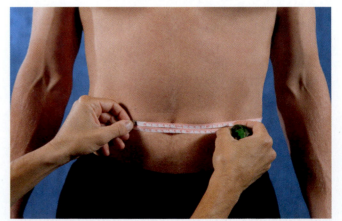

**Figure 23-3.** Measurement of abdominal circumference. With the subject standing upright and relaxed, a horizontal measure is taken at the greatest anterior extension of the abdomen, usually at the level of the umbilicus.

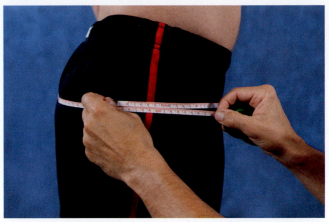

**Figure 23-4.** Measurement of hip circumference. With the subject standing erect with the feet together, a horizontal measure is taken at the maximal circumference of the buttocks.

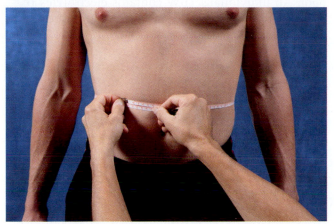

**Figure 23-5.** Measurement of waist circumference. With the subject standing, arms at the sides, feet together, and abdomen relaxed, a horizontal measure is taken at the narrowest part of the torso (above the umbilicus and below the xiphoid process).

motivation as clients see changes in their body dimensions. In the case of excess FM, clients will be inspired by a decline in girth measurements, whereas individuals who are interested in muscular hypertrophy will likely be motivated by increases in girth.

## Waist-to-Hip Ratio

Excess body fat poses significant health risks, and the location of the fat deposits may even be a better indicator of disease risk.[56] The waist-to-hip ratio (WHR) method helps differentiate android individuals, who carry excess fat in the abdominal area, from those who are gynoid and carry excess fat in the hips and thighs. Although any extra fat weight is detrimental to a person's health, individuals who are android and have a high WHR have a greater health risk. The waist measurement is divided by the hip measurement to determine WHR. See the Practice What You Know section later in this chapter for detailed protocols for determining WHR.

## Waist Circumference

Visceral fat contributes to android fat distribution and is very damaging, not only because it encroaches on the vital organs, but also because excess abdominal fat has been associated with insulin resistance. For every 1-inch (2.5-cm) increase in waist circumference in men, the following associated health risks are found[57]:

- Blood pressure increases by 10%
- Blood cholesterol level increases by 8%
- High-density lipoprotein decreases by 15%
- Triglycerides increase by 18%
- Metabolic syndrome risk increases by 18%

See the Practice What You Know section later in this chapter for detailed protocols for determining waist circumference.

## Skinfold Measurements

Subcutaneous body fat can be measured using a device called a **skinfold caliper** (Fig. 23-6). In an average person, approximately 50% of body fat is distributed just below the skin. For this reason, body composition can be easily calculated using the right tools and formulas. Skinfold formulas are derived from calculations based on extensive research involving hydrostatic weighing. In general, the skinfold caliper method produces a measurement that is ±2.0% to 3.5% of that obtained in hydrostatic weighing.[58,59] Further measurement error is likely if the health and fitness professional is inexperienced or uses poor technique, if the client is obese or extremely thin, or if the caliper is not properly calibrated. Before conducting skinfold measurements, health and fitness professionals must familiarize themselves with the exact site locations and proper grasping technique (see Figs. 23-7 through 23-12).

Given the variability in fat distribution from site to site, it is recommended that multiple sites be measured.[59] See the Practice What You Know section later in this chapter for detailed protocols for the skinfold method of body composition estimation.

## General Guidelines for Anthropometric Assessments

Many of the tests that measure body size and proportions can be used in conjunction with body-composition testing. Testing protocols are basically the same for all of the anthropometric tests:

- To become proficient, health and exercise professionals should train under an experienced technician and practice on a diverse group of individuals.
- These tests should be performed prior to exercise and under a state of normal hydration.
- Health and fitness professionals should explain the procedure for each test and ensure that the client is comfortable with the proposed measurement sites.
- Each measurement must be performed using precise landmarks and other standardized procedures.

## VIGNETTE continued

■ According to Suzanne's DEXA scan, her %BF is 32.1, which places her in the obese category. While difficult for Suzanne to accept, she admits that her poor nutrition habits and lack of physical activity have no doubt contributed to her current state of body composition and type 2 diabetes.

Experiences like Suzanne's are somewhat common among women who do not gain significant amounts of weight and who maintain the same size of clothing throughout their adult lives. Unfortunately, because of Suzanne's lack of exercise, she has relatively little FFM, which translates to lower muscle mass and potentially lower BMD compared with physically active women her age. As her body composition continued to change with advancing age, her body weight stayed relatively stable as FFM was replaced with FM, which is less dense, and therefore actually weighs less than FFM.

- Apply the appropriate population-specific or generalized equation to determine either body density or %BF.
- Health and fitness professionals should record values on the testing form, and evaluate and classify the client's measurements using normative data specific to the client's age, sex, ethnicity, and so on.
- Health and fitness professionals should discuss health and fitness concerns related to abnormal readings and educate clients on strategies to reduce personal risk and improve overall health.

### Bioelectrical Impedance Analysis

Based on a two-component body composition model, BIA measures the impedance or resistance to an electrical current as it travels through the body's water pool. An individual's TBW contains electrolytes (e.g., sodium and potassium), which are excellent conductors of electricity. Thus, when the volume of TBW is large, the electrical current flows more easily through the body with less resistance.[60] An estimate of TBW is acquired in the BIA process from which total body FFM

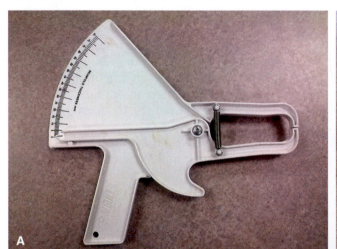
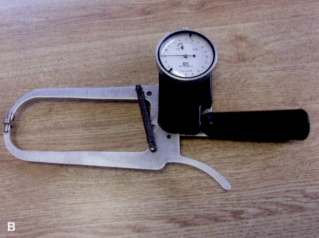
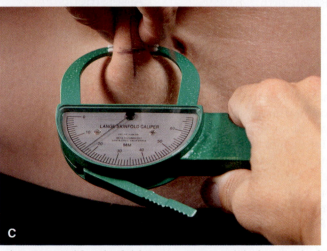

**Figure 23-6.** Common calipers that are used for skinfold measurements: (A) Slim Guide, (B) Harpenden, and (C) Lange.

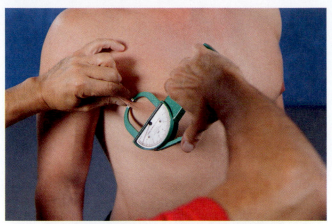

**Figure 23-7.** Demonstration of the chest skinfold measurement for male individuals. Locate the site midway between the anterior axillary line and the nipple. Grasp a diagonal fold and pull it away from the muscle.

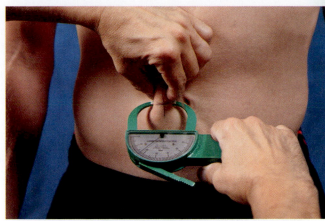

**Figure 23-9.** Demonstration of the abdominal skinfold measurement for male individuals. Grasp a vertical skinfold 1 inch to the right of the umbilicus.

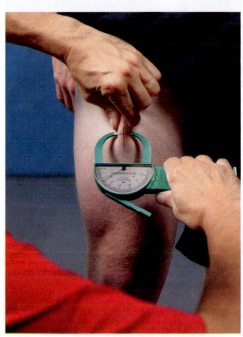

**Figure 23-8.** Demonstration of the thigh skinfold measurement for male individuals. Locate the inguinal fold of the hip with the hip flexed, and the superior border (top) of the patella, and find the midpoint on the top of the thigh. Grasp a vertical skinfold and pull it away from the muscle.

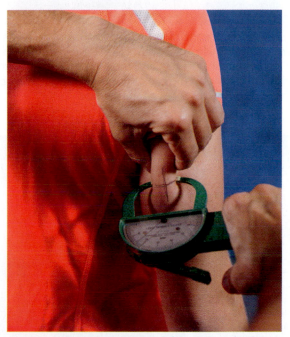

**Figure 23-10.** Demonstration of the triceps skinfold measurement for female individuals. Locate the site midway between the acromial and olecranon processes. Grasp a vertical fold on the posterior midline and pull it away from the muscle.

is calculated using the assumption that 73% of the body's FFM is water.[61] In one version, an imperceptible electrical current is passed through two pairs of electrodes, which are placed on one hand and one foot. In another technique, body weight is also measured while the individual is standing on a leg-to-leg pressure contact device,[62] which looks similar to a digital body-weight scale (Fig. 23-13).

BIA is based on the principle that the conductivity of an electrical impulse is greater through lean tissue, which contains water, than through fatty tissue. That is, individuals with a large amount of FFM and TBW have less resistance to an electrical current flowing

through their bodies compared with those with a smaller FFM. The analyzer, essentially an ohmmeter and a computer, measures the body's resistance to electrical current flow and computes body density and %BF.

The advantages of BIA include its portability, ease of use, and safety—although BIA is not recommended for individuals with a pacemaker. These advantages make it attractive for use in large-scale studies, but the application of the analysis can be problematic because of findings regarding relatively large intraindividual variability. The validity of BIA is influenced by hydration status, skin/room temperature, sex, age, disease state (e.g., HIV and conditions of water imbalance),

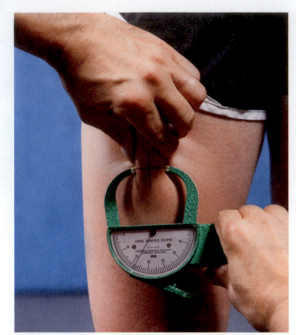

**Figure 23-11.** Demonstration of the thigh skinfold measurement for female individuals. Locate the inguinal fold of the hip with the hip flexed, and the top of the patella, and find the midpoint on the top of the thigh. Grasp a vertical skinfold and pull it away from the muscle.

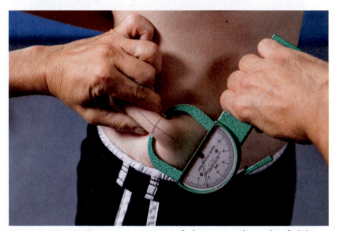

**Figure 23-12.** Demonstration of the suprailiac skinfold measurement for female individuals. Grasp a diagonal skinfold just above the iliac crest and equal with the anterior axillary line.

and ethnicity (e.g., prediction equations have been developed for non-Hispanic whites, non-Hispanic blacks, and Mexican American male and female individuals from 12 to 90 years of age).[63,64] Validity is also affected by level of fatness, because TBW and relative extracellular water are greater in obese individuals compared with normal-weight individuals.[65] Thus, the available BIA prediction equations are not necessarily applicable to overweight or obese children or adults.

Because BIA is essentially an assessment of TBW, individual elements that influence a person's whole-body resistance due to factors that alter hydration can also be a source of error (Table 23-7). In fact, between 3.1% and

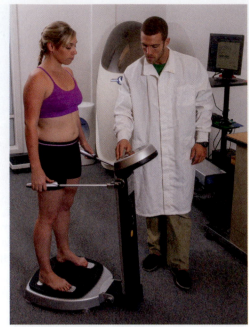

**Figure 23-13.** Example of a bioelectrical impedance analysis (BIA) machine used to measure %BF. BIA devices can conduct electrical current through the entire body from hand to foot, through the lower body from one foot to the other, or in the upper body from hand to hand.

3.9% of the variance in resistance may be attributed to daily fluctuations in TBW.[66]

To obtain the best possible BIA result, clients should adhere to the following guidelines[28]:
- No eating or drinking within 4 hours of the test.
- No exercise within 12 hours of the test.
- Urinate within 30 minutes of the test.
- No alcohol consumption within 48 hours of the test.
- No diuretic medications within 7 days of the test.
- No testing of female clients who perceive that they are retaining water because of a phase in their menstrual cycle.

## In Your Own Words

After meeting your client for the first time, it is agreed that you will assess her body composition using the BIA device available in the fitness facility when you meet with her next week. A day later, you see your new client after she finishes taking a 60-minute high-intensity indoor cycling class. She asks you if you could assess her body composition now, before she leaves the gym for the day. How would you respond to this client?

## Hydrostatic Weighing

Hydrostatic weighing, also called *hydrodensitometry* and *underwater weighing*, is considered the benchmark for computing body composition. This technique estimates

### Table 23-7. Individual Factors That Influence Whole-Body Hydration in BIA

| FACTOR | EFFECT ON BIA | CAUSE OF ERROR |
|---|---|---|
| Eating (2–4 hours before analysis) | Overestimates FFM | Decreases resistance of electrical current |
| Dehydrating practices (e.g., intentionally or unintentionally consuming an inadequate volume of fluids) | Underestimates FFM | Increases resistance of electrical current |
| Exercising (70% $\dot{V}O_2$max for 90–120 minutes) | Overestimates FFM | Losses in sweat and expired air during exercise decreases TBW (compared with relative loss of electrolytes) and increases the concentration of electrolytes, thereby decreasing resistance of electrical current |

BIA, bioelectrical impedance analysis; FFM, fat-free mass; TBW, total body water; $\dot{V}O_2$max, maximal oxygen consumption.
*Source:* Heyward and Wagner.[28]

body composition using measures of body weight, body volume, and residual lung volume. Historically, body density was converted to the percentage of body weight as FM using the two-compartment models of Siri[1] or Brozek et al.[2] More recently, a multicompartment model—combining body density with measures of bone density and TBW to calculate body fatness—has been used to calculate body fatness with hydrodensitometry.[67] Because multicompartment models take into account more individual factors, they are more accurate than two-compartment models.[68]

Because the hydrodensitometry margin of error is so low (there is only a 1.5%–2.0% margin of error when compared with cadaver assessments),[69] it is considered the gold standard of body composition estimation. Most of the other methods of computing body composition are based on formulas derived from underwater weighing research. The concept behind hydrostatic weighing is based on the Archimedes principle, which states that the upward buoyant force exerted on a body immersed in fluid is equal to the weight of the fluid the body displaces. This is measured by the amount body weight changes between on land and in the water, which gives the body volume of the object. Taking into account the weight or mass on land, we can then calculate body density: Density = mass/volume.

This technique measures the amount of water displaced when a person was completely submerged (Fig. 23-14) and exhaled all available air from the lungs (leaving only the residual volume [RV] and a small volume of air in the gastrointestinal tract). Fat tissue is less dense than lean tissue and displaces more water despite weighing less. The body is weighed on an underwater scale. As water buoyancy (i.e., the counterforce of water) reduces body weight significantly, and air and FM increase buoyancy, their respective contributions to underwater weight have to be determined. The RV should be measured in water to minimize error with

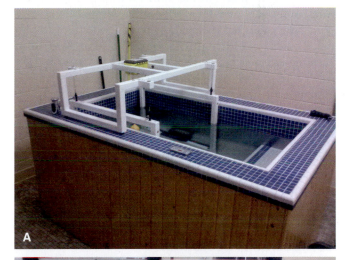

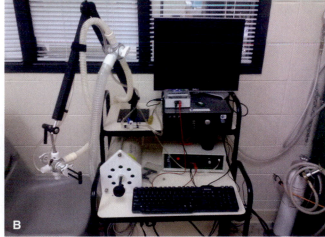

**Figure 23-14.** Main equipment needed to determine %BF through hydrodensitometry: (A) an underwater weighing tank with scale and (B) a machine to measure RV. If the subject performs the test appropriately and an accurate RV is obtained, hydrostatic weighing can estimate %BF for a client within 1% to 2% of the actual value. (Photos courtesy of Jeff Janot.)

this protocol. This volume can be 100 to 200 mL lower underwater because of the noncompressible nature of water that helps compact the lungs.

Given the costs, equipment, and expertise needed to accurately measure RV, mathematical calculations are often used to estimate RV, which may introduce a margin of error of 300 to 400 mL. For every 100-mL error in estimation of RV, the percent body fat error changes by approximately 0.7%.

Hydrodensitometry is highly dependent on subject performance, because many people feel uncomfortable remaining submerged underwater after they have exhaled all available air from their lungs. This is especially problematic in children or obese clients because it is difficult, if not impossible, for them to submerge completely underwater. In some cases, weight belts can be used to reduce buoyancy, but they cannot compensate for all aspects of performance problems.[69] A modified underwater-weighing procedure can be used to address problems of performance and/or the anxiety associated with the full-head submersion method. In this technique, subjects sit with the water level just below the chin. The modified method produces body density values that are nearly identical to the standard, full-head submersion procedure.[70] The modification can be useful for younger or older subjects, the infirm, handicapped, or other special populations.

Hydrostatic weighing is not a practical approach for the standard fitness environment. The apparatus is expensive, takes up a lot of room, and testing takes a considerable amount of time and expertise. This evaluation tool is often found in elite clinical settings and in many colleges and universities.

## Other Methods of Body-Composition Assessment

The science of body-composition assessment is a relatively young discipline, but it is evolving rapidly because of the use of advanced technologies, such as DEXA, air displacement plethysmography (ADP), and near-infrared interactance (NIR).

### Dual Energy X-ray Absorptiometry

A relatively new technology that has been found to be very accurate and precise (an error rate of less than 1.5%), DEXA is based on a three-compartment model that divides the body into three components—bone mineral, bone-free FFM, and FM. DEXA is so effective at assessing bone mineral content, it is the gold standard technique for the diagnosis of osteopenia and osteoporosis.

This technique is based on the assumption that bone mineral content is directly proportional to the amount of photon energy (radiation) absorbed by the bone being studied. DEXA uses a whole-body scanner that has two low-dose x-rays at different sources that read bone and soft tissue mass simultaneously. The radiation exposure from a whole-body DEXA scan ranges from 0.04 to 0.86 millirems (a measurement of radiation exposure), which is equivalent to between 1% and 10% of a chest radiograph.[61] The x-ray sources are mounted beneath a table with a detector overhead (Fig. 23-15). The scanner passes across a person's reclining body with data collected at 0.5-cm intervals. A typical whole-body DEXA scan takes between 10 and 20 minutes, depending on the specific type of scanner used.

DEXA has become the benchmark for body composition assessment techniques, because it has a higher degree of precision, while only involving one measurement, and has the ability to identify exactly where fat is distributed throughout the body (i.e., regional body-fat distribution), which is useful in cases where subjects have compromised nutrition status in disease states and growth disorders. In fact, most clinical studies use DEXA to evaluate the accuracy of other body-composition assessment techniques. This technique is safe and non-invasive, with little inconvenience to the individual (e.g., a person is not required to disrobe or monitor food or fluid consumption).

## FROM THEORY TO PRACTICE

### ■ BODY-COMPOSITION ASSESSMENTS FOR MORBIDLY OBESE CLIENTS

Body-composition assessment equipment and the associated prediction equations are limited in terms of use with severely obese clients. In addition, issues such as self-esteem and body image play a role in deciding when, if, and how to assess body composition in this population. In some situations, it is not practical or possible to assess body composition in severely obese clients. Alternatives to body-composition assessment include weight and circumference measurements. Before deciding on an assessment method, health and fitness professionals must ensure that published prediction equations are available, and that the equipment selected has been validated for use with a particular client.

BIA would seem like a good choice to use with obese clients, but most of the research published using BIA with this population tends to underestimate %BF. Carella and colleagues[71] measured body composition using BIA and hydrostatic weighing in obese patients who were enrolled in a weight-loss study and found that BIA tended to overestimate FFM (i.e., underestimate %BF) relative to hydrostatic weighing. In many cases, an accurate measurement of body composition is not needed, nor a priority, in severely obese clients.

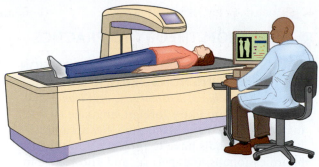

**Figure 23-15.** Dual-energy X-ray absorptiometry (DEXA) device for evaluating body composition. DEXA is the gold standard measure for evaluating bone density and content in the clinical setting. DEXA is also gaining increasing popularity in body composition research as the standard against which other methods are validated.

Disadvantages of DEXA include a small amount of radiation and the inability of the scanning bed to accommodate very large persons. For example, most obese adults and many obese children are often too wide, too thick, and too heavy to receive a whole-body DEXA scan.[72] DEXA estimates of FM are influenced by trunk thickness, with the error increasing as the individual's trunk thickness increases.[61]

In general, evidence suggests that DEXA is a very reliable and useful tool for measuring body-fat levels.[61,69] Although specific models have been tested and found to have certain biases that may overestimate FFM,[73] DEXA is a convenient method for measuring body composition in much of the population.[69] Given its successful application in clinical settings and the increased awareness of the inherent dangers of excess body fat, the use of DEXA in practical settings will undoubtedly become more commonplace in the near future.

## Air Displacement Plethysmography

ADP is a relatively new, noninvasive, and rapid way to assess body composition that predicts %BF within 1% to 3% of hydrostatic weighing results.[74] ADP is an alternative to the underwater weighing method—requiring no water submersion—and is better tolerated by individuals. ADP equipment, such as the BOD POD (COSMED, Rome, Italy), uses whole-body air displacement instead of water to measure body volume, and hence FM (Fig. 23-16). The BOD POD determines body volume by measuring the volume of air in the chamber while empty and then with a person inside.

In adults, high reliability has been reported for %BF and body density using the BOD POD.[75,76] ADP is considered a valid measurement technique in healthy older adults, although there is a tendency for an overestimation of FM by ADP compared with DEXA and a four-component model.[77] In infants younger than 6 months of age, body volume, and therefore FM, can be accurately acquired using the PEA POD (COSMED, Rome, Italy).[78] The principles of measurement of the PEA POD are similar to the BOD POD. Again, the

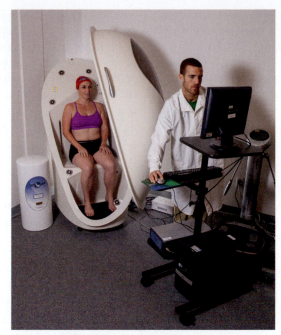

**Figure 23-16.** BOD POD air displacement plethysmography device. This method measures body volume much like the hydrostatic weighing technique, but instead of using water displacement theory, this machine uses air displacement to determine the body volume of the client. Generally, this method is a much more comfortable option for the client to perform compared with hydrostatic weighing.

advantages of using ADP methods include that they are noninvasive, fast, and carry no radiation exposure.

## Near-Infrared Interactance

NIR technology was developed by the U.S. Department of Agriculture to measure the amount of fat contained in beef and pork carcasses following slaughter. NIR uses a small probe that emits an infrared light through the skin, fat, and lean tissues, and then records their optical densities (changes in color and tone) as the light is reflected off bone and back to the probe.

NIR equipment that has been adapted for use with humans, such as the Futrex NIR model, is able to predict %BF based on the premise that optical densities of FM and FFM are proportional to the amount of subcutaneous fat. By comparing known optical density values for FM and FFM with the measured optical densities in subjects, one can estimate the amount of subcutaneous fat at the measured site. Most NIR equipment uses the anterior aspect of the biceps as the common NIR measurement site. Once the test is finished, NIR data are entered into a prediction equation based on the person's height, weight, frame size, and level of activity to estimate %BF.

Although NIR is an inexpensive and rapid way to measure %BF in humans, there has been significant debate over its reliability and validity.[28,79,80] Factors such as probe pressure, skin color, and hydration status can affect results. Numerous studies using NIR produced mixed results. Mclean and Skinner[81] found that skinfolds more accurately predicted body fat than NIR when underwater weighing was used as the criterion measure. When using NIR to estimate body composition, it is critical that an experienced technician who follows the manufacturer's recommended procedures perform the test. At best, NIR is a rough estimate of %BF, with an inherently high error rate.

## CALCULATING IDEAL BODY WEIGHT

Determination of body composition is essential for an allied health or fitness professional who is designing a personalized exercise program, especially if the primary goal is either weight loss or weight gain. Body composition values can also be used to determine a goal weight. This calculation is based on the assumption that throughout the fitness program, FFM will not change. Notably, with any weight loss or gain, there is typically a change in the amount of both FFM and FM.

## FOLLOW-UP ASSESSMENTS

During subsequent reassessments, body composition will likely change because of a loss of body fat and an increase in lean tissue. Between measurements, a client may notice changes in the way his or her clothes fit. These subjective observations will be motivating to the client. Objective reassessments of body composition will be especially important for a client who has not

### DOING THE MATH
**Calculating Desired Body Weight**

Desired body weight =
(FFM/[100% – desired % fat]) × 100

*Sample goal weight calculation*
To determine a goal weight based on body composition, a few simple calculations are necessary.
　　Starting information: Female client's current weight is 168 pounds, with 28% body fat
　　Initial goal: To achieve 24% body fat without losing lean tissue
* *Determine FM in pounds.*

　　Body weight × BF%: 168 lb × 28% = 47 lb fat

* *Determine FFM.*

　　Total weight – FM: 168 lb – 47 lb = 121 lb FFM

* *Calculate goal weight.*

　　Divide current FFM by 76% (100% – goal BF%): 121/0.76 = 159 lb

## FROM THEORY TO PRACTICE

### ■ DISCUSSING BODY COMPOSITION USING NONSCIENTIFIC LANGUAGE

Terms such as *mass, densitometry*, and *lean body tissue* may sound like a foreign language to many people. At the same time, health and fitness professionals have to project a strong sense of professionalism, expertise, and knowledge in what they say and do to attract and keep good clients. The key is in learning how to communicate with clients based on their education levels, fitness knowledge, and previous exercise experiences. A good rule is to assume that new clients have little, if any, fitness and exercise background, and proceed from there.

　　Before defining body composition, make certain that clients understand that weight scales, height–weight charts, and BMI charts only consider total body weight, or total body weight in proportion to height, to indicate if individuals are of ideal weight, overweight, or obese. Anyone trying to lose weight needs to understand that he or she is really trying to lose fat, not necessarily weight. Charts are not a good indication of ideal body weight for general health or for athletic performance. During a weight-loss program combining diet and exercise, there are going to be times when the rate or amount of weight loss slows, stops, or even reverses, and yet individuals can still be losing fat and gaining FFM. The only way to know for sure is through periodic body-composition assessments.

　　There are several ways to define body composition using nonscientific language. Clients should continually be reeducated about exercise science principles and terminology as they become more comfortable and experienced with their training. Using the classic two-component model, body composition is defined as the ratio of FM or FFM to total body mass. Lean body mass is sometimes used in place of FFM. Both versions are correct, with the only difference being that lean body mass includes a small amount of essential lipids, whereas FFM does not.

　　The following examples are ways to explain body composition in lay terms:
* "Body-composition testing measures how much body fat you have in proportion to the weight of your muscles, bones, and other tissues."
* "Body-composition testing is an estimate of the percentage of your weight that is fat, compared with 'fat-free' weight, which makes up muscles, bones, and organs."

noticed any significant change on the bathroom scale. Clients may need to be reminded that as lean mass increases and body fat decreases, the scale cannot differentiate between the two.

Assessing body composition on a frequent basis does not necessarily improve accuracy, and it may cause more apprehension than motivation once people figure out that changes in body composition occur slowly. There are no definitive guidelines on how often body composition should be performed in a given population, because there are simply too many variables to consider.

Practically speaking, there is little value in having it performed more frequently than monthly. For most people, two or three times a year should be adequate. Body composition may need to be assessed on a more frequent basis with a client who has a chronic disease or an eating disorder. In such cases, monitoring weight and lean body mass is essential to the medical therapy and treatment goals.

## VIGNETTE conclusion

■ Armed with the knowledge of her high %BF, Suzanne hires a personal trainer to help her improve her body composition. This included a focused program of cardiorespiratory endurance exercise to expend calories and lose excess body fat, and resistance training to improve, or at least maintain, muscle mass and BMD. Both of these types of exercise will also facilitate Suzanne in her goal to combat her type 2 diabetes and eventually reduce or eliminate her need for prescribed medications (based on her physician's evaluation and recommendations).

After 3 months of training, Suzanne has lost a few pounds of body weight and decreased her body fat by 3%. She is looking forward to further reductions. She reports that she feels stronger and has more energy, and her doctor confirms that she is on the right track for controlling her type 2 diabetes without the use of medications.

Suzanne is an example of an individual who is of normal weight, but who is also obese. For reasons such as this, it is important to confirm measures of height and weight against body-composition assessment values so that a determination can be made about a person's FM versus FFM. Tracking body-composition values throughout the course of a physical-activity or weight-management program provides a clearer explanation of the changes that might be occurring on the scale.

## CRITICAL THINKING QUESTIONS

1. Your new client, Mr. Jones, is ready for his physical-fitness assessment, which includes an estimation of his body composition. Upon first sight, it is evident that Mr. Jones is very obese. How should you handle this situation with Mr. Jones?

2. What are some of the reasons that estimating an individual's body composition using the two-component model might result in error?

3. How does body composition affect performance in sports or other physical activities?

## ADDITIONAL RESOURCES

Online BMI calculators are available where an individual can simply key in his or her height and weight and be given the BMI: http://acefitness.org/calculators and http://apps.nccd.cdc.gov/dnpabmi/Calculator.aspx

American College of Sports Medicine. *ACSM's Guidelines for Exercise Testing and Prescription.* 9th ed. Philadelphia, PA: Wolters Kluwer/Lippincott Williams & Wilkins; 2014.

American College of Sports Medicine. Position Stand: The female athlete triad. *Med Sci Sports Exerc.* 2007;39:1867–1882. Available at: http://journals.lww.com/acsm-msse/Fulltext/2007/10000/The_Female_Athlete_Triad.26.aspx

Heyward VH, Wagner DR. *Applied Body Composition Assessment.* 2nd ed. Champaign, IL: Human Kinetics; 2004.

Jackson AS, Pollock ML. Practical assessment of body composition. *Physician Sportsmed.* 1985;13:76–90.

National Heart, Lung and Blood Institute; Obesity Education Initiative Expert Panel. *Clinical Guidelines on the Identification, Evaluation, and Treatment of Overweight and Obesity in Adults: The Evidence Report* [NIH Publication No. 98-4083]. Bethesda, MD: National Institutes of Health; 1998.

The Female Athlete Triad Coalition: http://femaleathlete-triad.org

## REFERENCES

1. Siri WE. Body composition from fluid spaces and density. In: Brozek J, Henschel A, eds. *Techniques for Measuring Body Composition.* Washington, DC: National Academy of Sciences; 1961.
2. Brozek J, Grande F, Anderson J, Keys A. Densitometric analysis of body composition: Revision of some quantitative assumptions. *Ann N Y Acad Sci.* 1963; 110:113–140.
3. Friedl KE, DeLuca JP, Marchitelli LJ, Vogel JA. Reliability of body-fat estimates from a four-component model by using density, body water, and bone mineral measurements. *Am J Clin Nutr.* 1992;55:764–770.
4. Fuller NJ, Jebb SA, Laskey MA, Coward WA, Ellis M. Four-compartment model for the assessment of body composition in humans: Comparison with alternative methods and evaluation of the density and hydration of fat-free mass. *Clin Sci.* 1992;82:687–693.
5. Baumgartner RN, Heymsfield SB, Lichtman S, Wang J, Pierson RN. Body composition in elderly people: Effect of criterion estimates on predictive equations. *Am J Clin Nutr.* 1991;53:1345–1353.
6. Wang J, Heymsfield S, Aulet M, Thornton J, Pierson R. Body fat from body density: Underwater weighing vs. dual-photon absorptiometry. *Am J Physiol.* 1989; 256:E829–E834.
7. Williams DP, Going SB, Massett MP, Lohman TG, Bare LA, Hewitt MJ. Aqueous and mineral fractions of the fat-free body and their relation to body fat estimates in men and women aged 49–82 years. In: Ellis KJ, Eastman JD, eds. *Human Body Composition: In Vivo Methods, Models, and Assessment.* New York: Plenum; 1993:109–113.
8. Cote K, Adams WC. Effect of bone density on body composition estimates in young adult black and white women. *Med Sci Sports Exerc.* 1993;25:290–296.
9. Ortiz O, Russell M, Daley TL, et al. Differences in skeletal muscle and bone mineral mass between black and white females and their relevance to estimates of body composition. *Am J Clin Nutr.* 1992;55:8–13.
10. Schutte JE, Townsend EJ, Hugg J, Shoup RF, Malina RM, Blomqvist CG. Density of lean body mass is greater in blacks than in whites. *J Appl Physiol.* 1984;56:1647–1649.
11. Lohman TG. Applicability of body composition techniques and constants for children and youth. In Pandolf KB, ed. *Exercise and Sport Sciences Reviews.* New York: Macmillan; 1986:325–357.
12. Heymsfield SB, Wang J, Lichtman S, Kamen Y, Kehayias J, Pierson RN. Body composition in elderly subjects: A critical appraisal of clinical methodology. *Am J Clin Nutr.* 1989;50:1167–1175.
13. Slaughter MH, Lohman TG, Boileau RA, et al. Skinfold equations for estimation of body fatness in children and youth. *Hum Biol.* 1988;60:709–723.
14. Jackson AS, Pollock ML, Ward A. Generalized equations for predicting body density of women. *Med Sci Sports Exerc.* 1980;12:175–182.
15. Jackson AS, Pollock ML. Practical assessment of body composition. *Physician Sportsmed.* 1985;13:76–90.
16. Ramachandrappa S, Farooqi IS. Genetic approaches to understanding human obesity. *J Clin Invest.* 2011; 121:2080–2086.
17. Lohman TG. Advances in body composition assessment. *Current Issues in Exercise Science Series.* Monograph No. 3. Champaign, IL: Human Kinetics; 1992.
18. Singhal A, Wells J, Cole TJ, Fewtrell M, Lucas A. Programming of lean body mass: A link between birth weight, obesity, and cardiovascular disease? *Am J Clin Nutr.* 2003;77:726–730.
19. Lohman TG, Boileau RA, Slaughter MH. Body composition in children and youth. In Boileau RA, ed. *Advances in Pediatric Sport Sciences.* Champaign, IL: Human Kinetics; 1984:22–26.
20. Kuczmarski RJ. Need for body composition information in elderly subjects. *Am J Clin Nutr.* 1989;50: 1150–1157.
21. Chumlea WC, Baumgautner RN. Status of anthropometry and body composition data in elderly subjects. *Am J Clin Nutr.* 1989;50:1158–1166.
22. Kuk J, Saunders T, Davidson L, Ross R. Age-related changes in total and regional fat distribution. *Ageing Res Rev.* 2009;8:339–348.
23. Lang T, Cauley JA, Tylavsky F, Bauer D, Cummings S, Harris TB. Computed tomographic measurements of thigh muscle cross-sectional area and attenuation coefficient predict hip fracture: The health, aging, and body composition study. *J Bone Miner Res.* 2010;25:513–519.
24. Katch FI, Katch VL. The body composition profile: Techniques of measurement and application. *Clin Sports Med.* 1984;3:31–63.
25. Janssen I, Katzmarzyk PT, Ross R. Waist circumference and not body mass index explains obesity-related health risk. *Am J Clin Nutr.* 2004;79:379–384.
26. Tuck SP, Pearce MS, Rawlings DJ, Birrell FN, Parker L, Francis RM. Differences in bone mineral density and geometry in men and women: The Newcastle Thousand Families Study at 50 years old. *Br J Radiol.* 2005;78:493–498.
27. Eurich AD, Brown LE, Coburn JW, et al. (2010). Performance differences between sexes in the pop-up phase of surfing. *J Strength Cond Res.* 2010;24: 2821–2825.
28. Heyward VH, Wagner DR. *Applied Body Composition Assessment.* 2nd ed. Champaign, IL: Human Kinetics; 2004.
29. Centers for Disease Control and Prevention. *Early release of selected estimates based on data from the January–September 2011 National Health Interview Survey.* March 21, 2012. Available at: http://cdc.gov/nchs/nhis/released201203.htm#11.
30. Hagiwara S, Miki T, Nishizawa Y, Ochi H, Onoyama Y, Morri H. Quantification of bone mineral content using dual-photon absorptiometry in a normal Japanese population. *J Bone Miner Res.* 1989;4:17–22.
31. Sugimoto T, Tsutsumi M, Fujji Y, et al. Comparison of bone mineral content among Japanese, Koreans, and Taiwanese assessed by dual-photon absorptiometry. *J Bone Miner Res.* 1992;7:153–159.
32. Tsai KS, Huang KM, Chieng PU, Su CT. Bone mineral density of normal Chinese women in Taiwan. *Calcified Tissue Res.* 1991;48:161–166.
33. Cohn SH, Abesamis C, Zanzi I, et al. Body elemental composition: Comparison between black and white adults. *Am J Physiol.* 1988;234:E419–E422.
34. Nelson DA, Feingold M, Bolin F, Parfitt AM. Principal components analysis of regional bone density in black and white women: Relationship to body size and composition. *Am J Phys Anthropol.* 1991;86:507–514.
35. Kuczmarski RJ. Prevalence of overweight and weight gain in the United States. *Am J Clin Nutr.* 1992; 55:S495–S502.
36. Bosy-Westphal A, Mast M, Eichhorn C, et al. Validation of air-displacement plethysmography for estimation of body fat mass in healthy elderly subjects. *Eur J Nutr.* 2003;42:207–216.
37. Wilmore JH. Body composition in sport and exercise: Directions for future research. *Med Sci Sports Exerc.* 1983;15:21–31.

38. Kallings LV, Johnson JS, Fisher RM, et al. Beneficial effects of individualized physical activity on prescription on body composition and cardiometabolic risk factors: Results from a randomized controlled trial. *Eur J Cardiovasc Prev Rehabil.* 2009;16:80–84.

39. Beck BR, Snow CM. Bone health across the lifespan—exercising our options. *Exerc Sports Sci Rev.* 2003;31:117–122.

40. Aloia JF, Cohn SH, Babu T, et al. Skeletal mass and body composition in marathon runners. *Metabolism.* 1978;12:1793–1796.

41. Nilsson BE, Westlin NE. Bone density in athletes. *Clin Orthop.* 1971;77:179–182.

42. Creighton DL, Morgan AL, Boardley D, Brolinson PG. Weight-bearing exercise and markers of bone turnover in female athletes. *J Appl Physiol.* 2001;90:565–570.

43. Barry DW, Kohrt WM. Exercise and the preservation of bone health. *J Cardiopulm Rehabil Prev.* 2008; 28:153–162.

44. Bea JW, Lohman TG, Cussler EC, Going SB, Thompson PA. Lifestyle modifies the relationship between body composition and adrenergic receptor genetic polymorphisms, ADRB2, ADRB3 and ADRA2B: A secondary analysis of a randomized controlled trial of physical activity among postmenopausal women. *Behav Genet.* 2010;40: 649–659.

45. Kohrt WM, Bloomfield SA, Little KD, Nelson ME, Yingling VR; American College of Sports Medicine. American College of Sports Medicine Position Stand: Physical activity and bone health. *Med Sci Sports Exerc.* 2004;36:1985–1996.

46. Morseth B, Emaus N, Lone Jørgensen L. Physical activity and bone: The importance of the various mechanical stimuli for bone mineral density. A review. *Nor J Epidemiol.* 2011;20:173–178.

47. Sanborn CF, Wagner WW. Response to Nelson and Evans. *Med Sci Sports Exerc.* 1987;19:621–622.

48. Arasheben A, Barzee KA, Morley CP. A meta-analysis of bone mineral density in collegiate female athletes. *J Am Board Fam Med.* 2011;24:728–734.

49. Wolf AM. Economic outcomes of the obese patient. *Obes Res.* 2002;10:S58–S62.

50. Lohman TG, Pollock ML, Slaughter MH, Brandon LJ, Boileau RA. Methodological factors and the prediction of body fat in female athletes. *Med Sci Sports Exerc.* 1984;16:92–96.

51. Frisch RE, Wyshak G, Vincent L. Delayed menarche and amenorrhea in ballet dancers. *N Engl J Med.* 1980;303:17–19.

52. Frisch RE, Wyshak G, Albright NL, et al. Lower lifetime occurrence of breast cancer and cancers of the reproductive system among former college athletes. *Am J Clin Nutr.* 1987;45:328–335.

53. American College of Sports Medicine. Position Stand: The female athlete triad. *Med Sci Sports Exerc.* 2007; 39:1867–1882.

54. Metropolitan Life Insurance Company. New weight standards for men and women. *Stat Bull Metropolitan Life Insurance Co.* 1959;40:1–4.

55. Metropolitan Life Insurance Company. 1983 Metropolitan height and weight tables. *Stat Bull Metropolitan Life Insurance Co.* 1983;64:1–19.

56. Chobanian AV. *JNC 7 Express: The Seventh Report of the Joint National Committee on Prevention, Detection, Evaluation, and Treatment of High Blood Pressure* [NIH Publication No. 03-5233]. Washington, DC: National Institutes of Health and National Heart, Lung, and Blood Institute; 2003.

57. Janssen I, Heymsfield SB, Wang Z, Ross R. Skeletal muscle mass and distribution in 468 men and women aged 18–88 years. *J Appl Physiol.* 2000;89:81–88.

58. Lohman TG. Assessment of body composition in children. *Pediatr Exerc Sci.* 1989;1:19–30.

59. American College of Sports Medicine. *ACSM's Guidelines for Exercise Testing and Prescription.* 8th ed. Philadelphia, PA: Wolters Kluwer/Lippincott Williams & Wilkins; 2010.

60. Thomasett A. Bioelectrical properties of tissue impedance measurements. *Lyon Med.* 1962;207:107–118.

61. Lee SY, Gallagher D. Assessment methods in human body composition. *Curr Opin Clin Nutr Metab Care.* 2008;11:566–572.

62. Nunez C, Gallagher D, Visser M, et al. Bioimpedance analysis: Evaluation of leg-to-leg system based on pressure contact footpad electrodes. *Med Sci Sports Exerc.* 1997;29:524–531.

63. Chumlea WC, Guo SS, Kuczmarski RJ, et al. Body composition estimates from NHANES III bioelectrical impedance data. *Int J Obes Relat Metab Disord.* 2002;26:1596–1609.

64. Rush EC, Chandu V, Plank LD. Prediction of fat-free mass by bioelectrical impedance analysis in migrant Asian Indian men and women: A cross validation study. *Int J Obes.* 2006;30:1125–1131.

65. Pateyjohns IR, Brinkworth GD, Buckley JD, et al. Comparison of three bioelectrical impedance methods with DXA in overweight and obese men. *Obesity.* 2006;14:2064–2070.

66. Jackson AS, Pollock ML, Graves JE, Mahar MT. Reliability and validity of bioelectrical impedance in determining body composition. *J Appl Physiol.* 1988;64:529–534.

67. Guo SS, Chumlea WC, Roche AF, Siervogel RM. Age- and maturity-related changes in body composition during adolescence into adulthood: The Fels Longitudinal Study. *Int J Obes Relat Metab Disord.* 1997;21:1167–1175.

68. Sun SS, Chumlea WC, Heymsfield SB, et al. Development of bioelectrical impedance analysis prediction equations for body composition with the use of a multi-component model for use in epidemiological surveys. *Am J Clin Nutr.* 2003;77:331–340.

69. Duren DL, Sherwood RJ, Czerwinski SA, et al. Body compositions methods: Comparisons and interpretations. *J Diabet Sci Technol.* 2008;2:1139–1146.

70. Donnelly JE, Brown TE, Israel RG, Smith-Sintek S, O'Brien KF, Caslavka B. Hydrostatic weighing without head submersion: Description of a method. *Med Sci Sports Exerc.* 1988;20:66–69.

71. Carella MJ, Rodgers CD, Anderson D, Gossain VV. Serial measurements of body composition in obese subjects during a very-low-energy diet (VLED) comparing bioelectrical impedance with hydrodensitometry. *Obes Res.* 1997;5:250–256.

72. Tataranni PA, Ravussin E. Use of dual-energy X-ray absorptiometry in obese individuals. *Am J Clin Nutr.* 1995;62:730–734.

73. Schoeller DA, Tylavsky FA, Baer DJ, et al. QDR 4500A dual-energy X-ray absorptiometer underestimates fat mass in comparison with criterion methods in adults. *Am J Clin Nutr.* 2005;81:1018–1025.

74. Fields D, Goran M, McCrory M. Body composition assessment via air-displacement plethysmography in adults and children: A review. *Am J Clin Nutr.* 2002;75:453–467.

75. Noreen EE, Lemon PW. Reliability of air displacement plethysmography in a large, heterogeneous sample. *Med Sci Sports Exerc.* 2006;38:1505–1509.

76. Anderson DE. Reliability of air displacement plethysmography. *J Strength Cond Res* 2007;21:169–172.
77. Borud LG, Flegal KM, Looker AC, Everhart JE, Harris TB, Shepherd JA. Body composition data for individuals 8 years of age and older: U.S. population, 1999-2004. *Vital Health Stat.* 2010;250:1–87.
78. Ellis KJ, Yao M, Shypailo RJ, et al. Body composition assessment in infancy: Air-displacement. *Am J Clin Nutr* 2007;85:90–95.
79. Moon JR, Hull HR, Tobkin SE, et al. Percent body fat estimations in college men using field and laboratory methods: A three-compartment model approach. *Dyn Med.* 2008;7:7–15.
80. Moon JR, Hull HR, Tobkin SE, et al. Percent body fat estimations in college women using field and laboratory methods: A three-compartment model approach. *J Int Soc Sports Nutr.* 2007;4:16–23.
81. Mclean KP, Skinner JS. Validity of Futrex-5000 for body composition. *Med Sci Sports Exerc.* 1992;2:253–257.

# *Practice What You Know:* Body-Composition Assessment Techniques

Most adults initiate an exercise program in an attempt to lose weight. Accordingly, it is important to be able to accurately assess a person's body composition to determine a reasonable body-weight goal and to develop a safe and effective exercise program to reach it. An accurate body-composition assessment measures the relative percentages of FFM and FM within a particular individual.

## ANTHROPOMETRIC MEASURES

Anthropometric measures include measurements of height, weight, and/or circumference to assess body size or dimension. They are easy to administer and require minimal equipment. Examples of this approach include:

- Circumference measurements
  - WHR
  - Waist circumference
- Skinfold measurements

Although these measurements demonstrate strong correlations to health, morbidity, and mortality, they provide only estimations of body composition and fitness level.

## CIRCUMFERENCE MEASUREMENTS

When taking circumference measurements, precision is necessary to validate the results. To ensure accuracy, the technician must use exact anatomical landmarks for taking each measurement (see Table 1). In addition, procedures must be followed in accordance with established guidelines:

- When measuring body circumference, it is important to measure precisely and consistently.
- All measurements should be made with a nonelastic, yet flexible tape.
- The tape should be snug against the skin's surface without pressing into the subcutaneous layers. Individuals should wear thin, form-fitting materials that allow for accurate measurements.
- Technicians should rotate through the battery of sites, initially measuring each site only once.
- Duplicate measurements should be taken of each site. If recorded values are not within 5 mm, it is necessary to remeasure.
- Technicians should wait 20 to 30 seconds between measurements to allow the skin and subcutaneous tissue to return to its normal position.

## Table 1. Standardized Description of Circumference Sites and Procedures

| | |
|---|---|
| Abdomen | With the subject standing upright and relaxing, a horizontal measure is taken at the greatest anterior extension of the abdomen, usually at the level of the umbilicus. |
| Arm | With the subject standing erect and arms hanging freely at the sides with hands facing the thighs, a horizontal measure is taken midway between the acromion and olecranon process. |
| Buttocks/hips | With the subject standing erect with the feet together, a horizontal measure is taken at the maximal circumference of the buttocks; this measure is used for the hip measure in a hip–waist measure. |
| Calf | With the subject standing erect (feet apart ~20 cm [8 in.]), a horizontal measure is taken at the level of the maximum circumference between the knee and the ankle, perpendicular to the long axis. |

*Continued*

## *Practice What You Know:* Body-Composition Assessment Techniques–cont'd

### Table 1. Standardized Description of Circumference Sites and Procedures–cont'd

| | |
|---|---|
| Forearm | With the subject standing, arms hanging downward but slightly away from the trunk, and palms facing anteriorly, a measure is taken perpendicular to the long axis at the maximal circumference. |
| Midthigh | With the subject standing with one foot on a bench so the knee is flexed 90 degrees, a measure is taken midway between the inguinal crease and the proximal border of the patella, perpendicular to the long axis. |
| Upper thigh | With the subject standing, legs slightly apart (~10 cm [4 in.]), a horizontal measure is taken at the maximal circumference of the hip/upper thigh, just below the gluteal fold. |
| Waist | With the subject standing, arms at the sides, feet together, and abdomen relaxed, a horizontal measure is taken at the narrowest part of the torso (above the umbilicus and below the xiphoid process). The National Obesity Task Force (NOTF) suggests obtaining a horizontal measure directly above the iliac crest as a method to enhance standardization. Unfortunately, current formulae are not predicated on the site suggested by the NOTF. |

**Procedures**
- All measurements should be made with a flexible yet inelastic tape measure.
- The tape should be placed on the skin surface without compressing the subcutaneous adipose tissue.
- If a Gulink spring-loaded handle is used, the handle should be extended to the same marking with each trial.
- Take duplicate measures at each site, and retest if duplicate measurements are not within 5 mm of each other.
- Rotate through measurement sites or allow time (about 20-30 seconds) for skin to regain normal texture.

Adapted from the American College of Sports Medicine.[59] Modified from Callaway CW, Chumlea, WC, Bouchard, C, et al. Circumferences. In: Lohman TG, Roche AF, Martorell R, eds. *Anthropometric Standardization Reference Manual.* Champaign, IL: Human Kinetics; 1988.

### Body-Composition Equations for Estimating Body Fat Percentage From Circumference Measurements

In situations where other methods of body-composition assessment are either not available or not appropriate (e.g., with severely obese clients), circumference measurements can be used. Following are the equations for men and women.

**Men:**

% BF = 10.8336 + 0.031457 (mean abdomen in cm) – 0.10969 (body weight in kg)

Mean abdomen: Average of the following two measurements:
- The smallest circumference of the waist (natural waist)
- The circumference at the level of the umbilicus
Example: Rick weighs 120 kg and has the following circumference measurements:
- Natural waist: 102 cm
- Umbilicus: 127 cm

## *Practice What You Know:* Body-Composition Assessment Techniques–cont'd

Mean abdomen circumference: (102 cm + 127 cm)/2 = 114.5 cm

Rick's %BF = 10.8336 + 0.031457 (115 cm) − 0.10969 (120 kg) = **27.6**

**Women:**

% BF = 51.03301 + 0.11077 (mean abdomen) − 0.17666 (height in meters) + 0.14354 (body weight in kg)

Mean abdomen: Average of the following two measurements:
• The smallest circumference of the waist (natural waist)
• The circumference at the level of the umbilicus
Example: Joy is 1.37 m tall, weighs 100 kg, and has the following circumference measurements:
• Natural waist: 110 cm
• Umbilicus: 89 cm

Mean abdomen circumference: (110 cm + 89 cm)/2 = 99.5 cm

Joy's %BF = 51.03301 + 0.11077 (100 cm) − 0.17666 (1.37 m) + 0.14354 (100 kg) = **47.5**

### Waist-to-Hip Ratio
To determine a subject's WHR, the waist measurement is divided by the hip measurement. Table 1 describes the waist and hip circumference sites, and Table 2 lists the relative risk ratings for WHRs.

### Waist Circumference
There is a strong correlation between excess abdominal fat and a number of health risks, including type 2 diabetes, hypertension, and hypercholesterolemia. Table 1 describes the waist circumference site, and Table 3 presents the risk categories associated with various waist circumferences for men and women.

### Table 2. Waist-to-Hip Ratio Norms

| SEX | WHR NORMS | | | |
| --- | --- | --- | --- | --- |
| | EXCELLENT | GOOD | AVERAGE | AT RISK |
| Men | <0.85 | 0.85–0.89 | 0.90–0.95 | ≥0.95 |
| Women | <0.75 | 0.75–0.79 | 0.80–0.86 | ≥0.86 |

WHR, waist-to-hip ratio.
Data from Bray GA, Gray DS. Obesity: Part I: Pathogenesis. *Western J Med.* 1988;149:429–441.

### Table 3. Criteria for Waist Circumference in Adults

| RISK CATEGORY | WAIST CIRCUMFERENCE | |
| --- | --- | --- |
| | WOMEN | MEN |
| Very low | <27.5 in. (<70 cm) | <31.5 in. (<80 cm) |
| Low | 27.5–35.0 in. (70–89 cm) | 31.5–39.0 in. (80–99 cm) |
| High | 35.5–43.0 in. (90–109 cm) | 39.5–47.0 in. (100–120 cm) |
| Very high | >43.5 in. (>110 cm) | >47.0 in. (>120 cm) |

*Source:* Bray GA. Don't throw the baby out with the bath water. *Am J Clin Nutr.* 2004;79:347–349.

## *Practice What You Know:* Body-Composition Assessment Techniques–cont'd

### SKINFOLD MEASUREMENTS

For men, the Jackson and Pollock three-site skinfold locations are as follows[15]:

- Chest: a diagonal skinfold taken midway between the anterior axillary line (crease of the underarm) and the nipple
- Thigh: a vertical skinfold taken on the anterior midline of the thigh between the inguinal crease at the hip and the proximal border of the patella
- Abdominal: a vertical skinfold taken 2 cm (~1 in.) to the right of the umbilicus

For women, the Jackson and Pollock three-site skinfold locations are as follows[15]:

- Triceps: a vertical fold on the posterior midline of the upper arm taken halfway between the acromion (shoulder) and olecranon (elbow) processes
- Thigh: a vertical skinfold taken on the anterior midline of the thigh between the inguinal crease at the hip and the proximal border of the patella knee
- Suprailiac: a diagonal fold following the natural line of the iliac crest taken immediately superior to the crest of the ilium and in line with the anterior axillary line

Body composition can be determined by adding the three skinfold measurements and plugging the values into the conversion tables (see Tables 4 and 5), or by calculating body density from which body composition can be computed.[15] It is important to remember that body density should be recorded using five decimal places to ensure accuracy in measurement.

**Table 4.** Percent Body Fat Estimations for Men: Jackson and Pollock Formula

| SUM OF SKINFOLDS (mm) | AGE GROUPS | | | | | | | | |
|---|---|---|---|---|---|---|---|---|---|
| | <22 | 23–27 | 28–32 | 33–37 | 38–42 | 43–47 | 48–52 | 53–57 | >57 |
| 8–10 | 1.3 | 1.8 | 2.3 | 2.9 | 3.4 | 3.9 | 4.5 | 5.0 | 5.5 |
| 11–13 | 2.2 | 2.8 | 3.3 | 3.9 | 4.4 | 4.9 | 5.5 | 6.0 | 6.5 |
| 14–16 | 3.2 | 3.8 | 4.3 | 4.8 | 5.4 | 5.9 | 6.4 | 7.0 | 7.5 |
| 17–19 | 4.2 | 4.7 | 5.3 | 5.8 | 6.3 | 6.9 | 7.4 | 8.0 | 8.5 |
| 20–22 | 5.1 | 5.7 | 6.2 | 6.8 | 7.3 | 7.9 | 8.4 | 8.9 | 9.5 |
| 23–25 | 6.1 | 6.6 | 7.2 | 7.7 | 8.3 | 8.8 | 9.4 | 9.9 | 10.5 |
| 26–28 | 7.0 | 7.6 | 8.1 | 8.7 | 9.2 | 9.8 | 10.3 | 10.9 | 11.4 |
| 29–31 | 8.0 | 8.5 | 9.1 | 9.6 | 10.2 | 10.7 | 11.3 | 11.8 | 12.4 |
| 32–34 | 8.9 | 9.4 | 10.0 | 10.5 | 11.1 | 11.6 | 12.2 | 12.8 | 13.3 |
| 35–37 | 9.8 | 10.4 | 10.9 | 11.5 | 12.0 | 12.6 | 13.1 | 13.7 | 14.3 |
| 38–40 | 10.7 | 11.3 | 11.8 | 12.4 | 12.9 | 13.5 | 14.1 | 14.6 | 15.2 |
| 41–43 | 11.6 | 12.2 | 12.7 | 13.3 | 13.8 | 14.4 | 15.0 | 15.5 | 16.1 |
| 44–46 | 12.5 | 13.1 | 13.6 | 14.2 | 14.7 | 15.3 | 15.9 | 16.4 | 17.0 |
| 47–49 | 13.4 | 13.9 | 14.5 | 15.1 | 15.6 | 16.2 | 16.8 | 17.3 | 17.9 |
| 50–52 | 14.3 | 14.8 | 15.4 | 15.9 | 16.4 | 17.1 | 17.6 | 18.2 | 18.8 |
| 53–55 | 15.1 | 15.7 | 16.2 | 16.8 | 17.4 | 17.9 | 18.5 | 19.1 | 19.7 |
| 56–58 | 16.0 | 16.5 | 17.1 | 17.7 | 18.2 | 18.8 | 19.4 | 20.0 | 20.5 |
| 59–61 | 16.9 | 17.4 | 17.9 | 18.5 | 19.1 | 19.7 | 20.2 | 20.8 | 21.4 |
| 62–64 | 17.6 | 18.2 | 18.8 | 19.4 | 19.9 | 20.5 | 21.1 | 21.7 | 22.2 |
| 65–67 | 18.5 | 19.0 | 19.6 | 20.2 | 20.8 | 21.3 | 21.9 | 22.5 | 23.1 |
| 68–70 | 19.3 | 19.9 | 20.4 | 21.0 | 21.6 | 22.2 | 22.7 | 23.3 | 23.9 |
| 71–73 | 20.1 | 20.7 | 21.2 | 21.8 | 22.4 | 23.0 | 23.6 | 24.1 | 24.7 |
| 74–76 | 20.9 | 21.5 | 22.0 | 22.6 | 23.2 | 23.8 | 24.4 | 25.0 | 25.5 |
| 77–79 | 21.7 | 22.2 | 22.8 | 23.4 | 24.0 | 24.6 | 25.2 | 25.8 | 26.3 |
| 80–82 | 22.4 | 23.0 | 23.6 | 24.2 | 24.8 | 25.4 | 25.9 | 26.5 | 27.1 |

# Practice What You Know: Body-Composition Assessment Techniques–cont'd

## Table 4. Percent Body Fat Estimations for Men: Jackson and Pollock Formula–cont'd

| SUM OF SKINFOLDS (mm) | AGE GROUPS | | | | | | | | |
|---|---|---|---|---|---|---|---|---|---|
| | <22 | 23–27 | 28–32 | 33–37 | 38–42 | 43–47 | 48–52 | 53–57 | >57 |
| 83–85 | 23.2 | 23.8 | 24.4 | 25.0 | 25.5 | 26.1 | 26.7 | 27.3 | 27.9 |
| 86–88 | 24.0 | 24.5 | 25.1 | 25.7 | 26.3 | 26.9 | 27.5 | 28.1 | 28.7 |
| 89–91 | 24.7 | 25.3 | 25.9 | 26.5 | 27.1 | 27.6 | 28.2 | 28.8 | 29.4 |
| 92–94 | 25.4 | 26.0 | 26.6 | 27.2 | 27.8 | 28.4 | 29.0 | 29.6 | 30.2 |
| 95–97 | 26.1 | 26.7 | 27.3 | 27.9 | 28.5 | 29.1 | 29.7 | 30.3 | 30.9 |
| 98–100 | 26.9 | 27.4 | 28.0 | 28.6 | 29.2 | 29.8 | 30.4 | 31.0 | 31.6 |
| 101–103 | 27.5 | 28.1 | 28.7 | 29.3 | 29.9 | 30.5 | 31.1 | 31.7 | 32.3 |
| 104–106 | 28.2 | 28.8 | 29.4 | 30.0 | 30.6 | 31.2 | 31.8 | 32.4 | 33.0 |
| 107–109 | 28.9 | 29.5 | 30.1 | 30.7 | 31.3 | 31.9 | 32.5 | 33.1 | 33.7 |
| 110–112 | 29.6 | 30.2 | 30.8 | 31.4 | 32.0 | 32.6 | 33.2 | 33.8 | 34.4 |
| 113–115 | 30.2 | 30.8 | 31.4 | 32.0 | 32.6 | 33.2 | 33.8 | 34.5 | 35.1 |
| 116–118 | 30.9 | 31.5 | 32.1 | 32.7 | 33.3 | 33.9 | 34.5 | 35.1 | 35.7 |
| 119–121 | 31.5 | 32.1 | 32.7 | 33.3 | 33.9 | 34.5 | 35.1 | 35.7 | 36.4 |
| 122–124 | 32.1 | 32.7 | 33.3 | 33.9 | 34.5 | 35.1 | 35.8 | 36.4 | 37.0 |
| 125–127 | 32.7 | 33.3 | 33.9 | 34.5 | 35.1 | 35.8 | 36.4 | 37.0 | 37.6 |

*Source:* Jackson and Pollock.[15]

## Table 5. Percent Body Fat Estimations for Women: Jackson and Pollock Formula

| SUM OF SKINFOLDS (mm) | AGE GROUPS | | | | | | | | |
|---|---|---|---|---|---|---|---|---|---|
| | 22 | 23–27 | 28–32 | 33–37 | 38–42 | 43–47 | 48–52 | 53–57 | >57 |
| 23–25 | 9.7 | 9.9 | 10.2 | 10.4 | 10.7 | 10.9 | 11.2 | 11.4 | 11.7 |
| 26–28 | 11.0 | 11.2 | 11.5 | 11.7 | 12.0 | 12.3 | 12.5 | 12.7 | 13.0 |
| 29–31 | 12.3 | 12.5 | 12.8 | 13.0 | 13.3 | 13.5 | 13.8 | 14.0 | 14.3 |
| 32–34 | 13.6 | 13.8 | 14.0 | 14.3 | 14.5 | 14.8 | 15.0 | 15.3 | 15.5 |
| 35–37 | 14.8 | 15.0 | 15.3 | 15.5 | 15.8 | 16.0 | 16.3 | 16.5 | 16.8 |
| 38–40 | 16.0 | 16.3 | 16.5 | 16.7 | 17.0 | 17.2 | 17.5 | 17.7 | 18.0 |
| 41–43 | 17.2 | 17.4 | 17.7 | 17.9 | 18.2 | 18.4 | 18.7 | 18.9 | 19.2 |
| 44–46 | 18.3 | 18.6 | 18.8 | 19.1 | 19.3 | 19.6 | 19.8 | 20.1 | 20.3 |
| 47–49 | 19.5 | 19.7 | 20.0 | 20.2 | 20.5 | 20.7 | 21.0 | 21.2 | 21.5 |
| 50–52 | 20.6 | 20.8 | 21.1 | 21.3 | 21.6 | 21.8 | 22.1 | 22.3 | 22.6 |
| 53–55 | 21.7 | 21.9 | 22.1 | 22.4 | 22.6 | 22.9 | 23.1 | 23.4 | 23.6 |
| 56–58 | 22.7 | 23.0 | 23.2 | 23.4 | 23.7 | 23.9 | 24.2 | 24.4 | 24.7 |
| 59–61 | 23.7 | 24.0 | 24.2 | 24.5 | 24.7 | 25.0 | 25.2 | 25.5 | 25.7 |
| 62–64 | 24.7 | 25.0 | 25.2 | 25.5 | 25.7 | 26.0 | 26.7 | 26.4 | 26.7 |
| 65–67 | 25.7 | 25.9 | 26.2 | 26.4 | 26.7 | 26.9 | 27.2 | 27.4 | 27.7 |
| 68–70 | 26.6 | 26.9 | 27.1 | 27.4 | 27.6 | 27.9 | 28.1 | 28.4 | 28.6 |
| 71–73 | 27.5 | 27.8 | 28.0 | 28.3 | 28.5 | 28.8 | 29.0 | 29.3 | 29.5 |
| 74–76 | 28.4 | 28.7 | 28.9 | 29.2 | 29.4 | 29.7 | 29.9 | 30.2 | 30.4 |
| 77–79 | 29.3 | 29.5 | 29.8 | 30.0 | 30.3 | 30.5 | 30.8 | 31.0 | 31.3 |
| 80–82 | 30.1 | 30.4 | 30.6 | 30.9 | 31.1 | 31.4 | 31.6 | 31.9 | 32.1 |
| 83–85 | 30.9 | 31.2 | 31.4 | 31.7 | 31.9 | 32.2 | 32.4 | 32.7 | 32.9 |
| 86–88 | 31.7 | 32.0 | 32.2 | 32.5 | 32.7 | 32.9 | 33.2 | 33.4 | 33.7 |
| 89–91 | 32.5 | 32.7 | 33.0 | 33.2 | 33.5 | 33.7 | 33.9 | 34.2 | 34.4 |
| 92–94 | 33.2 | 33.4 | 33.7 | 33.9 | 34.2 | 34.4 | 34.7 | 34.9 | 35.2 |
| 95–97 | 33.9 | 34.1 | 34.4 | 34.6 | 34.9 | 35.1 | 35.4 | 35.6 | 35.9 |

*Continued*

## *Practice What You Know:* Body-Composition Assessment Techniques–cont'd

### Table 5. Percent Body Fat Estimations for Women: Jackson and Pollock Formula–cont'd

| SUM OF SKINFOLDS (mm) | AGE GROUPS | | | | | | | | |
|---|---|---|---|---|---|---|---|---|---|
| | 22 | 23–27 | 28–32 | 33–37 | 38–42 | 43–47 | 48–52 | 53–57 | >57 |
| 98–100 | 34.6 | 34.8 | 35.1 | 35.3 | 35.5 | 35.8 | 36.0 | 36.3 | 36.5 |
| 101–103 | 35.3 | 35.4 | 35.7 | 35.9 | 36.2 | 36.4 | 36.7 | 36.9 | 37.2 |
| 104–106 | 35.8 | 36.1 | 36.3 | 36.6 | 36.8 | 37.1 | 37.3 | 37.5 | 37.8 |
| 107–109 | 36.4 | 36.7 | 36.9 | 37.1 | 37.4 | 37.6 | 37.9 | 38.1 | 38.4 |
| 110–112 | 37.0 | 37.2 | 37.5 | 37.7 | 38.0 | 38.2 | 38.5 | 38.7 | 38.9 |
| 113–115 | 37.5 | 37.8 | 38.0 | 38.2 | 38.5 | 38.7 | 39.0 | 39.2 | 39.5 |
| 116–118 | 38.0 | 38.3 | 38.5 | 38.8 | 39.0 | 39.3 | 39.5 | 39.7 | 40.0 |
| 119–121 | 38.5 | 38.7 | 39.0 | 39.2 | 39.5 | 39.7 | 40.0 | 40.2 | 40.5 |
| 122–124 | 39.0 | 39.2 | 39.4 | 39.7 | 39.9 | 40.2 | 40.4 | 40.7 | 40.9 |
| 125–127 | 39.4 | 39.6 | 39.9 | 40.1 | 40.4 | 40.6 | 40.9 | 41.1 | 41.4 |
| 128–130 | 39.8 | 40.0 | 40.3 | 40.5 | 40.8 | 41.0 | 41.3 | 41.5 | 41.8 |

*Source:* Jackson and Pollock.[15]

### Body Density Formulas

Men (chest, thigh, and abdominal):

Body density = 1.10938 – 0.0008267 (sum of three skinfolds) + 0.0000016 (sum of three skinfolds)$^2$ – 0.0002574 (age)

Women (triceps, thigh, and suprailium):

Body density = 1.099421 – 0.0009929 (sum of three skinfolds) + 0.0000023 (sum of three skinfolds)$^2$ – 0.0001392 (age)

Body density of fat tissue equals 0.9 g/cc, and the density of fat-free tissue is approximately 1.1 g/cc, although these figures vary slightly by age, sex, and ethnicity. Once body density is determined, it needs to be converted to body composition. Two of the most commonly used prediction equations to estimate percent body fat are as follows:

- Brozek et al.[2]: % Fat = (457/body density) – 414
- Siri[1]: % Fat = (495/body density) – 450

These calculations provide generalized measurements of subcutaneous fat for an average person based on the populations that were used to establish these coefficients. Tables P-4 and P-5 provide a quick reference for use with the three-site protocol for both men and women, based on the age of the individual.

### Skinfold Measurement Protocol
#### Equipment

- Skinfold caliper, properly calibrated (e.g., Slim Guide, Lange, Harpenden)
- Marking pencil (optional)

#### Pretest Procedures

- To ensure testing accuracy, the subject should be optimally hydrated and always be measured prior to exercise.
- Because this particular test can feel intrusive to a first-time subject, the technician should make sure the subject is familiar and comfortable with the protocol.
- If a marking pencil is to be used, it should be washable; an eyeliner pencil works well.

## *Practice What You Know:* Body-Composition Assessment Techniques–cont'd

### Test Protocol and Administration

- To ensure accuracy in assessing body composition using the skinfold caliper method, it is important to measure each skinfold in the appropriate location and use standardized techniques.
- All measurements are taken on the right side of the body while the subject is standing.
- Skinfold locations should be properly identified using anatomical landmarks and measurements. Use of a marking pencil will help ensure precise landmarks and consistency.
- Hold the calipers in the right hand, grasping the skinfold site with the left hand. (Left-handed calipers are available, which reverses the hand position.)
- The thumb and index finger of the left hand are opened to about 8 cm (~3 in.) and positioned 1 cm (~0.5 in.) above the measurement site.
- Grasp or pinch the skinfold site making a fold line (double fold of skin) that corresponds to the site instructions.
- The skin and underlying fat are simultaneously pulled firmly away from the underlying muscle tissue to accurately assess subcutaneous fat.
- The pinch is maintained while the calipers are positioned perpendicular to the site and on the site location (1 cm below the thumb and index finger), midway between the top and the base of the fold.
- Slowly release the caliper trigger, reading the dial to the nearest 0.5 mm approximately 2 or 3 seconds after release.
- After taking the skinfold reading, gently squeeze the trigger to remove the caliper before releasing the skinfold pinch.
- Moving on to the next site, repeat the earlier steps. Each site should be measured a minimum of two times to ensure consistency between measurements. If subsequent readings do not agree within 10% of each other, a third measurement is necessary and the average of the two acceptable scores should be taken (i.e., within 10% of each other). It is recommended that the technician wait 20 to 30 seconds between measurements to allow the skin and fat to redistribute.
- Record all measurements on a testing form.
  - Evaluate and classify the subject's body composition using normative data (see Table 23-2).

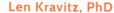

Len Kravitz, PhD

CHAPTER 24

# Weight-Management Strategies

## CHAPTER OUTLINE

## LEARNING OUTCOMES

1. Describe weight-management strategies for overweight and obese individuals.

2. Explain the application of behavior-change techniques for successful weight loss in overweight and obese individuals.

3. Describe the importance of an appropriate dietary intervention in a successful weight-management program.

4. Identify the steps involved in a behavior-modification intervention for weight management.

5. Explain some exercise considerations for overweight men and women completing cardiorespiratory and resistance training.

6. Design a weight-loss intervention for an overweight client.

## ANCILLARY LINK

Visit Davis*Plus* at http://davisplus.fadavis.com for study and practice resources, including online quizzes, animations that help explain physiological processes, podcasts concerning news and career trends in exercise physiology, and practice references.

## VIGNETTE

■ In her first meeting with the certified health coach at her local health club, 36-year-old Sarita expresses frustration with her constant battles with weight loss. She has tried numerous fad diets over the years, most recently "The 17 Day Diet", which she tried with some friends after reading about it on Facebook. She has never really exercised and has come to the realization that she needs to adopt a more realistic and comprehensive approach to addressing her weight and improving her health.

After 17 days of adhering to a 1,200-calorie daily diet, Sarita lost 7 pounds, but spent much of that time "starving and grumpy." She quickly gained the weight back after returning to her normal diet. It is this most recent "failure" that drove Sarita to seek the help of Opal, a health coach whom Sarita met at a health fair at her office building.

What would be an appropriate first step for Sarita's weight-management program, and how can Opal best introduce her to a more well-rounded approach to weight loss?

Weight management is often a challenging task, given that modern culture generally supports behavior patterns in which less energy is expended via physical activity and calorie-dense, inexpensive foods are heavily advertised and readily available. However, according to evidence-based research, there appears to be several achievable approaches in lifestyle, diet, activity, and behavioral change that can reverse or reduce these environmental tendencies. All health and fitness professionals can do their part in supporting the efforts of clients in terms of weight management. Using the content presented in this chapter, each professional can help individuals overcome the challenges of obesity, sustain weight that is lost by using appropriate weight regain prevention, and enjoy increased health and quality of life.

resulted in experimental subjects having a 58% lowered risk for development of type 2 diabetes, as compared with a control group, and was also much better than the **metformin** (prescription medication used to treat people with type 2 diabetes) group (Fig. 24-1).[3] In addition, this preventive effect was seen to hold for the 3,200 men and women of all racial and ethnic backgrounds in this study.

It is clear that the cornerstone of treatment for overweight and obese individuals is lifestyle modification.[3] Commonly, the three major components of a successful obesity treatment program are:

1. Lifestyle and behavioral modifications (including physical activity)
2. Nutritional programming
3. Exercise programming

## WEIGHT-MANAGEMENT STRATEGIES FOR OVERWEIGHT AND OBESE INDIVIDUALS

Losing weight, and maintaining the weight loss, is often very difficult, if not elusive, because of the multifactorial nature of obesity. Still, it is important to emphasize that even small changes in body weight can result in consequential health benefits. Studies show that a 5% to 10% loss of initial body weight is associated with meaningful improvements in cholesterol levels, hypertension, and glucose metabolism.[1] Successful weight-loss maintenance programs strive to attain intentional weight loss of at least 10% of one's weight and maintain that loss for a minimum of 1 year,[2] which is a realistic goal.[3]

The Diabetes Prevention Program study showed that a 4-year lifestyle intervention of physical activity and diet designed to induce a loss of 7% in body weight

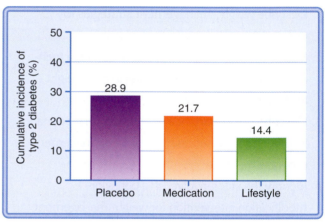

**Figure 24-1.** The Diabetes Prevention Program study showed that a 4-year lifestyle intervention of physical activity and diet resulted in experimental subjects having a 58% lowered risk for development of type 2 diabetes. It was also more effective than medication.

## RESEARCH HIGHLIGHT

### Misconceptions and Facts About Obesity

In a study funded by the National Institutes of Health (NIH), Casazza and colleagues[4] set out to study numerous beliefs about obesity that persist in the absence of supporting scientific evidence (presumptions), as well as those that persist despite contradicting evidence (myths). The researchers used Internet searches of popular media and scientific literature to identify, review, and classify obesity-related myths and presumptions. What they found were seven obesity-related myths concerning the effects of small, sustained increases in energy intake or expenditure, establishment of realistic goals for weight loss, rapid weight loss, weight-loss readiness, physical education classes, breast-feeding, and energy expended during sexual activity. They also identified six presumptions about the purported effects of regularly eating breakfast, early childhood experiences, eating fruits and vegetables, weight cycling, snacking, and the built (i.e., human-made) environment. Lastly, the authors reported nine evidence-supported facts that are relevant for the formulation of sound public health, policy, or clinical recommendations.

The following myths of obesity were found to persist, even though there are contradictory data that do not support them:

- Small, sustained changes in energy intake or expenditure result in significant, long-term weight changes.
- Setting realistic weight-loss goals is important so that obese individuals do not become frustrated and, therefore, lose less weight.

## RESEARCH HIGHLIGHT–cont'd

- Large, rapid weight loss results in poorer long-term weight outcomes than slow, gradual weight loss.
- Assessing the stage of change or diet readiness is important in helping patients who seek weight-loss treatment.
- The way that physical education classes are taught today plays an important role in preventing or reducing childhood obesity.
- Breast-feeding protects against obesity.
- The calorie expenditure of one bout of sexual activity equates to 100 to 300 kcal for each person involved.

The following presumptions about obesity were reported, even though there is a lack of evidence to support them:

- Regularly eating (rather than skipping) breakfast protects against obesity.
- The exercise and eating patterns that we learn in early childhood become habits that influence our weight throughout life.
- Eating more fruits and vegetables protects against obesity, regardless of whether any other intentional behavioral or environmental changes are made.
- Weight cycling (i.e., yo-yo dieting) is associated with increased mortality.
- Snacking contributes to weight gain and obesity.
- The built environment (i.e., accessibility to sidewalks and parks) influences obesity.

The following list presents obesity-related facts that are supported by sufficient evidence to consider them empirically proved:

- Although genetic factors play a large role, genes do not fully dictate a person's destiny.
- Diets effectively reduce weight, but they generally do not work well in the long term.
- Exercise increases health levels, regardless of body weight or weight loss.
- Sufficient doses of physical activity or exercise aids in long-term weight maintenance.
- Continuation of conditions that promote weight loss promotes maintenance of lower weight.
- Greater weight loss or maintenance is achieved for overweight children with programs that involve the parents and the home setting.
- Provision of meals and use of meal-replacement products promote greater weight loss.
- The continued use of some pharmaceutical agents can help patients achieve clinically meaningful weight loss and maintain the reduction.
- In appropriate patients, bariatric surgery results in long-term weight loss and reductions in the rate of incident diabetes and mortality.

Fitness professionals are encouraged to read Casazza and colleagues'[4] entire article because it sheds light on the numerous myths and presumptions about obesity that reflect unsupported beliefs held by many people, including academics and the general public. Casazza and colleagues were careful to conclude that any of the aforementioned myths and presumptions might one day be justifiably proved correct with appropriate scientific research. They also note that the facts about obesity, of which professionals may be reasonably certain, are facts that are useful today.

Casazza K, Fontaine KR, Astrup A, et al. Myths, presumptions, and facts about obesity. *N Engl J Med.* 2013;368:446–454.

## LIFESTYLE AND BEHAVIORAL MODIFICATION

The common course of weight-loss interventions indicates that weight is lost rapidly at first, with the point of maximum loss often occurring 6 months after beginning treatment.[2] Once the treatment period is over, however, weight is slowly regained until body weight returns to near the original level. Thus, it is central that weight-management strategies present lifestyle modifications that represent sustainable changes in the way a person lives his or her life.

All too often, individuals view a weight-loss program as an isolated period during which a person goes on a diet, takes exercise classes, or employs a personal trainer to get in shape. Others may attempt diet strategies with unrealistic expectations for weight loss and then give up when these goals are not met. It is important to educate clients that they are launching a new (or modified) way of life, not just a short-term quick fix to attain some loss of weight. In addition, it is important to emphasize that the overall health benefits of increasing physical activity with a balanced approach to eating and meal planning can improve quality of life and reduce the risks for development of **coronary heart disease**, **hypertension**, colon cancer, and diabetes, while also improving mental well-being and musculoskeletal function in **activities of daily living**.[5]

## Transtheoretical Model of Behavioral Change

To empower clients to make true behavioral changes, it is essential that health and fitness professionals understand what actually determines an individual's behavior. Although several models offer different approaches to understanding behavior and behavioral change, the most widely used in the health and fitness industry is the **transtheoretical model of behavioral change (TTM)**, which is sometimes referred to as the stages-of-change model (Fig. 24-2). According to the TTM, people who change their behavior go through several stages, from precontemplation (not thinking about changing), to contemplation (weighing the pros and cons of changing), preparation (getting ready to make a change), action (practicing the new behavior), and finally, maintenance (incorporating the new behavior into one's lifestyle). These stages of change constitute the first component of the TTM and are outlined in Table 24-1 (note the addition of lapse to the stages).

Applying the TTM in a weight-management program requires addressing different behaviors simultaneously. For example, a client may be entering the action stage in terms of reducing empty-calorie foods, but have doubts about his or her ability to maintain an exercise program. It is important to assess a client's stage of change for exercise and diet readiness separately, then use appropriate intervention strategies accordingly.

In addition to the stages of change, health and fitness professionals should be aware of three other components of the TTM: processes of change, self-efficacy, and decisional balance.

## Processes of Change

The second component of the TTM consists of the **processes of change** that are used to pass from one stage to the next. Each transition has a unique set of processes and is based on specific individual decisions and mental states, such as individual readiness and motivation. The most effective change strategies are stage-specific interventions that target the natural processes people use as they move from one stage to the next. Examples of the processes of change for the different stages are presented in the From Theory to Practice feature later in this chapter.

## Self-efficacy

The third component of the TTM is **self-efficacy**. In the lifestyle-modification context, self-efficacy is the belief in one's capabilities to be physically active and to maintain healthful nutrition.[6,7] A circular relationship exists between self-efficacy and behavioral change, such that a person's self-efficacy is related to whether he or she will participate in activity, and a person's participation in activity influences his or her self-efficacy level. Therefore, self-efficacy acts as both a determinant and an outcome of behavioral change.

In addition, a reliable relation exists between self-efficacy for activity and stage of behavior change, such that precontemplators and contemplators have significantly lower levels of self-efficacy than people in the action and maintenance stages. This is a logical relation. Individuals who are in the precontemplation and contemplation stages are not exercising at all or are doing so very infrequently, which may reflect the belief that they do not have the ability or knowledge required to be active, whereas individuals in the action and maintenance stages are engaged in regular activity programs, thus demonstrating a belief in the ability to be active.

So how does a person develop self-efficacy? The most important and powerful predictor of self-efficacy is past performance experience. This means that an individual who has had past success in adopting and maintaining a physical-activity program will have higher self-efficacy regarding his or her ability to be active in the future. It also means that those individuals with no exercise experience will have much lower self-efficacy regarding their abilities to engage in an exercise program. Therefore, it should be the exercise professional's primary goal to get these nonexercisers some sort of positive exercise experience. The self-efficacy has to come from somewhere, so those initial

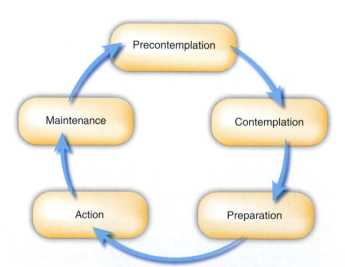

**Figure 24-2.** According to the transtheoretical model of behavioral change, people who change their behavior go through several stages, including precontemplation, contemplation, preparation, action, and maintenance.

## Table 24-1. Stages of Behavior Change

| STAGE | TRAITS | GOALS | STRATEGIES |
|---|---|---|---|
| **Precontemplation** | Unaware or under-aware of the problem, or believe that it cannot be solved (e.g., latent pain) | Increase awareness of the risks of inactivity and of the benefits of activity<br>Focus on addressing something relevant to them<br>Have them start thinking about change | Validate lack of readiness to change and clarify that this decision is theirs.<br>Encourage reevaluation of current behavior and self-exploration while not taking action.<br>Explain and personalize the inherent risks.<br>Use general sources, including media, Internet, and brochures to increase awareness. |
| **Contemplation** | Aware of the problem and weighing the benefits vs. risks of change<br>Have little understanding of how to go about changing | Inform them of available options<br>Provide cues to action and some basic structured direction | Validate lack of readiness to change and clarify that this decision is theirs.<br>Encourage evaluation of the pros and cons of making change.<br>Identify and promote new, positive outcome expectations and boost self-confidence.<br>Offer invitations to become more active (e.g., free trials). |
| **Preparation** | Seeking opportunities to participate in activity (combine intent and behavior with activity) | Structured, regular programming with frequent positive feedback and reinforcements on their progress | Verify that the individual has the underlying skills for behavior change and encourage small steps toward building self-efficacy.<br>Identify and assist with problem-solving obstacles.<br>Help the client identify social support and establish goals. |
| **Action** | Desire for opportunities to maintain activities<br>Changing beliefs and attitudes<br>High risk for lapses or returns to undesirable behavior | Establish exercise as a habit through motivation and adherence to the desired behavior | Implement behavior-modification strategies.<br>Focus on restructuring cues and social support toward building long-term change.<br>Increase awareness to inevitable lapses and bolster self-efficacy in coping with lapses.<br>Reiterate long-term benefits of adherence.<br>Require continual feedback on progress. |
| **Maintenance** | Empowered, but desire a means to maintain adherence<br>Good capability to deal with lapses | Maintain support systems<br>Maintain interest and avoid boredom or burnout | Reevaluate strategies currently in effect.<br>Plan for contingencies with support system, although this may no longer be needed.<br>Reinforce the need for a transition from external to internal rewards.<br>Plan for potential lapses.<br>Encourage program variety. |
| **Lapse** | Encounter lapses that they are unable to overcome | Return to action | Identify reasons for lapse.<br>Identify current stage of change to progress once again toward action.<br>Maintain existing systems and relationships, and offer appropriate support. |

encounters with exercise are extremely critical for promoting and triggering change.

## Decisional Balance

The final component of the TTM is **decisional balance**, which refers to the numbers of pros and cons an individual perceives regarding adopting and/or maintaining an activity program.[8] Precontemplators and contemplators perceive more cons (e.g., sweating, sore muscles, time, cost, unwanted physical changes, and boredom) related to being regularly active than pros. The perceived cons do not have to be logical or realistic to prevent an individual from being active. As people progress through the stages of change, the balance of pros and cons shifts, such that people in the action and maintenance stages perceive more pros about being active than cons. The active behavior of people in these later stages reflects this change in decisional balance. The decisional balance worksheet presented in Figure 24-3 can be used to help clients weigh the perceived benefits against the potential losses involved with making a change. Although this worksheet is a valuable tool to help health and exercise professionals and clients work together to clarify potential barriers or psychological roadblocks, avoid becoming overly reliant on worksheets. The most effective approach is to use worksheets in conjunction with continued communication and observation to build a complete understanding of client needs and to develop appropriate programming.

The natural change in decisional balance that occurs as people progress through the stages of change suggests that exercise professionals can influence their perceptions about being active and help encourage people to start an activity program. When working on shifting decisional balance, it is important to remember the processes of change related to moving from one stage to the next. For example, when working with a precontemplator or contemplator, it is important to emphasize a wide variety of benefits of being physically active and avoid arguing about the cons they perceive about exercise. Often, the cons that nonexercisers perceive about physical activity are a result of misinformation and a lack of experience. In addition, it is important that the discussed benefits are both short and long term. For example, emphasizing only the long-term weight-loss benefits of an activity program can be overwhelming and may make those benefits seem unattainable. Focusing on the short-term benefits, such as increased energy and mastery of the exercise itself, will give the client something to look forward to immediately.

**Instructions:**
- Work with the client to document the gains and potential losses that he or she might experience when making a lifestyle change.
- Identify and list the recommended implementation stages needed to achieve the gains, and list coping strategies that can be used to deal with the potential losses or obstacles associated with the change.

### DECISIONAL BALANCE WORKSHEET

Perceived gains associated with adopting desired behaviors:

1. _____
2. _____
3. _____
4. _____

Perceived losses associated with adopting desired behaviors:

1. _____
2. _____
3. _____
4. _____

Strategies to maximize potential for achieving gains:

1. _____
2. _____
3. _____
4. _____

Strategies to minimize potential of perceived losses:

1. _____
2. _____
3. _____
4. _____

**Figure 24-3.** The decisional balance worksheet is a valuable tool to help health and fitness professionals and clients work together to clarify potential barriers or psychological roadblocks.

# FROM THEORY TO PRACTICE

### ■ EXAMPLES OF THE PROCESSES OF CHANGE IN THE TRANSTHEORETICAL MODEL OF BEHAVIORAL CHANGE FROM A FITNESS PROFESSIONAL'S PERSPECTIVE

## PRECONTEMPLATION

A fitness professional is having a discussion with his uncle, who is questioning how anyone can make a living by helping people exercise. The uncle is sedentary and thinks that exercise is for women who take aerobics or for bodybuilder types who are looking to bulk up. He views exercise as completely irrelevant to his life. The fitness professional's initial thought is to argue with his uncle and to tell him that he is completely misinformed, but this would be counterproductive. The fitness professional needs to educate his uncle without lecturing or arguing with him. The fitness professional decides to pull up his website, which contains videos of some of his workouts. He shows his uncle how exercise has transformed over the years and the diversity of his clientele. In addition, he shares some of the successes of his clients, including weight loss and changes in blood pressure and cholesterol. The fitness professional presents and shares this information in a general context that is not specific to, or directed at, his uncle. As the discussion continues, he answers his uncle's questions and even invites him into the gym to meet a couple of his clients and to watch him go through a few workouts.

## CONTEMPLATION

A fitness professional receives a phone call at the gym from a woman who saw an advertisement for a free trial week. She says that she does not currently work out and that she has never exercised in a gym before. She seems very apprehensive and nervous on the phone; says that she is not sure if it is for her, but that she knows she needs to be more active. She asks the fitness professional whether there is any programming for beginners and whether someone will be available to help her if she comes in, because she does not know what she is doing. The fitness professional talks to the woman for a few minutes and then invites her into the gym for a tour and a meeting, during which they can talk and he can answer any questions she may have. They set an appointment for the next day. During the meeting, the fitness professional serves as a sounding board for the woman's questions and concerns. He introduces her to the gym staff members that they encounter and describes the various options for activity. He even talks about what people typically wear when they work out. The woman has a lot of doubt about starting a program, and the fitness professional emphasizes the benefits of being active. To help her learn more about the different options, he invites her to a beginner-level group fitness class and introduces her to the instructor of that class. He then gives her a pass for an introductory training session that will teach her the basics of strength training and how she could start a program. Before she leaves, he invites her to the facility's health fair, which is taking place the following weekend. He explains that it will be a good opportunity to meet more people and get additional information about exercise options.

## PREPARATION

A fitness professional is approached by a member at the gym who comes in a few times a month and goes through a basic workout. He tells the fitness professional that he wants to be more consistent and lose weight, but that he is having a difficult time finding the motivation. He says that he is not really sure what he needs to be doing and that he needs help. The fitness professional talks with the member and ensures him that he is off to a great start. He emphasizes that he just needs a little more direction and accountability in his workouts. The fitness professional asks if he would like some help setting new goals. As they talk, the fitness professional casually introduces the member to a couple of the staff at the gym whom he has never met. The fitness professional offers to show him a couple of new exercises and goes over the different programming options at the club. The member comments that he had no idea there were so many activities. The fitness professional then tells him about a group of men he trains 2 days a week who are also trying to lose weight. He invites the member to join them for their next workout.

## ACTION

A fitness professional has a female client who has been consistently training 3 days a week for a couple of months. She is seeing great results and loves her workouts. She is always happy to come in and never misses an appointment. The client has two children, and with the school year coming to an end, she knows her schedule will change. She really wants to continue to train. The fitness professional encourages the client by telling her how great she has done, reminding her how much she has accomplished. They then talk about the challenges she will face trying to stick to her workouts when her children are out of school. He tells her that she will likely be less consistent with her workouts and proposes developing a plan to help her stay with the program. The fitness professional teaches her the importance of flexibility in her program

*Continued*

## FROM THEORY TO PRACTICE–cont'd

and offers a couple of exercise options she can do outside of the gym with her children. They also look at changing the times of her workouts to accommodate her new schedule. The fitness professional tells the client that he knows she can do it and not to hesitate to ask for help if she is having challenges with her schedule.

### MAINTENANCE

A longtime client of a fitness professional has lost more than 60 lb (27 kg) and feels great. He has reached his goals and loves being physically active. He has even started taking his family for hikes on the weekends. He rarely misses an appointment and is one of the fitness professional's easiest clients to deal with. The fitness professional understands, however, that this state of consistency may not last forever, so she plans a sit-down session with the client to evaluate the program and set new goals. The fitness professional tells her client that she wants to switch up his program a bit and introduce some more functional training. She also recommends switching to a group-training session for one of his sessions each week. The fitness professional explains that she thinks he would really enjoy the group activity, which will give him an opportunity to meet more people in the gym. They also talk about the client's upcoming schedule, work activities, and travel plans, and discuss strategies to help him stay active during any inconsistencies in his schedule. The fitness professional also emphasizes to the client that he should keep her posted if he starts to get bored or lose motivation. Finally, the fitness professional praises the client for his continued success and dedication to the program.

Relapse can occur at any stage of the TTM, including during the maintenance stage. Any change that may occur in an individual's life, such as moving, starting school, changing jobs, or suffering an injury, can trigger a relapse into irregular activity or even no activity, or a return to unhealthful eating.

## VIGNETTE continued

■ During their first session together, Opal explores Sarita's history with weight loss and notes that it is marked by large fluctuations as Sarita started and stopped fad diets over the years in a quest for a quick fix. They discuss the need for true lifestyle change, and Opal attempts to redirect Sarita's focus on appearance by explaining the many health benefits of very moderate weight loss. At 160 pounds, Sarita is surprised to learn that losing as little as 8 to 16 pounds and maintaining that weight loss would significantly improve her overall health. Sarita admits that her goal has always been to lose 40 pounds as quickly as possible.

Opal recognizes that Sarita is in the preparation stage of behavioral change, so she uses some very specific strategies to move her into the action stage. First, she helps Sarita identify obstacles and develop solutions to overcome them before they actually confront her. In addition, Opal finds that Sarita's self-efficacy for adhering to dietary changes appears to be fairly high, but that when it comes to exercise, her self-efficacy is extremely low. Therefore, the focus of their first several exercise sessions will be on building confidence in the gym setting and getting used to using the various machines.

## Principles of Lifestyle Modification

Health psychology research has clarified many helpful principles of lifestyle modification, including operant conditioning, the principle of limited self-control, the false-hope syndrome, the planning fallacy, stress management and negative mood, and lifelong sustainability and relapse prevention. Although many of these principles seem like simple common sense, it is important for health and fitness professionals to use these concepts when evaluating and guiding their clients' lifestyle-modification efforts.

### Operant Conditioning

**Operant conditioning** examines the relations between behaviors and consequences. Behaviors followed by a reward are likely to repeated, whereas behaviors followed by a punishment are less likely to be repeated. Eating behaviors in particular are often wrapped up with a complex system of punishments (feeling guilty for overeating) and reward (enjoyment of eating and feeling nourished and satisfied). When working with clients seeking weight control, it is best to focus on factors that reward exercise and healthful eating behaviors, keeping in mind that autonomous forms of motivation work best.

### Limited Self-control

Self-control is a limited resource. Although some people have more self-control than others, no one has an unlimited supply of self-control. The more that health and fitness professionals can minimize the amount of self-control needed to maintain lifestyle modifications, the more successful their clients will be. In addition, because habits are comfortable and require little self-control, the more quickly lifestyle modifications can become habits, the happier and more successful a client will be. It is important to recognize that coping with stress requires a certain level of self-control, which explains why it is more difficult to change a habit when the person is under a lot of stress. Finally, self-control appears to be renewed daily, which is why many people are more successful when performing exercise in the morning rather than later on, when self-control has been depleted by the events of the day.

## False-Hope Syndrome

People's tendency to set unrealistic goals is called the **false-hope syndrome**.[9] Setting ambitious goals makes people feel good, but clients can become disappointed in themselves and ultimately discontinue their efforts if they fail to reach these goals.

## Planning Fallacy

The **planning fallacy** states that people consistently underestimate the time, energy, and other resources required to complete a given task.[10] Clients often say they will spend more time exercising than they really can, or that they will change their eating habits more drastically than they can really tolerate.

## Stress Management and Negative Mood

Stress is the most common reason people abandon their plans to change behavior. Stress depletes self-control, lowers feelings of self-efficacy, and decreases energy and motivation. Too much stress triggers negative emotions such as anxiety, anger, and sadness. Some people respond to feelings of stress by eating when they are not hungry (i.e., emotional eating). Controlling stress is a key to successful lifestyle modification.

## Lifelong Sustainability and Relapse Prevention

The lifestyle modifications and behavioral changes that lead to weight loss must be maintained to prevent weight regain. A hectic lifestyle offers many opportunities for disruption to lifestyle-modification programs, even for people with the best of intentions. Relapse-prevention discussions with clients can encourage them to anticipate and visualize occasions during which they may experience lapses in their behavior-change programs. Lapses are normal and should be accepted and taken in stride. Although feelings of disappointment may arise when lapses occur, it is important for clients to avoid feelings of failure or guilt, because these negative thoughts and emotions can deplete self-control and energy, increase feelings of stress, and lead to total relapse and motivational collapse.

## Behavioral Approaches

The behavioral approaches to weight loss are multifaceted. The behavioral therapy evidence suggests that several techniques may be successfully incorporated to help clients attain long-term weight control[11]:

- *Proper assessment of the client's readiness to change:* Weight-loss achievement and maintenance in the long term depends on the individual being ready (Fig. 24-4) and able to build new attitudes and behaviors about physical activity and food consumption into his or her daily life. Table 24-1 presents different stages in a client's readiness to change and offers strategies for how to address the various barriers to change.

- *Teaching accurate self-monitoring of food consumption:* Obese individuals tend to underestimate how much they eat by approximately 30% to 50%.[1] Thus, teaching clients to accurately self-monitor is vital for long-term success of the weight-management intervention.

- *Realistic goal-setting:* Unrealistic goal-setting may set up a client for failure and cause her or him to self-blame (e.g., "I have no willpower."), when it may actually be the treatment that is flawed.[11] Help clients identify modest, achievable goals and the potential barriers that need to be overcome. **SMART goals** are specific, measurable, achievable, relevant, and time bound. This goal-setting process should be followed with a written and personalized action plan. Establish rewards along the way for desired outcomes.

- *Dietary change:* Costain and Croker highlight the following key dietary messages for adults managing body weight[11]:
  √ Include a variety of foods from the main food groups.
  √ Consider portion size.
  √ Reduce the proportion of fat, particularly **saturated fat**.
  √ Substitute saturated fat with **omega-3 fats** such as from salmon and trout.
  √ Increase fruit and vegetable consumption to at least five portions daily.
  √ Make low glycemic index, whole-grain, high-fiber, carbohydrate-rich foods part of meals.
  √ Reduce sugar intake.
  √ Limit salt intake.
  √ Follow a structured meal pattern, starting with breakfast.

- *Increased physical activity:* Physical activity to increase energy expenditure can be achieved via programmed activity in which exercise is performed during a discrete period via activities like swimming, jogging, and biking. In addition, energy expenditure can be increased with lifestyle activity by including more spontaneous movement in daily activities (e.g., standing, moving, and walking). Much more on the role of physical activity in weight management is presented in the Exercise Programming for Overweight and Obese Clients section later in this chapter.

## Weight-Loss Readiness Quiz

Are you ready to lose weight? Your attitude about weight loss affects your ability to succeed. Take this Weight-Loss Readiness Quiz to learn if you need to make any attitude adjustments before you begin. Mark each item true or false. Please be honest! It's important that these answers reflect the way you really are, not how you would like to be. A method for interpreting your readiness for weight loss follows:

1. _____ I have thought a lot about my eating habits and physical activities to pinpoint what I need to change.
2. _____ I have accepted the idea that I need to make permanent, not temporary, changes in my eating and activities to be successful.
3. _____ I will only feel successful if I lose a lot of weight.
4. _____ I accept the idea that it's best if I lose weight slowly.
5. _____ I'm thinking of losing weight now because I really want to, not because someone else thinks I should.
6. _____ I think losing weight will solve other problems in my life.
7. _____ I am willing and able to increase my regular physical activity.
8. _____ I can lose weight successfully if I have no "slip-ups."
9. _____ I am ready to commit some time and effort each week to organizing and planning my food and activity programs.
10. _____ Once I lose some initial weight, I usually lose the motivation to keep going until I reach my goal.
11. _____ I want to start a weight-loss program, even though my life is unusually stressful right now.

## Scoring the Weight-Loss Readiness Quiz

To score the quiz, look at your answers next to items 1, 2, 4, 5, 7, and 9. Score "1" if you answered "true" and "0" if you answered "false."

For items 3, 6, 8, 10, and 11, score "0" for each true answer and "1" for each false answer.

To get your total score, add the scores of all questions. No one score indicates for sure whether you are ready to start losing weight. However, the higher your total score, the more characteristics you have that contribute to success. As a rough guide, consider the following recommendations:

1. If you scored 8 or higher, you probably have good reasons for wanting to lose weight now and a good understanding of the steps needed to succeed. Still, you might want to learn more about the areas where you scored a "0" (see "Interpretation of Quiz Items").
2. If you scored 5 to 7, you may need to reevaluate your reasons for losing weight and the methods you would use to do so.
3. If you scored 4 or less, now may not be the right time for you to lose weight. While you might be successful in losing weight initially, your answers suggest that you are unlikely to sustain sufficient effort to lose all the weight you want, or keep off the weight that you do lose. You need to reconsider your weight-loss motivations and methods and perhaps learn more about the pros and cons of different approaches to reducing.

## Interpretation of Quiz Items

Your answers to the quiz can clue you in to potential stumbling blocks to your weight-loss success. Any item score of "0" indicates a misconception about weight loss, or a potential problem area. While no individual item score of "0" is important enough to scuttle your weight-loss plans, you should consider the meaning of those items so that you can best prepare yourself for the challenges ahead. The numbers below correspond to the question numbers.

1. It has been said that you can't change what you don't understand. You might benefit from keeping records for a week to help pinpoint when, what, why, and how much you eat. This tool also is useful in identifying obstacles to regular physical activity.
2. Making drastic or highly restrictive changes in your eating habits may allow you to lose weight in the short-run but be too hard to live with permanently. Similarly, your program of regular physical activity should be one you can sustain. Both your food plan and activity program should be healthful and enjoyable.
3. Most people have fantasies of reaching a weight considerably lower than they can realistically maintain. Rethink your meaning of "success." A successful, realistic weight loss is one that can be comfortably maintained through sensible eating and regular activity. Take your body type into consideration. Then set smaller, achievable goals. Your first goal may be to lose a small amount of weight while you learn eating habits and activity patterns to help you maintain it.
4. If you equate success with fast weight loss, you will have problems maintaining your weight. This "quick fix" attitude can backfire when you face the challenges of weight maintenance. It's best—and healthiest—to lose weight slowly while learning the strategies that allow you to keep the weight off permanently.
5. The desire for, and commitment to, weight loss must come from you. People who lose and maintain weight successfully take responsibility for their own desires and decide the best way to achieve them. Once this step is taken, friends and family are an important source of support, not motivation.
6. While being overweight may contribute to a number of social problems, it is rarely the single cause. Anticipating that all of your problems will be solved through weight loss is unrealistic and may set you up for disappointment. Instead, realize that successful weight loss will make you feel more self-confident and empowered and that the skills you develop to deal with your weight can be applied to other areas of your life.
7. Studies have shown that people who develop the habit of regular, moderate physical activity are most successful at maintaining their weight. Exercise does not have to be strenuous to be effective for weight control. Any moderate physical activity that you enjoy and will do regularly counts. Just get moving!
8. While most people don't expect perfection of themselves in everyday life, many feel that they must stick to a weight-loss program perfectly. This is unrealistic. Rather than expecting lapses and viewing them as catastrophes, recognize them as valuable opportunities to identify problem triggers and develop strategies for the future.
9. Successful weight loss is not possible without taking the time to think about yourself, assess your problem areas, and develop strategies to deal with them. Success takes time. You must commit to planning and organizing your weight loss.
10. Do not ignore your concerns about "going the distance," because they may indicate a potential problem. Think about past efforts and why they failed. Pinpoint any reasons, and work on developing motivational strategies to get you over those hurdles. Take your effort one day at a time; a plateau of weight maintenance within an ongoing weight-loss program is perfectly okay.
11. Weight loss itself is a source of stress, so if you are already under stress, it may be difficult to successfully implement a weight-loss program at this time. Try to resolve other stressors in your life before you begin a weight-loss effort.

**Figure 24-4.** Weight-loss–specific readiness quiz that health and exercise professionals can administer to clients to obtain information about a client's knowledge and attitudes about his or her willingness to start the process of losing weight.

- *Stimulus control:* **Stimulus control** involves learning how to avoid triggers such as the sight of food and wanting to eat, or dealing with cravings for food. For example, clients can be taught to avoid purchasing unhealthful food so that it is not available in the home. Stimulus control could also include exposing oneself to reminders to perform a healthy behavior. An example is a client who frequently leaves the office late, is therefore late for his workout, and is getting only half of his scheduled workout time. To help with this problem, he sets an alarm on his computer for the days of his workouts to remind him 5 minutes before it is time to leave. This reminder triggers him to prepare to leave his office and head to the gym, resulting in a full workout session. Lastly, for clients who are carefully monitoring their caloric intake, it is best not to go on a strict diet of specific food deprivation. In fact, satisfying some food cravings by eating in moderation may quell the craving and prevent overeating. In addition, creating workable diversions to food cravings, such as going on a walk or drinking a large glass of water, may be viable solutions.
- *Cognitive restructuring:* **Cognitive restructuring** is a behavioral technique that involves learning how to replace unhealthy or negative thoughts and "self-talk" about weight loss with positive affirmations.
- *Relapse management:* Relapse-management education attempts to make clients aware that lapses and relapses are a normal part of behavior change. This strategy helps to relieve the stress of "being a diet failure" that some individuals experience when they miss an exercise session or overindulge in a meal.
- *Establish ongoing support:* Ongoing support involves creative communication techniques such as e-mail, phone, and websites that provide maintenance support to clients in an effort to sustain the lifestyle changes that have been made.

Wing and Phelan[12] have studied and identified the key attributes of successful weight-loss maintainers from the National Weight Control Registry, the largest database in the world of persons who are sustaining long-term weight loss. Despite using various approaches to lose weight, these weight-loss maintainers share some chief behavioral characteristics, including the following:

- Frequent self-monitoring of body weight and food intake
- Eating a diet low in fat and higher in carbohydrate
- Eating breakfast and regular meals
- Limiting fast-food consumption
- Accepting realistic weight-loss goals
- Performing high levels of physical activity (≥1 hr/day)

## FROM THEORY TO PRACTICE

### ■ SETTING SMART GOALS

Clients often express fairly general health and fitness goals, such as wanting to "tone muscles" or "lose some weight." Health and exercise professional can help clients define goals in more specific and measurable terms so that progress can be evaluated. Effective goals are commonly said to be SMART goals (Fig. 24-5):

- *Specific:* Goals must be clear and unambiguous, stating specifically what should be accomplished.
- *Measurable:* Goals must be measurable so that clients can see whether they are making progress. Examples of measurable goals include performing a given strength-training workout two times a week or losing 5 lb (2.3 kg).
- *Attainable:* Goals should be realistically attainable by the individual client. The achievement of attaining a goal reinforces commitment to the program and encourages the client to continue exercising. Attaining goals is also a testimony to the fitness professional's effectiveness.
- *Relevant:* Goals must be relevant to the particular interest, needs, and abilities of the individual client.
- *Time bound:* Goals must contain estimated timelines for completion. Clients should be evaluated regularly to monitor progress toward goals. Fitness professionals should err on the conservative side of goal-setting in terms of what might be realistically achieved by the client. Lofty goals feel good and sound inspirational, but clients can be disappointed when progress is slow.

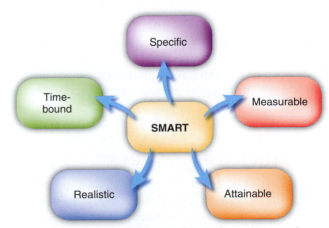

**Figure 24-5. SMART goals.** Health and exercise professionals can help clients define goals in more specific and measurable terms so that progress can be evaluated.

## FROM THEORY TO PRACTICE

### ■ GUIDING CLIENTS IN PROBLEM-SOLVING THROUGH COGNITIVE RESTRUCTURING

Problem-solving often evolves naturally from self-monitoring, as clients become aware of the situations in which they overeat, eat the wrong things, or skip their exercise sessions. Although it may be tempting for fitness professionals to solve the problems themselves, problem-solving must be client driven, so that solutions are more congruent with clients' needs and lifestyles. Consciously changing the way one perceives or thinks about something is called *cognitive restructuring*. Cognitive restructuring requires developing a mindful awareness of one's automatic thoughts, or self-talk, and consciously changing counterproductive thoughts. Over time, and with practice, clients can learn to change the way they think, and thus the ways they feel and behave. Thinking is intimately tied to behavior, so it is important for clients to be aware of their thought patterns as they work on changing specific behaviors.

Fitness professionals can help clients apply cognitive restructuring when weighing the pros and cons of starting a weight-control program. While educating clients about the benefits of exercise, the goal should be to make physical exercise appealing to them. This will be a continued effort while working with clients. For example, clients who say they "hate" exercise should try to see physical activity in a more positive light. Cognitive restructuring may make them more aware of the things they say to themselves about exercise. This can be part of their self-monitoring routine. For example, they can make a note of the thoughts and feelings that occur as they get ready to participate in physical activity.

To continue this example, suppose a client who was overweight as a child associates exercise with being teased in school. Fitness professionals should explore this association and help the client understand that there are ways to be active that do not involve teasing. They should strive to help clients adopt new ways of thinking and create more positive feelings about physical activity. This means steering them away from any negative automatic thoughts relating to exercise and then creating more positive associations.

Clients may uncover other automatic thoughts that produce feelings of stress and weaken self-efficacy. For example, many clients feel that if they are not perfect, they are failures. They may judge themselves as always falling short or discount positive results because they have not reached unrealistic expectations. When automatic thoughts are brought into the light of day, they often sound silly. For example, "I must be perfect in my weight-control behaviors," will sound unreasonable for most clients. The fitness professional can guide clients to rephrase such thoughts to be more supportive and realistic; for example, "Nobody is perfect. I am making improvements in several areas (list), and I am getting healthier and stronger every day."

Especially harmful is all-or-nothing thinking. Many clients develop the attitude that they are either "on" or "off" the diet. "On" means being perfect; "off" can mean destructive behaviors such as overeating and not exercising. The beauty of lifestyle-modification programs is that they help clients learn to think about lifelong behavior change, rather than being on or off diets. Hopefully, as clients become aware of counterproductive thinking, they can learn to replace negative thoughts with more positive and realistic ones.

Cognitive restructuring requires a great deal of practice and self-monitoring. It also requires the ability to observe one's own thinking and not to accept one's immediate thoughts as "reality." Positive thinking alone is not enough; clients must restructure thoughts in ways that are believable, as well as positive. "I love exercise" may not ring true to a client, but "I don't mind walking on the treadmill while I watch TV" might *become* true.

---

- Recognizing that weight control is an ongoing process and commitment

Once an individual has maintained a weight loss for 2 to 5 years, the chances of longer-term success greatly improve.

## NUTRITIONAL PROGRAMMING

Over the past five decades, there has been a remarkable increase in the various types of diets. In essence, the goal of the weight-loss dietary intervention is to keep the dietary content nutritionally correct for health concerns, while also introducing some reasonable means of reducing calorie intake. This is referred to as a portion-control approach to dietary intervention. Modern society has influenced food consumption so dramatically that attainment of this goal can be very difficult.

The following criteria for safe and responsible weight loss should be followed (also see Chapters 3 and 20):

- The diet should meet the **Recommended Dietary Allowances (RDAs)** for vitamins, minerals, and proteins, and provide adequate amounts of fiber.
- The diet should be low in energy to induce weight loss, but not in essential nutrients.
- The weight-loss program should be directed toward a slow, steady weight loss unless a health condition of the client suggests a different approach.

- The diet should be pleasant and satisfactory for the client, for the client to sustain the new eating style.
- The program should include a strategy for weight maintenance, because there are no health benefits to be achieved from losing weight only to regain it.
- Clinical assessment of the client and identification of any conditions that may be affected by dieting and weight loss should be recognized and addressed appropriately.

According to the Position Statement on the Appropriate Intervention Strategies for Weight Loss and Prevention of Weight Regain for Adults by the American College of Sports Medicine (ACSM),[13] the absolute dietary energy intake should be adjusted (via portion control in food consumption and physical activity to expend more calories) to elicit an energy deficit of approximately 500 to 1,000 **kilocalories** per day.[14] In addition, ACSM recommends reducing dietary fat intake to less than 30% of total energy intake.[14] Therefore, with this deficit, a minimum weight loss of 1 to 2 lb (0.5–0.9 kg) per week would be realistic. A caloric deficit of 3,500 kilocalories is needed to lose approximately 1 lb (0.5 kg) of fat.

The NIH suggests that a healthful eating plan include the following healthful foods[15]:

- Fruits, which can be canned (in juice or water), fresh, frozen, or dried
- Vegetables, which can be canned (without salt), fresh, frozen, or dried
- Fat-free and low-fat milk and milk products such as low-fat yogurt, cheese, and milk
- Lean meat, poultry, fish, peas, and cooked beans
- Whole-grain foods such as oatmeal, brown rice, whole-wheat bread and grain foods like bagels, bread, pasta, cereal, tortillas, and crackers
- Canola or olive oils and soft margarines made from these oils in small amounts because they are high in calories
- Unsalted nuts, like walnuts and almonds, in small amounts because of their high caloric value

Health and exercise professionals should be familiar with the *Dietary Guidelines for Americans,* which are published every 5 years by the U.S. Department of Agriculture (USDA) and ChooseMyPlate (http://ChooseMyPlate.gov). The *2010 Dietary Guidelines for Americans*[16] provide science-based advice aimed at promoting health and reducing the risk for major chronic diseases through diet and physical activity. These guidelines encourage most Americans to eat fewer calories, be more active, and make informed food choices. The complete guidelines can be found online (http://dietaryguidelines.gov). With the release of the *2010 Dietary Guidelines for Americans,*[16] the USDA introduced http://ChooseMyPlate.gov, which presents a simplified approach to nutrition and food group recommendations, and breaks down food groups by balancing the correct portions of each food group on a plate for an easy visual (Fig. 24-6). By logging on to the

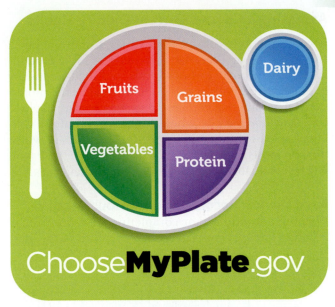

**Figure 24-6.** The ChooseMyPlate website (http://ChooseMyPlate.gov) provides individuals with personalized nutrition recommendations in their "Daily Food Plan" based on age, sex, weight, height, and physical activity level.

website, individuals can receive personalized nutrition recommendations in their "Daily Food Plan" based on age, sex, weight, height, and physical activity level.

Most lifestyle-modification diet programs use a high-carbohydrate, low-fat plan.[3] Other dietary approaches that may be used to produce greater initial weight loss include meal replacements (e.g., bars, cereals, and prepared entrees), portion-controlled prepared meals (i.e., lower-calorie meals of conventional foods), low-carbohydrate and high-fat diets (usually about 50–100 g carbohydrate daily without restrictions in fat), and low **glycemic index** diets (although the research is inconclusive on this strategy).

### VIGNETTE *continued*

■ A few sessions into Sarita's program, she and Opal have established a comfortable rapport, and Sarita is gaining confidence in her ability to adhere to a nutrition and exercise program for the long haul. Opal has used ChooseMyPlate (http://ChooseMyPlate.gov) to help Sarita with her nutritional needs, and Sarita is completing a food log each day to share at their sessions.

Opal also introduces Sarita to the concept of adding small bouts of movement throughout her day, as opposed to waiting to get to the gym to "exercise." Sarita begins walking the 1 mile to work a few days each week and makes a conscious effort to get up and move around the office throughout the day.

## Assessing a Client's Current Dietary Habits

Several methods can be used to learn more about a client's eating and lifestyle patterns, including food diaries/food records, 24-hour recall, and food-frequency questionnaires. With practice, a fitness and health professional may find that certain clients may be very likely to complete food records, whereas others may only be willing or able to give a 24-hour recall. Regardless of which method is used, the information gleaned from these tools will be invaluable in helping clients meet their goals.

### Food Diaries, Records, and 24-Hour Recall

Keeping a food diary or completing a 24-hour recall involves having clients describe a "typical" eating day, including all foods and beverages (Fig. 24-7). Food diaries and records are completed during the day as each food or beverage is consumed, whereas a 24-hour recall is completed the following day by memory. Be sure to discuss difference in eating behavior on weekends versus weekdays when individuals are not in their normal routines. One thing to consider is that people generally underestimate or under-report their caloric intake and tend to eat more salads, vegetables, and lower-calorie foods when using a food diary than their weight might suggest. Experience with probing the client, asking nonjudgmental questions, and offering a supportive environment is likely to reveal a more truthful picture of a client's eating pattern.

|  | Meal/snack time | Food/beverage & amount | Food group servings | Hunger level | Mood/ thoughts | Location | Challenges |
|---|---|---|---|---|---|---|---|
| **BREAKFAST** |  |  |  |  |  |  |  |
|  |  |  |  |  |  |  |  |
|  |  |  |  |  |  |  |  |
|  |  |  |  |  |  |  |  |
|  |  |  |  |  |  |  |  |
| **SNACK** |  |  |  |  |  |  |  |
|  |  |  |  |  |  |  |  |
|  |  |  |  |  |  |  |  |
| **LUNCH** |  |  |  |  |  |  |  |
|  |  |  |  |  |  |  |  |
|  |  |  |  |  |  |  |  |
|  |  |  |  |  |  |  |  |
|  |  |  |  |  |  |  |  |
| **SNACK** |  |  |  |  |  |  |  |
|  |  |  |  |  |  |  |  |
|  |  |  |  |  |  |  |  |
| **DINNER** |  |  |  |  |  |  |  |
|  |  |  |  |  |  |  |  |
|  |  |  |  |  |  |  |  |
|  |  |  |  |  |  |  |  |

**Figure 24-7.** Sample format for a food diary.

## Food Frequency Questionnaire

Food frequency questionnaires, which list foods that clients rate as eating, for example, a certain number of times per day, week, or month, may be challenging for clients, because it can be difficult to truly estimate the number of times an individual food is eaten. However, the benefit of this tool is that the client is less likely to forget foods because they are listed on the chart. It is also easy to identify the type of diet the client typically follows (e.g., low-fat/high-fiber or high-protein/high-fat).

## Food Models and Portion Estimates

A portion is the amount of food a person chooses to eat, whereas a serving is a standardized amount of a food used to estimate and/or evaluate one's intake. Increases in portion sizes have been frequently cited as an important contributing factor to the growing rates in obesity seen over the past several decades.[17] Portions are difficult for some to estimate, and correct estimates could mean the difference between a 1,400-calorie diet and a 2,200-calorie diet (Fig. 24-8).

Fitness professionals can assist clients in a number of ways when estimating their portions. The guidelines presented in Table 24-2 can be used to help clients more accurately determine the amount of food that they are consuming.

## Estimating Caloric Needs

A variety of methods can be used to estimate a client's daily calorie needs. Daily energy needs (caloric requirement) are determined by three factors (Fig. 24-9):

- **Resting metabolic rate (RMR)**
- **Thermogenesis** (calories required for heat production)
- Physical activity

RMR is the amount of energy (measured in calories) expended by the body during quiet rest. RMR makes up between 60% and 75% of the total calories used

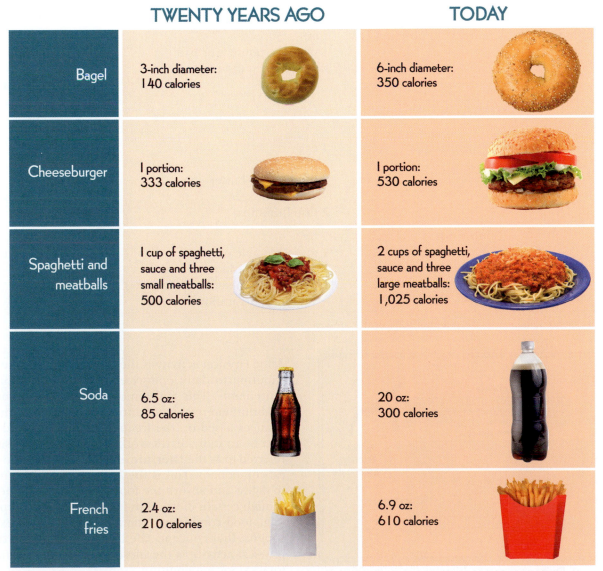

| | TWENTY YEARS AGO | TODAY |
|---|---|---|
| Bagel | 3-inch diameter: 140 calories | 6-inch diameter: 350 calories |
| Cheeseburger | 1 portion: 333 calories | 1 portion: 530 calories |
| Spaghetti and meatballs | 1 cup of spaghetti, sauce and three small meatballs: 500 calories | 2 cups of spaghetti, sauce and three large meatballs: 1,025 calories |
| Soda | 6.5 oz: 85 calories | 20 oz: 300 calories |
| French fries | 2.4 oz: 210 calories | 6.9 oz: 610 calories |

**Figure 24-8.** Increases in portion sizes have been frequently cited as an important contributing factor to the growing rates in obesity seen over the past several decades.

## Table 24-2. Estimating Portion Size

| FOOD GROUP | KEY MESSAGE | WHAT COUNTS? | LOOKS LIKE... |
| --- | --- | --- | --- |
| Grains | Make half your grains whole. | *1 oz equivalent:*<br>1 slice of bread<br>1 cup ready-to-eat cereal<br>½ cup cooked rice, pasta, or cooked cereal<br>5 whole-wheat crackers | <br>CD cover<br>A baseball<br>½ a baseball |
| Vegetables | Vary your veggies.<br>Make half your plate fruits and vegetables. | *1 cup:*<br>1 cup raw or cooked vegetables<br>2 cups raw leafy salad greens<br>1 cup vegetable juice | <br>Baseball<br>Softball |
| Fruits | Make half your plate fruits and vegetables. | *1 cup:*<br>1 cup raw fruit<br>½ cup dried fruit<br>1 cup 100% fruit juice | <br>Tennis ball<br>2 golf balls |
| Milk | Switch to fat-free or low-fat (1%) milk. | *1 cup:*<br>1 cup milk, yogurt, or soy milk<br>1.5 oz natural cheese or 2 oz processed cheese | <br>Baseball<br>1½ 9-volt batteries |
| Protein foods | Choose lean proteins. | *1 oz:*<br>1 oz meat, poultry, or fish<br>¼ cup cooked dry beans<br><br>1 egg<br><br>1 tbsp peanut butter<br>½ oz nuts or seeds<br>2 tbsp hummus | Deck of cards (3 oz) for lean meats; checkbook (3 oz) for fish<br>½ golf ball<br>½ of a Post-It note<br>Golf ball |
| Oils | Choose liquid oils and avoid solid fats. | *3 tsp:*<br>1 tbsp vegetable oils<br>½ medium avocado<br>1 oz peanuts, mixed nuts, cashews, almonds, or sunflower seeds | Tip of thumb |

For more specific amounts, please visit http://ChooseMyPlate.gov.

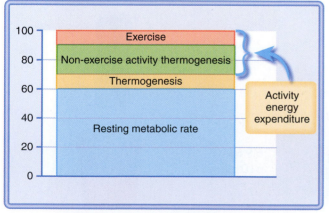

**Figure 24-9.** Daily energy needs (caloric requirement) are determined by three factors: resting metabolic rate (RMR), thermogenesis (calories required for heat production), and activity energy expenditure.

daily. Physical activity is the second largest factor contributing to daily energy expenditure or calorie requirements. This is the most variable component of 24-hour energy expenditure, because this number changes based on the frequency, intensity, and duration of an individual's workouts. Thermogenesis, also referred to as the **thermic effect of food**, is the smallest component. This is the amount of calories needed to digest and absorb the foods that are consumed. Although certain diets claim to enhance this component (e.g., food-combining programs), no research exists to support that concept. The bottom line is that regular physical activity is the most effective way to increase total caloric expenditure.

The following section reviews methods for determining a client's energy needs. This information does not, however, take into account a client's disease risk in relation to his or her weight or nutritional habits. For more information on how to use tools such as **waist-to-hip ratio** and **body mass index (BMI)**, see Chapter 23

There are numerous ways to calculate a client's daily caloric needs. The simplest method is to multiply the client's weight (in pounds) by the appropriate conversion factor (Table 24-3). This calculation will yield an approximation of how many calories the individual needs to maintain his or her current weight, based on activity level and sex.

Another useful method for calculating energy needs is to estimate RMR, taking into account weight, height, age, and sex, and then multiply that value by a conversion factor that takes into account physical activity. The Mifflin-St. Jeor equations[18–20] are commonly used for this purpose in overweight and obese individuals because they are more accurate for this population than for normal-weight individuals.

Use of the Mifflin-St. Jeor equations requires two steps:
- Step 1: Calculate RMR.
- Step 2: Calculate thermic effect of physical activity (TEPA), which includes the thermic effect of food (TEF).

RMR represents the energy needed by the body to perform its vital bodily functions (e.g., respiration, heart rate, brain activity, etc.). TEF represents the energy needed to chew, swallow, digest, absorb and store food. TEPA represents the energy used for exercise, activity and non-exercise activity thermogenesis (NEAT). NEAT denotes the energy expended for everything we do that does not include sleeping, eating, physical activity or exercise; and ranges from simple standing to fidgeting and moving about.

**Mifflin-St. Jeor Formulas:**
- For men: RMR = $(9.99 \times kg) + (6.25 \times cm) - (4.92 \times age) + 5$
- For women: RMR = $(9.99 \times kg) + (6.25 \times cm) - (4.92 \times age) - 161$

*Example:* Calculate RMR for an inactive 35-year-old woman participating in ~60 minutes of moderate-intensity activity 4×/week, who stands 5'4" (165 cm) and weighs 155 lbs. (70.45 kg):
- RMR = $(9.99 \times kg) + (6.25 \times cm) - (4.92 \times age) - 161$
- RMR = $703.8 + 1,031.2 - 172.2 - 161$

- RMR = 1,402 Kcal (energy needed to keep her body alive and functioning)

To calculate **Total Daily Energy Expenditure (TDEE)**, multiply the calculated RMR score by the selected **Standard Activity Factor Score (SAF)** presented in Table 20-4. These SAF scores provide a general estimate of the individual's activity level (primarily reflecting exercise activity). In this example, the activity level of our 35-year old would best be represented by the SAF score of 1.55. Her TDEE therefore equals:

$$TDEE = 1,402 \text{ kcal} \times 1.55 = 2,173 \text{ kcal per day}$$

*Note:* One inaccuracy that arises when using these mathematical formulas and SAF scores is that estimation of daily activity is based primarily upon the quantity and intensity of exercise, which may only represent a few hours of the week. Ideally, an activity factor score would weigh all activities of daily living and not simply exercise. For example, a person who exercises four 4 hours/ per week, but spends the balance of his or her waking hours seated at a computer terminal may expend fewer daily calories than if that person stood and actively moved about for eight 8 to 10 hours a day.

In addition to the previous estimation equations, another method called **indirect calorimetry** is used to predict RMR. Because oxygen is used in the metabolic process to create energy, a person's metabolic rate can be determined by measuring how much oxygen he or she consumes when breathing. A relation exists between the body's use of oxygen and the energy it expends, so scientists use formulas to convert gas usage into energy (calories) used. Historically, oxygen consumption measurements were only performed with a medical device called *metabolic cart,* which can cost between $20,000 and $50,000. Newer technology has made it possible to measure oxygen consumption using handheld devices, making the analysis more accessible and affordable.

## Simple Solutions

In light of this potential for significant error using quantitative measures to estimate a client's caloric/energy needs, it may be prudent to shift the focus away from outcomes (caloric balance and numbers) to the change process. Using simpler approaches to achieve goals empowers individuals to take charge of their own actions and decisions.

**Table 24-3. Conversion Factors for Estimating Daily Caloric Requirements Based on Gender and Activity Level**

| GENDER | ACTIVITY LEVEL* | | |
| --- | --- | --- | --- |
| | LIGHT | MODERATE | HEAVY |
| Male | 17 | 19 | 23 |
| Female | 16 | 17 | 30 |

*Light activity level: walking (level surface, 2.5–3.0 miles/hr), housecleaning, child care, golf; moderate activity level: walking (3.5–4.0 mph), cycling, skiing, tennis, dancing; heavy activity level: walking with a load uphill, basketball, climbing, football, soccer

## Table 24-4. Standard Activity Factor Scores to Estimate Total Daily Energy Expenditure

| ACTIVITY SCORE | ACTIVITY LEVEL | DESCRIPTION |
|---|---|---|
| 1.200 | Sedentary | Little or no physical activity (54% of U.S. population) up to ~30 minutes of moderate-intensity physical activity daily |
| 1.375 | Lightly active | Sedentary criteria + light-intensity exercise 1–3 days/week |
| 1.550 | Moderately active | Sedentary criteria + moderate-intensity exercise 3–5 days/week |
| 1.725 | Very active | Sedentary criteria + moderate- to vigorous-intensity exercise 6–7 days/week |
| 1.900 | Extremely active | Sedentary criteria + vigorous daily training or job that requires hard physical work/labor |

### DOING THE MATH:
### Mifflin-St. Jeor Equations for Estimating Daily Caloric Needs

- Men: $RMR = (9.99 \times weight) + (6.25 \times height) - (4.92 \times age) + 5$
- Women: $RMR = (9.99 \times weight) + (6.25 \times height) - (4.92 \times age) - 161$

Multiply the RMR value derived from the prediction equation by the appropriate activity correction factor:

- 1.200 = sedentary (little or no exercise)
- 1.375 = lightly active (light exercise/sports 1–3 days/week)
- 1.550 = moderately active (moderate exercise/sports 3–5 days/week)
- 1.725 = very active (hard exercise/sports 6–7 days/week)
- 1.900 = extra active (very hard exercise/sports and a physical job)

*Note:* This equation is more accurate for obese than nonobese individuals.

Using the Mifflin-St. Jeor equation for estimating RMR, help the following clients estimate the appropriate daily caloric intake range to support their moderately active lifestyles (1.550 × the calculated RMR).

**Client: William**
- Body weight: 176 lb (80 kg)
- Height: 6 feet (183 cm)
- Age: 40 years

$(9.99 \times 80 \text{ kg}) + (6.25 \times 183 \text{ cm}) - (4.92 \times 40) + 5 = 1,751$

$1,751 \times 1.550 = 2,714$ calories

**Client: Abby**
- Body weight: 135 lb (61 kg)
- Height: 5'7" (170 cm)
- Age: 37 years

$(9.99 \times 61 \text{ kg}) + (6.25 \times 170 \text{ cm}) - (4.92 \times 37) - 161 = 1,329$

$1,329 \times 1.550 = 2,060$ calories

Dr. James Levine[21] introduced a concept of a metabolic profile aimed at increasing nonexercise activity thermogenesis (NEAT), or spontaneous physical activity. This profile suggests that NEAT associated with occupation and leisure (e.g., going to work or school, performing household tasks, and ambulation) could increase energy expenditure and thus hold significant promise in combating the obesity epidemic. Dr. Levine's metabolic profile tool asks individuals to list their typical Monday through Friday and/or weekend schedule. This information is used qualitatively and not quantitatively to help individuals identify problematic areas throughout their day when they are sedentary and could consider making changes (i.e., increasing awareness to the type and amount of sedentary activities in a day).

Through this method, individuals can be encouraged to include simple, yet manageable tasks that increase overall expended calories. More importantly, this method allows individuals to identify problematic areas and then find their own solutions, building self-efficacy and intrinsic motivation while strengthening commitment for change. The idea is to help individuals develop a process to evaluate the efficacy of these NEAT challenges on a weekly basis.[22] For example, during a 4-hour bout at a computer terminal, explore opportunities to increase NEAT during bathroom and water/coffee breaks (walking to bathrooms or break rooms that are farther away) or with company meetings (walking meetings). Visit http://www.letsmove.gov for a variety of excellent ideas for improving NEAT. Greater levels of NEAT promote greater weight loss.[21]

## Using Caloric Information to Affect Weight

Once the client's daily calorie needs have been estimated, this information can be used to help the client lose, gain, or maintain weight. To change weight by 1 lb (0.45 kg), caloric intake must be decreased or increased by 3,500 calories. For weight loss, it is advisable to reduce caloric intake by 250 calories per day and to increase daily expenditure (through physical activity) by 250 calories. This 500-calorie difference, when multiplied by 7, creates a weekly negative

## RESEARCH HIGHLIGHT

### Obesity Related to Energy Expenditure from NEAT

The notion that obesity may be more related to energy expenditure related to NEAT than to energy expenditure related to exercise is supported by the literature. When positive energy balance is imposed through overfeeding, Levine and colleagues[23] demonstrated that obese subjects sat 2.5 hr/day more than lean subjects. The lean sedentary volunteers stood and walked for more than 2 hr/day longer than obese sedentary subjects, even though all subjects lived and worked in similar environments. Therefore, those who voluntarily increase their NEAT the most (primarily through walking) gain the least fat, and those who consume excess calories but do not increase their NEAT gain the most fat.[23] These researchers also calculated that if the obese subjects were to adopt the same activity patterns as the lean subjects, they could expend an additional 350 kcal/day because of their larger size. Thus, NEAT and specifically walking are of substantial energetic importance in obesity. It might seem obvious that because people with obesity are heavier, they sit more than lean people. However, these differences are not due to greater body weight alone, because when lean subjects gained weight through overfeeding, their tendency to stand/ambulate persisted, and when obese subjects became lighter, their tendency to sit did not change.[5] Research in this area supports the notion that perhaps peoples' environments need to be reengineered to promote NEAT. This argument makes sense, especially given the fact that despite the best efforts nationally, participation in physical activity is at an all-time low and obesity rates are at an all-time high.

In addition to promoting obesity, being sedentary throughout the day also has significant negative health implications. Research by Katzmarzyk and colleagues[24] examined the relation between mortality and the amount of time spent sitting (Fig. 24-10). After a 12-year period examining 17,013 subjects, they discovered that even in physically active individuals, a strong correlation exists between the amount of time spent sitting and mortality risk. They concluded that physical activity and exercise is insufficient in canceling out all of the ill effects of being sedentary. The authors suggest that too much sitting reduced high-density lipoprotein levels in the blood and decreased levels of lipoprotein lipase activity in body cells. These elevated circulating levels of fat in the blood resulted in an increased risk for cardiovascular risk.

Levine JA, Lannigham-Foster LM, McCrady SK, et al. Interindividual variation in posture allocation: Possible role in human obesity. *Science*. 2005;28:584–586.

Levine JA, Eberhardt NL, Jensen MD. Role of nonexercise activity thermogenesis in resistance to fat gain in humans. *Science*. 1999;283:212–214.

Katzmarzyk PT, Church TS, Craig CL, Bouchard C. Sitting time and mortality from all causes, cardiovascular disease and cancer. *Med Sci Sports Exerc*. 2009;41:998–1005.

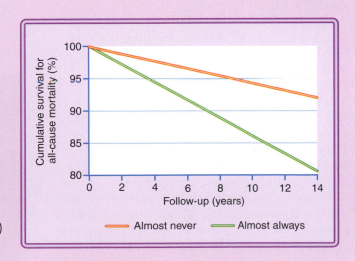

**Figure 24-10.** A dose–response relation exists between sitting time (almost never vs. almost always) and risk for mortality from all causes.

caloric balance that results in a loss of 1 lb (0.45 kg). These numbers can be doubled to achieve a weight loss of 2 lb (0.91 kg) per week, but that may be too great a goal for some clients. Most health organizations recommend a weight-loss rate of 1 to 2 lb (0.45–0.91 kg) per week.[12,16]

## EXERCISE PROGRAMMING FOR OVERWEIGHT AND OBESE CLIENTS

Most studies showing clinically significant weight loss (≥5% of body weight) demonstrate this with energy restriction (i.e., eating fewer calories) combined with physical activity to create a larger negative energy balance (i.e., more calories expended than consumed).[25] Research has found that physical activity lasting longer than 150 min/week has a minimal effect on weight loss.[25] In studies ranging from 12 weeks to 16 months in duration, physical activity lasting more than 150 min/week usually resulted in modest weight loss (defined as ~2–3 kg, or ~4.5–6.6 lb), with physical activity between 225 and 420 min/week resulting in the greatest weight loss (5–7.5 kg, or 11–16.5 lb).[25] The data indicate that moderate-intensity exercise is the preferred level of exertion. This correlates to 60% to 70% of maximal oxygen uptake and 11 to 13 on the ratings of perceived exertion scale (6–20 scale).

## Exercise Guidelines

Programming exercise for overweight and obese clients must take into consideration their unique needs because many of these individuals may be severely deconditioned and/or have orthopedic limitations. ACSM[26] and Donnelly[25] et al have published the following guidelines for overweight and obese clients[1]:

- Establish a reduction in initial body weight of at least 5% to 10% over 3 to 6 months.
- The primary mode of exercise should be aerobic activities with resistance exercise included as a supplemental activity.
- Non–weight-bearing activities are encouraged (to avoid orthopedic risk).
- Initial emphasis of the exercise training should be on duration and frequency (keeping intensity moderate and progressing gradually).
- Frequency of training should be 5 to 7 days per week.
- Progressively accumulate 250 to 300 min/week (~2,000 kcal/week) of moderate-intensity exercise for weight loss and prevention of weight gain.
- Create a negative energy balance of 500 to 1,000 kcal/day (which is equivalent to a 0.5–1 kg loss of weight per week). This reduction should be combined with a reduction in dietary fat to less than 30% of total energy intake.
- Include the use of behavior-management techniques (including relapse prevention).

The concept of **periodization**, which has its foundations in resistance training, is also encouraged when planning aerobic exercise for weight reduction. Periodization is based on an inverse relation between intensity (how hard) and volume (total repetitions) of training (see Chapter 16). With aerobic exercise, intensity can be individualized with percentage of maximal heart rate (%MHR), **maximal aerobic capacity (%VO$_2$max)**, or ratings of perceived exertion, where volume is differentiated by the duration of the session, as well as the frequency of sessions.

Following are some specific periodization suggestions that can be used to individualize the exercise design for optimizing weight loss during aerobic exercise:

- Incorporate frequent cardiorespiratory workouts that are low intensity for a longer duration.
- Include some cardiorespiratory workouts that are of higher intensity for a shorter period. This may best be realized with high-intensity, continuous training or with interval training. To avoid physiological and orthopedic stress and injury, complete only one higher-intensity workout per week.
- Incorporate various modes of training, often referred to as cross-training. The theory of multimode training (using two or more different modes of cardiorespiratory exercise) implies that by doing so the body is averted from getting overly fatigued and from overuse of the same muscles in the same movement patterns.[27] This helps to limit the occurrence of musculoskeletal system stress and aids in the prevention of muscle soreness and injuries. Therefore, theoretically, a person will be able to safely do more work, more frequently, which equates to higher total energy expenditure and fat utilization.[27]
- Vary the workout designs regularly (Fig. 24-11). Attempt to find a satisfactory method for each client or group exercise participant, so that cardiorespiratory workouts vary within each week, weekly, biweekly, or in any combination. Varying the workouts provides a new stimulus to the body's cardiorespiratory system in an effort to avoid the consequences of overuse exercise fatigue. Hans Selye demonstrated this "change the stimulus" concept, which he coined the **general adaptation syndrome**.[28]

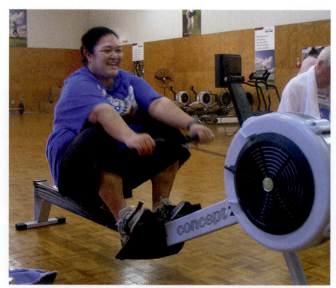

**Figure 24-11.** Varying the workouts provides a new stimulus to the body's cardiorespiratory system in an effort to avoid the consequences of overuse exercise fatigue.

## Biomechanical Considerations for Cardiorespiratory Exercise

The preferred type of cardiorespiratory exercise for overweight and obese individuals is a combination of weight-bearing (such as walking and elliptical exercise) and non–weight-bearing (such as cycling and swimming) modes. Exercise choices should be based on an individual's preferences and exercise history. Fitness professionals can help clients find modes of exercise with which they have a perceived comfort level with few (if any) negative barriers. The majority of the time exercising should be at a low intensity level to avoid joint stress and injury. Therefore, running, jumping, and high-impact types of movements are not recommended. These physical activities may lead to some musculoskeletal problems associated with body weight and impact forces from the repeated (and forceful) foot strikes on the ground surface.

The emphasis of the cardiorespiratory exercise programs should be on performing longer and/or more frequent bouts of exercise. It is important to monitor muscle soreness from the exercise and always ask the client if he or she is experiencing any orthopedic problems or discomfort. Stationary cycling is preferable to road cycling, because it eliminates any balance-related problems while also avoiding the hazards of traffic. Walking is considered a very good initial exercise because it requires no extra skill.

When beginning a walking or weight-bearing exercise regimen with a client, it is important to keep a few things in mind. Make sure the person has good fitness shoes. Obese and overweight individuals need high-quality fitness shoes with good shock-absorbing qualities.

Swimming and aquatic exercise programs provide total-body exercise with little to no weight-bearing due to the buoyancy of water. Buoyancy is also a benefit for overweight and obese people who may have joint problems (such as arthritis of the knee, hip, or ankle or structural problems of these three joints).

Fitness facilities now have a variety of exercise equipment for use. Personal trainers and other fitness professionals are encouraged to help clients find exercise devices that are easy to use and that do not cause any back, knee, or ankle discomfort. For instance, recumbent bikes are good cycling options for obese individuals as compared with stationary or road cycling. However, make sure the bike seat is comfortable for the overweight or obese client. Elliptical machines are also good choices for obese clients who can tolerate weight-bearing load because the nonimpact nature of elliptical training may be less punitive to knees compared with other forms of weight-bearing exercise such as walking. For some obese clients, balance will be an additional challenge with some modes of exercise. If this is the case, select exercise devices that have handrails to avoid falling.

## Resistance Training

The increase in muscle mass from resistance exercise has been shown to elevate RMR in some individuals. Most resistance-training programs elicit an increased fat **oxidation** (burning) after the workout (as the body uses additional energy to restore cell processes to homeostasis).[25] Exercise programs that combine aerobic training and resistance exercise exhibit superior results in weight and fat loss. In "diet plus resistance training" programs, the addition of resistance training promotes the preservation and/or increase in fat-free mass (FFM).[25]

Thus, one of the noteworthy benefits of resistance exercise as it relates to body composition in overweight populations is the positive impact of maintaining, or increasing, fat-free body mass while encouraging the loss of fat body weight in a progressive overload resistance-training program. Therefore, any resistance-training program design for overweight and obese persons should be meaningful to the overall health and goals of the client, and an adjunct to the cardiovascular program for weight loss.

## RESEARCH HIGHLIGHT

### Walking Effort of Obese Compared with Nonobese Women

Mattsson, Larsson, and Rossner[29] have presented some useful data about walking among the obese female population. The most interesting finding of this study was that level walking was much harder work for obese women as compared with normal-weight women. On average, obese women used as much as 56% $VO_2$max during walking as compared with 36% $VO_2$max for normal-weight women. The authors noted that even though obese women do not necessarily walk with a waddle or straddled legs, they do walk with an abnormal gait pattern that increases their relative oxygen cost. The authors conclude that walking for some obese individuals may be too exhausting (and sometimes painful) because of these biomechanical differences in gait, and they recommend incorporating alternative training modes of exercise in the workout design.[29]

Mattsson E, Larsson UE, Rossner S. Is walking for exercise too exhausting for obese women? *Int J Obes Metab Disord.* 1996;21:380–386.

## In Your Own Words

As part of your fitness facility's orientation to new members, an initial fitness evaluation is offered, which includes a skinfold body composition assessment. Jarrod, a new member, has signed up with you for the orientation and has just arrived for the appointment. By observation, it is clear that Jarrod is obese, and he confides in you that he is uncomfortable being assessed. How would you talk with Jarrod about his concerns?

## Biomechanical Considerations for Resistance Training

There are some biomechanical concerns to note with resistance exercise and overweight and obese persons. For some overweight and obese individuals, as well as older individuals and those with mobility and/or balance challenges, seated exercises are good options. These types of exercises can be useful in building basic muscle strength. While seated in a chair, individuals are able to do a variety of arm raises, leg lifts, and "bending" stretches. However, the seats on some exercise machines were not designed for large persons, which may limit the feasibility of using some strength-training equipment. In addition, weight benches are typically quite narrow, which could result in the loss of balance for some clients.

Another concern involves getting into and out from some resistance-training devices, which may be difficult because of the size of a client's belly. Sometimes it is preferable not to use exercise devices that are close to the floor (such as some abdominal devices) because an overweight person may have great difficulty getting down to and up from the floor.

In addition, certain supine exercises may cause breathing difficulty for some obese clients (inhibiting the passage of air); always check that a client's breathing is regular and uninterrupted during all exercises.

Prudence should be taken in doing too much lunge and squat work with overweight persons, because of possible knee and back discomfort and injury.

## Realistic Goals and Realistic Obstacles

In any type of programming, realistic goals can only come from a realistic examination of the obstacles to health-behavior change. The two main steps to this process are:

1. Discover the potential obstacles to achieving the client's goals.
2. Help the client find solutions to navigate the obstacles before he or she faces them.

Common obstacles to health-behavior change can be either internal or external. Internal obstacles relate to a client's attitudes, opinions, thoughts, feelings, and self-talk about health, fitness, exercise, or nutrition. External obstacles can include time, family, and work responsibilities.

The key to success, regardless of the obstacles in the way, is to develop solutions before problems appear. That way, the client develops improved reactions to challenges that are more in line with health goals. Another reason this is essential in the initial stages of a program is that this provides the client with the opportunity to think of solutions when not actually facing the obstacle. When facing an obstacle that has historically thrown the client off course from his or her health goals, the most familiar path will be the one that is taken unless a different response has been planned.

Through facilitation by health and fitness professionals, the client can gain confidence from the knowledge that there has been a different solution created in collaboration with a competent, caring professional. Often the boost to morale that comes from this is enough to provide the client with the motivation to successfully work through an obstacle. Simply altering the familiar path of facing obstacles alone with effective coping strategies is enough to enhance the client's ability to

---

### RESEARCH HIGHLIGHT

#### Resistance Training Can Promote Increased Resting Metabolic Rate

In as soon as 6 months, a program of regular resistance exercise training can contribute to significant increases in RMR, even in previously sedentary, deconditioned individuals. Hunter et al[30] conducted a 26-week resistance-training study with beginning, sedentary, older (61–77 years) men (n = 7) and women (n = 8).[31] Subjects completed supervised workouts consisting of 2 sets of 10 repetitions (with 2 minutes of rest between each set). The resistance exercises were elbow flexion, elbow extension, lateral pull-down, seated row, chest press, leg extension, leg curl, seated press, back extensions, bent-leg sit-ups (15–25 repetitions), and squats or leg presses (as determined by the supervising exercise physiologist). The subjects trained at an intensity within 65% to 80% of their one-repetition maximum. Progressive overload was carefully integrated in the program after reviewing daily training logs and retesting of the one-repetition maximum every 3 weeks. At the end of this 6-month investigation, male and female subjects increased their RMR by 7%, which was approximately an additional 100 calories per day.[31]

Hunter RR, Wetzstein CJ, Fields DA, Brown A, Bamman MM. Resistance training increases total energy expenditure and free-living physical activity in older adults. *J Appl Physiol.* 2000;89:977–984.

successfully navigate challenges that had previous derailed his or her efforts.

## Preventing Weight Regain

Many individuals are capable of losing weight, but maintaining a reduced body weight is a long-standing challenge. Consistent physical activity is the best predictor of sustained weight management after weight loss[25]; and when it comes to preventing weight gain, "more is better." Some research specifies that individuals who lost more than 10% of their body weight in 24 months were participating in 275 minutes of physical activity a week.[25] For best practices and outcomes, Donnelly et al[25] recommend 250 to 300 min/week (~2,000 kcal/week) of moderate-intensity exercise for prevention of weight gain.

## MEDICAL TREATMENT OF OBESITY

In an effort to decrease the health impact of obesity and provide individuals with medical options for weight loss, medications have been developed to block fat absorption, increase energy expenditure, and suppress appetite. Surgical procedures have also been created to treat morbid obesity. The following sections provide a brief review of weight-loss medications and bariatric procedures.

## Medications and Physiological Responses

Hickey and Israel[33] note that nearly 300 clinical trials are researching some aspect of obesity.[13] However, currently, only two drugs have been approved by the U.S. Food and Drug Administration for long-term treatment of obesity: sibutramine (Meridia) and orlistat (Xenical, or over the counter as alli).

Sibutramine prevents the removal of norepinephrine and serotonin in the brain, thereby prolonging some of their effects. For example, serotonin and norepinephrine act as appetite suppressants in the brain. Thus, sibutramine acts to prolong these hunger-suppressing effects. Research on sibutramine shows that it averages about 10 lb (~4.45 kg) greater weight loss compared with a placebo over the course of 1-year treatments.[21] The research on sibutramine suggests that it is relatively safe, minimally elevating heart rate (4 beats/min) and blood pressure (2–4 mm Hg for both systolic and diastolic pressure). A minor increase of high-density lipoprotein (the healthy cholesterol) and a small decrease in triglycerides have also been shown. No research exists beyond 2 years with the use of sibutramine.

The primary function of orlistat is to prevent the absorption of fats from the diet, thereby reducing caloric intake. It is intended for use in combination with a physician-supervised, reduced-calorie diet. Orlistat is successful at blocking approximately 30% of dietary fat absorption.[13] Over the course of a year, the use of orlistat averages about a 6.5 lb (~2.89 kg) greater weight

## FROM THEORY TO PRACTICE

### ■ CREATE A WAKING DAY "METABOLIC PROFILE"

One new way for exercise professionals to integrate lifestyle movement into the life of a client is to create a waking day "metabolic profile." A waking day metabolic profile timeline is an awareness index for the client to realize how much sitting he or she is doing on a daily basis. The goal of this process is to incorporate episodes of lifestyle physical activity during sustained sitting times in a person's daily life.[32] Health and exercise professionals can help the client identify the sustained seated times of the day and then provide interventions to add physical activity during those periods.

For example, the waking day metabolic profile of a client indicates that she works (Monday–Friday) at a desktop computer workstation for 4 hours in the morning and 4 hours in the afternoon, and watches TV and reads for 2 hours each night. Some lifestyle physical activity options to try to break up the sustained sitting periods at work might include:

- Stand up and walk around the office every 30 minutes.
- Stand up and move every time the client needs to get some water.
- Stand and/or walk around the room when talking on the telephone.
- Take a 5-minute walk break with every coffee break.

Some lifestyle physical activity intervention suggestions to break up the 2-hour time frame of watching TV and reading are as follows:

- Get up and move during every commercial.
- Get up and move around the room every 30 minutes.
- Stand up and do some easy (i.e., not strenuous) lunges or squats at least once per half hour.
- Stand up and move for the opening segment of each TV show.
- At the end of reading every 10 to 12 pages, get up to walk around the room or house.

loss compared with a placebo.[13] However, orlistat has been shown to have considerable gastrointestinal adverse effects, including abdominal pain, diarrhea, flatulence, bloating, and upset stomach.[13] The long-term research on orlistat is yet to be published.

Clearly, a great deal more needs to be learned about the interplay of food intake and the complex biological, neuroendocrine, and physiological mechanisms of the human body. Although much research is being conducted in this area, simple solutions do not appear to be forthcoming in the near future. In addition, Hickey and Israel[33] note that the **pathogenesis** (disease development) of obesity is multifaceted and likely to vary between individuals.[13] This suggests that the idea of one "super pill" for overweight and obesity treatment is fairly unlikely. In addition, it is hoped that any obesity medications be administered along with lifestyle changes that involve behavior modification, exercise, and healthful food consumption.

## Surgical Interventions

**Bariatrics** is the branch of medicine that deals with the causes, prevention, and treatment of obesity. The term *bariatrics* comes from the Greek root *baro* (weight) and suffix *iatrics* (a branch of medicine). Surgical treatment of obesity is suggested to be appropriate only for those individuals with BMIs ≥40 kg/m² or with BMI ≥35 kg/m² in the presence of **comorbidities** (one or more disorders [or diseases] in addition to a primary disease—obesity).[1]

The **gastric bypass** and **vertical banded gastroplasty** are two procedures that have been performed to treat obesity. In the vertical band procedure, a band mechanically restricts food intake, creating an early sense of satiety that limits intake. Because of the higher-than-expected complication rate, vertical banded gastroplasty is no longer routinely performed. The gastric bypass involves separating a small pouch of the stomach with a line of staples and reconnecting it to the small intestine to dramatically limit food intake. Bariatric surgery results in a 30% (gastric bypass) and 25% (vertical banded gastroplasty) average reduction of initial weight.[34] Improvements of mood, hypertension, asthma, sleep apnea, and diabetes have also been observed.[1] Clinical trials suggest that gastric bypass surgery is associated with much better weight-loss maintenance than vertical banded gastroplasty. This is because patients who eat high-fat or high-sugar meals tend to have more stomach cramping and gastrointestinal distress (with gastric bypass surgery), and thus avoid these foods to evade this discomfort. Naturally, before any type of bariatric procedure, patients need to be rigorously screened to determine whether there are any medical or behavioral contraindications to the surgery.

## FROM THEORY TO PRACTICE

### ■ STEPS TO ATTAIN A HEALTHY BODY WEIGHT

#### CLIENT 1

Your client is a 35-year-old woman who has no cardiovascular disease risk factors. She is currently a sedentary person who would like to start exercising to lose some body fat. Her body weight is 150 lb. Her height is 5'4".

#### STEPS TO ATTAIN A HEALTHY BODY WEIGHT

- Determine the client's percent body fat (%BF) using an accessible body composition assessment method (i.e., skinfold measurements, hydrostatic weighing, or bioelectrical impedance). Client 1's %BF was estimated with bioelectrical impedance to be 30%. *Note:* This tells us that 70% of this person's weight is FFM.
- Calculate the client's FFM in pounds: FFM = 150 lb × 0.70 = 105 lb
- Establish your initial %BF target goal for this client's weight-management program. For an initial goal, try to guide the client to attain 27% body fat, which is a goal of 73% FFM.
- Divide the client's present FFM by %FFM goal to obtain the target body weight: 105 lb/0.73 = 144 lb
- Calculate the weight-loss goal by subtracting target body weight from present body weight: 150 lb – 144 lb = 6 lb. Assuming that the lost weight will be fat, the goal for this client is to lose 6 lb of fat to be 27% body fat.
- Because l lb of body fat is 3,500 calories, determine how much of a caloric deficit to create on a daily basis. *Note:* The absolute dietary energy intake should be adjusted (with dietary restriction and increased physical activity) based on the body to elicit an energy deficit of approximately 500 to 1,000 kcal/day.[14] You can begin by establishing a 250-kilocalorie restriction for the client's diet and a 250-kilocalorie expenditure/day physical activity program. This creates a 500-kilocalorie deficit total each day.
- How long will it take for the client to lose the initial goal of 6 lb? 500 kcal/day × 7 days/week = 3,500 kcal/week or 1 lb/week. Therefore, in 6 weeks the client will have lost 6 lb of fat.

#### CLIENT 2

Client 2 is 42-year-old male who has prehypertension (138/88 mm Hg). He is currently a sedentary person and his doctor wants him to lose some weight and start exercising. His body weight is 180 lb. His height is 5'6".

## FROM THEORY TO PRACTICE–cont'd

### STEPS TO ATTAIN A HEALTHY BODY WEIGHT

- Determine the client's %BF using an accessible body-composition assessment method (i.e., skinfold measurements, hydrostatic weighing, or bioelectrical impedance). This individual's %BF was calculated with skinfold measurements to be 32%. What percentage of this person's body weight is FFM?
- Calculate the client's FFM in pounds.
- Establish the initial target %BF goal for this client. For this example, set the target %BF goal at 28% body fat. What then is the goal % for FFM?
- Divide the client's present FFM by %FFM goal to obtain the target body weight.
- Calculate target weight loss by subtracting the target body weight from present body weight.
- Because l lb of body fat is 3,500 calories, determine how much of a caloric deficit (with diet and exercise) to create on a daily basis.
- Establish a 350-kilocalorie restriction to the client's diet and a 300-kilocalorie expenditure through a daily physical activity program.
- After establishing this 650-kilocalorie deficit, how long will it take the client to attain this goal weight?

### CHECK YOUR ANSWERS

- What % of this person's body weight is FFM? 100% – 32% = 68% FFM
- Calculate the client's FFM in pounds. FFM = 180 lb × 0.68 = 122 lb
- What then is the goal % for FFM? With an initial target goal of 28% BF, the goal % of FFM is 100% – 28% = 72%, or 0.72.
- Divide the client's present FFM by the goal %FFM to obtain the target body weight. 122 lb/0.72 = 169 lb
- Calculate target weight loss by subtracting the target body weight from present body weight. 180 lb – 169 lb = 11 lb to lose
- Establish a 350-kilocalorie restriction to the client's diet and a 300-kilocalorie expenditure through a daily physical activity program.
- After establishing this 650-kilocalorie deficit, how long will it take the client to attain this goal weight? 650 kcal/day × 7 days/week = 4,550 kcal/week; 4,550 kcal/3,500 kcal = 1.3 lb to be lost each week. So in 8.5 weeks (11 lb × 1 wk/1.3 lb = 8.5 wk), the client will have attained the new healthy goal weight of 169 lb.

## VIGNETTE *conclusion*

■ After 12 weeks of working with Opal, Sarita is thrilled to have met her initial 16-pound weight-loss goal. She still fills out her daily nutrition log, but now also completes a physical-activity log that she and Opal review at their weekly sessions. Only 12 weeks earlier, Sarita struggled to walk for 15 minutes on the treadmill during her first session. She is now walking for 30 minutes 4 days a week, performing total-body resistance-training workouts twice each week, and just recently added a Saturday morning yoga class to her routine. She loves the camaraderie of the class setting, and her confidence is higher than ever. While Sarita's self-determination and perseverance are certainly the primary reasons for her success, she attributes Opal's attention to detail, willingness to start slowly, and individualized programming with getting her started in the right direction.

## CRITICAL THINKING QUESTIONS

1. Vincent is an overweight 38-year-old who wants to work with a fitness professional to help him overcome his frustration with becoming more physically active and losing weight. He has a difficult time sticking with a fitness program because as he puts it, "I never felt accepted in PE classes or sports activities as a kid because other students would make fun of my weight, and I've never been able to achieve my goal of losing 50 pounds." What would a prudent fitness professional do to help Vincent improve his self-efficacy with exercise?

2. Gemma is a 45-year-old recently divorced mother of two who just moved to a new city to start a new job. She just found out that one of her children will need special medical therapy to deal with a chronic health condition and that her new job requires that she is "on call" during three 24-hour blocks at a time. Gemma is also considering changing her eating habits and starting a new exercise program to help her deal with the mounting stress she is experiencing. According to the theory of limited self-control, what are the factors in Gemma's situation that may or may not help her achieve her nutrition and exercise goals?

3. Louis is a computer programmer who sits at his desk at least 9 hours each day and enjoys playing video games during his time away from work. Essentially, he gets no physical activity and reports that he has no time in his schedule to exercise. How can Louis increase his daily physical activity without making a commitment to a structured exercise program?

## ADDITIONAL RESOURCES

*Dietary Guidelines for Americans,* which are published every 5 years by the USDA, encourage most Americans to eat fewer calories, be more active, and make informed food choices. The complete guidelines can be found at http://dietaryguidelines.gov.

ChooseMyPlate (http://ChooseMyPlate.gov) presents a simplified approach to nutrition and food group recommendations, and breaks down food groups by balancing the correct portions of each food group on a plate for an easy visual.

http://www.letsmove.gov offers excellent ideas for improving NEAT.

## REFERENCES

1. Fabricatore AN, Wadden TA. Treatment of obesity. *Clin Diabet.* 2003;21:67–72.
2. World Health Organization. *Overweight and obesity.* Available at: http://who.int/mediacentre/factsheets/fs311/en. Accessed July 4, 2011.
3. Van Gaal LF. Dietary treatment of obesity. In: Bray G, Bouchard C, James WPT, eds. *Handbook of Obesity.* New York: Marcel Dekker, 2003; 875–890.
4. Casazza K, Fontaine KR, Astrup A, et al. Myths, presumptions, and facts about obesity. *N Engl J Med.* 2013;368:446–454.
5. Levine JA, Lannigham-Foster LM, McCrady SK, et al. Interindividual variation in posture allocation: Possible role in human obesity. *Science.* 2005;28:584–586.
6. Bandura A. *Social Foundations of Thought and Action: A Social Cognitive Theory.* Englewood Cliffs, NJ: Prentice Hall; 1986.
7. Bandura A. Self-efficacy: Toward a unifying theory of behavioral change. *Psychol Rev.* 1977;84:191–215.
8. Janis IL, Mann L. *Decision Making.* New York: Macmillan; 1979.
9. Polivy J, Herman CP. The false-hope syndrome: Unfulfilled expectations of self-change. *Curr Dir Psychol Sci.* 2000;9:128–131.
10. Buehler R, Griffin D, Ross M. Exploring the "planning fallacy": Why people underestimate their task completion times. *J Pers Soc Psychol.* 1994;67:366–381.
11. Costain L, Croker H. Helping individuals to help themselves. *Proc Nutr Soc.* 2005;64:89–96.
12. Wing RR, Phelan S. Long-term weight loss maintenance. *Am J Clin Nutr.* 2005;82(suppl):222S–225S.
13. Jakicic JM, Clark K, Coleman E, et al; American College of Sports Medicine. American College of Sports Medicine position stand. Appropriate intervention strategies for weight loss and prevention of weight regain for adults. *Med Sci Sports Exerc.* 2001;33:2145–2156.
14. Kravitz L. Multi-mode training for optimal exercise performance. *Austr Fitness Netw.* 2003;16:43–46.
15. Srikanthan P, Seeman TE, Karlamangla AS. Waist-hip-ratio as a predictor of all-cause mortality in high-functioning older adults. *Ann Epidemiol.* 2009;19:724–731.
16. U.S. Department of Agriculture. *Dietary Guidelines for Americans.* 2010. Available at: http://dietaryguidelines.gov
17. Ello-Martin JA, Ledikwe JH, Rolls BJ. The influence of food portion size and energy density on energy intake: Implications for weight management. *Am J Clin Nutr.* 2005;82(1 Suppl.):236S–241S.
18. Frankenfield D, Roth-Yousey L, & Compher C. Comparison of predictive equations for resting metabolic rate in healthy nonobese and obese adults: A systematic review. *J Am Diet Assoc.* 2005;105:775–789.
19. Mifflin MD, St Jeor ST, Hill LA, Scott BJ, Daugherty SA, Koh YU. A new predictive equation for resting energy expenditure in unhealthy individuals. *Am J Clin Nutr.* 1990;51:241–247.
20. Frankenfield DC, Rowe WA, Smith JS, Cooney RN. Validation of several established equations for resting metabolic rate in obese and non-obese people. *J Am Diet Assoc.* 2003; 103: 1,152-1,159.
21. Levine J. *Move a Little, Lose a Lot.* New York: Three Rivers Press; 2009.
22. Miller WR, Rollnick S. *Motivational Interviewing.* 2nd ed. New York: The Guilford Press; 2002.
23. Levine JA, Eberhardt NL, Jensen MD. Role of nonexercise activity thermogenesis in resistance to fat gain in humans. *Science.* 1999;283:212–214.

24. Katzmarzyk PT, Church TS, Craig CL, Bouchard C. Sitting time and mortality from all causes, cardiovascular disease and cancer. *Med Sci Sports Exerc.* 2009;41:998–1005.

25. Donnelly JE, Blair SN, Jakicic JM, Manore MM, Rankin JW, Smith BK. Appropriate physical activity intervention strategies for weight loss and prevention of weight regain for adults. *Med Sci Sports Exerc.* 2009;41:459–471.

26. American College of Sports Medicine. *ACSM's Guidelines for Exercise Testing and Prescription.* 9th ed. Philadelphia, PA: Wolters Kluwer/Lippincott Williams & Wilkins; 2014.

27. Loos RJF, Bouchard C. Obesity—is it a genetic disorder? *J Int Med.* 2003;254:401–425.

28. Selye H. Forty years of stress research: Principal remaining problems and misconceptions. *Can Med Assoc.* 1976;115:53–56.

29. Mattsson E, Larsson UE, Rossner S. Is walking for exercise too exhausting for obese women? *Int J Obes Metab Disord.* 1996;21:380–386.

30. Hunter RR, Wetzstein CJ, Fields DA, Brown A, Bamman MM. Resistance training increases total energy expenditure and free-living physical activity in older adults. *J Appl Physiol.* 2000;89:977–984.

31. Kravitz L. The 25 most significant health benefits of physical activity and exercise. *IDEA Fitness J.* 2007;4:54–63.

32. Hamilton MT, Healy GN, Dunstan DW, Zderic TW, Owen NO. Too little exercise and too much sitting: Inactivity physiology and the need for new recommendations on sedentary behavior. *Curr Cardiovasc Risk Rep.* 2008;2:292–298.

33. Hickey MS, Israel RG. Obesity drugs and drugs in the pipeline. *ACSM Health Fitness J.* 2007;11:20–25.

34. Karmali S, Stoklossa CJ, Sharma A, et al. Bariatric surgery: A primer. *Can Fam Physician.* 2010;56:873–879.

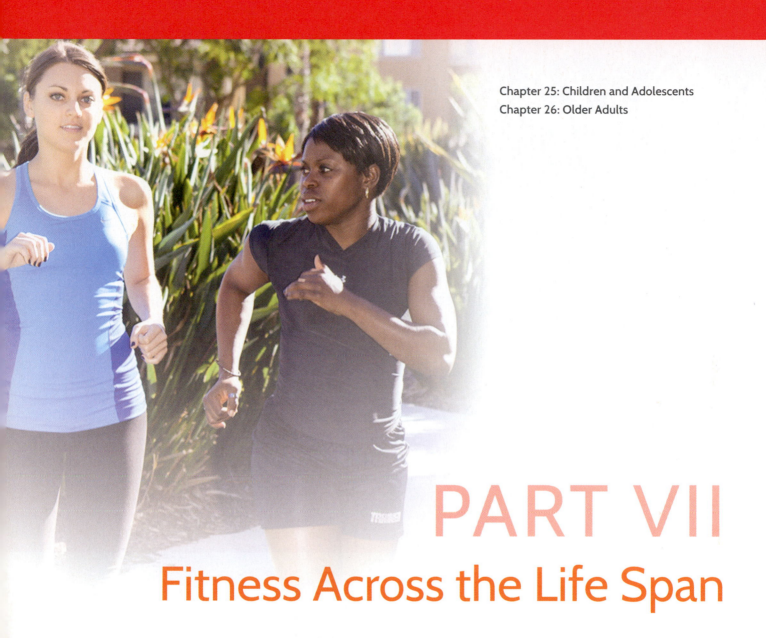

# PART VII
## Fitness Across the Life Span

This portion of the text provides information relative to exercising during all decades of life. Chapter 25 covers the growth and maturation processes in young exercisers and how they impact many of the training principles presented earlier in the book. Program design considerations for young exercisers are presented, especially as they relate to health and safety issues. Chapter 26 deals specifically with the physiological changes associated with aging that can impact the acute and chronic adaptations to exercise training in older adults. Specific programming guidelines for older adults are presented that focus on maximizing the enjoyment, safety, and effectiveness of training programs for this population.

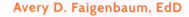

Avery D. Faigenbaum, EdD

CHAPTER 25

# Children and Adolescents

## CHAPTER OUTLINE

## LEARNING OUTCOMES

1. Describe the problem of physical inactivity and obesity in today's youth.
2. Explain the influence of growth and development on physiological functions.
3. Describe the differences in the metabolic and cardiorespiratory responses to exercise between children and adults.
4. Describe the neuromuscular adaptations to resistance training in children and adolescents.
5. Identify the health- and fitness-related benefits of regular physical activity in youth.
6. Describe program design considerations for children and adolescents.
7. List age-appropriate strategies to promote physical activity in youth with different needs, goals, and abilities.

## ANCILLARY LINK

Visit DavisPlus at http://davisplus.fadavis.com for study and practice resources, including online quizzes, animations that help explain physiological processes, podcasts concerning news and career trends in exercise physiology, and practice references.

## VIGNETTE

■ Jennifer is a group fitness instructor who specializes in working with children. In the after-school program she runs at a local recreation center, Jennifer leads children of all ages and physical capabilities through group exercise routines, small-group personal training, and noncompetitive games that foster teamwork and involve aerobic activity. During enrollment, Jennifer meets Mr. and Mrs. Greenberg, the parents of an obese 12-year-old boy named Jacob. They have been reading a lot about the long-term risks of childhood obesity and are eager to enlist Jennifer's help in getting their child on track to a healthier lifestyle.

The first thing Jennifer does is conduct an interview with Jacob's parents, during which she learns that Mr. and Mrs. Greenberg have been trying to address his lack of physical activity at home by having Jacob complete 30 minutes of walking on the treadmill every day after school. He has been complaining that this is "boring," and his behavior has been adversely affected by the constant arguing about exercise.

What should Jennifer do to help Jacob and his parents address the important issue of Jacob's long-term health and well-being?

Over the past quarter century, the prevalence of overweight and obesity among children and adolescents has become a major public health concern, and weight-related health problems are being diagnosed with increasing frequency in younger populations. The economic costs associated with escalating medical expenses are mounting, and the deleterious effects of childhood obesity and physical inactivity on lifelong health and well-being are incalculable.

Physical inactivity is recognized as the fourth leading risk factor for global mortality for noncommunicable diseases after hypertension, tobacco use, and high blood glucose.[1] Clearly, an infrastructure must be created and sustained that promotes healthy lifestyles for all individuals, particularly children and adolescents who need to develop the competence and confidence in their abilities to be physically active. This chapter describes the basic growth and development cycles of youth, as well as this population's physiological responses to exercise. Program design considerations for children and adolescents, and strategies for implementing youth-centered programming are also presented.

## PHYSICAL ACTIVITY IN THE YOUTH POPULATION

In 2010, the American Council on Exercise joined forces with the White House, the U.S. Department of Health and Human Services, the U.S. Department of Education, and the U.S. Department of Agriculture to reduce childhood obesity and promote regular physical activity among younger populations. This type of collaboration highlights the magnitude of this public health concern and emphasizes the importance of health-care providers, government officials, pediatric researchers, school teachers, and health and fitness professionals working together to improve the health and well-being of children and adolescents.

But how much physical activity do children really need, and what type of physical activity may prevent the development of risk factors and pathological processes later in life? How does the cardiorespiratory and musculoskeletal machinery of youth differ from that of adults, and how do these differences influence the design of pediatric fitness programs? Finally, what factors motivate boys and girls to be physically active (Fig. 25-1), and how

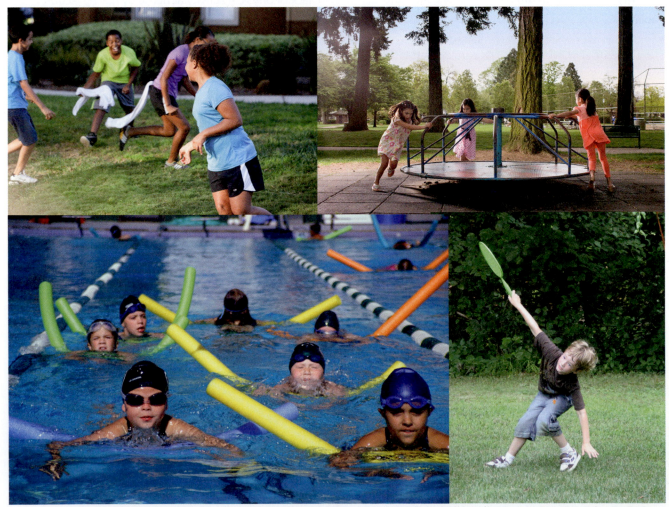

**Figure 25-1.** Youth physical activity is characterized by short, vigorous bouts of play followed by brief rest periods as needed. Having fun is a primary motivator for children.

can health and fitness professionals develop youth programs that promote physical activity as an ongoing lifestyle choice? Watching boys and girls on a playground supports the premise that youth are active in different ways and for different reasons than adults. Youth physical activity is characterized by short, vigorous bouts of play followed by brief rest periods as needed, and having fun is a primary motivator for children. Consequently, the adult exercise programming paradigm and coaching philosophy are inappropriate and at times inconsistent with the needs, interests, and abilities of children and most adolescents.

The physiology of children is dynamic, and youth are in a constant state of change. Throughout childhood and adolescence, the developing body is evolving physically, psychologically, and socially into a mature adult. All markers of physical fitness, including peak oxygen consumption ($\dot{V}O_2$), muscle strength, and sprint speed, are in a constant state of transformation during this temporal journey. Although some physiological markers (e.g., maximal cardiac output) reflect an increase in size of the left ventricle, other measures (e.g., glycolytic capacity) are independent of changes in body dimensions. Moreover, children of the same chronological age can exhibit striking differences in their rates of biological maturation.

Health and fitness professionals who work with children and adolescents need to be cognizant of the physical and psychosocial uniqueness of youth, and be attentive to the developmental diversity among younger participants. These issues are critically important for optimizing training adaptations, creating an enjoyable experience, and sparking a lifelong interest in physical activity. In addition, an understanding of pediatric exercise science has preventative implications. The promotion of regular physical activity during childhood and adolescence has become an attractive strategy for ameliorating future health risks later in life. Such efforts, however, have become more challenging as fitness practitioners continue to define effective age-appropriate strategies for altering sedentary behaviors among contemporary youth.

Important terms used in this chapter are defined in Box 25-1.

## VIGNETTE continued

■ Jennifer establishes two primary goals for the first few weeks of Jacob's participation in her after-school program. The first is to develop a program that increases Jacob's confidence in his ability to be physically active. The second—and this should be the ultimate objective of any health and fitness professional working with children—is to help establish a pattern of fun and effective physical activity that will spark a lifelong interest in exercise.

It is clear to Jennifer that Jacob's parents, although they certainly have the best intentions, do not understand how children typically perform physical activity. Walking for 30 consecutive minutes is simply not something most children enjoy. In addition, because most of the games that the children play during her group sessions involve walking or running, Jennifer decides to modify games and activities during small-group personal training to enhance motor skill proficiency while having fun. After a few weeks of replacing his treadmill walking with age-appropriate games and skill-building activities, Jacob has enhanced his activity level and seems to enjoy playing with his friends.

## GROWTH AND DEVELOPMENT

Children and adolescents have different needs than adults and are active in different ways. No matter how big, strong, or coordinated a child is, boys and girls are still growing and are typically experiencing many activities for the very first time. Moreover, measures of health and fitness are in a constant state of change during childhood and adolescence, which makes it more challenging to distinguish maturational differences in physiological measures from training-induced gains in physical fitness.

Sprint speed, for example, normally improves throughout childhood and adolescence even without participation in a structured training program. Comparing the 100-meter dash time of an 8-year-old child with a 16-year-old adolescent supports the premise

### Box 25-1. Terms and Definitions

*Adolescence:* A period between childhood and adulthood that includes girls aged 12 to 18 years and boys aged 14 to 18 years

*Children:* Boys and girls who have not yet developed secondary sex characteristics (roughly up to the age of 11 in girls and 13 in boys)

*Exercise:* A type of physical activity that is planned and regular (*Note:* The term *exercise* in this chapter does not suggest that free play during childhood is inconsequential, but rather emphasizes the premise that habitual physical activity needs to be programmed for children and adolescents.)

*Pediatric:* Both children and adolescents

*Physical activity:* Any bodily movement produced by skeletal muscle that results in energy expenditure

*Youth:* Both children and adolescents

that physical measures will improve over time as a result of growth and maturation. But if an 8-year-old child participates in a well-designed fitness program that includes plyometrics and resistance training, it is likely that sprint performance will improve beyond gains due to growth and development.

## Age, Maturation, and Training

Figure 25-2 illustrates the possible outcomes of fitness training in younger populations. The blue line represents normal development as a result of growth and maturation, whereas the orange line illustrates training-induced gains that are possible with fitness training. A child who participates regularly in a fitness program will have better performance at any age when compared with an age-matched peer who does not engage in fitness training or sports conditioning. Furthermore, it is reasonable to assume that children who develop confidence and competence in their abilities to be physically active are building a foundation for even greater gains during adulthood.

The green line is an example of what could happen if the cumulative stress from fitness training, sports practice and competition, and other physical activities exceed the physical abilities of a young participant. For example, if a young athlete is not given enough time to recover from the physical and psychological stress of regular vigorous training, a decrease in performance and an increase in sports-related injuries are likely.[2] An understanding of the possible outcomes of fitness training will assist in the design, implementation, and progression of developmentally appropriate programs for children and adolescents.

## Pubertal Effects on Physical Fitness

Considerable interindividual differences in physical development exist among youth of the same age. For example, a 12-year-old girl can be taller and more

physically skilled than a 12-year-old boy, and two 14-year-old adolescents can have considerable differences in height, body mass, and muscle strength. These differences are related to the timing of puberty, which can vary from 8 to 13 years of age in girls and from 9 to 15 years of age in boys. Although the onset of puberty is typically 2 years later in males than females, the age at which puberty begins is influenced by genetics and environmental factors including nutrition, exercise habits, and socioeconomic conditions.[3]

The process of puberty is initiated by hormonal signals from the brain to the gonads (i.e., ovaries and testes). It is characterized by developmental changes in reproductive function and growth in body size and composition. The actions of the sex hormones estrogen (in females) and testosterone (in males) produce sex-specific outcomes that are characteristic of this developmental process. For example, during puberty, physical changes in boys include an increase in muscle mass, whereas adipose tissue tends to accumulate in girls. The expression of puberty in girls is also characterized by breast development (beginning about age 11 years) and menarche, or first menstrual bleeding, approximately 2 years later.[4] Menarche denotes the start of a female's reproductive capacity.

Although it is not possible to assess puberty with body measurements, longitudinal data for height can provide useful information to mark the age at onset of the adolescent growth sport and the age at the maximum rate of growth, which is termed *peak height velocity* (PHV).[3] On average, the age of PHV is about 12 years in girls and 14 years in boys (Fig. 25-3). Youth can grow more than 10 cm (4 in.) in 1 year during this

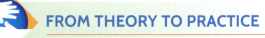

## FROM THEORY TO PRACTICE

### ■ PUBERTY AND PHYSICAL FITNESS

Puberty is not a discrete event, but rather a process of physical changes related to sexual maturation in which a child's body matures into an adult body. During this period, the broad spectrum of changes that occur can influence various measures of physical fitness. For example, during puberty, sex-related changes in physical fitness begin to diverge.[4] Boys continue to increase their aerobic fitness, whereas absolute values for maximal oxygen consumption ($\dot{V}O_2max$) in girls begin to plateau around age 16 years. In terms of muscular fitness, a clear "spurt" in strength and power occurs with puberty in boys, but not in girls because of hormonal influences. These findings are important for health and fitness professionals who work with youth. These findings also highlight the significance of encouraging young female individuals to participate in well-designed fitness programs that include exercises that enhance muscular fitness.

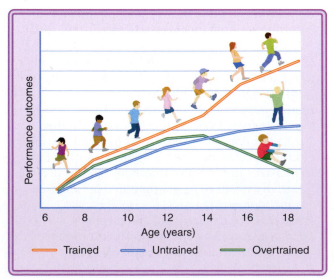

**Figure 25-2.** Possible outcomes of exercise training during childhood and adolescence: untrained, trained, and overtrained.

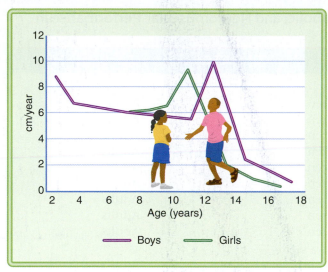

**Figure 25-3.** Growth curve for height in boys and girls (in centimeters). *(Source: Tanner JM, Whitehouse RH, Takaishi M. Standards from birth to maturity for height, weight, height velocity, and weight velocity: British children, 1965. Arch Dis Child. 1966;41:454.)*

growth period. The age at PHV is an indicator of somatic (physique) maturity and can also provide a landmark for other measures of sexual maturation. For example, menarche occurs after PHV in girls, and peak strength development occurs after PHV in boys and girls.[3] Because considerable variability exists in the age at which youth pass through this developmental stage, health and fitness professionals need to be sensitive to interindividual differences in physical appearance and abilities when working with children and adolescents.

## Stages of Maturation

Stages of maturation or pubertal development can be assessed in terms of skeletal age, somatic maturity, or sexual maturation. In female individuals, menarche is a marker of sexual maturation. In male individuals, the best indicators of sexual maturity are physical features called *secondary sex characteristics* (e.g., facial hair, pubic hair, and deepening of the voice). Secondary sex characteristics, which include breast development in female individuals, can be used to describe pubertal maturation in terms of different stages. Developmental milestones such as independent walking (about age 13 months) can be used to assess neuromuscular maturity but are not indicators of pubertal development.[3] That is, a youth's neuromuscular development does not necessarily coincide with his or her pubertal maturation. Therefore, health and fitness professionals should not judge a child's or adolescent's physical ability based on visible characteristics of maturation.

The most common staging system was described by and named for J.M. Tanner. It includes a sequence of stages that progress from Tanner stage 1 (preadolescence) to Tanner stage 5 (mature adult).[5] Criteria for each stage are based on pubic hair growth and breast and genital maturation, and ratings are ordinarily made by observation at a clinical examination.[3] As previously noted, considerable variability exists in the age at which youth pass through these stages. For example, two young participants in an exercise class can have the same chronological age but differ by several years in their biological age or degree of maturation. Sensitivity to interindividual differences in abilities and physical appearance is especially important when working with children and adolescents in a fitness program.

## PHYSIOLOGICAL RESPONSES TO EXERCISE

An understanding of the metabolic, cardiorespiratory, and neuromuscular responses to exercise in youth is essential for designing developmentally appropriate pediatric fitness programs. Children are not miniature adults, and physiological differences between younger and older populations can influence acute and chronic adaptations to exercise training. The emphasis of the following section is on the principles of pediatric exercise science that have practical implications for health and fitness professionals who design youth exercise programs. Table 25-1 provides a comparison of metabolic, cardiorespiratory, and neuromuscular performance in children and adults.

### Metabolic Responses

Perhaps the most visible difference between children and adults is that children tend to be "metabolic nonspecialists" in regard to fitness performance.[6] Unlike adults, who tend to specialize in sports such as weightlifting or long-distance running, the strongest child in a class is likely to be a leader in an endurance run as well. These observations are supported by laboratory data that suggest that children with a relatively high level of aerobic fitness tend to perform well during anaerobic tests as well.[4] Although factors related to body size and training adaptations could explain, at least in part, the observed link between different forms of physical fitness in youth, health and fitness professionals should appreciate the relative lack of metabolic specialization in younger populations.

The metabolic uniqueness of children is one reason it is important for youth to be exposed to a variety of sports and activities before the age of 15 years.[7] Youth who specialize in a single sport or activity year-round tend to suffer more overuse injuries and are more likely to encounter psychosocial issues.[8] Conversely, youth who participate in several sports seem to be protected from the harmful effects of single-sport risk.[9] Participating regularly in different sports and activities can yield many physical and psychosocial benefits related to both short- and long-term development, provided the training program and coaching philosophy are consistent with the needs, interests, and abilities of younger populations.[10]

### Anaerobic and Aerobic Metabolism

As described in Part II: Fueling Physical Activity of this textbook, energy needed by skeletal muscle is provided

**Table 25-1.** Comparison of Cardiorespiratory, Metabolic, and Neuromuscular Performance in Children and Adults

| MEASURE | COMPARISON | | |
|---|---|---|---|
| **Cardiorespiratory** | | | |
| Resting heart rate | Children | = | Adults |
| Maximal heart rate | Children | > | Adults |
| Stroke volume | Children | < | Adults |
| Cardiac output | Children | < | Adults |
| Tidal volume | Children | < | Adults |
| Breathing frequency | Children | > | Adults |
| a-vO$_2$ difference | Children | = | Adults |
| Peak $\dot{V}O_2$ (L/min) | Children | < | Adults |
| Endurance performance | Children | < | Adults |
| **Metabolic** | | | |
| ATP storage/kilogram muscle | Children | = | Adults |
| Phosphocreatine resynthesis | Children | ≥ | Adults |
| Glycolytic activity | Children | < | Adults |
| Exercise lactate | Children | < | Adults |
| Exercise fatty acid oxidation | Children | > | Adults |
| Anaerobic performance | Children | < | Adults |
| Exercise recovery | Children | > | Adults |
| **Neuromuscular** | | | |
| Muscle fiber number | Children | = | Adults |
| Muscle fiber size | Children | < | Adults |
| Absolute muscle strength | Children | < | Adults |

ATP, adenosine triphosphate; a-$\dot{V}O_2$ difference, arterial-venous oxygen difference, or the difference in the oxygen content of the blood between the arterial blood and the venous blood; it represents how much oxygen is removed from the blood in capillaries as the blood circulates in the body; $\dot{V}O_2$, oxygen consumption.

by adenosine triphosphate (ATP), which can be generated by anaerobic or aerobic processes. The ATP-phosphocreatine (ATP-PC) system and glycolysis are anaerobic pathways and do not require oxygen, whereas the resynthesis of ATP within the mitochondria by a series of reactions that ultimately require oxygen is referred to as aerobic metabolism. The replenishment of ATP is essential, because performance of any physical activity is dependent on ATP, which is needed for muscle contraction. Anaerobic pathways resynthesize ATP at a very rapid rate and are critical for short, high-intensity activities, but the supply of energy from these sources is limited. Conversely, energy from aerobic metabolism is released at a slower rate, but much more energy can be generated from this source, which is better suited for longer, less intense activities.

Although our relative understanding of exercise metabolism in youth is limited, a review of early findings based on muscle biopsy data suggest that ATP and PC levels at rest are similar to adults.[11] In terms of exercise-related differences in anaerobic metabolism, preadolescents appear to have a faster rate of intramuscular PC resynthesis than adults, which suggests that the capacity of children to perform high-intensity exercise for less than 10 to 15 seconds is not impaired.[12]

However, evidence indicates that glycolytic activity is limited in children as compared with adults.[13] Glycolysis is the anaerobic breakdown of glucose to pyruvate. As energy demands increase and glycolysis proceeds, lactate begins to accumulate in the muscle and some diffuses into the blood, where it is often measured. Because the rate of muscle lactate production is dependent on the balance between aerobic and anaerobic metabolism, less lactate is produced when pyruvate is oxidized in the tricarboxylic acid cycle to carbon dioxide and water. Although additional research is needed, the available data indicate limited glycolytic activity in youth as compared with adults. Thus, less mature subjects should not be expected to perform as well as adults on short-burst, high-energy activities lasting 30 to 120 seconds. Also, exercise programming for this population should be more geared to aerobic versus anaerobic activities.

Because the ability to generate and maintain anaerobic power is lower in children than in adults, performance on short-burst activities is worse in younger participants. The Wingate anaerobic test is a popular cycle test of short-term power because it allows for the determination of peak power, usually over 1 to 5 seconds, and mean power over a 30-second test. A consistent finding is that both peak power and mean power increase with age, although after age 12 years the nonlinear increase in short-term power is more marked in boys than in girls.[13] It is likely that age-related differences in muscle characteristics (e.g., muscle mass) and muscle enzyme activity could explain these observations.

Although age-related differences in metabolism are more noticeable during short-burst anaerobic activities than longer-duration aerobic events, differences in cellular aerobic function between children and adults have been reported.[4] Findings suggest that children have enhanced oxidative enzymes, which enable them to oxidize free fatty acids at a higher rate than adults.[14] From a metabolic perspective, children appear to be well-equipped for aerobic-type sports and activities. However, this difference seems to diminish during adolescence, which suggests that hormonal changes during puberty influence the regulation of energy metabolism.[15]

## VIGNETTE continued

■ In addition to the fact that most children do not like performing continuous exercise, Jennifer recognizes two other issues related to Jacob's parents pushing him to perform 30 minutes of exercise each day after school. During the education sessions she conducts with the children each week, she decides to address these concerns in a group setting without singling out Jacob. The first issue she discusses with the kids is the fact that exercise should be fun—and it is important to find sports and activities you enjoy. Some kids like basketball and soccer, and others like outdoor games and free play activities.

The second issue involves the development of intrinsic motivation. Extrinsic motivation, as attempted by Jacob's parents, is not effective in the long run. Exercising to satisfy one's parents or avoid fights at home will not help a child overcome the inevitable obstacles that face anyone trying to sustain a lifestyle change. In contrast, exercising for the mere enjoyment of participation, as exemplified when a person is motivated intrinsically, is important for long-term program adherence. It is Jennifer's job to help the kids in her program develop the intrinsic motivation—along with perceived confidence in their physical abilities—to adhere to the program over the long haul.

## Exercise Lactate and Recovery

Children typically demonstrate lower levels of blood lactate than adults during submaximal and maximal exercise, which supports the contention that youth have a depressed capacity for glycolytic metabolism.[15] Whereas levels of blood lactate during maximal exercise tend to increase throughout childhood and adolescence, blood lactate values during the growing years

tend to be lower than those typically observed in exercising adults. Thus, at the same lactate concentration, a child is exercising at a relatively higher exercise intensity than an adult. It is likely that differences in muscle mass and muscle enzyme activity are responsible for the better performance in more mature individuals. The early work of Eriksson and Saltin[16] revealed muscle lactate concentrations following a peak $\dot{V}O_2$ test of 8.8, 10.7, 11.3, and 15.3 mmol/kg wet muscle weight for boys aged 11.6, 12.6, 13.5, and 15.5 years, respectively. By comparison, muscle lactate concentrations of 25 mmol/kg wet muscle weight are common in adults following maximal exercise.

Although the rate of elimination of lactate after exercise is the same in youth and adults, children tend to recover faster from physical exertion.[12] Although factors related to muscle mass and energy metabolism may explain, in part, child–adult differences in recovery, it is possible that youth may recover faster from high-intensity bouts of physical exertion because they have less to recover from. That is, a lower level of peak power or absolute strength in children as compared with adults may yield less potential for an absolute reduction in performance.[17,18] When organizing fitness activities for school-aged youth, health and fitness professionals should be aware of the greater ability of children to resist fatigue.

## Cardiorespiratory Responses to Exercise

Differences in the cardiorespiratory responses to exercise between children and adults are easily observable when adults play with children. At the same exercise or play intensity, children breathe a little harder and have higher heart rates. This is a normal physiological response to an acute bout of physical activity that should be expected in younger populations.

### Acute Cardiorespiratory Responses

Although resting heart rates are similar between youth and adults, children and adolescents exhibit higher heart rates and lower stroke volumes (amount of blood ejected per ventricular contraction) at all exercise intensities than do older populations.[4] Cardiac output, defined as the volume of blood pumped by the heart per minute, is a function of heart rate and stroke volume. Because children and adolescents have smaller hearts, and therefore smaller ventricles, than adults, it is not surprising that youth have lower stroke volumes. Consequently, the higher heart rates children typically exhibit when exercising with an adult are probably an attempt to compensate for the smaller ventricular size and lower stroke volume. However, the heart-rate compensation during exercise is somewhat incomplete, because youth show smaller increases in cardiac output at all exercise intensities as compared with adults.[4]

Maximal heart rates do not change appreciably during childhood and early adolescence, and it is not uncommon for a child's heart rate to exceed 200 beats/min during a bout of vigorous physical activity.[4] Therefore, the estimation of maximal heart rate by age-based equations (e.g., 220 – age; 208–(0.7 × age) is inappropriate for youth between 7 and 15 years of age. If heart-rate monitors are used during aerobic workouts or fitness testing, the expected heart-rate response to vigorous exercise should be discussed in advance with the participants to reduce any unwarranted concerns that may arise from high heart-rate values. Also, children with a higher peak $\dot{V}O_2$ tend to recover faster than those with a lower peak $\dot{V}O_2$.[19] Health and fitness professionals should be aware of the interindividual variability in the recovery from aerobic exercise, which may be a useful marker of aerobic fitness.

The total amount of air a person breathes per minute is called *minute ventilation*. This measure is a product of tidal volume (volume of each breath) and respiratory rate (number of breaths per minute). For example, if an adult has a tidal volume of 700 mL and a respiratory rate of 16 breaths/min, the minute ventilation would be 11,200 mL/min (700 mL/breath × 16 breaths/min), or 11.2 L/min. Children and adolescents have a higher breathing frequency and a lower tidal volume than adults at all exercise intensities.[4] Therefore, it is normal for healthy children and adolescents to breathe rapidly during a vigorous fitness activity because they process a relatively smaller amount of air in absolute terms per minute. However, during maximal exercise, minute ventilation expressed per kilogram of body weight is equal between youth and adults.[4] Although additional research on ventilation kinetics in pediatric populations is warranted, no data suggest that the respiratory responses to exercise in young, healthy populations limit exercise performance.

## VIGNETTE continued

■ During the third week of Jacob's participation in the program, his parents contact Jennifer because they are very concerned that Jacob is talking about dropping out of the program. The next day, Jennifer asks Jacob why he is feeling this way. He tells her that he gets tired during the games and admits that he got really scared one day while running because he felt like his heart was racing and he could not catch his breath. Jennifer reassures Jacob by explaining to him the normal sensations that can be expected during and after exercise. She also gives Jacob options to try during the workout sessions to modify the intensity so that he does not feel concerned about catching his breath and feeling too tired. In addition, Jennifer encourages Jacob to let her know if he is feeling uncomfortable during their sessions so that she can address his concerns immediately and modify the lesson plan for the remaining activities.

The difference between the oxygen content of arterial blood and venous blood is called the *arteriovenous oxygen difference*. Children and adolescents seem to extract the same amount of oxygen from the blood as adults at rest and during exercise.[4] Furthermore, no compelling data suggest that aerobically trained youth extract more oxygen from the blood than untrained youth.

## In Your Own Words

The parents of a healthy 8-year-old child in your after-school fitness program inform you that they have reviewed a few fitness websites and noticed that many of them recommend using a target heart rate formula to monitor exercise intensity. They want to know why you do not use that method to program the appropriate aerobic exercise intensity for their son. What explanation would you provide to address their question?

### Aerobic Fitness in Youth

A widely recognized criterion measure of aerobic fitness in youth is termed *peak $\dot{V}O_2$*. This measure reflects the limits of the oxygen delivery system during aerobic exercise in youth. Peak $\dot{V}O_2$ can be expressed in absolute (L/min) or relative (mL/kg/min) terms. When peak $\dot{V}O_2$max is expressed in absolute terms, the value increases steadily from 6 to about 18 years of age, although values for girls are about 0.2 L/min lower than those of boys at the same chronological age.[20] When peak $\dot{V}O_2$max is expressed relative to body mass, the value for boys remains relatively stable during childhood and adolescence at 48 mL/kg/min, whereas the value for girls shows a decline from approximately 45 to 35 mL/kg/min because of sex-related changes in body composition.[21]

Cross-sectional and longitudinal data show that peak $\dot{V}O_2$ increases with age and maturation in both sexes and is highly correlated with body size.[13] Data analysis of about 5,000 peak $\dot{V}O_2$ values from 8- to 16-year-olds indicate that peak $\dot{V}O_2$ increases in girls and boys by 80% and 150%, respectively, during this developmental period.[21] Physiological explanations for sex-related differences in peak $\dot{V}O_2$ during the growing years include greater muscle mass and higher hemoglobin concentrations in boys as compared with girls.

In adults, peak $\dot{V}O_2$ is closely linked to cardiorespiratory fitness and is an established measure of one's ability to perform prolonged periods of endurance exercise. In children, peak $\dot{V}O_2$ reflects the physiological functioning of the cardiorespiratory system, but it is only weakly related to objectively measured physical activity and endurance performance.[4,22] That is, during childhood and adolescence, peak $\dot{V}O_2$ per kilogram remains relatively stable, whereas performance in standard field tests such as the 1-mile run consistently improves over time.

For example, during the growing years, the 1-mile (1.6-km) run time will improve by roughly 5 minutes, but peak $\dot{V}O_2$ per kilogram will remain relatively stable in boys or decrease somewhat in girls during this period.[23] Moreover, during preadolescence, training-induced gains in peak $\dot{V}O_2$ (~5%–10%) are significantly less than gains typically observed in adults (~15%–30%), which suggests that physiological adaptations to aerobic training in children are maturity dependent.[4,24] The relatively small gains in peak $\dot{V}O_2$ after aerobic training in youth appear to be a function of enhanced stroke volume.[25]

Smaller children and adolescents are also less economical than adults while walking or running.[4] That is, they are less metabolically efficient during weight-bearing motor activities, so they have higher energy requirements per kilogram of body mass. If a child and an adult jog at the same pace, the child will be jogging at a significantly higher relative intensity than the adult. Throughout childhood and adolescence, the progressive improvement in running economy will typically translate into a progressive decline in the percentage of one's aerobic capacity at a given exercise intensity. Although factors such as stride frequency and running performance need to be considered when examining the association between energy cost and maturity, these are important considerations for health and fitness professionals who monitor changes in endurance performance in younger populations as well.

## Thermoregulation in Younger Populations

A related concern involves thermoregulation for the exercising child or adolescent. During exercise, heat production increases and the body must increase blood flow to the skin for heat removal. Children and adolescents have a larger surface area-to-mass ratio than adults, which allows for a greater heat exchange. When the environmental temperature is lower than body temperature (e.g., in a swimming pool), more heat is dissipated. However, when the environmental temperature is higher than body temperature (e.g., during summer sports practice), less heat will be lost. Children and adolescents also produce less sweat per gland, primarily because they have less muscle mass than adults, which contains more water than fat mass; this results in reduced heat dissipation via evaporation. Failure to effectively remove body heat during strenuous exercise in conditions of high ambient temperature and humidity would result in a decrement in performance and an increased risk for heat-related illness.[26]

Factors including level of aerobic fitness, clothing, body composition, wind velocity, and hydration can influence thermoregulation during exercise.[27] Of note, a participant's state of hydration is critically important because increasing levels of dehydration incurred via sweating during exercise can result in undesirable changes in circulatory efficiency and an increase in body temperature.[26] Because children

sweat less efficiently than adults,[28] young participants may have less tolerance for exercise in the heat.

Youth tend to underestimate the amount of fluid they need to stay hydrated during prolonged periods of exercise. Because thirst is a poor indicator of fluid needs, health and fitness professionals need to be aware of thermoregulatory concerns and encourage adequate fluid intake before, during, and after exercise. Researchers found that voluntary fluid intake replaced 78% of fluid loss with water, but more than 100% with a glucose and electrolyte solution in boys with ad libitum drinking (allowed to drink with a frequency and volume of their own choosing).[29] Of practical importance, the addition of flavor to a carbohydrate–electrolyte drink can help to reduce voluntary dehydration in children.[29] Although cultural factors can influence taste and food preferences, in one report that examined children's thirst and drink preferences during exercise-induced hypohydration, the magnitude of rehydration was statistically greater with grape- and orange-flavored beverages.[30]

## Neuromuscular Factors and Strength Development

Because of growth and maturation, it can be expected that healthy children and adolescents will show noticeable gains in muscular fitness (i.e., muscular strength, muscular power, and local muscular endurance). Although all youth do not follow the same rate of change, variables such as grip strength, sit-up performance, and jumping performance increase from childhood through the early teenage years.[3] While growth-related increases in muscle size influence gains in muscular performance, developmental neurological changes can also contribute to observed gains in muscular performance during childhood and adolescence.[3,13] Therefore, health and fitness professionals who work with youth need to consider size-independent factors when evaluating the acute and chronic responses to fitness programs that include resistance training.[31,32]

Although some debate persists whether muscle strength per cross-sectional area increases with age, absolute levels of muscular strength increase between 8 and 16 years of age without specialized training.[13] Moreover, muscle mass increases linearly with age in both sexes during the growing years, although androgenic hormones cause an increase in the rate of muscle growth in boys at puberty. In male individuals, the amount of muscle mass as a percentage of total body mass increases from 43% at age 5 years to 53% at age 17 years, whereas this change is not observed in female individuals, who have values of 41% and 42%, respectively, at these ages.[4]

In addition to gains in muscle size, qualitative changes in muscle tissue and neuromuscular maturation can influence the expression of voluntary strength.[4] Unlike male adults, who typically respond to resistance-training protocols with an increase in myofibrillar protein and muscle hypertrophy, factors other than muscle size are involved in the development of muscle strength in preadolescent youth. Most notably, neuromuscular changes in motor unit firing rate, recruitment, or conduction velocity and growth-related alterations in muscle pennation angle can contribute to qualitative changes in muscle function in children.[4,33]

Following regular participation in a resistance-training program, children and adolescents can improve their strength above and beyond gains due to growth and maturation. Although relative or percent gains in muscular strength achieved by untrained children are similar to untrained adults (about 30% in 8–12 weeks), training-induced gains in muscle strength during preadolescence are primarily due to the aforementioned neuromuscular factors.[32] During puberty, testicular testosterone secretion in male individuals is associated with gains in fat-free mass following resistance training, whereas smaller amounts of testosterone in female individuals limit the magnitude of training-induced increases in muscle hypertrophy. Knowledge of qualitative and quantitative changes in muscle tissue and neuromuscular function, along with an understanding of realistic outcomes from resistance training, are important considerations for health and fitness professionals who develop resistance-training programs for children and adolescents.

## VIGNETTE continued

■ After 1 month of Jacob's regular participation in the after-school program, Jennifer decides to introduce resistance training to his routine. Not only does Jacob love the new form of exercise, he is proud of his considerable strength compared with other participants. Some of the younger children even gather around when Jacob performs certain exercises, amazed at how much he can lift.

Although it is important to downplay competition in the weight room and focus on developing proper exercise technique, Jennifer knows that many heavier children excel at resistance training, giving them a rare opportunity to shine in front of their peers. The ego boost, combined with the weight loss Jacob has experienced in the first month, boosts his self-esteem.

## In Your Own Words

A 15-year-old girl asks you if she will get "big muscles" if she lifts weights. She is worried that she will look too "bulky." How would you answer this question, and what might you suggest to address her concern?

## PHYSICAL ACTIVITY AND PEDIATRIC HEALTH

Regular participation in physical activity offers observable health and fitness value to children and adolescents.[1,34] Gains in physical fitness, as well as positive improvements in a child's psychosocial well-being, are typically reported following regular participation in exercise programs.[35,36] In addition, substantial evidence indicates that physical activity, including physical education, can help improve cognitive skills, student concentration, and classroom behavior in school-aged youth.[37,38] Physical activity is now recognized as a powerful marker of health in younger populations.[39,40]

### Health-Related Benefits

Health and fitness professionals have the information to justify physical-activity programs for youth because of the numerous benefits that have been documented through research.[1,4] Regular participation in moderate-to-vigorous physical activity (MVPA) helps to reduce body fat, improve blood lipids, build skeletal tissue, strengthen muscles, improve aerobic fitness, and reduce symptoms of anxiety and depression.[1,41,42] More recent observational and experimental evidence has found that children who engage regularly in adequate amounts of physical activity at the desired intensity are more likely to have healthy cardiometabolic biomarkers (e.g., improved insulin sensitivity and endothelial function).[43] Perhaps of equal importance to health and fitness professionals is the observation that health-related behaviors that are acquired during childhood and adolescence tend to carry over into adulthood.[44]

Participation in free play, recreational activities, and structured games also provides school-aged youth with an opportunity to develop fundamental movement skills (FMS), which provide the foundation for an active lifestyle.[45] FMS include locomotor (e.g., jumping and hopping), object control (e.g., kicking and catching), and stability (e.g., balancing and twisting) skills. Longitudinal research has found that FMS proficiency observed early in life predicts subsequent fitness levels later in life[46–48] (Fig. 25-4). That is, children who develop competence and confidence in their abilities to kick, throw, jump, and run during the primary school years are more likely to be active during adolescence. Youth who enhance their physical fitness and acquire FMS proficiency also tend to be better prepared for participation in a variety of sports and activities.[49,50] An inactive lifestyle is a risk factor for sports-related injuries, and conditioning programs that improve physical fitness can reduce sports-related injuries in young athletes.[51,52] Even though the total elimination of sports-related injuries is an unrealistic goal, more than half of overuse injuries in young athletes may be preventable with straightforward approaches that include coaching education and preparatory fitness conditioning.[50]

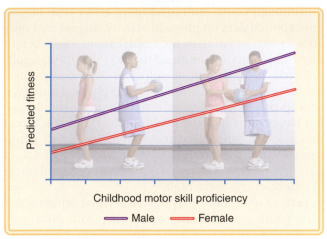

**Figure 25-4.** Children who develop competence and confidence in their abilities to kick, throw, jump, and run in childhood are more likely to have increased levels of fitness during adolescence.

## Physical Activity Guidelines

A youngster who enjoys physical activity and learns how to live a physically active life is more likely to become an active, healthy adult. Thus, the primary goal of youth fitness programs is not only to engage boys and girls in a variety of enjoyable physical activities, but for all youth to become aware of the intrinsic values and benefits of regular physical activity so they become adults who engage in desirable patterns of habitual physical activity. Children and adolescents with disabilities should work with their health-care providers to establish a safe and effective fitness program that is consistent with individual needs and abilities.

Pediatric guidelines state that school-aged youth should accumulate at least 60 minutes of MVPA daily.[1,34] These guidelines indicate that children and adolescents can achieve substantial health-related benefits by performing a variety of physical activities that include aerobic and strength-building exercises.[1,34] Although physical activity of amounts greater than 60 min/day will provide additional benefits, it is also important to consider the intensity as well as the mix of health- and skill-related activities that are part of youth fitness programs.

Participation in physical activity should not begin with competitive sport, but should evolve out of participation in a variety of structured (i.e., physical education) and unstructured (i.e., free play) activities. The musculoskeletal system of sedentary children and adolescents is not prepared for the demands of regular sports practice and competition. The International Olympic Committee states that the ideal system for preventing sports injuries in inactive youth should involve a preparticipation evaluation followed by an individualized exercise program to address fitness deficits.[53]

Regular participation in physical activity also promotes feelings of well-being, enhances self-esteem, and simply makes boys and girls feel better about themselves.[38] Well-organized youth activity programs characterized by caring and competent health and fitness professionals give children and adolescents the opportunity to make new friends and gain confidence in their ability to be physically active. Numerous studies have also shown positive relationships between physical activity and academic achievement.[37]

## Health- and Skill-Related Fitness

Health-related activities typically require endurance, strength, or flexibility, whereas skill-related activities require agility, balance, coordination, speed, power, and reaction time.[38] Although most contemporary youth programs focus on health-related components of physical fitness, youth who are exposed to an environment with opportunities to enhance their

## RESEARCH HIGHLIGHT

### Is Physical Activity During Youth Sports Practices Enough?

Millions of boys and girls participate in youth sports, and limited data suggest that youth sports can contribute to the recommended amount of MVPA. However, direct observations of youth sports practice have shown that a significant amount of time is spent being inactive, and some organized youth programs focus more on competition than physical activity. Researchers in California documented the physical activity patterns during organized youth soccer and baseball/softball practices in 200 young athletes aged 7 to 14 years.[54] Accelerometers were used to objectively measure time in sedentary, light, moderate, and vigorous physical activity.

Results of the study indicate that less than one fourth of youth obtained the recommended 60 minutes of MVPA during sports practice. Substantial MVPA differences by sport, sex, and age were noted, with soccer players, boys, and younger subjects spending more time in MVPA. Although participation in youth sport can offer physical and psychosocial benefits, these findings suggest that youth sports practice makes a less-than-optimal contribution to current physical activity goals. Improved policies and practices, which include coaching education and extending short sessions, may help to improve the potential health-enhancing effects of youth sport.[54]

Leek D, Carlson J, Cain K, et al. Physical activity during youth sports practices. *Arch Pediatr Adolesc Med.* 2011;165: 294-299.

skill-related proficiency tend to be more active later in life.[46–48] Thus, youth programs that balance FMS acquisition with health-related physical activities may offer the best approach for promoting lifetime physical activity.

Children who do not develop competence and confidence in their abilities to perform FMS early in life may not be able to break through a hypothetical "proficiency barrier" later in life that would allow them to participate in a variety of health-enhancing sports and activities with confidence and vigor.[55] Thus, health- and skill-related components of physical fitness are not mutually exclusive, but rather closely linked for promoting life-long physical activity.

## Hypoactivity and Disease Risk

Despite the detrimental effects of hypoactivity (i.e., inadequate physical activity) on the health and well-being of young people,[56] recent epidemiological reports indicate that contemporary youth are not as active as they should be. Physical activity seems to progressively decrease after age 6 years.[57–59] The eventual decline and disinterest in physical activity that appears to be a contemporary corollary of low FMS proficiency starts even earlier in overweight children.[60]

Because many chronic diseases that become clinically manifest during the adult years are influenced by lifestyle habits established during the growing years, participation in meaningful physical activities early in life may prevent the development of risk factors and pathological processes later in life. This view is supported by the growing prevalence of overweight and obesity in sedentary children and the troubling diagnosis of type 2 diabetes (formerly referred to as adult-onset) in adolescents who for the most part are obese.[36,61,62]

Although youth tend to be more active than adults, self-reported data on physical activity suggest that only 30% to 40% of youth in the United States meet current physical activity recommendations.[63,64] Although self-reported data may not be sufficient to evaluate cross-cultural differences in young people's physical activity, it appears that lack of physical activity among schoolchildren has become a global health problem. In one report that assessed physical activity habits in 72,845 youth from 34 countries, only 23.8% of boys and 15.4% of girls met current activity recommendations, and levels of sedentariness were high.[65]

Instead of outdoor play and structured fitness activities, youth are spending more time with electronic media (e.g., television and video games), which may displace more active pursuits.[66] Moreover, only a few states in the United States require physical education in every grade (K–12). Also, only 12% of high school students achieved public health objectives for participation in aerobic and muscle-strengthening activities.[67,68] In the aforementioned report from the Centers for Disease Control and Prevention, the prevalence of meeting physical activity objectives was found to be lower among female students, students in upper grades, and students with obesity.[67]

The impact of a sedentary lifestyle during the growing years on lifelong pathological processes and associated health-care costs has created a need for health-care providers and fitness professionals to provide opportunities for all children and adolescents to be physically active during this vulnerable period of life.[36,69,70] Because sedentary behaviors of young people tend to track into adulthood,[71] some observers suggest that the term *exercise deficit disorder* should be used to describe a condition characterized by reduced levels of physical

---

## RESEARCH HIGHLIGHT

### Does Skill-Related Fitness Matter?

Physical fitness tests for school-aged youth typically consist of health-related fitness components that measure endurance, flexibility, and strength. However, a growing body of evidence indicates that fitness measures that involve locomotor, manipulative, and stability skills may be associated with important long-term health benefits for children and adolescents. To examine the relation between motor skill proficiency in childhood and subsequent adolescent physical activity, researchers measured motor proficiency in a group of children (age range, 7.9–11.9 years) and then assessed their physical activity habits during adolescence 6 to 7 years later.[47] Motor skill measurements included kicking, catching, throwing, hopping, galloping, and jumping.

Results of the study indicate that the amount of time adolescents spent in MVPA was positively associated with motor skill proficiency, particularly object control proficiency, during childhood. Although children should be encouraged to participate in a variety of age-appropriate activities, these findings suggest that object control skills such as catching, throwing, and kicking should be practiced and reinforced early in life. Because children with poor motor skills may choose not to participate in physical activities later in life, school- and community-based youth fitness programs that target motor skill proficiency are needed to increase physical activity participation during the growing years.[47]

Barnett L, Van Beurden E, Morgan P, et al. Childhood motor skill proficiency as a predictor of adolescent physical activity. *J Adolesc Health.* 2009;44:252–259.

activity that are inconsistent with positive health outcomes.[72] As such, youth who are not meeting the current recommendations for physical activity could be identified and treated early in life with specific exercise recommendations for achieving physical activity goals and encouraging positive behavior change within the family structure.

## Overweight and Obesity

It is becoming more apparent that the lack of regular physical activity, along with the greater accessibility to energy-dense foods, is contributing to the increasing prevalence of overweight and obesity among children and adolescents. Over the past three decades, the prevalence of childhood obesity has more than doubled for adolescents and has more than tripled for children.[62] Data from a national survey using body mass index as a main outcome measure indicate that, among American youth aged 2 through 19 years, 31.7% are at risk for becoming obese (defined as ≥85% but <95% of the sex-specific body mass index for age) and 16.9% are obese. Unfortunately, this trend is likely to get worse, because 9.5% of infants and toddlers are already obese.[62]

These trends have significant ramifications for health-care providers and health and fitness professionals because of the increased prevalence of cardiovascular disease risk factors and obesity-related comorbidities such as type 2 diabetes, heart disease, and certain cancers.[39,61] For American children born in the year 2000, the lifetime risk for being diagnosed with diabetes is estimated to be 30% for boys and 40% for girls.[61] Health and fitness professionals who work with youth should also be aware that pediatric obesity may be associated with psychosocial abnormalities including depression and low self-esteem.[73] Obese youth have fewer friends, miss more school days, and are often ostracized and teased about their weight.[74] Furthermore, researchers observed that obese children and adolescents have a lower health-related quality of life than youth who are at a healthy weight and a similar quality of life as those diagnosed with having cancer.[75]

### VIGNETTE continued

■ During another education session, Jennifer addresses nutrition, enlisting the help of Roberto, a local registered dietitian, to discuss the importance of making healthy choices. Roberto says, "I'm going to describe the typical dinner of many families in our community. Mom or Dad picks up fast food on the way home from a long day at work, the family sits in the TV room to eat dinner, and then stay there for most of the evening until it's time to get ready for bed."

Some of the kids start laughing, so Roberto asks why. Jacob speaks up: "That sounds exactly like my family!" Many of the other kids express the very same thing. Jennifer and Roberto spend the next hour discussing quick, healthy meals that the kids can make with their parents, even when time is limited. Jacob leaves that day excited to help his Mom make a healthy dinner for the family.

## PROGRAM DESIGN CONSIDERATIONS

Children and adolescents have different fitness goals than adults and are active for different reasons. Enhancing one's level of aerobic fitness and improving

## FROM THEORY TO PRACTICE

### ■ TRAINING OVERWEIGHT YOUTH

The prevalence of childhood obesity continues to increase, and effective strategies are needed to enhance the health and well-being of obese youth. Although all youth need to be physically active daily, obese youth often lack the motor skills and confidence to be physically active, and they often perceive prolonged periods of aerobic exercise to be boring or discomforting. Conversely, obese youth tend to enjoy resistance training because it is typically characterized by short periods of physical activity interspersed with brief rest periods as needed.

However, when working with obese youth, the goal of the program should not be limited to increasing muscle strength or improving body composition. It is also important to teach new skills, have fun, make friends, and offer a stimulating program that gives participants a positive attitude about physical activity. Although there is not one optimal combination of sets, repetitions, and exercises, beginners should start with one or two sets of 10 to 15 repetitions on a variety of exercises for the upper body, lower body, and torso. It may be reasonable for obese youth to start resistance training on weight machines and gradually progress to free weights and medicine ball exercises that require more coordination and skill to perform correctly. Regular resistance training offers many benefits to obese youth while exposing them to an enjoyable form of exercise that can be carried over into adolescence and adulthood.

one's blood lipid profile may be important motivating factors for adults, but most children want to have fun, build friendships, and improve physical skills. The importance of creating an enjoyable experience should not be overlooked, as enjoyment has been found to mediate the effects of youth physical activity programs.[76] Also, the exercise environment should be safe, well-lit, and free of any hazards that could cause injury.

Because young children are concrete thinkers, they need to enjoy the process of being physically active and see little value in monotonous workouts or prolonged periods of high-intensity exercise. Health and fitness professionals should not forget about the importance of play, which provides children with an opportunity to feel good about their accomplishments, build friendships, and experience the mere enjoyment of physical activity.[77] Moreover, the long-lasting value of creating physically educated individuals should not be overlooked, because positive attitudes and behaviors established early in life are the building blocks for a healthy lifestyle later in life.

Although the choice of activity and intensity of the exercise program are important considerations, physical activity experiences need to be positive and consistent with the needs, abilities, and activity patterns of children and adolescents. To make physical activity a lifelong habit, youth should gain confidence in their perceived abilities, enhance their FMS competence, and experience the mere enjoyment of movement. Even sedentary youth can achieve the recommended amount of physical activity with a modest commitment and support from their parents and schoolteachers. Sedentary youth can increase the amount of time they have for physical activity by reducing sedentary leisure pursuits such as television viewing, computer use, and video games.

The goal should be to accumulate at least 60 minutes of MVPA throughout the day rather than perform a continuous bout of activity at a predetermined intensity. Although continuous activity is not physiologically harmful, it is not the most appropriate method of exercise for youth, who tend to enjoy nonsustained activities or games.[78] Researchers have observed that the majority of intense activities in youth fitness programs typically last less than 15 seconds.[79] Continuous MVPA lasting more than 5 or 10 minutes without rest or recovery is rare among children, because they have short attention spans and do not enjoy this type of training. Health and fitness professionals should carefully design and sensibly progress youth programs that are characterized by alternate bouts of low, moderate, and vigorous physical activity with brief periods of rest and recovery as needed.

Qualified professionals who understand pediatric training guidelines and genuinely appreciate the physical and psychosocial uniqueness of children and adolescents should provide supervision and instruction. Basic education on warm-up procedures, proper exercise technique, skill-based progression, and fundamental training principles should be part of all youth fitness programs. Although no preventive trials have focused specifically on measures to prevent fitness-related injuries in youth, modifiable risk factors associated with exercise-related injuries in younger populations that can be reduced or eliminated with qualified supervision and instruction are outlined in Table 25-2. General guidelines for prescribing health- and skill-related fitness are discussed in the following sections.

## Aerobic Exercise

Adults typically perform continuous aerobic (or endurance) exercise to increase their $\dot{V}O_2max$ and improve their cardiovascular disease risk profile. Although this type of training can be beneficial, most youth view prolonged periods of aerobic exercise as monotonous, boring, and discomforting. Health and fitness professionals who work with children and adolescents should modify aerobic exercise guidelines for adults to better match the physical and psychosocial characteristics of youth. Stop-and-go games or circuit-training activities that alternate higher-effort and lower-effort segments are recommended because they increase children's likelihood of completing the exercise session.

**Table 25-2. Modifiable Risk Factors Associated With Youth Exercise-Training Injuries That Can Be Reduced (or Eliminated) With Qualified Supervision and Instruction**

| RISK FACTOR | MODIFICATION BY QUALIFIED PROFESSIONAL |
|---|---|
| Unsafe exercise environment | Adequate training space and proper equipment layout |
| Improper equipment storage | Proper and secure storage of exercise equipment |
| Unsafe use of equipment | Instruction on safety rules in the exercise area |
| Excessive load and volume | Gradual progression of exercise program |
| Poor exercise technique | Clear instruction and feedback on exercise movements |
| Poor trunk control | Targeted core training |
| Previous injury | Communicate with treating clinician and modify program |
| Growth process | Modify training to address specific needs and abilities |
| Inadequate recuperation | Include less intense training sessions |
| Chronic fatigue | Consider lifestyle factors such as proper nutrition and adequate sleep |

The standard means of assessing aerobic exercise intensity in adults is heart-rate monitoring (e.g., 60%–75% of heart rate reserve). In one respect, heart-rate monitoring is problematic for children who have great difficulty finding and counting their pulse rate during exercise. Moreover, there is little need for healthy children to monitor their heart-rate response because adult target heart-rate formulas are inappropriate for youth younger than 16 years. Generally, simple observations may be sufficient for determining children's physical exertion during their training sessions.

The aerobic segment of youth programs should include FMS (e.g., skipping, jumping, hopping, kicking, and throwing), as well as activities that involve apparatus including hoops, cones, playground balls, and beach balls. In addition, physically active but less competitive games can keep children moving and motivated without fear of failure. Inactive youth should begin with 20 or 30 minutes and gradually progress to 60 minutes or more on all or most days of the week. When appropriate, vigorous bouts of activity should be incorporated into youth programs, because a lack of this type of activity is a significant predictor of fatness, whereas performance of vigorous exercise is positively correlated to fitness in youth.[80]

## Resistance Training

Resistance training refers to a specialized method of conditioning that involves the progressive use of a wide range of resistive loads and a variety of training modalities. For decades, youth were discouraged from participating in structured resistance training (or strength training). The primary reason for this precaution was a belief that resistance training would be harmful to the developing musculoskeletal system of a child. However, research clearly demonstrates that resistance training can be a safe, effective, and worthwhile activity for children and adolescents provided that age-appropriate training guidelines are followed[81–83] (Fig. 25-5).

Although there is no scientific evidence to suggest that the risks and concerns associated with youth resistance training are greater than those of other sports and recreational activities in which children and adolescents regularly participate, youth resistance-training programs must be competently supervised, properly instructed, and appropriately designed.[31,32] If established youth resistance-training guidelines are not followed, there is the potential for injury. In one report, two thirds of resistance-training–related injuries sustained by 8- to 13-year-old patients who reported to emergency departments in the United States were to the hand and foot, and most were related to "dropping" and "pinching" in the injury descriptions.[84] Health and fitness professionals must be aware of the inherent risk associated with resistance training and should attempt to decrease this risk by following established training guidelines. These guidelines include qualified supervision, safe exercise equipment, and appropriate training resistance levels or weights.

Although there is no minimum age for participating in a youth resistance-training program, children and adolescents should have the emotional maturity to accept and follow directions, and should appreciate the benefits and concerns associated with this type of training.[32] In general, if a child is ready for participation in some type of sport activity (generally age 7 or 8 years), he or she may be ready to resistance train. Different types of equipment, including free weights (i.e., barbells and dumbbells), child-size weight machines, elastic bands,

## RESEARCH HIGHLIGHT

### Dispelling Myths About Youth Resistance Training

The qualified acceptance of youth resistance training by medical and fitness professionals is becoming universal, yet misperceptions regarding the safety and effectiveness of this type of exercise for youth still persist. Of note, some observers still believe that resistance training will stunt the growth of children, and others consider resistance training to be ineffective during childhood. Furthermore, there is a lingering concern that resistance exercise will make young muscles big and bulky.

A review of the scientific evidence indicates that resistance exercise will not stunt the growth of children.[83] In fact, participation in weight-bearing physical activities such as resistance training may actually increase the bone strength of school-aged youth. Also, children can make impressive gains in strength without observable gains in muscle size because training-induced strength gains during preadolescence are primarily due to neuromuscular factors.[82] That is, with proper instruction and practice time, children become better at recruiting and coordinating muscle fibers for greater force production. A compelling body of scientific evidence indicates that resistance training can be a safe, effective, and worthwhile method of conditioning for children and adolescents, provided the training program is well designed and supervised by qualified fitness professionals.[82,83]

Faigenbaum A, Myer G. Resistance training among young athletes: Safety, efficacy and injury prevention effects. *Br J Sports Med.* 2010;44:56–63.

Malina R. Weight training in youth-growth, maturation, and safety: an evidence-based review. *Clin J Sport Med.* 2006;16:478–487.

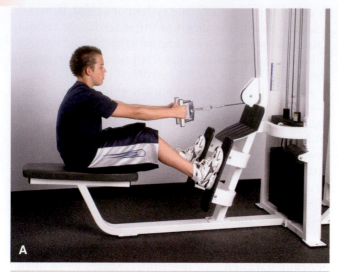

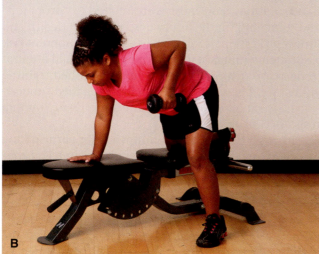

**Figure 25-5.** Resistance training is a safe, effective, and worthwhile activity for children and adolescents. (A) Seated row. (B) Dumbbell one-arm row.

and medicine balls, can be used in youth resistance-training programs in addition to the performance of body-weight exercises.[85]

Both single-joint (e.g., dumbbell curl) and multi-joint exercises (e.g., squat) can be incorporated into a youth resistance-training program. In is important to include multijoint movements in youth programs because these exercises require the coordinated action of many muscle groups. Also, the importance of strengthening the core musculature (i.e., abdominals, hips, and lower back) should not be overlooked because of the potential for lower-back pain in sedentary youth.[86] That is, prehabilitation strengthening exercises for the abdominals, hips, and lower back should be included as part of a preventative health measure. Depending on individual needs and the demands of specific sports, other prehabilitation exercises (e.g., internal and external rotation) can be incorporated into youth resistance-training sessions.

Of practical relevance, resistance training may offer observable health value for overweight youth who often perceive prolonged periods of aerobic exercise to be boring or discomforting.[87] Overweight youth seem to enjoy resistance training because it is characterized by short periods of physical activity interspersed with rest periods as needed. Moreover, resistance training gives overweight youth a chance to shine and gain confidence in their abilities to be physically active. In addition to enhancing muscular fitness, regular participation in a resistance-training program has been found to result in favorable changes in body composition and insulin sensitivity in overweight youth.[88,89]

The following list provides general youth resistance-training guidelines:

- Provide qualified instruction and close supervision.
- Focus on developing correct exercise technique.
- Begin with one to two sets of 10 to 15 repetitions using light-to-moderate loads.
- Increase the resistance gradually (5%–10%) as strength improves.
- Progress to multiple sets of 6 to 15 repetitions on selected exercises.
- Perform exercises for the upper body, lower body, and core musculature.
- Resistance train two to three times per week on nonconsecutive days.
- Systematically vary the training program over time to optimize adaptations.
  - Avoid competitive lifting and bodybuilding.

## Flexibility Exercise

Although flexibility is a well-recognized component of health-related fitness, long-held beliefs regarding the traditional practice of warm-up static stretching have been questioned.[91–93] An acute bout of static stretching can have a negative influence on strength and power performance, and research findings suggest that static stretching immediately before exercise has no significant effect on injury prevention.[92,94,95] This is not to suggest that children and teenagers should avoid regular static stretching, but rather that health and fitness professionals should consider the immediate impact of an acute bout of static stretching on performance.

The cool-down may actually be the ideal time to perform static stretching exercises because the muscles are already warmed up and participants need to recover from the exercise session with less intense activities. Youth should perform a variety of static stretches for the upper body, lower body, and midsection. Each stretch should be held for 10 to 30 seconds and repeated two to four times.[38]

### VIGNETTE continued

■ Three months after first meeting the Greenberg family, Jennifer asks Jacob and his parents to stay late one day for a quick chat about Jacob's progress. Although she did not perform any health or fitness

## RESEARCH HIGHLIGHT

### Is Low Muscle Fitness Associated With Metabolic Risk in Youth?

Although the clinical symptoms of cardiovascular disease do not become apparent until later in life, atherosclerosis has its roots during the pediatric years, and clustering of risk factors (e.g., elevated serum cholesterol, blood pressure, body fatness, and cardiopulmonary fitness) has been reported in younger populations. Prior research has shown that aerobic fitness is a strong predictor for clustering of cardiovascular risk factors in youth. However, it is unclear whether muscular strength is associated with cardiovascular risk in children and adolescents.

Researchers from Norway examined the independent associations of muscular fitness and cardiorespiratory fitness with clustered metabolic risk in 2,818 participants between 9 and 15 years of age.[90] The results revealed that low levels of muscle fitness were associated with clustered metabolic risk, independent of cardiorespiratory fitness (Fig. 25-6). An inverse association was also reported between cardiorespiratory fitness and clustered metabolic risk. The results of this study demonstrate that muscular fitness and cardiorespiratory fitness are independently and inversely associated with clustered metabolic risk in youth. The results also highlight the need to promote participation in both aerobic and strength-building activities.[90]

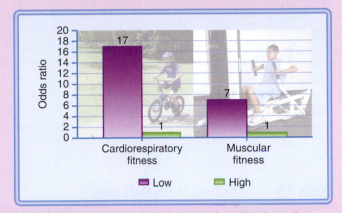

**Figure 25-6.** The odds of metabolic risk in youth are greatest for those individuals with low levels of cardiorespiratory and muscular fitness. Conversely, those individuals with high levels of cardiorespiratory and muscular fitness have much lower odds of metabolic risk.

Steene-Johannessen J, Anderssen S, Kolle E, Andersen LB. Low muscle fitness is associated with metabolic risk in youth. *Med Sci Sports Exerc.* 2009;41:1361-1367.

assessments at the outset of this community-based intervention, there is plenty of evidence that Jacob is truly benefitting from the program. Some objective changes are evident. Jacob has lost weight and has grown considerably stronger in only 3 months. He is watching less television at home and enjoys playing outside with his friends. More importantly, he has undergone a positive transformation. His self-esteem has improved, along with his behavior at home and even his grades in school. He loves the program and is very motivated to continue.

## Dynamic Warm-up

Sufficient scientific evidence does not exist to endorse pre-event static stretching in youth physical activity programs. Therefore, there has been increasing interest in warm-up procedures that involve the performance of dynamic movements designed to elevate core body temperature, enhance motor unit excitability, improve kinesthetic awareness (the body's ability to coordinate motion and the body's awareness of where it is in time and space), maximize active ranges of motion, and develop FMS skills.[96–98] This type of pre-event protocol is referred to as dynamic exercise and typically includes low-, moderate-, and high-intensity hops, skips, jumps, lunges, and various movement-based exercises for the upper and lower body. Dynamic activities do not involve the bouncing-type movements that are characteristic of ballistic stretching, but rather a controlled elongation of specific muscle groups.

From a practical perspective, getting youth ready for fitness activities or sports practice is not just about low-intensity aerobic exercise and static stretching. A well-designed, dynamic warm-up can set the tone for the session and establish a desired tempo for the upcoming activities. If the first few minutes of the class are up-tempo, exciting, and possess variety, performance will likely meet or exceed expectations. This concept of instant activity satisfies the need for children to move when they enter the gymnasium and helps to focus their attention on listening and learning.[99] In addition, dynamic warm-up activities that are active, engaging, and challenging provide an opportunity for participants to gain confidence in their abilities while practicing FMS.

## Fundamental Movement Skills

In addition to enhancing health-related fitness, health and fitness professionals should also include games and activities that enhance skill-related fitness, such as those that involve balloons or medicine balls (Tables 25-3 and 25-4).

Although children and adolescents should be encouraged to participate in a variety of physical activities, if they choose to do so, health and fitness professionals must be sure that youth develop the necessary prerequisite FMS before facing the difficulties of more demanding fitness programs or sports training sessions. Youth who achieve a broad repertoire of FMS are more likely to experience success and participate in physical activities as a lifetime choice.[45,49] Because children

## FROM THEORY TO PRACTICE

### ■ DYNAMIC WARM-UP

Because the current practice of warm-up static stretching has been based more on intuition than scientific evidence, there is a growing interest in dynamic warm-up procedures that include low-, moderate-, and high-intensity hops, skips, and jumps, and various movement-based exercises for the upper and lower body. Dynamic movements are not only more enjoyable to perform than static stretching, this type of movement preparation sets the tone for the class and better prepares boys and girls for the demands of fitness workouts and sports training. And because equipment is not needed, dynamic warm-up protocols are a cost-effective method for enhancing FMS that are the basic components of games and sports.

A 10-minute dynamic warm-up typically consists of 10 to 12 drills that progress from less intense to more intense. Participants perform each dynamic movement for about 10 yards, rest about 5 to 10 seconds, and then repeat the same exercise for 10 yards as they return to the starting point. Examples of these drills include high knee walk, lunge walk, lateral lunge, glute kicks, stepping trunk twists, hand walk, carioca, and speed skips.

## Table 25-3. Activities With Balloons

| ACTIVITY | INSTRUCTIONS |
|---|---|
| Squat jump | Hold a balloon near the chest, squat down slowly, then jump up off the ground. |
| 90-Degree jump | Hold a balloon near the chest, squat down slowly, then jump up off the ground turning 90 degrees clockwise. Complete one circle and then repeat in the opposite direction. |
| Forward lunge | Hold the balloon against the chest and lunge forward the moving balloon to the right and left. |
| Balloon tap | Start in the push-up position with a balloon on the floor in front of the head. Lightly touch the top of the balloon with the right hand. Return to the starting position and repeat with the left hand while keeping the body in a straight line. |
| Crab walk | Place the balloon between the knees in the crab position. Walk forward, side to side, and backward. |
| Plank walk | Place a balloon between the knees/lower legs in the push-up position. Move forward, keeping the body straight and the balloon off the ground. |
| Curl-up | Hold a balloon against the chest while in the curl-up starting position. Lift the shoulder blades off the floor and press the balloon toward the ceiling. For additional challenge, toss the balloon in the air during the curl-up, then catch the balloon and return to the starting position. |
| Knee tap and catch | In the standing position with arms extended, drop the balloon, tap the balloon with the right knee, and catch the balloon. Then repeat with the left knee. For additional challenge, make one complete 360-degree body circle after each tap. |
| Single-leg balance | While standing on the right foot, place the left foot near the right knee. Press the balloon overhead, in front, and to the right and left. For additional challenge, toss the balloon in the air during the overhead press, then catch the balloon and return to the starting position. |
| Get up and catch | Sit on the floor with the balloon in front of the chest. Toss the balloon in the air and quickly stand up and catch it before it lands on the ground. |

## Table 25-4. Medicine Ball Games and Activities

| ACTIVITY | INSTRUCTIONS |
| --- | --- |
| ABC ball | Stand and hold a medicine ball, and spell all the letters in a word or name by moving the ball in different directions to draw large letters. |
| Blind ball drop | Stand with arms extended in front of body, holding a ball with eyes closed. Drop the ball, then attempt to catch it as close to the floor as possible. |
| Target practice | Stand holding a ball against the chest with both hands. Dip about 3–4 inches, then return to the starting position as the ball is released. Aim toward a target on the floor (e.g., a hula hoop) about 10–15 feet away. This game should not require maximal effort, but rather the ability to adjust muscular effort to achieve a desired result. |
| Spin and catch | From a standing position with the ball near the chest, toss the ball into the air, then spin 180 degrees and catch it. Progress to full 360-degree spin and catch moving clockwise, then counterclockwise. |
| Stepping stones | Set up a line of leather medicine balls across the floor. The goal is to walk across the balls and get to the other side without falling. |
| Cat and mouse | A group of children stand in a circle in the athletic stance with two children holding balls that represent a "cat" and a "mouse." The balls are then passed quickly around the circle so the "cat" does not catch the "mouse." For additional challenge, add another ball (e.g., a "dog"). Periodically change directions. |
| Bocce ball | Roll a ball and then attempt to roll another ball as close as possible to the first ball rolled. |
| Wall ball | Sit on floor about 6 feet from the wall. Toss a ball with an overhead throw against the wall, then stand up and catch it on one bounce. |

do not naturally know how to hop, skip, jump, and throw properly, health and fitness professionals need to provide competent instruction and quality practice time for learning FMS that are characteristic of how children move and play.

Although an understanding of the importance of health- and skill-related fitness for youth is valuable, a key issue is to know how to provide youth with the skills, knowledge, attitudes, and behaviors that lead to a lifetime of physical activity. Instead of isolating fitness components, youth programs should integrate health- and skill-related fitness components into every session.[100] The integration of health- and skill-related fitness components will help youth master FMS, improve movement mechanics, and enhance their physical fitness while participating in a program that includes variety, progression, and proper recovery intervals.[52] This can be accomplished by ensuring that each exercise session includes health-related fitness exercise activities including aerobic, resistance, and flexibility training and skill-related fitness movements including functional activities required during games and play. Combining the synergistic activities of resistance exercise and motor skills can be accomplished by sandwiching the resistance-training program between purposeful sessions of warm-up and cool-down activities. More specifically, the children perform approximately 10 minutes of dynamic warm-up exercises, followed by about 20 to 30 minutes of resistance training, followed by approximately 15 minutes of games and 5 minutes of cool-down activities.

Exercise programs should be consistent with individual needs and abilities, and the initial volume and intensity should be low enough to allow time for proper adaptation. Youth should be taught how to perform each exercise correctly and should receive constructive feedback from health and fitness professionals (Fig. 25-7). Once youth become proficient with a series of exercises, they can advance to the next successive phase (e.g., increasing the duration of a functional movement skill interval or adding appropriate load to a resistance training exercise). There is no one combination of exercises, sets, and repetitions that

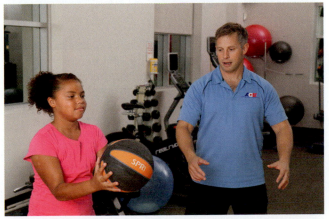

**Figure 25-7.** It is important for youth to be taught how to perform each exercise correctly and receive constructive feedback from health and exercise professionals.

optimizes training adaptations in all youth, but integrative fitness programs that include FMS development may provide the best opportunity to spark an interest in lifelong physical activity.

## Motivation and Leadership

The challenges associated with promoting youth fitness should be met with enthusiastic leadership, creative programming, and developmentally appropriate teaching strategies. Health and fitness professionals need to respect children's feelings while appreciating the fact that their thinking is different from that of adults. For example, attitude is everything as far as young people are concerned. Children prefer teachers who are encouraging and supportive, and have a caring attitude toward each student's personal progress (Fig. 25-8). In addition, health and fitness professionals should develop an appropriate philosophy about training youth that is consistent with the physical and psychosocial uniqueness of younger populations. Health and fitness professionals who work with youth in advanced training programs (e.g., sports conditioning) should have additional knowledge and practical experience to properly instruct and progress this type of training.

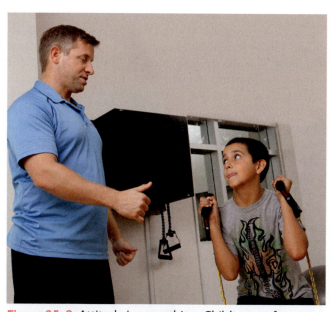

**Figure 25-8.** Attitude is everything. Children prefer teachers who are encouraging and supportive, and have a caring attitude toward each student's personal progress.

A major objective of youth fitness programming is for physical activity to become a habitual part of children's lives and hopefully persist into adulthood. With this objective in mind, health and fitness professionals must strive to increase participants' perceptions of their physical abilities and target deficiencies in specific movement patterns to foster participation in regular physical activity. This is particularly important for sedentary and overweight youth, who often lack the skills, confidence, and motivation to engage in health-enhancing aerobic exercise.[87,101] Thus, the focus of youth fitness programs should be on positive learning experiences in which all participants have an opportunity to make friends and feel good about their performances. Youth are not miniature adults, and the development of successful youth fitness programs requires an understanding of pediatric exercise science, sensitivity to growth-related differences in physical abilities, and a genuine interest in teaching children and adolescents.

## VIGNETTE conclusion

■ There is one last thing that Jennifer wants to discuss with the Greenbergs–the importance of social support and having good role models. She shares the story about the registered dietitian's visit, and the Greenbergs tell her that Jacob had already told them about it and that they have since made some changes to their evening routine. Jacob and his mom now cook dinner together an average of three nights each week, and the family enjoys a walk to the local playground every evening. Jennifer tells them how proud she is, not only of Jacob's progress, but also of the entire family. She encourages them to think about creating a "family fitness portrait" and to brainstorm ways for them to be active on the weekends. The Greenbergs leave that day excited about the important changes they have made in their lives. Jennifer is revitalized by their transformation and their newfound commitment to staying physically active as a family.

## CRITICAL THINKING QUESTIONS

1. You are the fitness director of a recreation center and want to start an after-school youth activity program for children between the ages of 7 and 12 years. You have access to an aerobic studio and different balls, bands, and exercise rings. Discuss the physical and psychological uniqueness of children, and highlight key program design considerations to ensure a safe, effective, and worthwhile experience for younger participants.

2. An 8-year-old competitive swimmer trains 5 days per week and her coach recently told her to avoid participation in other sports to allow more time for swimming. What factors influence sports performance during preadolescence, and what would you tell this youth coach about early sports specialization in young athletes?

3. The parents of an overweight adolescent are concerned that their son does not engage in any physical activity outside of school. What advice would you offer these parents, and what type of physical activity would you recommend for this 15-year-old adolescent?

## ADDITIONAL RESOURCES

President's Council on Fitness, Sports and Nutrition (http://fitness.gov): This site provides information for promoting good health through fitness, sports, and nutrition for people of all ages.

North American Society for Pediatric Exercise Science (http://naspem.org): This site provides information for the promotion of exercise science, physical activity, and fitness in the health and medical care of children and adolescents.

**Position Statements and Review Articles**

Armstrong N, McManus A. Physiology of elite young male athletes. *Med Sci Sports Exerc.* 2011;56:1–22.

Faigenbaum A, Kraemer W, Blimkie C, et al. Youth resistance training: Updated position statement paper from the National Strength and Conditioning Association. *J Strength Cond Res.* 2009;23:S60–S79.

McManus A, Armstrong N. Physiology of elite young female athletes. *Med Sci Sports Exerc.* 2011;56:23–46.

Mountjoy M, Andersen L, Armstrong N, et al. International Olympic Committee Consensus statement on the health and fitness of young people through physical activity and sport. *Br J Sports Med.* 2011;45:839–848.

Pate RR, O'Neill JR. Summary of the American Heart Association scientific statement: Promoting physical activity in children and youth: A leadership role for schools. *J Cardiovasc Nurs.* 2008;23:44–49.

Strong WB, Malina RM, Blimkie CJ, et al. Evidence based physical activity for school-age youth. *J Pediatr.* 2005; 146:732–737.

## REFERENCES

1. World Health Organization. *Global Recommendations on Physical Activity for Health.* Geneva: WHO Press; 2010.
2. American Academy of Pediatrics. Overuse injuries, overtraining and burnout in child and adolescent athletes. *Pediatrics.* 2007;119:1242–1245.
3. Malina R, Bouchard C, Bar-Or O. *Growth, Maturation and Physical Activity.* 2nd ed. Champaign, IL: Human Kinetics; 2004.
4. Rowland T. *Children's Exercise Physiology.* 2nd ed. Champaign, IL: Human Kinetics; 2007.
5. Tanner J. *Growth at Adolescence.* 2nd ed. Oxford, United Kingdom: Blackwell; 1962.
6. Bar-Or O. *Pediatric Sports Medicine for the Practitioner.* New York: Springer-Verlag; 1983.
7. National Association for Sport and Physical Education. *Guidelines for Participation in Youth Sport Programs: Specialization Versus Multi-sport Participation.* Reston, VA: Author; 2010.
8. Committee on Sports Medicine and Fitness. Intensive training and sports specialization in young athletes. *Pediatrics.* 2000;106:154–157.
9. Auvinen J, Tammelin T, Taimela S, et al. Musculoskeletal pains in relation to different sport and exercise activities in youth. *Med Sci Sports Exerc.* 2008;40: 1890–1900.
10. Cote J, Lidor R, Hackfort D. ISSP position stand: To sample or to specialize? Seven postulates about youth sport activities that lead to continued participation and elite performance. *Int J Sports Exerc Psychol.* 2009;7:7–17.
11. Eriksson B. Muscle metabolism in children: A review. *Acta Physiol Scand.* 1980;283:20–28.
12. Falk B, Dotan R. Child-adult differences in the recovery from high-intensity exercise. *Exerc Sport Sci Rev.* 2006; 34:107–112.
13. Armstrong N. *Paediatric Exercise Physiology.* Philadelphia, PA: Elsevier; 2007.
14. Riddell M. The endocrine response and substrate utilization during exercise in children and adolescents. *J Appl Physiol.* 2008;105:725–733.
15. Boisseau N, Delamarche P. Metabolic and hormonal responses to exercise in children and adolescents. *Sports Med.* 2000;30:405–422.
16. Eriksson B, Saltin B. Muscle metabolism during exercise in boys aged 11 to 16 years compared to adults. *Acta Paediatr.* 1974;28:257–265.
17. Faigenbaum A, Ratamess N, McFarland J, et al. Effect of rest interval length on bench press performance in boys, teens, and men. *Pediatr Exerc Sci.* 2008; 20:457–469.
18. Ratel S, Bedu M, Hennegrave A, et al. Effects of age and recovery duration on peak power output during repeated cycling sprints. *Int J Sports Med.* 2002;23: 397–402.
19. Singh T, Alexander M, Gauvreau K, et al. Recovery of oxygen consumption after maximal exercise in children. *Med Sci Sports Exerc.* 2011;43: 555–559.
20. Shvartz E, Reynolds R. Aerobic fitness norms for males and females aged 6 to 75 years: A review. *Aviat Space Environ Physiol.* 1990;61:3–11.
21. Armstrong N, Weisman J. Assessment and interpretation of aerobic fitness in children and adolescents. *Exerc Sport Sci Rev.* 1994;22:435–476.

22. Dencker M, Andersen L. Accelerometer measured daily physical activity related to aerobic fitness in children and adolescents. *J Sports Sci.* 2011;29:887–895.

23. Krahenbuhl G, Skinner J, Kohrt W. Developmental aspects of maximal aerobic power in children. *Exerc Sport Sci Rev.* 1985;13:503–538.

24. Payne V, Morrow J. The effect of physical training on prepubescent $\dot{V}O_2$ max: A meta analysis. *Res Q.* 1993; 64:305–313.

25. Obert P, Mandigout S, Nottin S, et al. Cardiovascular responses to endurance training in children. *Eur J Clin Invest.* 2003;33:199–208.

26. Armstrong L, Casa D, Millard-Stafford M, et al. Exertional heat illness during training and competition. *Med Sci Sports Exerc.* 2007;39:556–572.

27. Rowland T. Thermoregulation during exercise in the heat in children: Old concepts revisited. *J Appl Physiol.* 2008;105:718–724.

28. Inbar O, Morris N, Epstein Y, et al. Comparison of thermoregulatory response to exercise in dry heat among prepubertal boys, young adults, and older males. *Eur J Appl Physiol.* 2004;89:691–700.

29. Rivera Brown A, Gutierrez A, Gutierrez B, et al. Drink composition, voluntary drinking, and fluid balance in exercising, trained and heat-acclimatized boys. *J Appl Physiol.* 1999;86:78–84.

30. Meyer F, Bar-Or O, Salsberg A, et al. Hypohydration during exercise in children: Effect on thirst, drink preferences, and rehydration. *Int J Sports Nutr.* 1994;4:22–35.

31. Behm D, Faigenbaum A, Falk B, et al. Canadian Society for Exercise Physiology position paper: Resistance training in children and adolescents. *Appl Physiol Nutr Metab.* 2008;33:547–561.

32. Faigenbaum A, Kraemer W, Blimkie C, et al. Youth resistance training: Updated position statement paper from the National Strength and Conditioning Association. *J Strength Cond Res.* 2009;23:S60–S79.

33. Ramsay JA, Blimkie CJ, Smith K, et al. Strength training effects in prepubescent boys. *Med Sci Sports Exerc.* 1990;22:605–614.

34. U.S. Department of Health and Human Services. *2008 Physical Activity Guidelines for Americans.* Available at: http://health.gov/paguidelines.

35. Rowland T. Promoting physical activity for children's health. *Sports Med.* 2007;37:929–936.

36. Ruiz J, Castro-Pinero J, Artero E, et al. Predictive validity of health related fitness in youth: A systematic review. *Br J Sports Med.* 2009;43:909–923.

37. Centers for Disease Control and Prevention. *The Association Between School-Based Physical Activity, Including Physical Education, and Academic Performance.* Atlanta, GA: U.S. Department of Health and Human Services; 2010.

38. National Association for Sport and Physical Education. *Physical Education for Lifetime Fitness.* 3rd ed. Champaign, IL: Human Kinetics; 2011.

39. Ortega F, Ruiz J, Castillo M, et al. Physical fitness in children and adolescence: A powerful marker of health. *Int J Obes.* 2008;32:1–11.

40. Strong WB, Malina RM, Blimkie CJ, et al. Evidence based physical activity for school-age youth. *J Pediatr.* 2005;146:732–737.

41. Andersen L, Riddoch C, Kriemier S, Hills AP. Physical activity and cardiovascular risk factors in children. *Br J Sports Med.* 2011;45:871–876.

42. Larun L, Nordheim L, Ekeland E, et al. Exercise in the prevention and treatment of anxiety and depression among children and young people. *Cochrane Database Syst Rev.* 2006;3:CD004691.

43. Gutin B, Owens S. The influence of physical activity on cardiometabolic biomarkers in youths: A review. *Pediatr Exerc Sci.* 2011;23:169–185.

44. Telama R. Tracking of physical activity from childhood to adulthood: A review. *Obesity Facts.* 2009;2:187–195.

45. Lubans D, Morgan P, Cliff D, et al. Fundamental movement skills in children and adolescents. *Sports Med.* 2010;40:1019–1035.

46. Barnett L, Van Beurden E, Morgan P, et al. Does childhood motor skill proficiency predict adolescent fitness? *Med Sci Sports Exerc.* 2008;40:2137–2144.

47. Barnett L, Van Beurden E, Morgan P, et al. Childhood motor skill proficiency as a predictor of adolescent physical activity. *J Adolesc Health.* 2009;44:252–259.

48. Stodden D, Langendorfer S, Roberton M. The association between motor skill competence and physical fitness in young adults. *Res Q Exerc Sport.* 2009; 80:223–229.

49. Stodden D, Goodway J, Langendorfer S, et al. A developmental perspective on the role of motor skill competence in physical activity: An emergent relationship. *Quest.* 2008;60:290–306.

50. Valovich McLeod T, Decoster L, Loud K, et al. National Athletic Trainers' Association position statement: Prevention of pediatric overuse injuries. *J Athl Train.* 2011;46:206–220.

51. Hewett TE, Myer GD, Ford KR. Reducing knee and anterior cruciate ligament injuries among female athletes: A systematic review of neuromuscular training interventions. *J Knee Surg.* 2005;18:82–88.

52. Myer G, Faigenbaum A, Ford K, et al. When to initiate integrative neuromuscular training to reduce sports-related injuries and enhance health in youth? *Curr Sports Med Rep.* 2011;10:157–166.

53. Mountjoy M, Andersen L, Armstrong N, et al. International Olympic Committee Consensus statement on the health and fitness of young people through physical activity and sport. *Br J Sports Med.* 2011;45:839–848.

54. Leek D, Carlson J, Cain K, et al. Physical activity during youth sports practices. *Arch Pediatr Adolesc Med.* 2011;165:294–299.

55. Seefeldt V. Developmental motor patterns: Implications for elementary school physical education. In: Nadeau C, Holliwell W, Newell K, Roberts G, eds. *Psychology of Motor Behavior and Sport.* Champaign, IL: Human Kinetics; 1980:314–323.

56. Tremblay M, Colley R, Saunders T, et al. Physiological and health implications of a sedentary lifestyle. *Appl Physiol Nutr Metab.* 2010;35:725–740.

57. Nader P, Bradley R, Houts R, et al. Moderate to vigorous physical activity from ages 9 to 15 years. *J Am Med Assoc.* 2008;300:295–305.

58. Belcher B, Berrigan D, Dodd K, et al. Physical activity in US youth: Effect of race/ethnicity, age, gender, and weight status. *Med Sci Sports Exerc.* 2010;42:2211–2221.

59. Tudor-Locke C, Johnson W, Katzmarzyk PT. Accelerometer-determined steps per day in US children and adolescents. *Med Sci Sports Exerc.* 2010;42:2244–2250.

60. Dencker M, Thorsson O, Karlsson MK, et al. Daily physical activity and its relation to aerobic fitness in children aged 8-11 years. *Eur J Appl Physiol.* 2006;96:587–592.

61. Narayan K, Boyle J & Thompson T. Lifetime risk for diabetes mellitus in the United States. *J Am Med Assoc.* 2003;290:1884–1890.

62. Ogden C, Carroll M, Curtin L, et al. Prevalence of high body mass index in US children and adolescents, 2007-2008. *J Am Med Assoc.* 2010;303:242–249.

63. Li S, Treuth M, Wang Y. How active are American adolescents and have they become less active? *Obes Rev.* 2010;11:847–862.

64. Sisson S, Katzmarzyk P. International prevalence of physical activity in youth and adults. *Obes Rev.* 2008;9:606–614.

65. Guthold R, Cowan M, Autenrieth C, et al. Physical activity and sedentary behavior among schoolchildren: A 34 country comparison. *J Pediatr.* 2010;157:43–49.

66. American Academy of Pediatrics. Policy statement: Children, adolescents, obesity and the media. *Pediatrics.* 2011;128:201–208.

67. Centers for Disease Control and Prevention. Physical activity levels of high school students—United States, 2010. *Morb Mortl Wkly Rep.* 2011;60:773–777.

68. National Association of Sport and Physical Education and American Heart Association. *Shape of the Nation Report: Status of Physical Education in the USA.* Reston, VA: National Association of Sport and Physical Education; 2010.

69. Kones R. Is prevention a fantasy, or the future of medicine? A panoramic view of recent data, status, and direction in cardiovascular prevention. *Ther Adv Cardiovasc Dis.* 2011;5:61–81.

70. Trasande L, Liu Y, Fryer G, et al. Effects of childhood obesity on hospital care and costs. *Health Aff (Millwood).* 2009;28:751–760.

71. Biddle S, Pearson N, Ross G, et al. Tracking of sedentary behaviors of young people: A systematic review. *Prev Med.* 2010;51:345–351.

72. Faigenbaum A, Straccolini A, Myer G. Exercise deficit disorder in youth: A hidden truth. *Acta Paediatr.* 2011; 100:1423–1425.

73. Goodman E, Whitaker R. A prospective study of the role of depression in the development and persistence of adolescent obesity. *Pediatrics.* 2002;110:497–504.

74. Taras H, Potts-Datema W. Obesity and student performance at school. *J School Health* 2005;75:291–295.

75. Schwimmer J, Burwinkle T, Varni J. Health-related quality of life of severely obese children and adolescents. *J Am Med Assoc.* 2003;289:1813–1819.

76. Dishman R, Motl R, Saunders R, et al. Enjoyment mediates effects of a school-based physical activity intervention. *Med Sci Sports Exerc.* 2005;37:478–487.

77. Burdette H, Whitaker R. Resurrecting free play in young children. *Arch Pediatr Adolesc Med.* 2005; 159:46–50.

78. Ratel S, Lazaar N, Dore E, et al. High-intensity intermittent activities at school: Controversies and facts. *J Sports Med Phys Fit.* 2004;44:272–280.

79. Bailey R, Olsen J, Pepper S, et al. The level and tempo of children's physical activities: An observational study. *Med Sci Sports Exerc.* 1995;27:1033–1041.

80. Parikh T, Stratton G. Influence of intensity of physical activity on adiposity and cardiorespiratory fitness in 5-18 year olds. *Sports Med.* 2011;41:477–488.

81. Behringer M, vom Heede A, Yue Z, et al. Effects of resistance training in children and adolescents: A meta-analysis. *Pediatrics.* 2010;126:e1199–e1210.

82. Faigenbaum A, Myer G. Resistance training among young athletes: Safety, efficacy and injury prevention effects. *Br J Sports Med.* 2010;44:56–63.

83. Malina R. Weight training in youth-growth, maturation, and safety: An evidence-based review. *Clin J Sport Med.* 2006;16:478–487.

84. Myer G, Quatman C, Khoury J, et al. Youth vs. adult "weightlifting" injuries presented to United States emergency rooms: Accidental vs. non-accidental injury mechanisms. *J Strength Cond Res.* 2009;23: 2054–2060.

85. Faigenbaum A, Westcott W. *Youth Strength Training.* Champaign, IL: Human Kinetics; 2009.

86. Andersen L, Wedderkopp N, Leboeuf-Yde C. Association between back pain and physical fitness in adolescents. *Spine.* 2006;31:1740–1744.

87. Faigenbaum A, Westcott W. Resistance training for obese children and adolescents. *Pres Counc Phys Fit Sports Res Dig.* 2007;8:1–8.

88. Shaibi GQ, Cruz ML, Ball GD, et al. Effects of resistance training on insulin sensitivity in overweight Latino adolescent males. *Med Sci Sports Exerc.* 2006;38: 1208–1215.

89. Van der Heijden G, Wang Z, Chu Z, et al. Strength exercise improves muscle mass and hepatic insulin sensitivity in obese youth. *Med Sci Sports Exerc.* 2010;42:1973–1980.

90. Steene-Johannessen J, Anderssen SA, Kolle E, Andersen LB. Low muscle fitness is associated with metabolic risk in youth. *Med Sci Sports Exerc.* 2009; 41:1361–1367.

91. Stone M, O'Bryant HS, Ayers C, et al. Stretching: Acute and chronic? The potential consequences. *Strength Cond J.* 2006;28:66–74.

92. Behm D, Chaouachi A. A review of the acute effects of static and dynamic stretching on performance. *Eur J Appl Physiol.* 2011;111:2633–2651.

93. Faigenbaum A, McFarland J. Guidelines for implementing a dynamic warm-up for physical education. *J Phys Educ Recreat Dance.* 2007;78:25–28.

94. Shrier I. Stretching before exercise does not reduce the risk of local muscle injury: A critical review of the clinical and basic science literature. *Clin J Sports Med.* 1999;9:221–227.

95. Shrier I. Does stretching improve performance? A systematic and critical review of the literature. *Clin J Sports Med.* 2004;14:267–273.

96. Faigenbaum AD, Bellucci M, Bernieri A, et al. Acute effects of different warm-up protocols on fitness performance in children. *J Strength Cond Res.* 2005;19:376–381.

97. Faigenbaum AD, McFarland JE, Schwerdtman JA, et al. Dynamic warm-up protocols, with and without a weighted vest, and fitness performance in high school female athletes. *J Athl Train.* 2006;41: 357–363.

98. Siatras T, Papadopoulos G, Mameletzi D, et al. Static and dynamic acute stretching effect on gymnasts' speed in vaulting. *Pediatr Exerc Sci.* 2003;15: 383–391.

99. Graham G. *Teaching Children Physical Education.* Champaign, IL: Human Kinetics; 2001.

100. Myer G, Faigenbaum A, Chu D, et al. Integrative training for children and adolescents: Techniques and practices for reducing sports-related injuries and enhancing athletic performance. *Phys Sportsmed.* 2011;39:74–84.

101. Cliff D, Okely A, Morgan P, et al. Proficiency deficiency: Mastery of fundamental movement skills and skill components in overweight and obese children. *Obesity (Silver Spring).* 2012; 20:1024–1033.

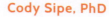

Cody Sipe, PhD

**CHAPTER 26**

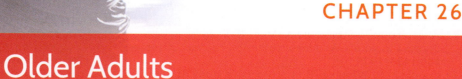

# Older Adults

## CHAPTER OUTLINE

## LEARNING OUTCOMES

1. Define *primary aging* and *secondary aging*.
2. Describe how aging contributes to declines in the body's physiological systems, including the neuromuscular, skeletal, and cardiometabolic systems.
3. List critical concepts related to physical function and disability with advancing age.
4. Identify considerations for conducting exercise testing with older individuals.
5. Explain the acute and chronic effects of exercise in aging individuals.
6. Describe safe and effective exercise training techniques.

## ANCILLARY LINK

Visit Davis*Plus* at http://davisplus.fadavis.com for study and practice resources, including online quizzes, animations that help explain physiological processes, podcasts concerning news and career trends in exercise physiology, and practice references.

## VIGNETTE

■ Danitza, a personal trainer, begins working with a new 67-year-old client named Julie. Danitza is a relatively new trainer whose typical clients have been women in their 30s who want to get back in shape after gaining weight from having children. She has very little experience working with older clients but feels that she is a good trainer and is confident she can adapt her strategies to be successful with Julie.

After 4 weeks of training, Danitza is feeling frustrated with her new client and is unsure of exactly what to do. Julie does not seem motivated to perform her quick-paced training routine, which consists of several supersets of resistance-training exercises interspersed with modified calisthenics and abdominal floor work. This routine is similar to what Danitza has used successfully with many clients, but she has modified it considerably in consideration of Julie's age. However, Julie complains often that many of the exercises hurt her knees or back, and Danitza constantly has to stop to re-teach movements that they have done before because Julie just cannot seem to remember them. Danitza feels that she has modified her exercise routine significantly to accommodate the needs of an older person and begins to think that Julie is simply lazy and whiny. She now dreads having to train Julie and wants to give her up as a client but cannot afford to do so. Danitza is feeling trapped.

How would a better understanding of the needs, interests, and motivations of mature individuals have helped Danitza avoid some of the frustrations she is now feeling? How would a more appropriate training program increase Julie's motivation while simultaneously easing the stress that she reports in her knees and back?

There have never, in human history, been more adults older than 55 years than there are today. The global population of mature adults has grown exponentially over the past several years and will continue to do so for the next 20 to 30 years (Fig. 26-1). The need to develop effective lifestyle interventions that have the potential to improve the quality of life for older persons is especially apparent when considering the growing proportion of older adults in today's society. The following statistics illustrate some aspects of the enormous demographic shift in the United States.[1]

- In the year 2014, nearly 44 million people, or 13.7% of the population, were 65 years and older.
- By 2030, 19.7% of the U.S. population, about 70 million people, will have passed their 65th birthday.
- The baby boomer generation began to turn 65 years in 2009, and the number of people aged 65 years and older is expected to nearly triple to 93 million within the next 50 years.
- The youngest members of the baby boomer generation will reach the age of 65 years in 2030.
- People aged 85 years and older currently represent the fastest-growing segment of the older population.
- By 2050, the size of the 85+ age group will increase to 19 million, almost 5% of the population.
- There were about 65,000 people aged 100 years or older in 2000, and the number of centenarians is projected to grow so quickly that there may be as many as 381,000 by 2030.

Thus, there has never been more of a need and opportunity for fitness professionals to specialize in working with this population.

However, mature adults typically have a different set of needs, interests, and desires than their younger counterparts and are often misunderstood.[2,3] Numerous myths, misconceptions, and negative stereotypes

about aging and what it means to grow old pervade society and the fitness industry (Box 26-1). These incorrect perspectives are barriers to working effectively with the mature population, especially with the aging baby boomer population. The boomers are the largest age cohort in history and are driving the growth of the mature population. Boomers began turning 65 in 2010. Perhaps more important than their sheer numbers are the different ideologies, perspectives, and collective experiences that they bring with them compared with the generation before them. It is vital that health and fitness professionals working with mature clients possess an understanding of the diverse physiological, psychological, emotional, and social needs of this ever-changing and fast-growing population.

This chapter examines some of the key issues that influence the relationship between physical activity and the aging process, beginning with a discussion of underlying biological mechanisms responsible for aging. The role that regular physical activity plays in healthy aging is also examined. The last portion of this chapter presents information on exercise testing and programming for older adults, and explains important health and safety issues unique to this population.

## COMMUNICATING WITH OLDER CLIENTS

It is not unusual for health and fitness professionals to have difficulty connecting and communicating with clients who are much older than themselves. Many potential barriers exist that can lead to misunderstanding and even conflict. Several areas should be addressed by health and fitness professionals who work with older adults, including stereotypes, generational gaps, value differences, and lack of professionalism.

### Stereotypes

Buying in to common myths and stereotypes associated with aging can have a negative effect on communication even before it starts. The truth about these stereotypes is that they do hold true for some individuals, but the old axiom "you can't judge a book by its cover" could not be more appropriate for this group. They are heterogeneous and very difficult to pigeonhole. Approaching older clients without preconceived ideas or judgments based on appearance alone will significantly increase a health fitness professional's ability to effectively communicate with them.

### Generational Gaps

The explosion of technological innovations has changed most aspects of society over the past 50 years. Communication technologies especially have significantly affected how people work, play, and interact with one another. E-mail, chat rooms, discussion groups, smartphones, text messaging, Facebook, and

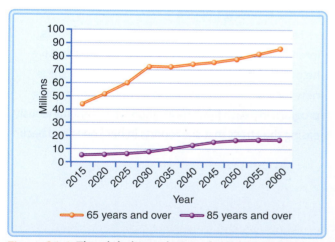

**Figure 26-1.** The global population of mature adults has grown exponentially in recent years and will continue to do so over the coming decades. (Data from Projections of the Population by Selected Age Groups and Sex for the United States: 2015 to 2060. U.S. Census Bureau, Population Division. December 2012.) http://www.census.gov/population/projections/data/national/2012.html

## Box 26-1. Common Negative Myths About Aging

Griffiths and Thinnes[50] described the following myths that health and fitness professionals would be wise to dispel:

- *Chronological age determines the way an older adult acts and feels.* The process of aging varies widely and is affected by many factors, including personality, experiences, health, and the natural responses to loss, aging, and death. Thus, health and fitness professionals should take this into account and treat their older clients as individuals within their own unique contexts, histories, and circumstances.
- *You can't teach an old dog new tricks.* Intelligence is both crystallized (from lived experiences that build wisdom) and fluid, which involves new skills and pieces of knowledge learned on the spot.
- *As one ages, one naturally becomes older and wiser.* Stereotyping, both positive and negative, can be detrimental. Believing that all older adult clients will be wiser is simply not accurate, just as it is not true that all older clients will be senile.
- *Older adults become more conservative as they age.* The fact is that many older clients will be very receptive to new ideas, especially if they involve their health, fitness, and well-being—depending in large measure on how the ideas are presented to them. Adults learn continuously from life experiences and, therefore, are often open to pursuing new interests and goals.[51]
- *Older adults are not productive, especially at work.* Between 2000 and 2015, the number of workers aged 55 years and older will have increased by 72%.[52] According to AARP,[53] 60% of older persons plan to work in some capacity during their retirement. Whether it is from economic need or the satisfaction derived from the work, many will take on part-time employment. In fact, only 11% of "boomers" are planning to stop working entirely when they reach retirement age.[54]
- *Older adults prefer quiet and tranquil daily lives.* It would be a mistake for health and fitness professionals to believe that older adults prefer a sedentary lifestyle. A hallmark of this generation is that boomers stay active as a key to health and well-being.
- *All older adults become senile.* There is confusion in using the term *senility* to describe psychosocial disorders that older adults deal with, such as anxiety, depression, grieving, or dementia. When an older adult appears confused, misunderstands, or needs more time to get directions, it is a mistake to assume this is a sign of senility.

Twitter have all had an impact on how people communicate. Most of these were more like science fiction than reality when older adults were growing up. Although some older adults have fully embraced these changes, others prefer more traditional forms of communication such as face-to-face conversations. They may even find some of these new forms of communication rude or inappropriate. Vast chasms can exist in values, beliefs about life, philosophies, worldviews, and so much more—and it is these differences that really make it difficult to connect with those much older or much younger than yourself.

## Value Differences

All individuals differ in their values, but some general commonalities have been identified. Understanding these values can help health and fitness professionals communicate more effectively with older adult clients.

- *Social connections and relationships:* The desire for social connections is strong. Health and fitness professionals may need to be open to building a relationship with older clients that might be more personal than is typical of a younger client.
- *Spirituality:* The later stages of life are characterized by recognition of one's own mortality and an opportunity for reflection of one's life. This often leads to a deeper, or even a resurgence of, spiritual connection and concern. Motivation for

exercise and healthy lifestyle habits are often linked to a spiritual awakening in older adults.

- *Quality without excess:* Retirees who have earned a good income and saved/invested well may be able to afford the finer things in life, but this does not mean that they are interested in being "flashy." In fact, many have learned that possessions mean very little.
- *Health and well-being:* Even mature adults who do not exercise are often interested in improving or maintaining their health by eating well, taking vitamin supplements, avoiding tobacco, and pursuing active hobbies.
- *Giving back:* The majority of retirees remain very active as volunteers to support community organizations, their church and neighborhood, and numerous worthy causes. This is important to them and even vital to their identity as a contributing member of society.

## Lack of Professionalism

Everyone has had a negative experience with an unprofessional employee, be it a clerk, manager, waiter, or cashier. The general lack of professionalism within the fitness industry often repels mature adults who see this behavior as juvenile and inappropriate. Whether it is a lack of attentiveness by front desk staff, a refusal to accept responsibility for a problem, poor exercise etiquette (e.g., not sharing equipment, wiping down equipment after use, or re-racking weights) that is either tolerated or even perpetuated by the staff, or health and fitness professionals discussing their wild weekend activities, these all create barriers with the mature adults the industry is trying to serve.

## In Your Own Words

Recently, your 72-year-old client Charles expressed an increased interest in making a commitment to eating healthier and tracking his workout sessions. However, Charles has confided in you that he feels intimidated by using the computer, and that in the past he gave up trying to use interactive technology because he found it difficult to navigate. What would you say to Charles to encourage him to use online technology, such as the USDA website Choose MyPlate (http://ChooseMyPlate.gov), to record his eating habits and track his physical activity? How would you communicate with this client about the various options in nutrition- and exercise-tracking software, while avoiding the stereotype that older adults have a hard time learning about or using modern technology?

## AGING CONCEPTS

Before considering exercise testing and training for older adults, it is essential to first grasp some key concepts pertaining to aging, as well as the factors involved in the process of aging. Key definitions are included in Box 26-2.

### Aging Basics

Organismal senescence (i.e., aging) is a natural and inevitable part of the life cycle. All living beings experience a period of growth and maturation followed by a period of decline, which is often accompanied by disease and which culminates eventually in death. Although the aging process is hardwired into our systems and cannot be stopped, this does not mean that people are completely at its mercy. On the contrary, individuals are able to significantly, and sometimes dramatically, influence how quickly or how well they age. The foods they eat, activities in which they choose to engage, environmental toxins to which they are exposed, and numerous other factors have been shown to either "accelerate" or "slow" the aging process. Yet, no one has found a way to stop the aging process altogether.

Master's athletes (i.e., older athletes) are often considered to be as ideal a model for studying aging, and

---

## Box 26-2. Aging Concepts

*Primary aging:* This is the innate process of maturation and subsequent decline that occur in the body's cells and physiological systems throughout the life span and make the organism more susceptible to disease, injury, and death. This process is considered to be "hardwired" into our genetic code and cannot be altered.

*Secondary aging:* This involves those age-related deteriorations that result from lifestyle behaviors (e.g., physical activity, nutrition, tobacco use, and alcohol consumption), disease processes (e.g., diabetes, cancer, and CVD), environment (exposure to toxins, air pollution, and ultraviolet radiation), injury, and illness. These factors are highly variable and can be significantly controlled by the individual to delay some age-related processes.

*Chronological aging:* This is simply the number of years a person has been alive. It has long been used as a way to categorize, and sometimes discriminate against, an individual. Chronological age, however, is a crude and often inaccurate means of determining how "old" an individual is from a biological or physiological perspective. The mature adult population is very diverse. Therefore, an individual who is older chronologically may be healthier, fitter, and more functional than his or her younger counterparts.

*Usual aging:* This term describes how the majority of individuals in a society "usually" or "typically" age. For example, the typical older adult is able to function independently but has an increased risk for disease or disability. The disability risk is due, in large part, to the reduced functional reserve capacity of the individual and his or her downward aging trajectory. That is, the individual has a reduced capacity for performing more intense activities.

*Successful aging:* Based on the research by Rowe and Kahn,[3] this is defined by the ability to maintain a low risk for disease and disease-related disability, high mental and physical function, and active engagement with life.

*Active aging:* This is a concept advanced by the International Council on Active Aging and adopted by the World Health Organization that encourages individuals to be "engaged in life" as fully as possible despite health status, disease conditions, or socioeconomic status. It recognizes the importance of each of the seven dimensions of wellness—physical, intellectual, emotional, spiritual, environmental, vocational, and social—to the overall well-being of an aging individual.

specifically quantifying **primary aging** (aging of the physiological systems throughout the life span), that we have available. These athletes have often lived pristine lives—eating well, exercising regularly, avoiding exposure to cigarette smoke, and having access to quality medical care. Yet, despite doing almost everything right, they still age. This is evidenced by the fact that performance records decrease with advancing age in virtually all individual competitive sports, including track and field, running, bicycling, and swimming.[4] The rates of decline are unique to each activity, but generally decrease after the age of 40 years, with an accelerated rate of decline after the age of 70 years. The question is not *if* they will age, but *how* they will age. Master's athletes tend to live longer, have fewer diseases, and possess higher levels of function than their less active peer counterparts, demonstrating the power of lifestyle to minimize the effects of **secondary aging** (i.e., age-related deteriorations that result from lifestyle behaviors, disease processes, environment, injury, and illness).

## Why Do People Age?

Many theories have been proposed to explain why or how people age from either a biological, physiological, or sociological perspective. Some have focused on primary aging, whereas others attempt to explain factors associated with secondary aging.[5] **Life course theory** is one of the prevailing perspectives of aging that recognizes the influence of past events on an older individual's current state of health and function. There is now a recognition that many factors that are out of an individual's control can have an impact on health, quality of life, and longevity, such as being born with a low birth weight, the birth mother smoking during pregnancy, being breast- or bottle-fed, not having access to quality health-care services, poor nutrition, and injuries during childhood.[6,7]

The more recent concept of active aging has been proposed as a way to promote the benefits of an active lifestyle for increasing longevity and quality of life. **Active aging** recognizes the importance of active engagement in life in multiple dimensions of wellness, such as physical, emotional, social, spiritual, and mental. It is important for fitness professionals who work with older adults to integrate these multiple dimensions of wellness into their programs.

## PHYSIOLOGY OF AGING

The typical physiological declines associated with aging have been well documented, and yet difficulty separating primary and secondary aging processes remains. Although the literature often reports average declines in physiological systems, a high degree of interindividual variability has been reported in the same literature. This means that, although studies may report that a particular component declines, on average, 30%

between the ages of 50 and 80 years, the actual range of decline among those individuals may be as large as 10% to 60%. Practically speaking, a 10% reduction in that particular component may have no significant effect on the individual, whereas a 60% reduction may cause significant problems and even lead to an active pathology.

When considering these physiological declines, it is important to recognize and appreciate the variability that exists among individuals. Assuming that mature adults of similar age are also similar in regard to health status, disease processes, or functional abilities fails to appreciate the diversity that exists within this population. Table 26-1 outlines the typical changes in physiological function and body composition with advancing age in healthy humans.

## Neuromuscular System

Muscular performance declines with advancing age in late life.[4] It is commonly reported that strength declines in sedentary older adults at a rate of about 1% per year beginning in their 40s and accelerates to approximately 3% per year once they reach their 70s.[4,8] However, a significant degree of variability exists within the literature that is dependent on such elements as the type of contraction used, muscle groups tested, sex, disease processes, and physical-activity status. The declines in muscular performance have been primarily attributed to the loss of muscle mass (**sarcopenia**) that results from the aging process,[9] because strength is highly correlated to muscle cross-sectional area. The average individual will lose approximately 40% of muscle mass between the ages of 20 and 70 years,[10] with a slightly greater loss in the lower extremities compared with the upper extremities.[8] It is estimated that anywhere from 22% to 53% of the older adult population will experience development of sarcopenia.[11] Although the loss of muscle mass is an independent risk factor for the development of disability, it alone does not fully explain the decline in strength associated with aging.[4,11]

Aging is associated with a preferential decrease in the size of type II (fast-twitch) muscle fibers compared with type I (slow-twitch) muscle fibers, an increase in connective tissue, altered muscle metabolism, and motor unit remodeling (approximately a 1% decrease in the number of motor units each year).[4,12] The loss of fast-twitch fibers has a major impact on a muscle's ability to generate the necessary force required of specific tasks. These changes can have negative implications for the individual's health and physical functioning, which can be at least partially reversed by exercise training. Resistance exercise can increase muscle mass, strength, power, and quality (i.e., muscular performance per unit muscle volume or mass), and improve muscle metabolism (e.g., glycemic control) even in the **oldest-old** adults (86–120 years old).[8] Aerobic exercise training can improve muscle metabolism but has little or no effect on muscle mass, strength, power, or quality.[8]

## Table 26-1. Summary of Typical Changes in Physiological Function and Body Composition With Advancing Age in Healthy Humans

| VARIABLES | TYPICAL CHANGES | FUNCTIONAL SIGNIFICANCE* |
|---|---|---|
| **Muscular function** | | |
| Muscle strength and power | Isometric, concentric, and eccentric strength decline from about age 40 years and accelerate after age 65–70 years. Lower-body strength declines at a faster rate than upper-body strength. Power declines at a faster rate than strength. | Deficits in strength and power predict disability in old age and mortality risk. |
| Muscle endurance and fatigability | Endurance declines. Maintenance of force at a given relative intensity may increase with age. Age effects on mechanisms of fatigue are unclear and task dependent. | Unclear but may impact recovery from repetitive daily tasks. |
| Balance and motility | Sensory, motor, and cognitive changes alter biomechanics (sit, stand, locomotion). These changes plus environmental constraints can adversely affect balance and mobility. | Impaired balance increases fear of falling and can reduce daily activity. |
| Motor performance and control | Reaction time increases. Speed of simple and repetitive movements slows. Altered control of precision movements. Complex tasks are affected more than simple tasks. | Impacts many IADL and increases risk for injury and task learning time. |
| Flexibility and joint ROM | Declines are significant for hip (20%–30%), spine (20%–30%), and ankle (30%–40%) flexion by age 70 years, especially in women. Muscle and tendon elasticity decreases. | Poor flexibility may increase risks for injury, falling, and back pain. |
| **Cardiovascular function** | | |
| Cardiac function | Maximum HR ($208 - 0.7 \times age$), stroke volume, and cardiac output decline. Slowed HR response at exercise onset. Altered diastolic filling pattern (rest and exercise). Reduced left ventricular ejection fraction percentage. Decreased HR variability. | Major determinant of reduced exercise capacity with aging. |
| Vascular function | Aorta and its major branches stiffen. Vasodilator capacity and endothelium-dependent dilation of most peripheral arteries (brachial, cutaneous) decrease. | Arterial stiffening and endothelial dysfunction increase CVD risk. |
| BP | BP at rest (especially systolic) increases. BP during submaximal and maximal exercise is higher in old vs. young, especially in older women. | Increased systolic BP reflects increased work of the heart. |
| Regional blood flow | Leg blood flow is generally reduced at rest, submaximal, and maximal exercise. Renal and splanchnic vasoconstriction during submaximal exercise may be reduced with age. | May influence exercise capacity, ADL, and BP regulation in old age. |
| $O_2$ extraction | Systemic: Same at rest and during submaximal exercise, same or slightly lower at maximal exercise. Legs: No change at rest or during submaximal exercise, decreased slightly at maximal exercise. | Capacity for peripheral $O_2$ extraction is relatively maintained. |
| Blood volume and composition | Reduced total and plasma volumes; small reduction in hemoglobin concentration. | May contribute to reduced maximal stroke volume via reduced cardiac preload. |
| Body fluid regulation | Thirst sensation decreases. Renal sodium- and water-conserving capabilities are impaired. Total body water declines with age. | May predispose to dehydration and impaired exercise tolerance in the heat. |
| **Pulmonary function** | | |
| Ventilation | Chest wall stiffens. Expiratory muscle strength decreases. Older adults adopt different breathing strategy during exercise. Work of breathing increases. | Pulmonary aging not limiting to exercise capacity, except in athletes. |

### Table 26-1. Summary of Typical Changes in Physiological Function and Body Composition With Advancing Age in Healthy Humans –cont'd

| VARIABLES | TYPICAL CHANGES | FUNCTIONAL SIGNIFICANCE* |
|---|---|---|
| Gas exchange | Loss of alveoli and increased size of remaining alveoli; reduces surface area of $O_2$ and $CO_2$ exchange in the lungs. | Arterial blood gases usually well maintained up to maximal exercise. |

**Physical functional capacities**

| VARIABLES | TYPICAL CHANGES | FUNCTIONAL SIGNIFICANCE* |
|---|---|---|
| Maximal $O_2$ uptake | Overall decline averages 0.4–0.5 mL/kg/yr (9% per decade) in healthy sedentary adults. Longitudinal data suggest rate of decline accelerates with advancing age. | Indicates a reduced functional reserve; disease and mortality risk factor. |
| $O_2$ uptake kinetics | Systemic $O_2$ uptake kinetics at exercise onset is slowed in old vs. young, but this may be task specific. Warm-up before exercise may normalize age difference. | Slow $\dot{V}O_2$ kinetics may increase $O_2$ deficit and promote early fatigue. |
| Lactate and ventilatory thresholds | Ventilatory thresholds increase with age. Maximal lactate production, tolerance, and clearance rate decline after exercise. | Indicative of reduced capacity for high-intensity exercise. |
| Submaximal work efficiency | Metabolic cost of walking at a given speed is increased. Work efficiency (cycling) is preserved, but $O_2$ debt may increase in sedentary adults. | Implications for caloric cost and $\dot{V}O_2$ prediction in older adults. |
| Walking kinematics | Preferred walking speed is slower. Stride length is shorter; double-limb support duration is longer. Increased gait variability. These age differences are exaggerated when balance is perturbed. | Implications for physical function and risk for falling. |
| Stair-climbing ability | Maximal step height is reduced, reflects integrated measure of leg length, coordinated muscle activation, and dynamic balance. | Implications for mobility and physically demanding ADL. |

**Body composition/metabolism**

| VARIABLES | TYPICAL CHANGES | FUNCTIONAL SIGNIFICANCE* |
|---|---|---|
| Height | Height declines approximately 1 cm per decade during the 40s and 50s, accelerated after 60 years (women > men). Vertebral disks compress; thoracic curve becomes more pronounced. | Vertebral changes can impair mobility and other daily tasks. |
| Weight | Weight steadily increases during the 30s, 40s, and 50s; stabilizes until about age 70 years; and then declines. Age-related changes in weight and BMI can mask fat gain/muscle loss. | Large, rapid loss of weight in old age can indicate disease process. |
| FFM | FFM declines 2%–3% per decade from 30–70 years of age. Losses of total body protein and potassium likely reflect the loss of metabolically active tissue (i.e., muscle). | FFM seems to be an important physiological regulator. |
| Muscle mass and size | Total muscle mass declines from about age 40 years, accelerated after age 65–70 years (legs lose muscle faster). Limb muscles exhibit reductions in fiber number and size (type II > I). | Loss of muscle mass and type II fiber size results in reduced muscle strength and power. |
| Muscle quality | Lipid and collage content increase. Type I MHC content increases; type II MHC content decreases. Peak-specific force declines. Oxidative capacity per kilogram of muscle declines. | Changes may be related to insulin resistance and muscle weakness. |
| Regional adiposity | Body fat increases during the 30s, 40s, and 50s, with a preferential accumulation in the visceral (intra-abdominal) region, especially in men. After age 70 years, fat (all sites) decreases. | Accumulation of visceral fat is linked to CVD and metabolic disease. |
| Bone density | Bone mass peaks in the mid-to-late 20s. BMD declines ≥0.5% per year after age 40 years. Women have disproportionate loss of bone (2%–3% per year) after menopause. | Osteopenia (1–2.5 SD below young control subjects) increases fracture risk. |

*Continued*

**Table 26-1.** Summary of Typical Changes in Physiological Function and Body Composition With Advancing Age in Healthy Humans—cont'd

| VARIABLES | TYPICAL CHANGES | FUNCTIONAL SIGNIFICANCE* |
|---|---|---|
| Metabolic changes | RMR (absolute and per kilogram FFM), muscle protein synthesis rates (mitochondria and MHC), and fat oxidation (during submaximal exercise) all decline with advancing age. | These may influence substrate utilization during exercise. |

Typical changes generally reflect age-associated differences on the basis of cross-sectional data, which can underestimate changes followed longitudinally.

*The strength of existing evidence for the functional associations ranges between A and D.

ADL, activities of daily living; BMD, bone mineral density; BMI, body mass index; BP, blood pressure; CVD, cardiovascular disease; FFM, fat-free mass; HR, heart rate; IADL, instrumental activities of daily living; MHC, myosin heavy chain; Peak, peak or maximal exercise responses; RMR, resting metabolic rate; ROM, range of motion; SD, standard deviation; $\dot{V}O_2$max, maximal oxygen consumption.

Reprinted from American College of Sports Medicine,[8] by permission.

The ability to coordinate muscular activity into functional movements also declines in old age. Significant declines in functional tasks such as putting on a shirt, managing buttons, zipping a garment, or cutting with a knife decline, as does performance on tests of coordination such as finger grasping or interfinger manipulation.[4] Sensorimotor information (collected from the visual and somatosensory systems) is critical to performing both simple and complex movements such as putting on a pair of glasses, dialing a phone, slicing food, or buttoning buttons. The visual system contributes spatial information from the environment such as location, direction, and speed of the individual.[4] Visual declines are common with aging and often include a reduced ability to detect contrasts, loss of depth perception, decreased illumination within the eye, increased sensitivity to glare (because of scattering of light within the eye), nearsightedness, and loss of peripheral vision.

The somatosensory system uses information about body contact (e.g., touch and vibration) and position (e.g., limbs of the body, head, and joint position) to help guide movements. Older individuals tend to have impaired distal lower-extremity **proprioception** (awareness of the body's position in relation to space and the environment), and vibration and discriminative touch. The ability to perceive motion of the joints appears to be impaired when movements are performed at slow speeds, but not when faster speeds are used.[4] These declines may contribute to poor balance and increased risk for falling, but these contributions have not been fully investigated.

It is said that "you can't teach an old dog new tricks," but research regarding motor learning with older adults shows that this is not true. Older adults are able to improve existing skill performance and learn new skills, although they may learn them at a slower rate than younger adults, and the manner in which they learn a new skill may be different.[13] Furthermore, they tend to adopt different muscle activation patterns and movement strategies to accomplish a task as a way to compensate for physical losses. For example, younger adults typically exhibit a sequential contraction of the tibialis anterior, quadriceps, and abdominals if they lose their balance and begin to fall backward. However, under the same circumstances, older adults show a delay in contracting the balance support muscles and sometimes exhibit an altered sequence of muscle contraction to prevent a backward fall.[4]

The loss of skeletal muscle is accompanied by an increase in fat mass. The data are not clear on how much fat is typically gained throughout middle adulthood, but fat mass appears to stabilize in the sixth decade of life.[4] Changes in body-fat distribution have been more clearly documented with older adults experiencing an increase in intra-abdominal fat accompanied by a decrease in subcutaneous fat on the limbs.[4] Abdominal obesity increases the risk for **cardiovascular disease (CVD)** and diabetes. These changes are due to a combination of factors, including genetics, physical activity levels, dietary habits, and hormonal changes. Both aerobic and resistance exercise training have been shown to be effective in reducing fat mass in older adults.[4,8] Conversely, excessive weight loss in older adults is more closely related to negative consequences for health and physical function (such as frailty), and should therefore be monitored when working with these clients.

## Skeletal System

Bone density declines at a rate of approximately 1% per year from age 40 to 50 years for both men and women. In women, bone density is reduced 2% to 3% per year during menopause, and every 5 to 10 years following menopause. Women often lose up to one third of their **bone mineral density (BMD)** during this time. The rate of bone loss increases for both men and women in the eighth and ninth decades of life.[4] The result is a weaker bone structure that is more susceptible to fracture. Physical activity level is one of many factors that influence peak bone development and the age-related loss of bone mass. Muscle strength is closely correlated with bone mass, indicating that the mechanical stimulus of movement is important in the development and maintenance of BMD. (Also see explanatory animation of the Physiology of Bone Formation on the DavisPlus site at http://davisplus.fadavis.com.)

**Osteoporosis** is a disease often associated with aging that is characterized by low bone mass and quality, which increases bone fragility and the risk of fractures. It is diagnosed through BMD testing. A BMD of 2.5 standard deviations below the mean for young women defines osteoporosis, whereas a BMD of 1.0 to 2.5 standard deviations below the mean for young women defines **osteopenia** (a loss of bone density that predisposes an individual for development of osteoporosis).[4] Approximately half of all women and 12% of all men older than 50 years will experience an osteoporosis-related fracture.[14] The most common fracture sites are the spine, hips, and wrists. Weight-bearing cardiovascular exercise, such as walking, jogging, or jumping rope, and high-intensity resistance exercise have been shown to either halt the loss of or even slightly improve BMD in older adults. Individuals with osteoporosis should avoid excessive spinal flexion (especially when accompanied with rotation) and activities that pose a high risk for falling, such as skiing, skating, and horseback riding.

Degenerative changes also occur in the joints with advancing age, including loss of lubrication and articular cartilage damage. **Osteoarthritis (OA)**, or degenerative joint disease, is characterized by pain and stiffness in the joints and is the most common form of arthritis.[14] Approximately 50% of adults older than 65 years and 85% of adults older than 75 years have OA.[4] It most often develops in the hips, knees, and back, and is the leading cause of disability in the United States.

The evidence shows that exercise training does not exacerbate pain or disease progression as once thought. Rather, aerobic and resistance exercise training are effective at decreasing pain and improving function in individuals with OA,[14] and should be included as essential components of a treatment plan for OA. Recommendations for individuals with OA include avoiding high-impact activities that may irritate or further damage joints; muscle strengthening using lower resistance levels and higher repetitions around the affected joints; low-impact aerobic exercise (land-based or aquatic); avoiding activities on days when the joint is inflamed (i.e., red, swollen, and painful); and stretching to improve pain-free joint range of motion.

If the condition progresses, a joint replacement may be warranted. OA is the most common reason for joint replacement surgery among older adults. Total knee and total hip replacement surgeries have a very high success rate for significantly reducing pain and increasing function. Advances in technology and surgical techniques are further increasing success rates and reducing recovery times. Depending on the location and type of surgery, individuals may have limitations in specific movements they are able to perform, such as deep squats and flexion of the hip past 90 degrees.

## VIGNETTE continued

■ Danitza reaches out to Blair, a more experienced trainer who has served as Danitza's mentor over the years. Blair is also an ACE-certified senior fitness specialist, having completed advanced continuing education in the topic of training this unique population. He agrees to help train Julie for a few sessions in an attempt to alleviate the frustration of everyone involved. Blair quickly notices that Julie has trouble moving up and down from the floor, so he replaced the abdominal floor work that Danitza had introduced with standing balance and core exercises that Julie finds much more comfortable. It is also evident that Julie is not quite ready for supersets and the other fast-paced exercises that Julie had been teaching. Together, Blair, Danitza, and Julie agree to a new approach that is more appropriate and comfortable for Julie, and that takes into account the needs associated with her current health status.

## Cardiometabolic System

The cardiometabolic system reflects the collective effects of the cardiovascular, pulmonary, and metabolic systems within the body. Maximal aerobic capacity, as measured by maximal oxygen consumption ($\dot{V}O_2$max), decreases with advancing age at a rate of about 30% to 40% per decade[15] (Fig. 26-2). This decrease is due to several factors, including reductions in cardiac output and arteriovenous oxygen difference. The reduction in maximum cardiac output is due primarily to the reduction in maximum heart rate, which decreases by about 1 beat/min/yr. The ejection fraction of the left ventricle during exercise also decreases from 85% for someone in their 30s to about 70% for someone in their 90s.[15] Blood vessels tend to become thicker and stiffer (known as **arteriosclerosis**), which makes them less compliant to accepting blood. Compliance of the common carotid artery decreases by as much as 50% from the age of 25 to the age of 75 years.[15] The stiffness of aging arteries increases the risk for hypertension, and the reduction of ejection fraction reduces the volume of blood that can be effectively pumped from the heart with each beat, resulting in higher heart rates at lower exercise intensities compared with younger adults. Thus, health and fitness professionals should be mindful of the fact that even at relatively low intensities, some older adults can experience cardiovascular fatigue.

Aerobic exercise training of sufficient intensity (>60% $\dot{V}O_2$max), frequency, and length ( ≥3 days/week for ≥16 weeks) can significantly improve $\dot{V}O_2$max in older adults by about 16%, although the

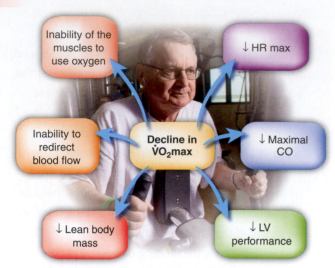

**Figure 26-2.** Factors that result in a decrease of maximal aerobic capacity, as measured by maximal oxygen consumption ($\dot{V}O_2max$). CO, cardiac output; HR, heart rate; LV, left ventricle.

magnitude of improvement is generally less in those younger than 75 years.[8] Interval training programs that use alternating periods of higher and lower intensities may improve $\dot{V}O_{2max}$ even more. Other cardiovascular adaptations include a lower heart rate at rest and at any submaximal exercise workload, smaller rises in blood pressures during submaximal exercise, increased maximal exercise stroke volume, and reductions in large-artery stiffness.

CVD is common among older adults, with about 84% of deaths related to CVD occurring in people 65 years or older. CVD can lead to a **myocardial infarction**, stroke, **transient ischemic attack**, and death. Active individuals of all ages have a lower prevalence of CVD than their inactive counterparts. Physical activity volume (including exercise) is inversely related to death from all causes in a dose–response manner. This means that the higher the volume of physical activity, the lower the risk for death. Moderate-intensity activity lasting at least 30 minutes on most, preferably all, days of the week is sufficient to reduce risk for premature death. This goal is attainable for many older adults.

**Hypertension** (blood pressure ≥ 140/90 mm Hg) is a risk factor for CVD and is a prevalent concern in the older population. Exercise training is recommended for the prevention and management of hypertension. Chronic aerobic exercise can decrease both systolic and diastolic blood pressure by approximately 5 to 7 mm Hg.[16] Individuals with controlled hypertension can safely exercise if some basic guidelines are followed:

- Individuals with severe or uncontrolled hypertension should be evaluated by a physician before initiating an exercise program.
- Avoid exercise if resting blood pressure is greater than 200/110 mm Hg.
- Perform an extended warm-up and cool-down, and monitor for post-exercise hypotension.

- Monitor blood pressure during exercise and discontinue if blood pressure exceeds 220/105 mm Hg.
- Avoid performing a **Valsalva maneuver** (holding the breath while bearing down on a closed glottis) during resistance training.
- Avoid high-intensity resistance exercise with high weights and low repetitions.

Common complications and comorbidities for individuals with CVD include diabetes, obesity, hypertension, dysrhythmias, angina, shortness of breath, reduced exercise capacity, and intermittent **claudication** (ischemic lower-extremity pain associated with **peripheral arterial disease**). Although it is outside the scope of practice for a health and fitness professional to prescribe exercise for the management of these conditions, it is prudent to be able to identify signs and symptoms associated with them and to be able to act quickly when they occur. In addition, individuals with CVD should obtain appropriate medical clearance before beginning an exercise program.

**Type 2 diabetes** (i.e., non-insulin–dependent diabetes mellitus) rates have increased considerably in the older adult population over the past decade.[14] Diabetes is an independent and strong risk factor for development of CVD. Diabetes is also the leading cause of adult-onset blindness, nontraumatic lower-limb amputations, and renal (kidney) failure. Diabetic older adults should engage in regular exercise and follow a heart-healthy diet to lose body fat, improve glycemic control, and reduce the need for medications.[4,14] Aerobic exercise training is the most effective method for improving insulin sensitivity and glycemic control, but resistance exercise training is also beneficial.

Individuals with diabetes should adhere to the following guidelines when starting and maintaining an exercise program:

- Monitor blood glucose before, during, and after exercise. Exercise should generally be avoided if pre-exercise blood glucose is less than 100 or more than 250 mg/dL.
- Exercising at the same time each day will allow easier tracking of the exercise effects on blood sugar control.
- Keep a quick-acting sugary snack on hand at all times, such as raisins or juice, in case of a hypoglycemic (low blood sugar) episode.
- Check feet regularly for cuts and/or ulcers that are not healing properly.
- Avoid exercising late at night to ensure that blood sugar is under control before sleeping.
- Adopt a low-to-moderate intensity program and avoid high-intensity exercise if relatively new to exercise.

Several age-related changes occur in the respiratory system, including changes in the structure of the lungs and airways, changes in lung volume, and impaired efficiency of gas exchange.[4] Although total lung capacity remains constant throughout life, residual volume and functional residual capacity increase by about 25%, whereas vital capacity decreases by about 25%. Disadvantages of having an enlarged chest volume combined with a reduced vital capacity include a decrease in mechanical efficiency of the respiratory muscles, which results in a tendency for dyspnea (difficulty breathing) and/or more rapid ventilation during exercise. Thus, for any given physical activity, older adults have a higher respiratory rate compared with younger adults. Despite these changes, it does not appear that the respiratory system limits exercise training.

## Cognition and Psychological Well-being

Although it is commonly believed that senility and dementia are normal aspects of aging, research indicates that age-related cognitive decline is attributable more to the secondary effects of lifestyle, specifically health and fitness levels, rather than the primary effects of the aging process.[4] There are numerous aspects to cognition, such as processing speed, visuospatial processing, controlled processing, and executive control, and each may be more or less affected by the aging process, health status, and physical activity participation. Evidence indicates that diseases such as diabetes, CVD, and cerebrovascular disease impair neuropsychological function. Hypertension has been linked very strongly to cognition, with evidence showing that it can slow sensorimotor speed and perceptual processing speed.[4]

Habitual physical activity is associated with a reduced risk for dementia and cognitive decline in older adults[8]; conversely, decreases in physical mobility are linked to cognitive decline. Even a single bout of aerobic exercise can improve memory, attention, and reaction time for a short period. Long-term participation in both aerobic and resistance-training programs leads to improvements in cognitive function, especially when combined. Programs that use cognitive challenges in combination with aerobic exercise typically lead to larger improvements.[8] The positive effects of regular exercise appear to be largest for tasks that are more complex and that require executive control. Exercise of low-to-moderate intensity conducted over a longer period appears to be more effective than short-term, higher-intensity programs.

## UNDERSTANDING FUNCTION

Functional capabilities vary significantly within the mature population, which is significantly heterogeneous. An individual's chronological age is only a rough guideline as to his or her **functional age** (i.e., his or her capabilities). Although functional capacity generally decreases with advancing age, the degree and rate of decline are highly variable so that individuals of the same age can exhibit highly variable levels of function, ranging from the physically dependent to elite athletes. Therefore, an 80-year-old may be able to outperform someone 10 or 20 years younger. Dr. Waneen Spirduso[4] described five functional categories of older adults[11] that are helpful to understanding the heterogeneity that exists within this group of individuals (Table 26-2).

## Table 26-2. Functional Categories of Older Adults

| CATEGORY | NAME | DESCRIPTION |
|---|---|---|
| 1 | Elite | The physically elite have achieved the highest level of physical function and are often more fit than sedentary individuals who are decades younger. They train rather intensely on a daily basis and typically compete in tournaments with others their age such as the Senior Olympics, Masters tournaments, or in other events. Because of their high levels of activity (and usually excellent dietary habits), they are also in excellent health. |
| 2 | Physically fit | Fit older adults exercise primarily for their health and well-being rather than for competition, and they do so anywhere from two to seven times per week. Their exercise programs are less intense and of shorter duration than those performed by the physically elite. They enjoy greater than average levels of health and are typically estimated to be much younger than their chronological age by their peers. |
| 3 | Independent | These individuals do not exercise but may be physically active. They are typically of average health and do not have any serious debilitating disease. However, because they do not focus as much on health, they are also at increased risk for disease and often possess multiple chronic disease risk factors. They have few functional limitations but are at greater risk for frailty and disability because of a reduction in physiological reserve capacity. |
| 4 | Frail | According to Campbell and Buchner,[55] frailty is a "condition or syndrome that results from a multisystem reduction in reserve capacity to the extent that a number of physiological systems are close to, or past, the threshold of |

*Continued*

## Table 26-2. Functional Categories of Older Adults—cont'd

| CATEGORY | NAME | DESCRIPTION |
|---|---|---|
| | | symptomatic clinical failure. As a consequence, the frail person is at increased risk of disability and death from minor external stresses." Frail older adults can perform ADL, such as bathing, dressing, transferring, toileting, and feeding, although they have a debilitating disease or condition. Because of their physical challenges they may be unable to perform all of the IADL, such as shopping, doing laundry, preparing meals, and doing light housework. It is also important to note that a single bout with an illness such as the flu or an injury such as a fall can quickly move frail individuals into the dependent category. |
| 5 | Dependent | These individuals are unable to perform all of the ADL and are dependent on others and/or physical aids (e.g., canes, walkers, or wheelchairs) to complete their daily tasks. The extent of their physical disability is determined by the degree to which they cannot perform ADL and IADL. Disability rates increase with chronological age and are higher in women, African Americans, and poor individuals. Individuals can move in and out of disablement, such as following a stroke (where function is lost) and during rehabilitation (where function is often regained). |

ADL, activities of daily living; IADL, instrumental activities of daily living.
Data from Spirduso et al.[4]

It is important to recognize that these categories represent a *continuum* of functional capacity, and individuals may move back and forth between the categories, depending on their current situation. For example, a physically fit individual who exercises regularly may experience some health problems or family issues that prevent him or her from training for an extended period. The lack of physical activity leads to a detraining effect so that this individual would now be considered independent rather than physically fit. The reverse could also happen so that an independent individual trains vigorously to move up to the physically fit or even elite category. It is helpful to recognize where individuals are on this continuum, but it may be even more important to understand their **aging trajectory**, (i.e., in which direction they are heading and how rapidly; Fig. 26-3).[17] As people get older, the tendency is to decline in functional ability (a downward trajectory) because of the effects of primary and secondary aging. The downward trajectory can be exacerbated by disease processes. If functional capacity declines to the point to where the individual can no longer fulfill his or her socially defined roles such as employee, caretaker, or volunteer, he or she is considered to be physically disabled.

The pathway to **disablement** (the process of becoming disabled) was first described by sociologist Saad Nagi[18] in 1965 and has since been expanded on by many others. Understanding this basic pathway can help health and fitness professionals develop a more effective approach to training. The steps in the pathway are:
- Active pathology and/or physical inactivity
- Impairments
- Functional limitations
- Disability

Over time, diseases such as diabetes, CVD, cancer, and osteoporosis can lead to physical impairments such

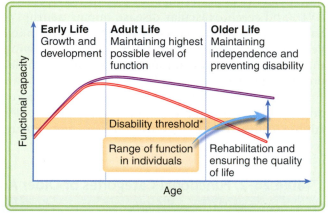

**Figure 26-3.** As people get older, the tendency is to decline in functional ability (a downward trajectory) because of the effects of primary and secondary aging. The downward trajectory can be exacerbated by disease processes. If functional capacity declines to the point where the individual can no longer fulfill his or her socially defined roles such as employee, caretaker, or volunteer, he or she is considered to be physically disabled. *(Adapted from Kalache and Kickbusch[17] by permission.)*

as muscle weakness, poor cardiorespiratory endurance, inflexibility, and poor reaction time. Depending on the specific pathology or mix of pathologies, these impairments may be a direct result of the disease processes or may be indirectly because of lower levels of physical activity. Individuals with disease often have lower levels of activity, which can exacerbate the disease process and lead to the impairments mentioned earlier.

Even in the absence of disease, physical inactivity can lead to impairments with advancing age. As impairments accumulate or worsen, eventually the individual will experience limitations in functional capabilities such as grasping and carrying objects, walking, and stair climbing. If these limitations become severe enough, the individual could lose the ability to perform duties that are essential to his or her socially defined roles (e.g., self-care and housekeeping tasks) and would then require assistance to perform these activities. Assistance could come from children, friends, social workers, or medical personnel. At this point, an individual would be considered disabled.

Exercise programs have shown modest success in improving functional capacity and delaying or avoiding disability in older adults with existing impairments.[19,20] Exercise has been consistently found to positively affect impairment-level factors such as muscle strength, muscle power, muscular endurance, cardiorespiratory endurance, flexibility, joint range of motion, and balance. However, evidence for the beneficial effects of exercise on functional limitations is less clear. This is likely due to the wide variety of subject characteristics (e.g., age, sex, functional capabilities, and disease processes) and exercise designs used (i.e., frequency, intensity, duration, and type), as well as the lack of specificity between the training intervention and the functional outcomes being assessed.

Reviews have indicated that although exercise interventions may significantly improve impairment-level factors, this does not always lead to similar gains in functional capacity. In addition, subjects who experience the greatest gains in impairment-level factors do not always experience the greatest gains in function. For example, an individual who performs a traditional progressive resistance-training program will significantly increase his or her strength, but may only minimally increase his or her ability to climb stairs, get out of a chair, or carry objects. Although muscular strength is an important component that is necessary for performing these tasks, it is not the only component. Function depends on a myriad of physiological components, as listed in Box 26-3.

## Box 26-3. Components Critical to Physical Function in Older Adults

- Muscular strength
  - Isometric
  - Concentric
  - Eccentric
- Muscular endurance
- Muscular power
- Muscular flexibility
- Joint range of motion
- Cardiorespiratory endurance
- Proprioception
- Coordination
- Motor control
- Reaction time
- Balance
- Stability
- Postural control
  - Anticipatory
  - Reactive

Evidence suggests that exercise interventions that challenge multiple components of fitness, such as aerobic, strength, power, flexibility, and balance, may lead to better functional improvements than programs that focus on a single component.[14,21,22]

### VIGNETTE continued

■ In their discussions with Julie, Blair and Danitza learn that she is less concerned about weight loss and more interested in improving her upper-body strength. The arthritis in her hands has made it difficult to perform some of her daily activities and she has trouble lifting her 5-year-old granddaughter. She also admits that the dumbbell exercises she had been doing have exacerbated the pain in her hands, but she was uncomfortable speaking up during the workouts. They also decide to incorporate balance and functional training into her routine.

During these team training sessions, Danitza realized that she has a lot to learn about training this diverse population, as making minor modifications to her usual routine is clearly not adequate. Blair agrees to help her identify the best continuing education options, as Danitza now enjoys working with Julie and finds helping her very rewarding.

## EXERCISE TRAINING

It is never too late to start exercising. The evidence strongly demonstrates that regular exercise can improve health and fitness for adults of all ages, and even after years of sedentary and unhealthy behaviors. Training studies with individuals in their 90s and beyond have demonstrated significant improvements (statistically and/or practically) in aerobic power, muscle strength, muscle power, flexibility, balance, physical function, and many aspects of health.

### Considerations

Because of the increased risk for, and prevalence of, chronic diseases and orthopedic limitations in the mature population, fitness professionals should fully evaluate their clients before beginning an exercise training program. The evaluation should include a comprehensive health-history questionnaire, goal-setting, and fitness testing. Although it is common for trainers to use the **Physical Activity Readiness Questionnaire (PAR-Q)** to screen clients (see Chapter 15: Cardiorespiratory Training), this is not always appropriate for older clients because the tool is validated only for use with clients up to the age of 69 years. In addition, the PAR-Q does not provide any specific information on the types and/or severity of existing diseases and conditions. It is more appropriate to instead evaluate clients using a health-history questionnaire that includes an assessment of the following:

- Current chronic diseases
- Current risk factors for disease (see coronary artery disease risk profile in Chapter 15)
- Current medications
- Prior surgeries and their dates
- Current musculoskeletal/orthopedic conditions
- Current illnesses and injuries
- Any history of physical activity and exercise

The health and fitness professional could also conduct some basic health-related data such as height/weight, body composition, resting heart rate, and resting blood pressure. This information will provide a well-rounded view of the client's physical needs. Following the health-history evaluation should be a discussion of the client's goals, remembering the diversity of the mature population. It is critical to understand what outcomes are important to him or her—improved health, quality of life, fitness, function, pain reduction, sports performance, disease management, stress reduction, social interaction, or something else.

Exercise testing to assess fitness is an extremely useful tool that should be a standard part of the client intake process, in addition to a comprehensive health-history questionnaire. Testing can help the health and fitness professional develop appropriate training programs, monitor outcomes more effectively, and make referrals for further medical evaluation when necessary. A wide variety of fitness assessment tools are available for professionals to use, but not all have been validated for use with older populations.

Health and fitness professionals should choose assessments for their older clients based on three basic criteria:

1. Existing health conditions and physical limitations of the client
2. Purposes for conducting the assessment
3. Expertise or skill of the professional who is conducting the test

Although numerous assessments have been developed and validated for use with older populations (Table 26-3), the health and fitness professional must choose wisely. Many assessments have either floor or ceiling effects that limit their use to clients within certain ranges of functional capacity.

## Table 26-3. Common Tests of Physical Function for Older Adults

| TEST | MEASURES | DESCRIPTION |
|---|---|---|
| **Senior Fitness Test Battery** | | |
| **8-Foot up and go** | Agility, dynamic balance | How quickly a person can walk around a cone 8 feet away and return to a sitting position |
| 30-Second chair stand | Lower-body strength | How many times a person can stand up from a seated position in 30 seconds |
| 2-Minute step test | Cardiorespiratory endurance | How many times a person can step in place in 2 minutes |
| 6-Minute Walk | Cardiorespiratory endurance | How far a person can walk in 6 minutes |
| Back scratch | Upper-body flexibility | How close a person can get their fingers when reaching one hand over the shoulder and the other hand behind the back |
| Sit and reach | Lower-body flexibility | How close to, or past, the toes a person can reach with both hands while in a seated position with both legs extended |
| 30-Second arm curl | Upper-body strength | How many times a person can curl a dumbbell (5 lb for women; 8 lb for men) in 30 seconds in a seated position |
| Continuous Scale Physical Functional Performance Test (CS-PFP) | Upper- and lower-body strength, upper-body flexibility, balance and coordination, and endurance | A battery of 15 everyday tasks such as pouring, sweeping a floor, and climbing stairs |
| Performance-Oriented Mobility Assessment (POMA) | Static and dynamic balance and gait | Composite score of a variety of functional tasks involving balance and gait |
| Dynamic Gait Index | Gait and dynamic balance | Composite score of several gait-related tasks such as walking with head turns, stepping over obstacles, and stair climbing |

**Table 26-3. Common Tests of Physical Function for Older Adults—cont'd**

| TEST | MEASURES | DESCRIPTION |
|---|---|---|
| Walkie-talkie test | Divided attentional demands | How well a person can talk and walk simultaneously |
| **Balance-specific tests** | | |
| Modified Clinical Test of Sensory Interaction in Balance | Visual, vestibular, and somatosensory system contributions to balance | How long (up to 30 seconds) an individual can stand under four conditions: eyes open/stable surface, eyes closed/stable surface, eyes open/unstable surface, eyes closed/unstable surface |
| Single-leg stand | Static balance | How long a person can stand on one leg (up to 30 seconds) |
| Berg Balance Scale | Static and dynamic balance | Composite score of 14 different tasks such as transferring from a chair, turning 360 degrees while standing, stepping up onto a bench |
| Fullerton Advanced Balance Scale | Static and dynamic balance | Composite score of 10 functional tasks such as tandem walk, stand on one leg, and two-foot jump |
| Tinetti Balance and Gait | Static and dynamic balance and gait | Composite score of nine functional tasks such as rising from a chair and standing with eyes closed |
| Functional reach test | Limits of stability | How far a person can reach forward in a standing position |
| Multidirectional reach test | Limits of stability | How far a person can lean to the front, sides, and rear in a standing position |

Elite and physically fit older adults can typically participate in many of the standard fitness tests that have been validated with younger populations that measure maximal aerobic capacity or muscle strength. Maximal tests of aerobic capacity can be conducted using motorized treadmills, cycle ergometers, or in the field (e.g., Cooper 12-minute test or the 1.5-mile test for time). The gold standard for measuring muscle strength is the one-repetition maximum (1 RM) test. This can be conducted using free weights, variable resistance machines, or specialized equipment such as isokinetic dynamometers following established protocols and guidelines.

Physically independent, frail, and dependent older adults should participate in targeted assessments appropriate for their level of function and health. For the independent adult, this could include measures of fitness that are commonly used with younger populations, such as the YMCA submaximal bicycle ergometer test, a standard sit-and-reach test, or abdominal curl-up test. Tests that rely on multiple repetitions of movements to assess muscular strength are commonly considered a safer alternative to 1 RM testing. However, predicting maximal strength with older populations is not as accurate and may therefore yield unreliable results. Functional fitness testing performed with an older adult can include assessments of static balance, dynamic balance, agility, mobility, gait, flexibility, whole-body function, and other components. Assessments can be single task, dual task, combinations of functional activities, or composite measures. A commonly used assessment tool is the Senior Fitness Test Battery, which consists of seven tests that measure muscular strength, flexibility, cardiorespiratory endurance, dynamic balance/agility, and body composition (see Table 26-3). Each test has been proven to be valid and reliable for use with older populations, is relatively safe, requires minimal equipment, requires minimal training for the tester, and can easily be performed with groups. Normative tables allow comparison of results with others of similar age and sex.

A number of questionnaires and scales have been developed to evaluate functional capacity, such as the Katz Index of Activities of Daily Living, Barthel Index, Instrumental Activities of Daily Living (IADL) Screening Questionnaire, and Medical Outcomes Study Short Form 36 (SF-36). However, the usage of these tools is typically limited to the clinical, nursing home, or retirement setting for use with frail and dependent populations. Health and fitness professionals can determine an older client's level of function through the pre-exercise health screen and interview process. Asking questions about current level of physical activity and limitations to movement can shed light on where the older adult client falls in respect to the functionality continuum.

## Aerobic Exercise

Mature adults engage in less physical activity than their younger counterparts. Aerobic exercise has been shown to be safe and beneficial for adults of all ages. By engaging in regular aerobic exercise, mature adults can decrease their risk for chronic diseases, manage their current diseases better, and increase aerobic exercise capacity.[8] Exercise should be of sufficient intensity ( $\geq 60\%$ $\dot{V}O_{2max}$ ), frequency ( $\geq 3$ days/week), and duration ( $\geq 20$ minutes) to elicit cardiovascular and health adaptations. Individuals without significant health risks or conditions can participate in more vigorous exercise and sports activity such as basketball or running. The mode of aerobic exercise is an important consideration and depends on the individual's orthopedic conditions, goals, and exercise history (Fig. 26-4). Those with significant arthritis of the knees, hips, or spine; joint replacements; osteoporosis; or other orthopedic conditions should avoid high-impact exercises such as jogging. Instead, these individuals should engage in low-impact or nonimpact exercises such as bicycling or swimming, or use cardiovascular equipment such as an upright bike, recumbent bike, recumbent stepper, treadmill, elliptical trainer, and rower. Clients with a history of falling or with balance deficits should avoid activities with an increased risk for falling such as skiing, horseback riding, or skating.

Typical techniques to monitor exercise intensity such as heart rate and the "talk test" can still be used with mature clients. However, it is also useful to use ratings of perceived exertion (RPE) to gauge intensity, especially if the client is taking medications that suppress heart rate such as beta blockers. An RPE of 12 to 13 on the Borg 6 to 20 scale corresponds to moderate-intensity aerobic exercise. RPE is often an easier tool for older clients to use when heart-rate monitors are unavailable and counting a pulse rate is difficult. Maximal heart rate has traditionally been calculated as "220 – age," but research indicates that a more accurate equation for determining maximal heart rate is "208 – (0.7 × age)" in healthy adults older than age 40 years.[23] The original formula tends to overestimate maximal heart rate in younger populations and underestimate it for older populations. Target heart rate should be calculated using either the direct or indirect heart-rate reserve methods according to the intensity desired. Although moderate-intensity exercise is generally recommended, the individual's health conditions and fitness status will determine the appropriate level of intensity that is both safe and effective.

## Resistance Exercise

By following traditional, progressive resistance training, older adults can increase their muscular strength by anywhere from 25% to more than 100%, depending on the exercise program being used, the duration of the training, age and sex of the client, and the specific muscle groups being trained.[8] Muscular power also increases following resistance exercise training, although evidence suggests that high-velocity training protocols may improve muscle power to a greater degree.[24,25] It is recommended that mature adults engage in at least

### FROM THEORY TO PRACTICE

#### ■ IS WALKING THE BEST EXERCISE FOR OLDER ADULTS?

What is the best exercise for older adults? Walking definitely offers many advantages. It requires no special equipment, can be performed indoors and outdoors, does not require any special skill or instruction, can be accomplished by the majority of older adults, and has been proved to be a healthy activity. However, is it really the best exercise for all older adults? To say yes is to accept the stereotype that all older adults are basically the same. Walking, unless performed on hilly terrain, is typically of rather low intensity. For deconditioned individuals, or for those with chronic conditions, this might be enough of a stimulus to improve their health and fitness levels. However, walking will likely provide too weak of a stimulus for a robust, vigorous, and active older adult who would benefit more from jogging, stepping, or cycling activities. For someone with severe knee OA, it might be too painful. For someone with balance deficits, it might be too risky. For individuals with orthopedic and/or balance problems, aquatic exercise could be a better option. The truth is that a single "best" exercise for older adults does not exist. What is best for one individual might be the worst for another. A competent health and fitness professional will always take into account the individual's unique needs, abilities, and goals when designing an exercise program.

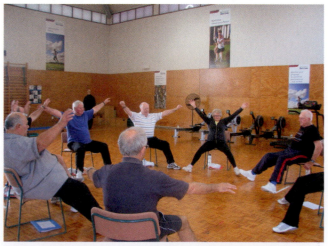

**Figure 26-4.** Chair-based exercise classes are also a good option for older adults. Clients with a history of falling or with balance deficits should avoid activities with an increased risk for falling. *(Courtesy of Lance Dalleck.)*

2 days/week of moderate-intensity strength training that includes 8 to 10 exercises involving the major muscle groups, 1 to 3 sets of 8 to 12 repetitions each.[8]

Mature adults can safely and effectively use a wide variety of resistance-training methods and equipment, such as resistance machines, resistance bands, free weights, body weight, and hydraulic and pneumatic equipment. Equipment selection is dependent on the individual's capabilities and goals. Each type has its advantages and disadvantages. It is a misconception that mature adults should only use light dumbbells or easy resistance bands because they might become injured. The muscles of older adults need to be challenged to grow stronger just as the muscles of younger adults do. Although this population has more orthopedic concerns, resistance exercise has been shown to be generally safe.[8]

## Functional Training

Novel methods of training are constantly being developed and evaluated for their ability to improve functional outcomes (e.g., performance of activities of daily living) as opposed to traditional measures of fitness (e.g., muscle strength) in older populations, because this is often the ultimate result that is being sought. Often referred to as multimodal, multicomponent, or functional task training, these programs are based on the concept of specificity and typically focus more on the replication of daily tasks with a much greater emphasis on including a broader range of functional components.

Special attention is often given to challenging motor control and coordination. There is a recognition that, as one researcher stated, there is a "complex interplay of cognitive, perceptual, and motor functions that are involved in the performance of daily tasks."[26] Functional task challenges are accomplished by using whole-body movements, often with environmental manipulations, and few, if any, traditional isolation-type exercises that focus on one body part (e.g., biceps curl or knee extension). Although extensive investigation remains in this area, the initial research appears to be very promising. Several studies have concluded that functional task training is more effective than traditional resistance exercise training for improving function, especially in older adults with disabilities.[27,28] Given the wide variety of training protocols and outcome measures that have been used, it is difficult to determine an optimal exercise program for maximizing functional outcomes. Because individuals also vary widely in their needs and abilities, an individualized approach is warranted. However, general guidelines have been developed based on the current research to help health and fitness professionals adopt a more functionally relevant approach with their mature clients (Box 26-4).[29]

Translational training, developed by researcher Joseph Signorile, uses a periodized model for improving function that uses two training cycles[22] (Fig. 26-5). The first cycle is similar to a standard periodized program where volume and intensity are manipulated to

### Box 26-4. Functional Training Principles

1. *Assess and prioritize.* Perform focused assessments to evaluate the needs and capabilities of the individual and then build the program around those results.

2. *Make purposeful decisions.* Each component included in the training routine (e.g., equipment, sets, repetitions, intensity level, speed, body position, and environmental demands) should play a purposeful role in improving functional outcomes. Eliminate exercise movements and methods that cannot be adequately justified.

3. *Train in three planes.* Human bodies are required to move in three planes (sagittal, frontal, and transverse) on a daily basis to complete tasks. To adequately prepare for these movement demands, older adults should train in all three planes to maximize the carryover of adaptations from the exercise room to the living room.

4. *Supplement and complement with isolation exercises.* Isolation-type exercises maximize gains in muscle mass and strength. For certain individuals who have experienced a significant degree of sarcopenia or are recovering from an injury, these methods would be appropriate to target specific muscle groups.

5. *Stand up whenever possible.* Mobility is an important component to the health and independence of older adults. Exercise movements performed in the standing position typically require more muscle activation, postural control, center of gravity control, proprioception, and balance than similar movements performed in a seated position. Seated movements should be used selectively or with clients who are either unable to stand or are fatigued.

6. *Order the exercise session according to energy level.* Complex, multicomponent movements that challenge coordination and motor control should be performed earlier in the exercise session before the individual becomes fatigued, to maximize performance and reduce risk for falling. Isolation-type or seated exercises can be reserved for later in the session.

7. *Maximize safety and success.* Whole-body, dynamic, and more complicated movements increase the risk for falling. Therefore, care must be given to monitor individuals closely and create an environment free of distractions and trip hazards.

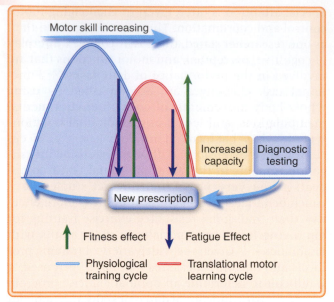

**Figure 26-5.** Translational training involves two cycles. The first cycle is similar to a standard periodized program where volume and intensity are manipulated to increase muscle mass and strength. The second cycle focuses on translating the newfound strength into functional task performance. *(Adapted from Signorile,[22] by permission.)*

increase muscle mass and strength. Throughout this cycle, exercise volume decreases, whereas exercise intensity (i.e., load) increases, just like a typical progressive resistance exercise program. The second cycle focuses on translating the newfound strength into functional task performance. This is accomplished by manipulating movement complexity to challenge motor control and coordination. For example, an individual may have used the leg press and leg extension machines to improve muscle mass and strength during the first cycle. At the beginning of the second cycle, he or she may perform lunges instead, which adds components of ankle stability, balance, postural control, and center of gravity control. This might progress into a telephone book transfer task that requires an individual to stand in the center of a square that has large phone books at each corner. The individual must lunge to a corner, pick up a phone book, then lunge to another corner and place the phone book in that corner. Movement complexity has increased by adding multiple directions and an upper-body task. Although translational training shows promise as an effective intervention, more research is needed to quantify its benefits.

## Training for Muscular Power

More focus is being given to the importance of **muscular power**, because it declines earlier and faster than muscular strength with advancing age.[8,25] Although muscle strength is essential to successfully complete many functional tasks in later life, studies show that muscular power is even more important for many tasks such as stair climbing and rising from a chair.[24]

Muscular, or mechanical, power is defined as the product of force and velocity (i.e., force × velocity). For muscles, this equates to muscular strength multiplied by contractile velocity or, practically speaking, how quickly a muscle can generate force. For older adults, muscular power has been identified as a critical component for the performance of many functional tasks, such as climbing stairs and rising from a chair, as well as participation in sporting events. Cross-sectional studies indicate that muscular power is much more highly correlated to functional task performance than muscular strength. Unfortunately, muscular power decreases even more rapidly than muscular strength with advancing age, indicating that movement velocity also decreases with advancing age. It has been suggested that this may be because of the preferential atrophy of fast-twitch (type II) muscle fibers.

Many studies indicate that power training may be more advantageous in improving function than traditional strength-training methods.[24,25] High-velocity (power-specific) training also increases muscle power to a greater degree than traditional low-velocity strength training. Interestingly, some data indicate that using lower loads (20%–40% 1 RM) and higher movement speeds may be more effective than higher loads (50%–70% 1 RM), which must be performed more slowly.[22]

Key concepts concerning power training include:

1. Power training often brings to mind images of Olympic power lifters performing snatches and clean-and-jerk movements with near-maximal weight. For mature adults, power training is typically accomplished by performing the concentric phase of standard resistance exercise movements much more rapidly (<1 second) and the eccentric phase at normal controlled speed (2–3 seconds). Studies have used a variety of equipment, including body weight, weighted vests, sandbags, medicine balls, resistance bands, free weights, aquatics, and pneumatic resistance exercise equipment safely and effectively.[30] A number of guidelines have been developed to help guide the health and fitness professional when designing a power training program; for example, training frequency, sets, and repetitions of power training appear to be similar to traditional strength training (2–3 sessions/week; 1–2 sets of 8–12 repetitions), although more investigation into the optimal training program is needed.[25,30] Repetitions as low as three to five per set have been recommended to maintain a greater velocity of movement and power output.[30]

2. Power training should be preceded by a conditioning phase that focuses on muscular strength and endurance, as well as proper technique.[30]

3. Muscular power can be maximally improved by using 60% 1 RM loads.[25]

4. Using lower loads (20%–40% 1 RM) and higher movement velocities may be more effective at improving balance and function than using higher loads.[31]

5. Concentric phases should be performed "as rapidly as possible," and the eccentric phase should be performed in a "slow and controlled" manner.[24]

6. A wide variety of equipment has been used, but selectorized weight machines are *not* recommended because of potential injuries that can occur at the end range of motion. The momentum developed by the weight stack during the movement may cause the foot or leg pad to lose contact with the limb. If this occurs, the individual must "catch" the weight when it returns. The force generated from this impact, especially if the limbs are not in proper position, may exceed the individual's capabilities and may lead to injury.

7. Plyometric-type exercises, such as squat jumps, must be used with caution because there is a greater risk for falling and joint injury during these movements. However, the true safety and/or danger of these ballistic methods needs further investigation.[30]

8. Power training appears to be as safe as traditional strength training with most clients. Minor musculoskeletal discomfort is the most commonly reported adverse event in the literature, although joint pain and falls are also concerns.[25]

9. Care must be taken when performing power training with frail clients or those with orthopedic conditions, as the safety of power training with these populations has not been adequately evaluated.[25]

10. The primary focus of power training should be on lower-body musculature and tasks related to mobility, but upper-body muscular power may also be important for the maintenance of function.[30]

## Balance and Fall Prevention

Falls are a major concern for older adults. Approximately one third of community-dwelling adults older than 65 years and 50% of those older than 80 years fall each year, with fall rates increasing for institutional residents.[32,33] Between 20% and 30% of these individuals suffer injuries that reduce their mobility and potentially compromise their independence. Falls are the leading cause of injury deaths for older adults. Approximately 5% of falls result in fractures, with hip fractures being the most common. Of those who suffer a hip fracture, 50% never regain their ability to walk and 20% die within 6 months.[32]

Falls are due to a number of intrinsic and extrinsic factors. Intrinsic factors that increase fall risk include a history of falls, age, living alone, certain medications, impaired mobility and gait, sedentary behavior, visual impairments, poor lower-extremity strength, and fear of falling.[33,34] Extrinsic risk factors include environmental hazards (e.g., poor lighting, slippery floors, and uneven surfaces), improper footwear and clothing, and the use of walking aids or assistive devices.[32,34] Exercise has been identified as the single best intervention to prevent falls in older adults, with up to 42% of falls being preventable by a well-designed exercise program.[32,34] Other effective interventions include home safety modifications, medication reduction or substitution with a physician's approval (especially psychoactive or central nervous system–depressant medications), reducing fear of falling through increasing self-efficacy in performing physical activity, and surgery to correct cataracts.[34]

Balance can be defined as control of the body's **center of mass** over the **base of support** and within the **limits of stability**.[14] Balance is a multidimensional concept, as it is controlled by multiple sensory (afferent) and motor (efferent) control systems. The visual, vestibular, and somatosensory systems send information about the environment to the central nervous system, which then determines which bodily movements to make to maintain balance (seated or standing). Deficits in either the afferent or the efferent pathways or in the processing of information can decrease balance performance and increase fall risk.

A scientific literature review makes the following recommendations for balance training[34]:

- Exercise must provide a moderate or high challenge to balance. Programs that do not challenge balance are not effective in preventing falls. Balance should be challenged in three ways: (1) reducing the base of support, (2) moving the center of gravity, and (3) reducing the need for upper-limb support during standing exercise.
- Exercise must be of a sufficient dose to have an effect. At least 2 hr/week of exercise for a 6-month period appears to be sufficient.
- Ongoing exercise is necessary. Balance improvements are lost quickly following the cessation of exercise.
- Fall-prevention exercise should be targeted at the general community, as well as those at high risk for falls.
- Fall-prevention exercise may be undertaken in a group or home-based setting.
- Walking training may be included in addition to balance training, but high-risk individuals should avoid performing brisk walking programs. Walking training is not a crucial feature of effective fall-prevention programs. Therefore, walking should only be included if it does not infringe on or decrease the effects of the balance training.
- Strength training may be included in addition to balance training. Strength training is not a crucial aspect of fall-prevention programs but may be included because of its many benefits for older populations.
- Health and fitness professionals should make referrals if other risk factors need to be addressed. As part of a comprehensive approach to fall reduction, evidence-based interventions that target specific risk factors should be provided by appropriate health/medical professionals.

## Fall-Reduction Strategies

A number of effective fall-reduction (i.e., balance-enhancement) exercise programs have been developed, studied, and implemented, such as the Otago Exercise Program, which consists of a set of leg muscle–strengthening and balance retraining exercises progressing in difficulty, and a walking plan. The FallProof Program is a model program that was developed at the University of California–Fullerton's Center for Successful Aging[14] (Table 26-4). This multidimensional program uses a variety of assessments to identify individual areas of deficit and tailors the exercise intervention strategies to address those deficits. It has been implemented successfully in a variety of individual and group settings. Qualified health and fitness professionals can become certified FallProof instructors.

Six critical issues are required for developing an all-inclusive strategy for optimizing balance training and fall prevention:

1. Employ multicomponent training, which is superior to single-component balance training.
2. Simulate loss of balance during training.
3. Couple resistance training with balance exercise training.
4. Correctly sequence balance exercises.
5. Create innovative balance exercise.
6. Change the availability of sensory cues.

## Multicomponent Training Is Superior to Single-Component Balance Training

The two explanations generally given for lack of a favorable adaptation from balance exercises are lack of specificity with training and performance of single-component compared with multicomponent training. It has been reported that training programs including only single-task activities fail to place individuals in environmental conditions similar to that experienced before and during a fall.[35] Importantly, although balance training focused on improving functional tasks (e.g., heel-toe walking or standing on one leg) will be successful for enhancing performance of that specific activity, it fails to adequately replicate activities of daily living that require maintaining balance while completing several activities simultaneously or while distracted. Health and fitness professionals must design regimens that entail concurrent performance of balance exercises and additional tasks. For example, in addition to performing heel-toe walking, individuals may simultaneously be requested to complete a cognitive task such as counting backward from 100 by increments of 3. An additional form of dual-component training may involve combining a balance exercise with another physical form of activity. For example, balance on one leg could be completed while playing catch with

## Table 26-4. FallProof Model of Balance Training

| DOMAIN | SUBDOMAINS | EXERCISE EXAMPLES |
|---|---|---|
| Center of gravity control (COG) | Seated COG | Forward and backward weight shifts while seated on a chair or stability ball |
| | Standing COG | Standing with one foot directly in front of the other (sharpened Romberg stance) |
| | Dynamic COG | Four-corner stepping |
| Multisensory | Visual | Focusing on a visual target while seated on a stability ball |
| | Vestibular | Standing on compliant surface with eyes closed |
| | Somatosensory | Weight shifts while standing on a firm surface with eyes closed |
| Postural strategy | Ankle strategies | Standing sways from the ankle |
| | Hip strategies | Reaching for objects while standing on a half-foam roller |
| | Step strategies | Resistance band release maneuver |
| Gait pattern enhancement and variation | | Side stepping |
| | | Braiding |
| | | Slalom walking |
| Strength and endurance | Upper body | Horizontal pulls, shrugs, triceps extensions, bicep curls |
| | Lower body | Wall squats, sit-to-stand squats, leg extensions, lateral leg lifts, calf raises |
| Flexibility | Upper body | Neck rotation, turtle stretch, chest stretch, lateral shoulder stretch, roll-down |
| | Lower body | Hamstrings stretch, hip abductor stretch, golf-ball roll, calf stretch |

Data from Rose.[14]

a light medicine ball. In summary, multitask balance training more closely replicates the activities of daily living that individuals will be performing, and whereby their balance performance will most likely be challenged by a disturbance.

## Simulate Loss of Balance During Training

Balance exercise training programs and fall-prevention interventions must include a focus on balance-recovery reactions.[36] Ultimately, it is the capability, or lack thereof, to recover from a balance perturbation (loss of balance) that eventually determines whether an individual falls. Balance disturbances can arise from collisions, slips, and trips. In addition, loss of balance can occur during voluntary movements, including bending, reaching, and turning. The body has a natural line of defense against balance disturbances that consists of rapid limb movements. For example, reaching out to grab a supporting object or quickly stepping forward with a lower limb are compensatory mechanisms aimed at preventing a fall. Accordingly, it is logical to address the balance-recovery skill levels of individuals; effective training programs will be those that replicate sudden and unpredictable balance disturbances. Importantly, to elicit the most favorable adaptations in a client's balance-recovery reaction capacity, health and fitness professionals should design exercises/activities that do not permit the individual to anticipate a balance perturbation.

## Couple Resistance Training With Balance Exercise Training

Despite the fact that poor balance is frequently associated with reduced muscular strength, the literature does not currently support resistance training alone as a successful strategy for enhancing balance performance and fall reduction. In a systematic review of the efficacy of resistance training as an isolated intervention for uniformly improving balance, it was reported that this approach was successful in only one of five instances.[37] Therefore, it is crucial to recognize that resistance training needs to also be *coupled* with balance exercise training for meaningful modifications to be conferred on postural stability. Indeed, the integrated exercise training approach has been found to be effective in the literature.[38]

## Correctly Sequence Balance Exercises

Aerobic, resistance, flexibility, and balance training are each critically important for the overall health, functional capacity, and quality of life of older adults. However, to fulfill the minimum frequency requirements of each form of activity, individuals will need to perform at least two (or more) activities the same day, and most likely within the same exercise session.[39] Balance training should precede both resistance and flexibility activities. Research has reported that participation in either resistance or flexibility activities before balance exercise can negatively impact performance.[40,41] For the older adult who may already face significant balance challenges, it would be inappropriate (and possibly harmful) to create additional perturbations because of improper activity sequencing. Balance training (when combined with resistance and flexibility activities) should be performed first or following aerobic activity when coupled alone with that mode.

## Create Innovative Balance Exercise

Conventional balance training programs include various sitting and standing activities, which for the motivated individuals has been shown to be effective over the long term. However, in less motivated individuals, the performance of repetitive, basic tasks can lead to poor adherence, less effective training, and ultimately cessation of training. Consequently, continuously designing novel and creative balance exercises is a requisite skill for health and fitness professionals.

Recent research has reported that incorporating interactive video games may be an effective strategy to use when designing balance activities for older adults.[42] For example, the Wii Fit has various balance modules, including soccer, skiing, and penguin, that can be performed at different skill levels, depending on the client's functional capacity (Fig. 26-6). Science has shown that progressively incorporating interactive video games into training can increase motivation and improve balance performance.[43]

## Change the Availability of Sensory Cues

Many falls occur during conditions in which an individual is unaccustomed. Poor lighting or uneven surfaces impair the sensory cues typically available, therefore temporarily compromising the balance performance. Challenges can be introduced into the training program

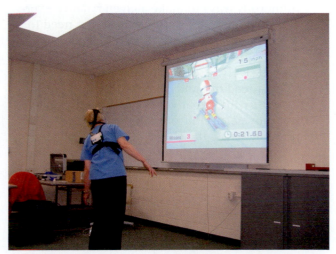

**Figure 26-6.** Research shows that incorporating interactive video games may be an effective strategy to use when designing balance activities for older adults.

as a means to better prepare individuals for circumstances where sensory cues are unavailable.[35] For instance, heel-toe walking may be performed with sunglasses worn (inside), eyes closed, or while slowly turning the head from side to side. In addition, standing balance exercises can be completed while standing on a foam pad or balance disk in an effort to disturb the surface conditions for which an individual is habituated. In conclusion, altering the sensory cues available is an important consideration when preparing the overall balance training program.

## Frequency, Intensity, Time, and Type Recommendations for Balance Exercise Training

The frequency, intensity, time, and type approach to exercise prescription used for cardiorespiratory fitness program design can also generally be applied to balance exercise programming.[44] Although research has yet to identify the optimal frequency, intensity, duration, and type of balance exercises, it has been recommended that balance training be performed 3 days per week for 10 to 15 minutes each session.[39] Intensity should be safe, but challenging. Balance training should be integrated into the overall physical-activity program according to the sequencing guidelines discussed earlier.

## Progression of Balance Training Exercises

A training program designed to optimize balance training and fall-reduction prevention should incorporate each of the key points discussed earlier. Individuals with no previous balance training experience should initially perform basic sitting and standing exercises as a means to improve balance performance. As these initial exercises become easier, an increase in difficulty can be accomplished in numerous ways[44]:

1. *Arm progressions.* Health and fitness professionals can vary the use and position of the arms in numerous ways to make a given balance exercise more difficult. Hands may at first need to be grasping or touching another object, such as a wall or back of a chair, to facilitate balance. Progressively, exercises can be performed with arms spread out and raised to shoulder height to assist with stability. Ultimately, individuals can move arms in from sides to a folded position across the chest.

2. *Surface progressions.* Health and fitness professionals can alter the surface or apparatus on which individuals perform balance exercises, progressively increasing the difficulty. For instance, foam pads, balance disks, and BOSU balls can be substituted for a hard, flat surface while performing multiple standing balance exercises. Similarly, physioballs can be exchanged for regular chairs when performing sitting exercises.

3. *Visual progressions.* Health and fitness professionals can mitigate the visual sensory cues provided to the individual during nearly all balance exercises. Various alternatives exist. Lighting of the room can be gradually dimmed, sunglasses may be worn inside, or eyes may be shut completely.

4. *Tasking progressions.* Health and fitness professionals should require individuals to initially master each balance exercise performed as a singular task. Although when this level of achievement is attained, additional tasks should be supplemented to the routine. Cognitive tasks or added physical tasks are a few of the readily available options.

Table 26-5 and Figure 26-7 summarize and illustrate balance exercises and training progression for older adults. Remember that it is also paramount to continuously seek novel and fun balance exercises. However, individuals should be cautioned about proceeding in difficulty without first demonstrating competency at the current level of balance exercise. Progressing too rapidly can actually contribute to a fall.

## Designing a Comprehensive Balance Training Program

The previous section has equipped readers with the most important balance training guidelines. Figure 26-8 outlines a sample weekly balance exercise program that combines each of these key considerations.

## Tai Chi for Fall Prevention

**Tai chi** is an ancient Chinese martial art with many different forms that incorporates mild strengthening, balance, postural alignment, and concentration by using slow, continuous movements of many body parts. It has positive effects on many components of balance and fall rates in older adults. Therefore, tai chi as a form of training to promote fall prevention has been the focus of numerous research studies on this population.[8,34,45] Studies report improvements in fear of falling, single-leg stance time, Berg balance scale, timed up and go, functional reach, and lower-body strength following tai chi.[45] The data indicate that the benefits are greater for independent and transitionally frail older adults compared with older frail individuals. In addition, tai chi training has demonstrated improvements in cardiovascular fitness and psychological well-being.[45] Because there are many tai chi forms and training programs used in the research literature, it is difficult to create an optimal prescription for older adults, although a minimum of two sessions a week for 12 weeks is necessary for improvements.[45]

## Vibration Training

Whole-body vibration training (WBV) is a relatively new form of exercise training that is increasing in

## Table 26-5. Balance Exercises and Training Progression for Older Adults

| POSITION | BALANCE EXERCISE |
|---|---|
| Sitting | Sit upright and complete the following progressions:<br>• Perform leg activities (heal, toe, or single-leg raises, marching). |
| Standing | • "Clock"—balance on one leg (45- or 90-degree angle), health and fitness professional calls out time, client moves nonsupport leg to time called (i.e., 5 o'clock, 9 o'clock), alternate legs.<br>• Perform leg activities (heal, toe, or single-leg raises—45- or 90-degree angle, marching).<br>• "Spelling"—balance on one leg, health and fitness professional asks client to spell word working with nonsupport leg (i.e., client's name, day of week, favorite food), alternate legs. |
| In motion | • Heel-to-toe walking along 15-foot line on floor (first with and then without partner)<br>• "Excursion"—alternating legs, lunge over a space separated by two lines of tape. Progress to hopping or jumping (using single-leg or double-leg) back and forth across the space.<br>• Dribble basketball around cones that require client to change direction multiple times. |
| Training progression | • Arm progressions—use surface for support, hands on thigh, hands folded across chest<br>• Surface progressions—chair, balance disks, foam pad, physioball<br>• Visual progressions—open eyes, sunglasses or dim room lighting, closed eyes<br>• Tasking progressions—single tasking, multitasking (i.e., balance exercise + pass/catch ball) |

Number of repetitions per exercise and rest intervals will be dependent on client conditioning and functional status.

popularity. A vibratory stimulus (either rotational or vertical) is applied to the entire body using specialized vibration units. Variations in frequency (Hz), amplitude (mm), magnitude (g), and duration are commonly used, and there is currently no consensus regarding the optimal settings to achieve specific outcomes. One review concluded that WBV is effective for older adults in improving bone density at the hip and tibia, but not the lumbar spine; it may be effective in improving muscular strength and power; and it may be effective in improving balance and functional mobility.[46] The authors noted that more high-quality studies are needed to determine the true effectiveness of WBV for this population, but that it has promise. Although the studies included in this review reported only minor adverse effects in their subjects from using WBV, it is important to carefully screen participants for comorbidities and chronic conditions that may preclude them from using WBV as a training tool.[46] Contraindications for WBV training include, but are not limited to, detached retina, acute deep vein thrombosis, severe CVD, and orthopedic conditions such as spinal disc herniation. Thus, if a health and fitness professional is considering incorporating WBV into an older adult's exercise program, it would be prudent to get a physician's clearance and recommendations for this specific activity before training.

## Yoga

Interest and participation in yoga is increasing among the general population and mature adults. A recent review on the benefits of yoga for older adults determined that although it may improve some components of fitness, more evidence is needed to determine its effectiveness.[47] The intensity of yoga is too low to enhance cardiovascular fitness and does not meet the American College of Sports Medicine's guidelines for moderate physical activity.[16] Modest improvements in gait, balance, upper- and lower-body flexibility, and lower-body strength were reported in the literature.[47] There is not enough evidence at this time to make a recommendation regarding the type or dosage of yoga for older adults.[47] Some yoga poses may be inappropriate for older adults with specific chronic diseases or orthopedic concerns.

## Aquatics

Aquatic exercise is often recommended as a suitable training method for older adults because of the reduction in joint forces that comes from the buoyancy of the water (Fig. 26-9). Water is a low-risk exercise environment that provides support to joints. In older adults, it has been shown to improve exercise adherence,

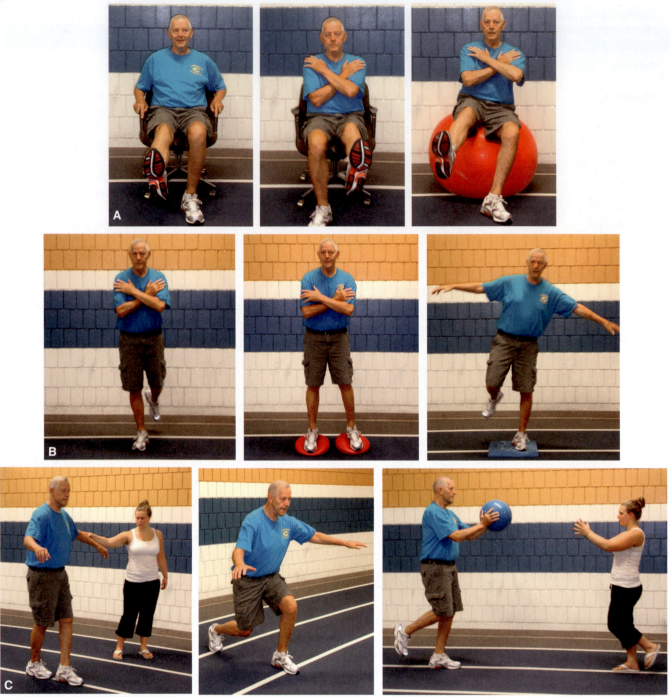

**Figure 26-7.** Sample balance exercises and training progression (from simple to complex). (A) sitting: closed eyes, arms crossed, physioball; (B) standing: arms crossed, balance disks, foam pad; (C) in motion: heel-to-toe, excursion, multitasking. *(Courtesy of Lance Dalleck and Jeff Janot.)*

step-test performance, knee and hip flexibility and strength, aerobic fitness, and physical functioning, while reducing the fear of falling.[48] It may be especially beneficial to individuals who have OA, are frail, have poor balance, or have osteoporosis.[48] During upright water exercise, such as aqua jogging or water aerobics, target heart rate is approximately 8 to 10 beats/min lower at a similar intensity of land-based exercise.[49] Therefore, it is recommended that heart rate and RPE both be used to monitor exercise intensity in the water.

**Client background and goals:** David, 66, attends a community fitness program offered through a local university 3 mornings per week. After several near falls in his home, David realized that initiating a balance training program would be in his best interest. He has been participating in the current program for 3 months and has progressed in difficulty on several exercises. A sample of the five exercises he completes each morning, along with a visual display, is presented below. Each exercise takes approximately 3 minutes, with the total program lasting 15 minutes.

| Exercise #1 | Exercise #2 | Exercise #3 | Exercise #4 | Exercise #5 |
|---|---|---|---|---|
| Single Leg Raises 10 right/left leg alternate 2 sets w/1-min rest arms crossed physioball | Catch use 4-lb medicine ball 15 tosses each set 2 sets w/30-sec rest rotate spot thrown to physioball | Spelling 2 words per leg alternate 2 sets w/30-sec rest arms extended hard flat surface | Heel Toe Walking 50 yds 2 sets w/30-sec rest walk w/partner arms crossed eyes closed | Stand arms crossed eyes closed nudge client 10 times 2 sets w/30-sec rest Bosu ball |

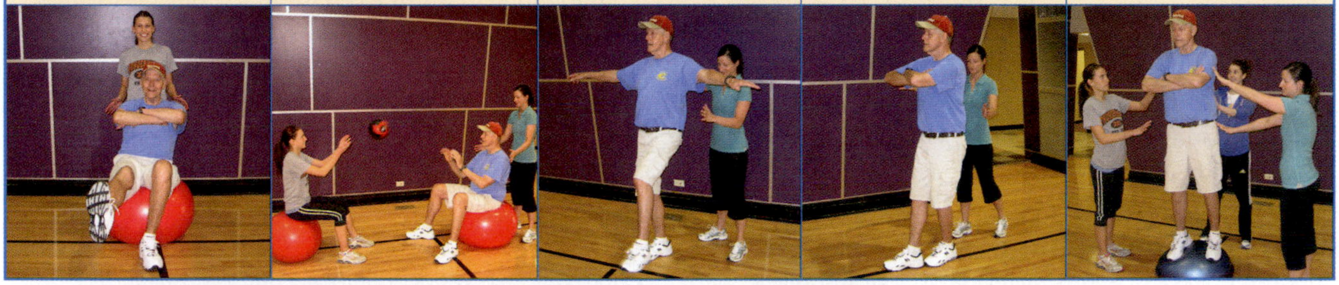

**Figure 26-8.** Case study approach to balance exercise training. *(Courtesy of Lance Dalleck and Jeff Janot.)*

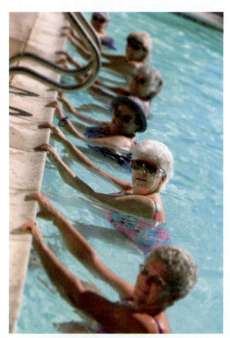

**Figure 26-9.** Aquatic exercise is often recommended as a suitable training method for older adults because of the reduction in joint forces that comes from the buoyancy of the water.

## VIGNETTE conclusion

■ If Danitza understood that older clients are not simply older versions of her younger clients, much of her frustration during the early sessions with Julie could have been avoided. Although some mature adults are similar to those 20 to 30 years younger, others are vastly different in their physiological, psychological, social, and emotional needs, as well as their interests, goals, and motivations for exercising. Using the same training program for all clients, as Danitza did, ignores their individuality and disregards the large variability that exists within the older population.

## CRITICAL THINKING QUESTIONS

1. You have your first appointment with a 72-year-old female client to start her on a training routine. What are some critical pieces of information that you should gather during this initial interview to develop a safe and effective exercise program for her?

2. You observe a mature client walking across the exercise floor. He has a slow, almost shuffling gait and stops periodically to steady himself by holding on to a piece of equipment. He sits down on the leg press machine and, to your surprise, lifts an impressive amount of weight. How do you reconcile these apparently contradictory observations in functional performance?

3. A 68-year-old healthy male client comes to you for a new exercise program. He has been following the same program (see later) for 6 months and is bored with it. In addition, he is not confident that the program is the best one for helping him achieve his primary goals—to be able to perform daily functional tasks optimally and to avoid disability. How might you modify this routine to better meet his goals?

   *Current routine:* Two sets of 15 repetitions on the following circuit of exercise machines performed 3 days per week: chest press, seated row, leg extension, leg curl, shoulder press, shoulder lateral raise, bicep curl, triceps pushdown, abdominal crunch, back extension

## ADDITIONAL RESOURCES

American College of Sports Medicine. American College of Sports Medicine position stand: Exercise and physical activity for older adults. *Med Sci Sports Exerc.* 2009;41:1510–1530.

American Council on Exercise. *ACE Senior Fitness Manual.* San Diego, CA: American Council on Exercise; 2013.

American Dietetic Association. Position of the American Dietetic Association, American Society for Nutrition, and Society for Nutrition Education: Food and nutrition programs for community-residing older adults. *J Am Dietet Assoc.* 2010;110:463–472.

Chodzko-Zajko WJ, Kramer AF, Poon LW. *Enhancing Cognitive Functioning and Brain Plasticity.* Champaign, IL: Human Kinetics; 2009.

Mullen SP, Wójcicki TR, Mailey EL, et al. A profile for predicting attrition from exercise in older adults. *Prev Sci.* 2013;14:489–496.

Rikli RE, Jones JC. *Senior Fitness Test Manual.* 2nd ed. Champaign, IL: Human Kinetics; 2012.

Signorile JF. *Bending the Aging Curve: The Complete Exercise Guide for Older Adults.* Champaign, IL: Human Kinetics; 2011.

## REFERENCES

1. Armstrong S, et al. National blueprint: Increasing physical activity among adults age 50 and older. *J Aging Phys Act.* 2001;9(Suppl.):5–13.
2. Palmore EB. *Ageism: Negative and Positive.* 2nd ed. New York: Springer Publishing Company; 1999:266.
3. Rowe JW, Kahn RL. *Successful Aging.* New York: Dell Publishing; 1998:265.
4. Spirduso W, Francis K, MacRae P. *Physical Dimensions of Aging.* 2nd ed. Champaign, IL: Human Kinetics; 2005.
5. Busse EW. Theories of aging. In: Busse E, Pfeiffer E, eds. *Behavior and Adaptation in Later Life.* Boston: Little Brown; 1969:11–32.
6. Elder Jr, GH, Johnson MK, Crosnoe R. The emergence and development of life course theory. In: Mortimer JT, Shanahan MJ, eds. *Handbook of the Life Course.* New York: Kluwer Academic/Plenum Publishers; 2003.
7. Bengston VL, Gans D, Putney N, Silverstein M. *Handbook of Theories of Aging.* 2nd ed. New York: Springer Publishing Company; 2009.
8. American College of Sports Medicine; Chodzko-Zajko WJP, Fiatarone-Singh DN, et al. Position stand: Exercise and physical activity for older adults. *Med Sci Sports Exerc.* 2009;41:1510–1530.
9. Vandervoot AS, Symons TB. Functional and metabolic consequences of sarcopenia. *Can J Appl Physiol.* 2001; 26:90–101.
10. Nair K. Aging muscle. *Am J Clin Nutr.* 2005;81:953–963.
11. Iannuzzi-Sucich M, Prestwood KM, Kenny AM. Prevalence of sarcopenia and predictors of skeletal muscle mass in healthy older men and women. *J Gerontol A Biol Sci Med Sci.* 2002;57A:M772–M777.
12. Rice C. Muscle function at the motor unit level: Consequences of aging. *Top Geriatr Rehabil.* 2000;15:70–82.
13. King BR, Fogel SM, Albouy G, Doyon J. Neural correlates of the age-related changes in motor sequence learning and motor adaptation in older adults. *Front Hum Neurosci.* 2013;7:142.
14. Rose DJ. *FallProof!™ A comprehensive balance and mobility training program.* 2nd ed. Champaign, IL: Human Kinetics; 2010:312.
15. Karavidas A, Lazaros G, Tsiachris D, Pyrgakis V. Aging and the Cardiovascular System. *Hellenic J Cardiol.* 2010;51:421–427.
16. *ACSM's Guidelines for Exercise Testing and Prescription.* 9th ed. Baltimore, MD: Lippincott Williams & Wilkins; 2014.
17. Kalache A, Kickbusch I. A global strategy for healthy ageing. *World Health.* 1997;50:4–5.
18. Nagi SZ. Some conceptual issues in disability and rehabilitation. In: Sussman MB, ed. *Sociology and Rehabilitation.* Washington, DC: American Sociological Association; 1965.
19. Chin A Paw MJ, van Uffelen JG, Riphagen I, van Mechelen W. The functional effects of physical exercise training in frail older people: A systematic review. *Sports Med.* 2008;38:781–793.
20. Keysor JJ, Jette AM. Have we oversold the benefit of late-life exercise? *J Gerontol A Biol Sci Med Sci.* 2001; 56A:M412–M423.
21. Latham NK, Bennett DA, Stretton CM, Anderson CS. Systematic review of progressive resistance strength training in older adults. *J Gerontol A Biol Sci Med Sci.* 2004;59A:48–61.

22. Signorile J. *Bending the Aging Curve: The Complete Exercise Guide for Older Adults*. Champaign, IL: Human Kinetics; 2011.

23. Tanaka H, Monahan KD, Seals DR. Age-predicted maximal heart rate revisited. *J Am Coll Cardiol*. 2001;37:153–156.

24. Porter MM. Power training for older adults. *Appl Physiol Nutr Metab*. 2006;31:87–94.

25. Tschopp M, Sattelmayer MK, Hilfiker R. Is power training or conventional resistance training better for function in elderly persons? A meta-analysis. *Age Ageing*. 2011;40:549–556.

26. de Vreede PL, Samson MM, van Meeteren NL, Duursma SA, Verhaar HJ. Functional-task exercise versus resistance strength exercise to improve daily function in older women: a randomized, controlled trial. *J Am Geriatr Soc*. 2005;53:2–10.

27. Kibele A, Behm DG. Seven weeks of instability and traditional resistance training effects on strength, balance and functional performance. *J Strength Cond Res*. 2009;23:2443–2450.

28. Krebs DE, Scarborough DM, McGibbon CA. Functional vs. strength training in disabled elderly outpatients. *Am J Phys Med Rehabil*. 2007;86:93–103.

29. Sipe C, Ritchie D. The Significant Seven. *IDEA Fitness J*. 2012;1:42–49.

30. Rice J, Keogh J. Power training: Can it improve functional performance in older adults? A systematic review. *Int J Exerc Sci*. 2009;2:131–151.

31. Sayers SP. High velocity power training in older adults. *Curr Aging Sci*. 2008;1:62–67.

32. Skelton D, Todd C. What are the main risk factors for falls among older people and what are the most effective interventions to prevent these falls? Copenhagen: WHO Regional Office for Europe; 2004.

33. Gillespie LD, Robertson MC, Gillespie WJ. Interventions for preventing falls in older people living in the community. *Cochrane Database Syst Rev*. 2009(2): CD007146.

34. Sherrington C, Tiedemann A, Fairhall N, Close JC, Lord SR. Exercise to prevent falls in older adults: An updated meta-analysis and best practice recommendations. *N S W Public Health Bull*. 2011;22:78–83.

35. Silsupadol P, Shumway-Cook A, Lugade V, et al. Effects of single-task versus dual-task training on balance performance in older adults: A double blind, randomized controlled trial. *Arch Phys Med Rehabil*. 2009;90:381–387.

36. Mansfield A, Peters AL, Liu BA, Maki BE. A perturbation-based balance training program for older adults: Study protocol for a randomized controlled trial. *BMC Geriatr*. 2007;7:12.

37. Orr R, Raymond J, Singh MF. Efficacy of progressive resistance training on balance performance in older adults. A systematic review of randomized controlled trials. *Sports Med*. 2008;38:317–343.

38. de Bruin ED, Murer K. Effect of additional functional exercises on balance in elderly people. *Clin Rehabil*. 2007;21:112–121.

39. Nelson ME, Rejeski WJ, Blair SN, et al. Physical activity and public health in older adults: Recommendation for adults from the American College of Sports Medicine and the American Heart Association. *Med Sci Sports Exerc*. 2007;39:1435–1445.

40. Behm DG, Bambury A, Cahill F, Power K. Effect of acute static stretching on force, balance, reaction time, and movement time. *Med Sci Sports Exerc*. 2004;36:1397–1402.

41. Moreland JD, Richardson JA, Goldsmith CH, Clase CM. Muscle weakness and falls in older adults: A systematic review and meta-analysis. *J Am Geriatr Soc*. 2004;52:1121–1129.

42. Nitz JC, Kuys S, Isles R, Fu S. Is the Wii Fit a new-generation tool for improving balance, health and well-being? A pilot study. *Climacteric*. 2010;13:487–491.

43. Betker AL, Szturm T, Moussavi ZK, Nett C. Video game-based exercises for balance rehabilitation: A single-subject design. *Arch Phys Med Rehabil*. 2006;87: 1141–1149.

44. American College of Sports Medicine. *Resources for the Personal Trainer*. 3rd ed. Baltimore, MD: Lippincott Williams & Wilkins; 2010.

45. Choi JH, Moon JS, Song R. Effects of Sun-style Tai Chi exercise on physical fitness and fall prevention in fall-prone older adults. *J Adv Nurs*. 2005;51:150–157.

46. Merriman H, Jackson K. The effects of whole-body vibration training in aging adults: A systematic review. *J Geriatr Phys Ther*. 2009;32:134–145.

47. Roland KP, Jakobi JM, Jones GR. Does yoga engender fitness in older adults? A critical review. *J Aging Phys Act*. 2011;19:62–79.

48. Devereux K, Robertson D, Briffa NK. Effects of a water-based program on women 65 years and over: A randomised controlled trial. *Aust J Physiother*. 2005;51: 102–108.

49. Van Norman K. *Exercise and Wellness for Older Adults*. 2nd ed. Champaign, IL: Human Kinetics; 2010.

50. Griffiths Y, Thinnes A. *Occupational Therapy with Elders*. New York: Mosby; 2011.

51. Atchley R. *Continuity and Adaptation in Aging: Creating Positive Experiences*. Baltimore, MD: Johns Hopkins University Press; 1999.

52. Dohm A, Shniper L. *Occupational Employment Projections to 2016: Monthly Labor Review*. 2007. Available at: http://www.bls.gov/opub/mlr/2007/11/art5full.pdf.

53. AARP. *Staying Ahead of the Curve: The AARP Work and Career Study*. 2003. Available at:http://www.aarp.org/work/working-after-retirement/info-2003/aresearch-import-417.html

54. U.S. Census Bureau. *Facts for Features*. 2006. Available at: https://www.census.gov/newsroom/releases/archives/facts_for_features_special_editions/

55. Campbell AJ, Buchner DM. Unstable disability and the fluctuations of frailty. *Age Ageing*. 1997;26:315–318.

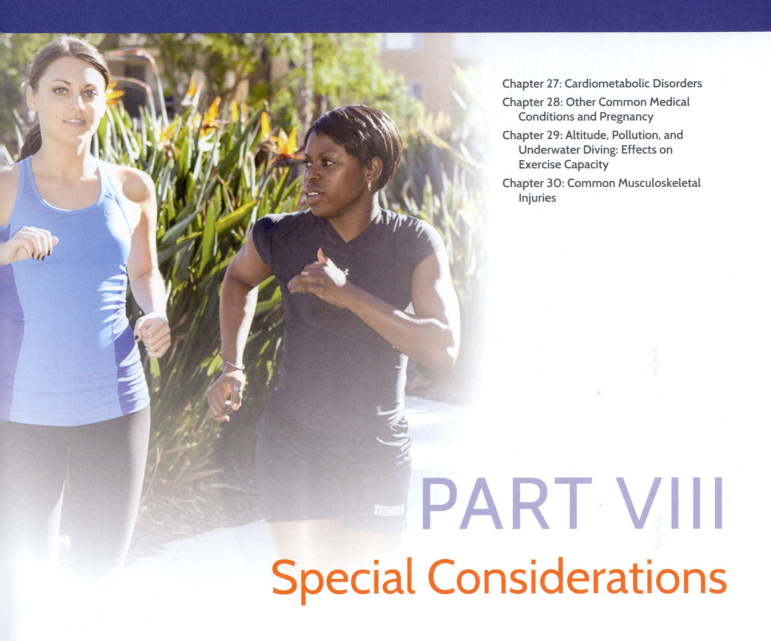

# PART VIII
## Special Considerations

The final section of this book provides information on a variety of medical conditions and environmental challenges that are likely to be encountered by health and fitness professionals as they work with clients. Chapter 27 describes many of the risk factors that predispose individuals to developing cardiovascular and/or metabolic disease. Collectively referred to as cardiometabolic disorders, research has shown that proper nutritional and exercise strategies are effective in helping to control or even reverse many of these conditions. Chapter 28 covers a variety of medical conditions for which it has been shown that properly supervised exercise can provide a therapeutic benefit. Exercising at altitude, underwater, and in a polluted environment are covered in Chapter 29. Each of these environmental challenges poses specific physiological changes that must be understood in order for you to safely program exercise for clients. The latest practical guidelines are presented so that clients can maximize their enjoyment when they exercise in these conditions.

Chapter 30 presents information relative to a wide variety of exercise-related injuries that are commonly seen in physically active individuals. Many of your clients are likely to have either acute or chronic injuries that must be taken into consideration as you develop and implement their workout programs. Steps to avoid injuries and ways in which to safely progress individuals through the recovery process are focuses of this chapter.

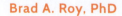

Brad A. Roy, PhD

# CHAPTER 27

# Cardiometabolic Disorders

## CHAPTER OUTLINE

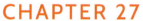

# CHAPTER OUTLINE—cont'd

## LEARNING OUTCOMES

1. Describe the current physical activity recommendations for adults as put forth in the *2008 Physical Activity Guidelines for Americans*.

2. Identify the common risk factors for cardiometabolic disorders.

3. Describe the following cardiometabolic and vascular disorders: hypertension, diabetes, metabolic syndrome, dyslipidemia, cardiovascular disease, and stroke.

4. Define *prehypertension* and *prediabetes,* and identify key lifestyle strategies for preventing the progression of these pre-states to full-blown hypertension and diabetes.

5. Identify the cluster of conditions that define metabolic syndrome.

6. Describe the role of exercise in treating cardiovascular and peripheral vascular disease.

7. Describe the common symptoms of coronary artery disease and steps to take when a person is experiencing these symptoms.

8. Explain the various types of exercise testing and their use in healthy individuals and people with chronic health conditions.

## ANCILLARY LINK

Visit Davis*Plus* at http://davisplus.fadavis.com for study and practice resources, including online quizzes, animations that help explain physiological processes, podcasts concerning news and career trends in exercise physiology, and practice references.

# VIGNETTE

■ Vincent Consolo is a successful computer programmer, developing and selling specialized software worldwide. He typically works long hours at his computer developing software programs and tends to spend his recreational time watching television and reading. Vincent's wife, concerned with his lack of physical activity, increasing weight, and shortness of breath with minimal exertion, had been pestering him to start an exercise program for a number of years. In the spring of 2011, Vincent finally gave in to her pressuring and decided to take up a home walking program to see if he could get some of the 225 pounds he now carried off his 5'10" frame. Because Vincent, now 46 years old, had not seen a health-care provider since college, he was unaware of his numerous underlying risk factors. Unknown to Vincent, he has a resting blood pressure (BP) of 148/102 mm Hg, total **cholesterol** (TC) of 259 mg/dL, **low-density lipoprotein (LDL)** cholesterol of 185 mg/dL, **high-density lipoprotein (HDL)** cholesterol of 38 mg/dL, and triglyceride level of 180 mg/dL.

What might be the result of Vincent's current level of health, and what preventive measures could he have taken to avoid the potential for adverse outcomes?

Since the 1970s, occupational, technological, and environmental advances have resulted in a significant decrease in daily physical activity and associated energy expenditure. Following closely behind the initial reduction in daily physical activity was an increase in America's available food supply, especially high-fat/energy-dense foods, a combination that has resulted in costly health consequences. Cancer and a variety of cardiometabolic disorders, such as **cardiovascular disease (CVD)**, diabetes, and the **metabolic syndrome (MetS)**, have dramatically increased over this same time period, to the point they are now the leading causes of death and disability in the United States. These health conditions are responsible for 7 of every 10 deaths in the United States and affect the quality of life of more than 130 million Americans.[1]

Although historically cardiometabolic disorders have been diseases of the aged, obesity, diabetes, and hypertension are becoming increasingly common in young adults and children. Allowing this trend to continue will only serve to further increase health-care spending and will have a dramatic impact on future American productivity. However, there is hope through the successful implementation of key lifestyle interventions that target three primary areas of risk: smoking, poor diet, and physical inactivity. Modification of these three key risk factors will dramatically decrease the future incidence of chronic disease and associated mortality, morbidity, and cost. For our purposes, the scope of this chapter focuses on cardiometabolic and vascular disease and physical activity.

Americans currently do not meet the minimum physical activity standard to promote health and well-being. As a result, obesity, heart disease, diabetes, MetS, and many other chronic health conditions continue to increase at an alarming rate. This chapter provides background information on the following cardiometabolic disorders and the role of exercise as a preventive strategy and therapeutic intervention:

- Hypertension
- Diabetes
- MetS
- **Dyslipidemia**
- **Stroke**
- Cardiovascular disorders
- **Peripheral vascular disease (PVD)** and **peripheral arterial occlusive disease (PAOD)**

The large prevalence of chronic disease makes it essential that exercise professionals have a basic understanding of the above conditions and the appropriate application of exercise training as a therapeutic intervention and preventive strategy. Generally speaking, people experiencing one or more of the earlier conditions will benefit from exercise training and are frequently referred to professionals, such as clinical exercise physiologists, who are appropriately trained to provide wellness coaching and exercise/lifestyle interventions.

Although the exact content of the lifestyle intervention program will depend on each person's current health status, physical condition, and other factors identified in the screening and referral process, the basic platform is somewhat similar across conditions. These lifestyle interventions typically include exercise, diet, smoking cessation, and behavioral change coaching that focuses on reducing risk factors and promoting wellness (Fig. 27-1). The exercise professional will individualize the intervention to accommodate the specific characteristics of each client, with appropriate modifications made to the activities to enhance safety and program effectiveness. It is also important to note that many people with chronic health conditions have comorbidities (e.g., a person with heart disease and diabetes who is overweight) that also impact the exercise program, and this further emphasizes the importance of individualizing each lifestyle intervention program.

## HYPERTENSION

Blood pressure, as defined in Chapter 7, is the force exerted by the blood against a vessel wall and is subject to a number of factors, including the volume of blood and the distensibility of the vessel wall. There are

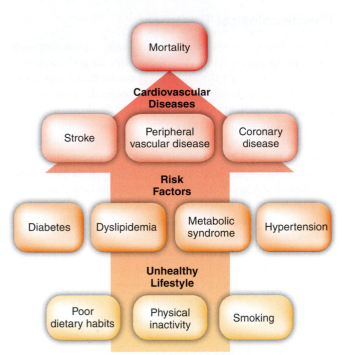

**Figure 27-1.** Relationships among an unhealthy lifestyle, risk factors, cardiovascular disease, and mortality. Lifestyle interventions typically include exercise, diet, smoking cessation, and behavioral change coaching that focuses on reducing risk factors and promoting wellness. In turn, long-term risk for the development of cardiovascular diseases and mortality is lessened.

two primary phases of BP: systolic and diastolic. **Systolic blood pressure** (SBP) is the pressure exerted during **systole**, or the contractile phase of the heart, and **diastolic blood pressure** (DBP) is the pressure in the vessel during **diastole** or the resting/filling phase of the cardiac cycle. The normal resting BP is 120/80 mm Hg or lower. During exercise, the systolic pressure increases with increasing workloads, whereas the diastolic pressure remains relatively constant.

Many Americans have elevated BP at rest, a condition referred to as **hypertension**. Hypertension, or high BP, is sometimes referred to as the "silent killer" and is one of the most prevalent chronic diseases in the United States, affecting more than 77.9 million people.[2] Hypertension is a powerful and independent risk factor for cardiovascular and renal diseases, especially coronary heart disease, **heart failure (HF)**, stroke, and

renal failure. Despite efforts to educate the public regarding hypertension and associated chronic health conditions, almost 30% of American adults are unaware of their hypertension, thus the term "silent killer." Approximately 40% of people with hypertension are not being treated, and of those who are undergoing treatment, 67% do not have their BP appropriately controlled. High BP is a significant health risk, with approximately 55,000 hypertension-related deaths occurring in the United States each year. Approximately 69% of people who have a first heart attack, 77% who have a first stroke, and 74% who have HF are hypertensive. It is estimated that each 20-mm Hg increase in SBP or 10-mm Hg increase in DBP doubles a person's risk for development of CVD.[3]

## VIGNETTE continued

■ Although Vincent's current BP is 148/102 mm Hg, a level considered to be hypertensive, he was unaware of the condition because he had not seen a medical provider in years and had not had his BP measured. His BP challenge began during college. When faced with a heavy academic load, Vincent began to forgo physical activity in favor of studying and challenging friends to computer games. By the end of his freshman year, Vincent's resting BP had increased to 135/86 mm Hg and his 5'10" frame was supporting 185 pounds, which resulted in a body mass index (BMI) of 26.5 kg/m² (overweight). Vincent's weight and declining physical activity were important factors affecting his increased resting BP.

## Diagnostic Criteria and National Heart, Lung, and Blood Institute Guidelines

Table 27-1 presents the classification of BP designated by the "Seventh Report of the Joint National Committee on Prevention, Detection, Evaluation and Treatment of High Blood Pressure."[4] The range between normal and stage 1 hypertension is considered **prehypertension**. Prehypertension is not a specific disease

**Table 27-1.** Joint National Committee VII Classifications of Blood Pressure

| CATEGORY | SYSTOLIC BLOOD PRESSURE (MM HG) | DIASTOLIC BLOOD PRESSURE (MM HG) |
|---|---|---|
| Normal | <120 | <80 |
| Prehypertension | 120–139 | 80–89 |
| Stage I hypertension | 140–159 | 90–99 |
| Stage II hypertension | ≥160 | ≥100 |
| Isolated systolic hypertension | ≥140 | <90 |

*Source:* Data from "The Seventh Report of the Joint National Committee on Prevention, Detection, Evaluation and Treatment of High Blood Pressure."[55]

category, but a designation that identifies people at increased risk for development of hypertension. It is estimated that 29.7 percent of the U.S. population 20 years of age and older fall into the prehypertension category. This is significant, because these individuals have twice the risk for development of hypertension compared with those with normal values.[2]

Hypertension may also be classified as "primary or essential" and "secondary." In people with essential hypertension, a specific cause is not identifiable, whereas secondary hypertension has an identifiable cause, such as renal vascular disease and endocrine disorders. Most hypertension cases, more than 95%, are categorized as essential.

## VIGNETTE continued

■ Vincent's BP during college was in the prehypertensive stage and should have been addressed with increased physical activity, dietary changes, and weight management. However, this did not occur, and over the years Vincent's resting BP continued to increase to a level of hypertension and increased risk for development of CVD. Because he refuses to see a medical provider, Vincent is unaware of his hypertensive state; left untreated, this level of BP may result in significant heart muscle hypertrophy and coronary artery damage. By becoming aware of the elevated BP, a number of treatment strategies could be implemented that would reduce his risk for development of chronic health conditions.

## Nonpharmacological Treatment

Although medications can be effective in lowering BP, they can have numerous negative side effects and are expensive. Thus, nonpharmacological lifestyle modifications are attractive and serve as the primary treatment focus for people diagnosed with prehypertension. These lifestyle interventions include dietary alterations, weight loss, exercise, smoking cessation, stress management/relaxation techniques, and moderation of alcohol intake. A low-fat diet rich in fruits and vegetables, such as the Dietary Approaches to Stop Hypertension (DASH) eating plan, is typically encouraged, together with a reduction in sodium intake and adequate intake of dietary potassium, calcium, and magnesium.[6] A large percentage of individuals with prehypertension and hypertension are overweight, and the increased body fat is associated with insulin resistance and hypertension. Weight loss has been shown to reduce BP by 5 to 20 mm Hg per 10-kg weight loss in people who are more than 10% over their ideal body weight.[6]

## Pharmacological Treatment

People diagnosed with stage 1 and stage 2 hypertension are also encouraged to make the earlier lifestyle changes in conjunction with the antihypertensive pharmacotherapy with which they may be treated. Commonly prescribed medications include thiazide diuretics, beta blockers, angiotensin-converting enzyme inhibitors, angiotensin II receptor blockers, calcium channel blockers, and others. Of these, thiazide diuretics are generally the first drug of choice for uncomplicated hypertension and are often used in combination with other drug classes for more complicated cases. The various types of medications used have different physiological effects that impact BP. For example, diuretics and angiotensin-converting enzyme inhibitors have a lowering effect on BP, because they decrease the volume of fluid pumped against the vessel wall. Vasodilators decrease peripheral resistance by increasing vessel diameter, and beta blockers lower BP by decreasing heart rate and contractility.

## Exercise and Hypertension

Exercise has both an acute and a chronic effect on BP, along with heart rate and various other physiological parameters. In both individuals with hypertension and those with normotension, a single exercise session can acutely lower BP during the post-exercise period (Fig. 27-2). However, the reduction is more pronounced in individuals with hypertension. This post-exercise decline in BP ranges from 5 to 15 mm Hg for SBP and up to 4 mm Hg for DBP, and in some people can persist for up to 22 hours.[13–16] Although the exact mechanism for this post-exercise effect is not fully understood, it appears to be related to a reduced peripheral vascular resistance that is not compensated for by an increase in cardiac output. This effect has also been documented

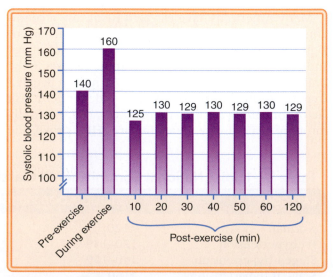

**Figure 27-2.** The post-exercise decline in blood pressure (BP) ranges from 5 to 15 mm Hg for systolic BP and up to 4 mm Hg for diastolic BP. In some people, this decline can persist for up to 22 hours.

## RESEARCH HIGHLIGHT

### Aerobic Fitness and Hypertension

Some people with normal resting BP will have an exaggerated SBP response during exercise (greater than 220 mm Hg), whereas others may have an abnormal increase in diastolic pressure (greater than 10-mm Hg change) with increasing workloads. People who are experiencing this exaggerated BP response are at greater risk for development of hypertension (1.7–2.4 times more likely) than those with a normal response. Regular participation in physical activity and other lifestyle changes such as weight loss and dietary modifications are highly encouraged in this population to decrease the likelihood of development of hypertension.[7-11]

Regular moderate-intensity aerobic exercise reduces the risk for development of hypertension and plays an important role in lowering SBP and DBP in people with hypertension. This preventive and therapeutic effect of exercise has been well demonstrated in the published literature. For example, findings from the Coronary Artery Risk Development in Young Adults (CARDIA) study showed that both physical activity and aerobic fitness are inversely related to BP and the future development of hypertension.[12] Research has also noted that the physiological measure of aerobic fitness (e.g., peak oxygen consumption [$\dot{V}O_2$]) appears to have a stronger association with a lowered incidence of hypertension than the actual behavior of physical activity. This finding may be due, in part, to the large variability in exercise intensity that is associated with measured physical activity across research studies. In some cases, the intensity may not be strong enough to elicit changes in aerobic fitness, resulting in a smaller impact on BP.

*Please see reference list at the end of the chapter.*

following resistance training, although the magnitude of BP change is not as great as following aerobic exercise. Combined aerobic and resistance exercise appears to produce a similar reduction in post-exercise BP as aerobic exercise alone.[17] Although additional research is needed to fully understand the underlying physiological mechanisms, the take-home message is that participation in regular exercise is important in reducing BP and maintaining a normotensive state.

The volume of regular aerobic exercise that has consistently been shown to reduce SBP and DBP is 150 minutes per week or more, with the greatest reductions occurring in individuals with hypertension.[18] This volume of activity is consistent with the *2008 Physical Activity Guidelines for Americans* and recommendations by the American College of Sports Medicine.[19,20] Both low- and high-intensity exercise training are effective at reducing BP at rest, during maximal or peak exercise, and during the post-exercise period.[21] Based on the current published literature and physical activity guidelines, it is recommended that both individuals with prehypertension and those with hypertension participate in regular exercise of moderate intensity for 30 minutes or more at least 5, if not more, days of the week. Aerobic activities such as walking, cycling, exercise ergometers, and swimming are excellent modes and should be supplemented with resistance training at least two times per week whenever possible. It is important that appropriate lifting and breathing technique (avoiding the Valsalva maneuver) is followed and avoidance of isometric exercise considered in those with known cardiac disease.

A number of the medications prescribed for the treatment of hypertension have a potential impact on the exercise and post-exercise response. Some medications

(e.g., beta blockers, calcium channel blockers) can blunt the heart rate response and cause orthostatic and post-exercise hypotension. These individuals should be taught to use ratings of perceived effort (RPE) to monitor exercise intensity, be advised to change positions slowly, and taught to follow each exercise session with a gradual and prolonged cool-down period. Diuretic medications are commonly prescribed and may place certain individuals at increased risk for dehydration and post-exercise hypotension, especially in warm environments. It is important that people on diuretic medications maintain their hydration status, and on very warm days moderate the intensity and/or duration of their activity.

Other forms of physical activity such as yoga and tai chi have also been shown to be beneficial for people with hypertension. These activities provide variety to the exercise program and promote relaxation, strength, and flexibility. The slow, mindful, and relaxing movements associated with yoga and tai chi may be especially effective at reducing BP in people who are experiencing high stress. Step pedometers or accelerometers are an excellent tool to raise an individual's awareness of their daily physical activity and to assist in gradually increasing their daily energy expenditure.

### In Your Own Words

As a best practices method, you routinely measure all new clients' BP before working with them as part of their initial fitness assessment. What would you say to a new client who wants to know why you are measuring his BP, even though he has never been diagnosed with hypertension in the clinical setting?

# DIABETES

**Diabetes** is a group of diseases characterized by high levels of blood glucose resulting from defects in **insulin** production, insulin action, or both. Diabetes causes abnormalities in the metabolism of carbohydrate, protein, and fat. When left untreated, or inadequately treated, diabetes results in a variety of chronic disorders and premature death. People with diabetes are at greater risk for development of a variety of chronic health problems that include heart disease, stroke, kidney failure, nerve disorders, eye problems, and others. Approximately 25.8 million children and adults (8.3% of the U.S. population) have diabetes, with only 18.8 million having been officially diagnosed. Unfortunately, because the symptoms associated with diabetes are not always present during the early stages of the disease, approximately 7.0 million people are unaware that they have diabetes. The prevalence of diabetes increases with advancing age, currently impacting nearly 27% of people older than 65 years.[22]

Historically, health-care providers have relied on a fasting plasma glucose (FPG) test or an oral glucose tolerance test (OGTT) to diagnose diabetes. With the FPG test, a fasting blood glucose level ≥126 mg/dL indicates diabetes. An FPG between 100 and 125 mg/dL signals **prediabetes**, a condition that occurs when levels are higher than normal but not in the diagnostic range of diabetes. Although FPG tests and OGTTs are still used as diagnostic tools, the **glycohemoglobin (HbA1c)** test, or simply the A1C test, has become the primary measurement used for managing diabetes. The basis of the A1C test is the attachment of glucose to hemoglobin, the protein in the red blood cell that carries oxygen to the tissues. Because red blood cells turn over approximately every 3 months, the A1C test represents an average blood glucose level over the previous 3-month period. The A1C measurement is reported as a percentage, and unlike the FPG test and OGTT, the A1C does not show day-to-day variations in blood glucose levels. A normal A1C level is less than 5.7%. The A1C test does not require the person to be in a fasting state, which is a significant advantage for medical providers who see patients throughout the day.

Approximately 97 million Americans have prediabetes, represented by an FPG test between 100 and 125 mg/dL, levels that are just below the diagnostic range of diabetes. People with prediabetes are at an increased risk for development of type 2 diabetes, **coronary artery disease (CAD)**, and stroke. A majority of people with prediabetes tend to be overweight and sedentary. Research has shown that individuals with prediabetes who engage in regular exercise and lose weight can prevent or delay the development of type 2 diabetes and other metabolic disorders.[22]

There are three primary types of diabetes. **Type 1 diabetes**, previously called *insulin-dependent diabetes mellitus*, develops when pancreatic beta cells that are responsible for producing insulin are destroyed by the body's immune system. The resulting decrement or cessation of insulin production (**hypoinsulinemia**) significantly impacts the body's ability to regulate blood glucose, thus exposing individuals to a higher-than-normal level of glucose in the blood (**hyperglycemia**). As a result, people with type 1 diabetes require regular insulin delivered by injections or a pump, to regulate blood glucose levels and prevent an accelerated use and incomplete breakdown of fatty acids that can result in **ketoacidosis**. Ketoacidosis occurs when a high level of ketones is produced as fat utilization increases because of the unavailability of carbohydrate to the tissues. This lack of glucose not only results in accelerated fatty-acid metabolism, but also in the incomplete breakdown of the fatty acid, which results in an accumulation of acidic ketones. The condition can be further exacerbated by dehydration that can result from increased urine production. Ketoacidosis is a serious medical condition that can deteriorate into a diabetic coma and even result in death. Box 27-1 presents the signs and symptoms of ketoacidosis.

Type 1 diabetes can occur at any age, but it most frequently occurs in children and young adults. In adults, type 1 diabetes accounts for 5% to 10% of all diagnosed cases of diabetes. The typical signs and symptoms of type 1 diabetes include excessive thirst and hunger, frequent urination, weight loss, blurred vision, and recurrent infections. During periods of insulin deficiency, a hyperglycemia occurs as a result of reduced glucose uptake and storage. A portion of the excess glucose is excreted in the urine, leading to thirst, dehydration, reduced appetite, and weight loss. Chronic, especially uncontrolled diabetes can result in a number of complications and chronic disease processes. Box 27-2 presents common complications associated with diabetes. (Also see explanatory animation of the Pathophysiology of Type 1 diabetes on the Davis*Plus* site at http://davisplus.fadavis.com.)

The most common form of diabetes is **type 2 diabetes**, previously referred to as **non-insulin–dependent diabetes mellitus**, which accounts for 90% to 95% of all diagnosed cases. Type 2 diabetes typically presents as **insulin resistance**, a disorder (affecting one third of adults aged ≥20 years) in

## Box 27-1. Signs and Symptoms of Ketoacidosis

- Thirst or dry mouth
- Frequent urination
- High blood glucose levels
- Increased levels of ketones in the urine
- Fatigue/lethargy
- Dry/flushed skin
- Nausea, vomiting, and/or abdominal pain
- Difficulty breathing, especially deep breaths
- Fruity odor of breath
- Confusion and difficulty paying attention

## Box 27-2. Common Complications Associated With Diabetes

- CVD, including CAD, stroke, and peripheral arterial occlusive disease
- High blood pressure
- Blindness
- Kidney disease
- Neuropathy and other neurological disorders
- Dental disease (periodontal or gum disease)
- Pregnancy complications
- Biochemical imbalances such as ketoacidosis
- Increased illness susceptibility
- Psychological challenges such as depression
- Amputation resulting from poor circulation and associated gangrene

which the cells do not use insulin properly. The inefficient utilization of insulin results in increased insulin demand, and over time the pancreas loses its ability to effectively produce insulin. The result is a combination of insulin resistance and impaired insulin production that leads to frequent states of hyperglycemia (Fig. 27-3). Initial treatment usually includes weight loss, diet modification, and exercise. Obesity, especially visceral obesity, is strongly associated with type 2 diabetes, making weight loss an important objective that will moderate and, in some cases, may even reverse the condition.[23] The initial treatment strategy usually focuses on lifestyle management (exercise, diet, and weight loss), but many individuals with type 2 diabetes are also placed on oral and, less frequently, injectable medications.

**Gestational diabetes** is a form of glucose intolerance that occurs during pregnancy and is present in approximately 2% to 10% of all pregnancies and 5% to 10% of women in the immediate post-partum period. It is more common among obese women, women with a history of gestational diabetes, and ethnic groups such as African Americans, Hispanic/Latino Americans, and American Indians. Immediate treatment is required to avoid complications in the developing fetus. Historically, women diagnosed with gestational diabetes have a 35% to 60% chance of development of diabetes over the subsequent 10 to 20 years, emphasizing the importance of maintaining regular exercise, appropriate nutritional habits, and weight in the post-partum years.[24]

### Treatment and Blood Glucose Control

The primary treatment goal for people with diabetes is threefold: (1) to normalize glucose metabolism, (2) to prevent diabetes-associated complications and disease progression, and (3) to prevent development of cardiovascular and other disease processes. Proper management of diabetes requires a team approach that includes physicians, diabetes educators, dieticians, exercise specialists, and perhaps most importantly, the diabetic person's self-management skills. Many people diagnosed with diabetes are referred to a diabetes self-management course taught by a certified diabetes educator. Diabetes self-management programs focus on self-care behaviors such as proper use of prescribed medications, healthy eating, physical activity, weight loss, blood sugar monitoring, and recognition of hypoglycemia and hyperglycemia signs and symptoms—skills that every person with diabetes should have.

### Benefits of Exercise With Type 1 Diabetes

A beneficial role of exercise at controlling blood glucose levels in type 1 diabetes has not been well demonstrated. A number of studies have been published that failed to show an independent effect of exercise training on improving glycemic control in people with type 1 diabetes. Even so, individuals with type 1 diabetes can improve their functional capacity, reduce their risk for CAD, and improve insulin receptor sensitivity with a program of regular physical activity. Thus, the primary focus of exercise training is on developing consistent, daily physical activity patterns that derive multiple health benefits, including decreased CVD risk and improved quality of life, with a secondary objective of enhancing glucose control.

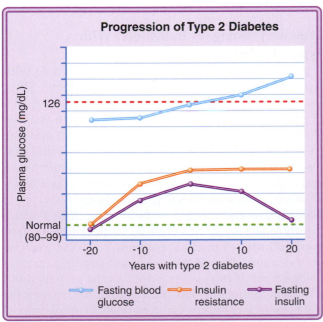

**Figure 27-3.** Progression from insulin resistance to type 2 diabetes. The inefficient utilization of insulin results in increased insulin demand, and over time the pancreas loses its ability to effectively produce insulin. The result is a combination of insulin resistance and impaired insulin production that leads to frequent states of hyperglycemia.

### Benefits of Exercise With Type 2 Diabetes

Regular exercise is essential for people with type 2 diabetes and the benefits are substantial, including

## VIGNETTE continued

■ Although Vincent has not been diagnosed with diabetes, his increased weight and lack of physical activity place him in a high-risk category for development of type 2 diabetes. Beginning a regular exercise program, modifying food choices, and gradually losing weight will significantly decrease his risk. This is extremely important, as progression to type 2 diabetes will further increase Vincent's overall risk for development of CVD, which could result in premature death.

prevention of CAD, stroke, PVD, and other diabetes-related complications. Regular exercise has consistently been shown to improve insulin resistance, blood lipid profiles, hypertension, impaired fibrinolysis, vascular inflammatory factors, and body weight. Each of these cardiometabolic risk factors can be present in type 2 diabetes and will significantly increase the person's risk for development of CAD. With excessive blood glucose elevation, blood fats increase to become the primary energy source for the body, putting individuals with diabetes at a greater risk for CAD, and the combination of exercise and weight loss can positively affect blood lipid levels, reducing the atherogenic risk. In addition, regular exercise can positively affect depression, anxiety, and other psychological conditions that are common to people with diabetes and other chronic comorbidities.

### Exercise and Diabetes

Because of potential adverse responses to an acute exercise session, physician clearance and guidance is recommended before people with diabetes begin an exercise training program. Proper medical guidance is important to ensure appropriate adjustment of medications and dietary intake are understood and followed, along with other important safety precautions. A gradual warm-up and cool-down period is an important part of every exercise session. Generally, the warm-up will consist of 5 to 10 minutes of light aerobic activity and a period of gentle stretching, whereas the cool-down phase will entail 5 to 10 minutes of gradually decreasing light-intensity activity that promotes a gradual reduction in heart rate to the pre-exercise level. It is important that individuals with diabetes are taught and encouraged to measure blood glucose levels before and after each exercise session. Exercise sessions should be delayed or postponed if the pre-exercise blood glucose level is less than 100 mg/dL. With additional carbohydrate consumption, the blood glucose level should normalize, allowing the individual to engage in the exercise session. Exercise should not be initiated when the pre-exercise blood glucose measurement is greater than 300 mg/dL or greater than 250 mg/dL with the presence of ketosis.

In the latter scenario, exercise is restricted until the person's blood sugar is under control, because exercise can exacerbate the situation. People with diabetes are encouraged to exercise with a partner and to wear a diabetes identification tag to alert responders to their diabetic condition should an adverse event occur.

### Exercise Training for Individuals With Type 1 Diabetes

The primary objective of exercise training for individuals with type 1 diabetes is the reduction of CVD risk and possible improvement in glucose regulation that can be achieved with regular or daily activity. Regular exercise training allows for more consistent diet and insulin regulation that will enhance and stabilize glucose control, decrease the risk for adverse events, and improve the exercise response. All levels of exercise including leisure activities, recreational sports, and competitive sports can frequently be performed by people with type 1 diabetes who do not have complications or comorbidities, and who are in good blood glucose control. Aerobic exercise activities and resistance training are beneficial and commonly prescribed at a moderate intensity between 55% and 75% of functional capacity or at an RPE of 11 to 13 (on a 6–20 scale). In people with advanced diabetes, the use of RPE is preferred because of the potential inaccuracies in heart-rate measurement that can result from diabetes-related complications such as autonomic and peripheral neuropathy. Long-duration and high-intensity exercise are generally avoided or carefully monitored. Long-duration activities increase the risk for hypoglycemia, and high-intensity exercise can increase the likelihood of hyperglycemia occurring.

### Exercise Training for Individuals With Type 2 Diabetes

A large percentage, more than 80%, of people with type 2 diabetes are either overweight or obese. Thus, the primary goal of exercise training for the majority of people with type 2 diabetes is not only to stabilize blood glucose levels, but also to burn calories and lose weight. Weight loss through appropriate diet and regular exercise may result in a decreased dependence on oral insulin medication to maintain appropriate levels of blood glucose. Generally, individuals with type 2 diabetes are encouraged to follow the *2008 Physical Activity Guidelines for Americans* by participating in 30 or more minutes of moderate-intensity aerobic exercise on 5 or more days of the week and strength training twice a week.[20] Regular exercise training in individuals with type 2 diabetes has been shown to improve insulin resistance, reduce diabetes-related complications, and reduce the risk for development of other chronic health conditions such as CVD.

### Precautions

People with diabetes are subject to a variety of potential adverse events during and after an exercise training session and should undertake precautions to avoid these complications. Exercise professionals, exercise partners, and other people working with individuals with diabetes must be aware of the potential complications associated with exercise and also know how to appropriately respond should such complications occur. Box 27-3 outlines preventive measures that are commonly taken to ensure a safe and effective exercise experience for individuals with diabetes.

## Box 27-3. Exercise Precautions for Individuals With Diabetes

1. Metabolic control before exercise
   a. Avoid exercise if fasting glucose levels are ≥250 mg/dL and ketosis is present, or if blood glucose levels are greater than 300 mg/dL and no ketosis is present.
   b. Ingest added carbohydrate if glucose levels are less than 100 mg/dL.
2. Blood glucose monitoring before and after exercise
   a. Identify when changes in insulin or food intake are necessary.
   b. Be aware of the glycemic response to different exercise conditions.
3. Food intake
   a. Consume added carbohydrate as needed to avoid hypoglycemia.
   b. Carbohydrate-based foods should be readily available during and after exercise.
4. Avoid injecting insulin into the primary muscle groups that will be used during exercise because it can easily be absorbed too quickly, resulting in hypoglycemia.
5. Avoid exercise during periods of peak insulin activity.
6. Exercise should be undertaken at the same time each day with a regular pattern of diet, medication, and consistent duration/intensity.
7. People with diabetes should exercise with a partner and wear a medical identification tag.
8. Proper hydration is essential, and fluids should be taken before, during, and after exercise to prevent dehydration. Extra caution should be taken on hot days because blood glucose levels can be impacted by dehydration.
9. Careful foot hygiene and proper footwear are important for people with diabetes. Cotton socks and good-fitting athletic shoes should be used, and the feet should be regularly checked for sores, blisters, irritation, cuts, and other injuries.
10. Pain should not be ignored, and exercise that results in unexpected pain should be immediately terminated.

## METABOLIC SYNDROME

MetS is a cluster of conditions that when occurring together increase a person's risk for development of CAD, type 2 diabetes, and stroke. Affecting more than 25% of the population, MetS is characterized by abdominal obesity, atherogenic dyslipidemia (especially high triglyceride levels and low levels of HDL), elevated BP, insulin resistance, and prothrombotic and proinflammatory states (Fig. 27-4). People with MetS have double the risk for development of CAD and are five times more likely to experience development of diabetes than those without the condition.[25] The risk for development of MetS is closely associated with physical inactivity, increased body weight, and insulin resistance along with genetic factors and advancing age. The prevalence is also higher in certain ethnic groups, such as African Americans, Hispanics, and Native Americans. Excess visceral (abdominal) fat is of particular concern and frequently is the result of physical inactivity and poor nutritional habits.

Although there are several working definitions of MetS, the American Heart Association (AHA) and the National Heart, Lung, and Blood Institute recommend that MetS be identified as the presence of three or more of the following components[26]:

- Increased waist circumference
  - Men: ≥40 inches (102 cm)
  - Women: ≥35 inches (88 cm)
- Elevated triglycerides level
  - ≥150 mg/dL
- Reduced HDL cholesterol
  - Men: less than 40 mg/dL
  - Women: less than 50 mg/dL
- Elevated BP
  - ≥130/85 mm Hg
- Elevated fasting blood glucose
  - ≥100 mg/dL

### Treatment

The primary treatment objective for MetS is to reduce the risk for development of CAD and type 2 diabetes.

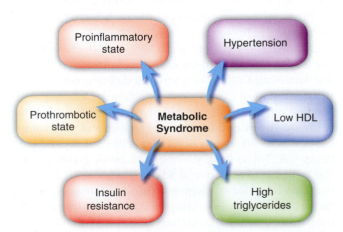

**Figure 27-4.** Various conditions associated with metabolic syndrome.

## VIGNETTE continued

■ Although Vincent does not meet the criteria for type 2 diabetes, he does have four of the primary components for MetS. Vincent's triglyceride level of 180 mg/dL, low HDL of 38 mg/dL, and resting BP of 148/102 mm Hg place him in the MetS category. In addition, with a BMI of 32.3 kg/m² (5'10" and 225 lb), his waist circumference most likely exceeds the criteria for MetS. MetS places him at an increased risk for development of type 2 diabetes and CAD, and appropriate intervention is critical to preventing future disabling and life-threatening events.

Lifestyle interventions, such as increased physical activity, healthy eating, weight loss, and tobacco cessation are essential treatment components. Some people with MetS are also placed on medications to treat hypertension, high blood sugar and elevated lipids (high LDL cholesterol or triglycerides, or both), and low HDL. In addition, some individuals are treated with medications such as aspirin that reduce the risk for blood clot formation.

## Exercise and Metabolic Syndrome

A variety of studies have shown that MetS is inversely associated with physical activity, with more active individuals having a lower incidence than those who are sedentary or less active.[27] Participants in the CARDIA study who remained active over a 13- to 15-year period were 51% less likely to develop MetS than their less active counterparts.[28] This finding is not surprising because physical inactivity has been shown to predispose people to a variety of health conditions, such as hypertension, insulin resistance, obesity, elevated lipids, low HDL, increased inflammatory markers, and coagulation factors, which are all major factors in MetS. An individual's level of cardiorespiratory fitness has also been shown to independently influence the risk for premature mortality in people with increased body weight or the presence of MetS, or both.[29]

Because most people with MetS are overweight or obese, the exercise program is usually designed around the American College of Sports Medicine guidelines for the treatment of overweight and obese individuals.[26,30] Dietary intervention combined with exercise training is important in enhancing weight loss and promoting other metabolic adaptations that reduce CAD and diabetes risk. Interestingly, weight changes generated by the removal of abdominal adipose tissue with liposuction do not appear to improve insulin resistance or risk factors for CAD, suggesting that the negative energy balance and other adaptations induced by diet and exercise are necessary for achieving the metabolic benefits that are associated with weight loss.[27] Lifestyle interventions, including exercise training, and other medical interventions are also based on the presence of other co-conditions the person may have, such as underlying CAD, hypertension, and dyslipidemia.

Most studies on exercise and MetS have evaluated the effect of various aerobic modes of activity, such as walking, elliptical training and other similar exercise ergometers, and stationary cycling. Both aerobic and resistance training are inversely associated with the prevalence of MetS and are effective components of the treatment strategy. Some obese individuals who have significant mobility limitations and/or joint discomfort may be better served with water exercise or other forms of non–weight-bearing activities. Pole walking (exerstriding or Nordic walking) is an excellent activity for people with mobility limitations and joint discomfort, and could easily be incorporated into the exercise program of a person with diabetes.

Individuals with MetS should be encouraged to develop an active lifestyle by looking for opportunities to avoid prolonged sitting and other sedentary activities, and to expend energy throughout their daily routine. Simple strategies such as taking the stairs, parking farther away, periodically getting up and moving about, and a variety of recreational and leisure-time physical activities will significantly reduce sedentary time and promote caloric expenditure. The contraction of skeletal muscle fiber stimulates an increase in the number and activity of GLUT-4 glucose transport proteins in skeletal muscle, and the increased GLUT-4 activity enhances glucose uptake by providing an insulin-like effect in the skeletal muscle, even in the presence of diminished insulin action.[21] Step pedometers and accelerometers are excellent tools for raising skeletal muscle activity awareness and promoting movement throughout the day. The goal is to gradually increase daily steps to 10,000 or more, which will place most individuals into the recommended range of physical activity for overweight and obese individuals.[31]

Exercise intensity will vary depending on each person's weight status, overall conditioning, and medical profile, at least initially, and may not be as important as total energy expenditure. Deconditioned individuals are usually advised to begin at a lower intensity and gradually progress to moderate levels (55%–75% of functional capacity or an RPE of 11–13 on the 6–20 scale). Because the primary goal is to burn calories and lose weight, daily activity is recommended and can consist of both continuous and intermittent activity. Similar to diabetes and other cardiometabolic disorders, the key to deriving long-term benefit is regular participation in daily physical activity, and step pedometers and accelerometers are frequently used to raise activity awareness and gradually progress daily energy expenditure.

## DYSLIPIDEMIA

**Dyslipidemia** refers to a disorder of lipoprotein metabolism that may be manifested by either overproduction (e.g., high cholesterol) or deficiency (e.g., low HDL). Dyslipidemia is strongly associated with a number of chronic health conditions including CAD, PVD, stroke, and diabetes. Causes may be primary (genetic factors) or secondary. Secondary causes include a sedentary lifestyle, poor diet (high consumption of saturated and trans fat and cholesterol), diabetes, chronic kidney disease, hypothyroidism, certain medications, use of oral contraceptive hormones such as estrogen and progestin, and other factors. The AHA estimates that 31.9 million American adults aged 20 and older have TC levels that are considered to increase the risk for the development of CVD (>240 mg/dL).[2]

Cholesterol is a waxy, fatlike substance that is found in all cell membranes and is transported in the blood plasma. It is manufactured by the liver and is found in certain foods such as dairy products, meat, and eggs. Cholesterol is an essential component of cell function and the production of hormones, vitamin D, and the bile acids that assist with fat digestion. However, high levels of cholesterol in the circulation are strongly associated with **atherosclerosis** and the development of a variety of cardiovascular disorders (Fig. 27-5).

Cholesterol travels through the body attached to a protein, referred to as a **lipoprotein**. The primary lipoproteins are classified as:

- *LDL:* LDL is the major carrier of cholesterol in the circulation, containing 60% to 70% of the body's total serum cholesterol. LDL is frequently referred to as the "bad" cholesterol because of its role in atherogenesis, the early stages of atherosclerosis.
- **Very low-density lipoprotein (VLDL)***: Synthesized in the liver, VLDL is the major carrier of triglyceride and cholesterol to the peripheral tissues. VLDL contains 10% to 15% of the body's total serum cholesterol.
- *HDL:* Often referred to as the "good" cholesterol, HDL is produced in the intestine and liver, and normally contains 20% to 30% of the body's TC. HDL levels are inversely correlated to CAD: the higher the level of HDL, the lower the risk for development of CAD.
- **Non-HDL cholesterol**: Non-HDL is defined as the TC minus HDL, or put another way, the sum of LDL, VLDL, and intermediate-density lipoprotein. Non-HDL cholesterol is strongly associated with the development of CVD, and non-HDL levels appear to be equal or better than LDL levels at identifying atherogenic particles.

Table 27-2 presents the classification of LDL, total and HDL cholesterol, and triglycerides. Historically, increased levels of TC and LDL have drawn the most attention, because they have a significant association to CVD, along with the TC to HDL ratio (**TC/HDL ratio**). A lower TC/HDL ratio indicates lower risk, with less than 3.5 being an ideal target. A second ratio derived by dividing the HDL cholesterol by the LDL cholesterol (**HDL/LDL ratio**) may be a more powerful predictor of CAD risk than the TC/HDL ratio. TC is derived by

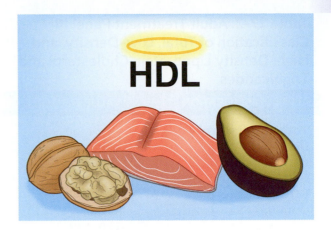

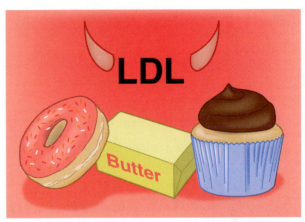

**Figure 27-5.** Often referred to as the "good" cholesterol, HDL levels are inversely correlated to coronary artery disease (CAD): the higher the level of HDL, the lower the risk for development of CAD. Conversely, LDL is frequently referred to as the "bad" cholesterol because of its role in atherogenesis, the early stages of atherosclerosis.

adding the HDL, LDL, and VLDL values; thus, TC can be elevated by increased HDL or good cholesterol, as well as the more atherogenic LDL and VLDL values. The HDL/LDL ratio compares the good HDL cholesterol with the atherogenic LDL with a goal of maintaining the ratio greater than 0.3. HDL is a key measure, and low levels of HDL are a significant contributor to the development of CAD.

Low HDL levels are an independent risk factor for CVD, *even among people with normal LDL and TC values*. The Third National Health and Nutrition Examination Survey indicates that just more than one third of U.S. adults have low HDL levels, defined as less than 40 mg/dL in men and less than 50 mg/dL in women.[32] It has been estimated that for every 1-mg/dL increase in HDL, there is a 2% decrease in CAD risk for men and a 3% decrease for women.[33] Thus, measurement of HDL and therapeutic interventions that raise low levels of HDL are key preventive measures in reducing the prevalence and impact of CVD.

## Table 27-2. Adult Treatment Panel III Classification of Total, Low-Density, and High-Density Lipoprotein Cholesterol and Triglycerides

| ATP III CLASSIFICATION | VALUES (MG/DL) |
|---|---|
| **Total cholesterol** | |
| Desirable | <200 |
| Borderline high | 200–239 |
| High | >240 |
| **LDL cholesterol** | |
| Optimal | <100 |
| Near optimal | 100–129 |
| Borderline high | 130–159 |
| High | 160–189 |
| Very high | ≥190 |
| **HDL cholesterol** | |
| Low | <40 |
| High | ≥60 |
| **Triglycerides** | |
| Normal | <150 |
| Borderline high | 150–199 |
| High | 200–499 |
| Very high | ≥500 |

ATP, Adult Treatment Panel; HDL, high-density lipoprotein; LDL, low-density lipoprotein.
*Source:* Data from the National Cholesterol Education Program.[35]

One of the most common dyslipidemias, **hypertriglyceridemia** (an elevated triglyceride level), is gaining increasing attention as a predictor of risk and interventional target for CVD, diabetes, and MetS.[34] Triglycerides are the most common form of fat stored in the body and play an important role in energy metabolism and as transporters of dietary fat. Formed by the combination of glycerol with three fatty acid molecules, triglycerides are a major component of VLDL and are also associated with low levels of HDL. A diet high in carbohydrates will increase triglyceride levels, especially in people with insulin resistance.

Hypertriglyceridemia is frequently found in people with diabetes and MetS, especially in those with an increased accumulation of fat mass and related obesity. High levels of adipose tissue can affect the process of sequestering free fatty acids for storage, resulting in an increased conversion of fatty acids to triglycerides. Chronic elevation of triglyceride levels is associated with both microvascular and macrovascular endothelial damage, and is associated with increased vessel wall inflammation, foam cell formation, and destruction of smooth muscle cells.[35] The resulting endothelial damage and dysfunction opens the door for cholesterol deposition, making chronically elevated triglyceride levels a significant risk factor for the development of CAD.

**VIGNETTE continued**

■ Vincent's TC level of 259 mg/dL and LDL level of 185 mg/dL place him in a high-risk category. In addition, his low HDL level of 38 mg/dL is very concerning, and it could, in part, be related to his lack of physical activity. According to his physician, Vincent is an excellent candidate for medical therapy using a lipid-lowering medication, such as a statin, and aggressive lifestyle changes to lower his elevated TC and LDL levels and increase his HDL. His triglyceride level of 180 mg/dL is considered borderline and would also benefit from increased physical activity and dietary modifications.

## Treatment

Treatment for elevated cholesterol and triglycerides and/or low HDL is based on the person's overall CVD risk profile and blood lipid levels. Treatment generally encompasses dietary modifications, exercise, and medications to alter abnormal lipid levels. National Cholesterol Education Program guidelines for people who have not had an acute CVD event recommend at least 6 months of nonpharmacological therapy before initiating a medication regimen. Those who have had a CVD event and/or are at high risk for one will be treated more aggressively than those who are at lower risk and without CVD. Both low-risk and higher-risk individuals may be placed on medication therapy.

Recent clinical research studies have demonstrated a significant reduction in CAD risk with the use of a class of medications referred to as statins (e.g., Lipitor [atorvastatin], Lescol [fluvastatin], Mevacor [lovastatin],

**DOING THE MATH:**
**What are Vincent's lipid ratios?**
- TC/HDL ratio
  - 259 mg/dL ÷ 38 mg/dL = 6.82
  - This is considered high risk. Ideally, the ratio should be less than 3.5.
- HDL/LDL ratio
  - 38 mg/dL ÷ 185 mg/dL = 0.205
  - This is also considered high risk. Ideally, the ratio should be more than 0.4.
- Triglycerides/HDL ratio
  - 180 mg/dL ÷ 38 mg/dL = 4.737
  - This is also considered high risk. Ideally, the ratio should be less than 2.0.

Pravachol [pravastatin], and Zocor [simvastatin]). Statin therapy has been associated with a significant risk reduction in all-cause mortality of 12%, in major coronary events of 30%, and in major cerebrovascular events of 19%, making statin medications a first-line treatment for people with elevated lipids, especially those with known CVD and those who are at high risk.[36] The downside to the utilization of statin medications is their associated expense and a variety of potential adverse effects such as muscle aches, soreness, and increased blood sugar.

Low HDL cholesterol, also a major concern, has typically been treated by increasing daily energy expenditure and modifying dietary intake. Niacin is also commonly prescribed to treat low HDL levels and can raise HDL by 15% to 35%. Niacin has also been shown to decrease VLDL levels via its action of blocking the breakdown of fats. However, more research on the long-term effects of niacin is required, especially in light of the 2011 AIM-HIGH study that was halted early because of an increased risk for stroke and its minimal impact on HDL in patients already taking statin medication.[2] Newer pharmaceutical medications are currently under investigation that also show some promise in increasing HDL levels.

## Exercise and Dyslipidemia

Participation in regular physical activity is essential for the primary and secondary prevention of CAD, a fact that has been well demonstrated in the published literature. Although the exact mechanisms by which regular physical activity protects against CAD are not fully understood, part of the benefit may be associated with a positive impact on lipoproteins. Because of this potential association, exercise and dietary modification have historically been included as part of the recommended treatment plan for people with high serum cholesterol and triglyceride levels, and for treating low HDL levels.

Combining exercise with dietary modification is effective at decreasing total elevated serum TC and LDL, especially when associated with weight loss. Data regarding the impact of exercise independent of weight loss on TC and LDL have been mixed, with the results not supporting a definitive improvement. Although regular exercise does not significantly decrease the total serum concentration, it does appear to increase the size of the LDL particles in the concentration. This impact of exercise on LDL particle size appears to occur independent of weight loss, and in some studies the result has also been irrespective of the intensity of exercise.[24] The typical value reported for LDL is the summed contribution of LDL particles (in milligrams) contained in a deciliter of plasma (mg/dL). However, LDL particles vary in size, with smaller particles being more dense and atherogenic than the larger, fluffy or buoyant particles. Thus, two people with the same standard LDL measurement (in mg/dL) may vary in their level of CAD risk depending on the proportion of small versus large particles

in the concentration. Exercise appears to increase the proportion of large particles present in a deciliter of plasma, thus reducing the risk for development of CAD.

Both HDL and triglyceride levels are also responsive to acute and chronic exercise training. A single acute session of exercise will reduce the level of circulating triglycerides, and this effect can persist for 24 to 72 hours. This acute effect emphasizes the importance of maintaining a regular pattern of exercise to derive long-term benefit. Improving a person's HDL level is important in reducing the individual's risk for cardiovascular morbidity and mortality. Whereas decreasing the LDL level reduces CAD risk by 1%, increasing the HDL level by 1 mg/dL results in a 2% risk reduction in men and a 3% reduction in women.[37]

People with abnormal lipid levels, who are free of other health conditions, are commonly encouraged to follow the general age-specific recommendations presented in the *2008 Physical Activity Guidelines for Americans* report.[20] Although the exact mechanisms by which exercise stimulates a favorable impact on lipoprotein levels are not fully understood, muscle contraction does increase **lipoprotein lipase (LPL)** activity. Increased LPL activity has a positive effect on fat metabolism and may be an initial step in increasing HDL and decreasing LDL, VLDL, and triglyceride levels (Fig. 27-6). Thus, the primary focus, especially initially,

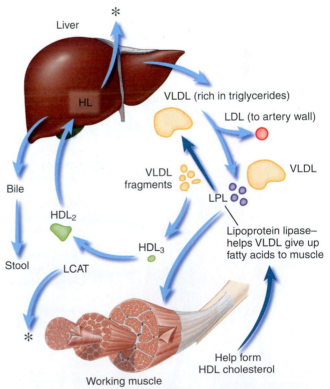

**Figure 27-6.** Physiological benefits of lipoprotein lipase (LPL). Increased LPL activity has a positive effect on fat metabolism and may be an initial step in increasing HDL and lowering LDL, VLDL, and triglyceride levels. Trained or active people tend to have greater concentrations of LPL.

is on the quantity of physical activity undertaken rather than increasing the level of fitness. Step pedometers and accelerometers are excellent tools that can be used by people who have abnormal lipid values to progressively increase the quantity of daily energy expenditure or "muscle contractions."

## CARDIOVASCULAR DISORDERS

CVD is the leading cause of death in the developed world. For more than 100 years, CVD has caused more deaths in the United States than any other major cause. On average, more than 2,150 Americans die of CVD each day—approximately 1 death every 40 seconds.[2] The AHA estimates that 83.6 million Americans have one or more types of cardiovascular disorders, including dyslipidemia, CAD, HF, hypertension, stroke, and PVD. In addition, the prevalence of CVD is expected to continue to increase as a result of the aging population and the accumulated effects of risk factors that occur over time.[3] Well-established risk factors that contribute to CVD include genetics, age, hypertension, smoking, diabetes, dyslipidemia, MetS, and lifestyle (diet and physical inactivity; Fig. 27-7).[2] The most common forms of CVD are high BP (77.9 million), coronary heart disease (15.43 million), heart failure (5.1 million), and stroke (6.8 million). Along with continuing to be the leading cause of mortality in the United States, CVD conditions are also top contributors

to the 45 million Americans living with a functional disability.[2]

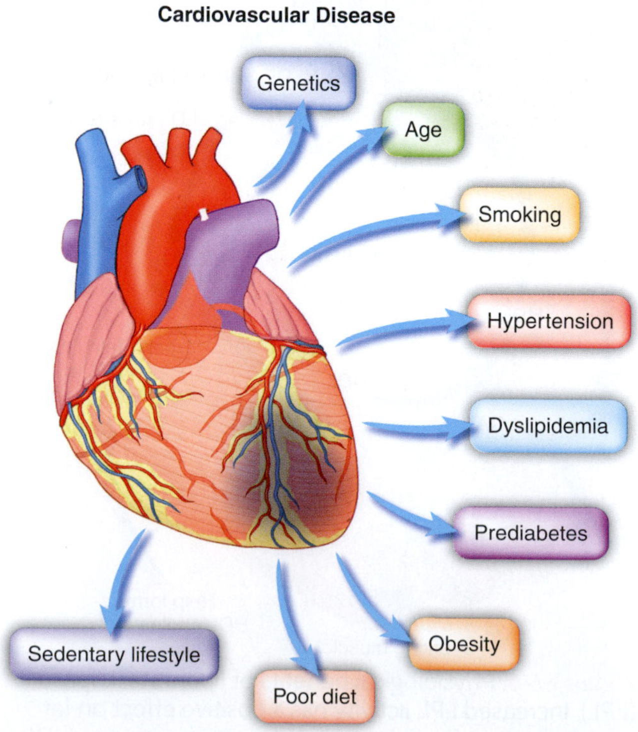

## Coronary Artery Disease

The heart muscle requires a constant flow of oxygen-rich blood that is supplied by the coronary arterial system. These small, torturous vessels are subject to numerous flow dynamics that can place strain on the vessel wall and, when combined with certain chemical (e.g., smoking), pressure (e.g., high BP), glucose, and lipid (cholesterol and triglycerides) impacts, can result in damage to the endothelium or innermost lining of an artery. Damage to the endothelium stimulates an inflammatory process and the deposition of lipid-rich plaque, calcified cholesterol, and accumulation of other substances that over time will narrow the vessel (Fig. 27-8). When this atherosclerotic process occurs in

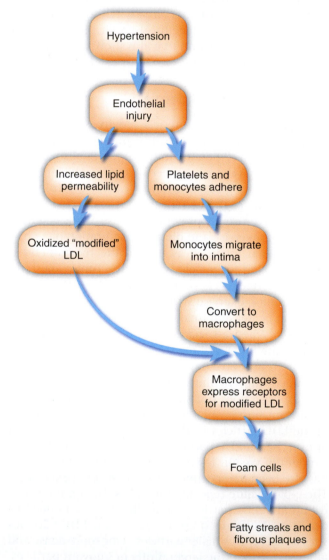

**Figure 27-8.** Key steps in the process of atherosclerosis. Damage to the endothelium stimulates an inflammatory process and the deposition of lipid-rich plaque, calcified cholesterol, and accumulation of other substances that over time will narrow the vessel.

**Figure 27-7.** Risk factors that contribute to cardiovascular disease include genetics, age, hypertension, smoking, prediabetes, dyslipidemia, obesity, and unhealthy lifestyle (poor diet and physical inactivity).

the coronary arterial system, it is referred to as CAD and is characterized by a narrowing of the coronary arteries that supply the heart muscle with blood and oxygen. The process of atherosclerosis can begin during childhood or the teen years and will slowly progress for many years before manifesting in symptoms, adverse events, or both. Although significant symptoms and events do not usually occur until after the fifth decade of life, in some people, the process may accelerate as early as the third decade. Over time the atherosclerotic process and associated plaque deposition narrows the arterial wall and eventually may impact blood flow to the heart muscle.

Atherosclerotic plaques (also referred to as atheromas or lesions) are typically placed into two categories, stable and unstable (or vulnerable) lesions, and most commonly occur in areas of vessel branching and turning that alter flow direction, velocity, and turbulence. Stable plaque tends to be characterized by an intact thick fibrous cap that consists of smooth muscle cells in a matrix rich in type I and II collagen. Vulnerable or unstable plaque consists of a lipid-rich core with foam cell infiltration, macrophages, smooth muscle cells, and cytokines.[38] This inflammatory environment releases proteolytic enzymes (e.g., tumor necrosis factor) that result in cap degradation or thinning. The thin fibrous cap is then subject to rupture and associated thrombosis (clot formation) that can rapidly close the artery, resulting in a heart attack or myocardial infarction (MI). Atherosclerosis is also the underlying cause of cerebral disease and PVD. Thus, manifestation of atherosclerosis may also include **transient ischemic attack (TIA)**, stroke, and **intermittent claudication**.

## Risk Factors

In the early 1940s, a landmark longitudinal epidemiological study was launched in Framingham, Massachusetts, that served to identify many of the primary risk factors for heart disease.[39] Numerous studies since the launch of this groundbreaking investigation have confirmed these risk factors, which are commonly grouped into modifiable and nonmodifiable categories. Historically, CAD has been considered and treated as a man's disease. However, current statistics indicate that CAD prevalence is also high in women, negating sex as one of the nonmodifiable risk factors. In fact, women are more likely than men to have a second heart attack, and a higher percentage of women die within a year of their initial MI. The common risk factors for CAD are listed in Box 27-4.

## Signs and Symptoms

Symptoms associated with CAD vary widely. For some people, the first sign of the disease is an **acute myocardial infarction** (MI or heart attack) or sudden cardiac death. Even people with advanced disease often do not manifest symptoms or functional impairment until a major event occurs. This is because blood flow to the heart muscle generally is not significantly compromised until the arterial narrowing occludes 50% to ≥70% of the vessel diameter. Most events (e.g.,

---

### Box 27-4. Risk Factors for Coronary Artery Disease

**Nonmodifiable Risk Factors**
- Advancing age
- Genetic abnormalities
- Close relatives with atherosclerosis disease manifestation (CAD, stroke, peripheral vascular occlusive disease)

**Modifiable Risk Factors**
- Tobacco smoking
- Hypertension
- Dyslipidemia
  - High concentration of LDL, VLDL, or both
  - Low concentration of HDL
  - An LDL/HDL ratio greater than 3:1
  - Elevated triglycerides
- Physical inactivity—sedentary lifestyle
- Obesity
- Diabetes or impaired glucose tolerance
- MetS
- Stress and/or significant clinical depression

**Other Risk Factors**
- Hypercoagulability
- Dietary factors
  - High intake of saturated fat and trans fat
  - High carbohydrate intake
  - Vitamin $B_6$ deficiency
- Elevated levels of
  - Homocysteine
  - Uric acid
  - Fibrinogen concentrations
  - Other inflammatory markers
- Hyperthyroidism
- Consistent sleep deprivation

---

## VIGNETTE continued

■ While too busy at work and not seeing a need to make an appointment with a medical provider, Vincent also did not recognize a few subtle signs of CAD that he was experiencing. He was becoming increasingly short of breath with minimal exertion, something he attributed to his elevated weight and age. However, over the past 6 to 8 weeks he periodically experienced what he suspected was indigestion and periodic wrist and elbow discomfort that was associated with climbing stairs.

MI or sudden cardiac death) do not happen because excessive plaque buildup closes off the artery, but because a fibrous cap in a marginally narrowed artery ruptures. The ruptured cap stimulates rapid clot formation and subsequent artery occlusion. The most common symptoms of CAD include:

- **Angina pectoris** (chest, neck, and jaw discomfort/pain; pressure or tightness/indigestion-like discomfort or pain that typically radiates to the left arm)
- Shortness of breath
- Weakness, fatigue, and reduced exertional endurance
- Light-headedness, dizziness
- Heart palpitations
- Leg swelling
- Numbness, loss of sensation, typically in the left arm, wrist, shoulder, or back

Symptoms are frequently exacerbated by physical exertion and relieved by rest. Some individuals are able to gradually walk through angina episodes with alternating exertion and rest, often referred to as window-shopping angina. Angina is also classified as "stable" and "unstable." **Stable angina** generally occurs with exertion and is reproducible at a given rate pressure product (heart rate × SBP). **Unstable angina** presents with periods of increasing frequency, low levels of intensity, and may even occur after meals and at rest. Many people are prescribed and taught to use **nitroglycerin** tablets when CAD symptoms occur. Nitroglycerin is a vasodilator that when absorbed sublingually will expand coronary artery diameter to increase blood flow and relieve symptoms. People with active symptoms that are not relieved by nitroglycerin are usually in a medical emergency and 911 should be called immediately.

## VIGNETTE continued

■ Vincent decided to start an exercise program that would consist of walking on the bike path that ran by his house. If nothing else, Vincent thought the fresh air and walk would help relieve some of the stress he had placed himself under with a new software design contract. He decided that he would do his walk before heading home from the office in the late afternoon. It was a beautiful, sunny spring day when Vincent began his initial walk. Shortly after reaching the bike path near his house, he began to experience the same wrist and elbow pain and shortness of breath that he got at home when climbing the stairs. Passing it off to deconditioning, he pushed on and before long was feeling a heavy

sensation in his chest that caused him to stop. He soon began to feel a fuzzy, light-headed sensation and suddenly passed out.

### Myocardial Infarction

An acute MI or heart attack often manifests as a sudden, crushing, squeezing chest tightness, pressure, and/or pain, and it is often accompanied by diaphoresis. The pain may radiate into the jaw, shoulder, neck, back, and down the left arm. Symptoms may also include unexplained shortness of breath, light-headedness, dizziness, and an upset stomach. However, some people only experience mild symptoms and others may be asymptomatic and simply pass out. In many women, the symptoms of an acute MI are only expressed by nausea, anxiety, palpitations, and a cold sweat or diaphoresis.

The acute MI is generally the result of unstable plaque rupture that results in rapid thrombus formation and significantly obstructs blood flow to the myocardium (Fig. 27-9). This is a serious medical emergency, and the person should be immediately transported to the nearest emergency department by emergency medical personnel. Lack of oxygen to the heart will result in the death of myocardial muscle, and rapid transportation and intervention will save critical muscle. Minimally invasive procedures can be used to re-open the obstructed artery, but generally there is a 4- to 6-hour window in which critical muscle can be preserved. Thus, early detection and treatment are paramount.

## VIGNETTE continued

■ Vincent was experiencing a heart attack or MI and had gone into a lethal heart rhythm called *ventricular fibrillation*. Fortunately for Vincent, he was walking by the ball field where spectators saw him pass out and immediately intervened. One spectator, a clinical exercise physiologist at the local hospital, began CPR while one of the coaches retrieved the league's automated external defibrillator (AED) and another called 911. Because of the quick response of the spectators and the presence of the AED, the clinical exercise physiologist was able to connect the AED and, following its instructions, shock Vincent back into a sinus rhythm. About that time the emergency medical team arrived and was able to stabilize Vincent and transport him to the local emergency department.

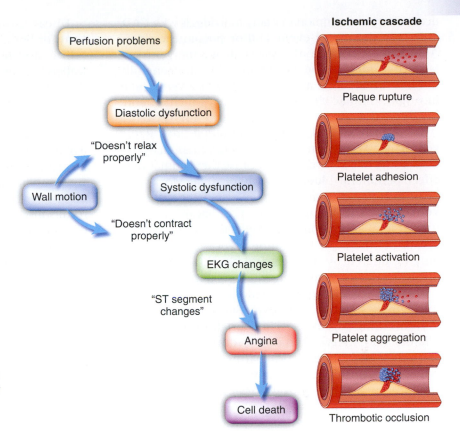

**Figure 27-9.** The ischemic cascade: a series of steps starting with plaque rupture that leads to thrombus and possibly cell death. An unstable plaque rupture that results in rapid thrombus formation sets in motion an ischemic cascade of events that can significantly obstruct blood flow to the myocardium and ultimately lead to an acute myocardial infarction.

## Heart Failure

HF results when the pumping ability of the left ventricle is compromised because of significant muscle damage resulting from an MI or, in some people, damage resulting from other factors such as genetic structural abnormalities, uncontrolled and prolonged hypertension, drug use, significant valvular disease, and infections. Heart failure can result from systolic or diastolic dysfunction and affect both the left and the right ventricles.

The cardiac cycle is split into two primary phases: systole and diastole. During systole, the ventricles contract, ejecting their blood out of the respective ventricle and into the arterial circulation. The right ventricle primarily supplies the pulmonary circulation and the left ventricle supplies the peripheral circulation. Diastole follows the systolic working phase, allowing the ventricles to relax and refill with blood. It is also during this phase that the coronary arteries supply blood to the heart muscle.

Systolic heart failure results from the inability of the right, left, or both ventricles to appropriately contract and pump blood from the respective ventricle to the arterial circulation. The incomplete emptying of the ventricles compromises circulatory flow and can result in the blood flow backing up and pressure increasing within the blood vessels. The increased pressure can force fluid from the blood vessels into body tissues. When the left ventricle is affected, fluid may collect in the lungs (pulmonary edema), compromising air exchange. Right-sided systolic failure results in fluid accumulation in the peripheral circulation, especially the ankles, legs, and abdomen.

In some people (the result of conditions such as high BP, hypertrophic cardiomyopathy, aortic stenosis, and others), the ventricular musculature becomes stiff and the ventricles are not able to fully relax during diastole.[40] The result is increased ventricular pressure and incomplete filling of the ventricle. Incomplete ventricular filling can result in blood backing up into the pulmonary and systemic circulation. The resulting compromise in blood flow through the lung and associated mismatching of ventilation significantly affects the delivery of oxygenated blood to the tissues. Symptoms of heart failure include resting and exertional dyspnea, leg and ankle swelling, bloating, fatigue/weakness, loss of appetite and associated weight loss, memory impairment, and confusion.

The number of people living with heart failure is on the rise, in part because of lifesaving interventional technology and the aging population. People with heart failure are prone to sudden death, with 10% dying within the initial year of diagnosis and more than 50% within 5 years because of lethal heart rhythm disturbances.[41] Because of these lethal rhythms, many people diagnosed with heart failure receive implantable defibrillators that are capable of detecting the life-threatening rhythm disturbance and converting it back to sinus rhythm with an electric shock. Use of these devices has significantly improved mortality outcomes in people with HF.

## Cardiac Dysrhythmia

**Cardiac dysrhythmias** are heart rhythm disturbances that may be benign or represent high risk for sudden death. They are common in many individuals with CAD, especially those post-event and/or post-intervention. Although atrial dysrhythmias, such as supraventricular tachycardia, can be quite rapid, they are generally not life-threatening, as are those that are ventricular in origin. Cardiac rhythm disturbances include both **bradycardia** (very slow rates) and **tachycardia** (very fast rates), and compromise blood flow. Rapid ventricular dysrhythmias such as ventricular tachycardia are especially worrisome, because they dramatically affect peripheral blood flow, myocardial work, and heart muscle perfusion. They can also deteriorate into **ventricular fibrillation** (sudden cardiac death). Ventricular fibrillation produces no effective cardiac output because of the rapid fibrillating myocardium and can only be altered by an electrical shock administered through a device such as an AED.

Modern technology has made it possible to effectively treat significant bradycardia and tachycardia rhythms using pacemakers, implantable cardiac defibrillators, and interventional procedures such as radio ablation of aberrant electrical pathways. Various medications are also frequently used to control heart rhythms, such as beta blockers that blunt both resting and exercise heart rates.

Cardiac dysrhythmias can be elicited by physical exertion, appearing during or shortly after exercise, especially sudden and high-intensity activity with an associated catecholamine surge. Prolonged warm-up and cool-down periods and low-to-moderate levels of exercise intensity are generally advised for people with rhythm disturbances who have been cleared to exercise. Although risk is increased during an acute exercise session, training adaptations to chronic exercise have been shown to decrease the risk for sudden death during submaximal exercise and while at rest.

## Valvular Heart Disease

The heart has four cardiac valves that regulate blood flow from the atria to the ventricles and from the ventricles into the pulmonary and peripheral circulation. The **mitral valve** regulates blood flow from the left atrium to the left ventricle, the **tricuspid valve** regulates flow from the right atrium to the right ventricle, the **pulmonary valve** regulates flow from the right ventricle to the pulmonary circulation, and the **aortic valve** regulates flow between the left ventricle and the peripheral circulation. The valves consist of an opening (orifice) and leaflets that function to open and close the valve. Some valves have chordate tendineae and papillary muscles that assist in the process. In some people, some or all of the components can become dysfunctional, obstructing flow or allowing blood to leak through the valve orifice. Valvular heart disease generally results from one of four primary causes: (1) acute rheumatic fever, (2) infection, (3) degenerative changes frequently associated with congenital abnormalities, and (4) myocardial ischemia/infarction that results in papillary muscle dysfunction.

Diseased valves are classified as **stenotic**, **regurgitant**, or both. Stenotic valves result from a narrowed orifice, and thickening and calcification of the valve leaflets or chordate tendineae. As stenosis progresses, additional pressure is required to effectively empty the atrial or ventricular chamber, and the heart responds by thickening the muscular walls of the affected chamber. This **cardiac hypertrophy** results in increased myocardial oxygen demand as the heart works to overcome the increased resistance caused by the narrowed valve.

Regurgitation or valvular leakage can gradually develop over time or have an acute onset. Regurgitation results in volume overload in the affected chamber as blood continues to flow through the valve following closure or is pumped backward during systole. Over time, the affected chamber compensates for the additional blood by dilating the chamber size and thickening the chamber walls.

Mild valvular regurgitation or stenosis generally produces no symptoms and individuals are able to perform moderate-to-vigorous levels of physical activity. Individuals with moderate-to-severe valve disease may experience significant shortness of breath, rhythm disturbances, angina, syncope, and decreased ability to exercise. These individuals are candidates for reconstructive or replacement surgery to prevent further myocardial remodeling and subsequent muscle damage. A synthetic or mechanical replacement valve may be used, or a biological valve made from animal or human tissue from a donated heart can be used. People with no or minimal myocardial damage generally go on to live very functional and active lives after surgical intervention.

## Interventional Treatment

People diagnosed with CAD and those experiencing an acute cardiac event are treated with a variety of noninvasive, minimally invasive, and invasive interventions. Noninvasive treatment usually consists of medications that control heart rate, contractility, and associated myocardial oxygen demand; exercise training; dietary counseling; and medications that improve abnormal lipid levels. Minimally invasive and invasive procedures are performed in both the acute or emergent setting and as elective procedures to prevent or reduce myocardial damage.

## Percutaneous Transluminal Coronary Angioplasty

A majority of people presenting to the emergency department with an acute MI will be taken directly to the cardiac catheterization laboratory and will undergo a minimally invasive interventional procedure to re-open the occluded vessel (Fig. 27-10). The most common of these procedures is percutaneous transluminal coronary angioplasty (PTCA), in which a balloon-tipped catheter is passed through the femoral or brachial artery into the coronary circulation to the blockage. The balloon is then inflated, expanding the

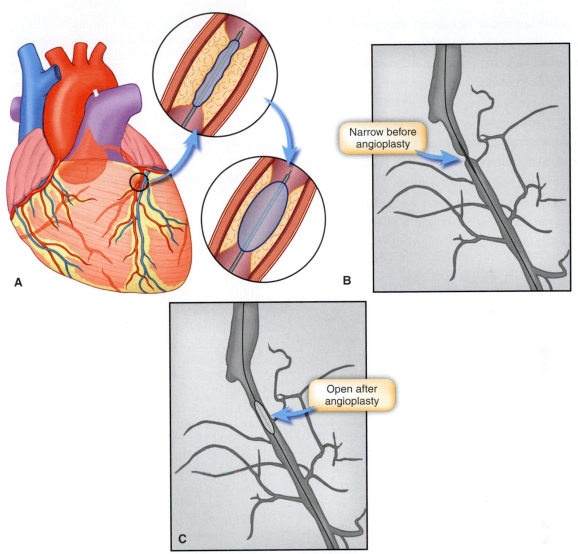

**Figure 27-10.** Percutaneous transluminal coronary angioplasty. A, In this procedure, a balloon-tipped catheter is passed through the femoral or brachial artery into the coronary circulation to the blockage. B, Before procedure. C, After procedure, when the arterial lumen is expanded and blood flow is re-established.

arterial lumen and re-establishing blood flow through the affected site.

## Stent Placement

Although PTCA is very effective at re-opening a blocked coronary artery, approximately 30% of people undergoing the procedure will experience a re-occlusion. Thus, many people will also undergo intracoronary stent placement where a wire mesh band is inserted via catheter into the coronary artery and expanded at the site of the lesion to enhance flow and maintain adequate lumen diameter. Early stent placement was also impacted by a high re-occlusion rate because of thrombus formation around the stent. However, drug-eluding stents have significantly reduced re-occlusion rates by emitting anticoagulant compounds that prevent clot formation.

## Coronary Artery Bypass Surgery

Individuals with complicated lesions or significant multivessel disease will frequently undergo **coronary artery bypass surgery (CABG)**. This highly invasive procedure requires opening of the chest cavity to place bypass grafts (vessels) on each side of the lesion to divert flow around the blockage. Typically, veins are harvested from the leg (e.g., saphenous vein), while the internal mammary artery can also be used to bypass the affected area of the coronary vessel. The success rate for CABG can extend to well more than 10 years when accompanied by appropriate lifestyle changes such as increased physical activity, smoking cessation, and appropriate nutritional intake.

## VIGNETTE continued

■ Upon arrival at the hospital emergency department, Vincent was immediately taken to the cardiac catheterization laboratory. He was found to have two occluded coronary arteries that were opened using balloon angioplasty, and stents were also placed. Vincent was admitted to the cardiac care unit for continued care and referred to the phase I cardiac rehabilitation team. During his short hospital stay, the **cardiac rehabilitation** team began to implement progressive physical activity, monitoring cardiovascular responses to activities of daily living such as combing hair, brushing teeth, and low-level walking. On day three, Vincent underwent a cardiopulmonary exercise test and was discharged from the hospital with a referral to the phase II cardiac rehabilitation program.

## Stress Testing

Exercise testing is commonly used to determine functional limitations and disease severity in people who are experiencing symptoms of CAD and those diagnosed with CAD (Fig. 27-11). The simplest form of graded exercise testing uses either a treadmill or bicycle ergometer to progressively increase exercise workloads and associated demand on the cardiovascular system. BP, heart rate, symptoms, and electrocardiogram (ECG) tracings are monitored to evaluate the exercise response and diagnose myocardial ischemia. In people with CAD, vasospasm and coronary artery narrowing occurs, which reduces the blood flow required to meet the increased myocardial oxygen demand during exercise, resulting in myocardial ischemia. In some people, the impaired myocardial blood flow will cause the ST segment of the ECG to become depressed, and this

pattern, especially when combined with symptoms, is indicative of myocardial ischemia. However, not all individuals with CAD will demonstrate these classic ECG changes, while some without disease will demonstrate mild levels of ST segment changes. In addition, some people with CAD, especially those who have experienced a previous MI and those with conditions such as chronic hypertension, may have abnormal resting ECGs that make the exercise ECG response difficult to interpret.

**Echocardiography** is frequently used with exercise stress testing to augment interpretation of the exercise response. Echocardiography uses sound waves to produce images of the heart muscle, valves, and blood flow through the chambers. Images taken at rest before exercise and then immediately after exercise are compared to evaluate changes in wall motion that may be indicative of myocardial ischemia. Heart muscle that lacks necessary blood flow and becomes ischemic will appear to be sluggish and not contracting as effectively as nonischemic muscle. Although echocardiography does not isolate vessel lesions, the involved vessels can be predicted by the area of muscle that appears to be ischemic.

Another form of exercise stress testing uses **myocardial perfusion studies** to identify areas of the heart that are not receiving adequate blood flow. Similar to stress echo, myocardial perfusion studies are undertaken at rest and following exercise stress. A radioactive isotope such as thallium or Cardiolite (sestamibi) is injected through a vein and taken up by the working heart muscle. A specialized camera is then used to image the heart and identify areas that have not taken up the isotope, indicating a lack of adequate perfusion. Areas of the heart not picking up the isotope at rest are indicative of damaged muscle, while decreased isotope perfusion after exercise is indicative of myocardial ischemia. As with stress echo, myocardial perfusion studies do not directly identify the involved vessels, but once again the portion of myocardium showing poor perfusion relates to the vessels supplying that area.

The clinical diagnostic information derived from exercise stress testing can be enhanced with the measurement of ventilatory gas exchange during the exercise test. Although **cardiopulmonary exercise testing (CPET)** has traditionally been used by physiologists for research and to evaluate and guide endurance athlete training, utilization of the technology in the clinical setting is becoming more common as an evaluation tool for patients with cardiovascular and/or respiratory disease. Similar to the standard ECG graded exercise test, CPET monitors BP and electrocardiography, but also includes the measurement of respiratory gas exchange. Typical measures during the symptom-limited exercise test include $\dot{V}O_2$, carbon dioxide output ($VCO_2$), and minute ventilation ($V_E$), together with pulse oximetry to measure oxygen saturation levels. Normal respiratory gas exchange response is dependent on both

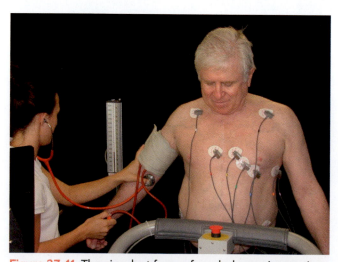

**Figure 27-11.** The simplest form of graded exercise testing uses either a treadmill or bicycle ergometer to progressively increase exercise workloads and associated demand on the cardiovascular system. Blood pressure, heart rate, symptoms, and electrocardiogram tracings are monitored to evaluate the exercise response and diagnose myocardial ischemia. *(Photo courtesy of Lance Dalleck)*

respiratory and cardiac function, referred to as ventilation to perfusion coupling. Thus, submaximal and peak exercise data derived from CPET can be used to differentiate cardiac and pulmonary disease, and to diagnose and quantify the functional impairment of conditions such as pulmonary hypertension, heart failure, and exercise-induced asthma.

Historically, maximal or peak $\dot{V}O_2$ and the ventilatory threshold have been the primary CPET measurements evaluated, both for athletes and in the clinical setting. Weber and coworkers[42] developed and published a heart failure severity scale based on the peak $\dot{V}O_2$ measurement that has been used to quantify functional limitations and as criteria for heart transplant decisions. Heart failure is generally broken into four functional classes using the New York Heart Association functional classification system. The four functional classes developed by Weber and coworkers[42] are based on measured $\dot{V}O_2$ and parallel the New York Heart Association classes. The classes are outlined in Table 27-3, as well as corresponding physical activity limitations.[43]

Numerous other respiratory gas exchange parameters that are strongly associated with cardiac- and pulmonary-related conditions and disease severity also can be elicited by submaximal exercise. One such parameter is the ventilatory equivalent for $CO_2$ expressed as $V_E/VCO_2$. The $V_E/VCO_2$ reflects the body's ability to eliminate $CO_2$ by comparing the breathing volume or $V_E$ with $VCO_2$ over the course of an exercise test. These submaximal data points are plotted as a graph, and the slope of the resulting line is calculated by linear regression. The derived slope is related to the severity of disease and risk for sudden death in patients with heart failure, with steeper slopes indicating greater functional limitation. In patients with heart failure, $V_E/VCO_2$ slope increases because of a mismatching of ventilation to perfusion in the lung as a result of compromised pump function. Similar to Weber's $\dot{V}O_2$ scale, Arena et al.[44] have developed a classification scale for patients with heart failure based on the $V_E/VCO_2$ slope.[45] Many other submaximal variables generated from CPET have diagnostic and prognostic value, including the ventilatory threshold, oxygen pulse ($HR/\dot{V}O_2$), end-tidal $CO_2$, respiratory rate, tidal volume, and others that can be calculated. CPET is also used to optimize cardiac resynchronization therapy (CRT) or pacemaker programming in patients with rate-responsive pacemaker implantations.

## Exercise and Cardiovascular Disease

Physical inactivity is a major independent risk factor for all forms of CVD, including CAD, in both men and women. People who participate in moderate amounts of physical activity have a 20% lower risk, whereas those who undertake higher amounts of exercise have a 30% or greater reduction in the risk for development of CAD.[46] The AHA has made improving America's cardiovascular health a primary objective for the year 2020, together with a 20% reduction in cardiovascular deaths. To meet these goals, the AHA has adopted seven ideal health metrics that have been shown by research to significantly reduce the risk for cardiovascular and all-cause mortality.[47–50] These metrics are broken down into two categories, as outlined in Table 27-4.

## Table 27-3. Classification of Heart Failure and Physical Activity Limitations

| NYHA CLASSIFICATION | WEBER CLASSIFICATION[42] | PEAK $\dot{V}O_2$ MEASURE (ML/KG/MIN) | PHYSICAL ACTIVITY LIMITATIONS |
|---|---|---|---|
| Class I (mild) | Functional class A | >20 | No physical activity limitation |
| Class II (mild) | Functional class B | 16–20 | Mild limitation; ordinary physical activity causes exertional fatigue, palpitation, and/or dyspnea |
| Class III (moderate) | Functional class C | 10–<16 | Marked limitation; low-level activity causes fatigue, dyspnea, and/or palpitations |
| Class IV (severe) | Functional class D | <10 | Symptomatic at rest; minimal physical activity causes marked increase in symptoms/discomfort |

NYHA, New York Heart Association.
*Source:* Data from the American Heart Association.[43]

## Table 27-4. American Heart Association Ideal Health Metrics

| CATEGORY | BEHAVIORS AND FACTORS |
|---|---|
| I: Four ideal health behaviors | a. Not smoking<br>b. Physical activity at recommended levels<br>c. BMI < 25 kg/m² <br>d. A diet that includes ≥3 servings of fruit and vegetables daily |
| II: Three ideal health factors | a. Systolic blood pressure < 120 mm Hg and diastolic blood pressure < 80 mm Hg<br>b. Total cholesterol < 200 mg/dL<br>c. Fasting plasma glucose levels < 100 mg/dL |

*Sources:* Data from Appel,[47] Ford et al.,[48,49] and Kvaavik et al.[50]

Research has shown that the number of ideal metrics a person has is significantly and inversely related to all-cause mortality and death from CVDs. Exercise is a powerful component to this risk-reduction strategy and can directly influence four of the AHA metrics: BMI, glucose, cholesterol, and BP. Numerous studies have shown a direct and inverse relation among physical activity, cardiorespiratory fitness, and all-cause and CVD mortality and morbidity.[51]

Cardiorespiratory fitness and exercise training are also strongly associated with survival in people with CVD. Therefore, exercise is considered a critical part of the treatment regimen for people diagnosed with CAD and for those who have experienced an acute event and/or interventional procedure. For many years, heart attack patients were restricted to bed rest for 6 weeks or longer. Unfortunately, this prolonged immobilization did not improve the healing process. In fact, it exposed the patient to additional risks of blood clots, lung infections, muscle wasting, and deconditioning. Since the early 1960s, many reports have been published that document the benefits of progressive physical activity in reducing mortality and morbidity among patients with CAD. Myers et al.[52] correlated a 1-MET increase in aerobic fitness with a 12% improvement in survival in men with CVD. Similarly, Moholdt et al.[53] demonstrated that all-cause mortality is decreased by as much as 33% when people with CVD participate in 30 minutes or more of moderate-to-vigorous intensity exercise one to three times per week.

### VIGNETTE continued

■ Two days after his discharge from the hospital, Vincent met with the clinical exercise physiologist in charge of the outpatient phase II cardiac rehabilitation program. The clinical exercise physiologist reviewed Vincent's medical history, current medical treatment, and the results of the cardiopulmonary exercise test in preparation for the initial meeting with Vincent. Vincent had been placed on a variety of medications, including beta blocker and statin therapy. Following an initial assessment, Vincent completed 12 weeks of progressively increased treadmill walking and light resistance training, and had the opportunity to work with a registered dietitian to modify his dietary intake. By the end of the program, Vincent's BP and cholesterol levels had normalized while his weight had minimally changed. However, he had developed a consistent pattern of exercise that Vincent was determined to maintain.

Historically, exercise programs for people with CAD have focused on low- to moderate-intensity aerobic

## RESEARCH HIGHLIGHT

### Cardiac Rehabilitation and Risk Stratification

Today, exercise training is an essential component of the recovery and ongoing therapeutic regimen for people with CAD. In almost all cases, a person recovering from a cardiac event and/or invasive intervention will benefit from an appropriately prescribed and monitored exercise program. The American Association for Cardiovascular and Pulmonary Rehabilitation (AACVPR), the AHA, and the American College of Cardiology Foundation (ACCF) recommend cardiac rehabilitation as a class or level 1 intervention for people with a recent MI, acute coronary syndrome, chronic stable angina, or heart failure, and after interventional procedures such as CABG, PTCA and

## RESEARCH HIGHLIGHT—cont'd

stent, valve surgery, and heart transplant.[54,55] Despite the AACVPR/AHA/ACCF recommendation and the strength of the published literature, cardiac rehabilitation and exercise training are highly underused, with only 14% to 35% of post-MI patients and 31% of post-CABG patients participating. The low participation levels are of great concern, because those completing a 36-visit cardiac rehabilitation program have been shown to have a 47% lower risk for death and a 31% lower risk for MI than those completing 1 or no sessions.[56]

Cardiac rehabilitation is a specialized program that provides supervised and nonsupervised exercise training, health education, and support for patients with heart disease. The program is generally broken into three phases:

- Phase I or inpatient: Phase I occurs during the patient's hospital stay and consists of early mobilization to prepare the patient for discharge and simple household activities.
- Phase II: Phase II is a multidimensional outpatient program that consists of ECG monitoring, supervised exercise training, and education focused on risk-factor reduction. This phase generally lasts for 12 weeks or 36 sessions but may be shorter or longer depending on individual patient needs.
- Phase III: This is an ongoing maintenance phase that consists of home and/or exercise facility-based physical activity and continued focus on risk-factor reduction.

Cardiovascular patients are also stratified into four risk classes based on guidelines published by the AHA.[57] These risk classes are:

- Class A: Apparently healthy individuals with no apparent clinical evidence of increased cardiovascular risk of exercise
- Class B: People with established CAD that is clinically stable and who are at low risk for cardiovascular complications of vigorous exercise
- Class C: Individuals with a history of multiple MIs or cardiac arrest who are at moderate or high risk for cardiac complications during exercise, and who have an exercise capacity of less than 6 METs and demonstrate ischemia on an exercise test
- Class D: People with unstable disease who require restriction of activity and for whom exercise is contraindicated

Generally, people referred to cardiac rehabilitation programs are class B and C, whereas those in class A are frequently cleared for independent exercise at home or at an exercise facility. It is in the scope of practice for clinical exercise physiologists, registered nurses with an exercise background, and physical therapists to work with high- and moderate-risk patients. Other exercise professionals, such as personal trainers, may work with people at low risk. The term *low risk* is generally applied to those patients who have all of the following characteristics: (1) an uncomplicated clinical course in the hospital, (2) no evidence of resting or exercise-induced ischemia, (3) functional capacity greater than 7 METs 3 weeks after any medical event or treatment that required hospitalization (e.g., angina, heart attack, or cardiac surgery), (4) normal ventricular function with an ejection fraction greater than 50%, and (5) no significant resting or exercise-induced arrhythmias (abnormal heart rhythms).[58]

*Please see reference list at the end of the chapter.*

activity for 30 or more minutes, three to five times per week. Recent research has shown that low- to moderate-risk patients may derive additional benefit by participating in interval sessions that include some vigorous-intensity exercise.[59] However, these sessions should be carefully monitored and appropriate warm-up and cool-down periods undertaken. In addition, people with CAD also benefit from the improvement of muscular strength and endurance that occurs with an appropriate program of resistance training. Many household and vocational activities require utilization of the upper-extremity musculature that has not traditionally been conditioned as part of cardiac rehabilitation programs. Generally, 1 to 2 sets of 12 to 15 repetitions are prescribed that consist of 8 to 10 exercises that work the major upper- and lower-extremity muscle groups, two times per week.

*Please see reference list at the end of the chapter.*

## PERIPHERAL VASCULAR DISEASE AND PERIPHERAL ARTERIAL OCCLUSIVE DISEASE

Similar to coronary atherosclerotic disease, PVD is caused by atherosclerotic lesions in one or more peripheral arterial and/or venous blood vessels, and is an important medical concern because there is a high risk for concurrent coronary and cerebral artery disease. Risk factors for PVD are similar to those for CAD, such as hyperlipidemia, smoking, hypertension, diabetes, family predisposition, physical inactivity, obesity, and stress. Nearly 35% of individuals diagnosed with PVD also have CAD, given the strong association of risk factors. It is not uncommon for individuals with CAD to experience symptoms of PVD following CABG, which serves to improve their cardiac function and subsequent ability to exercise.

The most prominent PVD risk factors are smoking and diabetes, with PVD occurring 11 times more frequently in individuals with diabetes than in those without diabetes. Diabetes accelerates the process of arteriosclerosis and atherosclerosis, affecting both the large vessels and microcirculation. Individuals with diabetes with PVD have been shown to have greater involvement of the smaller and more distal arteries than individuals without diabetes. The incidence of gangrene, a major complication of PVD, is estimated to be 40 times greater in individuals with diabetes.

A strong association exists between smoking and PVD,[60] and this risk factor should be addressed aggressively. Tobacco use not only impacts the arterial wall, but the effects of nicotine and carbon monoxide also reduce oxygen supply to the musculature. Nicotine stimulates the sympathetic nervous system, resulting in increased peripheral resistance and vasoconstriction, further compounding the already decreased blood flow and tissue oxygenation. In addition, nicotine increases platelet aggregation (promoting clot formation), whereas carbon monoxide readily binds with hemoglobin instead of oxygen, further impacting tissue oxygenation.

One of the most common forms of PVD is PAOD, resulting from atherosclerosis of the arteries of the lower extremities. This condition, characterized by intermittent claudication, results in exertional leg pain that dramatically alters quality of life and affects approximately 10% of the American population.[61] The most common sites for lower-extremity lesions include the abdominal aorta, iliac, femoral, popliteal, and tibial arteries. Consequently, blood flow distal to the lesion is reduced, resulting in ischemia and significantly impacting ambulation.

Normal blood flow to the peripheral musculature at rest generally averages close to 300 to 400 mL/min. With the onset of exercise, the combination of vasodilation and increased cardiac output stimulates up to a 10-fold increase in blood flow to the active tissue. This increase in blood flow returns to baseline levels within a few minutes of terminating the exercise activity.

Although resting blood flow in most people with PAOD is similar to that in healthy individuals, exercise blood flow is not. Whereas the metabolic demands of the working tissues significantly increase with activity, the arterial lesion affects the ability of the limbs to meet the metabolic demand by increasing blood flow. As a consequence, the reduced flow compromises tissue oxygenation, and the resulting ischemic condition stimulates pain in the affected limb.

Diagnosis of PAOD is made on the basis of the person's medical and symptomatic history, a physical examination, and information gathered from both noninvasive and invasive (arteriography) diagnostic tests. Patients typically present with diminished or nonpalpable pulses, decreased skin temperature, atrophy of the lower-leg musculature, toenail thickening, and hair loss in the affected extremity.[62]

The most common nondiagnostic test for PAOD measures ankle and arm systolic pressures at rest and post-exercise using a pneumatic cuff and Doppler ultrasonic flow detector. The ratio of ankle-to-arm systolic pressure (ankle–brachial index or ABI) is used to evaluate the severity of arterial narrowing. In a healthy individual, BP between the upper and lower extremities is similar, varying by only a few millimeters of mercury (mm Hg). However, in an atherosclerotic extremity, the systolic pressure distal to the lesion (typically taken at the ankle) will be reduced and the pressure reduction will accentuate with weight-bearing exercise. Thus, comparison of BPs between the arm (brachial) and ankle (ABI) at rest and after exercise are useful in assessing patients with PAOD. An ABI of less than 0.9 mm Hg is diagnostic of some degree of PAOD, with lower values indicating more severe disease.

The primary symptom associated with peripheral vascular occlusive disease (PVOD) is muscular pain caused by ischemia, or lack of blood flow to the muscle. Generally, this claudication pain is brought on by physical activity, but some people with more severe disease can also have pain at rest. Pain associated with PVOD is frequently described as a dull, aching, cramping pain and is reproducible at a given exercise workload. Many individuals with PVOD can only walk a limited distance before needing to stop and rest. Positional change is not required to bring symptomatic relief, and following the brief rest period, the individual usually is able to walk another short distance before stopping again. A subjective rating of pain can be made with the following five-point scale.[31]

- 0 = No pain
- 1 = Onset of pain
- 2 = Moderate pain
- 3 = Intense pain
- 4 = Maximal pain

## Treatment

Treatment of PAOD generally consists of a multicomponent approach, which involves cardiovascular risk reduction through pharmacology interventions and lifestyle coaching and symptom relief. Cardiovascular risk reduction includes controlling the most important modifiable risk factors for atherosclerosis: smoking, hypertension, diabetes mellitus, hyperlipidemia, and obesity. Furthermore, symptomatic patients are usually prescribed antiplatelet therapy in combination with a statin drug.[63] Symptom relief is largely targeted through exercise therapy, as described in the following section.

## Exercise and Peripheral Vascular Disease

People with PAOD typically reduce their daily walking because of claudication pain and a fear of exacerbating the symptoms by doing additional damage. Unfortunately, the resulting sedentary lifestyle leads to additional health challenges that may be even more debilitating. However, exercise plays an essential role in the treatment of people with PAOD and has been shown to be effective in improving ambulation distances in individuals with PVOD. Improvement has been associated with changes in blood viscosity, capillary density, and mitochondrial density, and increases in oxidative and glycolytic enzymes, all of which improve oxygen utilization. In addition, improvement in walking mechanics and pain perception also significantly influence exercise performance.[64] Because the risk factors for PVD are similar to those for CAD, one of the primary benefits of exercise is that it helps to reduce overall CAD risk and the risk for development of other chronic health conditions, along with improving overall cardiovascular endurance.

The objective of the exercise program is to stimulate improvement in arterial flow, oxygen extraction, and walking mechanics that ultimately serve to decrease oxygen demand at a given workload. Such changes will serve to improve the person's functional capacity, ability to ambulate with minimal or no pain, and ultimately quality of life. In addition, the treatment program should also focus on modifying underlying risk factors, such as smoking, and educating the person about PAOD (symptoms, foot care, nutrition, among others). Education is particularly important because of the anxiety associated with the pain that individuals with PVD experience.

Walking is the primary activity of choice, because it challenges the lower-leg muscles, effectively producing ischemia in the affected limb(s). This is important, because ischemia may be the primary stimulus for development of collateral circulation and other improvements in oxidative metabolism. Patients are typically encouraged to participate in 45 to 60 minutes of daily walking. The patient is instructed to walk to the point of intense pain (three to four on a five-point scale), rest until the pain subsides, and then repeat the ambulatory activity once again. The process should initially be repeated for a total of 20 to 30 minutes with gradual progression to 45 to 60 minutes per day. The initial workload intensity should stimulate claudication pain within 2 to 6 minutes of walking. When 8 to 12 minutes of continuous walking can be tolerated, the patient is encouraged to increase the walking pace or progress the total activity time.

Some people also may benefit by supplementing the walking program with other low-intensity, non–weight-bearing activities that further promote conditioning along with light upper-extremity resistance training. However, caution should be taken to ensure that patients are free of cardiovascular symptoms, stay within moderate intensities (RPE 9–13), and are taught appropriate lifting techniques.

It is important that exercise professionals are aware that people with PVD may also have underlying CAD. Some people with PAOD may experience CAD symptoms as walking distance and/or speed increases and may require additional medical evaluation.

## STROKE

Stroke, or brain attack, affects 795,000 Americans each year, and slightly more than 6.8 million Americans currently have a history of stroke. Strokes are the fourth leading cause of death in the United States behind heart disease, cancer, and chronic lower respiratory diseases. Approximately 30% of people who suffer a stroke die within the first year, and more than 50% are dead within 5 years after the initial stroke. Strokes occur more frequently in women than men and are more common among African Americans and Mexican Americans than whites.[2]

Strokes occur when the blood supply to the brain is cut off (**ischemic stroke**) or when a blood vessel in the brain bursts (**hemorrhagic stroke**). Approximately 87% of strokes are ischemic, many of which can be treated with the drug tissue plasminogen activator (tPA) if the person seeks immediate help. The drug tPA must be administered within the initial 3 hours of a stroke and can significantly reduce or eliminate the impairments that typically occur. Thus, it is imperative that all Americans are aware of and recognize the warning signs of a stroke:

- Sudden numbness or weakness of the face, arms, or legs
- Sudden confusion or trouble speaking or understanding others
- Sudden trouble seeing in one or both eyes
- Sudden walking problems, dizziness, or loss of balance and coordination
- Sudden severe headache with no known cause

Each year, approximately 200,000 to 500,000 Americans experience a TIA where the blood flow to a part of the brain stops for a brief period.[65] Unlike a stroke, the blockage is temporary and dissolves relatively quickly. However, the transient stoppage of blood flow does result in strokelike symptoms that may last from a few minutes to 1 to 2 hours. High BP, diabetes, elevated cholesterol, and atrial fibrillation are major risk factors for TIAs. The prevalence of TIA also increases with advancing age, and people with known heart disease and PVD are also at increased risk for TIA and stroke. People who experience TIA are at increased risk for stroke, with 3% to 10% having a stroke in the following 2 days and 9% to 17% within 90 days of the TIA event. In addition, individuals who have a TIA have a 10-year stroke, MI, or vascular mortality risk of 43%.[2]

Although a large number of people survive stroke, many experience physical limitations because of neurological damage, making stroke the leading cause of chronic disability. The length of time required to recover from a stroke is dependent on its severity. More than half of stroke survivors regain some level of functional independence, whereas 15% to 30% are permanently disabled. Strokes can dramatically reduce a person's quality of life—robbing them of their ability to speak and to use facial, arm, and leg muscles—and can cause other neurological impairments. In addition, people with stroke typically experience a significant decline in physical conditioning that leads to a variety of metabolic disorders and increased risk for recurrent stroke and MI. This is a downhill spiral, as the decline in functional capacity and associated metabolic changes, such as impaired glucose tolerance and type 2 diabetes mellitus, together with other risk factors, are further worsened by the ongoing physical inactivity that results from the stroke-related physical impairments.

Risk factors for stroke include hypertension, impaired glucose tolerance, smoking, heart disease and atrial fibrillation, previous stroke, TIA, physical inactivity, and depression. Hypertension is a powerful risk factor for both ischemic and hemorrhagic stroke. People with normal resting BP (<120/80>) have half the lifetime risk for stroke compared with those with hypertension. Impaired glucose tolerance and smoking double the risk for stroke, whereas depression has been associated with a 4.2-fold increased risk for TIA and stroke.[2]

## Exercise and Stroke

Research has demonstrated that there is an inverse relation between higher levels (vigorous) of physical activity and stroke risk. Most studies have placed this lower relative risk in the 14% to 50% range.[66–68] Lower levels of activity, such as walking, have also been shown to be related to lower stroke incidence.[69] As with other chronic health conditions, avoidance of physical inactivity is critical, and compliance with the 2008 Physical Activity Guidelines for Americans could dramatically decrease the future incidence of TIA and stroke.[20]

Physical rehabilitation following stroke typically focuses on optimizing the basic activity skills of daily living; regaining balance, coordination, and functional independence; and preventing complications and stroke reoccurrence. Unfortunately, this level of rehabilitation does not provide an adequate aerobic stimulus to reverse the physical deconditioning, muscular atrophy, and increased cardiovascular risk that result from stroke and its associated neurological impairment. Post-stroke patients can and have been shown to improve functional capacity using a variety of exercise modalities, such as bicycle ergometers, warm-water exercise, weight-supported treadmills, and pole walking. Gait, balance, and coordination training are also important aspects of the recovery program. Along with improving functional capacity, exercise also improves CVD risk factors (e.g., SBP, lipid profiles, insulin sensitivity,

glucose metabolism, and body composition) and fibrinolytic activity (the system responsible for dissolving clots), resulting in a reduced risk for CAD and recurrent stroke.

For many years, clinicians have considered the window for motor improvement following stroke to be 3 to 6 months. However, increasing clinical and experimental data show that exercise has the potential to improve selected motor performance even years after a stroke. Therefore, people with stroke should be encouraged to maintain and, when possible, progress their activity program to gain these potential additional benefits and associated improved quality of life. Today, many stroke patients transition into programs at medical fitness centers once released from the clinical care of their physical, occupational, and/or recreational therapist. Post-stroke exercise guidelines and recommendations are similar to those used for CAD and hypertension. Exercise activities may vary depending on the person's neurological deficit profile, current functional capacity, and risk factor status. Modalities previously mentioned such as cycle ergometer, walking/treadmill training, water exercise, and other exercise classes are frequently modified to accommodate clients who have had a stroke.

## VIGNETTE conclusion

Vincent was lucky in that he did not suffer significant damage to his heart muscle and gradually was able to drop his weight, BP, and lipid values into the normal range. His life was spared because of the quick response and CPR/AED intervention implemented by the clinical exercise physiologist and coaches at the ball field. However, this all could have been avoided had Vincent begun a habit of physical activity early in life and maintained a normal weight. Not only did Vincent not undertake any purposeful exercise, he also was sedentary throughout the day, placing him at increased risk for development of the conditions and resulting events he experienced. He was fortunate that the hospital had interventional cardiologists who could immediately treat the affected artery and a strong cardiac rehabilitation program that could guide him through the recovery phase.

## CRITICAL THINKING QUESTIONS

1. You are helping to coach a little league baseball team when one of the parents, who is also an assistant coach, becomes light-headed, short of breath, and describes a heavy feeling in his chest. What might be occurring and what should you do?

2. You are working as a personal trainer at a fitness facility with a client with type 2 diabetes. The client shows up for her midmorning workout feeling tired and a bit light-headed. She always carries a self-glucose monitor and carbohydrate sources. Should you get her right into the warm-up for the workout you have planned and see if the activity helps her fatigue and light-headedness?

3. You are working as a wellness coach for Glacier Transportation's employee wellness program. You have just completed an assessment on an employee and are now in the process of reviewing the results with him. He has the following findings:

   • Height: 69 inches

   • Weight: 180 pounds

• TC: 160 mg/dL

• HDL cholesterol: 30 mg/dL

• LDL cholesterol: 100 mg/dL

• Triglycerides: 150 mf/dL

• Glucose: 120 mg/dL

   Calculate the following ratios. What level of risk do they suggest? What recommendations might you have for him?

   • $BMI = (180/2.205) / 69 * 2.54 = 81.63 \ kg / 3.072m =$

   • $TC/HDL = 160/30 =$

   • $HDL/LDL = 30/100 =$

   • $TG/HDL = 150/30 =$

## ADDITIONAL RESOURCES

Exercise is Medicine: http://www.exerciseismedicine.org
Medicine and Science in Sports and Exercise (American College of Sports Medicine Position Statements): http://www.acsm-msse.org
Colberg SR, Albright AL, Blissmer BJ, et al.; American College of Sports Medicine; American Diabetes Association. Exercise and type 2 diabetes: American College of Sports Medicine and the American Diabetes Association: Joint position statement. *Med Sci Sports Exerc.* 2010;42:2282–2303.
Pescatello LS, Franklin BA, Fagard R, Farquhar WB, Kelley G, Ray CA. Exercise and hypertension. *Med Sci Sports Exerc.* 2004;36:533–553.

Kohrt WM, Bloomfield SA, Little KD, Nelson ME, Yingling VR; Physical Activity and Bone Health. *Med Sci Sports Exerc.* 2004;36:1985–1996.
*Advanced Health and Fitness Specialist Manual: The Ultimate Resource for Advanced Fitness Professionals.* San Diego, CA: American Council on Exercise; 2009.
Balady GJ, Arena R, Sietsema K, Myers J, et al. Clinician's guide to cardiopulmonary exercise testing in adults: A scientific statement from the American Heart Association. *Circulation.* 2010;122:191–225.

## REFERENCES

1. Kung HC, Hoyert DL, Xu JQ, Murphy SL. Deaths: Final data for 2005. *Natl Vital Stat Rep.* 2008;56:10.
2. American Heart Association: Heart disease and stroke statistics 2013 update: A report from the American Heart Association. *Circulation.* 2013;127:e6-e245.
3. Chobanian AV, et al. JNC 7 Express: The Seventh Report of the Joint National Committee on Prevention, Detection, Evaluation, and Treatment of High Blood Pressure. NIH Publication No. 03-5233. Washington DC: National Institutes of Health and National Heart, Lung and Blood Institute; 2003.
4. The Seventh Report of the Joint National Committee on Prevention, Detection, Evaluation and Treatment of High Blood Pressure. Washington, DC: US Department of Health and Human Services; National Institutes of Health; National Heart, Lung & Blood Institute; NIH Publication No. 04-5230; August 2004. Available at: http://www.nhlbi.nih.gov/files/docs/guidelines/jnc7full.pdf.
5. American Heart Association: Heart disease and stroke statistics 2009 update: A report from the American Heart Association Statistics Committee and Stroke Statistics Subcommittee. *Circulation.* 2009;119e;e21–e181.
6. Blumenthal JA, Babyak MA, Hinderliter A, et al. Effects of the DASH diet alone and in combination with exercise and weight loss on blood pressure and cardiovascular biomarkers in men and women with high blood pressure: The ENCORE study. *Arch Intern Med.* 2010;170:126–135.
7. Kayrak M, Bacaksiz A, Vatankulu MA, et al. Exaggerated blood pressure response to exercise—a new portent of masked hypertension. *Clin Exp Hypertens.* 2010;32:560–568.
8. Manolio TA, Burke GL, Savage PJ, Sidney S, Gardin JM, Oberman A. Exercise blood pressure response and 5-year risk of elevated blood pressure in a cohort of young adults: The CARDIA study. *Am J Hypertens.* 1994;7:234–241.
9. Miyai N, Arita M, Morioka I, et al. Response in subjects with high-normal BP: Exaggerated blood pressure response to exercise and risk of future hypertension in subjects with high-normal blood pressure. *J Am Coll Cardiol* 2000;36:1626–1631.
10. Sharabi Y, Ben-Cnaan R, Hanin A, Martonovitch G, Grossman E. The significance of hypertensive response to exercise as a predictor of hypertension and cardiovascular disease. *J Hum Hypertens.* 2001;15:353–356.

11. Singh JP, Larson MG, Manolio TA, et al. Blood pressure response during treadmill testing as a risk factor for new-onset hypertension: The Framingham heart study. *Circulation*. 1999;99:1831–1836.

12. Carnethon MR, Evans NS, Church TS, et al. Joint associations of physical activity and aerobic fitness on the development of incident hypertension: Coronary artery risk development in young adults. *Hypertension*. 2010;56:49–55.

13. Anunciacao PG, Polito MD. A review on post-exercise hypotension in hypertensive individuals. *Arq Bras Cardiol*. 2011;96:e100–e109.

14. Kelley GA, Kelley KA, Tran ZV. Aerobic exercise and resting blood pressure: A meta-analytic review of randomized, controlled trials. *Prev Cardiol*. 2001;4:73–80.

15. Kenney MF, Seals DR. Postexercise hypotension. Key features, mechanisms, and clinical significance. *Hypertension*. 1993;22:653–664.

16. Pescatello LS, Kulikowich JM. The after effects of dynamic exercise on ambulatory blood pressure. *Med Sci Sports Exerc*. 2001;33:1855–1861.

17. Keese F, Farinatti P, Pescatello L, Monteiro W. A comparison of the immediate effects of resistance, aerobic, and concurrent exercise on post exercise hypotension. *J Strength Cond Res*. 2011;25:1429–1435.

18. Kenny W, Holowatz LA. Hypertension. *ACE Advanced Health and Fitness Specialist Manual*. American Council on Exercise, San Diego, CA; 2008.

19. Haskell WL, Lee JM, Pate RR, et al.; American College of Sports Medicine; American Heart Association. Physical activity and public health: Updated recommendation for adults from the American College of Sports Medicine and the American Heart Association. *Circulation*. 2007;116:1081–1093.

20. *2008 Physical Activity Guidelines for Americans*. ODPHP Publication No. V0036. Washington, DC: U.S. Department of Health and Human Services. October 2008. Available at: http://www.health.gov/paguidelines.

21. Churilla JR. An evidence-based review of exercise and metabolic syndrome. *J Clin Exerc Physiol*. 2012;1:21–29.

22. American Diabetes Association. Centers for Disease Control and Prevention. National diabetes fact sheet: National estimates and general information on diabetes and prediabetes in the United States, 2011. Atlanta, GA: U.S. Department of Health and Human Services, Centers for Disease Control and Prevention; 2012. Available at: http://www.cdc.gov/diabetes.

23. Neeland IJ, Turer AT, Ayers CR, et al. Dysfunctional adiposity and the risk of prediabetes and type 2 diabetes in obese adults. *J Am Med Assoc*. 2012;308:1150–1159.

24. Ahmed HM, Blaha MJ, Nasir K, Rivera JJ, Blumenthal, RS. Effects of physical activity on cardiovascular disease. *Am J Cardiol*. 2012;109:288–295.

25. Ford ES. Risks for all-cause mortality, cardiovascular disease, and diabetes associated with the metabolic syndrome: A summary of the evidence. *Diabetes Care*. 2005;28:1769–1778.

26. American Heart Association/National Heart, Lung, and Blood Institute (AHA/NHLBI) Scientific Statement. Diagnosis and management of the metabolic syndrome. *Circulation*. 2005;112:e285–e290.

27. Meigs JB. The metabolic syndrome (insulin resistance syndrome or syndrome X). *UpToDate*. 2008. Available at: www.uptodate.com. Accessed January 19, 2009.

28. Carenthon MR, Loria CM, Hill JO, Sidney S, Savage PJ, Liu K; Coronary Artery Risk Development in Young Adults study. Risk factors for the metabolic syndrome: The Coronary Artery Risk Development in Young Adults (CARDIA) Study, 1985-2001. *Diabetes Care*. 2004;27:2707–2715.

29. Katzmareyk PT. Metabolic syndrome, obesity, and mortality: Impact of cardiorespiratory fitness. *Diabetes Care*. 2005;28:391–397.

30. American College of Sports Medicine. Position Stand: Appropriate physical activity intervention strategies for weight loss and prevention of weight regain for adults. *Med Sci Sports Exerc*. 2009;41:459–471.

31. American College of Sports Medicine. *ACSM's Guidelines for Exercise Testing and Prescription*. 9th ed. Philadelphia, PA: Lippincott Williams & Wilkins; 2014.

32. Ford ES, Giles WH, Dietz WH. Prevalence of the metabolic syndrome among U.S. adults: Findings from the Third National Health and Nutrition Examination Survey. *JAMA*. 2002;287:356–359.

33. Gordon DJ, Probstfield JL, Garrison FJ, et al. High-density lipoprotein cholesterol and cardiovascular disease. Four prospective American studies. *Circulation*. 1989;79:8–15.

34. Kohli P, Cannon CP. Triglycerides: How much credit do they deserve? *Med Clin N Am*. 2012;96:39–55.

35. National Cholesterol Education Program. Expert Panel on Detection, Evaluation and Treatment of High Blood Cholesterol in Adults. Summary of the 2nd Report of NCEP Expert Panel on Detection, Evaluation and Treatment of High Blood Cholesterol in Adults (Adult Treatment Panel III). NIH Publication No. 02-5213. Executive summary (2001). *J Am Med Assoc*. 2002;285:2486–2497.

36. Brugts JJ, Yetgin T, Hoeks SE, et al. The benefits of statins in people without established cardiovascular disease but with cardiovascular risk factors: Meta-analysis of randomised controlled trials. *Br Med J*. 2009;338:b2376.

37. Singh V. The effect of HDL levels on cardiovascular disease. eMedicine's Lipid Feature Series. 2006; Series 2, Issue 1. eMedicine from WebbMD. Available at: http://www.eMedicine.com. Accessed August 30, 2014.

38. Finn AV, Nakano M, Narula J, Kolodie FD, Virmani R. Concept of vulnerable/unstable plaque. *Arterioscler Thromb Vasc Biol*. 2010;30:1282–1292.

39. Dawber TR, Meadors CF, Moore FE. Epidemiological approaches to heart disease: The Framingham Study. *Am J Public Health Nations Health*. 1951;41:279–286.

40. Chatterjee K, Massie B. Systolic and diastolic heart failure: Differences and similarities. *J Card Fail*. 2007;13:569–576.

41. AIM-HIGH Investigators. Niacin in patients with low HDL cholesterol levels receiving intensive statin therapy. *N Eng J Med*. 2011;365:2255–2267.

42. Weber KT, Janicki JS, McElroy PA. Determination of aerobic capacity and circulatory failure. *Circulation*. 1987;76(Suppl. VI):VI40–VI45.

43. American Heart Association. Classes of heart failure. Available at: http://www.heart.org/HEARTORG/Conditions/HeartFailure/AboutHeartFailure/Classes-of-Heart-Failure_UCM_306328_Article.jsp. Accessed February 6, 2012.

44. Arena R, Myers J, Abella J, et al. Development of a ventilator classification system in patients with heart failure. *Circulation*. 2007;115:2410–2417.

45. Matsumoto A, Itoh H, Yoko E, et al. End-tidal CO2 pressure decreases during exercise in cardiac patients: Association with severity of heart failure and cardiac output reserve. *J Am Coll Cardiol*. 2000;36:242–249.

46. Haskell WL. *Physical Activity Guidelines Advisory Committee Report*. Atlanta, GA: U.S. Department of Health and Human Services. May 23, 2008. Available at: http://www.health.gov/paguidelines/Report.

47. Appel LJ. Empiric support for cardiovascular health: The case gets even stronger. *Circulation*. 2012;125:973–974.

48. Ford ES, Zhao G, Tasai J, Li C. Low-risk lifestyle behaviors and all-cause mortality: Findings from the National Health and Nutrition Examination Survey III Mortality Study. *Am J Public Health.* 2011;101:1922–1929.

49. Ford ES, Greenlund KJ, Hong Y. Ideal cardiovascular health and mortality from all causes and diseases of the circulatory system among adults in the United States. *Circulation.* 2012;125:987–995.

50. Kvaavik E, Batty GD, Ursin G, Huxley R, Gale CR. Influence of individual and combined health behaviors on total and cause-specific mortality in men and women: The United Kingdom health and lifestyle survey. *Arch Intern Med.* 2010;170:711–718.

51. Garber CE, Blissmer B, Deschenes MR, et al. American College of Sports Medicine Position Stand: Quantity and quality of exercise for developing and maintaining cardiorespiratory, musculoskeletal, and neuromotor fitness in apparently healthy adults: Guidance for prescribing exercise. *Med Sci Sports Exerc.* 2011;43:1334–1359.

52. Myers J, Prakash M, Froelicher V, Partington S, Atwood J. Exercise capacity and mortality among men referred for exercise testing. *N Eng J Med.* 2002;346:793–801.

53. Moholdt T, Wisloff U, Nilsen T, Slordahl S. Physical activity and mortality in men and women with coronary heart disease: A prospective population-based cohort study in Norway (the HUNT study). *Eur J Cardiovasc Prev Rehab.* 2008;15:639–645.

54. Smith SC Jr, Benjamin EJ, Bonow RO, et al. AHA/ACCF secondary prevention and risk reduction therapy for patients with coronary and other atherosclerotic vascular disease. 2011 update: A guideline from the American Heart Association and American College of Cardiology Foundation. *Circulation.* 2011;124:2458–2473.

55. Thomas RJ, King M, Lui K, Oldridge N, Pina IL, Spertus J. AACVPR/ACCF/AHA 2010 update: Performance measures on cardiac rehabilitation for referral to cardiac rehabilitation/secondary prevention services: A report of the American Association of Cardiovascular and Pulmonary Rehabilitation and the American College of Cardiology Foundation/American Heart Association task force on performance measures (writing committee to develop clinical performance measures for cardiac rehabilitation). *Circulation.* 2010;122:1342–1350.

56. Kawn G, Baldy GJ. Cardiac rehabilitation 2012: Advancing the field through emerging science. *Circulation.* 2012;125:e369–e373.

57. Fletcher GF, Balady GJ, Amsterdam EA, et al. Exercise standards for testing and training: A statement for healthcare professionals from the American Heart Association. *Circulation.* 2001;104:1694.

58. Roberts S. Special populations and health concerns. *ACE Personal Trainer Manual.* 3rd ed. San Diego, CA: American Council on Exercise; 2003.

59. Currie KD. Effects of acute and chronic low-volume high-intensity interval exercise on cardiovascular health in patients with coronary artery disease. *Appl Physiol Nutr Metab.* 2013;38:359.

60. Conen D, Everett BM, Kurth T, et al. Smoking, smoking cessation and risk of symptomatic peripheral artery disease in women: A prospective study. *Ann Intern Med.* 2011;154:719–726.

61. Dhaliwal G, Mukherjee D. Peripheral arterial disease: Epidemiology, natural history, diagnosis and treatment. *Int J Angiol.* 2007;16:38–44.

62. Hammond MC, Merli GJ, Zieler RE. Rehabilitation of the patient with peripheral vascular disease of the lower extremity. In: Delisa JA, ed. *Rehabilitation Medicine, Principles and Practice.* 2nd ed. Philadelphia, PA: J.B. Lippincott Co.; 1993.

63. Fokkenrood HJ, Lauret GJ, Scheltinga MR, Spreeuwenberg C, de Bie RA, Teijink JA. Multidisciplinary treatment for peripheral arterial occlusive disease and the role of eHealth and mHealth. *J Multidiscip Healthc.* 2012;5:257–263.

64. Hiatt RH, Wolfel EE, Meier RH, Regensteiner JG. Superiority of treadmill walking exercise versus strength training for patient with peripheral arterial disease: Implications for the mechanism of the training response. *Circulation.* 1994;90:1866–1874.

65. Kleindorfer D, Panagos P, Pancioli A, et al. Incidence and short-term prognosis of transient ischemic attack in a population-based study. *Stroke.* 2005;36: 720–723.

66. Lee IM, Paffenbarger RS Jr. Physical activity and stroke incidence: The Harvard Alumni Health Study. *Stroke.* 1998;29:2049–2054.

67. Willey JZ, Xu Q, Boden-Albala B, et al. Lipid profile components and risk of ischemic stroke: The Northern Manhattan Study (NOMAS). *Arch Neurol.* 2009;66: 1400–1406.

68. Williams PT. Reduction in incident stroke risk with vigorous physical activity: Evidence from 7.7 year follow-up of the National Runners' Health Study. *Stroke.* 2009;40:1921–1923.

69. Sattelmair JR, Kurth T, Buring JE, Lee I. Physical activity and risk of stroke in women. *Stroke.* 2010;41:1243–1250.

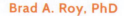

Brad A. Roy, PhD

CHAPTER 28

# Other Common Medical Conditions and Pregnancy

## CHAPTER OUTLINE

## LEARNING OUTCOMES

1. Describe the symptoms associated with exercise-induced asthma, as well as common treatments and preventive measures.
2. Identify the risk factors for developing cancer and lifestyle strategies that can minimize the risk for the development of cancer.
3. Define *osteoporosis* and *osteopenia*.
4. Describe the types of physical activity generally recommended as part of the treatment plan for people diagnosed with osteopenia and osteoporosis.
5. Compare and contrast rheumatoid arthritis, osteoarthritis, and fibromyalgia.
6. Explain the importance of physical activity for people diagnosed with arthritis and fibromyalgia.
7. Identify the common causes of low-back pain and strategies for preventing the development of chronic low-back conditions.
8. List the precautions that should be considered when developing exercise programs for prenatal and postpartum clients.

## ANCILLARY LINK

Visit Davis*Plus* at http://davisplus.fadavis.com for study and practice resources, including online quizzes, animations that help explain physiological processes, podcasts concerning news and career trends in exercise physiology, and practice references.

## VIGNETTE I

■ Luci is a personal trainer with advanced education and training in working with special populations. She splits her time between the medical fitness facility at a large hospital and her private practice training clients at a local gym. Rich, who has come to the gym to meet Luci for his first training session, was just beginning his freshman year of high school and was excited to try his first competitive sport by joining the cross-country team for the fall season. He had never run much, even in his middle school years. Physical education was an option that he really did not care for, and he chose instead to focus on music and drama opportunities. However, this year was different, because his best friend was joining the cross-country team and he wanted to share that experience with him. The first day of practice was not easy. The coach sent the team out for a 30-minute run. Rich was unable to complete the workout, as he quickly became short of breath and wheezy. He figured that he was just out of shape and things would get better as his conditioning improved.

How might Luci address Rich's situation, and what special considerations should she keep in mind?

Evidence continues to mount that daily choices and habits profoundly influence a person's short- and long-term health and well-being. This chapter introduces a number of medical conditions that health and fitness professionals encounter on a regular basis, including asthma, cancer, osteoporosis, arthritis, fibromyalgia, and low-back pain (LBP). In addition, relevant information about exercise during the prenatal and postpartum periods is provided.

In some instances, genetic and other non-lifestyle–related factors result in the development of chronic health conditions. However, in most people, these conditions are directly related to poor lifestyle choices and habits, especially physical inactivity, poor nutritional intake, and tobacco use.

Exercise is essential in preventing the development of most chronic conditions, and it has an important role as a therapeutic intervention. Health and fitness professionals, working in a variety of professional careers, frequently encounter opportunities to address these chronic conditions, using both primary and secondary prevention strategies and skills.

## ASTHMA

**Asthma** is a complex, chronic inflammatory response of the airways that is characterized by periodic episodes of reversible airway obstruction, increased bronchial reactivity, and airway inflammation (Fig. 28-1). In this clinical syndrome, many cells and cellular elements play a role, including interactions among inflammatory cells, their mediators, airway epithelium and smooth muscle, and the nervous system. In people who are susceptible, the inflammatory response results in recurrent symptoms of shortness of breath, wheezing,

coughing, and chest tightness. Asthma affects 5% to 12% of the population (approximately 23 million individuals) and is responsible for nearly 2 million annual emergency department visits, 500,000 hospitalizations, and 100 million days of restricted activity. Asthma is more common in children than in adults (10% of children and 5% of adults), and more than half of children with asthma experience symptoms before the age of 5 years.[1]

The inflammatory response and subsequent cascade of asthmatic events are typically set off by environmental triggers such as allergens (e.g., animal dander, dust mites, cockroaches, and mold), irritants (e.g., cigarette smoke, air pollution, strong odors and sprays, and pollens), viral respiratory illnesses, stress, cold air, and exercise. Allergies are responsible for triggering 60% to 90% of the asthma attacks in children and more than 50% of those experienced by adults. Approximately 3% to 10% of individuals with asthma are sensitive to aspirin and/or nonsteroidal anti-inflammatory drugs (NSAIDs), and 5% to 10% have occupation-induced airway reactivity. Other factors may include obesity, gastroesophageal reflux disease, chronic sinusitis, and perinatal factors such as maternal smoking, prematurity, and increased maternal age.

In people who are susceptible, endogenous and exogenous triggers can activate an inflammatory response that leads to airway hyperresponsiveness and airway obstruction caused by constriction of smooth muscle around the airways (Fig. 28-2), swelling of mucosal cells, and/or increased secretion of mucus. These periodic symptomatic episodes, which are associated with airflow obstruction, are generally reversible either spontaneously or with pharmacological treatment. Medication is typically centered on inhaled corticosteroids, short- and long-term bronchodilators, theophylline, anti-immunoglobulin E (anti-IgE), and others. These medications can reduce airway inflammation and smooth muscle constriction along with associated symptoms. However, in some people who experience chronic asthma attacks, the associated airflow limitation may be only partially reversible because of the airway remodeling that is associated with chronic untreated disease.

The primary goal of asthma treatment is to prevent or minimize symptoms to improve functional and psychological well-being.[2] Nonpharmacological therapy includes avoidance of environmental and occupational triggers, encouragement of regular exercise, and education regarding warning signs of an asthmatic attack and proper use of medications, such as inhalers.

Although genetic factors may control a person's predisposition to asthma, the full cause is likely to be multifactorial. Epidemiological evidence points to a reduction in asthma prevalence as a result of rural living, exposure to other children (e.g., siblings or early daycare), less frequent use of antibiotics, and some infections (e.g., measles and hepatitis A). These and other events may precipitate a gene–environment

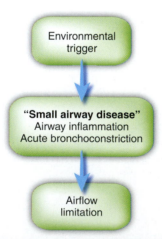

**Figure 28-1.** Basic process of an asthmatic episode. A variety of environmental triggers can instigate the process of airway inflammation and bronchoconstriction, which can then lead to reversible airway obstruction and airflow limitation. An asthmatic episode such as this can affect the person's ability to properly ventilate at rest and during exercise.

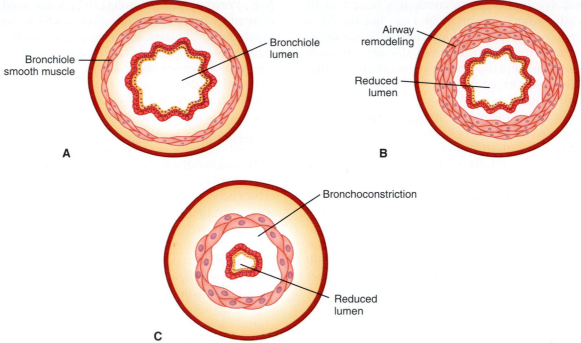

**Figure 28-2.** Bronchoconstriction. A, The normal bronchiole. B, Asthmatic episodes over time can cause permanent changes to the bronchiole, manifested by a thickening of the smooth muscle wall (remodeling) and narrowing of the airway lumen. This narrowing is only partially reversible and will limit airflow as a result. C, Bronchiole smooth muscle constricts in response to an internal or external trigger, causing narrowing of the airway lumen, leading to an obstruction of airflow in and out of the lung.

interaction that stimulates production of IgE and a resulting sensitization.[3]

Asthma is typically diagnosed by a detailed medical and family history, physical examination, and pulmonary function testing (**spirometry**) that evaluates forced vital capacity (FVC), the forced expiratory volume in 1 second ($FEV_1$), and the $FEV_1/FVC$ ratio before and after inhalation of a short-acting bronchodilator. When compared with predicted values, a reduced $FEV_1/FVC$ ratio indicates the presence of airway obstruction. The degree of reversibility after administration of a bronchodilator correlates with airway obstruction and provides an indication of the degree of severity. Some individuals may have exercise-induced respiratory symptoms without a formal diagnosis of asthma.

## VIGNETTE I continued

■ Subsequent practices produced a similar result for Rich, and he began to notice that his shortness of breath came on a bit more rapidly and intensely on the cold, dry fall days. It was particularly severe when he attempted to keep up with some of the older runners on an interval session, and the subsequent wheeziness lasted for 20 to 30 minutes after stopping the workout. Rich did his best to downplay his symptoms, but his coach was concerned and recommended to Rich's mother, Maria, that he be evaluated by his primary care physician. Maria is a member at Luci's gym; she gives Luci the background about Rich's illness and asks Luci about the condition. Luci states that she agrees with the coach that Rich should see his doctor for diagnosis and any relevant exercise recommendations.

### Exercise-Induced Asthma

Approximately 80% of people with asthma experience attacks during and/or after physical activity, which is referred to as **exercise-induced asthma (EIA)**. EIA typically occurs during or after aerobic exercise that requires the repetitive movement of large quantities of air through the airways. In some individuals, EIA may be brought on by sudden, intense exercise. Individuals with EIA are especially sensitive to dry, cold air that contains environmental allergens and/or pollutants that stimulate histamine release, drying of the airway, and/or airway cooling.

Common symptoms of EIA include cough, wheezing, chest tightness, excessive shortness of breath, and excess mucus. The severity of the response is related to the exercise ventilatory requirement and the environmental conditions. Symptoms of EIA commonly peak 5 to 10 minutes after stopping exercise and can last for 20 to 30 minutes. Although most people experience mild-to-moderate symptoms that gradually reverse with exercise cessation and medication administration, some individuals may experience severe bronchospasm resulting in death.[4]

Approximately 50% of individuals with an EIA episode experience a relative refractory period that begins less than 1 hour after exercise and lasts for up to 3 hours. During this refractory period, another exercise bout either will not produce an EIA attack or will result in a less intense reaction. Late asthmatic responses, 3 to 9 hours after the initial bronchospasm, also occur in approximately half of the EIA population. These late responses are typically more common in children and tend to be mild in nature. In addition, some people will also develop a hacking cough 2 to 12 hours after exercise that can last for 1 to 2 days.

## VIGNETTE I continued

■ Dr. Jefferson carefully quizzed Rich regarding his symptoms and the activities that were associated with them. He recommended doing baseline pulmonary function tests and an **exercise challenge test**. The exercise test showed that Rich has reactive airways, and he was officially diagnosed with EIA. Rich was prescribed a Ventolin inhaler and was instructed to use it 20 to 30 minutes before exercising. In a letter to Luci, Dr. Jefferson also discussed the importance of doing a slow, gradual warm-up before his more intense training sessions.

EIA is generally diagnosed by the individual's clinical presentation and medical history. In some cases, an exercise challenge test with pre-spirometry and post-spirometry is conducted to diagnose and quantify the severity of the condition. The U.S. Olympic Committee requires a positive exercise challenge test to be documented for an athlete to be cleared for the use of controlled substances that prevent and alleviate EIA symptoms. Following baseline spirometry measurements, the athlete exercises on a treadmill or, in some cases, a bicycle ergometer, incrementally increasing the workload to 70% to 85% of the maximum predicted heart rate and then maintaining that workload for 6 to 10 minutes. Spirometry is then repeated at 2- to 10-minute intervals for 15 to 30 minutes and compared with baseline values. A 10% or greater reduction in $FEV_1$ or the $FEV_1/FVC$ ratio is diagnostic of EIA, with greater decrements indicating increased severity.

First-line medication treatment for EIA is use of short-acting $beta_2$-agonist medications, such as albuterol (e.g., Proventil and Ventolin), which are used to both treat and prevent symptoms. Individuals are frequently taught to prophylactically use a prescribed medication inhaler 20 to 30 minutes before beginning their exercise session. Some individuals may also be treated with long-acting $beta_2$ agonists (Salmeterol) and mast cell stabilizers such as cromolyn sodium (NasalCrom).

## Exercise and Asthma

Although asthma is not a contraindication to exercise, many people with asthma choose to avoid physical exertion because of the discomfort of shortness of breath and associated symptoms. Unfortunately, this avoidance of exercise results in significant deconditioning, increased risk for other chronic health conditions, and possible exacerbation of EIA symptoms when they do occur. A survey of adults with asthma reported that they had lower self-health ratings and greater perceived activity limitations than their nonasthmatic counterparts. Close to half of the adults with asthma reported that they avoid activities because of their symptoms. In addition, the number of overweight and obese individuals was greater in the asthma group, consistent with the lower level of reported physical activity. The survey also noted that less than one quarter of the respondents with EIA used a prophylactic therapy, such as an albuterol inhaler, before exercise.[5]

Furthermore, some people with EIA choose to deny symptoms and do not seek medical care because of embarrassment, peer pressure, fear of not being allowed to participate in the sport of their choice, and a variety of other reasons. Thus, the actual prevalence of EIA may be underreported.[6]

Although exercise and strenuous physical activities can trigger bronchoconstriction, regular exercise provides a number of benefits. Acute exercise stimulates the withdrawal of parasympathetic vagal tone and increased sympathetic nervous system stimulation. The resulting effect on airway smooth muscle is **bronchodilation**. Thus, brief intervals of acute exercise can lead to bronchodilation and be effective in reducing/reversing bronchoconstriction.[7] Because EIA is brought on by hyperventilation, individuals with asthma should be encouraged to undertake a gradual and prolonged intermittent warm-up and extended cool-down period. The prolonged, gradual warm-up period will allow some people to use the refractory period to lessen the bronchospastic response during subsequent higher-intensity exercise. In addition, it is important that people with asthma follow their medical provider's instructions for the use of prophylactic medications before exercise sessions.

## VIGNETTE I conclusion

■ The inhaler and prolonged warm-up session provided significant relief from Rich's EIA, and he was gradually able to increase his training intensity. Over the course of the season, Rich significantly improved his times and moved up to the number three spot on the team. With Luci's help, he learned to stay well hydrated and to reduce the intensity of his workouts or move indoors on days when the air quality was poor.

## Exercise Guidelines

Most people with controlled asthma will benefit from regular exercise and can follow exercise guidelines for the general population (Table 28-1). Exercise conditioning can help to reduce the ventilatory requirement for various tasks, making it easier for individuals with asthma to participate in normal daily activities, recreational events, and competitive sports. Regular exercise has been shown to improve exercise capacity, reduce exercise-induced bronchoconstriction and associated medication consumption, and improve psychosocial factors.[8,9]

There is also some evidence that increased physical fitness, resulting from exercise training, may decrease the risk for exacerbation and reduce the severity of exercise-induce asthma attacks.[10,11] Regular exercise training has been shown to have an anti-inflammatory effect in many chronic conditions, such as heart disease, chronic pain syndromes, rheumatological conditions, and others. Although this effect on the inflammatory response in individuals with asthma is less clearly defined, a recent study documented a reduction in airway inflammation following aerobic exercise training in a group of patients with asthma.[12,13] The results of these and other studies indicate that regular exercise training should be an important component of the treatment regimen for individuals with asthma.

As with all chronic conditions, people with asthma should be cleared by their physicians before beginning an exercise program. This allows the physician to provide the individual with a medication/treatment plan to prevent EIA attacks and a response plan to lessen the effects should an asthma attack occur. Only people with stable asthma should exercise without medical supervision. General activity guidelines for people with asthma include:

- Individuals diagnosed with asthma should have rescue medication with them at all times and be instructed on how to use it should symptoms occur. Some physicians will also instruct the person to use a bronchodilating inhaler before beginning an exercise session.
- People with asthma should be encouraged to drink plenty of fluids before, during, and after exercise to prevent dehydration.
- Asthma triggers should be avoided during exercise and consideration given to moving indoors on extremely hot or cold days, or when pollen counts and/or air pollution is high. Some individuals may benefit by wearing a face mask during exercise to help keep inhaled air warmer and humid.
- Gradual and prolonged warm-up and cool-down periods should be utilized.
- The initial intensity should be kept low and gradually increase over time. The peak exercise intensity should be determined according to the client's state of conditioning and asthma severity. Exercise intensity should be reduced if asthma symptoms begin to occur and the exercise session terminated if symptoms worsen.
- If an asthma attack is not relieved by medication, the emergency medical system should be activated.
- People with asthma often respond best to exercise in mid-to-late morning.
- Individuals with well-controlled asthma can typically use the exercise guidelines for the general population for cardiovascular and strength training.

## Table 28-1. General Beginner Exercise Program Guidelines for Individuals With Controlled Asthma

| MODE OF EXERCISE | FREQUENCY | INTENSITY | TIME/VOLUME | TYPE |
|---|---|---|---|---|
| Aerobic | 3–5 days/week | 40%–60% HRR/$\dot{V}O_2R$ RPE 3–5/10 scale | 30 min/day Intermittent, multiple bouts/day as needed | Walking, running, cycling, elliptical, swimming |
| Resistance | 2–3 days/week | 50%–60% 1RM RPE 5–6/10 scale | 2 sets 10–15 repetitions | Free weight or machine Functional may be best |
| Flexibility | Minimum 3 days/week | Mild discomfort | 15–60 sec/stretch 3–4 exercises/joint | Static/PNF/Dynamic |

HRR, heart rate reserve; PNF, proprioceptive neuromuscular facilitation; RPE, rating of perceived exertion; 1RM, one repetition maximum; $\dot{V}O_2R$, oxygen consumption reserve.

*Source:* Data from Durstine JL, Moore G, Painter P, Roberts S. *ACSM's Exercise Management for Persons With Chronic Diseases and Disabilities.* 3rd ed. Champaign, IL: Human Kinetics; 2009.

See Chapter 6 for additional information about asthma.

## In Your Own Words

Sam, a high school lacrosse player, has been coping with asthma since his childhood. He has become very tentative during preseason practice after experiencing an EIA attack when working out on his own during the summer. He is worried that he will not be adequately prepared for the upcoming season, but is scared to push himself too hard. How can you put Sam's mind at ease and help him become better prepared to avoid future episodes and to respond to episodes that do occur?

## CANCER

**Cancer** is the common term for a group of more than 100 diseases characterized by uncontrolled growth of abnormal cells that are capable of invading other tissues through the blood and lymph systems. Continued uncontrolled spread of these abnormal cells can result in death. As the second leading cause of death in the United States, cancer, or **malignant neoplasms**, caused 567,628 deaths in 2010 (these figures do not include the more than 1 million basal and squamous cell skin cancers that also occurred), a 0.06% decline from 2009. The combined total of deaths from heart disease and cancer represented 47% of all deaths in 2010. There are currently 12 million cancer survivors in the United States (5.5 million male and 6.5 million female survivors). It is estimated that 41% of individuals born in 2010 will be diagnosed with one or more cancer types in their lifetime.[14]

Since 2000, overall cancer rates have been gradually declining. Between 2004 and 2008, the rate of new cancer diagnosis decreased by an average of 0.6% per year for male individuals, whereas female individuals experienced a 0.5% decline per year from 1998 to 2006. Rates for female individuals leveled off from 2006 through 2008.[15] Although this is good news, the incidence of some cancer types has trended upward from 1999 through 2008. These cancer types include melanoma of the skin, kidney and renal, thyroid, pancreatic, liver, esophageal, adenocarcinoma, and human papillomavirus–related oropharynx.[15] Furthermore, because cancer is strongly associated with age, it has been estimated that the number of Americans diagnosed with cancer may significantly increase in the next 50 years because of the aging population. Concurrently, the number of cancer survivors will also significantly increase because of earlier detection and advanced treatment technology.

Cancer is characterized by uncontrolled growth and spread (**metastasis**) of cells within the body. Cancer begins in the cell, the body's basic unit of life. Normal cells grow and divide in an orderly, controlled fashion to produce new cells that replace old and/or damaged cells. Cancer cells develop when the DNA of normal cells is damaged, producing mutations that affect this orderly, controlled process. The damaged DNA and associated mutations result in uncontrolled cell growth, formation of tissue masses called **tumors**, and in some cases, metastasis to other areas of the body through the blood and lymph systems.

The growth of cancer tumors and spread of metastasized cells can eventually interfere with organ and organ system function, possibly leading to death. Although **malignant** cells typically metastasize, **benign** cells do not spread throughout the body and invade other tissues. However, like malignant neoplasms, benign tumors can pose a challenge when they grow too large and compress and/or interfere with vital organs, organ systems, and their important bodily functions.

## VIGNETTE II

■ Trinity is a 40-year-old mother of four boys who recently completed a year-long battle with breast cancer. Over the past 20 years, Trinity has gained quite a bit of weight as she has worked hard to raise her children. Over this period, Trinity has been physically inactive and has eaten a lot of high-calorie fast-food dinners while getting her boys to various activities. Trinity is concerned that the hormone medications she will be taking for the next several years are known to cause weight gain. Therefore, she sought out the help of Luci after hearing her speak at a support group for women coping with the aftermath of cancer treatment.

Assuming Trinity's oncologist has provided the clearance necessary for Trinity to work with Luci, how might Luci be able to help Trinity shed some weight without overdoing it in the early stages of recovery?

## Types and Causes of Cancer

Colon, pancreatic, prostate, and breast cancer are the most common forms of cancer in men and women. However, lung cancer accounts for more than 28% of cancer-related deaths and continues to be the leading cause of cancer death for both sexes. The most common types of cancer cases and causes of death for men and women are listed in Table 28-2. The 5-year survival rate for all cancers is currently estimated at 67%.[16] African Americans have lower survival rates (58%) for all cancers compared with other groups. However, the range of 5-year survival rates varies significantly

### Table 28-2. 2012 Estimated Top Cancer Types and Deaths

| ESTIMATED NEW CASES | | ESTIMATED DEATHS | |
|---|---|---|---|
| **MALE** | **FEMALE** | **MALE** | **FEMALE** |
| Prostate | Breast | Lung and bronchus | Lung and bronchus |
| Lung and bronchus | Lung and bronchus | Prostate | Breast |
| Colon and rectum | Colon and rectum | Colon and rectum | Colon and rectum |
| Urinary bladder | Uterine corpus | Pancreas | Pancreas |
| Melanoma of the skin | Thyroid | Liver and intrahepatic bile duct | Ovary |
| Kidney and renal | Melanoma of the skin | Leukemia | Leukemia |
| Non-Hodgkin's lymphoma | Non-Hodgkin's lymphoma | Esophagus | Non-Hodgkin's lymphoma |
| Oral cavity and pharynx | Kidney and renal | Urinary bladder | Uterine corpus |

Source: Data from the American Cancer Society.[16]

among cancer types, from a low of 6% for pancreatic cancer to 99% for prostate cancer that has not spread to distant parts of the body.

The cause of cancer is complex, because it is linked to many factors such as environmental exposures (e.g., pollutants, ultraviolet light, and chemicals), lifestyle practices (e.g., smoking, physical inactivity, alcohol use, and diet), medical interventions, viral infections, genetic traits, gender, and aging. In particular, smoking, obesity, and physical inactivity are associated with numerous cancer types. Thus, improving lifestyle practices by not smoking, being physically active each day, healthful eating, and minimizing alcohol intake and exposure to ultraviolet light are essential to decreasing a person's risk for cancer.

## V I G N E T T E   I I   continued

■ The first step in working with Trinity was to obtain some key information from her oncologist, Dr. Harkness. Luci wrote a note to Dr. Harkness asking the following questions:

• Are there any signs or symptoms that I should be aware of that would indicate a problem or need for immediate referral back to your office?

• What exercises are contraindicated? Is Trinity at any increased risk for fractures, anemia, bleeding, etc.?

• What are the long-term goals for Trinity?

• What is Trinity's long-term prognosis? What type of progress should I expect?

• Is Trinity on any medications that will affect her performance?

Not only does asking these questions improve the individualized care that Luci can provide to

Trinity, but it enhances Luci's credibility with the cancer care team. Dr. Harkness responds quickly, giving Luci the green light to begin training Trinity right away with a few restrictions, the most important of which is the need to be understanding of Trinity's low fitness level and the tendency to become severely fatigued after even mild exercise. The treatment has taken a tremendous toll on Trinity, so a very slow progression will be necessary.

## Treatment

A variety of invasive and noninvasive treatments for cancer are available, which are frequently used in combination. Common primary treatments include surgery, chemotherapy, radiation therapy, pharmacologic therapy, immunotherapy, hyperthermia, transplant therapy (bone marrow and stem cell), and targeted therapy using specialized chemotherapy agents that are designed to attack specific targets on cancer cells.

The primary treatment of cancer is frequently associated with significant negative side effects, both physical and emotional. Pain is relatively common and can be caused by the cancer itself or by treatments such as surgery and radiation. Medications, both over-the-counter NSAIDs and prescription narcotics such as opioids, may be prescribed to treat pain. Other common adverse effects to treatment interventions include nausea and vomiting, fatigue, anemia, lymphedema, infections, mental fogginess, peripheral neuropathy, skin irritation, hair loss, and weight loss.

Frequently, primary treatments are used in conjunction with each other (e.g., surgery and chemotherapy) to attack the tumor(s). Dietary counseling and exercise are also important components of the treatment program for most patients with cancer. In addition, secondary or complementary therapies may also be incorporated into the treatment regimen. These may include approaches such as acupuncture, aromatherapy, massage therapy, meditation, music therapy, prayer, and spirituality.

## VIGNETTE II *continued*

■ Luci starts Trinity on a low-intensity exercise program that consisted of walking and utilization of the facility's cross trainers, along with participating in the therapeutic yoga class that was specifically designed for people with chronic health conditions and those recovering from cancer interventions. Luci is also helping Trinity accept the current state of her physical abilities, because Trinity has been very upset about the medication-induced weight gain and her poor stamina even during slow walking. For Trinity, the focus should be on the process of becoming physically active without much concern for intensity or immediate weight loss.

## Exercise and Cancer

Research studies over the past two decades have shown that physical activity can help protect active people from acquiring some cancers (e.g., colon, prostate, endometrium, and breast cancer), either by balancing caloric intake with energy expenditure or by other means. An increased risk for development of cancer of the colon, prostate, endometrium, breast, and kidney has been linked to weight gain and obesity.[17–21] Although exercise has not been definitively shown to prevent other forms of cancer, an increasing body of literature indicates that it does play a significant role in improving the risk factors associated with cancer development.[17,20,22] There is some evidence that physical activity improves immune function,[23] and that improvement may be an additional benefit of exercise in the prevention and treatment of some forms of cancer. However, current research is not conclusive.

A growing body of literature supports the use of exercise to treat, reduce, and, in some cases, prevent some of the mental and physical challenges that cancer survivors frequently face. Traditionally, people being treated for, or recovering from, cancer were told to rest and to limit their physical activity. This reduction in activity and resulting loss of strength, endurance, and mobility only served to intensify the deterioration of physical and mental function, and accentuated the signs and symptoms related to cancer and associated treatments.

Research suggests that exercise training is not only safe and possible during cancer treatment, but also serves to maintain and/or improve physical function,

mental outlook, and quality of life.[24] Exercise benefits include preservation and improvement of muscle strength and endurance; improved balance and overall physical function; reductions in fatigue, nausea, anxiety, and depression; and decreased risk for heart disease, osteoporosis, and diabetes. Exercise training has also been associated with reduced risk for recurrence and increased survival in some types of cancer, particularly breast and colon cancer.[25,26] Exercise may positively impact survival in other types of cancer as well because of its effect on cardiovascular disease, diabetes, obesity, and other health risk factors. The primary objectives of exercise in the treatment of cancer include:

1. Avoid inactivity.
2. Maintain and improve cardiovascular conditioning.
3. Prevent musculoskeletal deterioration by maintaining and improving strength, balance, and mobility.
4. Improve body composition and associated body image.
5. Reduce/attenuate symptoms such as nausea and fatigue, and improve the individual's mental health outlook and overall quality of life.
6. Reduce or delay recurrence and/or the development of an additional primary cancer.
7. Improve physiological, psychological, and cognitive outcomes, and potentially lower morbidity and mortality associated with cancer.

## VIGNETTE II *conclusion*

■ As Trinity's base of conditioning improved, Luci gradually introduced some light resistance training. Over the course of the next few months, Trinity's strength and endurance continued to improve, and she was able to resume her normal activities with more vigor than before the cancer interventions. She chose to attend a special surfing camp in Hawaii for cancer survivors and was surprised to see how much more energy and vigor she had than other participants who had not been through a program similar to the one she participated in with Luci.

## Exercise Guidelines

In general, the physical activity guidelines adopted by the U.S. Department of Health and Human Services are applicable to cancer patient's pretreatment and posttreatment intervention.[27] However, basic conditioning, comorbidities, treatments, and treatment effects will vary widely among patients with cancer, necessitating an individualized approach. Thus, the specific exercise program undertaken will be tailored to the person's needs, cancer type, the specific treatments he or she is undergoing, and current medical and physical fitness status. Currently, treatment options for patients with cancer include surgery, radiation, and/or chemotherapy. These and other treatment regimens, such as hormonal and targeted therapies, have potential adverse effects that health and fitness professionals must be cognizant of to take the appropriate precautions.

Because treatment therapies are constantly changing, participation of the patient's health-care provider(s) in developing an exercise program is important so the potential effects of the various interventions on the patient are fully understood and appropriate adaptations are made. Such individualization is important, because activity that may be of low intensity for one client with cancer may be high intensity for another of the same age and sex.

Generally, the training protocol will center on aerobic activities, light strength training, and stretching, and be supplemented with recreational activities (Table 28-3). Some people undergoing chemotherapy and/or radiation can become anemic and require reduced exercise intensity, whereas others may have compromised skeletal integrity that may prevent weight-bearing activities. Thus, each patient is always individually assessed and a specific individualized program developed.

General guidelines for patients with cancer include (also review the American College of Sports Medicine Roundtable on Exercise Guidelines for Cancer Survivors for additional information)[20]:

1. People with cancer should obtain physician clearance before starting an exercise program. Physicians may choose to refer the patient to a physical therapist and/or clinical exercise physiologist for initial program development and monitoring. The referral should include any specific exercise recommendations, activities that should be avoided, and other precautions.
2. It is important that the patient with cancer starts slowly and builds gradually, with a primary focus on duration more than intensity. Intermittent activity with frequent rest breaks may be most appropriate.
3. Intensity should be light-to-moderate depending on the patient's condition and responses to treatment and activity. Intensity may vary day to day based on treatments and related fatigue.
4. Patients with cancer that is in remission may be able to exercise at higher intensities with physician approval.
5. Resistance training will generally use light weights with 1 or 2 sets of 10 to 15 repetitions. Proper technique is essential, and movements should be slow and purposeful.
6. Proper warm-up and cool-down periods that include light stretching and range-of-motion activities should be performed.
7. Patients with cancer who are experiencing numbness in the feet and/or balance challenges are at greater risk for falls. Uneven surfaces and/or any weight-bearing exercise that could cause a fall and injury should be avoided. Stationary equipment, such as elliptical trainers and cycles, may be better than treadmills or outdoor walking.
8. To avoid irritation, patients with cancer should not expose skin that has had radiation to the chlorine in swimming pools.
9. Patients with cancer should be encouraged to eat a balanced diet and drink plenty of fluids. Patients may benefit from counseling provided by a registered dietician and should discuss this with their physician.

## Exercise Precautions

The following precautions should be taken with regard to exercise in individuals with cancer:

1. Women undergoing treatment for breast cancer who experience arm or shoulder discomfort should be cleared by their physician before beginning upper-body exercise training.

## Table 28-3. General Beginner Exercise Program Guidelines for Individuals With Cancer

| MODE OF EXERCISE | FREQUENCY | INTENSITY | TIME/VOLUME | TYPE |
|---|---|---|---|---|
| Aerobic | 3–5 days/week | 40%–50% HRR/$\dot{V}O_2R$ RPE 3–5/10 scale | 20–60 min/day | Walking, cycling, rowing elliptical, water exercise |
| Resistance | 2–3 days/week | 30%–40% 1RM RPE 3–4/10 scale | 1–2 sets 10–15 repetitions | Free weight or machine Resistance bands Functional may be best Include balance training |
| Flexibility | Daily | Mild discomfort | 15–60 sec/stretch 3–4 exercises/joint | Static/PNF/Dynamic |

HRR, heart rate reserve; PNF, proprioceptive neuromuscular facilitation; RPE, rating of perceived exertion; 1RM, one repetition maximum; $\dot{V}O_2R$, oxygen consumption reserve.
*Source:* Data from Durstine JL, Moore G, Painter P, Roberts S. *ACSM's Exercise Management for Persons With Chronic Diseases and Disabilities.* 3rd ed. Champaign, IL: Human Kinetics; 2009.

2. Patients with anemia should not exercise without physician clearance and may require reduced intensity levels.

3. Patients with low white blood cell counts and those taking medications that may reduce their ability to fight infection should consider avoiding public gyms and places, and exercise at home.

4. Caution should be taken when working with patients with bone metastases who are at increased risk for skeletal fractures. Adjustments should be made to intensity, duration, and the type of exercise to minimize fracture risk. Certain medication treatments may also increase fracture risk.

5. Patients with colon cancer with an ostomy should have physician clearance before beginning weight training and should also refrain from contact activities/sports.

6. Patients who have experienced frequent vomiting and/or diarrhea may be dehydrated and in mineral imbalance, and should be encouraged to drink lots of fluids and check with their physicians before resuming exercise training.

7. Swollen ankles, unexplained weight gain, and/or shortness of breath at rest or with limited exertion are abnormal responses and should be reported to the patient's physician.

8. Patients should be cautioned to watch for bleeding, especially those taking blood thinners, and should avoid activities that increase the risk for fall and physical contact.

9. Patients with cancer should not exercise if they experience unrelieved pain, nausea/vomiting, or any other symptom of concern. Exercise should be postponed until their physicians can evaluate the situation and provide activity clearance.

10. Patients with cancer who have a catheter should avoid water exercise and other exposures that may cause infections. They should also avoid resistance-training exercises that involve the area of the catheter to protect against dislodging it.

11. Current guidelines recommend that people should not exercise within 2 hours of chemotherapy or radiation therapy treatment, because exercise-associated increases in circulation may impact the effects of therapy.

## In Your Own Words

Training clients who have cancer requires thoughtful preparation and working closely with their health-care providers. Although exercise is often recommended for individuals who are undergoing cancer treatment, physical activity is often curtailed because of fatigue and discomfort. How would you talk with a client who is being treated for cancer and feels discouraged by feelings of being physically drained? What considerations would you make to ensure that this client participates in appropriate exercise without overdoing it?

## OSTEOPOROSIS

Bone is a living tissue that consists of three primary components: (1) an organic component (type I collagen) that provides a flexible framework for bone, (2) an inorganic component (calcium-phosphate minerals) that provides strength and hardness, and (3) a water component. Bone continually goes through a process of bone resorption and formation. This process is coordinated by specialized cells called **osteoclasts** (bone resorption) and **osteoblasts** (bone formation). During the early growth years, the rate of bone formation is typically greater than the rate of bone resorption, resulting in an overall gain in bone mineral. This "remodeling" balance can be disrupted in children and young adults by smoking, poor nutrition, physical inactivity, certain medications, and conditions such as anorexia and bulimia. This disruption of the normal remodeling balance sets people up for early onset of **osteopenia** and **osteoporosis**, and places them at greater risk for fractures.

Osteoporosis is a preventable chronic and progressive disease that is characterized by low bone mass and disrupted microarchitecture (Fig. 28-3). Osteoporosis is one of the most prevalent public health issues in the United States and the most common metabolic bone disease (Fig. 28-4). Defined as a **bone mineral density (BMD)** that is 2.5 standard deviations (SDs) or more less than the mean for young adults, osteoporosis affects more women than men. It is estimated that 9.1 million women and 2.8 million men have BMD values 2.5 SDs or more below the mean.[28]

The World Health Organization criteria[29] reference T-scores in their guidelines for diagnosing osteoporosis, such that a T-score represents BMD compared with what is normally expected in a healthy, young adult of the same sex and an ideal BMD, with a normal value being more than −0.1. Therefore, when a T-score is greater than −1, BMD is considered normal. A T-score

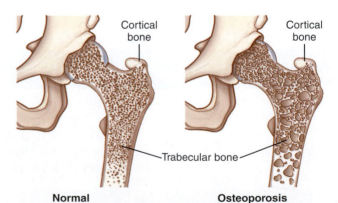

**Figure 28-3.** Normal bone and osteoporotic bone. Notice the differences within the bone architecture: The trabecular bone in this image is much different in osteoporotic bone compared with normal bone. This will significantly affect bone mass. Trabecular bone is more greatly affected as the severity of osteoporosis progresses with age.

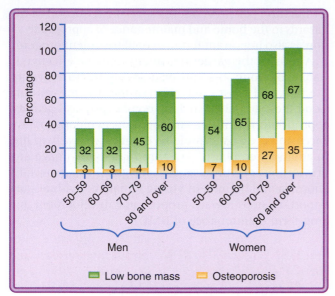

**Figure 28-4.** Relative percentage of men and women, aged 50 years and older, diagnosed with either osteoporosis or low bone mass (measured at the neck of the femur or lumbar spine) in the United States. *(Reproduced from Looker AC, Borrud LG, Dawson-Hughes B, Shepherd JA, Wright NC. Osteoporosis or low bone mass at the femur neck or lumbar spine in older adults: United States, 2005–2008. NCHS data brief no 93. Hyattsville, MD: National Center for Health Statistics; 2012.)*

## VIGNETTE III

■ Throughout her middle school and high school years, Mandy participated in gymnastics and was on the cheerleading squad. A thin, talented, and dedicated gymnast, Mandy trained hard to become successful. As she moved through puberty, Mandy began to gain weight, and her body began to demonstrate other physical changes that made some of her gymnastic activities more difficult. Her coaches began to criticize her about her weight gain. This caused Mandy, now 14 years old, to significantly cut back on her eating and add in a run each evening to try to keep her weight "under control." After a lot of pressure from her parents, Mandy finally agreed to meet with Luci for some help with getting her eating and exercise routine back into balance.

How might Luci be able to help, and what issues might Mandy be contending with as a result of her strict routine?

between −0.1 and −2.5 is a sign of osteopenia, a condition in which BMD is below normal and may lead to osteoporosis. Similar to prediabetes and prehypertension, people with osteopenia are at a greater risk for fracture and further bone deterioration to the level of osteoporosis. When the T-score is less than −2.5, it indicates osteoporosis.

Similar to hypertension being referred to as the "silent killer," osteoporosis is considered a "silent thief" in that the condition may not be recognized before bone deterioration is clinically significant. In some people, the occurrence of a fracture is the stimulating event for diagnosis of their osteoporotic condition.

Low BMD and associated deterioration in bone microarchitecture result in structural weaknesses and an increased risk for fractures. Each year, more than 2 million people suffer an osteoporotic fracture, and it is estimated that 50% of all women and 25% of all men older than 50 years will suffer an osteoporotic fracture within their lifetime.[30] Although fractures can occur in any bone, the most common sites are the proximal femur or hip, the vertebrae or spine, and the distal forearm or wrist. The consequences of hip and spine fractures are significant, especially in older Americans. Women with a hip fracture have a fourfold risk for incurring another fracture, and mortality in people older than 50 years during the first year following a hip fracture has been reported to be an average of 24% for both sexes combined.[28] Hip fractures increase exponentially with age because of bone density declines, loss of muscle strength, and poor balance. Falls are responsible for more than 90% of all hip fractures.[31]

Up to 90% of peak bone mass is acquired by age 18 years in girls and by age 20 years in boys, after which the amount of bone formation may not keep pace with the amount of bone being resorbed.[32] This imbalance between bone resorption and formation tends to accelerate as people age, resulting in a net loss of bone—approximately 5% to 10% per decade following achievement of peak bone mass. Bone loss is particularly pronounced in women following menopause and can also be affected by numerous other factors throughout the life span (Fig. 28-5). Age-associated bone loss is one reason why young female athletes must be particularly cautious about avoiding the **female athlete triad** (i.e., disordered eating, amenorrhea, and osteoporosis; for

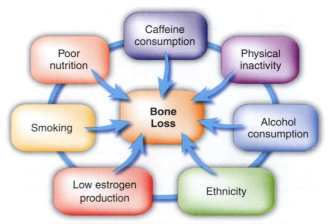

**Figure 28-5.** Common factors that affect the rate of bone loss with aging.

more information on the female athlete triad, see Chapter 23). Given the natural progression of decreasing BMD with age, young athletes should focus on attaining as much bone mineral as possible during their formative years so that they approach midlife with adequate stores of BMD.

The most common technology used to measure BMD is **dual-energy x-ray absorptiometry (DEXA)**. This technology uses a low-dose x-ray that emits photons at two different energy levels. These photons are subsequently absorbed by the various body tissues, and the amount of energy uptake by those tissues is used to calculate related densities. Along with bone density, DEXA is also frequently used to measure body composition. Other technologies are sometimes used, such as **quantitative computed tomography (QCT)** and **quantitative ultrasound (QUS)**, but DEXA is considered the gold standard.

Osteoporosis is both progressive and silent in that there are no typical symptoms that occur during the early and middle stages of the disease that alert a person of its presence. Frequently, the first sign of the disease is an unexpected fracture. As people age, the disease may become visually apparent with a loss of height and postural changes such as **Dowager's hump (hyperkyphosis)** (Fig. 28-6). In some people, bones can become so compromised that even minor movements, such as coughing, bending, sitting, standing, and hugging, result in painful fractures and increased immobility. This advanced level of osteoporosis may be associated with daily chronic pain and significantly reduced mobility and quality of life.

## Treatment

Lifestyle modifications, pharmacological interventions, and strategies to minimize fracture risk are the primary treatment components for people with osteopenia and osteoporosis. Lifestyle interventions include regular weight-bearing exercise, optimization of nutritional intake (especially calcium and vitamin D), smoking cessation, moderation of alcohol and caffeine intake, and strategies that minimize fracture risk. A variety of medications are also approved and used in the treatment of osteoporosis, including selected estrogen receptor modulators, bisphosphonates, calcitonin, and some injectable medications that are used in women at high risk

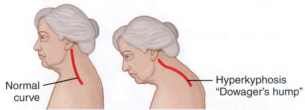

Normal curve — Hyperkyphosis "Dowager's hump"

**Figure 28-6.** Hyperkyphosis, or Dowager's hump, is a possible postural outcome of osteoporosis that can lead to problems with breathing, balance issues, and decreased functional mobility.

for fracture. Fall prevention, especially reduction of trip hazards in the home and maintenance of appropriate vision, is also important to the overall treatment program.

Although the earlier treatments may be effective in stabilizing bone loss and/or delaying fracture events, the best and most effective treatment is prevention. Good lifestyle habits such as regular physical activity, appropriate nutritional intake, and avoidance of tobacco and drug use should be emphasized early in life. In addition, emphasis on appropriate body image and prevention of unnecessary weight loss, especially anorexia and bulimia in young female individuals, are important steps toward proper bone development and long-term maintenance of BMD.

## VIGNETTE III continued

■ As a 14-year-old girl, Mandy's increased training and reduced eating place her at risk for development of osteopenia and eventually osteoporosis. Luci explains to Mandy and her parents that Mandy's skeleton is still growing and developing, and that she is 5 to 10 years away from reaching her peak bone mass. The reduced nutritional intake and increased training will significantly impact her body's ability to formulate additional BMD and, if continued over time, can result in a significant bone demineralization and osteoporosis.

## Exercise and Osteoporosis

Regular weight-bearing exercise is essential throughout a person's life span to optimize bone development and maintain balance in the bone remodeling process. Avoidance of physical inactivity should be stressed at all ages, because there is a direct link to the development of osteopenia, osteoporosis, and many other chronic health conditions. Regular aerobic exercise and resistance training, as recommended in the *2008 Physical Activity Guidelines for Americans,* will promote bone health and strengthen the musculoskeletal system to prevent falls and other potential fracture events. See Table 28-4 for a general physical activity program designed for individuals with osteoporosis.

Although the optimal strategy for preserving bone health remains unclear, it is known that physical stress determines the strength of bone. Mechanical stress applied to bone results in a small deformation, or bending, of bone, referred to as strain. This response to bone loading, known as "Wolff's Law," stimulates bone deposition and associated gains in bone mass and strength. Forces that result in bone strain are easily induced via impact with the ground. For this reason, weight-bearing exercise (such as jogging, hopping, skipping, jumping, and other plyometric exercises) is recommended and

**Table 28-4. General Beginner Exercise Program Guidelines for Individuals With Osteoporosis**

| MODE OF EXERCISE | FREQUENCY | INTENSITY | TIME/VOLUME | TYPE |
|---|---|---|---|---|
| Aerobic | 3–5 days/week | 40%–70% HRR/$\dot{V}O_2R$ RPE 3–5/10 scale | 30–60 min/day | Weight-bearing, low-impact exercise Water exercise for those with poor balance and high risk for fracture Jogging as tolerated |
| Resistance | 2–3 days/week | 60%–75% 1RM RPE 6–7/10 scale | 2 sets 8–12 repetitions | Free weight or machine Resistance bands Balance exercises included |
| Flexibility | Daily | Mild discomfort Care with stretch for those with high risk for fracture | 15–60 sec/stretch 3–4 exercises/joint | Static/Dynamic |

HRR, heart rate reserve; RPE, rating of perceived exertion; 1RM, one repetition maximum; $\dot{V}O_2R$, oxygen consumption reserve.
*Source:* Data from Durstine JL, Moore G, Painter P, Roberts S. *ACSM's Exercise Management for Persons With Chronic Diseases and Disabilities.* 3rd ed. Champaign, IL: Human Kinetics; 2009.

can be incorporated into a variety of games and activities. However, it is important to note that the type of activity chosen will depend on the physical and medical condition of each individual client.

The intensity of the loading force is a key determinant of the bone response to exercise. Bone-loading forces should be above those incurred with general activities of daily living, because higher stress results in greater strain. Bone's response to strain is also dependent on the frequency of loading, with higher-intensity loads requiring less frequency than lower-intensity loads. Shorter, frequent loading cycles have been shown to be more effective in increasing bone strength than longer single sessions. Improvement has been demonstrated with loading cycles ranging from 5 to 50 impacts per session.[33] Therefore, frequent sessions of multiple brief loading that are separated by a few hours of recovery may have the greatest impact on bone formation.

Resistance training is also an important component in the prevention of osteoporosis, depending on the person's physical condition and medical profile. Higher-intensity strength-training exercises (70%–80% one repetition maximum,1RM) may stimulate the most benefit to bone, and the associated improvements in strength assist in reducing the risk for falling.[34]

Other exercise activities such as tai chi and yoga, and other modalities such as stationary bicycling and rowing machines may also be beneficial. Because bone health is dependent on the regular forces placed on the musculoskeletal system, people of all ages should be encouraged to participate in regular, daily physical activity. This is especially important in the prevention of osteoporosis because of the lack of early symptoms associated with the condition and because it is challenging to reestablish optimal bone health once a person has progressed along the downward spiral of reduced BMD and loss of structural integrity.

## In Your Own Words

Your new middle-aged client hires you, prompted by her physician, to become more physically active to improve bone health and protect against osteoporosis. Upon reviewing your exercise plan, the client appears hesitant to continue, claiming that she understands the importance of the walking and balance-training components of the program, but she is not enthused about the resistance-training exercises you have recommended. How would you explain the importance of resistance exercise for bone health?

Because many individuals with osteoporosis are older, resistance exercises may need to be modified and some activities avoided, based on the individual's medical condition. For example, to prevent further injury and falls, some people with advanced osteoporosis (e.g., those with spinal and other fractures) may need to avoid:
- Spinal flexion, crunches, and rowing machines
- Jumping and high-impact aerobics
- Trampolines and step aerobics
- Abducting or adducting the legs against resistance
- Pulling on the neck with hands behind the head
- Other activities that have a high risk for falling

## VIGNETTE III *conclusion*

■ Mandy's coaches took the wrong approach by discussing their concern about her increasing body weight, which is a normal maturational process that she was undergoing. By doing so, they placed Mandy at risk for development of significant disordered eating patterns and increased her risk for bone loss and osteoporosis. Mandy is already participating in weight-bearing exercise. Luci points out that Mandy is exercising excessively and needs to reduce her training and meet with a dietitian to revamp her dietary habits. With the right approach, Mandy can continue to be a successful athlete and significantly decrease her risk for bone-related conditions. To work toward these goals, Mandy and her parents agree to have Mandy begin a training program with Luci while also consulting the registered dietitian whom Luci recommended.

## ARTHRITIS AND FIBROMYALGIA

**Arthritis**, a chronic condition that is characterized by inflammation and associated joint pain, affects more than 50 million adults in the United States, a number that is projected to increase to 67 million by 2030.[35] Arthritis is the most common cause of disability, with just more than 21 million people diagnosed with arthritis reporting significant activity limitations each year. Overall prevalence is higher in women (24.3%) than in men (18.7%), among obese and overweight individuals,

and in physically inactive people. Prevalence also increases with age in both sexes, and it is estimated that 294,000 children younger than 18 years have some form of arthritis or rheumatic condition.[36]

Although the term *arthritis* means "joint inflammation," it is typically used in a general sense to categorize more than 100 different types of diseases and conditions that affect the tissue surrounding the joints. The two primary forms of arthritis are **osteoarthritis (OA)**, a degenerative joint disease that leads to deterioration of cartilage and the development of bone growth (spurs) at the edges of joints and inflammation, and **rheumatoid arthritis (RA)**, a chronic and systemic inflammatory disease (Fig. 28-7). Other common conditions frequently classified under the arthritis "umbrella" are lupus, gout, and fibromyalgia.

Although it is considered an arthritis-related condition, fibromyalgia is not truly a form of arthritis, because it does not cause inflammation or associated damage to the joints, muscles, and/or soft tissues. However, it is considered a rheumatic condition because it impairs the joints and/or soft tissues and is associated with chronic pain.

Fibromyalgia is more common in women than in men (7:1 ratio) and typically strikes between the ages of 30 and 50 years. It is estimated that 3% to 5% of adult women and 0.5% of adult men have a fibromyalgia diagnosis.[37] It has been hypothesized that fibromyalgia results when a genetically susceptible individual comes in contact with some environmental trigger that sets symptoms in motion. However, the exact cause of fibromyalgia remains unclear. Many people with

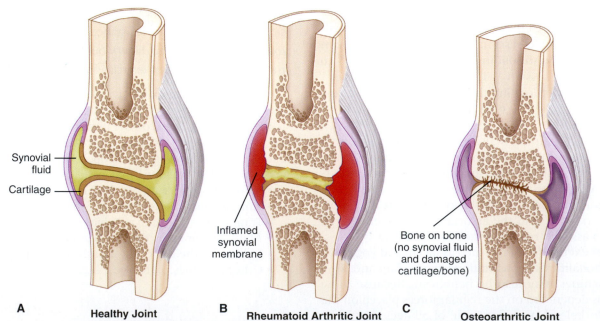

**Figure 28-7.** Rheumatoid arthritis and osteoarthritis. A, In a healthy joint, there is an appropriate amount of joint space, healthy cartilage, plenty of synovial fluid present, and no bone damage or inflammation. B, Rheumatoid arthritis is marked by an increased amount of inflammation in the synovial membrane, decreased joint space, and some bone and cartilage damage. This disorder can also cause deformity in the joint as well. C, In osteoarthritis, there is marked bone and cartilage damage and bony overgrowth. This disorder can progress to bone-on-bone contact, limiting appropriate joint space.

fibromyalgia attribute the onset to a stressor, such as an acute injury, illness, surgery, or long-term psychosocial stress.

## VIGNETTE IV

■ Giselle is a 58-year-old obese woman who suffers from significant joint pain, especially in her feet, knees, hips, and lower back. Her 5'8" frame supports 280 lb. Giselle has difficulty sleeping, leads a sedentary lifestyle, and has continued to stay at home now that her children are grown. She has been diagnosed with arthritis, fibromyalgia, type 2 diabetes, and hypertriglyceridemia.

How might exercise and weight loss positively affect Giselle's overall health?

## Rheumatoid Arthritis

RA, the most crippling form of arthritis, affects approximately 1% of the world's population. It is three times more common in women than in men, and although it most commonly affects people in their sixties, RA can strike at any age.[38] Classified as an autoimmune disease, RA is a systemic inflammatory condition or "polyarthritis" that affects multiple joints in the body and can also affect other organs. RA is characterized by an inflammatory process that primarily targets the synovial membrane of the affected joints, resulting in cartilage and bone erosion and, in some cases, joint deformity.

Although the exact cause of RA remains unknown, it may be the result of an abnormal immune response. Other genetic dispositions, infection, and hormonal changes may also be linked, but the definitive causes are currently still under investigation. Common symptoms include joint pain, redness, swelling, stiffness (especially morning stiffness), and, in more severe cases, contractures.

## VIGNETTE IV continued

■ Giselle's weight, high triglycerides, elevated blood glucose, and continued physical inactivity are major concerns and place her at high risk for the development of other chronic health conditions. After further evaluation, she was also diagnosed with both RA and OA. She was placed on a large variety of medications to treat her diabetes, chronic pain and inflammation, sleep issues, and depression/anxiety. She was also referred to the chronic disease program at the local medical fitness center, where she has begun working with Luci.

People with RA are also susceptible to a number of comorbidities, including coronary heart disease, serious infections such as tuberculosis, certain malignancies (e.g., multiple myeloma), and anxiety and depression. It is currently unclear whether the increased incidence of these conditions is directly related to the RA disease, other risk factors associated with the RA (e.g., hypertension, smoking, and immunosuppression), and/or the medications used to treat RA. However, it is important that these comorbidities are recognized and addressed as part of a comprehensive treatment plan.[39–41] Individuals with RA commonly undergo pharmaceutical treatment with nonbiological disease-modifying antirheumatic drugs (DMARDs), and in some cases, biological drugs are utilized. DMARDs work to suppress the immune system, which may slow the progression of the disease. Biological medications target a specific area of the immune system to reduce joint inflammation and are used to treat moderate-to-severe RA that cannot be controlled by DMARDs. These medications are prescribed to decrease disease activity and prevent joint deformity.[20] Exercise (including physical or occupational therapy, or both) and anti-inflammatory medications (e.g., NSAIDs, corticosteroids, and other analgesics) are also common elements of the treatment plan.

## Osteoarthritis

The most common type of joint disease, OA affects more than 27 million Americans.[28] This chronic condition is the result of articular cartilage breakdown that results in inflammation, bony overgrowth, and loosening and weakness of muscles and tendons. These changes limit movement, cause pain and swelling, and over time may progress to a level that allows bones in the affected joint to begin rubbing against each other. This joint degeneration is typically associated with overuse, trauma, obesity, and/or the degeneration of the joint cartilage that often occurs with aging. Other tissues can also be involved, such as ligaments, menisci, and muscles. Over time, the progressive damage may result in the need for joint replacement.

Despite the increasing prevalence of OA, the exact causes of the disease are not clearly understood, and currently there is no definitive cure for the condition. Some individuals will develop OA with no identifiable underlying cause or event, but the majority of cases are secondary to trauma, obesity, or both. Thus, OA has been divided into two types: (1) primary OA, which generally occurs later in life and is thus associated with age; and (2) secondary OA, which is associated with a traumatic event/injury and obesity, and occurs 10 or more years after the precipitating condition. Despite the association with age, not everyone experiences development of primary OA as they age. Although age does increase the likelihood or risk for development of OA, it is not a primary cause; OA is not part of the normal aging process, it is a disease.

OA primarily occurs in the knees, hips, and hands. However, it can also occur in other weight-bearing joints, such as the ankles, feet, and the cervical and lumbosacral spine, most commonly as the result of an injury. Increased body weight, a major global health issue, is strongly associated with the development of secondary OA, especially in the knees and hips. For every pound of weight gain, approximately 4 additional pounds of pressure are placed on the knees and close to 6 additional pounds of stress are placed on the hip joint.[42] Thus, it is not surprising that overweight individuals who lose weight also reduce their risk for development of OA.[43]

OA does not appear to be sex-specific, with both men and women equally affected. There does appear to be a genetic role in both the development and the progression of the disease. This is especially true in joints that do not fit together smoothly, affecting many, but not all, people who are double jointed and bow-legged. OA also appears to be more common in people who have weak musculature around joints, especially the knees.

The treatment of OA frequently includes nutrition counseling and weight control, physical and/or occupational therapy, warm-water exercise, medications, and surgery, depending on type and severity of arthritis.

## Fibromyalgia

**Fibromyalgia** is classified as a syndrome characterized by long-lasting widespread pain and tenderness at specific points on the body. The term *fibromyalgia* comes from the Latin roots "fibro" (connective tissue fibers), "my" (muscle), "al" (pain), and "gia" (condition of), and the term *syndrome* refers to a group of signs and symptoms that occur together and characterize an abnormality. Although they are not defining characteristics, sleep disturbances and fatigue are also integral symptoms of fibromyalgia.

Chronic pain syndromes such as fibromyalgia can present challenging and frustrating therapeutic dilemmas for physicians and patients. Fibromyalgia syndrome is not new. Centuries ago, Hippocrates described a condition he observed in patients with diffuse, musculoskeletal pain that resembled fibromyalgia. In 1816, William Balfour, a surgeon at the University of Edinburgh, described similar symptomatology in his patients. In 1904, William Gowers labeled this collection of symptoms "fibrositis," a somewhat misleading term because fibromyalgia is not characterized by inflammation as most types of arthritis are. In 1976, Dr. P. Kahler Hench coined the term "fibromyalgia syndrome" to better reflect the true nature of the condition.[38]

The most common symptoms of fibromyalgia include aches and pains similar to flu-like exhaustion, multiple tender points, stiffness, decreased exercise endurance, fatigue, muscle spasms, and paresthesias. Aches and pains are generally widespread and diffuse, fluctuating in intensity, and frequently are accompanied by marked stiffness. Other symptoms commonly described include excessive fatigue, disruptive sleep patterns, bowel and bladder irritability, anxiety, depression, cognitive difficulties, temporomandibular joint syndrome, sensitivity to loud noises, and "allergic" symptoms such as nasal congestion and rhinitis.

Accurately diagnosing fibromyalgia is challenging, because no definitive test or markers exist to make the diagnosis. Instead, the diagnosis is based on nonspecific, generalized symptoms such as pain, fatigue, and sleep disturbances. The American College of Rheumatology initially developed criteria for the diagnosis of fibromyalgia in 1990 that were characterized by a history of widespread pain occurring for longer than 3 months in combination with pain on palpation of 11 of 18 tender point sites.[44] However, the tender-point evaluation has been a bit problematic in that some physicians do not perform the evaluation correctly and others have chosen not to do it, but instead base the diagnosis strictly on symptoms. These challenges, as well as others, led to a multicenter study of patients with fibromyalgia and subsequent development of a simplified set of criteria. The new criteria, published in 2010 by Wolfe and colleagues,[45] do not require the tender-point evaluation, but instead use a widespread pain index and symptom-severity scale.

Because the primary cause of fibromyalgia remains unknown, there is no one definitive treatment for it. The typical treatment program includes a variety of modalities, including the following:

- Exercise
- Nutritional counseling
- Weight management
- Treatment of any underlying sleep disorder
- Allergy testing and treatment
- Stress management or relaxation techniques such as "mindful-based stress reduction"
- Massage therapy
- Medications such as analgesics, NSAIDs, selective serotonin reuptake inhibitors, tricyclic antidepressants, muscle relaxants, and others

People with fibromyalgia, like people with other arthritic and chronic pain conditions, are typically deconditioned and tend to shy away from exercise because of fear of exacerbating symptoms and the level of fatigue. Unfortunately, this lack of physical activity becomes a downhill spiral that produces further declines in fitness and results in lower levels of exertion that bring on fatigue and pain. Studies have shown that exercise is beneficial for people with fibromyalgia, easing symptoms and preventing the development of other chronic conditions associated with physical inactivity.[46] Aerobic exercise has an analgesic and antidepressant effect that can significantly reduce the pain, depression, and anxiety frequently associated with fibromyalgia.[47]

## Exercise and Arthritic and/or Inflammatory Conditions

Regular physical activity and exercise conditioning are an essential part of the therapy program for people with arthritis and fibromyalgia. In addition, physical inactivity increases the risk for coronary artery disease, diabetes, and other chronic health conditions, and the decreased bone loading that occurs with prolonged physical inactivity increases the risk for osteoporosis and associated bone fractures. See Table 28-5 for a general physical activity program for individuals with arthritis or other chronic inflammatory conditions.

Thus, people with arthritis and fibromyalgia should do everything they can to avoid inactivity. A consistent exercise program that promotes cardiovascular fitness, improved muscular strength and endurance, and stabilized joint mobility will break this downhill cycle and significantly improve daily function and associated quality of life. The *2008 Physical Activity Guidelines for Americans* emphasized the importance of physical activity for people with chronic conditions such as arthritis and fibromyalgia.[22] In 2010, "A National Public Health Agenda for Osteoarthritis" was released by the Centers for Disease Control and Prevention and the Arthritis Foundation that further emphasize the importance of regular physical activity. This call to action recommends that "low impact, moderate intensity aerobic physical activity and muscle strengthening exercise should be promoted widely as a public health intervention for adults with OA of the hip and/or knee."[48]

The safest and most effective activities for people with arthritis and fibromyalgia are low-impact, moderate-intensity aerobic activities that minimize stress on the affected joints. Activities such as walking on soft surfaces, pole walking, elliptical training, cycling, rowing, and water exercise (especially warm water) are generally recommended. In addition, muscle-strengthening activities are recommended at least 2 days a week to promote muscular strength and joint stability, and improve balance and coordination. People with hip or knee arthritis, or both, should avoid jarring exercises such as jogging and running, while those with elbow symptoms should avoid rowing.

Walking is an excellent activity, and the use of step pedometers or accelerometers can provide daily accountability for moving. After identifying the person's baseline daily step frequency, the device can be used to measure gradual increases in the number of daily steps taken. With or without the use of pedometers or accelerometers, the focus is on duration rather than the intensity of the activity, with a goal to gradually increase to 30 or more minutes on 5 or more days of the week.

Proper body alignment and exercise technique should be taught and emphasized at all times. Poor posture combined with reduced joint mobility and strength significantly impacts movement patterns, resulting in more rapid fatigue and greater risk for injury. In many cases, people with arthritis may be more limited by joint pain than by their cardiovascular function. Individuals with RA can experience periods of inflammatory flare-ups, and exercise is generally restricted during such times. Regular rest periods are also helpful during exercise sessions, making low-intensity interval training an exercise option.

Warm-water exercise can be especially beneficial for individuals with arthritis and fibromyalgia. The buoyant environment combined with the warm-water temperature is soothing to stiff and painful muscles and joints, and promotes physical conditioning. While gentle stretching is encouraged, it is very important that overstretching be avoided.

Although symptoms and fear may entice people with arthritic conditions to avoid physical activity, regular movement is a critical element of the treatment program and should be highly encouraged. Regular physical activity will improve function, pain, mood, and associated quality of life, and decrease the risk for development of other chronic conditions that may further impact the person's health and well-being.

**Table 28-5. General, Beginner Exercise Program Guidelines for Individuals With Osteoarthritis**

| MODE OF EXERCISE | FREQUENCY | INTENSITY | TIME/VOLUME | TYPE |
|---|---|---|---|---|
| Aerobic | 3–5 days/week | 40%–60% HRR/$\dot{V}O_2R$ RPE 3–5/10 scale | 30 min/day Intermittent, multiple bouts/day as needed | Low-impact exercise or non–weight bearing Warm-water exercise is very therapeutic |
| Resistance | 2–3 days/week | 40%–50% 1RM RPE 4–5/10 scale | 1 set 8–10 repetitions | Free weight or machine Resistance bands Functional exercises |
| Flexibility | Daily before regular exercise | Mild discomfort | 15–60 sec/stretch 3–4 exercises/joint | Static/Dynamic Pain-free ROM |

HRR, heart rate reserve; ROM, range of motion; RPE, rating of perceived exertion; 1RM, one repetition maximum; $\dot{V}O_2R$, oxygen consumption reserve.

*Source:* Data from Durstine JL, Moore G, Painter P, Roberts S. *ACSM's Exercise Management for Persons With Chronic Diseases and Disabilities.* 3rd ed. Champaign, IL: Human Kinetics; 2009.

## VIGNETTE IV conclusion

■ Giselle followed through with her physician's recommendation and enrolled in the chronic disease program with Luci at the medical fitness center. She began doing some warm-water exercise and over time progressed to pole walking. She found that the poles helped take some pressure off her joints and allowed her to gradually increase her walking distance. Giselle also worked with a dietitian to improve her eating habits, and the improved nutritional intake combined with the increased physical activity resulted in weight loss. Over the next year, Giselle remained consistent with her diet and exercise, and her weight dropped significantly to 214 pounds. She was also able to discontinue her oral diabetes medications.

## LOW-BACK PAIN

The lifetime prevalence rate of LBP has an average of 39% (±24% SD), with the variability depending on the surveyed population and the LBP definition (e.g., chronic vs. acute or nonspecific vs. specific).[49] One patient out of four presenting with an acute LBP episode is likely to experience a recurrence within 1 year.[49] Furthermore, approximately 10% of individuals with LBP will progress from acute to chronic LBP.[50]

LBP affects quality of life by interfering with recreational activities, daily living routines, and a person's ability to work productively. In the United States, healthcare costs among people with back pain increased by 65% from 1997 to 2005, which was more rapidly than the overall health-care costs, and accounted for 9% of the total health-care costs in 2005.[51] Today, the expenditures are likely higher. Back strain/sprain is one of the most common types of worker's compensation claims, and it significantly impacts an affected individual's productivity.[52] People with LBP are more likely to report symptoms of depression, anxiety, and sleep disruption. LBP is the number one disability for people younger than 45 years, and it is estimated that at any given time 1.2 million adults are disabled as a result of their LBP.[53] Thus, there is little wonder why reducing low-back injuries is a major safety focus of most employers.

Acute or short-term LBP typically lasts from a few days to a few weeks, and it is usually mechanical in nature. There are many causes of LBP, but no single explanation can be applied to everyone. Typical causes are trauma (e.g., sports injury, lifting, bending, reaching, or a sudden jolt such as in a car accident), certain disorders such as arthritis, and aging. Periodically, LBP occurs for no specific identifiable reason. Symptoms vary, ranging from muscle ache and tightness to shooting or stabbing pain that may radiate to other parts of the body, such as the legs. Although symptoms can be severe for a few days, they will often significantly improve within 2 to 4 weeks.

Chronic back pain is generally defined as pain that persists for 3 or more months. It is usually progressive and the exact cause can be challenging to determine. In some people, the spine becomes overly strained or compressed, resulting in a disc rupture or outward bulge that places pressure on 1 or more of the more than 50 nerves rooted to the spinal cord. Other specific causes include conditions such as spinal stenosis, osteoporosis and associated fractures, spinal degeneration, and spinal irregularities (such as scoliosis, kyphosis, and lordosis). In addition, medical conditions such as pancreatitis, pneumothorax, prostatitis, tumors, and infections can also manifest symptoms of LBP.

LBP most frequently occurs between the ages of 30 and 50 years, but it can affect people of all ages. Figure 28-8 illustrates some of the most common risk factors for the development of LBP or reasons for delayed recovery from LBP. It is extremely important that well-rounded exercise and lifestyle programs address these risk factors versus focusing only on pain management. Prevention and recovery programs are much more successful when the root causes of LBP are targeted. In addition, the incidence of LBP in children and teenagers has increased, in part because of overloaded school backpacks, improper lifting techniques, poor posture, and the increased incidence of overweight and obesity.

Diagnosis is generally made by taking an extensive history of the problem, especially in acute situations where back pain has occurred for less than 4 weeks. In most cases of LBP, the use of imaging technology such as x-rays, computed tomography, and magnetic resonance imaging scans do not provide additional information that will alter the treatment plan. Thus, the use of routine imaging technology for nonspecific LBP is generally not recommended, and its use is reserved for more complicated, specific cases where

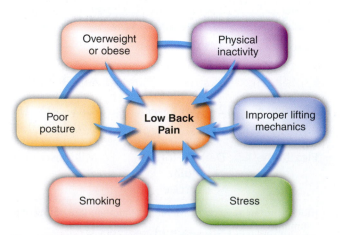

**Figure 28-8.** Common risk factors for development of low-back pain (LBP) and underlying factors that delay recovery from LBP.

## RESEARCH HIGHLIGHT

### Low-Back Pain and Obesity

Although the association between obesity and LBP is unclear, researchers have reported a linear correlation between increasing body mass index and LBP, especially in large-population studies.[54-56] There also appears to be a greater incidence of LBP in obese women versus obese men.[57,58]

Altered posture and a lack of spinal mobility could be underlying causes of LBP in obese individuals. Vismara et al[59] compared the spines of obese subjects with normal-weight control subjects and found significant differences at the lumbar, pelvic, and thoracic levels among the groups. Obesity seems to induce an increase in anterior pelvic tilt. The increased anterior pelvic tilt induces a greater flexion of the sacroiliac joints, which produces undue strain on the L5-S1 joint and surrounding intervertebral discs. This could lead to degenerative deterioration of those discs (i.e., degenerative disc disease). There have also been reports of increased lumbar lordosis in obese individuals with chronic LBP.[59,60] At the level of the thoracic spine, Vismara et al[59] found that range of motion during spinal forward flexion was significantly less in obese subjects and in obese subjects with chronic LBP as compared with normal-weight subjects. Stiffness in the thoracic spine translated to forward flexion performed mainly by the lumbar spine, which is most frequently involved in pain syndromes.

The postural differences noted earlier confirm the "kinetic chain" relationship of the musculoskeletal system. That is, if a joint experiences stiffness or immobility, nearby joints will sacrifice stability and become more mobile to ensure that important bodily movements occur. In the case of obesity, it appears that a rigid thoracic region along with a chronic anterior pelvic tilt forces the lumbar spine (the area located between the thoracic spine and the pelvis) to exceed its normal flexion capabilities, potentially leading to LBP. Vismara et al's[59] findings, along with others,[61,62] suggest that obese individuals should include strengthening of the lumbar and abdominal muscles, as well as mobility exercises for the thoracic spine and pelvis, to prevent or reduce chronic LBP.

Another biomechanical factor that could contribute to LBP in the obese population is increased abdominal circumference and its affect on the function of the muscles that support the spine. In fact, researchers have reported findings that suggest that abdominal obesity is the primary weight-related risk factor for LBP.[54,58] Increased abdominal mass shifts the body's center of gravity forward, farther away from the lumbar spine. The constant efforts of the erector spinae muscles to counteract the pull created by excess abdominal fat may jeopardize the muscles' function of reducing anterior shear forces on the lumbar spine.[63] Other effects of overworked erector spinae muscles include insufficient muscle force output, inappropriate neuromuscular activation, and muscular fatigue,[64] which are all detrimental to the stability of the spine.

A high concentration of abdominal adiposity could also indirectly increase the likelihood of LBP because it leads to the increased production of proinflammatory substances and is associated with dyslipidemia, which results in increased levels of circulating triglycerides and low-density lipoprotein. These factors play a major role in the development of atherosclerosis (the buildup of plaque in the arteries) in obese individuals.[65] Atherosclerosis could limit the amount of blood distributed to the spine and cause malnutrition of the disc cells,[66] which may contribute to disc degeneration. People with severe disc degeneration are more likely to have LBP.[67] These findings strengthen the argument for weight loss (especially the reduction of abdominal adiposity) in obese individuals as a treatment for LBP, because doing so can improve blood lipid profiles, allowing proper nourishment of the discs, and decrease the mechanical strain on the low back. In addition, strengthening the muscles of the trunk and performing regular aerobic endurance exercise are crucial for improving spine health.

*Please see reference list at the end of the chapter for cited references.*

interventional treatment (e.g., surgery or spinal injection) is being considered and for individuals who do not respond to conservative care.[68] Periodically, other tests such as an electromyogram and nerve conduction study will be used to evaluate potential muscle/nerve problems.

## VIGNETTE V

■ Howie is a 48-year-old customer service representative who spends much of his day seated at his computer. He has long struggled with LBP and has tried a number of back-strengthening programs over the years, most of which he heard about from friends or read in popular fitness magazines. Lately, he has been coping with tightness in his hips in addition to the LBP despite his ongoing attempts to work through the pain. He finally decided to seek out the help of a personal trainer.

How might Luci modify Howie's typical workouts to better address his back pain and hip tightness?

## Prevention and Treatment

Although there is no definitive evidence that LBP can be 100% prevented, certain lifestyle behaviors may reduce a person's chances of developing LBP and aid in fostering a more rapid recovery when acute situations arise. Regular physical activity and proper strength training that promotes good posture and core stability are important in maintaining good back health. Use of proper body mechanics (e.g., lifting techniques, sitting and standing posture, and avoiding sleeping positions that do not support the lower back) is vital. Many work-related LBP injuries are caused by repetitive lifting, twisting, and turning, especially with improper body mechanics. Proper nutritional intake, smoking cessation, minimizing the wearing of high-heeled shoes, and getting adequate rest are also important preventive strategies.

Treatment of LBP is typically based on the person's presenting condition and history. Conservative treatment is appropriate for most people diagnosed with acute nonspecific LBP. Approximately one third of these patients will experience improvement in less than 1 week and nearly two thirds will improve within the following 2 to 7 weeks. Treatment may include pain relievers such as acetaminophen and NSAIDs, ice application, massage, spinal manipulation, and light physical activity. Use of narcotics and muscle relaxants are also options, but generally are not recommended except in cases of severe pain. Treatment of chronic LBP lasting more than 3 months typically follows a similar pattern, although other modalities may be considered, such as spinal injections, transcutaneous electrical nerve stimulation, ultrasound, cognitive behavioral therapy, and acupuncture. Surgical intervention is generally reserved for the most severe cases, where conservative treatments have repeatedly failed and a specific cause has been identified (e.g., herniated disc or spinal stenosis).

### VIGNETTE V continued

■ Because most office workers tend to sit with poor posture, Luci spends her first meeting with Howie discussing ergonomics and teaching him how to modify his work station to improve his sitting posture and hopefully alleviate some of his back and hip issues. Howie has been focusing on improving back strength through resistance training, so Luci wants him to begin a more well-rounded routine. She therefore demonstrates stretches for the hip flexors and extensors, as well as several movements to address low-back stability and mobility, such as the unloaded cat/camel sequence exercise (Fig. 28-9). Other exercises, such as the

proper curl-up, the bird dog, and the plank, emphasize training of the muscles that support the spine while keeping the spine in a neutral position. It is important to perform the latter exercises with a neutral spine position to minimize compressive loads on the lumbar spine.

## Exercise and Low-Back Pain

Exercise is one of the cornerstones of both the prevention and the treatment of LBP. In fact, many medical professionals believe that a major cause of LBP is physical deconditioning, especially in large-muscle groups such as the back extensors.[69] Aerobic training and exercises for the low back and core musculature (i.e., spine-stabilizing musculature) should be performed on a regular basis, and proper technique for each exercise should be taught and practiced. Maintaining and improving muscle endurance (followed by strength) in the spine-stabilizing muscles is particularly important for people with LBP and will assist in developing and maintaining proper posture in all individuals.[70] Researchers have demonstrated that enhancing muscular endurance in the spine stabilizers is a better predictor

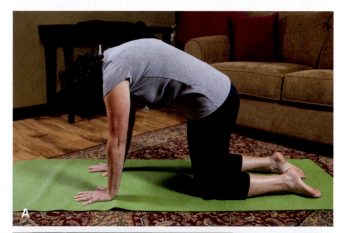

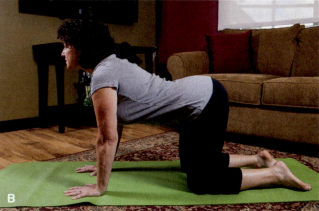

**Figure 28-9.** The unloaded cat/camel motion exercise is an example of an appropriate exercise to include in a low-back pain prevention or management program.

of successful recovery from LBP compared with strength capacity.[70] The reasoning may be that much of what these muscles are called on to do on a daily basis is to maintain spine position in an upright posture over the period of a normal day. This action directly speaks to endurance capacity, not strength, being most important to protect our spine day to day.

People who experience the pain and stiffness associated with LBP have a strong tendency to avoid physical activity and, in many cases, are advised to rest. However, in most cases, avoidance of movement only prolongs the recovery process; therefore, most people should be advised to stay active. Because there is no one single exercise program that fits all people with LBP, each person's symptomatic history and presenting condition is an important consideration in devising an appropriate individualized program. What is helpful for some people may exacerbate symptoms for another. Although medical providers typically refer patients with LBP to physical therapy, occupational therapy, and/or specialized programs in medical fitness centers, many people do not require specialized care and should be encouraged to begin with light exercise and gradually return to normal activity levels.

Cardiovascular (aerobic) training, resistance training, and basic core back exercises are the primary components of the exercise program and should be performed on a regular basis. Table 28-6 outlines a sample exercise prescription for the management of LBP and general guidelines to follow when designing these programs. Generally, people with LBP should avoid unsupported forward flexion; twisting at the waist with turned feet, especially when carrying or moving a load; lifting both legs and arms simultaneously when in a prone or supine position (e.g., the "Superman" exercise); and rapid movements, such as twisting, forward flexion, or hyperextension. Therapeutic aquatic exercise may be beneficial for some people with LBP, including those with pregnancy-related LBP.[71]

## VIGNETTE V conclusion

■ Howie had been performing his back-strengthening routine twice a week, but Luci advises him that he can safely perform the flexibility and stability program up to 7 days a week, as long as he uses good technique and follows the program they developed together. By combining a more ergonomic workstation with his new workout program, Howie is well on his way to overcoming the LBP that has long plagued him.

## PREGNANCY

For many years, the medical community encouraged pregnant women to reduce their physical activity and refrain from starting vigorous exercise programs because of concerns that exercise might harm the fetus. Early recommendations published in 1985 placed an upper heart rate limit of 140 beats/min on pregnant women, regardless of their current physical condition and exercise history.[72] Fortunately, since 1985, a large

**Table 28-6. General Beginner Exercise Program Guidelines for Individuals With Low-Back Pain**

| MODE OF EXERCISE | FREQUENCY | INTENSITY | TIME/VOLUME | TYPE |
|---|---|---|---|---|
| Aerobic | 3–5 days/week | 40%–60% HRR/$\dot{V}O_2R$ RPE 3–5/10 scale | 30 min/day Intermittent, multiple bouts/day as needed | Low-impact exercise (walking best) Warm-water exercise |
| Resistance | 2–3 days/week | 40%–60% 1RM RPE 4–6/10 scale | 2–4 sets 8–12 repetitions | Free weight or machine Core/spine stabilizer exercises Functional exercises |
| Flexibility | Daily | Mild discomfort | 15–60 sec/stretch 3–4 exercises/joint | Static/PNF/Dynamic Pain-free ROM Maintain neutral spine position Main focus on lower chain flexibility and less on lumbar spine ROM |

HRR, heart rate reserve; PNF, proprioceptive neuromuscular facilitation; 1RM, one repetition maximum; ROM, range of motion; RPE, rating of perceived exertion; $\dot{V}O_2R$, oxygen consumption reserve.
*Source:* Data from Durstine JL, Moore G, Painter P, Roberts S. *ACSM's Exercise Management for Persons With Chronic Diseases and Disabilities.* 3rd ed. Champaign, IL: Human Kinetics; 2009.

volume of research has shown that women who are pregnant can exercise safely, without harm to the fetus or themselves. The upper heart rate limit was relaxed by the American College of Obstetricians and Gynecologists (ACOG) in 1994, and a revision in 2002 encouraged all women who are experiencing healthy pregnancies to participate in regular physical activity.[72–74] Similar recommendations were published in Canada the following year, and in 2006, the American College of Sports Medicine released a Roundtable Consensus Statement providing evidence and recommendations in support of the safety of the **prenatal** (during pregnancy) and **postpartum** (after delivery) periods.[10,75] The expert panel made the following conclusions regarding exercise during pregnancy and the postpartum period:

- Exercise reduces the risk for **preeclampsia**.
- It treats or prevents gestational diabetes.
- Exercise helps manage or alleviate pregnancy-related musculoskeletal issues such as LBP, pregnancy-related incontinence, abdominal muscle disturbances, and joint and muscle injuries.
- It positively impacts mood and mental health. Many women experience mood changes during pregnancy and the postpartum period. Exercise has been shown to improve mood; increase vigor; reduce fatigue, stress, and anxiety; decrease depression; and improve self-concept.
- Exercise is safe and does not harm offspring health and development.

Women undergo a variety of physical changes during pregnancy that can limit the ability to exercise (Table 28-7). Total energy expenditure for a given workload is estimated by the resting energy expenditure plus the expenditure required to perform the workload. Resting energy expenditure significantly increases throughout pregnancy because of the increased metabolic demands of the uterus, placenta, and developing fetus, and the associated maternal body weight gain. Thus, a given workload will require a higher oxygen consumption ($\dot{V}O_2$) during pregnancy as compared with the nonpregnant state, and this increase in energy expenditure will gradually progress throughout the pregnancy term. The magnitude of the change in energy expenditure will be dependent on the exercise mode (weight-bearing or weight-supported), intensity, gestational age, and associated maternal weight gain.[76,77]

Along with impacting energy expenditure for a given workload, the average maternal weight gain of 25 to 40 pounds places additional stress on the joints of the back, pelvis, hips, and legs. As the fetus grows and weight gain occurs, the center of gravity moves upward and out, and these changes frequently result in low-back discomfort. Hormonal changes, particularly increased secretion of relaxin, result in joint laxity, creating an additional challenge to balance, coordination, and overall mobility, and further impacting the low back.

The increased resting $\dot{V}O_2$, or energy expenditure, parallels the increase in resting minute ventilation, primarily because of an associated increase in tidal volume. Generally, respiratory rate is minimally increased, but this can become more pronounced in some women as pregnancy advances. The increase in resting minute ventilation gradually rises throughout the pregnancy term as resting energy expenditure increases. Minute ventilation is also increased during submaximal exercise, with little to no increase at maximal exercise. Although the ventilatory threshold and respiratory compensation point occur at a similar percentage of peak $\dot{V}O_2$ as during nonpregnancy, the work rate may be reduced, especially during the second and third trimesters.[78–81] These respiratory changes are associated with increased resting and exercise dyspnea.

Although cardiovascular responses to exercise during pregnancy are similar to the nonpregnant state, the cardiac reserve, or the difference between resting and maximum cardiac function, is reduced in pregnant women. During the early months of pregnancy, hormonal signals stimulate increases in heart rate, blood volume, stroke volume, and cardiac output. As pregnancy progresses, blood volume increases 40% to 50%, stroke volume increases 10%, and heart rate increases 20%, resulting in just less than a 50% increase in cardiac output.[82] These cardiovascular changes enhance blood flow to the growing fetus and can make exercise more challenging for the pregnant mother. At submaximal workloads, stroke volume is increased, partly because of increased blood volume, and when combined with an increase in submaximal heart rate, this results in a higher cardiac output for a given workload. The increased cardiac output is necessary to meet the demand for increased $\dot{V}O_2$ associated with maternal weight gain and the developing fetus.

## Table 28-7. Physiological Changes From Pregnancy During Rest, Submaximal Exercise, and Maximal Exercise Conditions

| VARIABLE | RESTING | SUBMAXIMAL | MAXIMAL |
|---|---|---|---|
| Oxygen consumption ($\dot{V}O_2$) | Increased | Increased | Decreased |
| Minute ventilation ($V_E$) | Increased | Increased | No change |
| Cardiac output | Increased | Increased | Decreased |
| Heart rate | Increased | Increased | Increased |
| Stroke volume | Increased | Increased | Decreased |

After the first trimester, supine exercise activities are restricted or discouraged. Exercise in the supine position can potentially reduce venous return from the uterus caused by compression of the vena cava. The decreased blood flow and cardiac output can cause orthostatic hypotension.

The thermoregulatory system is also affected by pregnancy, resulting in a slight improvement in the women's ability to dissipate heat. This may be because of increased blood flow to the skin and increases in tidal volume. However, it is critical that the pregnant exerciser is aware of the ambient temperature before each workout and maintains appropriate hydration levels. Exercise increases body temperature, and increased ambient temperature and/or humidity may significantly affect a woman's ability to dissipate heat and could result in hyperthermia that could potentially harm the fetus. However, no reports have been published that hyperthermia associated with exercise causes malformations of the embryo or fetus.

## Exercise Guidelines for Pregnant Women

Recommendations from the American College of Sports Medicine, the Canadian Academy of Sport Medicine, the ACOG, the Society of Obstetricians and Gynaecologists of Canada, the Royal College of Obstetricians and Gynaecologists, and others have concluded that physician-guided exercise is beneficial during and after pregnancy, and poses minimal risk for the fetus and exercising woman.[10,74,83,84] See Table 28-8 for the ACOG and other guidelines for exercise during uncomplicated pregnancy.[74] High levels of exercise intensity and participation in activities that require a sudden burst of movement are generally discouraged. However, some highly trained, fit women without medical or obstetrical complications can safely undergo vigorous exercise under the advisement of their medical provider. Although research quantity is limited, current literature provides reassurance regarding athletes continuing their training during pregnancy with medical monitoring.[85]

Exercise provides a variety of potential benefits to pregnant women. Weight gain is a problem for most individuals, and pregnancy-related weight accumulation and postpartum weight retention is often the beginning of significant weight issues for many women. Research has shown that adherence to a regular program of exercise reduces the excess weight gain that is common during the childbearing years (ages 25–34 years).[86,87] Studies have also shown that both moderate aerobic exercise and resistance training during pregnancy and postpartum attenuates long-term weight gain in women.[86–89] Along with moderating weight gain during and after pregnancy, regular exercise has also been associated with an improved body image and lower incidence of mood disorders and depression associated with pregnancy-related hormonal changes.[90–93]

The bulk of the evidence appears to support exercise during pregnancy as being protective against development of gestational and postpartum diabetes, especially for women participating in vigorous exercise and those who were also active before pregnancy.[11,94] It has been estimated that women who exercise during pregnancy reduce their risk for development of gestational diabetes by as much as 59%.[95] However, some studies suggest that the protective effect of exercise against gestational diabetes may not be realized unless physical activity occurs both before and during pregnancy, and that it is more pronounced at greater levels of body mass index.[96–99]

Exercise has also been associated with reduced LBP, a common disorder during pregnancy. Prevalence rates between 61% and 88% of back pain with onset during pregnancy have been reported, as compared with 1-year prevalence rate of back pain, irrespective of onset, among women of the same age of approximately 40% in the general population.[100] Pregnancy-related LBP can be attributed, in part, to changes in body shape and weight gain that alter the center of gravity and impact

**Table 28-8.** General Beginner Exercise Program Guidelines for Pregnancy

| MODE OF EXERCISE | FREQUENCY | INTENSITY | TIME/VOLUME | TYPE |
|---|---|---|---|---|
| Aerobic | 3–4 days/week | RPE 3–5/10 scale | 30 min/day Intermittent, multiple bouts/day as needed | Low-impact exercise Avoid activities that increase risk for falls |
| Resistance | 2–3 days/week | 40%–50% 1RM RPE 4–5/10 scale | 1 set 8–10 repetitions | Upright or seated exercise past first trimester |
| Flexibility | 3 days/week | Mild discomfort | 15–60 sec/stretch 3–4 exercises/joint | Static/Dynamic Care to not exceed normal ROM |

HRR, heart rate reserve; 1RM, one repetition maximum; ROM, range of motion; RPE, rating of perceived exertion; $\dot{V}O_2R$, oxygen consumption reserve.

*Source:* Data from the American College of Obstetricians and Gynecologists.[74]

posture and lumbar curvature. These changes, especially when combined with hormonal changes, such as increased secretion of relaxin that results in ligament laxity and increased spinal mobility, lead to low-back discomfort.[101] Resistance training in general, and certain specific core exercises undertaken before pregnancy and during the first two trimesters (Fig. 28-10), may provide some benefit in reducing both the incidence and symptomatic intensity of LBP during pregnancy.[102–104]

Although concerns regarding the potential negative impact of exercise on fetal development are understandable, research has shown that the opposite may be true when appropriate exercise is undertaken during pregnancy. Studies have reported that children born to physically active women tend to be leaner and longer, demonstrate heightened attentiveness, and appear to be neuron developmentally advanced compared with children of physically inactive women.[105–110] Conversely, other studies have reported minimal to no added benefit on fetal development as a result of exercise training during pregnancy. However, there is currently no evidence that exercise training is harmful to the developing fetus in women undergoing an uncomplicated pregnancy.[22]

Certain conditions/complications may render exercise unsafe during pregnancy, making it important that exercise during pregnancy is physician guided. Complications can occur regardless of fitness and previous activity habits, and exercising under certain conditions could potentially place the fetus and/or woman

at further risk. A sampling of the conditions that may result in exercise restriction includes the following:

- Risk factors for preterm labor
- Premature labor
- Vaginal bleeding
- Premature rupture of membranes
- Preeclampsia
- Fetal growth restriction

Because exercise during pregnancy is not without some risk, it is important that pregnant exercisers be aware of the following warning signs. Should any of these occur, the exercise session should be postponed and the condition discussed with the woman's physician before resuming exercise training[74]:

- Vaginal bleeding
- Dizziness or feeling faint
- Increased shortness of breath
- Chest pain
- Headache
- Muscle weakness
- Calf pain or swelling
- Uterine contractions
- Decreased fetal movement
- Fluid leaking from the vagina

In general, the following guidelines are recommended when creating exercise programs for pregnant women[74]:

1. Light- to moderate-intensity exercise is recommended for untrained women. Beginning a vigorous exercise program shortly before or during pregnancy is not recommended.
2. Women who have been previously active may continue their exercise during the first trimester under medical advisement and as tolerated.
3. Women who have not previously been active should begin gradually—low-intensity exercise for 15 minutes with a gradual increase to 30 minutes is generally recommended. Some women may need to begin with even shorter durations and/or perform intermittent activity.
4. Gradually reduce the intensity, duration, and frequency of exercise during the second and third trimesters. For example, a woman who walks or runs an average of 40 minutes per session might reduce her time to 30 minutes during the first trimester and then further reduce duration and/or exercise intensity in the second and third trimesters.
5. Use of the rating of perceived exertion (RPE) scale rather than heart rate to monitor exercise intensity may be preferable for most pregnant women. Choose an intensity that is comfortable (e.g., RPE of 9–13). A pounding heart rate, breathlessness, or dizziness are indicators that intensity should be reduced.
6. Avoid the following exercises:
   - Activities that require extensive jumping, hopping, skipping, bouncing, or running

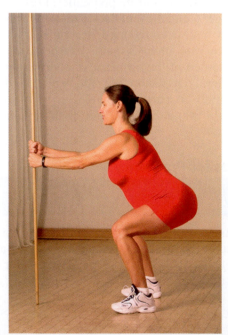

**Figure 28-10.** Supported body weight squat. This modification to the basic squat is an example of an appropriate resistance and core exercise for women to engage in during pregnancy. A dowel or body bar can be used as a prop to aid with balance. Take care to maintain neutral alignment through the pelvis and low back.

- Deep knee bends, full sit-ups, double leg raises, and straight-leg toe touches
- Contact sports such as softball, football, basketball, and volleyball
- Bouncing while stretching
- Activities where falling is likely (e.g., downhill skiing and horseback riding)

7. After the first trimester, consideration should be given to avoid exercises in the supine position.
8. Pregnant women should avoid long periods of standing and be encouraged to keep moving or sit and rest.
9. Exercise should be modified, moved indoors, or avoided when the temperature and/or humidity is high.
10. Proper fluid intake (1–1.5 mL water for each calorie consumed) is essential to balance loss of fluids from exercise and to prevent dehydration.[111]
11. Extended warm-up and cool-down periods should be used and some light stretching should be incorporated during the cool-down phase.
12. Pregnant women should avoid skiing, contact sports, scuba diving, jumping/jarring motions, and quick changes in motion.
13. Walking and running should occur on flat, even surfaces to reduce the likelihood of falls, especially as pregnancy progresses.

## Postpartum Exercise Guidelines

Following delivery, women require some recovery time to regain strength. Taking care of a newborn and the associated sleep interruption can easily lead to a fatigued state. Most women can resume exercising within a few days of an uncomplicated delivery. Generally, the initial focus is to gradually increase physical activity as a means for relaxation, personal time, and to regain a sense of control, rather than on improving physical fitness. Women who have had a cesarean delivery may require additional recovery time. Most women will gradually return to prepregnancy levels within 6 to 8 weeks. However, this timeframe is highly individualized.

Exercise following pregnancy is important and promotes a variety of benefits, including: (1) weight loss; (2) prevention of, or enhanced recovery from, postpartum depression; (3) improved cardiovascular and musculoskeletal fitness; (4) restoration of abdominal strength/support; and (5) increased energy and mood enhancement. Although there has been some concern regarding the impact of exercise on lactation, studies have not reported significant adverse effects.[112] High-intensity exercise may cause lactate to accumulate in breast milk, and some concern has existed that accumulation would sour the taste and affect infant milk consumption. However, in more recent research, no impact was observed on milk acceptance by infants 1 hour following high-intensity exercise despite increased lactate concentration in breast milk.[113] This study also demonstrated that moderate-intensity exercise does not significantly increase lactate concentration in breast milk post-exercise compared with pre-exercise levels.

Women should gradually build to a minimum of 150 minutes a week of moderate-intensity aerobic exercise and 2 days per week of resistance training as recommended by the *2008 Physical Activity Guidelines for Americans*.[27] The key is to gradually rebuild exercise duration and intensity, being careful to avoid excessive fatigue, and to drink plenty of fluids, especially if breast-feeding. General guidelines for exercise during the postpartum period are[114]:

- Begin slowly and gradually increase duration and intensity. The goal is to develop consistency, not see how hard one can work.
- Start with walking several times per week. Consider pool-based activities such as aqua aerobics.
- Avoid excessive fatigue and dehydration.
- Wear a supportive bra.
- Stop the exercise session if unusual pain is experienced.
- Stop the exercise session and seek medical evaluation if bright red vaginal bleeding that is heavier than a menstrual period occurs.
- Drink plenty of water and eat appropriately.

## CRITICAL THINKING QUESTIONS

1. For some individuals, physical activity is a trigger for an acute asthma episode, yet regular exercise is recommended for people with asthma. Explain how exercise can benefit people with asthma, even those diagnosed with EIA.

2. Clare is a 67-year-old retired bookkeeper who is seeking help with her "quickly worsening arthritis pain." She says that she used to do some light resistance training, but her wrists and hands have gotten so weak that gripping a dumbbell became impossible. In fact, she sometimes has trouble

turning doorknobs because of the weakness in her hands. Her hips are also becoming problematic, as they tighten up after prolonged sitting. What types of exercise would you recommended for Clare during the initial stage of a new exercise program?

3. As a stay-at-home mom, Becky has led a fairly sedentary lifestyle and has gained a significant amount of weight over the past 25 years. Her 5'6" frame now supports 225 pounds, and she presents to her physician with complaints of aching knees and hips, morning stiffness, and constant fatigue.

*Continued*

## CRITICAL THINKING QUESTIONS—cont'd

Some days, she just wants to sleep all day. She avoids exercise, perceiving that it will only serve to increase her fatigue and pain levels. What condition(s) might she have? When referred by her physician to a health and fitness professional, what should the health and fitness professional consider when developing a program?

4. You are working with a 22-year-old pregnant woman. What types of activities should be avoided, especially as her pregnancy progresses?

5. LBP is a common work-related complaint and injury. What type of strategies could be put into place at the worksite to minimize risk?

## ADDITIONAL RESOURCES

ACSM Current-Comments: http://www.acsm.org/access-public-information/brochures-fact-sheets/fact-sheets

American Council on Exercise. *ACE Advanced Health & Fitness Specialist Manual.* San Diego, CA: American Council on Exercise; 2008.

Barry DW, Kohrt WM. Exercise and the preservation of bone health. *J Cardiopulm Rehabil Prev.* 2008;28:153–162.

Chou R, Loeser JD, Owens DK, et al. Interventional therapies, surgery, and interdisciplinary rehabilitation for low back pain. *Spine.* 2009;34:1066–1077.

Conn VS, Hafdahl AR, Minor MA, Nielsen PJ. Physical activity interventions among adults with arthritis: Meta analysis of outcomes. *Semin Arthritis Rheum.* 2008;37:307–316.

Durstine JL, Moore G, Painter P, Roberts S. *ACSM's Exercise Management for Persons With Chronic Diseases and Disabilities.* 3rd ed. Champaign, IL: Human Kinetics; 2009.

Gunter KB, Almstedt HC, Janz, KF. Physical activity in childhood may be the key to optimizing lifespan skeletal health. *Exerc. Sport Sci. Rev.* 2012;40:13–21.

Jamtvedt G, Dahm KT, Christie A, et al. Physical therapy interventions for patients with osteoarthritis of the knee: An overview of systematic reviews. *Phys Ther.* 2008;88:123–136.

Lewis BA, Kennedy BF. Effects of exercise on depression during pregnancy and postpartum: A review. *Am J Lifestyle Med.* 2011;5:370–377.

Rippe JM. *Lifestyle Medicine.* Malden, MA; Blackwell Science; 1999.

Sabiston CM, Brunet J. Reviewing the benefits of physical activity during cancer survivorship. *Am J Lifestyle Med.* 2012;6:167–176.

U.S. Department of Health and Human Services. *Physical Activity and Health: A Report of the Surgeon General.* S/N 017-023-00196-5. Atlanta, GA: U.S. Department of Health and Human Services, Centers for Disease Control and Prevention, National Center for Chronic Disease Prevention and Health Promotion; 1996.

Wolfe F. The Natural History of rheumatoid arthritis. *J Rheumatol Suppl.* 1996;44:13–22.

## REFERENCES

1. National Heart, Lung, and Blood Institute Chartbook on Cardiovascular, Lung and Blood Diseases, U.S. Department of Health and Human Services, et al. National Asthma Education and Prevention Program (NAEPP) Expert Panel Report 3, 2009. Available at: http://www.nhlbi.nih.gov/research/reports/2012-mortality-chart-book.htm

2. Bousquet J, Jeffery PK, Busse WW, Johnson M, Vignola AM. Asthma. From bronchoconstriction to airways inflammation and remodeling. *Am J Respir Crit Care Med.* 2000;161:1720–1745.

3. Morris MJ, Schwarz AJ, Saglimbeni AJ, et al. Asthma: Medscape from WebMD, Diseases & Conditions; Allergy & Immunology; Asthma. Accessed February 5, 2012. http://emedicine.medscape.com/article/296301-overview

4. DiDario AG, Becker JM. Asthma, sports, and death. *Allergy Asthma Proc.* 2005;26:341–344.

5. Parsons JP, Craig DO, Stoloff SW, et al. Impact of exercise-related respiratory symptoms in adults with asthma: Exercise-induced bronchospasm landmark national survey. *Allergy Asthma Proc.* 2011;32:431–437.

6. Randolph C. The challenge of asthma in adolescent athletes: exercise induced bronchoconstriction (EIB) with and without known asthma. *Adolesc Med.* 2010;21:44–56, viii.

7. Ritz T, Rosenfield D, Steptoe D. Physical activity, lung function, and shortness of breath in the daily life of individuals with asthma. *Chest.* 2010;138:913–918.

8. Fanelli A, Cabral ALB, Neder JA, Martins MA, Carvalho CR. Exercise training on disease control and quality of life in asthmatic children. *Med Sci Sports Exerc.* 2007;39:1474–1480.

9. Mendes FAR, Goncalves RC, Nunes MPT, et al. Effects of aerobic training on psychosocial morbidity and symptoms in asthmatic patients: a randomized clinical trial. *Chest.* 2010;138:331–337.

10. American College of Sports Medicine. Impact of physical activity during pregnancy and postpartum on chronic disease risk. Special Communication Roundtable Consensus Statement. *Med Sci Sports Exerc.* 2006;989–1006.

11. Garcia-Aymerich J, Varraso R, Anto JM, Camargo CA Jr. Prospective study of physical activity and risk of asthma exacerbations in older women. *Am J Respir Crit Care Med.* 2009;179:999–1003.

12. Hallstrand TS. New insights into pathogenesis of exercise-induced bronchoconstriction. *Curr Opin Allergy Clin Immunol.* 2012;12:42–48.

13. Mendes FAR, Almeida FM, Cukier A, et al. Effects of aerobic training on airway inflammation in asthmatic patients. *Med Sci Sports Exerc.* 2011;43:197–206.

14. National Cancer Institute, National Institute of Health. 2012. Reducing Environmental Cancer Risk: What We Can Do Now. Available at: http://deainfo.nci.nih.gov/advisory/pcp/annualReports/pcp08-09rpt/PCP_Report_08-09_508.pdf

15. Eheman C, Henley SJ, et al. Annual report to the nation on the status of cancer, 1975-2008, Featuring cancers associated with excess weight and lack of sufficient physical activity. *Cancer.* 2012;118:2338–2366.

16. American Cancer Society. *Cancer Facts and Figures 2012.* Atlanta, GA: American Cancer Society; 2012.

17. American Cancer Society Guidelines on Nutrition and Physical Activity for Cancer Prevention. 2012. Available at: http://www.cancer.org/healthy/eathealthygetactive/acsguidelinesonnutritionphysicalactivityforcancerprevention/acs-guidelines-on-nutrition-and-physical-activity-for-cancer-prevention-intro. Accessed January 11, 2012.

18. Courneya KS, Mackey JR. Exercise during and after cancer treatment: Benefits, guidelines and precautions. *Int Sportmed J.* 2001;1:1–8.

19. Drouin J, Pfalzer L. *Cancer and Exercise.* The National Center on Physical Activity & Disability. Updated 2009. Available at: http://www.nchpad.org/163/1255/Cancer~and~Exercise. Accessed April 8, 2012.

20. Schmitz KH, Courneya KS, Matthews C, et al. American College of Sports Medicine roundtable on exercise guidelines for cancer survivors. Special communications: Roundtable consensus statement. *Med Sci Sports Exerc.* 2010:1409–1425.

21. World Cancer Research Fund/American Institute for Cancer Research. *Food, nutrition, physical activity, and the prevention of cancer: A global perspective.* Washington, DC: AICR; 2007.

22. U.S. Department of Health & Human Services; Physical Activity Guidelines Advisory Committee. *Physical Activity Guidelines Advisory Committee Report.* Washington, DC: U.S. Department of Health and Human Services; 2008.

23. Brolinson PG, Elliot D. Exercise and the immune system. *Clin Sports Med.* 2007;26:311–319.

24. Brown JC, Winters-Stone K, Lee A, Schmitz KH. Cancer, physical activity, and exercise. *Compr Physiol.* 2012;2:2775–2809.

25. Irwin ML, Mayne ST. Impact of nutrition and exercise on cancer survival. *Cancer J.* 2008;4:435–441.

26. Jankowski CM, Matthews EE. Exercise guidelines for adults with cancer: A vital role in survivorship. *Clin J Oncol Nur.* 2011;15:683–686.

27. U.S. Department of Health and Human Services. *2008 Physical Activity Guidelines for Americans: Be Active, Healthy and Happy.* 2008. Available at: http://www.health.gov/paguidelines/pdf/paguide.pdf.

28. National Osteoporosis Foundation. *Clinician's Guide to Prevention and Treatment of Osteoporosis.* 2013. Available at: http://nof.org/hcp/clinicians-guide

29. World Health Organization. Assessment of fracture risk and application to screening for postmenopausal osteoporosis. *WHO Technical Report Series,* 843. Geneva, Switzerland: WHO; 1984.

30. American Academy of Orthopaedic Surgeons. *United States Bone and Joint Initiative: The Burden of Musculoskeletal Diseases in the United States.* 2nd ed. Rosemont, IL: American Academy of Orthopaedic Surgeons; 2011.

31. Baumgaertner MR, Higgins TF. Femoral neck fractures. In: Bucholz RW, Heckman JD, Rockwood CA, Green DP, eds. *Rockwood and Green's Fractures in Adults.* Philadelphia: Lippincott Williams & Wilkins; 2002.

32. National Institutes of Health. *Osteoporosis: Peak Bone Mass in Women.* Bethesda, MD: National Institutes of Health National Resource Center; 2012.

33. Bassey EJ, Ramsdale SJ. Increase in femoral bone density in young women following high-impact exercise. *Osteoporos Int.* 1994;4:72–75.

34. Body JJ, Bergmann P, Boonen S, et al. Non-pharmacological management of osteoporosis: A consensus of the Belgian Bone Club. *Osteoporos Int.* 2011; 22:2769–2788.

35. Arthritis: Meeting the Challenge. Available at: http://www.cdc.gov/chronicdisease/resources/publications/aag/arthritis.htm. Accessed September 5, 2014.

36. Centers for Disease Control and Prevention. *Quick Stats on Arthritis.* Available at: http://www.cdc.gov/arthritis. Accessed January 25, 2009.

37. Lawrence RC, Felson DT, Helmick CG, et al; National Arthritis Data Workgroup. Estimates of the prevalence of arthritis and other rheumatic conditions in the United States, Part II. *Arthritis Rheum.* 2008;58:26–35.

38. Persson GR. Rheumatoid arthritis and periodontitis—inflammatory and infectious connections: Review of the literature. *J Oral Microbiol.* 2012;4.

39. Boonen A, Severens JL. The burden of illness of rheumatoid arthritis. *Clin Rheumatol.* 2011;30 (Suppl 1):s3–s8.

40. Dickens C, McGowan L, Clark-Carter D, Creed F. Depression in rheumatoid arthritis: A systematic review of the literature with meta-analysis. *Psychosom Med.* 2002;64:52–60.

41. Wasko MC. Comorbid conditions in patients with rheumatic diseases: an update. *Curr Opin Rheumatol.* 2004;16:109–113.

42. Arthritis Foundation. *Who Gets Osteoarthritis?* Available at: http://www.arthritis.org/who-gets-osteoarthritis.php. Accessed February 11, 2012.

43. Abbate LM, Stevens J, Schwartz TA, et al. The relationship between weight maintenance and incident radiographic knee osteoarthritis: The Johnston County Osteoarthritis Project. Presentation number 629. American College of Rheumatology Annual Scientific Meeting, 2009. October 19, 2009 in Philadelphia, PA.

44. Wolfe F, Ross K, Anderson J, et al. The prevalence and characteristics of fibromyalgia in the general population. *Arthritis Rheumatol.* 1995;38:19–28.

45. Wolfe F, Clauw DJ, Fitzcharles MA, et al. The American College of Rheumatology preliminary diagnostic criteria for fibromyalgia and measurement of symptom severity. *Arthritis Care Res.* 2010;62:600–610.

46. Mist SD, Firestone KA, Jones KD. Complementary and alternative exercise for fibromyalgia: A meta-analysis. *J Pain Res.* 2013;6:247–260.

47. Busch AJ, Webber SC, Brachaniec M, et al. Exercise therapy for fibromyalgia. *Curr Pain Headache Rep.* 2011;15:358–367.

48. Giles W, Klippel JH. *A National Public Health Agenda for Osteoarthritis.* Atlanta, GA: Centers for Disease Control and Prevention; 2010. Available at: http://www.cdc.gov/arthritis/docs/OAagenda.pdf.

49. Hoy DG, Bain C, Williams G, et al. A systematic review of the global prevalence of low back pain. *Arthritis Rheumatol.* 2012;14:2028–2037.

50. Johannes CB, Le TK, Zhou X, Johnston JA, Dworkin RH. The prevalence of chronic pain in United States adults: Results of an Internet-based survey. *J Pain.* 2010;14:1230–1239.

51. Martin BI, Deyo RA, Mirza SK, et al. Expenditures and health status among adults with back and neck problems. *JAMA.* 2008;299:656–664.

52. Lin CC, Haas M, Maher CG, Machado LA, van Tulder MW. Cost-effectiveness of general practice care for low back pain: A systematic review. *Eur Spine J.* 2011;20:1012–1023.

53. Wong D, Transfeldt E. *Macnab's Backache.* 4th ed. Philadelphia, PA: Lippincott Williams & Wilkins; 2007.

54. Han TS, Schouten JS, Lean ME, Seidell JC. The prevalence of low back pain and associations with body fatness, fat distribution and height. *Int J Obes Relat Metab Disord.* 1997;21:600–607.

55. Leboeuf-Yde C. Body weight and low back pain: A systematic literature review of 56 journal articles reporting on 65 epidemiologic studies. *Spine.* 2000;25:226–237.

56. Toda Y, Segal N, Toda T, Morimoto T, Ogawa R. Lean body mass and body fat distribution in participants with chronic low back pain. *Arch Intern Med.* 2000; 160:3265–3269.

57. Shiri R, Karppinen J, Leino-Arjas P, Solovieva S, Viikari-Juntura E. The association between obesity and low back pain: A meta-analysis. *Am J Epidemiol.* 2010;171:135–154.

58. Shiri R. Obesity and the prevalence of low back pain in young adults. *Am J Epidemiol.* 2008;167:1110–1119.

59. Vismara L, Menegoni F, Zaina F, Galli M, Negrini S, Capodaglio P. Effect of obesity and low back pain on spinal mobility: A cross sectional study in women. *J Neuroeng Rehabil.* 2010;7:3.

60. Gilleard W, Smith T. Effect of obesity on posture and hip joint moments during a standing task, and trunk forward flexion motion. *Int J Obes.* 2007;31:267–277.

61. Lehman GL. Biomechanical assessments of lumbar spinal function: How low back pain suffers differ from normals. Implications for outcome measures research. Part I: Kinematic assessments of lumbar function. *J Manipulative Physiol Ther.* 2004;27:57–62.

62. Nourbakhsh MR, Arab AM. Relation between mechanical factors and incidence of low back pain. *J Orthop Sports Phys Ther.* 2002;32:447–460.

63. McGill SM, Hughson RL, Parks K. Changes in lumbar lordosis modify the role of the extensor muscles. *Clin Biomech.* 2000;15:777–780.

64. Descarreaux M, Lafond D, Jeffrey-Gauthier R, Centomo H, Cantin V. Changes in the flexion relaxation response induced by lumbar muscle fatigue. *BMC Musculoskelet Disord.* 2008;9:1.

65. Howard BV, Ruotolo G, Robbins DC. Obesity and dyslipidemia. *Endocrinol Metab Clin North Am.* 2003;32:855–867.

66. Korkiakoski A, Niinimäki J, Karppinen J, et al. Association of lumbar arterial stenosis with low back symptoms: A cross-sectional study using two-dimensional time-of-flight magnetic resonance angiography. *Acta Radiologica.* 2009;50:48–54.

67. Cheung KM, Karppinen J, Chan D, et al. Prevalence and pattern of lumbar magnetic resonance imaging changes in a population study of one thousand forty-three individuals. *Spine.* 2009;34:934–940.

68. Wassenaar M. Magnetic resonance imaging for diagnosing lumbar spinal pathology in adult patients with low back pain or sciatica: A diagnostic systematic review. *Eur Spine J.* 2012;21:220–227.

69. Dugan SA. Role of exercise in prevention and management of acute low back pain. *Clin Occup En Med.* 2006;5:615–632.

70. McGill S. *Low Back Disorders.* 2nd ed. Human Kinetics Publishers: Champaign, IL; 2007.

71. Waller B, Lambeck S, Daly D. Therapeutic aquatic exercise in the treatment of low back pain: A systematic review. *Clin Rehabil.* 2009;23:3–14.

72. American College of Obstetricians and Gynecologists (ACOG). *Exercise During Pregnancy and the Postnatal Period.* Technical Bulletin. Washington, DC: ACOG; 1985.

73. American College of Obstetricians and Gynecologists (ACOG). *Exercise During Pregnancy and the Postnatal Period.* Technical Bulletin 189. Washington, DC: ACOG; 1994.

74. American College of Obstetricians and Gynecologists (ACOG). Exercise during pregnancy and the postpartum period. ACOG Committee Opinion 267. *Obstet Gynecol.* 2002;99:171–173.

75. Davies GA, Wolfe LA, Mottola MF, et al. Joint SOGC/CSEP clinical practice guideline: Exercise in pregnancy and the postpartum period. *Can J Appl Physiol.* 2003;28:330–341.

76. Artal R. Recommendations for exercise during pregnancy and the postpartum period. *UpToDate.* January 23, 2012. Available at: www.uptodate.com.

77. O'Toole ML. Physiologic aspects of exercise in pregnancy. *Clin Obstet Gynecol.* 2003;40:379–389.

78. Artal R, Fortunato V, Welton A, et al. Pulmonary responses to exercise in pregnancy. *Am J Obstet Gynecol.* 1986;154:378–383.

79. Khodiguian N, Jaque-Fortunato SV, Wiswell RA, et al. A comparison of cross-sectional and longitudinal methods of assessing the influence of pregnancy on cardiac function during exercise. *Semin Pernatol.* 1996;20:232–241.

80. Spinnewijn WE, Wallenburg HCS, Struijk PC, et al. Peak ventilator responses during cycling and swimming in pregnant and non-pregnant women. *J Appl Physiol.* 1996;81:738–742.

81. Wolfe LA, Walker RMC, Bonen A, et al. Effects of pregnancy and chronic exercise on respiratory responses to graded exercise. *J Appl Physiol.* 1994;76:1928–1936.

82. Martens D, Hernandez B, Strickland G, Boatwright D. Pregnancy and exercise: Physiological changes and effects on mother and fetus. *Strength Cond J.* 2006; 28:78–82.

83. Royal College of Obstetricians and Gynaecologists. *Exercise in Pregnancy.* RCOG Statement No. 4. January 2006. Available at: http://www.rcog.org.uk/womens-health/clinical-guidance/exercise-pregnancy

84. Canadian Academy of Sport Medicine, CASM/ACMS. *Position Statement: Exercise and Pregnancy.* 2008. Available at: http://www.casm-acms.org. https://secure.sirc.ca/newsletters/may08/documents/Pregnancy-PositionPaper.pdf Accessed 9/5/14

85. Pivarnik JM, Perkins CD, Moyerbrailean T. Athletes and pregnancy. *Clin Obstet Gynecol.* 2003;46:403–414.

86. Clapp JF. Exercise during pregnancy: A clinical update. *Clin Sports Med.* 2000;19:273–286.

87. Clapp JF, Little KD. Effect of recreational exercise on pregnancy weight gain and subcutaneous fat deposition. *Med Sci Sports Exerc.* 1995;27:170–177.

88. Barakat R, Lucia A, Ruiz JR. Resistance exercise training during pregnancy and newborn's birth size: A randomized controlled trial. *Int J Obes (Lond).* 2009;33: 1048–1057.

89. O'Toole ML, Sawicki MA, Artal R. Structured diet and physical activity prevent postpartum weight retention. *J Womens Health (Larchmt).* 2003;12:991.

90. Moore DS. The body image in pregnancy. *J Nurse Midwifery.* 1978;22:17–27.

91. Polman R, Kaiseler M, Borkoles E. Effect of a single bout of exercise on the mood of pregnant women. *J Sports Med Phys Fitness.* 2007;47:103–111.

92. Poudevigne MS, O'Connor PJ. A review of physical activity patterns in pregnant women and their relationship to psychological health. *Sports Med.* 2006;36:19–38.

93. Wise LA, Adams-Campbell LL, Palmer JR, Rosenberg L. Leisure time physical activity in relation to depressive symptoms in the Black Women's Health Study. *Ann Behav Med.* 2006;32:68–76.

94. Oken E, Ning Y, Rifas-Shiman SL, Radesky JS, Rich-Edwards JW, Gillman MW. Associations of physical activity and inactivity before and during pregnancy with glucose tolerance. *Obstet Gynecol.* 2006;108:1200–1207.

95. Liu J, Laditka JN, Mayer-Davis EJ, Pate RR. Does physical activity during pregnancy reduce risk of gestational diabetes among previously inactive women? *Birth.* 2008;35:189–196.

96. Dempsey JC, Butler CL, Sorensen TK, et al. A case-control study of maternal recreational physical activity and risk of gestational diabetes mellitus. *Diabetes Res Clin Pract.* 2004;66:203–215.

97. Dempsey JC, Sorensen TK, Williams MA, et al. Prospective study of gestational diabetes mellitus risk in relation to maternal recreational physical activity before and during pregnancy. *Am J Epidemiol.* 2004;159:663–670.

98. Dye TD, Knox KL, Artal R, et al. Physical activity, obesity, and diabetes in pregnancy. *Am J Epidemiol.* 1997;146:961–965.

99. Zhang C, Solomon CG, Manson JE, et al. A prospective study of pregravid physical activity and sedentary behaviors in relation to the risk for gestational diabetes mellitus. *Arch Intern Med.* 2006;166:543–548.

100. Thorell E, Kristiansson P. Pregnancy related back pain, is it related to aerobic fitness? A longitudinal cohort study. *BMC Pregnancy Childbirth.* 2012;12:30.

101. Kristiansson P, Svardsudd K, von Schoultz B. Back pain during pregnancy: A prospective study. *Spine.* 1996;21:701–709.

102. Piper TJ, Jacobs, E, Haiduke M, Waller M, McMillan C. Core training exercise selection during pregnancy. *Strength Cond J.* 2012;34:55–61.

103. Pujol TJ, Barnes JT, Elder CL. Resistance training during pregnancy. *Strength Cond J.* 2007;29:44–46.

104. Schoenfeld B. Resistance training during pregnancy: Safe and effective program design. *Strength Cond J.* 2011;33:67–75.

105. Clapp JF. Exercise and fetal health. *J Dev Physiol.* 1991;15:9–14.

106. Clapp JF III. The effects of maternal exercise on fetal oxygenation and feto placental growth. *Eur J Obstet Gynecol Reprod Biol.* 2003;110(Suppl. 1):S80–S85.

107. Clapp JF. Influence of endurance exercise on diet and human placental development and fetal growth. *Placenta.* 2006;27:527–534.

108. Clapp JF III. The effects of maternal exercise on early pregnancy outcome. *Am J Obstet Gynecol.* 1989;161:1453–1457.

109. Clapp JF, Kim H, Burciu B, Lopez B. Beginning regular exercise in early pregnancy: Effect on feto-placental growth. *Am J Obstet Gynecol.* 2000; 183:1484–1488.

110. Jackson MR, Gott P, Lye SJ. The effects of maternal aerobic exercise on human placental development: Placental volumetric composition and surface areas. *Placenta.* 1995;16:179–191.

111. Montgomery KS. Nutrition column: An update on water needs during pregnancy and beyond. *J Perinat Educ.* 2002;11:40–42.

112. Lovelady CA, Garner KE, Moreno KL, Williams JP. The effect of weight loss in overweight, lactating women on the growth of their infants. *N Engl J Med.* 2000;342:449–453.

113. Wright KS, Quinn T, Carey GB. Infant acceptance of breast milk after maternal exercise. *Pediatrics.* 2002;109:585–589.

114. Clapp JF, Cram C. *Exercising Through Your Pregnancy.* 2nd ed. Omaha, NB: Addicus Books; 2012.

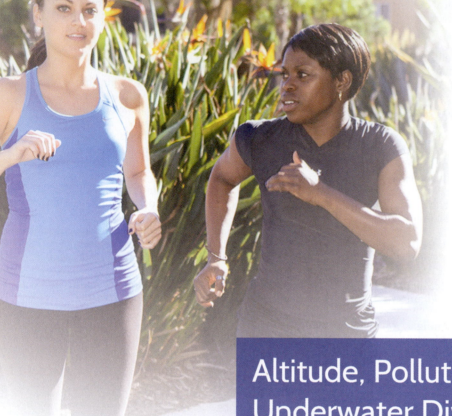

John Porcari, PhD
Scott Drum, PhD

CHAPTER 29

# Altitude, Pollution, and Underwater Diving: Effects on Exercise Capacity

## CHAPTER OUTLINE

# CHAPTER OUTLINE–cont'd

## LEARNING OUTCOMES

1. Describe environmental conditions at altitude, including percent air composition, solar radiation, changes in air temperature at various altitudes, wind speeds, and terrain effects on human effort.

2. Identify body/physiological changes related to acute altitude exposure.

3. Identify body/physiological changes related to chronic altitude exposure (acclimation).

4. Describe common changes in sea-level performance after altitude exposure or training.

5. Compare and contrast exercise performance at altitude with little to no acclimation with that after proper acclimation.

6. Identify the key elements of successful altitude training camps.

7. Describe changes in a person's general fitness level (positive and negative) and blood chemistry after a long sojourn to high altitude.

8. Identify notable health decrements/hazards that may occur with acute altitude exposure, such as acute mountain sickness.

9. Explain how exercise at altitude (vs. sea level) may aid in weight loss for overweight and obese individuals.

10. Describe the cardiopulmonary effects of air pollution.

11. Identify exercise performance inhibitors brought on by air pollution.

12. Explain why the risk for cardiovascular disease may increase with acute or chronic exposure to pollutants.

13. Briefly describe the history of diving.

14. Explain the physics of diving, specifically the concept of hydrostatic pressure, Boyle's law, and Henry's law.

15. Describe the major physiological responses during diving, including the diving reflex, ventilatory responses, hemodynamic responses, and the energy cost of diving.

16. Identify common diving equipment.

17. List possible complications during scuba diving.

## ANCILLARY LINK

Visit Davis*Plus* at http://davisplus.fadavis.com for study and practice resources, including online quizzes, animations that help explain physiological processes, podcasts concerning news and career trends in exercise physiology, and practice references.

## VIGNETTE I

■ Scott Jurek, a world-renowned ultra-running champion, had done it all. His seven consecutive Western States 100-Mile Endurance Run wins was unprecedented, especially because he did it all before his 30th birthday. Winning Western States was like winning the Super Bowl of 100-mile ultra-runs. Winning once makes a person a legend.

However, despite his overwhelming persona as a fierce competitor, Jurek lived at sea level in Seattle, Washington, and consequently tended to struggle during ultra-races at high altitudes because he lacked an acclimation strategy. He then decided to tackle the hardest and highest-altitude 100-mile run, the Hardrock 100 Endurance Run, which has an average running elevation of nearly 11,000 ft and about 33,000 ft of ascent.

How would a well-planned acclimation strategy improve Jurek's results in this high-altitude event?

Human adjustments to altitude are essential. Today, many nontraditional sport performers, such as extreme mountain bike racers and ultra-trail runners, need to be better informed about how to prepare for the environment, especially if they are arriving to race at altitude from a permanent sea-level training location. In order to get a better understanding of altitude and its effect on the human body, especially during exercise, it is essential to understand that exercise or exertion at elevation is harder compared with sea-level exercise. This chapter describes the acute and chronic biological differences, adjustments, and adaptations that the body makes to allow a person to alter his or her oxygen delivery and uptake in a manner that attempts to attenuate the deleterious effects of altitude on performance.

Another interesting environmental challenge involves exercising in areas of high air pollution. Increases in airborne **particulate matter (PM)**, primarily from the burning of fossil fuels, creates a variety of problems for both the cardiovascular and the pulmonary systems. Exercising under these conditions can have a significant impact on not only exercise performance, but overall health as well. The Air Pollution section in this chapter explores the acute and chronic responses to exercising under those conditions, and offers several practical suggestions for minimizing the consequences of living in those areas.

This chapter also reviews the topic of underwater diving. In the 1960s and 1970s, television shows such as *Sea Hunt* and *The Undersea World of Jacques Cousteau* were very popular, and people dreamed of diving for sunken treasure, exploring coral reefs in the Florida Keys, and diving for lobsters off the coast of Maine. A more recent program, *Bering Sea Gold,* centers on diving for gold in the waters off of Nome, Alaska, and highlights the adventure and dangers of underwater diving.

Today, it is estimated that more than 2.8 million individuals participate in the sport of scuba diving in such exotic locations as Cancun, Cozumel, and the Grand Cayman Islands.[1] Scuba diving is an excellent form of exercise, but it can be dangerous. Knowledge of proper equipment, understanding of a few basic physics principles, and awareness of how these factors affect underwater physiology can minimize the dangers of diving and make it an enjoyable and memorable experience.

Although there are many types of underwater diving, this chapter focuses on sport scuba diving, which is generally defined as diving in less than 120 ft of water. When diving at this depth, the diver does not need to breathe specialized gas mixtures and is not at risk for the dangers associated with being at depth for extended periods.

## ENVIRONMENTAL CONDITIONS AT ALTITUDE

When people travel to altitude, they not only face a decreased barometric/atmospheric pressure, but also enhanced solar radiation, diminished air temperature, varying wind speeds, and extreme ascent and descent terrain changes over the course of their stay. As you continue to read through this chapter, keep in mind the ever-changing environmental stresses that might occur over the course of a long, high-altitude backpacking trip, such as a multiple-night excursion in the Rocky Mountains (Fig. 29-1). Also keep in mind how environmental conditions at altitude might affect a person's ability to exercise or train if he or she is not accustomed to high elevations.

### Atmospheric Pressure Changes

From a standpoint of air composition, air always contains 20.93% $O_2$, 0.03% $CO_2$, and 79.04% $N_2$. However,

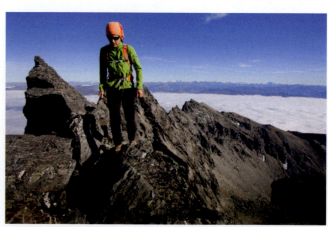

**Figure 29-1.** Environmental conditions at altitude can affect a person's ability to exercise or train if he or she is not accustomed to high elevations. *(Photo by Jakub Cejpak)*

atmospheric/barometric pressure ($P_B$) continuously drops as a person ascends to higher elevations, which results in a decreased availability of oxygen to the tissues. The pressure of a gas is defined as its **partial pressure ($P_x$)**, which is the pressure exerted by a specific gas within a defined volume or space (e.g., such as in the blood or lungs). Partial pressure of a gas is calculated using this equation: $P_x = P_B \times F_x$, where $F_x$ is fractional content of a gas and $P_B$ is the barometric pressure. For example, if $P_B$ at sea level is 760 mm Hg and the percentage of oxygen in the air is 20.93% (fractional percent of 0.2093), then the **partial pressure of oxygen ($P_{O_2}$)** at sea level is 760 mm Hg × 0.2093 = 159.1 mm Hg.

At the top of a 14,000-foot peak, the $P_B$ is only 447 mm Hg. The resultant $P_{O_2}$ is only 93.6 mm Hg (447 mm Hg × 0.2093). This pressure difference results in less oxygen transport/extraction by the tissues and can result in **hypoxia**. As a result of tissue hypoxia, speed of activity, such as running, also diminishes the higher a person trains or races above sea level.

Figure 29-2 shows the standard atmospheric model by the National Oceanic and Atmospheric Administration,[2] which illustrates air-pressure decrements with increasing altitude. It can be seen that as an individual travels to higher elevations, there is a reduced $P_{O_2}$, which results in a decreased pressure gradient or driving force for oxygen to diffuse from the blood into the tissues, such as to exercising skeletal muscle. This, in turn, results in diminished speed in a runner, for instance, because of hampered oxygen uptake to operate aerobic processes.

## Sun, Temperature, Wind, and Terrain Concerns

Aside from reduced oxygen availability at altitude, other environmental factors will impact a person's ability to perform—namely, solar radiation, air temperature, wind, and terrain issues.[3] Because a person is closer to the sun when at altitude, there is an increased exposure to ultraviolet light. This creates the need to wear appropriate protective clothing, such as long-sleeved, sun-reflective outerwear. The material should also be breathable and afford cooling properties when in motion and warming benefits when stationary. Many synthetic

**DOING THE MATH:**

Calculate the $P_{O_2}$ at 14,000 ft where the $P_B$ is 447 mm Hg:

$$P_{O_2} = 447 \text{ mm Hg} \times 0.2093 = 93.6 \text{ mm Hg}$$

This clearly illustrates a loss of oxygen partial pressure at altitude, which is the main driving force for loading oxygen into the bloodstream.

materials are currently on the market that will quickly dry while wicking away sweat.[3] By removing the sweat from the surface of the skin, the body is cooled by the process of evaporation, as discussed in Chapter 12.

In addition to solar radiation, for every 1,000 ft a person ascends above sea level, the air temperature decreases approximately 3.5°F.[4,5] Most high-altitude environments, then, are much cooler versus sea-level areas. Higher elevations are also typically windier than lower elevations. There may be winds caused by **orographic uplift**, which is forced lifting of air along a topographic barrier, such as a mountain range.[4] In addition, increased wind speeds are often observed in the mountains because of **katabatic wind**, which is normally any downslope wind, especially ones stronger than gentle mountain breezes.[4]

Finally, another environmental variation a person will experience in the mountains is highly erratic terrain. Athletes will often face not only the aforementioned weather changes, but also extreme ascents, such as 3,000- to 7,000-foot variations in elevations that will overload even the most well-trained individuals. The other end of the spectrum introduces the athlete or mountain traveler to severe, sometimes rocky descents in equal magnitude to the ascent. Thus, this type of exercise or cardiovascular overload not only affects biological systems, but also produces increased force production through joints and added friction to feet, leading to possible injuries.

### VIGNETTE I continued

■ As Scott Jurek prepared for the Hardrock 100 Endurance Run through the high elevations of the Rocky Mountains, he lived at elevation (i.e., Silverton, Colorado, the start and finish of the loop course) and ran on the course daily. While he trained and lived in the upper reaches of the Rockies, he experimented with different layers of clothing. He also became aware of the harsh and unpredictable nature of the sun, air temperature, wind, and terrain—yet another "real-life" advantage over competitors who were arriving directly from sea level just days before the race.

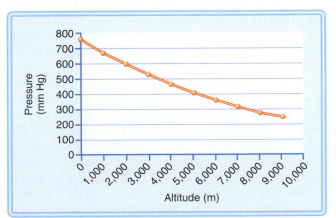

**Figure 29-2.** Standard atmospheric model by the National Oceanic and Atmospheric Administration, showing air pressure decrements with increasing altitude.

## Adjustments to Acute Altitude Exposure

Many acute adjustments take place in the body when traveling to altitude. In particular, cardiorespiratory decrements are typically evident at elevations from 580 m (1,900 ft) up to 4,300 m (14,110 ft) and beyond.[6] A person's **maximal oxygen consumption ($\dot{V}O_2$max)** is reduced by about 9% per 1,000-m (3,280-ft) increase in altitude above 1,050 m (3,445 ft).[6] The reason for these acute decrements stems from respiratory, cardiovascular, and metabolic adjustments that must be made to help the body adjust to its new environment. Therefore, while the body is adjusting, $\dot{V}O_2$max, for instance, will be decremented and remains low (vs. sea level) even after acclimation.

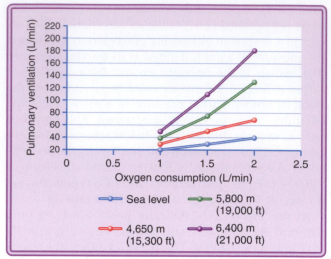

**Figure 29-3.** Relation of pulmonary ventilation ($\dot{V}_E$) to oxygen consumption (L/min) at sea level and various altitudes. Note that $\dot{V}_E$ progressively and nonlinearly increases as altitude increases.

## Respiratory Function

As a person ascends to higher elevations, especially 3,280 ft above sea level and beyond, the $Po_2$ of inspired air becomes progressively less. When the $Po_2$ of inspired air is lower, this results in a lower **arterial oxygen saturation ($Sao_2$)**. To compensate for this change in $Po_2$, **pulmonary ventilation ($\dot{V}_E$)** increases, commonly known as **hypoxic ventilatory response (HVR)**. HVR is a mechanism that helps maintain sufficient oxygen to the body's tissues and organs via increased air movement through the lung's terminal air sacs, called *alveoli*. Air movement specifically quantified throughout the alveoli is termed **alveolar ventilation ($Pao_2$)**.[6] By forcing more air (i.e., oxygen) through the alveoli and into the blood, $Sao_2$ is maintained. In general, the mechanism behind the HVR is enhanced sensitivity of peripheral chemoreceptors. Over a period of about 1 week at altitude, the HVR may subside a small amount, and the number of breaths taken per minute at rest should decrease and may even approach that of sea-level breathing. Also, $\dot{V}_E$ may slow, but most likely will not return to sea level values when acclimated. This is because of the enhanced sensitivity of receptors that help maintain $\dot{V}_E$ at a slightly greater rate.[6]

Figure 29-3 shows the effect of altitude on the ventilatory response to submaximal exercise. Note the greater magnitude of change in $\dot{V}_E$ as extreme altitude is reached (i.e., beyond 15,300 ft). Also, it may be helpful to remember that a normal resting $\dot{V}_E$ is about 5 L/min, and during intense exercise a person may reach upward of 200 L/min. Therefore, breathing capacity has the ability to change to a large magnitude from rest to peak or maximal exertion. Still, breathing adjustments during acute exposure to moderate-to-high altitudes are beneficial and necessary.

## Cardiovascular Function

With acute exposure to high altitude, heart rate (HR) tends to increase and there is a diminished stroke volume (SV). Thus, resting and exercise/training HRs may be higher at any given workload (e.g., a given running speed) to maintain cardiac output (Q). The reduction in SV is caused primarily by a reduction in blood

volume, which may be caused by dehydration.[7] All in all, the greater the altitude, the greater the cardiovascular strain on the heart. For instance, when the heart is pumping faster, the heart muscle itself needs more oxygen. However, because there is a lower $Sao_2$ with acute altitude exposure, heart function may be compromised.

The decreased arterial partial pressure of oxygen ($Pao_2$) causes less oxygen to be bound to hemoglobin, the primary oxygen-carrying protein in the blood. This results in a shortfall of oxygen available to the tissues during exercise. This oxygen shortfall requires that any individual exercising at altitude will have to decrease his or her intensity to maintain proper duration. Furthermore, because of unavoidable dehydration at altitude, blood volume remains low and tends to reduce the delivery of oxygen to muscle.

## Metabolic Function

Metabolically, individuals will most likely rely on carbohydrates during *acute* exposure to high altitude (i.e., the first few weeks), because carbohydrates require less oxygen to be converted into energy. **Basal metabolic rate (BMR)** is also typically elevated compared with sea level because of the increased work of breathing. Thus, increased caloric intake may be warranted to balance the elevated BMR.[8]

When discussing the use of carbohydrates (glucose) as a fuel during acute altitude exposure, keep in mind that the body is under heightened environmental stress. Thus, blood glucose may be reduced during acute altitude exposure. Consequently, there is an increase in skeletal muscle **glycogenolysis** (breakdown of muscle glycogen to glucose). This makes it vitally important to eat when initially exposed to altitude. Ingesting nutrients at regular intervals, especially carbohydrates, helps to maintain blood glucose and minimize the breakdown of muscle glycogen. Also, maintaining a relatively constant blood glucose level exerts an inhibitory effect on the breakdown of liver glycogen, which can then be used at a later time if needed.[9] In addition, because of the added reliance on glycolysis during acute exposure to altitude, there is increased blood lactate at rest and during submaximal exercise.[10] In general, acute altitude living temporarily enhances muscle glycogenolysis and glycolysis while decreasing the use of free fatty acids as fuel. Of course, substrate use is related to exercise intensity. Therefore, when exercising during acute elevation change, a person is cautioned to use less intensity with greater duration, noting that some form of activity or daily exercise speeds the acclimation process. Also, eating at regular intervals, even if not that hungry, speeds acclimation.

## Athletic Performance

With the earlier information about acute changes in respiratory, cardiovascular, and metabolic functions at altitude, it is no wonder that endurance performance is reduced, especially as elevation increases. Recall that HR and $\dot{V}_E$ will increase, whereas $\dot{V}O_2$max and SV will decline in response to the desaturation of arterial blood. In addition, a long-distance athlete will face a reliance on carbohydrate and increased lactate in the blood. In turn, this may dampen force production in skeletal muscle, reinforcing the advice for the athlete to slowly increase intensity and volume over a period of 2 to 6 weeks instead of trying to train at the same quantity/quality as when at sea level.[6]

## In Your Own Words

Your friend just got back from visiting a friend in Denver. He said that when he tried to go mountain biking up in the hills, he just did not have his usual energy level. Explain to him why he may have been feeling unusually fatigued when he tried to ride.

## Adjustments to Chronic Altitude Exposure

Many chronic adjustments take place in the body when living at altitude, beginning after about 4 weeks of altitude exposure.[6] For the most part, individuals will feel more comfortable at rest and during exercise because of these respiratory, cardiovascular, and metabolic adjustments that become more efficient and pronounced as time goes on. Performance at altitude will also get better, primarily because of increased circulating red blood cells (RBCs). This increase in RBCs is a result of the release of erythropoietin (EPO), which stimulates RBC production in the bone marrow. Increased RBCs carry and deliver more oxygen in the blood to working muscle and other tissue.

## Respiratory Function

As stated previously, increased circulating RBCs help deliver more oxygen to where it is required. In accordance with this, the hypoxic hyperventilatory response continues to be slightly elevated versus sea level. Therefore, $\dot{V}_E$ remains elevated even with chronic altitude exposure. This is manifested by an increased breathing frequency, which remains slightly elevated even when acclimated. These chronic changes confer benefit by maintaining $SaO_2$ and potentially oxygen extraction at the cellular (i.e., muscular) level.

## Cardiovascular Function

Mature erythrocytes (i.e., RBCs) begin to appear after about 7 days of altitude exposure. This is a result of the immediate release of the hormone EPO, stimulated by the low $P_B$. The production of RBCs is termed **erythropoiesis**.[8]

Because of persistent dehydration and the resultant loss of blood volume, Q remains depressed during exercise, except possibly at maximal exercise, where it may increase slightly. This increase at maximal exercise

### RESEARCH HIGHLIGHT

### Operation Everest II

Operation Everest II[11] was a study conducted by a group of researchers who suggested that the oxygen transport chain was composed of four main links: (1) moving oxygen from the atmosphere to the lung alveoli, (2) diffusion of oxygen from alveolar air to the bloodstream, (3) circulating that blood to the tissues, and (4) diffusion of the oxygen from the blood into the tissue mitochondria. Of these four links, 1 and 4 seemed to be the most adaptable and helped ensure the continuance of exercise, even at extreme elevations (i.e., above 20,000 ft). In addition, the researchers[11] observed a fourfold increase in alveolar ventilation after acclimation. Thus, the shift to maintain a greater ventilation rate versus sea level breathing persisted as an altitude dweller. This factor may have a deleterious effect on athletic performance, but it is a necessary mechanism to maintain $\%SaO_2$. In the end, the low $P_B$ coupled with the ability to never fully saturate arterial blood is the proverbial dagger in the lung of an endurance athlete training at altitude.

Sutton JR, Reeves JT, Wagner PD, et al. Operation Everest II: Oxygen transport during exercise at extreme simulated altitude. *J Appl Physiol.* 1988;64:1309–1321.

## RESEARCH HIGHLIGHT

### Lactate Paradox at Altitude

John B. West[12] helped perpetuate the term "lactate paradox" in 1986 in response to lower lactate levels after acclimation during submaximal to maximal exercise versus sea-level values and acute altitude exposure concentrations. The lactate paradox refers to the fact that there is less lactate appearance in blood during exercise *after* acclimation. Of course, during acute altitude exposure, blood lactate concentration is higher versus sea-level values for submaximal or maximal exercise. The paradox occurs with lower levels of blood lactate after acclimation despite a sustained low oxygen environment. The reasons for this vary and are still under great scrutiny, including some who defiantly deny the existence of a lactate paradox at altitude.[13,14] Readers are encouraged to read reports by West[13] and van Hall[14] to discover how the lactate paradox debate rages on. In summary, know that most individuals will elicit a greater blood lactate concentration during acute altitude exposure and, therefore, will not be able to sustain high workloads until acclimation occurs and blood lactate concentrations decline.

West JB. Lactate during exercise at extreme altitude. *Fed Proc.* 1986;45:2953–2957.

may be because of increased myocardial contractility and a well-maintained Frank-Starling curve, which links filling pressure to SV.[11] Therefore, despite a losing battle with regard to maintaining $\dot{V}O_2max$, cardiac adaptations remain strong and allow athletes to power through progressive workouts as they adapt to their new environment and somewhat impaired "pump and transport" system. In other words, cardiac function is well preserved at various altitudes, including extreme altitude, such as the summit of Mt. Everest, the highest peak in the world at 29,029 ft.[11]

### Metabolic Function

After acclimatization (of about 4 weeks)[6] to a new, high-altitude environment, especially greater than 2,100 m (6,800 ft), increased free fatty acid mobilization may occur, in conjunction with reductions in blood glucose concentration at rest and during exercise. However, some individuals may experience enhanced carbohydrate metabolism upon acclimation to altitude.[6] This indicates possible interindividual differences when it comes to assessing a person's ability to adapt to chronic altitude living. Therefore, physiologically, people should not take anything for granted when living at higher elevations. This section explores a few more metabolic adjustments to chronic altitude exposure.

Because of a highly stimulated sympathetic nervous system when at altitude, norepinephrine remains elevated on acclimation, whereas epinephrine declines to near sea level values after about 5 days. Despite the reported decrease in epinephrine, a net increase in catecholamines (i.e., epinephrine + norepinephrine) remains and helps preserve blood flow to the tissues through enhanced HR, SV, and Q. In addition, as mentioned previously, continued elevation of norepinephrine may help promote some fatty acid utilization during submaximal exercise. Even though the body uses fat as a fuel, anyone traveling to, and living at, altitude should be aware of the need for slightly greater carbohydrate consumption, especially during intense

exercise in a low oxygen environment. Recall that intense exercise primarily relies on stored sugar. Lastly, an interesting phenomenon after acclimation is less blood lactate appearance near $\dot{V}O_2max$, termed the **lactate paradox**.[6] This may be due, in part, to the decline in epinephrine after 5 days at altitude.[6]

### Athletic Performance

Normally, endurance performance will improve at altitude after acclimation, but may not approach the same status as at sea level. Because of the intact HVR and enhanced oxygen extraction, performance may improve as the oxygen transport chain is conserved. Still, athletes should be aware that their $\dot{V}O_2max$ will remain lower (vs. their sea level value) while at altitude. Also, their speed of activity may remain depressed. If the goal is to live, train, and race at high altitude, then the aforementioned chronic altitude adaptations to the respiratory, cardiovascular, and metabolic systems are beneficial. If the goal is to return to sea level for enhanced performance, research is equivocal regarding how beneficial altitude training will be to enhance endurance and improve race times.[6] Therefore, most athletes will only spend a limited amount of time living and training at altitude. Primarily, they want to boost their RBC count or total hemoglobin mass ($Hb_{mass}$) over about 4 to 6 weeks, then return to sea level for most of their training.

## VIGNETTE I continued

■ After overcoming the initial deleterious effects of acute altitude, Scott Jurek experienced chronic improvement in his training speed and ability to ascend tall peaks (up to 14,000 ft) with renewed vigor and strength over about a 5-week period. In addition, he had to be aware of consuming extra carbohydrate-rich meals while maintaining adequate hydration. Notably, he should have been feeling the effects of increased circulating RBCs and oxygen extraction in tissue for improved mitochondrial respiration right *before* his 100-mile race. Therefore, his oxygen-carrying ability, although not back to sea-level values, was much improved after a little over a month at altitude. He was ready to race the Hardrock 100 Endurance Run and go for a course record.

## Performance and Altitude Training

### Sea-Level Performance After Altitude Exposure

Contrary to many people's perceptions, the literature remains inconclusive regarding the effect of altitude training on improving sea-level performance.[6,15] One primary reason is that well-controlled research studies are still scarce, because many studies lack a sea-level control group.[6] Second, different "dosages" of hypoxia have been implemented in various research studies such that it is difficult to determine what the appropriate altitude, number of hours per day, and number of days at altitude should be.[6] Third, great individual variability occurs with altitude training. In fact, there may be responders and nonresponders to acclimatization, such that certain athletes or individuals will live and train at altitude but not improve their hematocrit (i.e., percent of RBCs) or ability to change oxygen delivery and extraction on return to sea level.[16] Thus, there remains a certain mystique surrounding altitude training. What is the best way, then, to use altitude as a positive training tool?

A promising trend, substantiated with well-designed research studies, is the **live high/train low (LHTL)** protocol.[6,17] With this protocol, an individual lives "high," up to 10,000 ft (~3,050 m) or greater, and trains "low" (i.e., near sea level). This can be accomplished one of two ways. One way is to live in an altitude tent at sea level. This enhances erythropoiesis and subsequently endurance performance because of improved oxygen delivery to, and extraction of oxygen in, muscle tissue. Interestingly, most nonelite athletes may "feel" an improvement in their endurance ability after only 2 to 4 weeks of living at "altitude" (i.e., sleeping in a hypoxic tent) and training low. Alternatively, athletes wishing to boost their sea-level performance may want to physically live at altitude, such as in Park City, Utah (altitude of 8,200 ft [2,500 m]), and train nearby at a lower elevation in Salt Lake, Utah (altitude of 4,100 ft [1,250 m]). This is convenient because Salt Lake City is only about a 30-minute drive from Park City. Several researchers[17] actually used the aforementioned cities for a 4-week period of LHTL endurance training. When compared with "high-high" (living and

training at 8,200 ft) and "low-low" (living and training in a mountain environment at sea level or about 492 ft), the LHTL individuals were the only runners to improve sea-level 5K time trial performance. The reason for this was an increase in RBC mass and $\dot{V}O_2$max. Subjects were able to maintain sea-level training velocities, which led to the faster 5K times. In other words, the best way to boost sea-level performance by using altitude is through "sleeping high and training low."

### Performance at Altitude After Acclimatization

Even if some athletes may be somewhat disappointed to learn that altitude training (i.e., living and training at altitude) does not necessarily improve sea-level endurance performance, especially in elite-level athletes, there is no doubt that performance at altitude is enhanced/improved following acclimatization and training at moderate-to-high elevations. Of course, a common theme throughout this chapter has been the boost in circulating RBCs (or hematocrit) and RBC mass that occurs with chronic altitude living. This usually takes up to 3 to 4 weeks or more. Furthermore, training or living for a period in a hypoxic environment induces better oxygen extraction, increased oxidative muscle enzymes, decreased blood lactate accumulation, and increased buffering capacity in the blood.[18] Thus, performance at altitude is certainly improved after chronic exposure to high elevations, especially as a strategy to race faster in high-altitude trail runs versus competitors who may not be acclimated when they show up the day before the race from sea level.

### Current Trends in Altitude Training

This section reviews possible trends in the area of altitude training for performance. The primary expert in this area is Dr. Randy Wilber, Senior Exercise Physiologist at the U.S. Olympic Training Center in Colorado Springs, Colorado, who has identified the following fads[6]: (1) normobaric (sea-level) hypoxia via nitrogen dilution or use of normobaric hypoxic apartments, (2) hypoxic sleeping units, (3) intermittent hypoxic exposure, and (4) supplemental oxygen use when living at altitude. The specifics of each trend are beyond the scope of this chapter, but Wilber's book, *Altitude Training and Athletic Performance*,[6] has more complete information.

In short, the continuous use of normobaric hypoxic apartments or sleeping in a hypoxic tent has been shown to increase the release of serum EPO and significantly boost reticulocyte (immature RBC) count, thus bolstering $\dot{V}O_2$max and endurance performance at sea level. Note that the aforementioned two techniques take place at sea level so that speed of training is maintained while the benefits of altitude on oxygen-carrying capacity (i.e., increased circulating RBC count) is realized. In addition, these two techniques are similar to the LHTL procedure pioneered by Levine and Stray-Gunderson.[17] In contrast, intermittent hypoxia use is less reliable and is not proved to promote better performance at sea level, especially because the hypoxic sessions are normally only for a few hours at a time during rest.

Lastly, high-intensity workouts using supplemental oxygen (~26%–60% inspired oxygen mixture) while *residing* at **moderate altitude** (i.e., 2,100–2,500 m or 6,890–8,200 ft) has been shown to boost sea-level performance. For example, an endurance athlete who is living in Gunnison, Colorado, at 7,703 ft (2,350 m) could run workouts (e.g., 3- to 5-min intervals or 15- to 20-minute tempo runs one or two times per week) on a treadmill while inspiring a gas mixture with ≥26% oxygen to simulate sea-level oxygen inhalation and pace.[6] This technique serves to provide "doses" of sea-level speed sessions. The end result is that while breathing the supplemental oxygen at elevation the athlete will be able to accomplish more work at a faster pace during the interval or tempo run (vs. doing the workout at elevation at a slower pace). Overall, greater muscular "speed" and "force" adaptations occur for sea-level racing.

In summary, current trends in altitude training revolve around the proven LHTL phenomenon, but conclusive evidence is still lacking to unequivocally state that all altitude training trends truly improve sea-level performance or altitude success. Moreover, when one considers the variable nature of each individual's response to altitude, with some people being "nonresponders" to altitude training, even LHTL strategies may not work for everyone.

## Altitude Training Programs of Successful Coaches

Over the years, altitude training has become a "go-to" training tool used by many coaches, including collegiate and elite athlete trainers. In general, endurance coaches use altitude training in doses. For instance, when first arriving at moderate altitude, former Cross Country Head Coach at Adams State College in Alamosa, Colorado (2,300 m/7,544 ft), Joe Vigil, PhD, recommends an acclimation period of about 1 week with low-volume and low-intensity aerobic training, coupled with general resistance training. During weeks 2 to 4 at altitude, training volume and intensity should approach that of sea-level values. After week 5 and by week 6 at altitude, a regeneration period occurs where overall training volume and intensity are decreased to ensure a smooth transition back to sea-level training. Finally, Vigil recommends racing after about 6 to 8 days on return to sea level for best results or the biggest boost in performance.[6]

Notably, Vigil's cross country running teams while at Adams State College were well-known for their aerobic conditioning and toughness, especially during Division II (D-II) National Cross Country Championship races. The 1992 national team won the D-II national cross country title in Slippery Rock, Pennsylvania, with an unprecedented perfect score of 15 points (i.e., with individual runners finishing first through fifth overall; top 5 runners score with their place finishes added together; the lowest score wins as a team). Notably, the team lived and trained "high" at 7,544 ft in Alamosa but raced exceptionally well, repeatedly, at sea level.

Several other well-known endurance coaches,[6] namely, Arturo Barrios, Cross Country and Track Coach for the World Class Athlete Program in Boulder, Colorado, and Ørjan Madsen, PhD, Director, Olympiatoppen Altitude Project with the Norwegian Olympic Committee, also recommend "doses" of altitude to improve sea-level performance. Barrios subscribes to approximately the same amount of time spent at altitude (i.e., up to 6 weeks) as Coach Vigil's suggestion. Madsen suggests several doses of 21 days at altitude in between national and international/world competitions. Again, refer to Dr. Randy Wilber's text, *Altitude Training and Athletic Performance,*[6] for complete information about these coaches and their altitude training programs. Tables 29-1, 29-2, and 29-3 summarize the altitude training programs of Vigil, Barrios, and Madsen.

## Gains and Decrements in General Fitness After Acclimatization

Notably, altitude training has pros and cons. In short, arriving at altitude stimulates the release of EPO to enhance the rapid production of circulating RBCs, giving the body an increased ability to deliver and extract oxygen at the tissue level. In addition, breathing rate increases to compensate for the lower atmospheric pressure and inspired oxygen density. Thus, over a period of about 3 to 4 weeks or even less, and training at moderate altitude, a person will experience about a 1% increase in hemoglobin concentration per week. Longer stays equal greater hemoglobin responses.[19] Furthermore, there may be a synergistic effect of hypoxia and physical training on the erythropoietic response during visits to high altitude.[19] This means that exercise at altitude potentially helps enhance the acclimation process.

It makes sense, therefore, to assume that exercising at altitude (i.e., in a hypoxic environment) ensures an adequate blood adaptation response to enhance fitness throughout the acclimatization period of about 4 weeks. In contrast, in some individuals, decrements in overall fitness may occur because of reduced caloric intake and sleep disturbances,[18] common adverse effects of living "high." Thus, athletes and exercisers should remain diligent in regard to eating a holistic (i.e., a variety of foods), nutrient-dense diet along with sufficient hydration (up to ≥5 L water with some sport drink per day). In addition, fitness may be compromised because of the decrement in $\dot{V}O_2$max; therefore, a person's ability to maintain a "fast" pace while at moderate altitude or greater may be diminished for several weeks or more. Be aware, then, while at altitude the body is under constant, general stress, and any exercise or "work" should be scaled back accordingly.

## Physiological Benefits to Altitude Training

The physiological benefits of altitude exposure/training are numerous (Table 29-4). They include respiratory,

**Table 29-1.** Altitude Training Program of Joe Vigil, PhD, former head cross country and track coach at Adams State College in Alamosa, Colorado (2,300 m/7,544 ft)

| PHASE | DURATION | TRAINING OBJECTIVES |
|---|---|---|
| Acclimatization | 1 week | • Slow endurance runs of 30-minute duration performed 2–3 times/day.<br>• Swimming, cycling, weight training, flexibility, and walking are included in the daily training schedule. |
| Primary training following acclimatization | 2–4 weeks | • Training volume is increased toward 100% of sea-level volume.<br>• For interval workouts the pace of the work interval is slower and the duration of the rest period longer versus sea-level pace and duration.<br>• Training intensity for both aerobic and anaerobic workouts is gradually increased. |
| Recovery and preparation for return to sea level | 1 week | • Fatigue should be avoided in the last 4–5 days before return to sea level.<br>• Training volume, training intensity, and general strength training are systematically decreased. |
| Return to sea level | | • First 4–5 days are used for recovery and reestablishment of the normal sea-level training pattern.<br>• Normal sea-level training continues for the next 2–3 days.<br>• The first competition should take place after 6–8 days at sea level.<br>• After the initial 6–8 days at sea level, training consists of a significant reduction in training volume in combination with a progressive increase in training intensity in preparation for key national and international competitions. |

*Source:* Reprinted from Wilber,[6] by permission.

**Table 29-2.** Altitude Training Program of Arturo Barrios, coach and former International Amateur Athletics Federation world champion in cross country and world record holder in the 10,000-m run

| PHASE | DURATION | TRAINING OBJECTIVES |
|---|---|---|
| Acclimatization | 1 week | • Long-distance runs of moderate intensity<br>• Reduction of sea-level volume by 20%<br>• Interval training not attempted |
| Primary training following acclimatization | 4–5 weeks | • Introduction of interval training:<br> - Pace of work interval must be slower than sea-level pace<br> - Duration of rest interval is doubled versus sea-level rest interval<br> - Gradual modifications are made to work interval pace (faster) and rest interval duration (shorter).<br>• Weekly hill workouts:<br> - 10 × 100 m<br> - 10-mile run at 2,560–2,590 m (8,400–8,500 ft) over rolling terrain |
| Return to sea level | 2–10 days | • Optimal schedule must be determined through trial and error:<br> - At 1–2 days before sea-level competition<br> - At approximately 7 days before sea-level competition<br> - At 7–10 days before sea-level competition<br> - Optimal schedule must be individualized for each athlete.<br> - Performance may be enhanced for up to 2 weeks following return to sea level. |

*Source:* Reprinted from Wilber,[6] by permission.

**Table 29-3.** Sample Altitude Training Program Prescribed by Ørjan Madsen, PhD, Director of Olympiatoppen Altitude Project, Norwegian Olympic Committee

| ALTITUDE CAMP 1 (21 DAYS) | SEA-LEVEL TRAINING (7–8 WEEKS) | NATIONAL CHAMPIONSHIPS (1–2 WEEKS BEFORE ALTITUDE CAMP 2) | ALTITUDE CAMP 2 (21 DAYS) | SEA-LEVEL TRAINING (15–21 DAYS) | WORLD CHAMPIONSHIPS (4–7 DAYS) |
|---|---|---|---|---|---|
| **Phase 1 = 2 days** Adaptation Initial adjustments **Phase 2 = 17 days** Application Increase in training load • **Basic training period = 7 days** - Endurance 1 - Sprints - Cross-training and strength training • **Specific training period = 10 days** - Endurance 1 - Endurance 2 - Sprints - Race pace/ anaerobic work - Cross-training and strength training **Phase 3 = 2 days** Regeneration Recovery | Similar to other sea-level period, just longer duration | Peaking = high intensity, low volume | Similar to Altitude Camp 1 | **Phase 1 = 2 days** Regeneration Recovery **Phase 2 = 13–19 days** Application Normal training increase • **Training period = 8 days** - Normal training - Taper - No competition • **Precompetition period = 5–11 days** - Stabilization of training - Taper - Mental preparation **Phase 3 = 4–7 days** Competition Maintain status | Peaking = high intensity, low volume |

*Note:* Madsen believes that altitude training should be performed at altitude (minimum altitude ≥ 1,800 m or 5,905 ft) and peak performance occurs about 16 to 24 days after return to sea level.
*Source:* Adapted from Wilber,[6] by permission.

heart, blood, muscle/metabolic, and buffering adaptations. In fact, lung muscles are potentially more trained because of marked hyperventilation, in addition to $Pao_2$ values rising and counteracting the decrement in $Sao_2$. The heart, although somewhat comprised because of decreased Q and HR during maximal and submaximal exercise after acclimation, has well-preserved contractility and may help induce increased capillary growth due to a lowered HR.[18] This underscores the variable nature of how the body responds, physiologically, to altitude exposure.

In relation to the blood, increased red cell volume, hemoglobin, and hematocrit values are observed, especially when training at more than 2,500 m (8,200 ft). This indicates that living at this elevation ensures adequate blood adaptations in most individuals as compared with living lower. Muscle metabolism also improves to a point, in that citrate synthase and other aerobic enzymes, such as 3-hydroxyacyl-coenzyme A, are likely to increase. Also, the oxygen-binding protein, myoglobin, which helps transport oxygen from blood to mitochondria, tends to increase.[20] However, because of poor study quality, the mechanisms behind muscle adaptation processes to altitude exposure remain elusive. Finally, muscle buffering capacity, most prominently with respect to hydrogen ion concentration from the production of lactic acid, is initially blunted when exposed to altitude. Upon acclimatization, the acid-base balance of the blood is restored and $Pao_2$ and $Sao_2$ also improve, improving a person's ability to deliver and extract oxygen.

## Table 29-4. Summary of Effects of Acute and Chronic Exposure to Altitude

| EFFECTS OF *ACUTE* EXPOSURE TO ALTITUDE | | EFFECTS OF *CHRONIC* EXPOSURE TO ALTITUDE | |
|---|---|---|---|
| CHANGE | EFFECT | CHANGE | EFFECT |
| ↑ Resting and submaximal HR | ↑ $O_2$ transport to tissue | ↓ Resting and submaximal HR (below ↑ of early altitude exposure) | Restoration of more normal circulatory homeostasis |
| ↑ Resting and submaximal $\dot{V}_E$ | ↑ $PaO_2$, ↓ $CO_2$, and $H^+$ in blood, AMS, left shift of oxyhemoglobin dissociation curve, predominance of hypoxic ventilatory drive | ↑ Pulmonary BP, ↑ pulmonary vascularity | Improved pulmonary perfusion |
| ↓ $\dot{V}O_2$max | ↓ Exercise capacity, ↓ speed of training | ↔ $\dot{V}O_2$max (does not decrement further) | Maintenance of oxygen delivery and extraction |
| Few acute changes in blood, muscle, or liver | | ↑ RBC 2,3-DPG<br>↓ Plasma volume, ↑ hemoglobin/RBC/ hematocrit values | Shifts $HbO_2$ curve to right<br>Improved $O_2$-carrying capacity of blood |
| | | ↑ Size and number of mitochondria, ↑ quantity of oxidative enzymes | Improved muscle biochemistry and ability to process oxygen in aerobic metabolism |
| | | ↑ Skeletal muscle vascularity | Improved $O_2$ transport |
| | | ↑ Tissue myoglobin | Improved cellular $O_2$ transport/storage capacity |

↑, increase; ↓, decrease; ↔, no change; AMS, acute mountain sickness; BP, blood pressure; HR, heart rate; $PaO_2$, alveolar partial pressure of oxygen; RBC, red blood cell; $\dot{V}O_2$max, maximal oxygen consumption.

## Health Risks and Altitude Exposure

More than 40 million tourists climb to altitudes greater than 2,500 m (8,200 ft) every year. Accordingly, health risks that are related to altitude sickness are increasing.[22] All nontraumatic health risks are due to altitude-induced atmospheric conditions, namely, low atmospheric pressure, including decreased $PO_2$, lower air temperature with increasing elevation, and decreased water vapor.[22]

Three primary health risks occur when exposed to altitude: **acute altitude sickness** (also known as acute mountain sickness [AMS]), **high-altitude pulmonary edema (HAPE)**, and **high-altitude cerebral edema (HACE)**. AMS is an altitude-induced illness with clinical symptoms of headache, nausea, vomiting, and weakness.[6] Although AMS is most prevalent at high altitude (>5,000 m/16,400 ft),[6] it has been reported in athletes and visitors to low or moderate altitude (i.e., as low as about 2,500 m/8,200 ft) as well. AMS may be exacerbated by aerobic exercise within the initial 6 to 10 hours of exposure in some individuals.[6,23] AMS persists for up to approximately 96 hours after arrival to altitude and disappears in about 4 or 5 days, peaking in severity on the second or third day.[23] If AMS does not

progress and subsides by the fifth day at altitude, then it may not reoccur. In general, AMS is not considered a life-threatening illness (Box 29-1).

HAPE and HACE are more life threatening and include the same symptoms as AMS. Furthermore, HAPE includes a disruption of normal breathing, blue lips and fingernails, mental confusion, and loss of consciousness. HACE further includes ataxia, irrationality, hallucinations, blurred vision, and blurring of consciousness.[23] In general, the severity of HAPE and HACE depends on altitude (i.e., higher elevations equal greater risk for and severity of onset of symptoms), rate of ascent, and susceptibility of the athlete or visitor to altitude (i.e., prior history of illness at altitude). Treatment for both maladies is simple and involves rapid descent to lower altitude and supplemental oxygen. Also, the Gamow bag is a form of treatment if rapid descent is not possible or a quick treatment method is needed to help alleviate symptoms of HAPE or HACE. The bag is essentially an inflatable pressure bag big enough to fit a whole person. The pressure inside the bag simulates sea level or possibly acts like a hyperbaric chamber (see the Climbing-High.com website for more details: http://www.climbing-high.com/the-gamow-bag.html).[24]

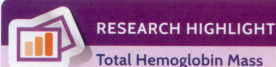

## RESEARCH HIGHLIGHT

### Total Hemoglobin Mass

When assessing how well a person acclimates to living at moderate-to-high altitude (simulated or actual environment), it is best to measure $Hb_{mass}$ in the blood versus only looking at hematocrit, for instance, which changes depending on hydration status of the body. Although the $Hb_{mass}$ measurement technique is cumbersome and involves testing in a laboratory, it is one of the best ways to measure actual adaptation to altitude living, which, in turn, should help improve performance at sea level or altitude[21] (Fig. 29-4).

For instance, researchers in Bobigny, France, found a 10.1% increase in $Hb_{mass}$ when elite middle-distance runners lived at a simulated high altitude (14 hr/day for 6 nights at 2,500 m and 12 nights at 3,000 m) and trained low (at 1,200 m) versus a control group sleeping and training in normoxia (i.e., sea level). The end result was that the LHTL group improved their maximal and submaximal aerobic performance by most likely boosting their oxygen transport ability when back racing at "sea level."[21] Mechanistically, this was due to the improved $Hb_{mass}$.

U.S. Air Force Academy Athletics. *Human performance laboratory.* Colorado Springs, CO: U.S. Air Force Academy Athletics. Available at: http://www.goairforcefalcons.com/genrel/120106aag.html. Accessed September 5, 2014.

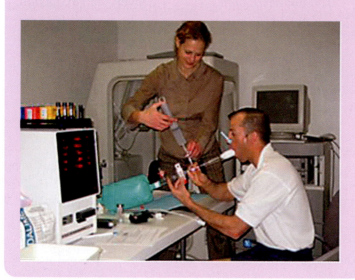

**Figure 29-4.** Demonstration of $CO_2$ rebreathing method to measure total hemoglobin mass in Olympic cross country ski athlete Liz Stephen. *(Photo courtesy of Noah Hoffman.)*

---

### Box 29-1. How to Avoid Acute Altitude Sickness

Following are some potential methods to avoid or treat the onset of AMS during acute altitude exposure:

- Take prescription acetazolamide or aspirin with adequate rest and recovery.
- Eliminate training or significantly modify training status until recovery or symptoms subside.
- Eat and drink at regular intervals, staying well-fed and hydrated.
- Progress to moderate or high elevation slowly, such as no more than about 1,500 ft/day.
- Arrive at altitude early and within 24 hours train or compete, then go back to sea level as soon as possible (i.e., this method assumes the exerciser will be gone from altitude before AMS strikes).

### VIGNETTE I conclusion

■ Scott Jurek arrived at the start of the Hardrock 100 Endurance Run in Silverton, Colorado, in mid-June, about 5 weeks before the race began in mid-July. The altitude in Silverton is nearly 9,305 ft. The course has a cumulative vertical gain of 33,992 ft of ascent (including a traverse over the 14,000-ft Handies Peak) and 33,992 ft of descent, for a total gain/loss of 67,984 ft. Because the nature of ultra-running is not "speed" but rather "time on feet," Jurek was attempting to effectively acclimate before the start while actively running most of the course and experimenting with clothing, hydration, and nutrient intake. During the initial week of his 5-week stay, he *slowly* trudged around the various trails to acclimate his mind, body, and eating habits while keeping a mind-set to gradually ramp up his mileage to accommodate high-altitude terrain by the fourth week. However, to save energy, he began a slight detraining process during the remaining 4 to 5 days before the start. Of note, his lung, heart, blood, muscle metabolic, and buffering adaptations were augmented in about 4 weeks, especially because he was specifically living and training high with an eye toward competing at an average elevation of about 11,000 ft during perhaps the most difficult 100-mile run in the world. Jurek accomplished his goal. On July 19, 2007, he set a new course record of 26 hours 8 minutes, beating the old course record by 27 minutes. Interestingly, Jurek opened the door for what was possible at Hardrock. The next race (in 2008), a young ultra-runner named Kyle Skaggs of Ashland, Oregon, smashed Jurek's record to finish in a still-unmatched course record time of 23 hours 23 minutes (at an age of 23 years). Notably, Skaggs emulated Jurek's pre-race training schedule and chose to live and train in Silverton for months before the race.

## AIR POLLUTION

Exposure to pollution or "smog" is generally a phenomenon of living in a large city and can have detrimental effects on health and exercise capacity—similar to acute altitude exposure (Fig. 29-5). In fact, epidemiological evidence indicates that air pollution adversely affects the cardiovascular (and pulmonary) system, leading to heightened cardiovascular morbidity and mortality. In addition, high levels of PM have been shown to adversely affect the respiratory lining, immune system, and blood coagulation processes.[27] Notably, about 60,000 deaths per year in the United States are attributed to air pollution.[27] The **Air Quality Index** (Fig. 29-6) measures the quality of air for five major air pollutants regulated by the Clean Air Act: ground-level ozone ($O_3$), particular matter, carbon monoxide (CO), sulfur dioxide ($SO_2$), and nitrogen dioxide. The color-coded chart has explanations for the numerical values.

Common microscopic and submicroscopic particles include $O_3$, $SO_2$, and CO.[10] Fine particles, with a mass median aerodynamic diameter less than 10 μm ($PM_{10}$), are emitted primarily from the combustion of fossil fuels and are related to increased mortality.[27] Mortality from the continued inhalation of fine particles may be caused by a reduced capacity of blood vessels to dilate and a concurrent increase in clotting activity. Moreover, lung capacity may decrease, and anyone with preexisting cardiovascular disease may be at heightened risk for a sudden cardiac event. Overall, physiological detriments

---

## RESEARCH HIGHLIGHT

### Altitude and Weight Loss in Obese Persons–A New Trend?

One new novel use of altitude training or exposure to altitude could be in aiding weight loss. In a recent article by Netzer et al,[25] the authors studied 20 obese individuals (average body mass index [BMI] and age were 33.1 kg/m$^2$ and 47.6 years, respectively) randomized to 1 of 2 groups: normobaric hypoxia (15 vol% $O_2$ equal to about 2,500 m or 8,200 ft) or normoxia (21 vol% $O_2$ equal to nearly sea level). Participants were unaware of their group assignment as they exercised in a special room built in normobaric conditions. Both groups trained in their individualized "fat burning zone" equal to moderate intensity (i.e., ~60% $\dot{V}O_2$max; HR of ~118 beats/min) for 8 weeks, 3 times per week for 90 minutes on a stepper, treadmill, and bicycle ergometer. The normobaric hypoxia group lost an average of 1.14 kg. The normoxia (control) group showed no weight loss from baseline to 8 weeks. Furthermore, although not significant versus the sham group, the normobaric hypoxic group tended to decrease their BMI to a greater extent.

Another study, conducted by Lippl et al,[26] also found that simulated altitude exposure may enhance weight loss. A 1-week stay in hypobaric hypoxia at 2,650 m (~8,700 ft) by 20 obese participants (mean age ± SD: 55.7 ± 4.1 years; mean BMI ± SD: 33.7 ± 1.0 kg/m$^2$) resulted in significant weight loss without increased exercise. Leptin levels also increased because of the 1-week altitude stimulus despite the reduction in body weight. Leptin is secreted by adipocytes and has the tendency to suppress appetite, although the mechanism is not well understood. Hypobaric hypoxia, which simulates high altitude, seems to stimulate leptin release,[26] and thereby has some regulatory effect on appetite. Subjects in this study lost weight (about 1.54 kg) over 1 week along with a concurrent, natural reduction in daily food intake of about 734 kcal/day, or 5,138 kcal/week, while maintaining normal everyday walking assessed via step counters. The authors attributed the weight loss to increased BMR and reduced food intake.

*Netzer NC, Chytra R, Kupper T. Low intense physical exercise in normobaric hypoxia leads to more weight loss in obese people than low intense physical exercise in normobaric sham hypoxia. Sleep Breath. 2008;12:129–134.*
*Lippl FJ, Neubauer S, Schipfer S, Lichter N. Hypobaric hypoxia causes weight reduction in obese subjects. Obesity. 2010;18: 675–681.*

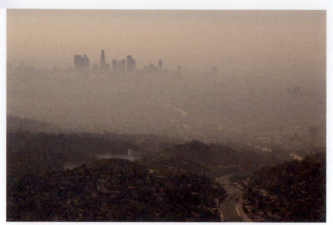

**Figure 29-5.** Air pollution adversely affects the cardio-vascular and pulmonary systems, leading to heightened cardiovascular morbidity and mortality. *(Photo by Tyler Oliver)*

to various pollutants depend on a "dose" response, including pollutant concentration, duration of exposure to PM, and the volume of air inspired.[10] During exercise, of course, an increase in ventilation rate increases exposure to PM; therefore, during peak pollution periods, exercise should potentially be limited.

## Cardiopulmonary Performance

In general, at any given workload, HR increases 5 to 10 beats above normal,[28] oxygen saturation remains steady or slightly declines,[28] and heart-rate variability (HRV) will be reduced[28] when exposed to air pollution. The latter effect, HRV reduction with increased PM, is a possible promoter of arrhythmogenic activity in the heart, especially in the elderly, possibly due to alteration of sodium, calcium, and potassium channels in the myocardium.[29] Thus, exercise intensity should be modified in this population when exposed to pollution.

Interestingly, even very short-term, acute exposure to air pollution may cause a decrement in exercise performance, especially at submaximal levels. Researchers[30] have shown that anaerobic threshold (AT), HR at ($AT_{HR}$), and percent $\dot{V}O_2max$ at ($AT\%\dot{V}O_2max$) will significantly decrease upon acute exposure to air pollution of 1 hour (Fig. 29-7). There was no change in $\dot{V}O_2max$, maximal HR, or velocity at AT ($AT_{vel}$). The primary reason for this was that at the highest levels of exertion, anaerobic processes, glycolytic muscle fibers, and the buffering of $H^+$ ions took over to maintain muscle power.[30] See Table 29-5 for a summary of the aforementioned study variables and how they changed in relation to air pollution. Again, note that maximal exertion levels were not affected by the exposure to air pollution for 1 hour. For instance, marathoners may have a harder time versus middle-distance runners competing in a polluted environment.

Remember, at lower or submaximal levels of exercise, the transport of oxygen to muscle and extraction of oxygen from blood are of primary importance to maintain aerobic energy production in working tissue. Whether an exerciser is acutely or chronically inhaling moderate to high amounts of PM, CO may be the most abundant pollutant. CO has about a 230 times greater affinity for hemoglobin than oxygen in the blood, and thereby reduces oxygen transport in the blood[31] (Fig. 29-8). This, in turn, decreases the ability to exercise at submaximal levels for long time periods.

On a more clinical level, acute exposure to air pollution lasting only 1 hour has the potential to severely limit individuals with acute or chronic cardiac or respiratory abnormalities during exercise. This holds true regardless of the severity of disease and consequently could lead to probable worsening of a person's condition.[30] Even healthy individuals with high functional capacities (i.e., military firemen) saw decrements in their submaximal workload after a 1-hour exposure to air pollution.[30]

In summary, air pollution and its effects on individuals may be hard to predict in any given environment.

| Air Quality Index Levels of Health Concern | Numerical Value | Meaning |
|---|---|---|
| Good | 0–50 | Air quality is considered satisfactory, and air pollution poses little or no risk. |
| Moderate | 51–100 | Air quality is acceptable; however, for some pollutants, there may be a moderate health concern for a very small number of people who are unusually sensitive to air pollution. |
| Unhealthy for sensitive groups | 101–150 | Members of sensitive groups may experience health effects. The general public is not likely to be affected. |
| Unhealthy | 151–200 | Everyone may begin to experience health effects; members of sensitive groups may experience more serious health effects. |
| Very unhealthy | 201–300 | Health alert: Everyone may experience more serious health effects. |
| Hazardous | 301–500 | Health warnings of emergency conditions. The entire population is more likely to be affected. |

**Figure 29-6.** The Air Quality Index. *(From Air Quality Index (AQI)–A guide to air quality and your health. AIRNow website. Available at: http://airnow.gov/index.cfm?action=aqibasics.aqi. Accessed September 5, 2014. http://www.airnow.gov/index.cfm?action=aqibasics.aqi.)*

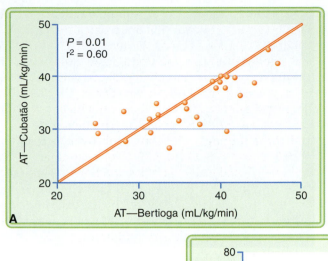

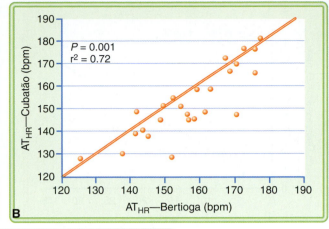

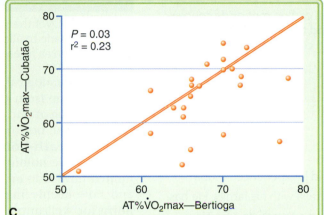

**Figure 29-7.** Biological impact of air pollution at Cubatão (polluted city) and Bertioga (low pollution) on cardiorespiratory parameters. Correlations were tested with the Pearson correlation method, and $p$ values (paired $t$ test) are reported in each panel. AT, anaerobic threshold; $AT_{HR}$, heart rate at anaerobic threshold; $AT\%\dot{V}O_2max$, percent maximal oxygen consumption at anaerobic threshold. *(Reprinted from Oliveira et al.24)*

**Table 29-5.** Cardiovascular performance variables of young adults in a polluted environment (Cubatão, Brazil) and in a relatively clean environment (Bertioga, Brazil)

| | BERTIOGA | | CUBATÃO | |
| --- | --- | --- | --- | --- |
| | MEAN ± SD | RANGE | MEAN ± SD | RANGE |
| $\dot{V}O_2max$ (mL/kg/min) | 54.82 ± 8.37 | 38.48–68.42 | 54.50 ± 7.31 | 44.09–66.30 |
| MHR (bpm) | 188.75 ± 10.33 | 173.00–206.00 | 189.12 ± 9.8 | 171.00–206.00 |
| AT (mL/kg/min) | 36.98 ± 5.62 | 25.10–46.93 | 35.04 ± 4.91 | 31.07–45.07 |
| $AT_{HR}$ (beats/min) | 157.44 ± 13.64 | 125.00–178.00 | 152.08 ± 14.86* | 129.00–180.00 |
| $AT_{vel}$ (km/hr) | 10.76 ± 1.51 | 8.00–14.00 | 10.56 ± 1.39 | 8.00–14.00 |
| $AT\%\dot{V}O_2max$ | 67.40 ± 5.35 | 52.00–78.00 | 64.56 ± 6.55* | 51.00–75.00 |

Data are reported for 25 healthy male adults who exercised in both cities. Note that Bertioga has a low level of pollution, whereas Cubatão has high levels of pollution.

*$p < 0.05$ compared with Bertioga (paired $t$ test).

AT, anaerobic threshold; $AT_{HR}$, heart rate at anaerobic threshold; $AT_{vel}$, velocity at anaerobic threshold; $AT\%\dot{V}O_2max$, percentage maximal oxygen consumption at anaerobic threshold; MHR, maximal heart rate; SD, standard deviation; $\dot{V}O_2max$, maximal oxygen consumption.
*Source:* Reprinted from Oliveira et al.[2]

Higher than normal amounts of CO in the blood seem to be one of the primary culprits when it comes to blunting exercise performance and possibly other cardiopulmonary parameters (except for HR, which is normally higher than usual) during exercise. Submaximal exercise seems to be most affected. Therefore, when exercising in regions with air pollution, take into account the following advice: (1) attempt to decrease exposure to pollutants before exercise (i.e., to reduce duration and dose of irritants); (2) refrain from exercising in areas with high amounts of CO (e.g., smoking areas, high-traffic spots, big city environments); and (3) abstain from exercise when pollutants may be near their greatest levels (i.e., 7–10 a.m. and 4–7 p.m.).[10]

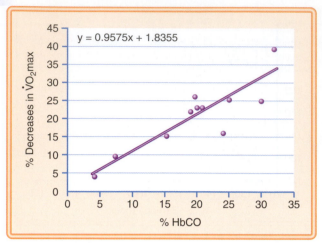

**Figure 29-8.** Relation between carbon monoxide concentration in the blood (HbCO) and the percent change or decrement in maximal oxygen consumption ($\dot{V}O_2$max).

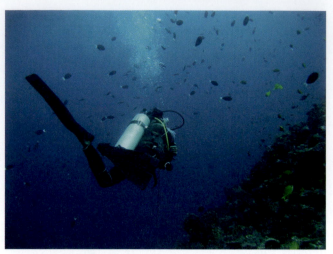

**Figure 29-9.** Over the years, many innovative attempts have been made to allow individuals to explore the ocean bottom as freely as possible. *(Photo by Zhu Difeng)*

## UNDERWATER DIVING

### VIGNETTE II

■ Andre is a 40-year-old inexperienced scuba diver on vacation in Australia with his family. He has taken lessons and gone on a few dives near his home in San Diego, and he is eager to experience the world-class dive sites in the area. He signs up for a few dives over the course of his 2-week trip. After his second dive, Andre tells Caroline, the dive instructor who works at the resort, that he is having terrible pain in his joints. He appears to be getting panicky and is actually doubled over in pain. What might be the cause of Andre's discomfort, and what can Caroline do to properly address the situation?

### Brief History of Underwater Diving

Since the beginning of time people have explored the depths.[32,33] Initially, the purpose of underwater diving was to forage for food and sponges. Over time, diving has evolved to include searching for pearls, salvaging sunken ships, conducting military operations, and/or simply the recreational pleasure of observing fish and the beauty of the underwater environment (Fig. 29-9). Over the years, many innovative attempts have been made to allow individuals to explore the ocean bottom as freely as possible. This section provides a brief overview of the landmark innovations that have changed how people can explore the underwater environment.

Dating back more than two thousand years, evidence suggests that humans explored the undersea world. Archeological digs uncovered shells that had to have come from the ocean bottom, and pictures within tombs of ancient civilizations depicted divers exploring the bottom of the ocean. All of this was done by **breath-hold diving** (i.e., diving from the surface while holding one's breath). Obviously, this limited how long individuals could stay underwater and how deeply they could explore. This was the norm for well into the 15th century, because there were no other alternatives for staying underwater for extended periods.

In the 1600s, diving bells were developed. These "bells" or chambers (caissons) were suspended from a ship and held vertically. The earliest diving bells would house a "bubble" of air. Divers would put their heads into the bell, breathe deeply to fill their lungs, and then explore away from the bell until they needed to take another breath. They would return to the bell and repeat this process. In this way, they could stay underwater until the air in the bell was exhausted.

The diving bell concept evolved into diving chambers. The most notable inventor was Edmond Halley, who is better known for discovering the comet named after him. Divers could explore away from the chamber while wearing a "cap of maintenance," which brought air to the diver through a leather hose. Air within the chamber could be replenished with weighted buckets lowered from the surface. These devices were very innovative in their design and were used fairly extensively to explore sunken ships and salvage booty.

In 1715, Englishman John Lethbridge developed a one-man, completely enclosed diving suit. The suit was essentially a leather-covered barrel of air equipped with a glass porthole for viewing. It had two armholes with watertight sleeves. This apparatus was lowered from a ship and provided more maneuverability than the diving bell. The operating depth of this apparatus was reported to be 60 ft, and it allowed Lethbridge and his colleagues to explore sunken ships.

The diving suit concept was expanded on in 1819 by German Augustus Siebe, who invented the first "diving dress." The diving dress consisted of a copper helmet and a leather jacket that allowed the diver to walk more freely on the bottom of the ocean.

These innovations allowed divers to explore deeper and stay underwater for longer periods. However, divers began to develop a variety of medical problems when they returned to the surface. In 1878, Paul Bert discovered that these problems were caused by nitrogen bubbles that had dissolved in the bloodstream. As the diver ascended from the depths, these bubbles would expand, often settle in the joints, and cause affected divers to walk with a bent over body position because of the pain. The term the **bends** was coined to describe this posture. It was suggested that, to dissipate these bubbles and avoid the bends, divers should ascend more slowly and stop at regular intervals. In 1908, J.S. Haldane published the first set of decompression tables for preventing the bends, a term that is often used interchangeably with **decompression sickness**.

Around this same time, the U.S. Navy developed the Mark V diving helmet. The diver wore an airtight helmet and suit, with air supply managed from the surface. This allowed the diver to move freely about the bottom. However, the helmet still required divers to be tethered to a ship or vessel on the surface and limited their mobility.

The next 40 years saw the evolution of a variety of devices that attempted to allow divers to carry their own air supply and be completely free from the surface. In 1943, Frenchmen Jacques Cousteau and Émile Gagnan invented the first "demand" regulator. The demand regulator allowed the diver to inhale compressed air from a tank on his or her back and exhale into the water. The device was called the Aqua Lung and allowed the diver to freely explore the bottom for as long as their air supply lasted. The Aqua Lung was a double-hose system, which was patented. Because the Aqua Lung was patented and difficult to obtain in Australia, Australian Ted Eldred designed a single-hose system called the "porpoise," which he began selling in 1952. This single-hose concept has become the most common tank-hose design in use today. These two devices led to development of the acronym **self-contained underwater breathing apparatus (SCUBA)** (coined by American physician Christian J. Lambertsen), which is used today to describe almost all underwater sport diving.

Since the advent of the Aqua Lung, many refinements have been made to diving equipment, with most of them designed to make the diving experience safer and more comfortable. The materials used for masks are now made out of form-fitting silicone, which is much more comfortable and durable than older rubber versions. Divers often now carry an "octopus," or extra regulator, attached to their tank as a safety measure in case their diving partner runs out of gas. A low-pressure hose is hooked up to an inflatable **buoyancy compensator** that can be adjusted with the push of a button. Fins are also lighter, more flexible, and easier to adjust, which makes the whole diving experience much more efficient and enjoyable.

Although the equipment for sport diving has undergone many stylistic changes, a great deal of time and energy has been spent on educating and certifying individuals on how to dive safely. The first scuba certification program was started by the YMCA in 1959. Quickly following, the National Association of Underwater Instructors was formed in 1960 and the Professional Association of Diving Instructors formed in 1966. National Association of Underwater Instructors and Professional Association of Diving Instructors are still actively certifying sport divers. To dive at most resorts and to refill scuba tanks, divers must show a certification card from one of these organizations.

## Physics of Diving

Diving below the surface of the water poses numerous challenges to the body, most of which are related to changes induced by properties related to physics. Failure to understand these properties and how to avoid diving-related injuries can cause serious injury and even death.

### Hydrostatic Pressure

The first challenge involves the increase in **hydrostatic pressure** as a person descends underwater. The increase in hydrostatic pressure is caused by the increased weight of the water from above. The deeper one dives, the greater the amount of water above the body, and hence the greater the pressure on the outside of the body. When a person dives into the deep end of a swimming pool and feels his or her ears start to hurt, this is largely due to the increase in hydrostatic pressure. The higher pressure pushes the ear drum in, resulting in pain.

Hydrostatic pressure is defined in terms of **atmospheres**, with the units being described in millimeters of mercury (mm Hg). Pressure on the outside of the body at sea level is 760 mm Hg, or 1 atmosphere. Every 33 ft below the surface of the water increases the pressure on the outside of the body by an additional 760 mm Hg, or 1 atmosphere. Table 29-6 outlines the relation between the depth of diving and the increase in hydrostatic pressure. The increase in hydrostatic pressure "pushes" on the outside of the body, which results in numerous physiological consequences.

### Boyle's Law

The increase in hydrostatic pressure also has a tremendous effect on the volume of air in the air-filled cavities of the bodies, especially the lungs. The relation between changes in pressure and changes in volume is described by **Boyle's law**, which states that, at a given temperature, the volume of a gas varies inversely with the pressure (Fig. 29-10).

**Table 29-6. Relation Between Depth of Diving and Increase in Hydrostatic Pressure**

| DEPTH | | PRESSURE | |
|---|---|---|---|
| FEET | METERS | ATMOSPHERES | MM HG |
| 11 | Sea level | 1 | 760 |
| 33 | 10 | 2 | 1,520 |
| 66 | 20 | 3 | 2,280 |
| 99 | 30 | 4 | 3,040 |
| 133 | 40 | 5 | 3,800 |
| 166 | 50 | 6 | 4,560 |
| 200 | 60 | 7 | 5,320 |
| 300 | 90 | 10 | 7,600 |
| 400 | 120 | 13 | 9,880 |
| 500 | 150 | 16 | 12,160 |
| 600 | 180 | 19 | 14,440 |

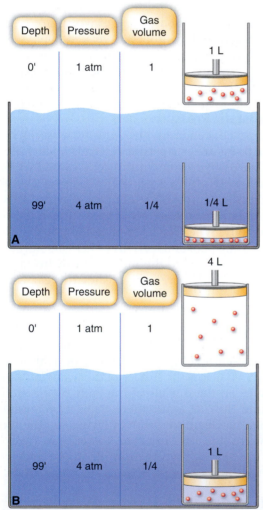

**Figure 29-10.** Boyle's law defines the relationship between the increase in hydrostatic pressure as a person descends below the surface and the impact that has on the volume of air in the air-filled spaces of the lungs. A, A volume equal to 1 L at sea level is reduced to one fourth of that volume (0.25 L) at a depth of 99 ft. B, A volume of 1 L inhaled at a depth of 99 ft will expand to 4 L at the surface.

For example, if the volume of air in the lungs on the surface is 5 L, this volume will be reduced to 2.5 L at a depth of 33 ft (2 atmospheres) and further reduced to 1.25 L at a depth of 99 ft (4 atmospheres). The converse of this relation becomes vitally important when ascending from depth. If a diver were to take a breath equal to 2 L at a depth of 99 ft and hold her breath as she came to the surface, that volume of air in the lungs would expand to 4 L at 33 ft and further to 8 L by the time she reached the surface. This expansion would most likely rupture the diver's lungs. This example illustrates why it is imperative that divers understand this basic law of physics and the relationship it has to safe diving.

## In Your Own Words

One of the most important things a person has to remember when scuba diving is to never hold your breath. Explain to a friend why it is so important *not* to hold in his or her breath when ascending from the bottom.

### Henry's Law

Another gas law that affects the safety of divers is **Henry's Law**, which describes the relation between pressure and how much gas can be dissolved in a liquid, namely, the blood. Henry's law states that, at a given temperature, the greater the partial pressure of a gas, the greater the amount of that gas that will be dissolved in solution (Fig. 29-11). Simply put, the deeper a diver descends (and pressure increases), the more gas that will be dissolved in the blood. When the diver ascends slowly (and pressure decreases), the dissolved gas is released from the blood and reabsorbed. However, if the diver ascends too rapidly, this gas does not have enough time to be reabsorbed and "bubbles" out of solution.

A good example of Henry's law is when you take the top off a bottle of soda pop and it "fizzes." This fizzing is caused by carbon dioxide ($CO_2$) bubbling out of

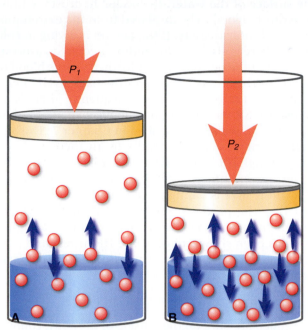

**Figure 29-11.** Henry's law describes the relationship between increases in the pressure of a gas and the amount of that gas that becomes dissolved in solution. The increase in pressure from A to B results in more gas molecules being dissolved into the solution.

solution. When soda is bottled, $CO_2$ is forced into solution (dissolved in the liquid) under high pressure. When the cap is on, there is higher pressure in the air above the liquid, which keeps the $CO_2$ in solution. When the cap is removed, this pressure is released, and the $CO_2$ is allowed to escape.

In divers, the same thing can happen with the various gases that are dissolved in the blood, particularly nitrogen. If a diver ascends too quickly, nitrogen can bubble out of solution and these bubbles can lead to a variety of problems, a phenomenon called decompression sickness. Guidelines for avoiding decompression sickness are described later in this chapter.

## VIGNETTE II continued

■ Caroline quickly recognizes that Andre is experiencing decompression sickness as a result of surfacing too quickly at the end of the dive and acts quickly to have an ambulance meet the boat at the hotel. Andre later admits that he was so overwhelmed by the beauty of the underwater terrain and wildlife that he lost sight of what he had learned in class. Andre and his family are staying at a resort that is famous for its scuba diving, and they are fortunate that the local hospital has the facilities to handle this type of emergency.

## Physiological Responses During Scuba Diving

The physiological responses to underwater diving are the result of a number of stressors on the body. These stressors include water temperature, increased hydrostatic pressure, the added weight of the scuba equipment, resistance of the water, resistance of breathing through the regulator, and the potential impact of the **diving reflex**. The diving reflex is a nervous system response that is exhibited when the face is submerged in cold water, which results in a slowing of the HR and a shunting of blood from extremities into the thorax. All of these factors can affect the cardiorespiratory responses of the body during diving and have an impact on the energy cost of exercising underwater.

It should be pointed at the outset that the exact physiological responses *during* scuba diving are not well documented, simply because of the technical difficulties in measuring cardiorespiratory parameters while underwater. Most of the measurements that have been made during exercise in the water have been done with the body submerged to neck level (with the head out of the water), or in a shallow water pool or swimming flume with the diver tethered to the laboratory equipment. Responses under these conditions are most likely very different than those that occur when a diver is swimming in open water, especially at depths below 100 to 120 ft.

### Diving Reflex

All mammals possess something called the diving reflex, which is designed to protect blood flow to the vital organs, while at the same time minimizing energy expenditure. By minimizing energy expenditure, aquatic mammals can extend the amount of time they can stay underwater before having to surface for air. Seals, for example, can stay submerged for periods of up to 30 minutes before they have to return to the surface. This allows them to chase fish for extended periods or avoid predators.

The diving reflex is not as developed in humans, but it still exists to some extent. For the diving reflex to be initiated, an individual's face must be submerged in water that is colder than 70°F (21°C). Because scuba diving is commonly performed in water that is below this temperature, the diving reflex may play a role in the hemodynamic responses to diving. If someone is diving in the Caribbean, however, where the water temperature is often warmer than 70°F, the diving reflex would not come into play.

The physiological responses to the diving reflex are a slowing of the HR (**bradycardia**), vasoconstriction of peripheral blood vessels (which shunts blood to the core of the body to maintain heart and brain blood flow), and a slowing of metabolism. This slowing of HR has been linked to an increased risk for cardiac dysrhythmias, specifically sinus bradycardia and sinus arrhythmia. Sinus bradycardia is simply a slowing of the HR to less than 60 beats/min, and sinus arrhythmia is an accentuated speeding up and slowing down of HR with inspiration and expiration, respectively. This is probably linked to the decrease in respiratory rate that typically occurs when breathing underwater. In any event, both of these dysrhythmias are considered benign and would have no adverse consequences on a diver.

## Ventilatory Reponses

$\dot{V}_E$ is lower during underwater exercise compared with exercising at similar workloads on land,[34,35] as is the ventilatory equivalent for oxygen ($\dot{V}_E/\dot{V}O_2$). The lower $\dot{V}_E/\dot{V}O_2$ indicates that less ventilation is needed to deliver 1 L oxygen to the tissues (see Chapter 8 for a refresher on $\dot{V}_E/\dot{V}O_2$). This phenomenon is thought to represent improved respiratory efficiency. The lower VE is a product of both a slower respiratory rate and a lower tidal volume. The slower respiratory rate is thought to be a product of the higher **partial pressure of inhaled oxygen**, which would result in more oxygen being carried in the blood. The higher $P_{O_2}$ is a result of the fact that the diver is breathing through a regulator, which adjusts the pressure of the inhaled air to be the same as the surrounding water pressure. Thus, a person would not have to breathe as frequently to deliver the same amount of oxygen to the working muscles. The decrease in tidal volume is most likely due to the added hydrostatic pressure on the outside of the chest, which makes the mechanics of chest expansion more difficult. The added work of breathing through a regulator could also limit the depth of inspiration. In either case, the diver would be taking shallower breaths than he or she typically would on land. The differences in $\dot{V}_E$ are evident at submaximal workloads and persist all the way up to maximal levels of exertion, so that maximal $\dot{V}_E$ is up to 40% lower in the water compared with land-based exercise.

Another factor that could lead to improved respiratory efficiency is a more effective distribution of blood flow within the lung while at depth. Because more blood is shunted to the thorax with the increased hydrostatic pressure, there is an enhanced ventilation/perfusion ratio within the lung. What that means is that more alveoli, especially at the top portion of each lung, will have a greater amount of blood distributed around them, which will enhance the transfer of oxygen from the air sacs into the bloodstream.

## Hemodynamic Responses

The hemodynamic responses to diving are different than land-based exercise and are related to three main factors: the diving reflex, the increase in hydrostatic pressure, and the fact that the diver is breathing oxygen at a higher partial pressure than on the surface.

### Heart Rate and Stroke Volume

One of the most profound cardiovascular changes with diving is a shunting of blood into the thorax as a direct result of the increase in external pressure on the outside of the body. As the diver descends below the surface of the water, the added hydrostatic pressure causes blood to be displaced from the extremities into the thoracic cavity. If the person is diving in cold water, there is also a diving reflex-mediated vasoconstriction in the periphery that further shunts blood to the core. This increases blood flow back to the heart (venous return or preload). Consequently, there is an increase in SV, mediated by an enhanced Frank-Starling mechanism, which is described in Chapter 7. This significant increase in SV results in an increase in Q, even though HR is somewhat lower in the water. The lower HRs are due to a combination of the diving reflex (if the dive is taking place in cold water) and the fact that the partial pressure of inhaled oxygen is higher than on land. Breathing oxygen at a higher $PO_2$ has been shown to decrease HR at rest and during submaximal exercise. This is called **hyperbaric bradycardia**.[34]

### Blood Pressure

The added pressure on the outside of the body, coupled with the diving reflex-mediated vasoconstriction, results in an increase in **total peripheral resistance (TPR)**. An increase in TPR will result in an increase in blood pressure compared with values on land. As discussed in Chapter 8, the normal response to dry-land aerobic exercise is for systolic blood pressure to increase and diastolic blood pressure to stay the same or decrease slightly. These changes are at least partially determined by TPR, which typically *decreases* with large-muscle aerobic exercise. In the water, if TPR *increases,* one would expect higher systolic and diastolic blood pressure values.

### Maximal Cardiac Output and Aerobic Capacity

Maximal cardiac output (Qmax) and $\dot{V}O_2max$ values are lower in the water compared with on land. Because Q is a product of HR and SV (Q = HR × SV), if either one of those values is decreased compared with land-based exercise, Q will be lower. Maximal HR has been shown to be approximately 7% lower in the water, whereas maximal SV is probably not affected. This 7% lower maximal HR results in a reduced Qmax.[34]

Because $\dot{V}O_2max$ is a product of Qmax and maximal oxygen extraction ($\dot{V}O_2max$ = Qmax × a-$\dot{V}O_2$ diff max), if either one of these values is decreased, $\dot{V}O_2max$ must also be reduced. Because Qmax is lower in the water compared with on land, $\dot{V}O_2max$ values are also lower by 7% to 10%. Another reason that $\dot{V}O_2max$ values are lower when scuba diving compared with swimming on the surface is that the primary means of locomotion when under the surface is by finning, which uses less muscle mass than freestyle swimming on the surface. The smaller muscle mass requires less total body oxygen ($\dot{V}O_2max$) compared with exercising using a larger muscle mass.

Another consequence of the increased shunting of blood into the thoracic cavity is an increase in blood flow to the kidneys. This results in an increase in urine production by the kidneys, with increased diuresis (urination). Anyone who has ever gone swimming, especially in cold water, has experienced this phenomenon. Soon after a person jumps into the water, he or she experiences the urge to urinate. The increase in hydrostatic pressure "pushes" blood from the extremities into the thorax, increasing blood flow to the kidneys, which increases urine production. The increased volume of urine in the bladder stimulates the receptors responsible for the urge to urinate.

One consequence of this pressure-induced diuresis is a loss of fluid, which can result in dehydration (similar to sweating). Dehydration is something that one would not normally connect to exercising in the water, but it is something that needs to be considered, regardless of the exercise environment.

## Energy Cost of Diving

A number of factors affect the energy cost of diving. These include swimming speed, current, buoyancy, weight of the equipment, body position, and size of the fins. Diving experience also plays a role, as more experienced divers are more efficient underwater and have less extraneous movements. The one overriding factor about scuba diving is that it is hard work. Water is 800 times more resistive than air, so it is harder to move through the water than it is to move on land. Any time it is harder to move, there is an increased energy cost. There is relatively little data on the energy cost of scuba diving, mainly because it is technically difficult to do. In a laboratory setting, energy cost is measured with a metabolic cart. To quantify oxygen consumption, you need to know the volume of expired air and the percentages of oxygen and $CO_2$ in the expired air. These measurements are virtually impossible to make underwater, which explains why a lot of the studies on scuba diving have been done in the shallow end of a swimming pool or in a swimming flume, where the subject is tethered to metabolic measuring equipment on the pool deck.

One factor that has a profound impact on energy cost is swimming speed.[35] A diver simply cannot go very fast underwater because of the increased drag of the water coupled with the added bulk of the diving equipment. On the surface, freestyle swimming speed in elite swimmers is in the neighborhood of 4.6 to 5.8 knots (4.0–5.0 miles/hr). Underwater, movement speed usually ranges from 0.6 to 1.2 knots (0.7–1.4 miles/hr). When swimming underwater, there is a curvilinear relation between swimming speed and energy cost. Even at 1 knot (1.2 miles/hr), the relative oxygen consumption is 25 mL/kg/min (7 metabolic equivalents [METs]). For someone with a 10-MET capacity, that represents 70% of their maximal capacity and puts a tremendous strain on the entire cardiorespiratory system. Current also plays a role when it comes to swimming speed, because any small increase in opposing current becomes a force that the diver must overcome.

Buoyancy also plays a role in the energy cost of diving. As divers descend from the surface, they have to let air out of their buoyancy compensator to sink to the bottom Once they achieve their desired depth, they strive to achieve a state of neutral buoyancy. Maintaining neutral buoyancy allows the diver to maintain a horizontal and more streamlined body position, which is more efficient than a more vertical body alignment. Once neutral buoyancy is reached, the diver can control going up and down over varying terrain by inhaling and exhaling.

The weight of diving gear has a large impact on energy cost. The combined weight of the diving equipment (e.g., tank, regulator, fins, and weight belt) can total between 50 and 75 lb, which is a lot of added weight (and bulk) to move through the water. Although the weight of the tank, regulator, and fins are relatively fixed, the thickness of the diver's wetsuit can impact how much weight the diver needs to carry on a weight belt to help him or her descend. A thicker wetsuit, which is needed in colder water, results in greater buoyancy, and hence the need for more weight to descend to the bottom.

In addition to the impact on energy cost, the weight of the diving gear makes a certain amount of strength a prerequisite for diving. Smaller and older individuals may struggle under the burden of carrying the added weight, especially when they are out of the water. Once they enter the water and adjust the air in their buoyancy compensator, the gear becomes almost weightless, and movement becomes easier.

Divers also wear fins to help move them through the water. With surface swimming, most of the propulsion comes from the arms; when scuba diving, most of the propulsion comes from the legs. Thus, high-quality fins are an essential item for divers of all levels of experience. Many types of fins are on the market, but research has shown that large, flexible fins result in approximately a 25% lower energy cost than rigid fins.[35] The various types of fins and their specific features are described in the next section.

## Diving Equipment

Common diving equipment includes a protective suit, mask, snorkel, fins, gas cylinder, regulator, diver computer, buoyancy compensator, and weight belt.

### Protective Suit

Most divers wear some sort of protective suit. The suit helps to protect their skin from sharp objects that may be on the bottom, but their main function is to prevent the loss of body heat. Water conducts heat away from the diver 20 times faster than air, so hypothermia can be a real problem for divers, even in relatively warm water. Protective suits are usually classified as either "wet suits" or "dry suits." **Wet suits** are made of neoprene, a spongy material that has trapped gas bubbles in its design. The suit provides an insulating barrier

## FROM THEORY TO PRACTICE

A common question that physicians have to answer, especially from scuba divers who have a history of heart disease (e.g., heart attack, coronary artery bypass surgery, or stent) is, "Can I scuba dive?" Although there are many complicating factors, including what medications the person is taking, a major determining factor is the fitness level of the individual. The widely publicized recommendation is that an individual should have a maximal capacity of at least 13 METs to scuba dive.[36] Certainly, not all scuba-diving activities require that level of fitness. However, by requiring that degree of cardiorespiratory endurance, instructors can be relatively sure that someone has an adequate reserve capacity to handle any emergency and physical stress that may occur. It has to be remembered that the person may be wearing upward of an extra 75 lb of diving gear. If he or she has to move quickly in an emergency situation, climb into the dive boat, or walk on the beach to get into the water, the diver must have the strength and fitness to safely do so.

Recently, this guideline has come under scrutiny as being too stringent.[37] Thirteen METs corresponds to a $\dot{V}O_2$max of 45.5 mL/kg/min, and enforcement of this guideline would exclude everyone except only the highly fit from diving. For instance, if a cutoff of 13 METs is used, 85% of men and 99% of women older than 50 years would be considered too deconditioned to scuba dive.[38] A goal of 10 METs has been suggested as a more realistic criterion. If individuals have an aerobic capacity below this level, it is recommended that they limit their diving to training in a pool and undertake a conditioning program to improve their fitness to a minimum of 10 METs. At that point they should be able to progress to open-water diving under supervision. Even though most diving activities do not require this level of fitness, having an adequate reserve capacity is essential if and when sudden and unexpected emergencies occur.

between the diver and the water. Wet suits also trap a thin layer of water between the diver and the suit. The body then warms up this thin layer of water, reducing the amount of body heat lost through the process of convection.

**Dry suits**, in contrast, are designed to keep the diver completely dry. The suits have watertight cuffs at the neck, wrists, and ankles, which keep water from entering the suit. Depending on the temperature of the water, the diver can wear either regular clothing or

insulated clothing under the suit to keep warm. In most cases, a low-pressure hose is attached from the diver's tank to the suit, so the diver can control the amount of air in the suit, which effectively makes it a buoyancy compensator. In addition to the protective suit, divers usually wear protective gloves and foot coverings (booties) to help protect and insulate the feet.

### Mask

Diving masks are designed so they cover the eyes and nose of the diver. The outer rim of the mask is typically constructed of a soft, silicon-based material, and the mask should fit snuggly enough so that it does not leak. Some masks may also have a "purge" valve located under the nostrils, so that exhaling through the nose helps to expel any water that has leaked into the mask. Masks with corrective lenses can also be custom made for individuals who wear glasses.

### Snorkel

A snorkel allows divers to swim on the surface, with their faces submerged in the water. Snorkels are usually a maximum of 15 inches in length, because below this depth the pressure is too great for divers to expand their chest and breathe air from the surface. In addition, snorkels are usually 0.75 to 1 inch in diameter. If they are narrower, it becomes too difficult to draw in air; if they are wider than this, they have too much dead-space air, which would limit the amount of fresh air that reaches the alveoli.

There are two basic types of snorkels: wet snorkels and dry snorkels. Wet snorkels consist of a mouthpiece and a straight tube that extends to the surface. A problem with a wet snorkel is that if the diver is swimming in rough water or momentarily dives below the surface, they must "blow out" any water that enters the tube. In contrast, a dry snorkel has a float valve mechanism on top that closes when the snorkel is submerged and then opens when the diver is on the surface. This helps to keep water out of the snorkel.

### Fins

Fins are another crucial piece of a diver's equipment, especially because the legs provide virtually all of the propulsive force when scuba diving. There are basically two types of fin designs and then classifications under each design. There are full-foot fins and open-heel fins. The full-foot designs slip on the diver's foot, similar to a shoe, and are usually worn barefoot or with thin neoprene stockings. The open-heel design, as the name suggests, has a strap that goes around the heel of the diver's foot and is worn with neoprene dive booties to prevent blisters.

Under each category of fin there are also paddle fins, split fins, and "force" fins. Paddle fins have been used the longest, but they are also the heaviest and least efficient. They are popular because they are the least expensive. Split fins have a gap in the middle and because of their design are the most efficient. Force fins are relatively new on the market and are V-shaped, similar to a fish's tail. They are the lightest and considered to be the fastest. Although there can be upward of a 25% difference in energy cost between the different fin designs (larger, more flexible fins being the most efficient), diver comfort is the overriding deciding factor when choosing fins.[35]

## Gas Cylinder

Most recreational divers dive with one tank attached to some sort of backpack-type harness. Tanks are typically made out of steel or aluminum, and a standard-sized tank holds 80 ft³ of air pressured to 3,000 pounds per square inch (psi). For perspective, this amount of air will last the average diver in the range of 30 to 60 minutes of diving time, depending on the depth of the dive, how hard the person is working or how fast he or she is swimming, and the size of the person.

The tank has a cylinder valve at the top, to which the regulator is attached. Because of the importance of having a reliable and safe air source when underwater, all tanks must be visually inspected every year for signs of corrosion and cracks, and be hydrostatically tested to check for cracks every 5 years. Approved tanks must be labeled as such before they can legally be refilled with air.

## Regulator

The regulator delivers the air from the tank to the diver. Remember, as the diver descends, air must be delivered at the same pressure as the ambient water pressure at that depth. At a depth of 33 ft, the pressure on the outside of the chest is 2 atmospheres (1,520 mm Hg). Thus, air must be delivered to the diver at this pressure so that he or she can inflate the lungs. The regulator does this in two stages.

The regulator is connected to the tank with the first stage of the regulator. The first stage of the regulator allows air to enter the hose at a lower pressure than the pressure in the tank. The pressure within the tank is usually 3,000 psi. The first stage reduces the pressure from 3,000 psi down to slightly above ambient water pressure.

The second stage of the regulator is within the mouthpiece. This stage of the regulator further reduces the air pressure so that it is delivered to the diver at a pressure that is equal to ambient water pressure. When the diver inhales, the negative pressure that is created within the lungs opens the diaphragm, and air is delivered to the diver. When the diver exhales, the diaphragm closes, stopping the flow of air, and the expired air is released into the water.

## Dive Computer

Usually a low-pressure hose is attached to the first stage of the regulator and is connected to a pressure gauge or dive computer. At a minimum, the gauge provides information on the remaining air in the tank, but it also may provide information about water depth, pressure, and estimated dive time remaining.

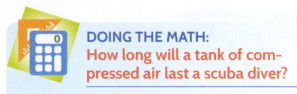

## DOING THE MATH: How long will a tank of compressed air last a scuba diver?

The standard-size scuba tank contains 80 ft³ of air (~2,300 L). If a person were to breathe from this tank on the surface, this tank would last approximately 329 minutes.

**How is this calculated?**
At rest, breathing frequency averages 14 breaths/min and tidal volume averages 500 mL (0.5 L). As discussed in Chapter 7, minute ventilation equals respiratory rate × tidal volume. Thus, minute ventilation = 14 breathes/min × 0.5 L/breath, which equals 7.0 L/min.

Dividing the tank volume (2,300 L) by minute ventilation (7 L/min) = approximately 329 minutes.

However, a scuba diver does not often sit on the surface and breathe from the tank; they descend underwater.

**If this person were to descend to 33 ft and just sit quietly, how long would the tank last?**
According to Boyle's Law, at 33 ft the pressure is 2 atmospheres (double the pressure on the surface). Thus, the 80 ft³ of available compressed air is reduced to 40 ft³, or 1,150 L. Assuming the same respiratory rate of 14 and tidal volume of 500 ml, how long will the tank last?

Minute ventilation = 14 × 0.5 L/min = 7 L/min

1,150 L ÷ 7 L/min = ~164 minutes

Realistically, however, when someone is scuba diving, he or she is not sitting still. Respiratory rate and tidal volume both increase as the diver moves through the water. Assuming a person is exercising moderately, respiratory rate increases to 20 breaths/min, and tidal volume increases to 1000 mL (1 L), how long will the tank last?

Minute ventilation = 20 × 1.0 L/min = 20 L/min

1,150 L ÷ 20 L/min = ~58 minutes

As you can see, the length of time a diver can stay underwater depends on such things as dive depth and level of exertion of the diver. However, it is also affected by the body size of the diver (e.g., women are smaller and breathe smaller volumes of air) and the experience of the diver (e.g., experienced divers are more efficient and use less air).

## Buoyancy Compensator

An essential part of diver gear is the buoyancy compensator, which regulates how much a diver either floats or sinks, depending on water depth. The buoyancy compensator is also attached to the first stage of the regulator by a low-pressure hose. The volume of air within the buoyancy compensator is usually adjusted by a push-button valve. On the surface, the diver fills the buoyancy compensator with enough air to allow him or her to float comfortably on the surface. When the diver wants to descend, he or she depresses a relief valve, which slowly releases air from the buoyancy compensator. As air is released, the diver descends. Once he or she reaches the desired depth, the diver can fine-tune the amount of air in the buoyancy compensator to achieve neutral buoyancy (this allows the diver to be almost weightless as he or she moves about the bottom and maximizes swimming efficiency).

When the diver wants to ascend, he or she depresses the inflow button, which adds air to the buoyancy compensator, and they *slowly* return to the surface. Once the diver starts to ascend, he or she will continually have to release air *out* of the buoyancy compensator, because as one moves toward the surface, the air in the buoyancy compensator will expand (Boyle's law), increasing buoyancy and causing the diver to ascend faster and faster.

## Weight Belt

Divers usually wear a weight belt around the waist to help them descend. Wet suits and dry suits, even though they are heavy when on land, become buoyant in the water, so divers need to wear additional weight to descend. The amount of weight can vary tremendously, depending on the thickness and buoyancy of the protective suit the diver is wearing. Someone who is diving in the Caribbean and only wearing a "shorty" suit may need only 5 to 8 lb of weight on the weight belt, whereas someone who is diving in extremely cold water and is wearing an 8-mm wet suit may need up to 30 lb to reach the bottom. As a general rule, a diver wears 10% of their body weight when diving in freshwater and 12% in saltwater.

## Complications During Scuba Diving

Scuba diving can be an enjoyable experience, but it also can be very dangerous. One study estimates that scuba diving is 96 times more dangerous than driving an automobile.[39,40] Most of the injuries associated with diving are a result of changes in pressure. Pressure-related injuries are collectively called **barotraumas** and can occur as one descends (when pressure increases) or ascends (pressure decreases).

## Mask Squeeze

Anyone who has ever tried to go to the bottom of a swimming pool while wearing swimming goggles has probably experienced "mask squeeze." Diving down as little as 10 ft increases the pressure on the outside of the body by more than 200 mm Hg. This increase in pressure pushes the lenses of the goggles inward, creating a vacuum between the lenses and the face. This vacuum can cause the eyes to bulge outward and may cause blood vessels in the eyes to rupture. When scuba diving, the mask covers the eyes and nose. Thus, breathing compressed air through the nose into the mask equalizes the pressure and eliminates mask squeeze.

## Ruptured Eardrum

In addition to the pressure on the outside of the mask, there is also pressure on the outside of the eardrum. The eardrum gets pushed inward and, unless the diver equalizes the pressure by pinching the nose and exhaling, the eardrum may rupture inward. The opposite can occur when a diver holds her breath while ascending. If the diver takes a breath in and holds it, the volume of air will expand (Boyle's law) and could rupture the eardrum in the outward direction.

## Nitrogen Narcosis

The compressed air that a diver breathes is composed primarily of nitrogen, oxygen, and $CO_2$. As mentioned earlier, as the diver descends, the regulator adjusts the partial pressure of the inhaled gases to the ambient water pressure. Thus, as the diver goes deeper, the partial pressure of all of the inhaled gases increases. Breathing nitrogen at a higher partial pressure than normal can lead to problems, which are referred to as the "rapture of the deep." Specifically, when higher levels of nitrogen dissolve in the fatty tissues of the brain, they have a **narcotic** effect. The feeling is similar to that a person experiences when taking narcotic drugs, namely, a decreased pain sensation and a general feeling of euphoria. Many people describe it as similar to being drunk. The problem is that this leads to a loss of

### FROM THEORY TO PRACTICE

Sometimes it is difficult to put a discussion of pressures into perspective because it is difficult to relate to what an increase in pressure feels like. To gain a better understanding of the pressures, try this exercise:

Have a friend put a blood pressure cuff on your arm and blow it up to 200 mm Hg. How does that feel? Probably not very good. That is the amount of pressure that is pushing on the outside of the body at a depth of approximately 10 ft underwater. At a depth of 33 ft, the pressure increase is 760 mm Hg. How do you think that would feel?

coordination and impaired judgment, which could be fatal at extreme depths. Fortunately, nitrogen narcosis is a reversible phenomenon that dissipates quickly when a diver ascends.

## Decompression Sickness

Decompression sickness was first described when subjects were diving or working at depth with the aid of underwater diving bells or caissons. As described earlier in this chapter, it was discovered when the divers returned to the surface, as they often experienced extreme joint pain and actually bent over because of the pain.

According to Henry's law, when a person dives to depth, more gas (all gasses) becomes dissolved in the bloodstream. Because of the high concentration of nitrogen in compressed air (~79%) and the high solubility coefficient for nitrogen, a great deal of nitrogen becomes dissolved in the blood. When a diver ascends too rapidly, the gas expands and "bubbles out" of solution. If these bubbles congregate in a joint, they may cause pain (the bends). If these bubbles occlude a blood vessel, they could cause a stroke or other organ damage, depending on which vessel they block. Decompression sickness can be avoided by following decompression tables published by the U.S. Navy (see Additional Resources). An explanation of these tables is beyond the scope of this text, but this skill requires advanced training and extra planning to avoid catastrophes.

In the event that decompression sickness does occur, divers can be placed in a decompression (hyperbaric) chamber. This chamber repressurizes the diver and forces the nitrogen bubbles to dissolve back into solution. The diver can then be slowly decompressed, and the nitrogen can leave the system in a very controlled manner.

## Oxygen Poisoning

Most people never think of oxygen as a "poison," but oxygen can become toxic if it is breathed at too high a partial pressure. When oxygen is breathed at extremely high partial pressures, too much oxygen gets dissolved in the plasma. At sea level, assuming a $P_B$ of 760 mm Hg and an oxygen concentration of approximately 21%, the $P_{O_2}$ in the lungs is 160 mm Hg (760 mm Hg × 0.21 = 160 mm Hg). Based on the oxygen dissociation curve described in Chapter 6, this results in a blood concentration of approximately 20 vol% (20 mL oxygen/ 100 mL blood). At a depth of 120 ft, the ambient pressure is 3,040 mm Hg (4 atmospheres). If the diver

is breathing compressed air, the $P_{O_2}$ in the blood is approximately 640 mm Hg (3,030 mm Hg × 0.21 = 636 mm Hg). At this $P_{O_2}$, the oxygen content in the blood rises to 29 vol%. This level of oxygen in the bloodstream can cause seizures and can quickly lead to death.[6]

Oxygen poisoning does not occur in scuba divers until they exceed a depth of 120 ft. This is why most recreational divers are advised not to descend beyond this depth for any length of time.

## Pneumothorax

One of the greatest dangers to inexperienced recreational divers involves holding the breath when ascending. Boyle's law states that the volume of a gas is inversely proportional to the pressure. For instance, a 3-L volume of air at sea level will equal 1.5 L at a depth of 33 ft. Conversely, 1.5 L of air inhaled at a depth of 33 ft would expand to 3.0 L at the surface. If a diver takes a deep breath when submerged to 33 ft and holds the breath on ascent, the expansion of the air may cause their lungs to overexpand and burst.

Similar to the lungs, air trapped in any enclosed cavity can expand, causing great pain and potential problems. This is particularly common in the sinuses, especially if the person has a cold and is congested. The mucus in the Eustachian tubes can interfere with the ability to equalize pressure on ascent, causing great discomfort.

## VIGNETTE 11 *conclusion*

■ Andre undergoes a series of hyperbaric oxygen therapy treatments at the hospital. Hyperbaric oxygen therapy involves breathing pure oxygen in a pressurized room or cylinder in which the air pressure is raised up to three times higher than normal air pressure. Although this was a frightening experience for Andre and his family, he is expected to fully recover after receiving the treatments. He is very fortunate that Caroline recognized his symptoms as those of decompression sickness and acted so quickly to get him to the hospital. Andre is a bit embarrassed and feels guilty for "ruining his family's vacation," but he has learned a tough lesson about the dangers of diving that will result in him being a lot more careful in the future.

# CRITICAL THINKING QUESTIONS

1. You live near sea level in La Crosse, Wisconsin. It is currently March. A client tells you she is planning to race the Leadville 50 Mile Trail Race in July in Colorado at an average elevation of 10,000 ft. What advice would you give the client about the change in $PO_2$, $PaO_2$, and $\dot{V}_E$ that should occur on *arrival* in Leadville at 10,225 ft? How will these changes affect $\dot{V}O_2max$ and pace at altitude versus sea level? What advice or racing strategy would you give your client if she told you she was racing for time and not to "just finish"?

2. You have been asked to be the expert for a talk at a local fitness center related to acclimatizing to altitude when living and training at sea level. First, discuss the reasons that may enhance sea-level performance related to blood and cardiopulmonary changes that occur with chronic altitude living/training. Next, what strategy will you suggest to gain blood and cardiopulmonary changes that are induced with "living" at altitude when residing at sea level?

3. As an emergency medical technician in the Rocky Mountains, you are held to a "higher" standard than other emergency medical technicians across the nation. It is your day off and you are hiking with a group of friends. You are hiking long distances from sea level to tag up to three 14,000-foot peaks in Colorado. You reach the first peak's summit and one of your buddies begins to tell you he feels nauseous, has a headache, and is a bit disoriented. He also seems to be spitting up fluid and you hear a rasp in his breathing. Explain what is occurring to your buddy and the best course of corrective action.

4. A friend of yours is planning to race the Los Angeles Marathon for a "good finish time." Your first thought is, *Wow, what a polluted city.* Your next thought is, *What a poor choice of venue*, especially if your friend wants to race "fast." Explain to your friend the possible physiological decrements he faces in a polluted city and suggest a different venue. Defend your suggestion.

5. You are diving in 60 ft of water with a friend. Suddenly, your friend indicates that she is having trouble breathing through her regulator. Her first instinct is to hold her breathe and surface as fast as possible. Using your knowledge of the gas laws, how should you respond in such a situation to help your friend? Why?

6. You and a friend have just flown to Cozumel, Mexico, to dive the Palancar Reef. On the day of your first dive you wake up with a runny nose and are very congested. What dangers does this pose for you as a diver?

7. A 65-year-old diver is recovering from a heart attack. He has recently had a graded exercise test and it was found that he has a maximal aerobic capacity of 7.5 METs. Do you think it is safe for him to dive? What sort of things would you want to know to make this decision, and what recommendations would you give this person?

8. You are a new diver and go into the dive shop to purchase an entire set of scuba diving gear. What will you need and what decisions do you need to make about each piece of equipment?

---

## ADDITIONAL RESOURCES

### Altitude and Pollution

Interactive altitude website: http://www.altitude.org/home.php. This website contains a plethora of information related to all things altitude, including a HAPE Database, calculators that explain the effect of ascent to high altitude, and interactive altitude facts.

Colorado Altitude Training (CAT): http://altitudetraining.com. CAT is a company based out of Colorado Springs, Colorado, and is a leading altitude simulation technology company that maintains one of the largest research and development divisions in the industry. Visit the website and view technology, such as altitude simulation tents, that may boost sea-level performance from sleeping "high" and training "low." Also, CAT manufactures hyperoxic (i.e., high oxygen) chambers that are built to house several treadmills for runners living and training "high" who wish to simulate "doses" of sea-level workouts when inside the chamber.

Acli-Mate Natural Sport Drinks: http://www.acli-mate.com/. This is a grass roots product line out of Gunnison,

Colorado, that may provide some relief from AMS when ascending to moderate altitudes from sea level. In addition, the Acli-Mate company produces Acli-Mate ENDURANCE for energy and hydration during exercise. All natural formulations are made by Dr. Roanne R. Houck, ND (Naturopathic Doctor), who lives and practices in Gunnison. (Disclosure: Dr. Drum endorses Acli-Mate, but has no monetary ties to the company.)

### Diving

Divers Alert Network: http://www.diversalertnetwork.org

National Association of Underwater Instructors: http://www.naui.org

Professional Association of Diving Instructors: http://www.padi.com/scuba-diving/

National Association of Rescue Divers: http://www.rescuediver.org/physics/divetabel.htm

U.S. Department of Commerce, National Oceanic and Atmospheric Administration: http://www.ndc.noaa.gov/dp_forms.html (see decompression tables)

## REFERENCES

1. Benso A, Broglio F, Aimaretti G, et al. Endocrine and metabolic responses to extreme altitude and physical exercise in climbers. *Eur J Endocrinol*. 2007;157:733–740.
2. National Oceanic and Atmospheric Administration. *US Standard Atmosphere*. Washington, DC: NOAA; 1976.
3. Graydon D, Hanson K, eds. *Mountaineering—The Freedom of the Hills*. 6th ed. Seattle, WA: The Mountaineers; 1997.
4. Ahrens DC. *Meteorology Today—An Introduction to Weather, Climate, and the Environment*. Pacific Grove, CA: Brooks/Cole, Thomson Learning; 2000.
5. Mees K, Olzowy B. Otorhinolaryngological aspects of high altitude medicine. *Laryngorhinootologie*. 2008;87: 276–287.
6. Wilber RL. *Altitude Training and Athletic Performance*. Champaign, IL: Human Kinetics; 2005.
7. Sawka MN, Convertino VA, Eichner ER, Schneider SM, Young AJ. Blood volume: Importance and adaptations to exercise training, environmental stresses, and trauma/sickness. *Med Sci Sports Exerc*. 2000;32:332–348.
8. Robergs RA, Roberts SO. *Exercise Physiology—Exercise, Performance, and Clinical Applications*. St. Louis, MO: Mosby-Year Book, Inc.; 1997.
9. Kelly KR, Williamson DL, Fealy CE, et al. Acute altitude-induced hypoxia suppresses plasma glucose and leptin in healthy humans. *Metabolism*. 2010;59:200–205.
10. Powers SK, Howley ET. *Exercise Physiology—Theory and Application to Fitness and Performance*. New York, NY: McGraw Hill; 2009.
11. Sutton JR, Reeves JT, Wagner PD, et al. Operation Everest II: Oxygen transport during exercise at extreme simulated altitude. *J Appl Physiol*. 1988;64:1309–1321.
12. West JB. Lactate during exercise at extreme altitude. *Fed Proc*. 1986;45:2953–2957.
13. West JB. Point: The lactate paradox does occur during exercise at high altitude. *J Appl Physiol*. 2007;102: 2398–2399.
14. van Hall G. Counterpoint: The lactate paradox does not occur during exercise at high altitude. *J Appl Physiol*. 2007;102:2399–2401.
15. Bailey DM, Davies B. Physiological implications of altitude training for endurance performance at sea level: A review. *Br J Sports Med*. 1997;31:183–190.
16. Chapman RF, Stray-Gundersen J, Levine BD. Individual variation in response to altitude training. *J Appl Physiol*. 1998;85:1448–1456.
17. Levine BD, Stray-Gunderson J. "Living high–training low": Effect of moderate-altitude acclimatization with low-altitude training on performance. *J Appl Physiol*. 1997;83:102–112.
18. Boning D. Altitude and hypoxia training—a short review. *Int J Sports Med*. 1992;18:565–570.
19. Berglund B. High-altitude training—aspects of hematological adaptation. *Sports Med*. 1992;14:289–303.
20. Terrados N. Altitude training and muscular metabolism. *Int J Sports Med*. 1992;13(Suppl. 1):S206–S209.
21. Brugniaux JV, Schmitt L, Robach P, et al. Eighteen days of "living high, training low" stimulate erythropoiesis and enhance aerobic performance in elite middle-distance runners. *J Appl Physiol*. 2006;100:203–211.
22. Mees K, Olzowy B. Otorhinolaryngological aspect of high altitude medicine. *Laryngorhinootologie*. 2008;87: 276–287.
23. Hoffman J. *Physiological Aspects of Sport Training and Performance*. Champaign, IL: Human Kinetics; 2002.
24. Climbing-High.com. *The Gamow bag*. Available at: http://www.climbing-high.com/the-gamow-bag.html. Accessed September 5, 2014.
25. Netzer NC, Chytra R, Kupper T. Low intense physical exercise in normobaric hypoxia leads to more weight loss in obese people than low intense physical exercise in normobaric sham hypoxia. *Sleep Breath*. 2008;12: 129–134.
26. Lippl FJ, Neubauer S, Schipfer S, Lichter N. Hypobaric hypoxia causes weight reduction in obese subjects. *Obesity*. 2010;18: 675–681.
27. Zareba W, Nomura A, Couderc JP. Cardiovascular effects of air pollution: What to measure in ECG? *Environ Health Perspect*. 2001;109(Suppl. 4):533–538.
28. Dockery DW, Pope CA 3rd, Kanner RE, Martin Villegas G, Schwartz J. Daily changes in oxygen saturation and pulse rate associated with particulate air pollution and barometric pressure. *Res Rep Health Eff Inst*. 1999;(83): 1–19; discussion 21–28.
29. Lux RL, Pope CA 3rd. Air pollution effects on ventricular repolarization. *Res Rep Health Eff Inst*. 2009;(141): 3–20; discussion 21–28.
30. Oliveira RS, Barros Neto TL, Braga ALF, et al. Impact of acute exposure to air pollution on the cardiorespiratory performance of military firemen. *Braz J Med Biol Res*. 2006;39:1643–1649.
31. Pottgiesser T, Umhau M, Ahlgrim C, et al. Hb mass measurement suitable to screen for illicit autologous blood transfusions. *Med Sci Sports Exerc*. 2007;39:1748–1756.
32. Edmonds C, Lowry C, Pennefather J. History of diving. *S Pac Underwater Med J*. 1975;5:1–7.
33. Lynch PR. Historical and basic perspectives of SCUBA diving. *Med Sci Sports Exerc*. 1996;28:570–572.
34. Doubt TJ. Cardiovascular and thermal responses to SCUBA diving. *Med Sci Sports Exerc*. 1996;28:581–586.
35. Pendergast DR, Tedesco M, Nawrocki DM, Fisher NM. Energetics of underwater swimming with SCUBA. *Med Sci Sports Exerc*. 1996;28:573–580.
36. Bove AA. Medical aspects of sport diving. *Med Sci Sports Exerc*. 1996;28:291–295.
37. Pollock NW. Aerobic fitness and underwater diving. *Diving Hyper Med*. 2007;37:118–124.
38. *ACSM's Guidelines for Exercise Testing and Prescription*. 8th ed. Philadelphia, PA: Lippincott Williams & Wilkins; 2010:84–89.
39. Lansche JM. Deaths during skin and SCUBA diving in California in 1970. *Calif Med J*. 1972;116:18–22.
40. Pendergast DR, Lundgren CEG. The underwater environment: Cardiopulmonary, thermal, and energetic demands. *J Appl Physiol*. 2009;106:276–283.

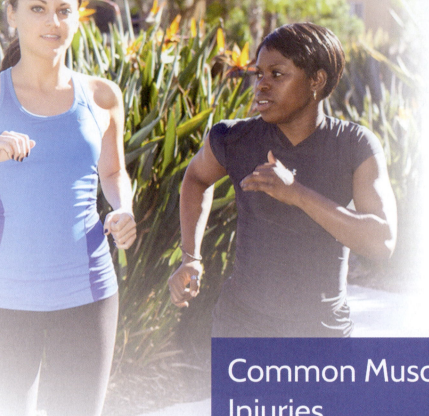

Scott Cheatham, DPT, PhD(c), ATC

CHAPTER 30

# Common Musculoskeletal Injuries

## CHAPTER OUTLINE

# CHAPTER OUTLINE–cont'd

## LEARNING OUTCOMES

1. Identify common tissue injuries associated with physical activity.
2. Explain the healing process of the body, including factors that affect how different tissues heal (e.g., muscles, ligaments, and bones).
3. Explain the difference between preexisting and acute injuries, and explain how to apply the P.R.I.C.E. method of treatment.
4. Explain the importance of flexibility and musculoskeletal injuries.
5. Describe common musculoskeletal injuries of the upper and lower extremities, and describe common treatments for each injury.
6. Describe the basic tenets of reconditioning common injuries to allow clients to return to activity safely.
7. Explain the importance of adhering to the scope of practice and accurate record-keeping.

## ANCILLARY LINK

Visit Davis*Plus* at http://davisplus.fadavis.com for study and practice resources, including online quizzes, animations that help explain physiological processes, podcasts concerning news and career trends in exercise physiology, and practice references.

## *VIGNETTE*

■ Rafael, a nationally ranked junior tennis player in the boys' 18 division, arrives at Marco's personal training studio with hopes of improving his overall fitness level and enhancing his game through sport-specific training, which is Marco's specialty. Specifically, Rafael is hoping to add speed to his serve, which he perceives as the greatest weakness in his game. Rafael mentions to Marco that he sometimes feels pain along the outside of his elbow after a long match or training session.

    What training techniques can Marco implement to strengthen Rafael's serve, and what might be the cause of Rafael's elbow pain? What actions can Marco take to address this pain while staying within his scope of practice as a personal trainer?

The number of people in the United States who are participating in some sort of physical activity or playing sports is extremely high. The Centers for Disease Control and Prevention estimate that more than 38 million boys and girls aged 5 to 18 years participate in youth sports,[1] and approximately 150 million adults participate in some form of physical activity.[2] With so many youths and adults participating in sports and physical activity, the needs for injury recognition, management, and prevention have grown. This chapter describes musculoskeletal injuries that are common in sports and physical activity for participants of all ages.

## COMMON TYPES OF INJURIES

When there is an injury to the human body, multiple structures can be damaged, including bone, cartilage, ligaments, and muscle. However, it is not uncommon for damage to the skin, nerves, blood vessels, and organs to occur at the same time. Having a basic knowledge of common injuries will help health and fitness professionals provide safe and effective exercises for individuals who have been injured. Following is a brief discussion of the structures that can be damaged as a result of some common types of injuries.

### Fractures

A **fracture** is a medical condition that results in a crack or actual break in a bone. The causes of fractures can be classified into low-impact or high-impact. **Low-impact trauma**, such as a fall on a level surface, can result in a minor fracture, and repeated **microtrauma** (small injuries) to a bone region can result in a minor stress fracture. **Stress fractures** occur from abnormal

or repeated stress and are common in distance runners and track athletes (Fig. 30-1). It is important not to confuse stress fractures with shin splints (see Lower-Extremity Injuries section later in this chapter). The signs and symptoms of stress fractures include[3]:

- Progressive pain that is worse with weight-bearing activity
- Focal pain
- Pain at rest in some cases
- Local swelling

**High-impact trauma** often occurs from motor vehicle accidents or high-impact sports such as football. Often these injuries are disabling and require immediate medical attention. Other medical conditions, such as infection, cancer, or osteoporosis, can weaken bone and increase the risks for fracture (also see Chapter 28).[3] Figure 30-2 illustrates examples of common fractures.

### Sprains

**Sprains** are injuries that occur to a joint and the surrounding ligaments. Ligament sprains often occur with trauma such as a fall or during contact sports. The most common joints for sprains include the ankle, knee, thumb/fingers, and shoulder. If a sprain occurs, the client often reports hearing a "popping" sound followed by immediate pain, swelling, instability, decreased **range of motion (ROM)**, and loss of function.[4] Table 30-1 provides a general grading system for ligament sprains. Of particular importance are injuries to the **anterior**

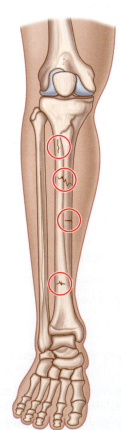

**Figure 30-1.** Common sites of stress fractures in the lower leg.

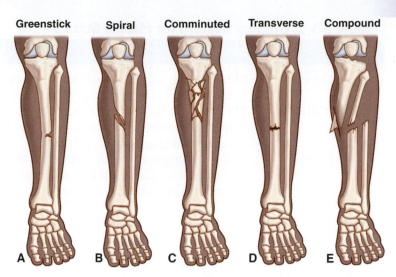

**Figure 30-2.** Common types of bone fractures. A, Greenstick, or incomplete. B, Spiral. C, Comminuted, or complex. D, Transverse. E, Compound, or open.

## Table 30-1. Grading System for Ligament Sprains

| SEVERITY | PHYSICAL EXAMINATION FINDINGS | IMPAIRMENT | PATHOPHYSIOLOGY | TYPICAL TREATMENT |
|---|---|---|---|---|
| Grade 1 | • Minimal tenderness<br>• Minimal swelling | Minimal | Microscopic tearing of collagen fibers | • Weight bearing as tolerated<br>• No splinting/casting<br>• Isometric exercises<br>• Full ROM<br>• Stretching/strengthening<br>• Exercises as tolerated |
| Grade 2 | • Moderate tenderness<br>• Moderate swelling<br>• Decreased ROM<br>• Possible instability | Moderate | Complete tears of some but not all collagen fibers in the ligament | • Immobilization with air splint<br>• Physical therapy<br>• ROM, stretching<br>• Strengthening exercises |
| Grade 3 | • Significant swelling<br>• Significant tenderness<br>• Instability | Severe | Complete tear/rupture of ligament | • Immobilization<br>• PT over a longer period<br>• Possible surgical reconstruction |

PT, physical therapy; ROM, range of motion.

cruciate ligament (ACL), medial collateral ligament (MCL) of the knee, and lateral ligaments of the ankle, which are described later.

## Strains

**Strains** are injuries that occur to a muscle or a muscle–tendon unit. Muscle strains are injuries in which the muscle works beyond its capacity, resulting in a tear of the muscle fibers. In mild strains, the client may report tightness or tension. In more severe cases, the client may report feeling a sudden "tear" or "pop" that leads to immediate pain and weakness in the muscle. Swelling, discoloration (**ecchymosis**), and loss of function often occur after the injury.[4] Strains of the lower extremity primarily occur in the hamstrings, groin, and calf. Table 30-2 outlines the grades of muscle strains.

Muscle strains of the hamstring group are often caused by a severe stretch to the muscle or a rapid, forceful contraction (e.g., during sprinting). The hamstrings have the highest frequency of strains in the body and are common in running and jumping sports. Risk factors include prior injury of the same muscle, age, poor flexibility, lower-extremity muscle imbalance, improper warm-up, and training errors.[4,5]

Groin or adductor strains are common in sports such as ice hockey and figure skating. These activities require explosive acceleration, deceleration, and change of direction. With injury, the client may report an initial "pull" of the groin muscles followed by intense pain and loss of function. Previous injury, preseason training errors, core muscle weakness, and muscle imbalance between the adductors and abductors are the most prevalent risk factors for injury.[6]

## Table 30-2. Grading System for Muscle Strains

| GRADE | DESCRIPTION |
| --- | --- |
| Grade I strain | This is a mild strain; a small number of muscle fibers are stretched or torn. The injured muscle is tender and painful but has normal strength. |
| Grade II strain | This is a moderate strain; a large amount of injured fibers and more severe muscle pain and tenderness are present. Mild swelling is present with noticeable loss of strength and possible bruising. |
| Grade III strain | This is a complete tear. Sometimes a "tear" or "pop" sensation is felt as the muscle tears. Grade III strains result in complete loss of muscle function, severe pain, swelling, tenderness, and discoloration. |

Calf muscle strains are common in most running and jumping sports. Risk factors include prior injury to the calf, age, muscle fatigue, fluid and electrolyte depletion, forced knee extension while the foot is dorsiflexed, or forced dorsiflexion while the knee is extended.[4,6]

## Cartilage Damage

Damage to joint articular **cartilage** often involves damage to both the **hyaline cartilage** (i.e., cartilage that covers the bone) and the **menisci** (i.e., shock absorbers). Of particular importance is damage to the structures of the knee joint (Fig. 30-3).

The most commonly reported knee injury is the meniscal tear. The menisci have an important role within the knee through their multiple functions. They assist with shock absorption, stability, joint congruency, lubrication, and proprioception.[7] **Meniscal injuries** often occur from trauma or degeneration. Acute injuries can occur from a combination of loading and twisting of the joint or with other traumatic injuries such as ACL tears (e.g., lateral meniscus) or MCL injury (e.g., medial meniscus).[7] Older individuals with degenerative joints are more predisposed to meniscal tears.[8] Individuals with meniscal tears may complain of stiffness, clicking or popping with joint loading, giving way, catching, and locking (more severe tears). Other signs include joint pain, swelling, and muscle weakness (e.g., in the quadriceps).[9]

The cartilage under the patella (i.e., the kneecap) can also become damaged, resulting in **chondromalacia patella (CP)** (Fig. 30-4). CP is a softening or wearing away of the cartilage behind the patella, resulting in inflammation and pain. This is caused by the posterior surface of the patella not properly tracking in the femoral groove. CP is commonly associated with improper training methods (e.g., overtraining, poor running style), sudden change in training surface (e.g., moving from grass to cement), lower-extremity muscle weakness and/or tightness, and foot overpronation (i.e., flat feet). The affected knee may appear swollen and warm, and pain often occurs behind the patella during activity.[4]

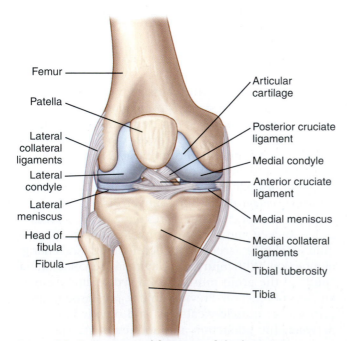

**Figure 30-3.** Anatomical features of the knee joint.

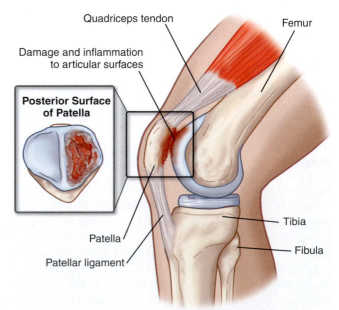

**Figure 30-4.** Chondromalacia patella, a softening or wearing away of the cartilage behind the patella, can be a likely cause of subpatellar pain during activity.

## Overuse Conditions

When the body is put through excessive demands during activity, overuse conditions such as bursitis, fasciitis, and tendinopathy often occur. Typically, clients begin new activities or exercise programs too fast. **Bursitis** is inflammation of the **bursa sac** (small, synovial fluid–filled sac between tissues) caused by acute trauma, repetitive overuse, muscle imbalance, or muscle tightness. Bursitis commonly affects the shoulder, hips, and knees.

**Fasciitis** is inflammation of the connective tissue called *fascia*.[4] It most commonly occurs in the foot and has been linked to various intrinsic and extrinsic factors. **Tendonitis** is a traditional term for inflammation of the tendon that often involves an overuse condition that commonly affects the elbows, knees, and ankles. The tendon cannot handle this new level of demand, resulting in pain and dysfunction.

A more current term that is replacing the term *tendonitis* is **tendinopathy**, which describes a degenerative disease process that occurs in a tendon. More recent research has found that repetitive use of a tendon leads to microtears and eventual fraying of the tissues if not properly addressed.[10–12] This is far from the traditional classification of tendonitis, which describes a pure inflammatory process. Although scientists are still studying the exact mechanisms, researchers have questioned the theory of a pure inflammatory response. More research is being conducted to support the idea that a degenerative cascade of events occurs.[13–15] In this chapter, the term *tendinopathy* is used to describe conditions of the lower extremity, and the term *tendonitis* is used to describe specific conditions in the upper extremity. This nomenclature follows the current classifications used in the literature.

## TISSUE REACTION TO INJURY

When an injury does occur, the healing process begins immediately. The body goes through a systematic process with three distinct phases: the inflammatory phase, the fibroblastic/proliferation phase, and the maturation/remodeling phase (Fig. 30-5).

The first phase is the **inflammatory phase**, which typically lasts from 0 to 6 days. The focus of the phase is to "close off" the injured area and begin the healing process. The local vessels constrict to stop bleeding, while other cells enter the wound to form a clot, fight infection, and begin the cleanup process.[16,17]

The second phase is the **fibroblastic/proliferation phase**, which begins at approximately day 3 and lasts to day 21. This phase begins by filling the wound with collagen and other cells that will eventually form a scar. Within 2 to 3 weeks, the wound can resist normal stresses, but wound strength continues to build for several months.[16,17]

The last phase is the **maturation/remodeling phase**, which can last up to 2 years. This phase begins the remodeling of the scar into a more organized

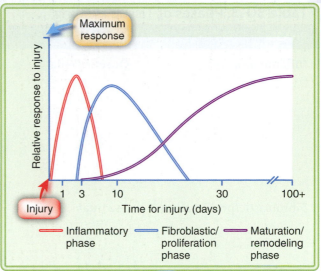

**Figure 30-5.** Different phases of tissue healing in reaction to injury. The inflammatory phase begins with clot formation followed by a general immune response to fight potential infection. The fibroblastic/proliferative phase involves the recruitment of fibroblasts that direct the creation of the collagen matrix to close the wound and form the scar. Formation of new blood vessels (angiogenesis) is also included in this phase. The remodeling phase involves refinement of the scar tissue to build strength and resistance to reopening of the wound. The total process can take up to 2 years to complete until full healing of the wound is realized.

structure that can regain up to 70% to 80% of its original strength. Table 30-3 summarizes the three phases of healing.[16,17]

When the tissues of the body (e.g., muscles, tendons, and ligaments) become inflamed, the individual will experience specific signs and symptoms of which the health and fitness professional needs to be aware. This is particularly important for post-injury or postsurgical individuals. The goal is to give these individuals a challenging exercise program that will not create inflammation. The signs and symptoms of tissue inflammation include pain, redness, swelling, warmth, and loss of function.[18]

## TREATMENT OF MUSCULOSKELETAL INJURIES

Health and fitness professionals need to understand different strategies in managing both preexisting and acute injuries. Both types of injuries can affect a client's physical performance and, if not properly managed, can lead to further injury. For each condition described in this section, common symptoms and recommended management strategies are explained.

### Preexisting Injuries

If a client suffers from an existing injury, proper management is essential. Often clients will approach health and fitness professionals seeking advice for present or

## Table 30-3. Phases of Tissue Healing

| PHASE | TIME FRAME | DESCRIPTION |
|---|---|---|
| Inflammatory | Onset to 6 days | The body responds quickly to any tissue disruption of the skin's surface. Within seconds of the injury, blood vessels constrict to control bleeding at the site. Platelets coagulate within minutes to stop the bleeding and begin clot formation. Platelets also release factors that attract other important cells to the injury. Neutrophils (white blood cells) enter the wound to fight infection and to attract macrophages. Macrophages break down necrotic debris and activate the fibroblast response. |
| Fibroblastic/proliferation | 3–21 days | 3 Days after the injury occurs, fibroblasts begin producing large amounts of collagen and proteoglycans. Collagen fibers are laid down randomly and are cross-linked into large, closely packed bundles. Within 2–3 weeks, the wound can resist normal stresses, but wound strength continues to build for several months. The fibroblastic phase lasts from 15–20 days and then wound healing enters the maturation phase. |
| Maturation/remodeling | Up to 2 years | During the maturation phase, fibroblasts leave the wound and collagen is remodeled into a more organized matrix. Tensile strength increases for up to 1 year following the injury. Although healed wounds never regain the full strength, they can regain up to 70%–80% of their original strength. |

past injuries. Health and fitness professionals must respect **scope of practice** and refrain from diagnosing the injury. A thorough medical history and assessment will help him or her make appropriate decisions regarding the client's exercise programming. The health and fitness professional should be able to answer the important questions: "Is exercise appropriate for the client, or should he or she first be cleared by a medical professional?" This will ensure client safety and provide the health and fitness professional with guidelines to follow.

If a client does have a preexisting condition, the exercise program may need to be modified. The client should be monitored for any changes in symptoms such as pain. Following are some commonly reported symptoms of overtraining after injury, surgery, or both[18]:

- Soreness that lasts longer than 4 hours
- Soreness or pain that occurs earlier or is increased from the prior session
- Increased stiffness or decreased ROM over several sessions
- Swelling, redness, and warmth in healing tissue
- Progressive weakness over several sessions
- Decreased functional usage

### Acute Injury Management

Acute injuries need to be handled in the best possible way to ensure a positive outcome. Client safety is paramount, and health and fitness professionals need to be prepared to refer the client out if the injury is serious enough. Remember, "When in doubt, refer out."

If an acute injury does occur, early intervention often includes medical management. The acronym **P.R.I.C.E.** (Protection, Restricted Activity, Ice, Compression, and Elevation) describes a safe, early intervention strategy for an acute injury (Fig. 30-6). Using the example of an ankle injury, *protection* includes protecting the injured ankle with the use of crutches and appropriate ankle bracing. *Restricted activity* includes limiting weight-bearing activity until cleared by the physician. *Ice* should be applied every 2 hours for 10 to 15 minutes. *Compression* can be done by using a compression wrap on the area, which helps to minimize local swelling. *Elevating* the ankle 6 to 10 inches above the level of the heart will also help to control swelling. This is done to reduce hemorrhage, inflammation, swelling, and pain.[4]

## In Your Own Words

One of your friends was playing basketball and rolled his ankle when he came down for a rebound. Explain to him how to acutely manage the injury using the elements of P.R.I.C.E.

## FLEXIBILITY AND MUSCULOSKELETAL INJURIES

Decreased flexibility has been associated with various musculoskeletal injuries, such as muscle strains and overuse conditions. When a muscle becomes

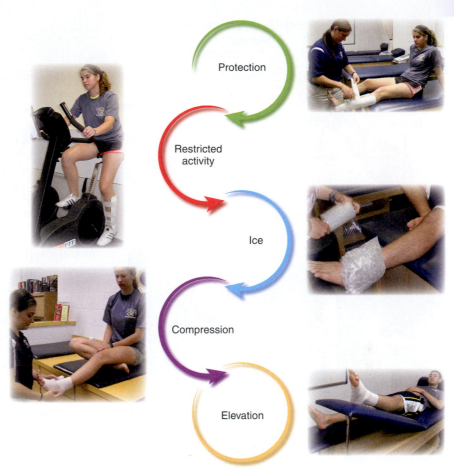

Figure 30-6. P.R.I.C.E. method for managing acute injuries. P = protection; R = restricted activity; I = ice; C = compression; E = elevation. *(Photos courtesy of Jeff Janot.)*

shortened and inflexible, it cannot generate adequate force or lengthen appropriately, which often leads to injury. In response, health and fitness professionals commonly recommend stretching programs to increase the client's flexibility (see Chapter 17).

Specific signs, symptoms, and other precautions may require the health and fitness professional to stop or avoid stretching activity to prevent injury[19]:

- Pain
- Restrictions by a medical doctor
- Prolonged immobilization of muscles and connective tissue
- Joint swelling (effusion) from trauma or disease
- Individuals with osteoporosis or rheumatoid arthritis
- Individuals with a history of prolonged steroid use

There are also specific contraindications to stretching[19]:

- A fracture site that is healing
- Acute soft-tissue injury
- Postsurgical conditions
- Joint hypermobility
- Area of inflammation or infection

If the client presents with any precautions or contraindications, further clearance from a medical professional is necessary before programming a stretching routine for this individual.

## COMMON UPPER-EXTREMITY INJURIES

Common upper-extremity injuries include shoulder impingement, rotator cuff injuries, and elbow tendonitis.

### Shoulder Impingement

**Shoulder impingement** occurs when the soft-tissue structures (e.g., bursa, rotator cuff tendons) get abnormally compressed (Fig. 30-7). This overuse can eventually lead to a rotator cuff tear if not managed properly. The condition is common in young athletes who participate in overhead activities such as tennis, baseball, and swimming. Middle-aged and older adults can also be at risk from doing repetitive overhead activity such as painting and lifting objects (Fig. 30-8).[20]

### Signs and Symptoms

Clients who suffer from shoulder impingement often complain of local pain at the front of the shoulder that radiates to the side of the arm. Aggravating activities may include lifting objects and reaching overhead or across the body. There may be swelling and tenderness in the front of the shoulder that causes pain and stiffness with movement.

### Early Management

Conservative treatment often includes avoiding aggravating activity (e.g., overhead and cross-body reaching,

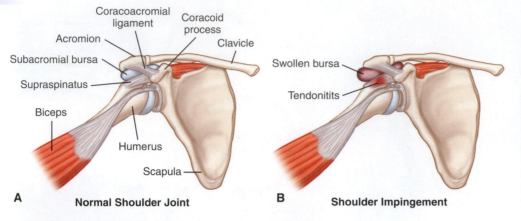

**Figure 30-7.** Anatomy of the shoulder joint. A, The normal shoulder joint has appropriate joint space with no impingement as the arm is abducted past 45 degrees. B, Notice decreased joint space, swollen and pinched bursa, and tendonitis of the supraspinatus muscle with the arm in the same position.

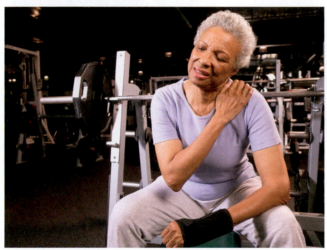

**Figure 30-8.** Shoulder impingement can be aggravated by a resistance-training exercise. *(Photo courtesy of Barry Austin.)*

placing a hand behind the back), physical therapy, modalities (e.g., ice or heat), oral anti-inflammatory medication, and cortisone injections.

## Exercise Programming

Health and fitness professionals should educate clients on avoiding aggravating activities and improving posture and body positioning. The exercise program should emphasize regaining strength and flexibility of the shoulder girdle. More specifically, strengthening the scapular stabilizers (e.g., rhomboids, mid-trapezius, and serratus anterior) and rotator cuff will help to restore proper scapulohumeral motion. The client should focus on stretching the major muscle groups around the shoulder to restore proper length to the anterior and posterior muscles (Fig. 30-9).

## Rotator Cuff Injuries

Injuries to the rotator cuff are common among athletes in "overhead" sports (e.g., volleyball, baseball, and tennis) and in middle-aged individuals. Figure 30-10 illustrates the four rotator cuff muscles that are used to stabilize the shoulder joint during activity. Injuries to the rotator muscles may be from an acute episode or be chronic in nature. Acute injuries are often related

to some type of trauma such as a fall on the shoulder or raising the arm against overwhelming resistance. Acute injuries commonly occur in individuals younger than 30 years and are often accompanied by severe loss of function. Consequently, chronic tears present as a gradual worsening of pain and weakness. Chronic tears are typically from some type of degenerative process in individuals older than 40 years, with male individuals and the dominant arm being most affected.[21–23]

### Signs and Symptoms

If an acute rotator cuff tear occurs, the client will primarily complain of feeling a sudden "tearing" sensation, followed by immediate pain and loss of motion. The client will typically have trouble lifting the arm above the head. Chronic tears show a gradual worsening, with more pain at night or after increased activity. Reaching overhead or behind the back is painful. Basic tasks such as putting on a shirt or grabbing a dish from a high shelf become difficult to impossible.[7,22,23] The cause of a rotator cuff tear is multifactorial, with common causes including overuse, postural dysfunction, joint degeneration, glenohumeral instability, dietary insufficiencies, and problems with the acromion or coracoid processes.[21]

### Early Management

Management of this condition includes modifying activity to avoid pain and reduce further damage. Avoiding aggravating activities and getting adequate rest will help relieve acute symptoms. Therapeutic modalities (e.g., ice or electrical stimulation), medication, and physical therapy may be beneficial to relieve symptoms.[4,22,23]

### Exercise Programming

The client may still be under restriction and treatment from the physical therapist or physician. Health and fitness professionals should follow these guidelines to avoid pain and further damage. Once cleared, the client can be progressed as tolerated.

Exercise modification and further injury recognition should be the focus of client education. Clients may typically want to push through the pain and dismiss any signs of further injury. Exercise and fitness professionals

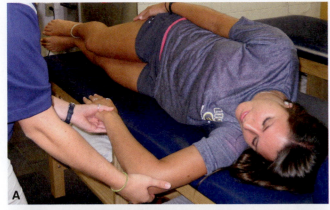

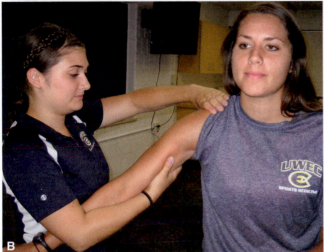

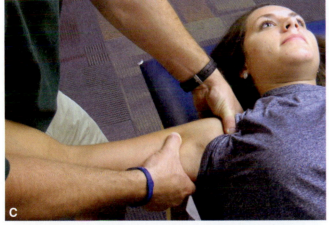

**Figure 30-9.** Examples of assisted exercises to help relieve and manage shoulder impingement. A, For the sleeper stretch, the allied health professional is applying a gentle stretch to the shoulder by pushing downward on the wrist. B, For traction, the allied health professional is applying light traction by pulling downward on the arm. C, For traction with small oscillations, the allied health professional is applying force down on the arm and up on the shoulder joint to improve joint space at the shoulder. (Note that these maneuvers are outside the scope of practice of fitness professionals.) *(Photos courtesy of Jeff Janot.)*

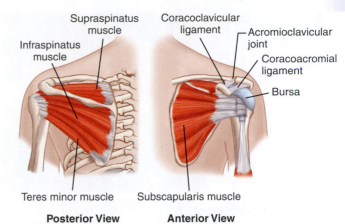

**Figure 30-10.** The anatomy of the rotator cuff from both an anterior and a posterior view.

Stretching should focus on restoring muscle balance across the whole upper body. Stretching should target the pectoralis group and latissimus dorsi. A general stretching program for the upper body can be added to maintain overall mobility.

The strengthening program should follow guidelines from the medical professional. The program should target the scapular musculature and the rotator cuff, and progress what has been done in physical therapy. The client may show poor scapulohumeral rhythm that is demonstrated by the shoulder hiking up during elevation activity. Thus, the client may still need isolated strengthening of specific muscles before beginning functional movements (Fig. 30-11). Health and fitness professionals can use a variety of training methods such as repetitions, speed of movement, and time intervals to challenge the client. However, all exercises should be pain-free and adhere to physician guidelines. Clients with a rotator cuff tear are commonly told to avoid overhead activity, painful movements, repetitive tasks, and lifting of heavy loads.[22,23]

As with the other pathologies mentioned earlier, low-loading cardiovascular activity with minimal upper-extremity involvement is preferred. Activities performed on the stationary bike and elliptical trainer are preferred over activities that involve the upper extremity such as rowing and swimming.

Proper clearance by the medical professional should be obtained before progressing any physical activity. A gradual return is important, especially with overhead activity. The client may still have residual pain that may limit certain movements. With these clients, basic **activities of daily living (ADLs)** should be mastered first, then progressed to more advanced activity. The client may have been limited with motion and function because of pain and muscle guarding. This can create a weakened shoulder because of the prolonged disuse and affect overall scapular motion. ROM and neuromuscular control should be restored to ensure pain-free activity. This is why a slow return is important to avoid an exacerbation or re-injury.

should help their clients understand their limitations and how to modify the training program. Specific movements such as repetitive overhead and cross-body movements should be avoided until cleared by a medical professional.

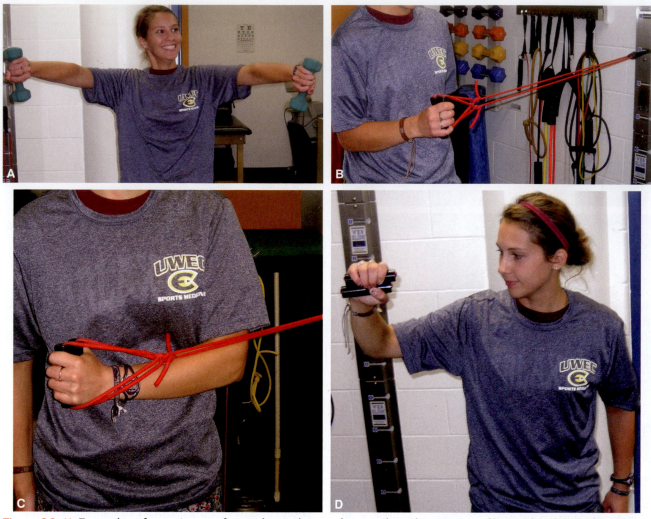

**Figure 30-11.** Examples of exercises performed to isolate and strengthen the rotator cuff complex: (A) weights, (B) external rotation with band, (C) internal rotation with band, and (D) internal rotation with shoulder joint abducted 90 degrees. *(Photos courtesy of Jeff Janot.)*

## Elbow Tendonitis

Tendonitis of both the flexors and extensors of the elbow can occur with overuse of the upper extremity. This condition has been classified as either lateral epicondylitis or medial epicondylitis to signify the area of tissue trauma (Fig. 30-12).

**Lateral epicondylitis**, often termed "tennis elbow," is defined as an overuse or repetitive trauma injury of the wrist extensors at their origin on the lateral epicondyle of the humerus. **Medial epicondylitis** is often called "golfer's elbow" and is also a repetitive overuse injury of the wrist flexors at the origin at the medial elbow. Common causes for both conditions include overuse, repetitive trauma, or muscle imbalance. This condition is common in adults 30 to 55 years old.[24,25]

## Signs and Symptoms

Clients will often complain of local nagging pain at the lateral epicondyle or medial epicondyle during aggravating activities. Pain will diminish with rest but tends to get worse over time if not addressed properly.

## Early Management

Conservative treatment often includes avoiding aggravating activity, physical therapy, therapeutic modalities (e.g., ice or heat), assistive devices (e.g., wrist or elbow splints), oral anti-inflammatory medication, and cortisone injections.

## Exercise Programming

The exercise program should emphasize educating the client on avoiding aggravating activities and improving posture and body positioning. Regaining strength and flexibility of the wrist/elbow flexors and extensors is important. The client should wear a wrist or elbow splint or elbow support wrap during activity, and the health or fitness professional should monitor for increased symptoms, such as pain and progressive forearm muscle weakness.

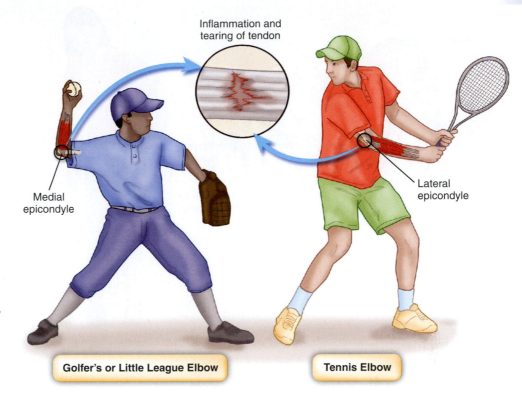

Inflammation and tearing of tendon

Medial epicondyle

Lateral epicondyle

Golfer's or Little League Elbow

Tennis Elbow

**Figure 30-12.** Tendonitis of the elbow at the sites of the lateral and medial epicondyles. Medial epicondylitis, sometimes referred to as "Little League elbow," is also caused by overuse from general throwing and pitching activities.

## VIGNETTE continued

■ Marco suspects that Rafael is suffering from lateral epicondylitis, which is commonly referred to as "tennis elbow." This overuse injury often results from poor mechanics during a backhand swing. Marco tells Rafael that he should avoid activities that aggravate the pain and ice his elbow if the pain flairs up. Marco also recommends that Rafael seek the help of Eleanor, the athletic trainer at the tennis academy, because treating this condition is outside of Marco's scope of practice. The athletic trainer will likely prescribe a wrist or elbow splint and provide guidelines for modifying Rafael's workouts. Rafael is clearly distressed by Marco's feedback regarding his elbow injury, but Marco reminds him that this type of injury will only get worse over time if not addressed properly.

## LOWER-EXTREMITY INJURIES

Common lower-extremity injuries include trochanteric bursitis, iliotibial band friction syndrome (ITBFS), patellofemoral pain syndrome (PFPS), infrapatellar tendinopathy, meniscal injuries, ACL injuries, ankle sprains, shin splints, Achilles tendinopathy, and plantar fasciitis.

## Trochanteric Bursitis

**Trochanteric bursitis** is characterized by painful inflammation of the trochanteric bursa between the greater trochanter of the femur and the gluteus medius/iliotibial complex (Fig. 30-13).[26,27] This condition is more common in female runners, cross-country skiers, and ballet dancers. Inflammation of the bursa may be caused by an acute incident or repetitive (cumulative) trauma. Acute incidents may include trauma from falls, contact sports (e.g., football), and other sources of impact.[28,29] Repetitive trauma may be caused by excessive friction from prolonged running or an increase or change in activity.

### Signs and Symptoms

Trochanteric pain and/or **paresthesias** (e.g., tingling, prickling, and numbness) often radiate from the greater trochanter to the posterior lateral hip, down the iliotibial tract, to the lateral knee.[30] Symptoms are most often related to an increase in activity or repetitive overuse.

### Early Management

Conservative treatment often includes avoiding aggravating activity, physical therapy, therapeutic modalities (e.g., ice or heat), assistive devices (e.g., a cane), oral anti-inflammatory medication, and cortisone injections.

### Exercise Programming

When the client is ready to return to gym activity, a written clearance from his or her physician may be necessary. The client may walk with a limp because of pain and weakness. This often results in decreased muscle length (e.g., quadriceps or hamstrings), myofascial tightness (e.g., iliotibial band [ITB] complex), and weak or inhibited muscles. The client should slowly return to

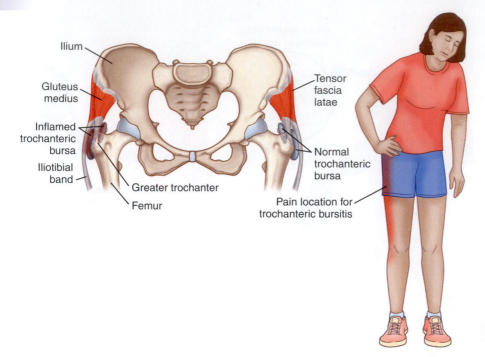

**Figure 30-13.** Trochanteric bursitis in the hip region.

activity with an emphasis on proper training techniques (e.g., training schedule), proper equipment (e.g., shoe wear), and early injury recognition. The exercise program should include regaining flexibility, strength, and neuromuscular control at the hip.

## Iliotibial Band Friction Syndrome

**Iliotibial band friction syndrome (ITBFS)** is a repetitive overuse condition that occurs when the distal portion of the ITB rubs against the lateral femoral epicondyle.[18] ITBFS is common among active individuals 15 to 50 years of age and is primarily caused by training errors in runners, cyclists, volleyball players, and weight lifters.[27] Risk factors may include overtraining (e.g., increase speed, distance, or frequency), improper shoe wear or equipment, changes in running surface, muscle imbalance (e.g., weakness or tightness), structural abnormalities (e.g., flat feet, bow-legged, and leg length discrepancy), and failure to correctly stretch.[18,31]

### Signs and Symptoms

Clients often report a gradual onset of tightness, burning, or pain at the lateral aspect of the knee during activity (Fig. 30-14). The pain may be localized but generally radiates to the outside of the knee and/or up the outside of the thigh. Snapping, popping, or pain may be felt at the lateral knee when it is flexed and extended.[18,31] Aggravating factors may include any repetitive activity such as running (e.g., downhill) or cycling. Symptoms often resolve with rest but can increase in intensity and frequency if not properly treated.

### Early Management

Conservative treatment of ITBFS often includes avoiding aggravating activity, physical therapy, therapeutic

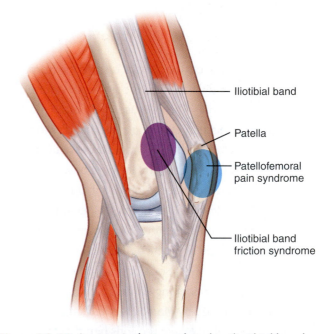

**Figure 30-14.** Anatomical sites related to iliotibial band friction syndrome and patellofemoral pain syndrome.

modalities (e.g., ice or heat), assistive devices (e.g., a cane), oral anti-inflammatory medication, and cortisone injections.

### Exercise Programming

The client may present with weakness in the hip abductors, ITB shortening, and tenderness throughout the ITB complex. As with trochanteric bursitis, this can cause a limp because of pain. A slow return to activity is recommended, with an emphasis on proper training techniques (e.g., training schedule), proper equipment (e.g., shoe wear), and early injury recognition. The exercise program should include regaining flexibility, strength, and neuromuscular control at the hip.

## Patellofemoral Pain Syndrome

**Patellofemoral pain syndrome (PFPS)** is often called "anterior knee pain" or "runner's knee" (Fig. 30-14). This syndrome has been found to have the highest prevalence among runners. In fact, PFPS makes up 16% to 25% of all running injuries.[32]

The cause of PFPS is often considered multifactorial and can be classified into three primary categories:

1. **Overuse**: PFPS can occur when repetitive loading activities cause abnormal stress to the knee joint, which leads to pain and dysfunction. The excessive loading exceeds the body's physiological balance, which leads to tissue trauma, injury, and pain.[32,33] Recent changes in intensity, frequency, duration, and training environment (e.g., surface) may contribute to this condition.

2. **Biomechanical**: Misalignment of the kinetic chain during activity can lead to biomechanical abnormalities that can alter patellar tracking and/or increase patellofemoral joint stress. Pes planus or flat foot has been associated with PFPS by altering the alignment of the knee.[34,35] Loss of the medial arch flattens the foot, which may cause a compensatory internal rotation of the tibia and/or femur that alters the tracking of the patellofemoral joint. This abnormal tracking may cause excessive stress to the patella, which can eventually lead to pain. Conversely, pes cavus or high arches causes less cushioning compared with a normal foot. The lower extremity has less ability to absorb stress during demanding activities. This leads to excessive stress to the patellofemoral joint, particularly with loading activities such as running. Lastly, an abnormally large **Q-angle** has been associated with PFPS.[35,36] The Q-angle is the angle formed by lines drawn from the anterior superior iliac spine to the central patella and from the central patella to the tibial tubercle (Fig. 30-15). The Q-angle is an estimate of the effective angle at which the quadriceps group pulls on the patella.[18] A normal Q-angle is considered to be less than 12 degrees, and angles greater than 15 degrees are considered pathological.[18]

3. **Muscle dysfunction**: Lower-extremity muscle weakness, tightness, and length deficits have been associated with PFPS. Because of its fascial connection with the patella, tightness and shortening of the ITB complex can cause the patella to improperly track laterally, creating excessive patellofemoral contact pressure.[33,37] Also, tightness in the hamstrings and gastrocnemius/soleus complex can cause a posterior force to the knee, which results in increased patellofemoral contact pressure.[18,37] Muscle

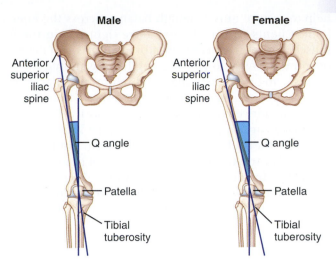

**Figure 30-15.** The Q-angle in males and females.

weaknesses in the quadriceps, hip abductors, and external rotators have been associated with PFPS.[38–41] In particular, quadriceps weakness has been associated with abnormal patellofemoral tracking. If the quadriceps cannot activate efficiently during activity, the patella will track abnormally. Also, weakness of the hip abductors and external rotators can cause femoral adduction/internal rotation, abnormal knee valgus, and compensatory foot pronation.[18,37,42] This can affect patellofemoral tracking, which may lead to pain and dysfunction.

### Signs and Symptoms

Commonly reported symptoms of PFPS include pain with running, stair climbing, squatting, or prolonged sitting. The client will typically describe a gradual "achy" pain that occurs behind or underneath the knee cap but may be immediate if trauma has occurred.[32] Clients may also report knee stiffness, giving way, clicking, or a popping sensation during movement.[18,37]

### Early Management

Early management for PFPS includes avoiding aggravating activities (e.g., prolonged sitting, deep squats, and running), modifying training techniques (e.g., frequency and intensity), proper shoe wear, physical therapy, patellar taping, knee bracing, foot orthotics, patient education, oral anti-inflammatory medication, and modalities (e.g., ice and heat).

### Exercise Programming

The focus of the gym program is to progress what has been done in the early stages. Health and fitness professionals must remember that restoring proper flexibility and strength is the key with PFPS. Addressing tightness in the ITB complex through stretching and myofascial release (e.g., on a foam roller) can have a major impact on the dynamics of the patellofemoral joint. Stretching of the hamstrings and calves will also help to restore muscle-length balance across the knee joint. Clients with PFPS may have tightness in these muscle groups from compensatory patterns that developed in response to pain. Strengthening should focus on restoring proper strength and neuromuscular control throughout the hip, knee, and ankle. Strengthening the quadriceps group should be a priority. Exercises for the hip and ankle complex should be included because of their effects on the knee joint. Improving femoral control through strengthening of the hip muscles will help to control the forces imposed on the knee joint. The muscles that control the ankle complex may need to be strengthened to have distal control.

## Infrapatellar Tendinopathy

**Infrapatellar tendinopathy**, or "jumper's knee," is an overuse syndrome characterized by a degenerative process of the patellar tendon at the insertion into the distal pole of the patella (Fig. 30-16). This injury is more common in sports such as basketball, volleyball, and track and field because of the repetitive loading from jumping.[43] In fact, approximately 20% of jumping athletes will suffer from this problem. Male and female athletes are equally affected with bilateral problems. With single-limb problems, male athletes are affected two times more than female athletes.[44,45]

### Signs and Symptoms

Commonly reported symptoms of patellofemoral pain syndrome include pain at the distal knee cap into the infrapatellar tendon. Pain has also been reported with running, walking stairs, squatting, or prolonged sitting (i.e., theater sign).[18,37]

### Early Management

Early management includes avoiding aggravating activities (e.g., plyometrics, prolonged sitting, deep squats, and running), modifying training techniques (e.g., frequency and intensity), proper shoe wear, physical therapy, patellar taping (Fig. 30-17), knee bracing, arch supports, foot orthotics, patient education, oral anti-inflammatory medication, and therapeutic modalities (e.g., ice and heat).

### Exercise Programming

As with PFPS, the focus should be to restore proper flexibility and strength in the lower extremity. Addressing tightness in the quadriceps through stretching and myofascial release (e.g., on a foam roller) can have a major impact on the dynamics of the infrapatellar tendon. Stretching and self-myofascial release of the ITB, hamstrings, and calves will also help to restore muscle-length balance across the knee joint. Strengthening should focus on restoring strength and neuromuscular control throughout the hip, knee, and ankle. Strengthening the quadriceps group should be a priority. Exercises for the hip and ankle complex should be included because of their effects on the knee joint. The muscles that control the ankle complex may need to be strengthened to have distal control.

## Meniscal Injuries

Meniscal tears are one of the most commonly reported knee injuries. The menisci have an important role

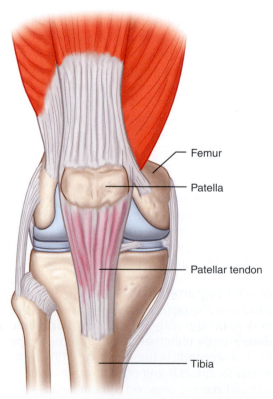

**Figure 30-16.** Anatomy of "jumper's knee" (patellar tendon irritation).

Femur
Patella
Patellar tendon
Tibia

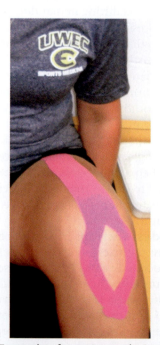

**Figure 30-17.** Example of a taping technique to support the patella and improve patellar tracking to manage patellofemoral pain syndrome and infrapatellar tendinopathy. *(Photo courtesy of Jeff Janot.)*

within the knee through their multiple functions. First, both the medial and the lateral menisci act as shock absorbers and assist with load bearing of the joint. Second, the menisci work together to assist with joint congruency of the femur and tibia during motion. Third, they act as secondary restraints to give the joint more stability. Fourth, the menisci assist with joint lubrication by helping to maintain a synovial layer inside the joint. Fifth, nerve endings within the menisci are thought to give proprioceptive feedback during motion and compression.[7,46] Notably, the menisci receive blood in only 10% to 25% of the outer periphery, called the *vascular zone*. Because of its blood supply, this region may heal better than the nonvascular inner region of the meniscus.[7,46] This can be a factor when surgery is necessary.

Meniscal injuries often occur from trauma or degeneration. Traumatic injuries can occur from a combination of loading and twisting of the joint. For example, a tear can occur when an individual suddenly decelerates and twists on a flexed knee during running. The combination of axial loading with pivoting of the femur on the tibia causes a shear force across the meniscus. This exceeds the strength of the tissue, resulting in injury.[7] Older individuals with degenerative menisci are more predisposed to meniscal tears.[8] Meniscal tears can also occur with other traumatic injuries such as acute ACL tears (e.g., lateral meniscus) or MCL injury (e.g., medial meniscus).[7]

## Signs and Symptoms

When a client has a meniscal tear, he or she may complain of symptoms during activity. Commonly reported symptoms include stiffness, clicking or popping with joint loading, giving way, catching, and locking (in more severe tears). Other signs include joint pain, swelling, and muscle weakness (e.g., quadriceps).[7,47]

## Precautions

Frequently, with nonoperative management, the client will be cleared to resume activity once symptoms have diminished, but will be encouraged to avoid deep squats, cutting, pivoting, or twisting for as long as symptoms are present.[7] Postsurgical procedures have specific precautions that are discussed later.

## Nonoperative Management

Indications for nonoperative management include absent or diminished symptoms and small or degenerative tears.[7] Typically, the client will be sent to physical therapy to improve strength and ROM. Therapeutic modalities (e.g., ice and heat), compression, bracing, and oral anti-inflammatory medication often accompany physical therapy. If conservative management fails, then surgical intervention may be the next step.

## Surgical Considerations

In the past, total meniscectomy (removal of the greater part of the meniscus) was commonly done to relieve symptoms of meniscal injuries. Over time, this procedure has become less popular because of the progressive joint degeneration that it causes. Currently, arthroscopic (e.g., with a camera) partial meniscectomy and meniscal repairs are the two most common procedures. When choosing which procedure is appropriate, the surgeon must consider several factors, including age, location, severity, associated ligament injury, and type of tear.[47]

With a partial meniscectomy, the surgeon removes only the unstable, torn fragments and leaves the viable, healthy tissue intact. This is typically done when there is a large tear that enters the avascular inner zone.[47] The goal is to preserve as much as possible and allow the remaining meniscus to still serve its function without causing early degeneration.

A meniscal repair involves suturing the torn fragment back in place. The ideal location is a tear that occurs in the outer vascular zone. This procedure preserves the meniscal tissue but requires a slower rehabilitation because of healing of the repair versus extracting the torn tissue. The ideal candidate is an active individual younger than 50 years with a small tear in the outer vascular zone.[8,47]

## In Your Own Words

A college football player (running back) who suffered a right knee medial meniscal tear and may have surgery asks you to explain the difference between a meniscectomy and meniscal repair. How would you answer this client's question?

## Early Management

Early management after partial meniscectomy or meniscal repair may involve specific precautions for the first 2 to 8 weeks depending on the surgeon's preference. With partial meniscectomy, there is no anatomical structure that needs to be protected, so rehabilitation can be progressed more aggressively with immediate partial or full weight bearing. The client still may have to use crutches and a brace. The meniscal repair often involves a slower progression with partial or non–weight bearing with crutches and a brace. The client may also have ROM restrictions for knee flexion (e.g., 60 degrees) for the first 4 to 6 weeks to protect the healing tissue.[7,18]

For both procedures, the client is typically sent to outpatient physical therapy for 6 to 12 weeks depending on the physician's plan of care and insurance constraints. During this time, the goal is to increase ROM, improve lower-extremity strength (e.g., quadriceps), control pain and swelling, and progress into more functional activity.

## Exercise Programming

Health and fitness professionals may begin to see clients for gym activity as soon as 4 weeks for meniscectomy and 8 to 12 weeks for meniscal repair.[7,18] The client may do a combination of physical therapy and gym activities. As noted earlier, it is important to consult with the physician or physical therapist regarding exercise precautions or contraindications. The following strategies take into account clearance by the physician and the client's ability to load the knee with no symptoms.

At this point, the client will have done stretching for a period of time. However, gym activity can be more demanding on a weakened lower extremity than general rehabilitation. With both the partial meniscectomy and meniscal repair, progressive stretching of the muscle groups that cross the knee should be done. Specifically, stretching of the quadriceps and hamstrings should be emphasized to help maintain adequate flexibility.

When programming exercises for both the meniscectomy and the meniscal repair, exercises that require deep squatting, cutting, or pivoting should be avoided until cleared by the doctor. Examples of exercises to avoid include bar squats, leg presses, or lunges greater than 90 degrees of flexion, full ROM on the leg extension machine, and plyometric or agility drills that include cutting or pivoting. These exercises may cause high shear forces to the healing tissues, which can result in re-injury. In fact, deep squatting and hyperflexion of the knee is discouraged for the first 6 months with a meniscal repair.[7]

Most gym exercises are safe if progressed appropriately by the health and fitness professional. Common exercises include both closed kinetic chain (CKC) exercises (i.e., foot or hand fixed on the ground) and open kinetic chain (OKC) exercises (i.e., foot or hand not fixed on the ground or surface). CKC activities such as squats, leg presses, and lunges can be performed initially from 0 to 45 degrees and progressed to 90 degrees once cleared by the physician. OKC activities such as the straight-leg raise, side-lying abduction, and side-lying adduction are encouraged to isolate the hip musculature. Initially, knee extensions are advised from 90 to 60 degrees and progressed once cleared. More advanced, multiplanar activity should be safe once adequate healing has taken place and proper clearance is obtained.

Functional integration back into athletic activity should be relatively easy for these clients. In general, the client with partial meniscectomy can return to basic activity after 2 to 4 weeks and return to athletic and sports activity between 6 to 12 weeks after surgery. For the client with a meniscal repair, running may begin at 3 to 4 months after surgery, and full return to athletic and sports activity may begin 5 to 6 months after surgery.[7]

As mentioned earlier, deficits in general balance may be evident because of disuse of the kinetic chain. Basic progression of balance activities would be appropriate at this stage.

## Anterior Cruciate Ligament Injuries

ACL injuries are the most common sports-related injury of the knee. Most ACL injuries (i.e., 70%–80%) are noncontact, with the remaining 20% to 30% resulting from some sort of direct impact to the knee or lower leg.[48] ACL injuries most often occur in relatively young athletic individuals 15 to 45 years of age.[48] The ACL has a primary role to prevent anterior translation of the tibia on the femur. The ACL and posterior cruciate ligament work together to control excessive rotary motion.[7] An intact ACL can resist forces between 1,725 and 2,195 Newtons (N) before failing. Typical running and cutting maneuvers create only approximately 1,700 N of force.[7,18] However, injury will occur if the forces imposed on the knee exceed its strength.

### Signs and Symptoms

When an ACL injury occurs, it is often traumatic, involving the mechanisms mentioned earlier. The client will often report hearing a "pop" during the activity with immediate swelling, instability, decreased ROM, and pain. This typically requires immediate medical care to immobilize and protect the joint, followed by a visit to the orthopedic physician for further diagnosis and intervention (e.g., nonoperative vs. operative).[47]

### Nonoperative Management

Nonoperative treatment for older, sedentary individuals may be beneficial, but it may be problematic for younger, active individuals. The ACL-deficient knee may still cause instability with activity and may lead to further injury to knee structures such as the menisci or articular cartilage.[18] The focus of treatment is to maintain adequate ROM, gait, proprioception, and strength of the muscles around the knee. Specifically, strengthening the hamstrings has been shown to help prevent anterior translation of the tibia. Modalities including ice and compression wrapping may be used to control swelling.[18]

With nonoperative management the client may be cleared to slowly resume activity once symptoms have diminished, but may be restricted from jumping, cutting, pivoting, or twisting motions.[7] Wearing a protective knee brace is recommended to protect the deficient knee during activity. After rehabilitation, some individuals attempt to return to their activity or sport despite the presence of instability. If this proves unsuccessful, surgery may be the next option. Postsurgical procedures have specific precautions that are discussed later. Before surgery, the physician may prescribe preoperative rehabilitation to restore ROM, muscle strength, and proper gait.

### Surgical Considerations

Several procedures are currently used by surgeons to repair the ACL. Surgeries involving the medial one third of the patellar tendon and the medial hamstring (semitendinosus) are the two most common procedures. Both of the procedures have good short- and long-term functional outcomes.[55–58]

### Patellar Tendon Graft

The patellar tendon graft procedure involves taking the middle third of the individual's patellar tendon

## SEX DIFFERENCES

### Noncontact Female Anterior Cruciate Ligament Injuries

Female noncontact knee ACL injury rates have increased in recent years, especially in the sports of soccer and basketball. For soccer, female athletes are two times more likely to injure their ACL than male athletes.[49,50] Also, female basketball players are three times more likely to injure their ACL than their male counterparts.[49,50] The exact reasons for these high incidences are still being studied.[51] Several risk factors have been identified that include, but are not limited to, sex, poor lower-body strength, hormonal influences, joint ROM, poor core strength and proprioception, poor mechanics with running and jumping, different knee joint geometry (i.e., shallower medial knee joint, small and narrow intercondylar notch width), increased knee joint laxity, prior ACL surgery, and familial predisposition.[52-54] Currently, two knee ACL injury prevention programs have preliminary evidence to reduce injury rates and improve performance. These programs are discussed further in the Research Highlights feature later in this chapter.

The mechanism of injury often involves a maneuver of deceleration combined with twisting, pivoting, or sidestepping (Fig. 30-18). The combined multiplanar movements cause a traumatic shearing force that exceeds the tensile strength of the ACL, resulting in injury.[48]

Sex influences are also involved with various intrinsic and extrinsic variables for both male and female individuals, although a comprehensive discussion on these variables is beyond the scope of this chapter.

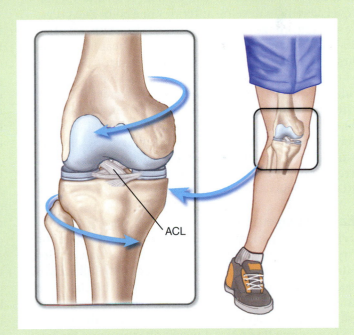

ACL

**Figure 30-18.** The mechanism of injury for most ACL tears is a rapid deceleration followed by a quick change of direction through sidestepping or pivoting.

(autograft) to replace the damaged ACL. This procedure has been performed since the 1920s.[47] This procedure has consistently demonstrated excellent surgical outcomes, with a 90% to 95% success rate in individuals returning to pre-injury level of activity.[58] This procedure is recommended for athletes in high-demand sports.[59] This procedure may not be indicated for people with a history of patellofemoral pain, arthritis, or patellar tendonitis, or smaller individuals with a narrow patellar tendon.[60] Reported problems with the procedure include postoperative pain behind the knee cap and pain with squatting.[61,62] The patellar graft has an initial failure rate of 2,300 Newtons (Ns, a unit of force equal to the amount needed to accelerate 1 kilogram of mass at the rate of 1 meter per second squared), which is stronger than a healthy, intact ACL.[7,18]

### Hamstring Tendon Graft

The hamstring semitendinosus procedure is also used because of the high tensile strength of the hamstring tendon. Surgeons typically harvest strands of tendons from the medial semitendinosus to reconstruct the ACL. Surgeons also may use additional tendons from the gracilis muscle, which creates a combined four-strand tendon graft that has an estimated failure rate of 4,108 N.[7,18] This truly creates a stronger repair than the patellar tendon graft. This procedure may be beneficial for younger patients who still have open growth plates. With the hamstring tendon graft there are no graft bone ends like in the patellar graft that could violate the growth plate and stimulate early closure.[63] This procedure has fewer problems with pain behind the kneecap, better cosmesis (no anterior incision), decreased postoperative stiffness, and faster recovery.[7] Reported problems with the procedure include increased laxity of the new ligament because of graft elongation (stretching), slower healing of the tendon graft, and loosening of the graft at the anchoring site in the bone.[7]

### The Allograft

Surgeons are also using cadaveric or allograft grafts from the Achilles tendon, tibialis anterior, and patellar tendon to replace the torn ACL.[63] Allografts are recommended for patients who have had unsuccessful prior ACL reconstruction or who have multiple ligaments that need repair. Advantages include decreased morbidity at the donor site, decreased surgical time, and less postoperative pain. Problems with the allograft procedure include risk for infection and graft elongation.[63,64]

### Postoperative Precautions

It is not uncommon for clients who return to higher-level activity to develop anterior knee pain. The prevalence rate ranges from 15% to 25%, with reported incidence rates as high as 55%.[7] The healing patellar graft has been linked to anterior knee pain. The knee should be gradually introduced to activity to allow adaptation and adequate healing. To protect the graft, the physician may have the client wear a protective brace for the first year after surgery or may have him or her permanently wear it during activity. Activity should be stopped if any of the following occur: increased pain at surgical site, increased swelling, loss of ROM, and increased exercise pain.[7]

### Early Management

Typically, the patient will be in physical therapy for the first 3 to 4 months depending on the physician and insurance constraints. The client is generally full weight bearing with crutches and a brace for the first 2 to 6 weeks. The client may also get a custom brace later on to wear during workouts and athletic activity.[7]

During the first 6 to 12 weeks after surgery, the fixation of the graft into the bone is the weakest point.[7,18] Exercise programming during this time must take into account this weakness. Also, the graft goes through a sequence of avascular necrosis (breakdown), revascularization, and remodeling. This sequential process helps to change the properties or "ligamentize" the graft that will eventually resemble the original ACL that was replaced. The implanted graft begins to resemble the original ACL in about 6 months to 1 year. Full maturation has been reported to occur after 1 year.[7,18]

A vast amount of protocols on ACL rehabilitation have been published. Early protocols developed in the 1970s and 1980s stressed more protection of the knee with limited weight bearing and immobilization with a cast or brace for the first 6 to 12 weeks. The client was then slowly progressed with strength and ROM, then to running between 9 and 12 months.[7] As experts began to understand more about the ACL, the protocols began to mature between the late 1980s to 1990s. This led to the development of the "accelerated protocol" in which early mobility is stressed while still protecting the graft through bracing. Researchers found that early, safe activities that loaded the graft site helped to stimulate healing.[60] Today, most protocols are based on milestones that the individual must meet before continuing to the next phase. For example, the individual needs to have adequate quadriceps strength, proprioception, and ROM before being able to unlock the brace and walk without crutches. Common among protocols is a return to functional activity between 12 and 16 weeks and a return to sporting activities around 6 months.[7,18,26] Most orthopedic surgeons have developed their own protocols based on the type of surgery, preference, experience, and available research. Reviewing specific protocols is beyond the scope of this textbook. The following section discusses recommendations within each category that are based on the idea that the client has been cleared to do gym activity.

### Exercise Programming

Health or fitness professionals may begin to see the client as soon as 12 to 16 weeks after surgery. The patient may do a combination of physical therapy and gym activities. It is important for the professional to consult the physician or physical therapist regarding what procedure was done, the postoperative protocol, and obtaining clearance for gym activity.

Stretching the muscles around the knee is a priority for the client. One important principle is that weak muscles can become tight, and tight muscles can become weak. Weakened muscles may not be able to generate adequate force because of poor strength and endurance. This may create tightness because of the inability to generate the needed force for movement. A tight muscle has a poor length–tension relationship and cannot generate adequate force for movement. Specifically, the quadriceps, hamstrings, and calves should be targeted to maintain adequate flexibility around the knee.

The choice between CKC and OKC activity is of utmost importance for the client who is postsurgical. The goal is to progressively strengthen the leg without risking injury to the graft site. It is recommended that OKC knee extension be limited to 90 to 30 degrees of extension, and flexion can be full ROM. With CKC exercise, 0 to 60 degrees is recommended as a safe range.[7] It is important to understand that limiting the ROM helps protect the healing graft by preventing excessive force to the joint. OKC exercises with the knee straight and CKC exercises within the ranges mentioned earlier are recommended to protect the surgical site. The ROM precautions can be lifted once adequate healing has taken place.

Strengthening of the quadriceps, hamstrings, and hip musculature is important. Both the hamstrings and the quadriceps play a key role in prevention of further injury. Training should focus on developing symmetrical strength between muscle groups, which has been shown to be effective in preventing ACL tears.[7] Hip strengthening should be implemented because of its effect on the knee joint during CKC exercises.

Functional integration may begin as early as 12 weeks with basic activity and can be progressed toward athletic activity between 4 and 6 months. The goal during this time (12 weeks to 6 months) is to safely load the knee in all planes of motion without compromising the graft site.

Clients who have undergone ACL reconstruction will have deficits in balance. Balance activity should have been implemented in the early stages of rehabilitation (Fig. 30-19). At the time of gym activity, the client should have good balance with basic single-leg activity. Progressively challenging the knee in multiples planes will help prepare the joint for higher-level activity.

Low-loading cardiovascular activity such as water aerobics, the stationary bike, and the elliptical trainer is preferred over higher-loading activity until the client is cleared.

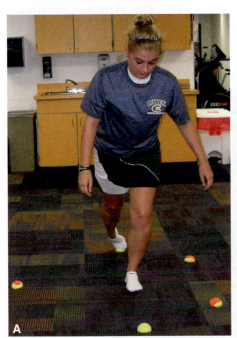
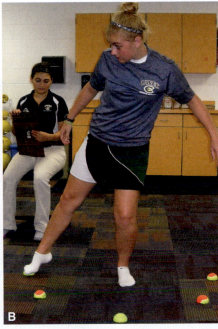
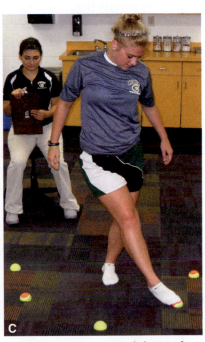

**Figure 30-19.** The star excursion balance test is a potential way to assess the stability and proprioceptive abilities of the knee after anterior cruciate ligament reconstruction surgery. Activities that are involved in this test can also be used to train balance in these individuals. In this test, the client is asked to touch the points of the star as indicated by the examiner while maintaining proper balance and posture. Here, the client is extending the hip (A) to touch the posterior mark, abducting the hip (B) to touch a mark on the right side, and adducting the hip (C) to touch a mark on the left side. *(Photos courtesy of Jeff Janot.)*

## RESEARCH HIGHLIGHT

### Anterior Cruciate Ligament Prevention Programs for Female Soccer Players

Currently, two popular programs, Sportsmetrics and the Prevent Injury and Enhance Performance program (PEP), have preliminary evidence that they help prevent ACL injuries and improve performance.[51,65] Both these programs last about 20 to 30 minutes and focus on various aspects of training including warm-ups, stretching, muscle strengthening, plyometrics, landing and running mechanics, and agility drills.[66] The goal of these programs is to address potential deficits in strength and coordination in the abdominal core and lower extremity to prevent further injury. Researchers are still looking for answers, and more high-quality studies are needed to fully validate these programs.[59] The other challenge is to develop a global consensus among coaches and organizations on how to implement these types of programs. Currently in the United States, there is no national consensus, with only a minority of coaches implementing such programs.[67] As understanding grows, there will likely be more support for the implementation of these programs to decrease the incidences of noncontact knee ACL injuries among female athletes globally.

*Please see reference list at the end of the chapter.*

## Ankle Sprains

Ankle sprains are common in the athletic population. They account for 10% to 30% of sports-related injuries in young athletes.[68] Ankle sprains are most common in sports such as basketball, volleyball, soccer, and ice skating.[69] There are little data regarding risk factors for ankle sprains. However, a history of ankle sprains has been found to be a risk factor. Foot type, general laxity, and sex have also been linked to incidents of ankle sprains.[69]

Lateral or inversion ankle sprains are the most common ankle sprain (Fig. 30-20). In fact, 85% of ankle sprains are to the lateral structures of the ankle.[70,71] The mechanism is typically inversion with a plantar-flexed foot. The lateral ankle ligaments are the most common structures involved, which include the anterior talofibular ligament, calcaneofibular ligament, and posterior talofibular ligament.

Medial or eversion ankle sprains account for less than 10% of all ankle injuries and result from forced dorsiflexion and eversion of the ankle. The medial deltoid ligament is the most common structure involved, and injury often requires further examination to rule out a fracture.[4]

### Signs and Symptoms

With lateral ankle sprains, the individual can often recall the mechanism and hearing a "pop" or "tearing" sound. Specific signs and symptoms for ligament sprains are described in Table 30-1. Medial ankle sprains rarely happen in isolation. The individual is often unable to recall the specific mechanism but can reproduce discomfort by dorsiflexing and everting the ankle. There may be medial swelling with tenderness over the deltoid ligament.[4]

### Early Management

Most often, individuals with lateral and medial ankle sprains are referred to a medical doctor for further diagnosis and treatment. Grade I and II lateral sprains are often immobilized with an ankle brace for several days. Grade III lateral sprains are often immobilized with a removable cast boot for up to 3 weeks.[18] Early management can begin 1 to 3 weeks after injury unless a severe ankle sprain has occurred, which may require further immobilization.[18] The client may be sent to physical therapy to improve strength, flexibility, proprioception, and endurance, and to control swelling.

### Exercise Programming

The health or fitness professional may begin to see the client for gym activity as soon as 1 to 2 weeks for grade I, 2 to 3 weeks for grade II, and 3 to 6 weeks for grade III.[18] During this time, the client may still be in physical therapy and is ready to transition to gym activity. Restoring proper balance, flexibility, and strength is the key with these injuries.

Clients who have suffered ankle sprains may have deficits in balance. The ligaments are a major source of proprioceptive feedback for balance and joint position sense.[19] Stretching of the gastrocnemius and soleus may be beneficial if the client has tightness and decreased length after immobilization. General stretches for the lower extremity should be included to maintain adequate flexibility. Strengthening the lower leg will be beneficial with particular emphasis on the muscles that control the foot and ankle. Targeting the peroneal group for inversion ankle sprains is important for prevention. Clients with eversion ankle sprains may have more global deficits because of the fact that eversion ankle sprains are rarely in isolation; often they follow other trauma such as a fracture. Strengthening programs for these injuries are often individual and are determined by the injury.

## Shin Splints

**Shin splints** is a general term used to describe exertional leg pain. Shin splints account for 10% to 15% of all injuries caused by running activity and 60% of lower-leg pain.[18,72] Shin splints are typically classified into two specific conditions: **medial tibial stress syndrome (MTSS)** and **anterior shin splints** (Fig. 30-21).

MTSS, or posterior shin splints, is an overuse injury that occurs in the active population. MTSS is an exercise-induced condition that is often triggered by a sudden change in activity.[73] MTSS is actually periostitis, or inflammation of the periosteum (connective tissue covering) of the bone. Pain is often local at the tendon–bone interface. This condition is considered a traction injury, which often occurs

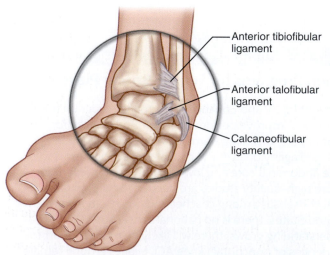

- Anterior tibiofibular ligament

- Anterior talofibular ligament

- Calcaneofibular ligament

**Figure 30-20.** The most common mechanism of injury to the ankle: lateral or inversion movement. The major ligaments frequently involved in this injury are the calcaneofibular and anterior talofibular.

## FROM THEORY TO PRACTICE

You are a health and fitness professional working with a 19-year-old male basketball player (guard position) who suffered a grade II inversion ankle sprain 3 months ago after landing wrong on an opponent's foot during a game. The athlete has been discharged from rehabilitation and referred to you by the physician to design a sports-specific training program. The physician wants the client to wear an external ankle brace during activity with no other restrictions. What factors need to be considered to design a safe and effective basketball-specific program for this athlete? Think about the following factors:

1. *Prior injuries and medical issues:* It is recommended to do a review of the patient's medical history to screen for any prior injuries or current medical issues that could impede the athlete's exercise program.
2. *Previous rehabilitation:* Consider what the athlete was doing in rehabilitation at discharge. As a general rule, it is good to continue where the athlete left off in rehabilitation to provide a smooth transition into sports-specific training.
3. *Athlete's goals:* This may be the most important aspect of designing an effective program. Understanding the athlete's goals based on his or her perceived strengths and weaknesses will help guide the overall program.
4. *Demands of the sport:* Consider the athlete's position and what type of metabolic and musculoskeletal demands can occur during play. Consider what physiological parameters should be stressed to progress the athlete's fitness level.
5. *Pretesting before exercise:* Based on all of the information gathered, it is important to conduct the appropriate baseline testing such as muscular strength, muscular endurance, flexibility, balance, and basketball-specific testing to get an accurate assessment of the client's current level of fitness. This will help guide the overall program design including exercise selection, sets, reps, rest periods, and any precautions during activity.

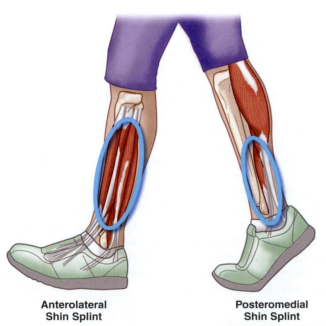

**Anterolateral Shin Splint**          **Posteromedial Shin Splint**

**Figure 30-21.** Common sites for shin splints to occur in an individual.

at the distal insertion of the soleus or flexor digitorum longus muscle. More recently, MTSS has been linked to other lower-extremity pathology including tendinopathy, anterior and posterior tibialis dysfunction, tightness in the gastrocnemius and soleus, and tibial stress fractures.[74]

Anterior shin splints are also common in the active population, and pain often occurs in the anterior compartment. The cause of anterior shin splints is not completely known, but it is often associated with exertional activity.[18] The anterior compartment muscles (e.g., tibialis anterior, extensor digitorum longus, and extensor hallucis longus), fascia, and periosteal attachments are most commonly affected. Anterior shin splints are also common in runners and the military.[18]

### Signs and Symptoms

Clients commonly complain of a "dull ache" along the distal two thirds of the posterior medial tibia for MTSS and the distal anterior shin for anterior shin splints.[18] The pain is elicited by initial activity but diminishes as activity continues. Hours after activity, the pain typically returns. If the condition progresses, the pain may become constant and restrict physical performance.

### Early Management

Management of both MTSS and **anterior shin splints** includes modifying training with lower-impact conditioning and cross-training (e.g., introducing aquatic exercise). However, the best intervention may just be to rest. Therapeutic modalities (e.g., ice or ultrasound), oral anti-inflammatory medication, cortisone injections, heel pads, and bracing may also be beneficial to relieve symptoms. The client may be referred to physical therapy to address these issues.

## Exercise Programming

The client may be restricted with activity or may be limited because of pain. The role of the health and fitness professional should be to slowly introduce the client back to full unrestricted activity without exacerbating the symptoms. Cross training to maintain adequate levels of fitness is indicated in the early stages. For both conditions, stretching and strengthening have been shown to be beneficial. Pain-free stretching of the calf muscles, especially the soleus, has been shown to be effective in relieving symptoms related to MTSS. Stretching the anterior compartment has been shown to help relieve symptoms in anterior shin splints.[4,18]

A general lower-body stretching program should accompany more specific stretching to address any secondary muscle length deficits that may affect the foot and ankle. Rest and modified activity are the primary interventions for symptom relief. However, there may be some residual strength deficits in the muscles that control the ankle. Targeting the muscles that control the ankle is the goal, especially the calf and anterior tibialis muscles.

## Achilles Tendinopathy

Injury to the Achilles tendon is common in athletes and in the active population. The prevalence of the condition is most common in runners, gymnasts, and dancers. Other common sports include track and field, volleyball, and soccer. Typically, older athletes are more affected by the condition than teens or children.[14] This condition can eventually lead to rupture if not addressed appropriately.

Various intrinsic and extrinsic factors are associated with this condition. Intrinsic factors include age, body weight, pes cavus, pes planus, leg-length discrepancies, and lateral ankle instability. Extrinsic factors include errors in training, prior injuries, poor footwear, muscle weakness, and poor flexibility.[11–14] The extrinsic factors are typically responsible for acute tendon trauma. Overuse and chronic injuries are often multifactorial and include a combination of intrinsic and extrinsic factors.[12]

### Signs and Symptoms

Individuals often complain about pain that is 2 to 6 cm above the tendon insertion into the calcaneus (Fig. 30-22). The typical pattern is initial morning pain that is "sharp" or "burning" and pain with more vigorous activity. Rest will often alleviate the pain, but as the condition becomes worse the pain becomes more constant and begins to interfere with the performance of ADLs.[14,18]

### Early Management

Early management includes controlling pain and inflammation by using therapeutic modalities (e.g., ice), rest, and oral anti-inflammatory medication.[14] Proper training techniques, losing weight, proper shoe wear,

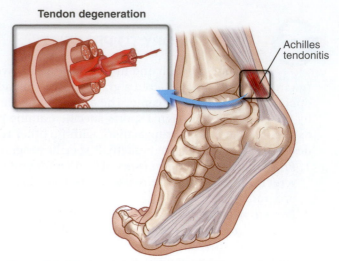

**Tendon degeneration**

Achilles tendonitis

**Figure 30-22.** Anatomical site of Achilles tendonitis or tendinopathy. The cutout image shows the microscopic view of the tendon and how it can degenerate and cause tearing or rupture of the structure.

orthotics, strengthening, and stretching can help alleviate pain and prevent progression of the condition.[12,14] Also, the client may be sent to physical therapy to address the factors mentioned earlier.

### Exercise Programming

The client may be cleared to exercise immediately to tolerance or may have some activity restrictions. A gradual, pain-free return to activity is indicated for this condition. Modifications in training techniques and environment should be addressed with emphasis on client education. The goal is to design a program that helps to meet their overall goals but does not exacerbate their condition.

Restoring proper length to the calf muscles can reduce strain to the muscle–tendon unit and decrease symptoms.[11] The client should be cautioned to stretch to tolerance and to avoid overexertion. Overstretching of the Achilles can cause irritation to the muscle–tendon unit and should be avoided.

Eccentric strengthening of the calf complex has been shown in the literature to be beneficial for relieving symptoms. Eccentric exercise may reduce pain and improve strength in Achilles tendonitis.[75] Progressively loading the Achilles with eccentric activity can benefit the client but may be even more beneficial when combined with other interventions.

## Plantar Fasciitis

**Plantar fasciitis** is an inflammatory condition of the plantar aponeurosis or fascia of the foot (Fig. 30-23). This condition has been reported to be the most common cause of heel pain and heel spur formation, and it accounts for 10% of running injuries.[76] Plantar fasciitis is more common in obese individuals and people who are on their feet for long periods.[77] Several intrinsic and extrinsic risk factors are associated with this

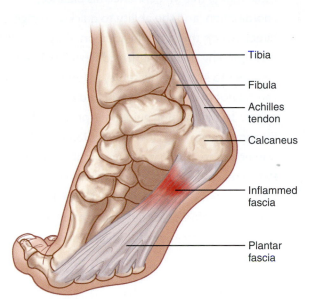

**Figure 30-23.** Plantar fasciitis. The pain associated with plantar fasciitis is located at the base of the calcaneus bone of the foot.

Tibia

Fibula

Achilles tendon

Calcaneus

Inflammed fascia

Plantar fascia

condition. Intrinsic factors include pes planus (excessive pronation or low arch height), pes cavus (high arch height), decreased strength, and poor flexibility of the muscles of the calf and hip. Extrinsic factors include overtraining, improper shoe wear, obesity, and unyielding surfaces.[76]

## Signs and Symptoms
Typically, individuals report pain on the plantar, medial heel at its calcaneal attachment that worsens after rest but improves after 10 to 15 minutes of activity.[76] In particular, clients will commonly report excessive pain during the first few steps in the morning.

## Early Management
Conservative treatment of this condition may include therapeutic modalities (e.g., ice), oral anti-inflammatory medication, heel pad or plantar arch, stretching, and strengthening exercises. The medical doctor may prescribe physical therapy, a night splint, or orthotics, or inject the area with cortisone.[76,77]

## Exercise Programming
The client may be cleared to exercise immediately to tolerance or may have some restrictions. The goal is to design a program that challenges the client but does not excessively load the foot. Integrating specific foot exercises into the general fitness program often provides the best results. This allows clients to work toward their fitness goals, as well as address their foot problems.

Stretching of the muscles in the lower chain (e.g., quadriceps, hamstrings, gastrocnemius, and soleus) and the plantar fascia is beneficial and has been shown to help relieve symptoms. Often, plantar fasciitis is the symptom of tight hip and knee flexors and extensors; thus, particular attention should be shown in these areas during the management process. Self-myofascial release techniques, including rolling the foot over a baseball, golf ball, or dumbbell, may help to break up myofascial adhesion in the plantar fascia.

Strengthening the foot intrinsic muscles may help to improve arch stability of the feet and help to unload the stresses imposed across the plantar fascia. Strengthening of the gastrocnemius, soleus, peroneals, tibialis anterior, and tibialis posterior may be needed to help improve strength at the ankle.

## RECORD-KEEPING

Keeping current and accurate records for every client is essential for the health and fitness professional. The important principle to remember is that if it is not written down, it does not exist. Important areas of documentation include the medical history, exercise record, incident report, and correspondence.

### Medical History

The health and fitness professional must maintain current records for each client's medical conditions. This includes present and past medical conditions and current medications. It is advisable for the professional to update each client's records every 3 months, including medical clearances.

### Exercise Record

The client's exercise record needs to stay current with specific notations for any changes such as a new onset of pain. This will provide the health and fitness professional with an accurate record of any program changes when the incident occurred.

### Incident Report

If an injury does occur during a workout session, it needs to be handled appropriately. First, the client's injury will need immediate medical attention. This may include minor first aid or activation of EMS. Client safety is the number one priority. Second, after the client is safe, a formal written account of the incident needs to be documented. Most organizations will have a specific incident report that is filled out after an accident has occurred. Third, the health and fitness professional needs to keep his or her own account of what occurred and keep any pertinent documentation. This will ensure accurate accounts of the incidents.

### Correspondence

Because of the 1996 Health Insurance Portability and Accountability Act (HIPAA), all clients' medical records are confidential. The health and fitness professional must obtain written permission before discussing this information with an outside party. If outside consultation is necessary, obtaining a written clearance by the client is advisable. The goal is to keep the client's information private. The health and fitness professional should document all conversations and sharing of information. This will ensure protection of the client's personal information.

## VIGNETTE conclusion

■ Rafael is worried that his elbow injury will keep him from playing tennis for an extended period. However, Marco assures him that this is not necessarily the case, as they can still work on overall fitness by improving his cardiovascular conditioning and adding sport-specific movements that will enhance his balance, coordination, and the ability to quickly change directions on the court. In addition, they can work on improving the strength and flexibility in Rafael's shoulder to improve his serve, as long as they are careful not to overwork the injured elbow and adhere to the training guidelines provided by Eleanor. By working closely with Rafael's athletic trainer and tennis coach, Marco is able to help Rafael reach his goals while still addressing his injury concerns. In the long run, they can work on improving Rafael's racquet-swing mechanics to avoid future flare-ups of this condition.

## CRITICAL THINKING QUESTIONS

1. Explain the difference between a strain and a sprain, and discuss early intervention strategies.

2. Explain the physiological actions that occur within each of the three phases of healing, and discuss safe CKC and OKC exercises that can be done within each phase. Pick two of the nonsurgical pathologies discussed as examples.

3. Develop a safe exercise program for one of the upper-extremity pathologies discussed in this chapter. Be sure to list specific exercises, sets, repetitions, frequency, and any precautions.

4. Develop a safe exercise program for one of the lower-extremity pathologies discussed in this chapter. Be sure to list specific exercises, sets, repetitions, frequency, and any precautions.

5. A 28-year-old female soccer player who underwent a knee ACL reconstruction (i.e., patellar tendon) 4 months ago is coming to you for a sports-specific exercise program. Before administering the program, you need to take a health history. List specific questions that should be asked to determine any health risks or medical issues that could affect the exercise program.

## ADDITIONAL RESOURCES

### Websites
Web MD, Consumer Resources from the Medical Field: http://www.webmd.com
Gatorade Sports Science Institute: http://www.gssiweb.org
E-Medicine Health: http://www.emedicinehealth.com
The Mayo Clinic: http://www.mayoclinic.com/health/DiseasesIndex/DiseasesIndex
LiveStrong.com: http://www.livestrong.com

### Textbooks
Anderson MK, Hall SJ, Martin M. *Foundations of Athletic Training: Prevention, Assessment, and Management*. 5th ed. Baltimore, MD: Lippincott Williams & Wilkins; 2012.
Brotzman B, Wilk K. *Clinical Orthopedic Rehabilitation*. 2nd ed. St. Louis, MO: Mosby; 2003.
Kisner C, Colby L. *Therapeutic Exercise: Foundations and Techniques*. 5th ed. Philadelphia, PA: F.A. Davis Company; 2002.

## REFERENCES

1. Centers for Disease Control and Prevention. Heads Up: Concussion in Youth Sports. Available at: http://www.cdc.gov/concussion/pdf/heads_up_activity_report_final-a.pdf. Accessed August 5, 2012.

2. Centers for Disease Control and Prevention. Nonfatal sports- and recreation-related injuries treated in emergency departments—United States, July 2000-June 2001. *MMWR Morb Mrtl Wkly Rep*. 2002;51:736–740.

3. Cosca DD, Navazio F. Common problems in endurance athletes. *Am Fam Physician*. 2007;76:237–244.

4. Anderson MK, Hall SJ, Martin M. *Foundations of Athletic Training: Prevention, Assessment, and Management*. Philadelphia, PA: Lippincott Williams & Wilkins; 2004.

5. Orchard JW. Intrinsic and extrinsic risk factors for muscle strains in Australian football. *Am J Sports Med*. 2001;29:300–303.

6. Maffey L, Emery C. What are the risk factors for groin strain injury in sport? A systematic review of the literature. *Sports Med*. 2007;37:881–894.

7. Manske RC. *Postsurgical Orthopedic Sports Rehabilitation: Knee & Shoulder*. St. Louis, MO: Mosby; 2006.

8. Goldstein J, Zuckerman JD. Selected orthopedic problems in the elderly. *Rheum Dis Clin North Am*. 2000;26:593–616.

9. Logerstedt DS, Snyder-Mackler L, Ritter RC, Axe MJ. Knee pain and mobility impairments: meniscal and articular cartilage lesions. *J Orthop Sports Phys Ther*. 2010;40:A1–A35.

10. Abate M, Silbernagel KG, Siljeholm C, et al. Pathogenesis of tendinopathies: Inflammation or degeneration? *Arthritis Res Ther.* 2009;11:235.

11. Kader D, Saxena A, Movin T, Maffulli N. Achilles tendinopathy: Some aspects of basic science and clinical management. *Br J Sports Med.* 2002;36:239–249.

12. Paavola M, Kannus P, Jarvinen TA, Khan K, Jozsa L, Jarvinen M. Achilles tendinopathy. *J Bone Joint Surg* 2002;84-a:2062–2076.

13. Maffulli N, Khan KM, Puddu G. Overuse tendon conditions: Time to change a confusing terminology. *Arthroscopy.* 1998;14:840–843.

14. Mazzone MF, McCue T. Common conditions of the Achilles tendon. *Am Fam Physician.* 2002;65:1805–1810.

15. Paavola M, Kannus P, Järvinen TAH, Khan K, Józsa L, Järvinen M. Achilles Tendinopathy. *J Bone Joint Surg.* 2002;84:2062-2076.

16. Cooper DM. Wound healing: New understandings. *Nurse Pract Forum.* 1999;10:74–86.

17. Hunt TK, Hopf H, Hussain Z. Physiology of wound healing. *Adv Skin Wound Care.* 2000;13(2 Suppl.):6–11.

18. Brotzman SB, Wilk KE. *Clinical Orthopaedic Rehabilitation.* St. Louis, MO: Mosby, Incorporated; 2003.

19. Kisner C, Colby LA. *Therapeutic Exercise: Foundations and Techniques.* Philadelphia, PA: F.A. Davis Company; 2007.

20. Fongemie AE, Buss DD, Rolnick SJ. Management of shoulder impingement syndrome and rotator cuff tears. *Am Fam Physician.* 1998;57:667–674, 680–682.

21. Ainsworth R, Lewis JS. Exercise therapy for the conservative management of full thickness tears of the rotator cuff: A systematic review. *Br J Sports Med.* 2007;41:200–210.

22. Burbank KM, Stevenson JH, Czarnecki GR, Dorfman J. Chronic shoulder pain: Part I. Evaluation and diagnosis. *Am Fam Physician.* 2008;77:453–460.

23. Burbank KM, Stevenson JH, Czarnecki GR, Dorfman J. Chronic shoulder pain: Part II. Treatment. *Am Fam Physician.* 2008;77:493–497.

24. Johnson GW, Cadwallader K, Scheffel SB, Epperly TD. Treatment of lateral epicondylitis. *Am Fam Physician.* 2007;76:843–848.

25. Whaley AL, Baker CL. Lateral epicondylitis. *Clin Sports Med.* 2004;23:677–691, x.

26. Hospital for Special Surgery, Department of Rehabilitation; Cioppa-Mosca JM, Cahill JB, Tucker CY. *Postsurgical Rehabilitation Guidelines for the Orthopedic Clinician.* St. Louis, MO: Mosby Elsevier; 2006.

27. Dougherty C, Dougherty JJ. Managing and preventing hip pathology in trochanteric pain syndrome. *J Musculoskel Med.* 2008;25:521–525.

28. Lievense A, Bierma-Zeinstra S, Schouten B, Bohnen A, Verhaar J, Koes B. Prognosis of trochanteric pain in primary care. *Br J Gen Pract.* 2005;55:199–204.

29. Segal NA, Felson DT, Torner JC, et al. Greater trochanteric pain syndrome: Epidemiology and associated factors. *Arch Phys Med Rehabil.* 2007;88:988–992.

30. Little H. Trochanteric bursitis: A common cause of pelvic girdle pain. *Can Med Assoc J.* 1979;120:456–458.

31. Martinez JM, Honsik K, Lorenzo CT. Physical medicine and rehabilitation for iliotibial band syndrome. 2006. http://emedicine.medscape.com/article/307850-overview. Accessed September 9, 2014.

32. Dixit S, DiFiori JP, Burton M, Mines B. Management of patellofemoral pain syndrome. *Am Fam Physician.* 2007;75:194–202.

33. Piva SR, Fitzgerald K, Irrgang JJ, et al. Reliability of measures of impairments associated with patellofemoral pain syndrome. *BMC Musculoskelet Disord.* 2006;7:33.

34. Barton CJ, Levinger P, Webster KE, Menz HB. Walking kinematics in individuals with patellofemoral pain syndrome: A case-control study. *Gait Posture.* 2011;33:286–291.

35. Gross MT, Foxworth JL. The role of foot orthoses as an intervention for patellofemoral pain. *J Orthop Sports Phys Ther.* 2003;33:661–670.

36. Waryasz GR, McDermott AY. Patellofemoral pain syndrome (PFPS): A systematic review of anatomy and potential risk factors. *Dyn Med.* 2008;7:9.

37. Juhn MS. Patellofemoral pain syndrome: A review and guidelines for treatment. *Am Fam Phys.* 1999;60:2012–2022.

38. Fredericson M, Cookingham CL, Chaudhari AM, Dowdell BC, Oestreicher N, Sahrmann SA. Hip abductor weakness in distance runners with iliotibial band syndrome. *Clin J Sports Med.* 2000;10:169–175.

39. Fredericson M, Yoon K. Physical examination and patellofemoral pain syndrome. *Am J Phys Med Rehabil.* 2006;85:234–243.

40. Ireland ML, Willson JD, Ballantyne BT, Davis IM. Hip strength in females with and without patellofemoral pain. *J Orthop Sports Phys Ther.* 2003;33:671–676.

41. Powers CM. The influence of altered lower-extremity kinematics on patellofemoral joint dysfunction: A theoretical perspective. *J Orthop Sports Phys Ther.* 2003;33:639–646.

42. Robinson RL, Nee RJ. Analysis of hip strength in females seeking physical therapy treatment for unilateral patellofemoral pain syndrome. *J Orthop Sports Phys Ther.* 2007;37:232–238.

43. Ferretti A, Ippolito E, Mariani P, Puddu G. Jumper's knee. *Am J Sports Med.* 1983;11:58–62.

44. Almekinders LC, Vellema JH, Weinhold PS. Strain patterns in the patellar tendon and the implications for patellar tendinopathy. *Knee Surg Sports Traumatol Arthrosc.* 2002;10:2–5.

45. Blazina ME, Kerlan RK, Jobe FW, Carter VS, Carlson GJ. Jumper's knee. *Orthop Clin North Am.* 1973;4:665–678.

46. De Smet AA, Tuite MJ. Use of the "two-slice-touch" rule for the MRI diagnosis of meniscal tears. *AJR* 2006;187:911–914.

47. Maxey L, Magnusson J. *Rehabilitation for the Postsurgical Orthopedic Patient.* St. Louis, MO: Mosby; 2001.

48. Griffin LY, Agel J, Albohm MJ, et al. Noncontact anterior cruciate ligament injuries: Risk factors and prevention strategies. *J Am Acad Orthop Surg.* 2000;8:141–150.

49. Agel J, Arendt EA, Bershadsky B. Anterior cruciate ligament injury in national collegiate athletic association basketball and soccer: A 13-year review. *Am J Sports Med.* 2005;33:524–530.

50. Arendt EA, Agel J, Dick R. Anterior cruciate ligament injury patterns among collegiate men and women. *J Athl Train.* 1999;34:86–92.

51. Wojtys EM. The ACL dilemma. *Sports Health.* 2012;4:12–13.

52. Alentorn-Geli E, Myer GD, Silvers HJ, et al. Prevention of non-contact anterior cruciate ligament injuries in soccer players. Part 1: Mechanisms of injury and underlying risk factors. *Knee Surg Sports Traumatol Arthrosc* 2009;17:705–729.

53. Smith HC, Vacek P, Johnson RJ, et al. Risk factors for anterior cruciate ligament injury: A review of the literature—part 1: Neuromuscular and anatomic risk. *Sports Health.* 2012;4:69–78.

54. Smith HC, Vacek P, Johnson RJ, et al. Risk factors for anterior cruciate ligament injury: A review of the literature—part 2: hormonal, genetic, cognitive function, previous injury, and extrinsic risk factors. *Sports Health.* 2012;4:155–161.

55. Aglietti P, Buzzi R, D'Andria S, Zaccherotti G. Long-term study of anterior cruciate ligament reconstruction for chronic instability using the central one-third patellar

tendon and a lateral extraarticular tenodesis. *Am J Sports Med.* 1992;20:38–45.

56. Eriksson K, Anderberg P, Hamberg P, et al. A comparison of quadruple semitendinosus and patellar tendon grafts in reconstruction of the anterior cruciate ligament. *J Bone Joint Surg Br.* 2001;83:348–354.

57. Marder RA, Raskind JR, Carroll M. Prospective evaluation of arthroscopically assisted anterior cruciate ligament reconstruction. Patellar tendon versus semitendinosus and gracilis tendons. *Am J Sports Med.* 1991;19:478–484.

58. Spindler KP, Kuhn JE, Freedman KB, Matthews CE, Dittus RS, Harrell FE, Jr. Anterior cruciate ligament reconstruction autograft choice: bone-tendon-bone versus hamstring: Does it really matter? A systematic review. *Am J Sports Med.* 2004;32:1986–1995.

59. Grimm NL, Shea KG, Leaver RW, Aoki SK, Carey JL. Efficacy and degree of bias in knee injury prevention studies: A systematic review of RCTs. *Clin Orthop Relat Res.* 2013;471:308–316.

60. Tyler TF, McHugh MP, Gleim GW, Nicholas SJ. The effect of immediate weightbearing after anterior cruciate ligament reconstruction. *Clin Orthop Relat Res.* 1998: 141–148.

61. Freedman KB, D'Amato MJ, Nedeff DD, Kaz A, Bach BR Jr. Arthroscopic anterior cruciate ligament reconstruction: A metaanalysis comparing patellar tendon and hamstring tendon autografts. *Am J Sports Med.* 2003; 31:2–11.

62. Sachs RA, Daniel DM, Stone ML, Garfein RF. Patellofemoral problems after anterior cruciate ligament reconstruction. *Am J Sports Med.* 1989;17:760–765.

63. Noyes FR, Barber-Westin SD. Reconstruction of the anterior cruciate ligament with human allograft. Comparison of early and later results. *J Bone Joint Surg Am.* 1996;78:524–537.

64. Nikolaou PK, Seaber AV, Glisson RR, Ribbeck BM, Bassett FH 3rd. Anterior cruciate ligament allograft transplantation. Long-term function, histology, revascularization, and operative technique. *Am J Sports Med.* 1986;14:348–360.

65. Noyes FR, Barber Westin SD. Anterior cruciate ligament injury prevention training in female athletes: A systematic review of injury reduction and results of athletic performance tests. *Sports Health.* 2012;4:36–46.

66. Voskanian N. ACL Injury prevention in female athletes: Review of the literature and practical considerations in implementing an ACL prevention program. *Curr Rev Musculoskeletal Med.* 2013;6:158–163.

67. Joy EA, Taylor JR, Novak MA, Chen M, Fink BP, Porucznik CA. Factors influencing the implementation of anterior cruciate ligament injury prevention strategies by girls soccer coaches. *J Strength Cond Res.* 2013;27: 2263–2269.

68. Perlman M, Leveille D, DeLeonibus J, et al. Inversion lateral ankle trauma: Differential diagnosis, review of the literature, and prospective study. *J Foot Surg.* 1987; 26:95–135.

69. Ivins D. Acute ankle sprain: An update. *Am Fam Physician.* 2006;74:1714–1720.

70. Balduini FC, Tetzlaff J. Historical perspectives on injuries of the ligaments of the ankle. *Clin Sports Med.* 1982;1:3–12.

71. Garrick JG. Epidemiologic perspective. *Clin Sports Med.* 1982;1:13–18.

72. Bates P. Shin splints—a literature review. *Br J Sports Med.* 1985;19:132–137.

73. Moen MH, Tol JL, Weir A, Steunebrink M, De Winter TC. Medial tibial stress syndrome: A critical review. *Sports Med.* 2009;39:523–546.

74. Galbraith RM, Lavallee ME. Medial tibial stress syndrome: Conservative treatment options. *Curr Rev Musculoskelet Med.* 2009;2:127–133.

75. Wasielewski NJ, Kotsko KM. Does eccentric exercise reduce pain and improve strength in physically active adults with symptomatic lower extremity tendinosis? A systematic review. *J Athl Train.* 2007;42:409–421.

76. Buchbinder R. Clinical practice. Plantar fasciitis. *N Engl J Med.* 2004;350:2159–2166.

77. Cole C, Seto C, Gazewood J. Plantar fasciitis: Evidence-based review of diagnosis and therapy. *Am Fam Physician.* 2005;72:2237–2242.

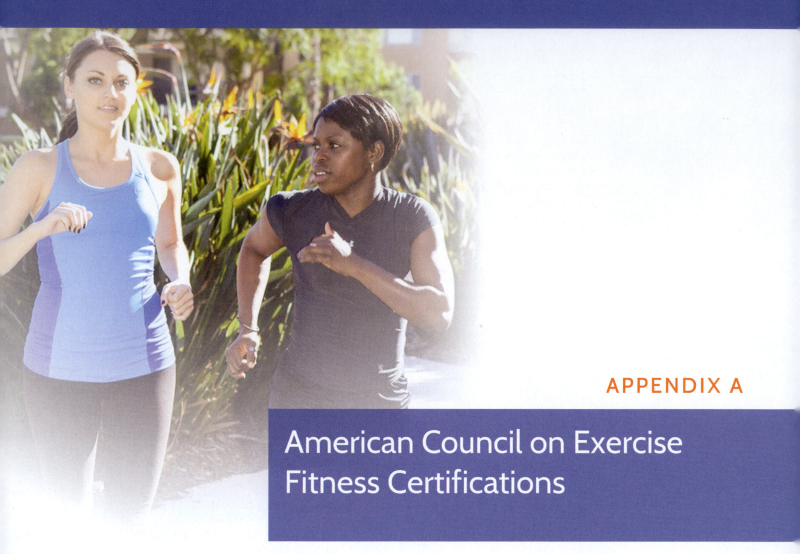

# American Council on Exercise Fitness Certifications

The American Council on Exercise (ACE) offers four primary certifications, and there are currently more than 55,000 ACE-certified professionals in the United States and around the world. After earning a certification, you can choose to focus your studies with a specialty certification in topics ranging from youth fitness and mind–body exercise to fitness nutrition and senior fitness. To learn more about ACE and its many educational offerings, visit the ACE website: http://ACEfitness.org/fitness-certifications.

## PERSONAL TRAINER

The ACE Personal Trainer Certification is designed for fitness professionals who provide one-on-one or small-group fitness instruction to people who are apparently healthy or have medical clearance to exercise.

## GROUP FITNESS INSTRUCTOR

The ACE Group Fitness Instructor Certification is designed for fitness professionals who teach any form of exercise to apparently healthy individuals in a group setting.

## HEALTH COACH

The ACE Health Coach Certification prepares professionals from fitness, health care, workplace wellness, and a variety of other fields to lead clients to long-term, healthy lifestyle change using in-depth behavior-change strategies and a knowledge of fitness and nutrition. The certification equips professionals with insight on behavioral psychology, the physiology of obesity, techniques for lifestyle coaching, development of weight-management programs, and the relationship between exercise and nutrition for weight control.

## ADVANCED HEALTH & FITNESS SPECIALIST

The ACE Advanced Health & Fitness Specialist Certification provides in-depth knowledge for health and fitness professionals working with individuals at risk for or recovering from a variety of cardiovascular, pulmonary, metabolic, and musculoskeletal diseases and disorders, as well as special population groups including older adults, youth, and prenatal and postnatal women.

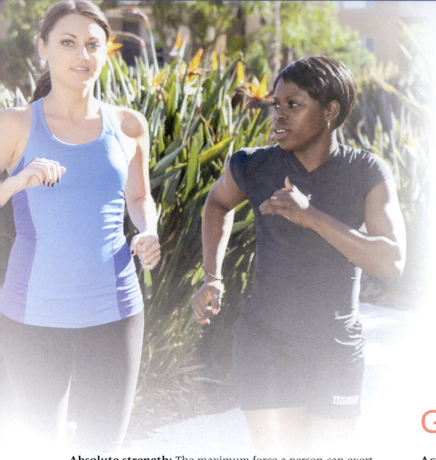

# Glossary

**Absolute strength:** The maximum force a person can exert with his or her whole body, or part of the body, irrespective of body size or muscle size.

**Acceleration:** The rate of change in velocity.

**Accessory muscles of ventilation:** The muscles other than the diaphragm and intercostal muscles that may be used for labored breathing.

**Acetylcholine:** A neurotransmitter and derivative of choline that is released at the ends of nerve fibers in the somatic and parasympathetic nervous systems, and is involved in the transmission of nerve impulses in the body.

**Acetyl-Coenzyme A:** A molecule produced from either carbohydrate or free fatty acid catabolism that enters into the Krebs cycle.

**Actin:** Contractile protein that makes up the thin filament in the sarcomere of a myofibril.

**Action potential:** The transmission of a nerve impulse along the length of the membrane of a muscle cell or nerve cell due to changes in electrical potential.

**Active aging:** A concept advanced by the International Council on Active Aging and adopted by the World Health Organization that encourages individuals to be "engaged in life" as fully as possible despite health status, disease conditions, or socioeconomic status. It recognizes the importance of each of the seven dimensions of wellness—physical, intellectual, emotional, spiritual, environmental, vocational, and social—to the overall well-being of an aging individual.

**Active isolated stretching (AIS):** A technique that blends portions of active and passive stretching that was originally used during rehabilitation for surgery patients.

**Active stretching:** The process of enhancing the stretch of a muscle by actively contracting its antagonist.

**Active system:** Consists of the muscular system, and through its action it provides the necessary stiffness to a joint to aid in maintaining its stability.

**Activities of daily living (ADL):** Activities normally performed for self-care and include personal hygiene (e.g., bathing), performing household chores, walking, shopping, and other similar activities.

**Acute altitude sickness:** Illness that results from changes in the body's responses to lowered levels of oxygen and air pressure changes.

**Acute myocardial infarction:** Sudden heart attack.

**Adaptability:** The ability of an organism to adjust and enhance its ability to tolerate stressors like environmental changes to the demands of exercise.

**Adenosine diphosphate (ADP):** A molecule that combines with inorganic phosphate to resynthesize adenosine triphosphate (ATP).

**Adenosine triphosphate (ATP):** Refers to a high-energy phosphate molecule. The breakdown (or hydrolysis) of ATP results in the release of free energy that can be harnessed to support muscle action. The design of cellular metabolism is to maintain ATP and three energy systems exist to regenerate ATP at different maximal rates for differing durations.

**Adherence:** The extent to which people follow their plans or treatment recommendations, for example, exercise adherence is the extent to which people follow an exercise program.

**Adipogenesis:** The process of cell differentiation by which preadipocytes become adipocytes.

**Adipose tissue:** Fatty tissue; connective tissue made up of fat cells.

**Adrenal glands:** Triangle-shaped endocrine glands that sit atop each kidney; produce and secrete various hormones like epinephrine from the adrenal medulla, and glucocorticoids and aldosterone from the adrenal cortex.

**Adrenocorticotropin hormone (ACTH):** Hormone produced by the anterior pituitary lobe that stimulates the adrenal cortex to release cortisol.

**Aerobic:** With, or in the presence of, oxygen.

**Aerobic exercise:** Exercise that increases the need for oxygen to fuel the effort.

**Aerobic fitness:** The capacity of the cardiopulmonary systems to increase the amount of oxygen delivered to the muscles, enabling them work longer or harder.

**Afferent:** Conducting or conducted inward or toward something, such as a nerve carrying an impulse toward the central nervous system.

**Afferent (Ia) pathways:** In the nervous system, the pathways of afferent neurons that carry nerve impulses from receptors or sense organs toward the central nervous system.

**Afterload:** The pressure within the aorta and pulmonary trunk that the left and right ventricles of the heart, respectively, must overcome in order to eject blood out of the heart.

**Agility:** The ability to rapidly and accurately change the position of the body in space.

**Aging trajectory:** The conceptualization of an individual's (self) or population group's course of aging, including psychological and physiological variables.

**Agonist:** The muscle directly responsible for observed movement; also called the *prime mover.*

**Air Quality Index:** A number used by government agencies to communicate to the public the amount of pollutants currently held by the air or how polluted it is forecast to become.

**Albumin:** A water-soluble protein molecule that is coagulable by heat, such as that found in egg white, milk, and (in particular) found in blood serum where it is used to transport various fats.

**Aldosterone:** A hormone released from the adrenal cortex gland in response to reduced blood sodium concentrations, and decreased blood volume and blood pressure.

**All-or-none law of action potential:** A principle that states that the strength of a response of a nerve cell or muscle fiber is not dependent on the strength of the stimulus. Essentially, there will either be a full response or there will be no response at all.

**All-or-none principle:** The principle of muscle contraction that states that when a motor unit is activated, all of the muscle fibers will maximally contract.

**Alpha cells ($\alpha$ cells):** Endocrine cells in the islets of Langerhans of the pancreas that produce and secrete glucagon.

**Alveolar ducts:** Tiny ducts that connect the respiratory bronchioles to alveolar sacs, each of which contains a bunch of alveoli.

**Alveolar interdependence:** The process that occurs when an alveolus collapses and the surrounding alveoli recoil to pull open the collapsed alveolus.

**Alveolar sacs:** Terminal endpoints of the alveolar ducts, which give rise to alveoli in the lung.

**Alveolar ventilation ($\dot{V}_A$):** The volume of gas per unit time that reaches the alveoli, the respiratory portions of the lungs where gas exchange occurs.

**Alveoli:** Spherical extensions of the respiratory bronchioles and the primary sites of gas exchange with the blood.

**Amenorrhea:** The absence of menstruation.

**Amino acids:** Nitrogen-containing compounds that represent the building blocks of protein.

**Amortization phase:** The transition period between the eccentric and concentric actions during any muscle action, especially modalities like plyometrics that plays a crucial role within the stretch-shortening cycle that contributes to power development.

**Amylopectin:** A soluble polysaccharide and highly branched polymer of glucose found in plants that can be digested fairly rapidly.

**Amylose:** The crystallizable form of starch, consisting of long unbranched polysaccharide chains that is digested more slowly.

**Anabolic:** The synthesis of compounds into more complex materials like building muscle.

**Anabolic steroid:** Synthetic derivatives of the male sex hormone testosterone; used for their muscle-building characteristics.

**Anaerobic fitness:** The ability to use the energy systems not dependent on oxygen and are used to fuel any immediate change in activity or intensity, or to sustain short bouts of higher-intensity activity.

**Anatomical dead space:** The volume of air that is inhaled that does not take part in the gas exchange because it remains in the conducting airways of the pulmonary system.

**Android:** Adipose tissue or body fat distributed in the abdominal area (creating the characteristic apple-shaped individual).

**Angina pectoris:** Chest, neck, jaw discomfort/pain, pressure, or tightness/indigestion-like discomfort or pain that can be experienced in many regions of the upper extremity, but typically radiates down the left arm.

**Anorexia nervosa:** A potentially harmful eating disorder characterized by refusal to maintain body weight of at least 85% of expected weight; coupled by an intense fear of gaining weight or becoming fat; and body image disturbances that include a disproportionate influence of body weight on self-evaluation. In women this is typified by the absence of normal menses for at least three consecutive cycles.

**Antagonist:** The muscle that acts in opposition to the contraction produced by an agonist or prime mover muscle.

**Anterior cruciate ligament (ACL):** A primary stabilizing ligament of the knee that travels diagonally from the notch of the distal femur and the medial border of the lateral femoral condyle of the femur to its point of insertion in front of the intercondyloid eminence or medial tibial spine of the tibia.

**Anterior shin splints:** Pain in the anterior compartment muscles of the lower leg, fascia, and periosteal lining. Often induced by exertional or modality changes in activity.

**Anthropometric:** Relating to the measurement and study of the human body and its parts and capacities.

**Anthropometry:** The measurement and study of the human body and its parts and capacities.

**Antidiuretic:** A substance that inhibits urine production, thereby aiding in the retention of plasma volume.

**Antidiuretic hormone (ADH):** Hormone released by the posterior pituitary as a result of increased osmolality of the plasma; reduces urinary excretion of water to reduce the potential for dehydration.

**Antioxidants:** Substances that prevent or repair oxidative damage; includes vitamins C and E, some carotenoids, selenium, ubiquinones, and bioflavonoids.

**Aortic bodies:** Several small clusters of chemoreceptors, baroreceptors, and supporting cells located along the aortic arch.

**Aortic pressure:** The blood pressure in the root of the aorta.

**Aortic valve:** The valve that regulates blood flow between the left ventricle and the peripheral circulation.

**Arginine vasopressin:** Also known as vasopressin, argipressin, or antidiuretic hormone; a hormone found in most mammals that functions to retain water in the body and to constrict blood vessels to preserve blood pressure.

**Arterial oxygen saturation ($SaO_2$):** The percentage of oxygen-binding sites on hemoglobin in the blood that are combined with oxygen.

**Arterioles:** Small-diameter blood vessels that extend and branch out from an artery and lead to capillaries; the primary site of vascular resistance.

**Arteriosclerosis:** A chronic disease in which thickening, hardening, and loss of elasticity of the arterial walls result in impaired blood circulation; develops with aging, and in hypertension, diabetes, hyperlipidemia, and other conditions.

**Arteriovenous oxygen difference (a-vO$_2$ diff):** The difference in the oxygen content of the blood between the arterial blood and the venous blood. It is an indication of how much oxygen is removed from the blood in capillaries as the blood circulates throughout the body.

**Arthritis:** Inflammation of a joint; a state characterized by joint degeneration and inflammation.

**Asthma:** A complex chronic inflammatory response of the airways that is characterized by periodic episodes of reversible airway constriction (obstruction), increased bronchial reactivity, and airway inflammation.

**Atherosclerosis:** A specific form of arteriosclerosis characterized by the accumulation of fatty material on the inner walls of the arteries, causing them to harden, thicken, and lose elasticity.

**Athletic heart syndrome:** A nonpathological condition commonly seen in endurance athletes, in which the heart is enlarged, and the resting heart rate is lower than normal.

**Atmospheres:** On Earth, units of air pressure based on the internationally recognized standard atmosphere (atm), which is defined as 101,325 Pa (or 1,013,250 dynes/cm$^2$). One (atm) equals 14.696 lb per square inch (psi). One atm is equivalent to the pressure of air exerted upon the earth's surface at sea level.

**Atrioventricular node (AV node):** The specialized mass of conducting cells in the heart located at the atrioventricular junction.

**Atrioventricular valves:** Either of two heart valves through which blood flows from the atria to the ventricles; prevents the return of blood into the atria when the ventricles contract.

**Atrophy:** A reduction in muscle size (muscle wasting) because of inactivity, aging or immobilization.

**Autogenic inhibition:** An automatic reflex reduction in muscle action and force production, and in muscle spindle activity caused by stimulation of the Golgi Tendon Organ (GTO).

**Automaticity:** The capacity of a cell to initiate an impulse without an external stimulus.

**Axons:** Long slender projection of an individual nerve fiber that conducts nerve impulses away from the neuron's cell body.

**Balance:** The ability to maintain center of gravity (COG) or center of mass (COM) over a static or dynamically changing base of support (BOS).

**Ballistic flexibility:** Refers to the amount of unrestricted movement present during bobbing, bouncing, or jerking motions (e.g., ballistic stretching).

**Ballistic stretching:** Dynamic stretching characterized by rhythmic bobbing or bouncing motions representing relatively high-force, short-duration movements.

**Bariatrics:** The branch of medicine that deals with the causes, prevention, and treatment of obesity.

**Baroreflex:** The reflex mechanism by which baroreceptors regulate blood pressure that produces vasodilation and a decrease in heart rate when blood pressure increases, and vasoconstriction and an increase in heart rate when blood pressure decreases.

**Barotraumas:** Pressure-related injuries.

**Basal metabolic rate (BMR):** The energy required to complete the sum total of life-sustaining processes, and is very similar to resting metabolic rate, which represents the total rate of energy expenditure or calories expended at true rest (fasted state).

**Base of support (BOS):** The space under and between one's feet.

**Bends:** *See* Decompression sickness.

**Benign:** A noncancerous growth or tumor; mild disease or condition that is not life threatening.

**Beta cells (β cells):** Endocrine cells in the islets of Langerhans of the pancreas responsible for synthesizing and secreting the hormone insulin, which decreases the glucose levels in the blood.

**Beta-oxidation:** A series of reactions in the mitochondria whereby free fatty acid molecules are oxidized to acetyl-coenzyme A.

**Bicarbonate:** A salt of carbonic acid that contains the anion HCO$_3$ in which a single hydrogen atom has been replaced.

**Bioavailability:** The degree to which a nutrient can be digested, absorbed, and used by the body.

**Bioelectrical impedance analysis (BIA):** Measures the impedance or resistance to an electrical current as it travels through the body's water pool.

**Bioenergetics:** A component of the larger field of the study of the science of energy transfer called *thermodynamics*. The study of energy transfer in chemical reactions within living tissue.

**Biological value (BV):** An estimate of protein quality determined by dividing the nitrogen used for tissue formation by the nitrogen absorbed from food and then multiplying by 100.

**Blocked practice sessions:** Primarily focus on closed or pre-determined skills performed repeatedly to improve movement mechanics and efficiency.

**Blood pressure (BP):** The pressure exerted by the blood on the walls of the arteries; measured in millimeters of mercury (mm Hg) with a sphygmomanometer (blood pressure cuff).

**Body composition:** The proportion of fat and fat-free mass in the body, given the knowledge that a lower proportion of body fat generally leads to a healthier body.

**Body mass index (BMI):** A relative measure of body height to body weight used to determine levels of health, from underweight to extreme obesity.

**Bohr effect:** A decrease in the amount of oxygen associated or bound with hemoglobin and other respiratory compounds in response to a lowered blood pH that results from an increased concentration of carbon dioxide in the blood.

**Bone mineral density (BMD):** A measure of the amount of minerals (mainly calcium) contained in a certain volume of bone.

**Boyle's law:** States that, at a given temperature, the volume of a gas is inversely related to pressure exerted by or upon the gas.

**Bradycardia:** A low resting heart rate; typically less than 60 beats per minute.

**Breath-hold diving:** Diving from the surface while holding one's breath.

**Bronchial tree:** The branching system of bronchi and bronchioles conducting air from the windpipe into the lungs.

**Bronchioles:** The smallest tubes that supply air to the alveoli (air sacs) of the lungs.

**Bronchoconstriction:** The constriction of the airways in the lungs caused by the tightening of surrounding smooth muscle, with consequent coughing, wheezing, and shortness of breath.

**Bronchodilation:** Expansion of the bronchial air passages.

**Bulimia nervosa:** An eating disorder characterized by recurrent episodes of uncontrolled binge eating; recurrent inappropriate compensatory behavior such as self-induced vomiting, laxative misuse, diuretics, or enemas (purging type), or fasting and/or excessive exercise (nonpurging type); episodes of binge eating and compensatory behaviors occur at least twice per week for 3 months; self-evaluation is heavily influenced by body shape and weight; and the episodes do not occur exclusively with episodes of anorexia.

**Buoyancy compensator:** An inflatable vest used to control a person's buoyancy underwater or to rest at the surface.

**Bursa sac:** Small, synovial fluid-filled sac located between structures or tissues.

**Bursitis:** Inflammation of the bursa sac caused by acute trauma, repetitive overuse, muscle imbalance, or muscle tightness.

**Calcitonin:** Hormone secreted by the thyroid gland that has the effect of lowering blood calcium by enhancing greater uptake into the bones or removal via the kidneys.

**Calorie:** *See* Kilocalorie.

**Calorimetry:** Measurement of the amount of heat liberated or absorbed through a chemical reaction, formation of a solution or through a change of physical state. As all energy ultimately degrades to heat, this process is utilized to measure the caloric content of foods.

**Cancer:** The common term for a group of more than 100 diseases characterized by uncontrolled growth of abnormal cells that are capable of invading other tissues through the blood and lymph systems.

**Capillaries:** The smallest blood vessels that supply blood to the tissues, and the site of all gas and nutrient exchange in the cardiovascular system. They connect the arterial and venous systems.

**Carbaminohemoglobin:** A compound of hemoglobin and carbon dioxide which represents one of the methods by which carbon dioxide is transported in the blood.

**Carbohydrate loading:** A method of attempting to increase muscle glycogen stores by consuming a high-carbohydrate diet in the days preceding an endurance event. Strategy consists of two stages: a glycogen depletion stage involving bouts of higher-intensity exercise coupled with low-to-moderate carbohydrate intakes (<55% of total kilocalories) to deplete glycogen, followed by a glycogen loading stage where exercise is tapered (low intensity to no exercise), coupled with a high carbohydrate intake (>70% of total kilocalories).

**Carbohydrates:** A hydrocarbon containing carbon, hydrogen and oxygen which is the body's preferred source of energy and a metabolic primer that enables complete metabolism of fats. Dietary sources include sugars (simple) and grains, rice, potatoes, and beans (complex). Carbohydrates are as glucose in blood and as glycogen in muscles and liver.

**Cardiac acceleration center:** *See* Cardiovascular control center.

**Cardiac cycle:** The period from the beginning of one heartbeat to the beginning of the next heartbeat.

**Cardiac dysrhythmias:** Heart rhythm disturbances that may be benign or represent a high risk for sudden death.

**Cardiac hypertrophy:** The thickening of the walls in the heart. Although left ventricular hypertrophy is more common, enlargement can also occur in the right ventricle, both ventricles, or atria.

**Cardiac inhibitory center:** A vasomotor center in the medulla oblongata that exerts an inhibitory influence on the heart.

**Cardiac muscle:** A type of involuntary, striated muscle tissue that makes up the walls of the heart and provides the continuous rhythmic action known as heart contractions.

**Cardiac output ($\dot{Q}$):** The amount of blood pumped by the heart per minute; usually expressed in liters of blood per minute.

**Cardiac rehabilitation:** A branch of rehabilitation medicine dealing with optimizing physical function in patients with cardiac disease or recent cardiac surgeries.

**Cardiometabolic disease:** A condition that puts an individual at increased risk for heart disease and diabetes, and includes the following factors: elevated blood pressure, triglycerides, fasting plasma glucose, and C-reactive protein, and decreased levels of high-density lipoprotein.

**Cardiopulmonary exercise testing (CPET):** A noninvasive test that provides assessment of the integrative exercise responses involving the pulmonary, cardiovascular, hematopoietic, neuropsychological, and skeletal muscle systems, which are not adequately reflected through the measurement of individual organ system function.

**Cardiorespiratory endurance:** The capacity of the heart, blood vessels, and lungs to deliver oxygen and nutrients to the working muscles and tissues during sustained exercise and to remove metabolic waste products that would result in fatigue.

**Cardiorespiratory fitness:** The ability to perform large-muscle movement over a sustained period; related to the capacity of the heart-lung system to deliver oxygen for sustained energy production. Also called *cardiorespiratory endurance* or *aerobic fitness.*

**Cardiovascular control center:** A part of the brain responsible for the regulation of the rate at which the heart beats through the nervous and endocrine systems.

**Cardiovascular disease (CVD):** A general term for any disease of the heart, blood vessels, or circulation.

**Cardiovascular drift:** A cardiovascular phenomenon that represents a gradual increase in heart-rate response during a steady-state bout of exercise.

**Cardiovascular system:** Includes the heart and the blood vessels, and is responsible for the transport of blood throughout the body.

**Carotid bodies:** A small mass of receptors in the carotid artery that is sensitive to chemical changes in the blood.

**Cartilage:** A smooth, semi-opaque material that absorbs shock and reduces friction between the bones of a joint.

**Casein:** An insoluble milk protein or the curdled portion of milk; a protein that empties from the stomach slowly and allows for a sustained release of amino acids into the bloodstream.

**Catabolism:** The aspect of metabolism involving the breakdown of complex molecules, resulting in the release of free energy.

**Catecholamines:** Hormones released from the adrenal medulla (epinephrine and norepinephrine) as part of our sympathetic response to a stressor.

**Center of gravity (COG):** The point at which the distribution of our body weight would be considered equal in all directions; generally located slightly anterior to the S1-S2 joint at the sacrum.

**Center of mass (COM):** Defines the location in which the majority of an individual's weight is concentrated.

**Central chemoreceptors:** Any of the sensory nerve cells or chemical receptors that are located in the medulla of the brain.

**Central nervous system (CNS):** The brain and spinal cord.

**Cerebral cortex:** The outer region of the brain, and the most highly developed region responsible for thinking, perceiving, rationalizing, decision making, and producing and understanding language.

**Chemoreceptors:** Neural receptors that respond to some local chemical change; usually refers to those that influence the respiratory and cardiovascular control centers in the brainstem.

**Chloride shift:** The movement of chloride ions from the plasma into red blood cells as a result of the transfer of carbon dioxide from tissues to the plasma; an exchange process that serves to maintain blood pH.

**Choice reaction:** Requires an individual to pick an appropriate response when presented with several possible stimuli.

**Cholesterol:** A fatlike substance found in the blood and body tissues and in certain foods. Can accumulate in the arteries and lead to a narrowing of the vessels (atherosclerosis).

**Chondromalacia patella (CP):** Inflammation of the underside of the patella (kneecap) and softening of the cartilage that is associated with knee pain.

**Chronic disease:** Any disease state that persists over a certain period.

**Chronic hypertrophy:** An increase in muscle size that results from repeated long-term resistance training.

**Chronic obstructive pulmonary disease (COPD):** A condition, such as asthma, bronchitis, or emphysema, in which flow within the upper or lower pulmonary airways become chronically obstructed.

**Chronological aging:** The number of years a person has been alive; has long been used as a way to categorize, and sometimes discriminate against, an individual. Chronological age, however, is a very crude and often inaccurate means of determining how "old" an individual is from a biological or physiological perspective. The mature adult population is very diverse; therefore, an individual who is older chronologically may be healthier, fitter, and more functional than his or her younger counterparts.

**Circuit training:** Also known as vertical load training, involves organizing multiple exercises into a sequence with shorter or no recovery intervals between each station.

**Circumflex:** Bending around something else; curved.

**Claudication:** Ischemic lower-extremity pain associated with peripheral arterial disease.

**Closed drills:** Preprogrammed training drills that are performed in a predictable and unchanging environment.

**Cocontraction:** Occurs when muscles surrounding joints (agonist and antagonists) contract together either through dynamic (concentric/eccentric) or isometric action.

**Cognitive restructuring:** A behavioral technique that involves learning how to replace unhealthy or negative thoughts and "self-talk" about weight loss with positive affirmations.

**Collagen:** The main constituent of connective tissue, such as ligaments, tendons, and muscles.

**Colonic tone:** Reflects the functionality of the colon in absorbing and moving food along its length. During exercise, as blood flow to the colon is reduced, colonic tone decreases, reducing the rate of absorption and passage of foods through the gut.

**Comorbidities:** The presence of one or more additional disorders (or diseases) co-occurring with a primary disease or disorder.

**Complete protein:** A protein source that contains all of the essential amino acids in the exact ratios needed by the body.

**Compound sets:** Involves completion of two exercises emphasizing the same muscle groups before taking a rest interval (e.g., one set of body-weight pull-ups followed immediately by one set of lat pull-downs for the back).

**Concentric:** A type of dynamic (isotonic) muscle contraction involving shortening of the sarcomeres as the muscle develops tension.

**Concentric muscle action:** Production of tension in the muscle while the muscle fibers are shortening.

**Conducting zone:** In the respiratory system, it represents air that never reaches the alveoli, and includes the nose, pharynx, larynx, trachea, bronchi, bronchioles, and terminal bronchioles; it functions to filter, warm, and moisten air and conduct it into the lungs.

**Conduction:** The direct flow of heat through a medium or material resulting from direct physical contact. Examples include immersion in water or lying on a cold solid surface.

**Contamination:** To make impure by the introduction of unwholesome or undesirable elements.

**Contractility:** The ability of muscle tissue (cardiac or skeletal) to contract when stimulated.

**Contraindications:** Any condition that renders some particular movement, activity, or treatment improper or undesirable.

**Control system:** Refers to the neurological system that provides both conscious and subconscious (reflexive) control in contributing to stability.

**Convection:** The transfer of heat created by the passage of molecules over a surface. Examples include a fan blowing air currents or water washing over the body.

**Coordination:** The ability to process and execute appropriate actions or motor responses with proper sequence (timing) and magnitude to produce smooth, flowing movement; requires adequate levels of proprioception and spatial awareness.

**Core body temperature:** The temperature of deep structures of the body, such as the visceral organs, as compared with that of peripheral tissues.

**Cori cycle:** The cycle of lactate-to-glucose between the muscle and the liver.

**Coronary artery bypass grafting (CABG):** A highly invasive procedure that requires opening of the chest cavity to place bypass grafts (vessels) on each side of the lesion to divert flow around the blockage.

**Coronary artery disease (CAD):** The major form of cardiovascular disease; results when the coronary arteries are narrowed or occluded, most commonly by atherosclerotic deposits of fibrous and fatty tissue; also called *coronary heart disease.*

**Cortex (Adrenal):** Outer portion of the adrenal gland.

**Corticosteroids:** Hormones released by the adrenal cortex that play a major role in maintaining blood glucose and fluid and electrolyte balance, and support the development of secondary sex characteristics. Generally, corticosteroids are categorized as mineralocorticoids, glucocorticoids, and gonadocorticoids.

**Coupled reactions:** A catch-all term for a variety of reactions where two hydrocarbon fragments are coupled with the aid of a metal catalyst.

**C-reactive protein:** A protein found in the blood, the levels of which rise in response to inflammation.

**Creatine phosphate:** Naturally occurring molecule synthesized in the liver and kidneys from amino acids, and is an integral part of the Phosphagen energy system forming phosphocreatine; 95% of creatine in the body is located within skeletal muscle.

**Creep:** The lengthening that occurs when a stretch force is applied to connective tissue.

**Crimp:** The zigzag structure of collagen, which gradually straightens out when subjected to high-tensile forces.

**Current Good Manufacturing Practices (CGMPs):** Regulations as specified by the U.S. Food and Drug Administration that describe the methods, equipment, and quality control procedures required for food processing, medical device manufacturing, and related industries.

**Cyclic adenosine monophosphate (cyclic AMP):** A second-messenger molecule derived from adenosine triphosphate (ATP) that transfers the effects of hormones like glucagon and epinephrine, which are first messengers, to the intracellular environment.

**Cytochromes:** Any of a number of compounds consisting of heme bonded to a protein; function as electron transfer agents in many metabolic pathways, especially cellular respiration.

**Cytokines:** Hormone-like low molecular weight proteins, secreted by many different cell types, which regulate the intensity and duration of immune responses and are involved in cell-to-cell communication.

**Dalton's law:** Total pressure of a gas mixture is equal to the sum of the partial pressures of each individual gas.

**Dead space ventilation ($V_D$):** The amount of air that is in the conducting zone (to terminal bronchioles), not used in respiration; usually equal to one third of minute respiration.

**Decisional balance:** Refers to the weighting of the pros and cons an individual perceives regarding adopting and/or maintaining an activity program.

**Decompression sickness:** A condition that results when sudden decompression causes nitrogen bubbles to form in the tissues of the body; common in divers, who often call it "the bends."

**Deep fascia:** A layer of fascia that can surround individual muscles and divide groups of muscles into compartments.

**Deformation:** The action or process of changing in shape or distorting, especially through the application of pressure or force.

**Dehydration:** A state of decreased total body fluid that is categorized as mild (<2% loss of body weight), moderate (2%–7%), and severe (>7%).

**Delayed-onset muscle soreness (DOMS):** Soreness that occurs 24 to 48 hours after strenuous exercise, the exact cause of which is unknown.

**Dendrites:** The portion of nerve fibers that transmits impulses toward a nerve cell body; also known as the receptive portion of nerve cells that picks up sensory information.

**Denervation muscle atrophy:** A progressive shrinkage of muscle fibers when the nerve supply to the muscle is severed, resulting in strength loss and muscle wasting.

**Deoxyhemoglobin:** The form of hemoglobin without bound oxygen.

**Deoxyribonucleic acid (DNA):** A self-replicating material present in nearly all living organisms that is the carrier of genetic information.

**Depolarization:** A change in a cell's resting membrane potential where the interior becomes less negative relative to the outside as positively-charged sodium ions move into the cell.

**Depression:** A condition of general emotional dejection and withdrawal; sadness greater and more prolonged than that warranted by any objective reason.

**Depressor area:** A region of the brain that exerts a strong inhibitory effect on sympathetic nervous system activity when stimulated.

**Detraining:** The partial or complete loss of training-induced adaptations in response to an insufficient training stimulus.

**Diabetes:** A disease involving dysfunctional carbohydrate metabolism in which either an absolute deficiency of insulin production or resistance to recognize insulin results in the inability to properly metabolize carbohydrates.

**Diastole:** The period of filling of the heart between contractions; also known as the recoil or recovery phase of the heart contraction cycle.

**Diastolic blood pressure (DBP):** The pressure in the vessel during diastole or the filling phase of the cardiac cycle.

**Dietary Reference Intakes (DRI):** The general term used to denote a set of reference values used to plan and assess nutrient intakes of healthy people. These values, which vary by age and sex, include: (1) Recommended Dietary Allowance (RDA)—average daily level of intake sufficient to meet the nutrient requirements of nearly all (97%–98%) healthy people; (2) adequate intake (AI)—established when evidence is insufficient to develop an RDA and is set at a level assumed to ensure nutritional adequacy (approximately 50%); and (3) tolerable upper intake level (UL)—maximum daily intake unlikely to cause adverse health effects.

**Dietary Supplement Health and Education Act (DSHEA):** A bill passed by Congress in 1994 that sets forth some regulations and guidelines for dietary supplements.

**Dietary supplements:** Any product other than tobacco that is taken by mouth and contains a dietary ingredient intended to supplement the diet—may include vitamins, minerals, herbs or other botanicals, amino acids, or a combination of those and/or other substances.

**Dilutional hyponatremia:** Abnormally low blood sodium level that results from excessive intake of low-sodium fluids such as water.

**Direct calorimetry:** A method of determining a body's energy use by measuring the amount of heat released from the body; usually measured using an insulated chamber.

**Disablement:** The process of becoming disabled.

**Disaccharides:** Short chains of double sugar units; the nutritionally important ones in human diet are called *sucrose*, *lactose*, and *maltose*.

**Discrete task:** A task with a clear beginning and an end, and should be the focus of drill selection during the initial stage of learning new motor skills.

**Diuretic:** Any substance that increases the excretion of water from bodies by producing larger volumes of urine, doing so in a variety of ways like removing sodium from the body.

**Diving reflex:** A nervous system response exhibited when the face is submerged in cold water, which results in a slowing of the heart rate and a shunting of blood from extremities into the thorax.

**Doping:** The practice of ingesting a banned substance in an effort to improve athletic performance.

**Dorsal:** Of, on, or relating to the upper side or back of an animal, plant, or organ.

**Dose-response relationship:** Direct association between the amount of a stimulus and the magnitude of the desired outcome (e.g., amount of physical activity and good health).

**Dowager's hump (hyperkyphosis):** An exaggerated outward curve of the thoracic spine, often associated with vertebral fractures and osteoporosis.

**Downregulation:** A process in which the number or activity of hormone receptors decreases, typically in response to abnormally high hormonal activity.

**Dry suits:** Provide thermal insulation or passive thermal protection to the wearer while immersed in water, and are worn by divers, boaters, water sports enthusiasts, and others who work or play in or near cold water.

**Dry-bulb temperature:** The actual air temperature.

**Dual-energy X-ray absorptiometry (DEXA):** An imaging technique that uses a very low dose of radiation to measure bone density; can also be used to measure overall body fat and regional differences in body fat.

**Dynamic balance:** The ability to maintain balance while moving; requires an individual to lose, manipulate, and regain control of his or her center of mass over a changing base of support, such as when walking, marching, running, skipping, and jumping.

**Dynamic (or active) stretching:** Form of stretching that involves taking the joints through their ranges of motion while continuously moving. Often beneficial when warming up for a particular sport or activity that involves the same joint movements, it prepares the neuromuscular system for movement.

**Dyslipidemia:** A condition characterized by abnormal blood lipid profiles; may include elevated cholesterol, triglyceride, or low-density lipoprotein (LDL) levels and/or low high-density lipoprotein (HDL) levels.

**Dyspnea:** Difficult or labored breathing.

**Eating disorder:** A severe alteration in eating patterns linked to psychological or emotional changes. Eating disorders are usually more evident in young female athletes but can affect any segment of the population.

**Eccentric muscle action:** Production of tension within the muscle by lengthening the muscle fibers.

**Eccentric phase:** A type of isotonic or dynamic muscle contraction in which the muscle undergoes lengthening against a resistance; sometimes called *negative work* or *negative reps*.

**Ecchymosis:** The escape of blood into the tissues from ruptured blood vessels marked by a black-and-blue or purple discolored area.

**Eccrine glands:** The major sweat glands of the human body, found in virtually all skin.

**Echocardiogram:** A test that uses sound waves to produce images of the heart and is used for the diagnosis or monitoring of heart disease.

**Echocardiography:** The use of ultrasound waves to investigate the action of the heart.

**Edema:** Swelling resulting from an excessive accumulation of fluid within the tissues of the body.

**Efferent:** Conducting or conducted outward or away from something, such as a nerve carrying an impulse away from the central nervous system.

**Efferent pathway:** The pathway in which efferent nerves, otherwise known as motor or effector neurons, carry nerve impulses away from the central nervous system to effectors such as muscles or glands.

**Ejection fraction (%EF):** The percentage of the total volume of blood within the left ventricle that is pumped out during the systolic contraction of the heart.

**Elastic limit:** The maximum extent to which a tissue may be stretched without permanent alteration of size or shape.

**Elasticity:** The ability of tissue to regain its original shape and size after being deformed; also known as elastic deformation.

**Elastin:** A protein, similar to collagen, found in connective tissue that has elastic properties.

**Electrocardiogram:** A recording of the electrical activity of the heart.

**Electrolyte:** A mineral that exists as a charged ion in the body and that is extremely important for normal cellular function.

**Electron transport chain (ETC):** A series of electron receivers located along the inner mitochondrial membrane; the electron receivers sequentially receive and pass electrons along the chain to the final receiver—molecular oxygen.

**End-diastolic volume:** The volume of blood present within the ventricle at the end of the cardiac filling cycle or diastole.

**Endergonic:** Accompanied by, or requiring the absorption of energy; the products being of greater free energy than the reactants.

**Endocardium:** The thin, smooth membrane that lines the inside of the chambers of the heart and forms the surface of the valves.

**Endocrine gland:** A specialized gland that produces and/or secretes hormones.

**Endocrine system:** A physiological system made up of glands and tissues that release hormones to maintain homoeostasis of many bodily functions.

**Endogenous sources:** Produced from within the body.

**Endomysium:** A layer of connective tissue that surrounds individual muscle fibers and contains capillaries, nerves, and lymphatics.

**End-systolic volume:** The volume of blood remaining within the ventricle at the end of contraction, or systole, which represents the beginning of cardiac filling or diastole.

**Energy availability:** The ability of the body to obtain energy to fuel exercise; decreased when an athlete increases his or her physical activity without appropriately increasing caloric intake or even restricting caloric intake. When this happens, the body attempts to restore energy balance by using less energy for growth, reproduction, and various other important bodily functions.

**Energy expenditure:** The amount of energy a person uses in the form of calories.

**Entropy:** Consists of the portion of energy released from a reaction that cannot be harnessed to perform work such as muscle contraction, because of its function in increasing disorder or randomness.

**Enzyme:** A unique protein structure that speeds up a specific chemical reaction.

**Epicardium:** A serous membrane that forms the innermost layer of the pericardium and the outer surface of the heart.

**Epiglottis:** The cartilage located in the throat that guards the entrance to the trachea and prevents fluid or food from entering it during the act of swallowing.

**Epimysium:** A layer of connective tissue that encloses the entire muscle and is continuous with fascia and other connective-tissue wrappings of muscle, including the endomysium and perimysium.

**Epinephrine:** Hormone released as part of the sympathetic response to exercise; also called *adrenaline*.

**Ergogenic:** Intended to enhance physical performance, stamina, or recovery.

**Erythropoiesis:** The production of red blood cells.

**Essential amino acid:** Amino acids that cannot be made by the body and must be attained through the diet.

**Essential fat:** Fat thought to be necessary for maintenance of life and reproductive function.

**Essential fatty acids (EFAs):** Fatty acids that the body needs, but cannot synthesize; includes linolenic (omega-3) and linoleic (omega-6) fatty acids.

**Essential nutrients:** A nutrient required by the body for normal body functioning that cannot be synthesized by the body or cannot be synthesized in adequate amounts to support good health; must therefore be obtained through dietary sources.

**Estradiol:** The most potent naturally occurring estrogen hormone in humans, which is released from the ovary; greatest level exist during a female's reproductive years.

**Estrogen:** Generic term for estrous-producing steroid compounds produced primarily in the ovaries, but also within fats cells and the adrenal gland; the female sex hormones.

**Evaporation:** The process by which molecules in a liquid state (e.g., water) spontaneously become gaseous (e.g., water vapor).

**Excess post-exercise oxygen consumption (EPOC):** A measurably increased rate of oxygen uptake following strenuous activity. This additional amount of oxygen is used in the processes (hormone balancing, replenishment of fuel stores, cellular repair, innervation, and anabolism) to restore the body back to its resting state, and in the process of adaptation to the exercise stimulus.

**Excitation-contraction coupling:** The process by which myosin heads bind to the exposed active sites on the actin filaments to initiate a muscle contraction.

**Excretion:** The process of eliminating or expelling compounds like waste material from the body.

**Exercise:** Physical activity that is planned, structured, repetitive, and is performed with the intention of improving or maintaining one or more components of physical fitness; a subcategory of physical activity.

**Exercise challenge test:** An exercise test used to make a diagnosis of asthma, which includes a controlled run on a treadmill followed by scheduled multiple spirometry maneuvers.

**Exercise-induced asthma (EIA):** Transient and reversible airway narrowing triggered by vigorous exercise.

**Exercise-induced hypoxemia:** A significant decrease in oxygen saturation (<95%) during maximal and submaximal exercise observed in moderately and highly trained athletes.

**Exercise physiology:** The study of the acute responses and chronic adaptations to a wide range of physical exercise conditions, including environmental exposure to heat, cold, altitude, and pollution.

**Exergonic:** A metabolic or chemical process accompanied by the release of energy.

**Exhalation:** The process or action of exhaling or expiring air.

**Exocrine gland:** A gland or tissue that secretes substances through a duct or system of ducts; saliva and sweat glands are examples.

**Exogenous sources:** Produced outside the body.

**Expiration:** The act of expelling air from the lungs; exhalation.

**Expiratory reserve volume (ERV):** The additional amount of air that can be expired from the lungs after normal expiration.

**External respiration:** The process of inhalation and exhalation; where inhalation represents the process of taking in air to extract oxygen and exhaling air to remove carbon dioxide.

**Extrafusal fibers:** Standard muscle fibers that produce tension and skeletal movement by contraction, and innervated by alpha motor neurons.

**Facilitation:** The process of increasing motor nerve excitability.

**False-hope syndrome:** The tendency of people to set unrealistic goals.

**Fartlek training:** A form of training during which the exerciser randomly changes the aerobic intensity based on how he or she is feeling. Also called *speed play.*

**Fascia:** Plural = fasciae; strong connective tissues that perform a number of functions, including developing and separating the muscles within the body, and providing structural support and protection.

**Fasciae:** *See* Fascia.

**Fascicles:** Small bundles or clusters, especially of nerve, tendon, or muscle fibers.

**Fasciitis:** Inflammation of the connective tissue called *fascia.*

**Fast-twitch motor unit:** A motor unit composed of fast-twitch muscle fibers; characterized as having a low oxidative capacity and high glycolytic capacity; recruited for rapid, powerful movements such as jumping, throwing, and sprinting.

**Fast-twitch muscle fibers:** One of several types of muscle fibers found in skeletal muscle tissue; characterized as having a low oxidative capacity and high glycolytic capacity; recruited for rapid, powerful movements such as jumping, throwing, and sprinting; also called *type II fibers.*

**Fat loading:** A strategy of progressively increasing the quantity of fat ingested in order to increase fatty acid oxidation, and thus preserve glycogen stores during prolonged exercise.

**Fat mass (FM):** The actual amount of essential and nonessential fat in the body.

**Fat-free mass:** That part of the body composition that represents everything but fat—composed of blood, bones, connective tissue, organs, and muscle; sometimes used interchangeably with *lean body mass,* although they are not technically the same as lean mass also contains fat.

**Fatty acid oxidation:** The metabolism of fatty acids that are broken down to provide adenosine triphosphate (ATP) in the presence of oxygen; fuels low- to moderate-intensity activity of longer durations.

**Female athlete triad:** A set of three symptoms experienced by nearly 25% of female endurance athletes—amenorrhea, osteoporosis, and disordered eating.

**$FEV_1$/FVC ratio:** Represents the proportion of a person's vital capacity that he or she is able to expire within the first second of expiration.

**Fiber:** Carbohydrate chains present in a block formation that the body cannot break down (digest) nor absorb, and pass through the body undigested.

**Fibrils:** Small or slender fibers, such as those found in muscle and connective tissues.

**Fibroblastic/proliferation phase:** The stage of wound healing characterized by new blood vessel formation, collagen deposition, granulation tissue formation, epithelialization, and wound contraction.

**Fibromyalgia:** A syndrome characterized by long-lasting, widespread pain and tenderness at specific points on the body.

**Fibrous pericardium:** The most superficial layer of the pericardium in the heart; made up of dense connective tissue, which acts to protect the heart, anchoring it to the surrounding walls and preventing it from overfilling with blood.

**Fick's law for diffusion:** The property that governs the transfer rate of gases through tissue membranes.

**Filtration:** The action or process of filtering something, such as small particles from a liquid.

**First messenger:** An extracellular substance (such as a hormone) that binds to a cell-surface receptor and initiates intracellular activity.

**First ventilatory threshold (VT1):** Intensity of aerobic exercise at which ventilation starts to increase in a nonlinear fashion in response to an accumulation of metabolic by-products in the blood.

**Flavin adenine dinucleotide (FAD):** A coenzyme that transfers hydrogen and the energy associated with the hydrogens.

**Flavin adenine dinucleotide hydroquinone (FADH):** A coenzyme that is important in electron transport in mitochondria; the reduced form of flavin adenine dinucleotide (FAD).

**Flexibility:** The range of motion (ROM) available around a joint or the degree of tissue extensibility available at a joint.

**Follicle-stimulating hormone (FSH):** A gonadotropic hormone secreted by the anterior pituitary lobe that stimulates the ovaries to release eggs and produce estrogen, and stimulates the testes to produce sperm.

**Force couples:** Muscles working as a group to provide opposing, directional, or contralateral pulls to achieve balanced movement.

**Force transmission:** The act of transmitting force, such as transmission of muscle forces to the skeleton.

**Forced expiratory volume ($FEV_1$):** The amount of air exhaled within the first second of maximal exhalation.

**Forced vital capacity (FVC):** The total amount of air that can be forcibly exhaled after a maximal inhalation.

**Force-velocity relationship:** Refers to the inverse relationship between velocity of concentric contraction and the resulting force production, such that, as the velocity of a concentric contraction increases, the force produced decreases.

**Fracture:** A medical condition that results in a crack or actual break in a bone. The causes of fractures can be classified into low-impact or high-impact.

**Frank-Starling law of the heart:** The stroke volume of the heart increases in response to an increase in the volume of blood filling the heart when all other factors remain constant.

**Free energy:** Refers to the fraction of energy released from a reaction that can be used to perform work, such as muscle contraction.

**Free fatty acid (FFA):** A fatty acid that is only loosely bound to plasma proteins in the blood. Fatty acids are used by the body as a metabolic fuel.

**Free nerve endings:** An unspecialized, afferent nerve ending; they function as cutaneous receptors and are essentially used by vertebrates to detect pain.

**Full-body stability:** Refers to the overall stability of the body and implies the sum of all the local stability links within the kinetic chain.

**Functional age:** A measure of aging using various indications beyond chronological age; these indices include biological age, social age, and psychological age.

**Functional residual capacity (FRC):** The total volume of air present in the lungs at the end of passive expiration and includes residual volume (RV) plus expiratory reserve volume (ERV).

**Fundamental movement skills (FMS):** Gross motor skills that are the foundational movements for more complex and specialized skills required by children throughout their lives to competently and confidently participate in different games, sports, and recreational activities offered at school and in the community.

**Gait:** The manner by which locomotion is achieved by humans using the limbs; walking.

**Galactose:** A monosaccharide; a component of lactose.

**Ganglia:** A group of nerve cell bodies usually located in the peripheral nervous system.

**Gastric bypass:** A surgical procedure used for treatment of morbid obesity that reduces stomach capacity and allows food to bypass part of the small intestine.

**Gastric emptying:** The passage of food and fluid from the stomach to the small intestines for further digestion and absorption.

**General adaptation syndrome (GAS):** A three-stage (alarm, adaptation, and exhaustion) universal process first defined by researcher Hans Selye in 1936 that describes the body's response to stress.

**Gestational diabetes:** A form of glucose intolerance that occurs during pregnancy and is present in approximately 2% to 10% of all pregnancies and 5% to 10% of women in the immediate postpartum period.

**Global muscle:** Larger muscles that are located more superficially and often cross two or more joints.

**Globe temperature:** Reflects radiant heat and is normally higher than the dry-bulb temperature.

**Glucagon:** Hormone released from the alpha cells of the pancreas when blood glucose levels are low or during exercise; stimulates glycogen breakdown, and glucose release from the liver to increase blood glucose. Also supports the release of free fatty acids from adipose tissue to be used as fuel.

**Glucocorticoids:** Steroid hormones produced by the adrenal cortex that are important in regulating the metabolism of carbohydrates, fats, and proteins.

**Glucogenic:** A metabolic pathway that results in the generation of glucose from noncarbohydrate carbon substrates.

**Gluconeogenesis:** The production of glucose in the liver from nonsugar substrates such as pyruvate, lactate, glycerol, and glucogenic amino acids.

**Glucose:** A simple sugar; the form in which all carbohydrates are used as the body's principal energy source.

**Glucose-alanine cycle:** Involves muscle protein being degraded to provide more glucose to generate additional adenosine triphosphate (ATP) for muscle contraction.

**Gluten:** Protein compound made of two proteins called *gliadin* and *glutenin* that are found joined together with starch in the grains wheat, rye, and barley; exposure to gliadin can lead to immunologic distress for some sensitive individuals and those with celiac disease.

**Glycemic index (GI):** A ranking of carbohydrates on a scale from 0 to 100 according to the extent to which they increase blood sugar levels.

**Glycemic load (GL):** A measure of glycemic response to a food that takes serving size into consideration; GL = (glycemic index × grams of carbohydrate)/100.

**Glycogen:** The storage form of glucose found in animal tissue composed of many glucose molecules bound together. It is located almost exclusively within muscle and liver tissue.

**Glycogen-depletion stage:** Moderate- to high-intensity exercise to deplete glycogen stores, coupled with low-to-moderate carbohydrate intakes (<55% of total kcal).

**Glycogen-loading stage:** Tapered exercise (low-intensity, short-duration), coupled with high carbohydrate intakes (>70% of total kcal).

**Glycogenolysis:** The breakdown of glycogen to glucose to be further metabolized to produce energy.

**Glycohemoglobin (HbA1c):** A blood test that measures the amount of sugar (glucose) bound to hemoglobin; a measure of how much glucose has been in the blood during the past 2 to 4 months. Also called *glycosylated hemoglobin.*

**Glycolysis:** A series of enzyme-controlled reactions that degrade glucose to two pyruvate molecules.

**Glycolytic:** Pertaining to the metabolic process that breaks down carbohydrates and sugars through a series of reactions to either pyruvic acid or lactic acid (lactate) and releases energy for the body in the form of adenosine triphosphate (ATP).

**Golgi tendon organ (GTO):** A sensory organ within a tendon that, when stimulated, results in a reduced stimulus to the alpha and gamma motor neurons within the same muscle or muscle group to protect against the accumulation of excessive tension from stretching or loading under force.

**Golgi-Mazzoni corpuscles:** A specialized mechanoreceptor located in the joint capsule that is responsible for detecting joint compression. Any weight-bearing activity stimulates these receptors.

**Gonadocorticoids:** Steroid hormones secreted by the adrenal cortex in small amounts that facilitate reproductive function.

**Ground reaction forces (GRFs):** The force exerted by the ground upon the body.

**Growth hormone (GH):** Hormone secreted by the anterior pituitary lobe that facilitates protein synthesis, fat metabolism and overall growth; also known as human growth hormone (HGH).

**Gynoid:** Adipose tissue or body fat distributed on the hips and in the lower body (pear-shaped individuals).

**Haldane effect:** The promotion of carbon dioxide dissociation by oxygenation of hemoglobin.

**Haldane transformation:** Multiplication of inspired oxygen concentration by the ratio of expired to inspired nitrogen concentrations in the calculation of oxygen consumption or respiratory quotient by the open circuit method.

**Hatha yoga:** A yoga system of physical exercises and breathing control.

**Heart failure (HF):** Inability of the heart to pump blood at a sufficient rate to meet the metabolic demand or the ability to do so only when the cardiac filling pressures are abnormally high, frequently resulting in lung congestion.

**Heart rate:** The number of heart beats per minute.

**Heart rate reserve (HRR):** The reserve capacity of the heart to perform biological work; the difference between maximal heart rate and resting heart rate. It reflects the heart's ability to increase its rate of beating to increase cardiac output above its resting level to maximal intensity.

**Heart rate threshold:** The heart rate during exercise that corresponds with the anaerobic or lactate threshold.

**Heat cramps:** A mild form of heat-related illness that generally occurs during, or after strenuous physical activity and is characterized by painful muscle spasms attributed to excessive loss of fluid and/or electrolytes.

**Heat exhaustion:** A serious heat-related illness; usually the result of intense exercise in hot, humid environments and is characterized by profuse sweating, which results in fluid and electrolyte loss, blood pressure reductions, light-headedness, nausea, vomiting, decreased coordination, and often syncope (fainting).

**Heat stress index:** A heat index of how hot a given climate temperature "feels" based on heat and humidity.

**Heat stroke:** A medical emergency that is the most serious form of heat illness because of heat overload and/or impairment of the body's ability to dissipate heat; characterized by high body temperature (>105° F [>40.5° C]); dry, red skin; altered level of consciousness; seizures; coma; and possibly death.

**Heat syncope:** A sudden dizziness experienced after exercising in the heat.

**Hematocrit:** A measure of the number of red cells found in the blood, stated as a percentage of the total blood volume. The normal range is 43% to 49% in men and 37% to 43% in women.

**Hemoconcentration:** A decrease in plasma volume due to fluid losses resulting in an increase in the concentration of red blood cells within the blood.

**Hemodynamics:** Pertaining to the forces involved in the circulation of blood (e.g., heart rate, stroke volume, and cardiac output).

**Hemoglobin:** The protein molecule in red blood cells specifically adapted to carry oxygen molecules (by bonding with them).

**Hemorrhagic stroke:** When a blood vessel in the brain bursts.

**Henry's law:** Describes the ability of gas to dissolve itself within a liquid (i.e., blood), which is determined by the pressure of the gas above the fluid, the solubility of the particular gas within that fluid, and the temperature of that fluid.

**Herbal supplements:** Plant-derived substances used for medicinal purposes.

**Hering-Breuer reflex:** Inflation and deflation reflexes that help regulate the rhythmic ventilation of the lungs, thereby preventing overdistension and extreme deflation.

**High-altitude cerebral edema (HACE):** A potentially fatal form of altitude sickness where the brain swells and stops functioning in the normal way.

**High-altitude pulmonary edema (HAPE):** A life-threatening form of pulmonary edema (fluid accumulation in the lungs) that occurs in otherwise healthy mountaineers at altitudes typically above 2,500 meters (8,200 ft).

**High-density lipoprotein (HDL):** A plasma complex of lipids and proteins that contains relatively more protein and less cholesterol and triglycerides. High HDL levels are associated with a lower risk for coronary heart disease.

**High-fructose corn syrup (HFCS):** A man-made, inexpensive sweetener derived from corn starch that is composed of glucose and fructose and found in a wide range of processed foods.

**Homeometric regulation:** Intrinsic mechanisms that control the strength of ventricular contractions that depend on the length of myocardial fibers at the end of diastole.

**Homeostasis:** An internal state of physiological balance.

**Homeothermic:** Describes the fact that regardless of the environment in which people exist or the effects of other influences that may alter body temperature (e.g., heat generated during activity or exercise), humans possess the capacity to maintain a relatively constant internal or core body temperature.

**Hormones:** Chemical messengers produced and released by an endocrine gland or tissue and transported through the blood to a target organ.

**Humidification:** The process of making the air more humid; raising the water vapor content of a gas.

**Hyaline cartilage:** Cartilage that covers the bone.

**Hydrocarbons:** A compound composed of hydrogen and carbon, such as any of those that are the chief components of petroleum and natural gas.

**Hydrophobic:** Tending to repel or fail to mix with water.

**Hydrostatic pressure:** The pressure equivalent to that exerted on a surface by a column of water of a given height.

**Hydrostatic weighing:** Weighing a person fully submerged in water. The difference between the person's mass in air and in water is used to calculate body density, which can be used to estimate the proportion of fat in the body.

**Hyperbaric bradycardia:** Slowing of the heart rate in high-oxygen environments.

**Hyperglycemia:** An abnormally high content of glucose (sugar) in the blood (>100 mg/dL).

**Hyperhydration:** Excessive water intake or water intoxication, also known as water poisoning or dilutional hyponatremia.

**Hypermobile:** Having joints that demonstrate greater mobility or stretching than normal.

**Hyperplasia:** An increase in the number of cells or the proliferation of cells that may result in a gross enlargement of an organ or tissue.

**Hypertension:** a state of elevated blood pressure, or the elevation of resting blood pressure above 140/90 mm Hg.

**Hypertensive response:** A systolic blood pressure (SBP) greater than 220 mm Hg for men and SBP greater than 190 mm Hg for women, or an increase in diastolic blood pressure (DBP) greater than 10 mm Hg, or DBP greater than 90 mm Hg during exercise echocardiography.

**Hypertonic:** Having a concentration that is greater than the concentration of human blood.

**Hypertonicity:** Altered nerve activity within a shortened muscle that only requires a smaller or weaker nerve impulse to stimulate a contraction.

**Hypertriglyceridemia:** An elevated triglyceride level.

**Hypertrophic cardiomyopathy:** A disorder in which the heart muscle has hypertrophied to the point that it does not relax enough to fill the heart with blood and thus has reduced pumping ability.

**Hypertrophy:** An increase in the cross-sectional size of a cell.

**Hypoglycemia:** A deficiency of glucose in the blood commonly caused by too much insulin, too little glucose, or too much exercise where glycogen stores become depleted. It is most commonly found in individuals with insulin-dependent diabetes and is characterized by symptoms such as fatigue, dizziness, confusion, headache, nausea, or anxiety.

**Hypohydration:** Dehydration; excessive loss of body water.

**Hypoinsulinemia:** An abnormally low concentration of insulin in the blood.

**Hypomobile:** Decreased ability to move a joint of the body.

**Hypotension:** Abnormally low blood pressure.

**Hypotensive response:** A progressive decline in systolic blood pressure.

**Hypothalamus:** An organ in the brain situated below the thalamus that coordinates both autonomic nervous system function and pituitary activity.

**Hypothermia:** Abnormally low body temperature.

**Hypothyroidism:** Underactivity of the thyroid gland, leading to reduced secretion of thyroid hormones and a reduction in resting metabolic rate.

**Hypoxia:** A condition in which there is an inadequate supply of oxygen to tissues.

**Hypoxic ventilatory response:** The increase in ventilation induced by hypoxia.

**Iliotibial band friction syndrome (ITBFS):** A repetitive overuse condition that occurs when the distal portion of the iliotibial band rubs against the lateral femoral epicondyle.

**Impulse:** The electrochemical process propagated along nerve fibers.

**Inadvertent doping:** Occurs when an athlete consumes a supplement or uses a medication to treat an illness, without realizing that it contains a banned substance, and consequently returns a positive drug test result.

**Incomplete protein:** A protein that does not contain all of the essential amino acids in the ratios needed by the body.

**Indirect calorimetry:** Used to predict resting metabolic rate. Because oxygen is used in the metabolic process to create energy, a person's metabolic rate can be estimated by measuring how much oxygen he or she consumes when breathing.

**Inflammatory phase:** An immediate tissue reaction to injury, trauma or an antigen that may include pain, swelling, itching, redness, heat, and loss of function.

**Infrapatellar tendinopathy:** An overuse syndrome characterized by a degenerative process of the patellar tendon at the insertion into the distal pole of the patella.

**Inhalation:** The action of inhaling or breathing in.

**Inhibiting factors:** Substances produced by the hypothalamus that are capable of inhibiting the secretion of a given hormone by the anterior pituitary lobe.

**Inhibition:** Designed to decrease excitability, or promote relaxation.

**Inorganic phosphate:** A molecule that combines with adenosine diphosphate (ADP) to resynthesize adenosine triphosphate (ATP).

**In-season:** The period or time frame in which athletes are actually competing in their sport.

**Insoluble:** A substance that is incapable of being dissolved within an aqueous solution.

**Inspiration:** The mechanical process of drawing air into the lungs; inhalation.

**Inspiratory capacity (IC):** The maximum amount of air that can be inhaled into the lungs after a normal exhalation.

**Inspiratory reserve volume (IRV):** The maximal amount of additional air that can be drawn into the lungs after normal inspiration.

**Insulin:** Hormone released from the beta cells of the pancreas that allows peripheral cells (e.g., the muscle cells) to take up glucose.

**Insulin-like growth factor I (IGF-I):** A polypeptide structurally similar to insulin released from muscle cells following resistance training that is the primary mediator of growth hormone. IGF-I stimulates systemic body growth through stimulation of protein synthesis and has growth-promoting effects on almost every cell in the body, especially skeletal muscle, cartilage, bone, liver, kidney, nerves, skin, hematopoietic cell, and lungs.

**Insulin-like growth factor II (IGF-II):** A polypeptide structurally similar to insulin that is secreted primarily during fetal development; its major role is as a growth-promoting hormone during gestation. IGF-II is much less active in the adult body.

**Insulin resistance:** A disorder (affecting one third of adults aged ≥20 years) in which the cells do not use insulin properly.

**Integration:** Training all parameters of physical fitness (health- and skill-related) to improve overall functional strength, ability and neuromuscular efficiency to produce force, reduce force, and dynamically stabilize the kinetic-chain segments body during movements.

**Intensity:** Level of physical exertion or effort.

**Interleukin-6:** A protein that acts to stimulate the immune response during infection and after trauma, which ultimately leads to inflammation.

**Intermittent claudication:** Muscle pain (e.g., ache, cramp, numbness, or sense of fatigue), classically in the calf muscle, which occurs during exertion or exercise, such as walking, and is relieved by a short period of rest.

**Intermuscular coordination:** The ability to activate certain muscles, or muscle groups, in a specific order to perform skilled movements or actions.

**Internal respiration:** The metabolic processes that take place in the cells and tissues during which oxygen is utilized to produce energy and carbon dioxide which is then released to the blood to be transported to the lungs.

**Interneuron:** A neuron that is found entirely in the central nervous system and connects the afferent and efferent pathways.

**Interventricular septum:** The thick wall separating the ventricles of the heart from one another.

**Intrafusal fibers:** Contractile muscle fibers located within the muscle spindle that are innervated by gamma motor neurons.

**Intramuscular coordination:** Refers to the number of motor units within a muscle that a person can simultaneously activate.

**Ions:** Atoms or molecules with a net electric charge due to the loss or gain of one or more electrons.

**Ischemia:** A decrease in the blood supply to a bodily organ, tissue, or part caused by constriction or obstruction of the blood vessels.

**Ischemic stroke:** When the blood supply to the brain is cut off.

**Isovolumetric contraction:** An event occurring in early systole, during which the ventricles contract with no corresponding volume change.

**Isovolumetric relaxation:** The part of the cardiac cycle between the time of aortic valve closure and mitral opening, during which the ventricular muscle decreases its tension without lengthening so that ventricular volume remains unaltered.

**Katabatic wind:** Normally any downslope wind, especially ones stronger than gentle mountain breezes.

**Ketoacidosis:** A metabolic state marked by the accumulation of ketone bodies (ketones) attributed to incompletely metabolized fatty acids or amino acids on account of inadequate amounts of available carbohydrates; results in lowering of blood pH which can be potentially harmful and presence of ketones (acetone) on a person's breath.

**Ketogenic:** Related to the accumulation of excessive amounts of ketone bodies in the body tissues and fluids as a result of incompletely metabolized fatty acid or amino acid breakdown.

**Kilocalorie (kcal):** A measurement of the amount of energy in a food that is available after digestion. The amount of heat required to raise the temperature of 1 kg water 1°C between 14.5 and 15.5 degrees Celsius. Also called a *calorie.*

**Kilojoule (kJ):** 1,000 joules or 238.8459 calories. A Joule is a unit of work and energy, equal to the work done when a force of 1 Newton moves through a distance of 1 m in the direction of the force. One kcal = 4.184 kj.

**Kinesthetic awareness:** The body's ability to coordinate spatial and temporal awareness with movement.

**Kinetic chain:** The body and its extremities consist of bony segments linked by a series of joints. The kinetic chain concept likens these segments and their linkages to a chain.

**Krebs cycle:** Refers to one of the energy systems within the mitochondria whereby energy is primarily transferred from derivatives of amino acid, carbohydrate, and lipid oxidation to the electron carriers nicotinamide adenine dinucleotide (NAD) and flavin adenine dinucleotide (FAD) for subsequent regeneration of adenosine triphosphate (ATP) in the electron transport chain.

**Lactate:** Refers to a product manufactured from the reduction of pyruvate by adding hydrogen.

**Lactate paradox:** The observation that for individuals fully acclimatized to high altitudes, deeper rates of ventilation flush greater quantities of carbon dioxide from the lungs, consequently lowering the peak post-exercise blood lactate levels during a given exercise protocol.

**Lactate threshold (LT):** The point during exercise of increasing intensity at which blood lactate begins to accumulate above resting levels, where lactate clearance is no longer able to keep up with lactate production.

**Lactic acid:** A metabolic by-product of carbohydrate metabolism during high-intensity physical activity.

**Lacto-ovo-vegetarian:** A vegetarian who also consumes dairy and eggs.

**Lacto-vegetarian:** A vegetarian who also consumes dairy products.

**Larynx:** The organ of the voice; located between the trachea and the base of the tongue.

**Lateral epicondylitis:** An overuse or repetitive trauma injury of the wrist extensor muscles that occurs near their origin on the lateral epicondyle of the humerus.

**Lean body mass:** The components of the body (apart from fat), including muscles, bones, nervous tissue, skin, blood, and organs; although it generally is used in practical terms to reflect muscle mass.

**Left anterior descending coronary arteries:** One of the heart's coronary artery branches from the left main coronary artery, which supplies blood to the left ventricle.

**Left bundle branch:** The bundle of cardiac nerves that feeds the left ventricle.

**Length-tension relationship:** Refers to the relationship between the length of the sarcomere or muscle fiber and the ability to produce force/tension. An optimal length of the muscle fiber for producing force exists. Lengths that are above or below this optimal length result in a reduced amount of force produced when stimulated.

**Leptin:** A hormone released from fat cells that acts on the hypothalamus to regulate energy intake. Low leptin levels stimulate hunger and subsequent fat consumption.

**Life course theory:** An approach for analyzing people's lives within structural, social, and cultural contexts.

**Ligaments:** Strong, fibrous tissues that connect one bone to another.

**Limiting amino acid (LAA):** The essential amino acid that is present in limited supply from a food to support growth and maintenance, and because it cannot be synthesized by the body, it must be supplied by foods providing better sources of this compound.

**Limits of stability:** The degree of allowable sway from the line of gravity without a need to change the base of support.

**Linear speed:** Straight-line speed; determined by the combination of stride frequency (the number of strides per unit time) and stride length (the distance covered in a single stride).

**Lipolysis:** The breakdown of triglycerides in adipose tissue to free fatty acids (FFAs) and glycerol.

**Lipoprotein:** An assembly of a lipid and protein that serves as a transport vehicle for fatty acids and cholesterol in the blood and lymph.

**Lipoprotein lipase (LPL):** An enzyme attached to the endothelial surface of capillaries that stimulates the breakdown of circulating triglycerides into fatty acids for cellular uptake into cells.

**Live high/train low (LHTL):** The training concept that supports living at higher altitudes to experience the physiological adaptations that occur, while maintaining the same exercise intensity during training at sea level.

**Load training:** Phase 3 of the Functional Movement & Resistance Training component of the ACE Integrated Fitness Training Model where the exercise program is advanced with the addition of an external resistance, placing emphasis on muscle force production, and the variables of training can be manipulated to address a variety of exercise goals.

**Local muscle:** The deep muscles located directly next to the joint.

**Local stability:** Refers to individual joint stability within the body.

**Low-density lipoproteins (LDL):** The major carrier of cholesterol in the circulation, containing 60% to 70% of the body's total serum cholesterol; frequently referred to as the "bad" cholesterol because of its role in atherogenesis, the early stages of atherosclerosis.

**Luteal phase:** The second half of the menstrual cycle, after ovulation.

**Luteinizing hormone (LH):** A gonadotropic hormone secreted by the anterior pituitary that stimulates ovulation in female mammals, and stimulates testosterone and androgen release in male mammals.

**Macrocycle:** Constitutes the timeframe of an entire training program, ranging from a few months to a few years.

**Macronutrient:** A nutrient that is needed in large quantities for normal growth and development like carbohydrates, fats and proteins.

**Macrotrauma:** Refers to a specific event within the body where the force placed on the body exceeds its stability levels; includes events such as accidents where the impact from hitting the ground creates the injury.

**Malignant:** Tending to be severe and become progressively worse.

**Malignant neoplasms:** Cancer; a broad group of diseases involving unregulated cell growth.

**Maltodextrin:** A partially hydrolyzed starch converted to an oligosaccharide that is used as a food additive.

**Maturation/remodeling phase:** A cyclical process by which bone maintains a dynamic steady state through resorption and formation of a small amount of bone at the same site.

**Maximal force production:** How much force a muscle fiber produces per unit of fiber cross-sectional area.

**Maximal heart rate (HRmax):** The highest heart rate a person can attain.

**Maximal oxygen consumption ($\dot{V}O_2$max):** Considered a good indicator of cardiovascular endurance and represents the maximum amount of oxygen (mL) a person utilizes over unit of time (usually expressed within one minute). Also called *maximal oxygen uptake,* peak $\dot{V}O_2$ or maximal *aerobic capacity.*

**Maximal velocity:** The highest speed attained during an event or performance.

**Mean arterial pressure (MAP):** Equals the product of cardiac output and total peripheral resistance, and represents the average pressure within an artery over a complete heartbeat cycle.

**Mechanical efficiency:** Applies to any system of moving parts; its goal is to minimize mechanical stress and energy expenditure.

**Mechanoreceptor:** A specialized sensory end organ that responds to mechanical stimuli such as tension, pressure, or displacement.

**Medial collateral ligament (MCL):** One of four ligaments that are critical to the stability of the knee joint; spans the distance from the medial end of the femur to the top of the medial tibia.

**Medial epicondylitis:** An overuse or repetitive trauma injury of the wrist flexors or forearm pronators that occurs near the origin on the medial epicondyle of the humerus.

**Medulla oblongata:** The lower portion of the brainstem.

**Meissner's corpuscle:** A specialized mechanoreceptor located in the superficial aspect of the skin that is responsible for detecting light touch; occurs abundantly in the skin of the fingertips, palms, soles, lips, tongue, and face.

**Menarche:** The first menstrual period of an individual.

**Meniscal tears:** A tear in the rubbery, C-shaped cartilage disc that cushions the knee.

**Menisci:** Shock absorbers within the knee located between the femoral and tibial condyles.

**Mesocycle:** The training timeframe identified to achieve a distinct training objective; usually organized into months or weeks.

**Messenger ribonucleic acid (mRNA):** A nucleic acid present in all living cells with the main function of carrying instructions from deoxyribonucleic acid (DNA) for controlling the synthesis of proteins.

**Metabolic equivalents (METs):** A simplified system for classifying physical activities where 1 MET is equal to true resting oxygen consumption, which is approximately 3.5 mL oxygen per kilogram of body weight per minute (3.5 mL/kg/min).

**Metabolic syndrome (MetS):** A cluster of factors associated with increased risk for coronary heart disease and diabetes— abdominal obesity indicated by a waist circumference ≥ 40 in. (102 cm) in men and ≥35 in. (88 cm) in women; levels of triglyceride ≥ 150 mg/dL (1.7 mmol/L); HDL levels less than 40 and 50 mg/dL (1.0 and 1.3 mmol/L) in men and women, respectively; blood pressure levels ≥ 130/85 mm Hg; and fasting blood glucose levels ≥ 110 mg/dL (6.1 mmol/L).

**Metabolism:** The physical and chemical processes of the body by which material substance is produced (e.g., cell regeneration), maintained, and destroyed, and by which energy is made available.

**Metastasis:** The spreading of a disease (especially cancer) to another part of the body.

**Metformin:** Prescription medication used to treat people with type 2 diabetes.

**Microcycle:** The smallest training time frame for organizing the longer-term programming variables, usually organized into daily or weekly training programs.

**Micronutrient:** A nutrient that is needed in small quantities for normal growth and development.

**Microtrauma:** Unnoticed injuries that occur as a result of repetitive overuse.

**Mineral:** An inorganic substance needed in the diet in small amounts to help regulate bodily functions.

**Mineralocorticoids:** Steroid-based hormones produced by the adrenal cortex that regulate the balance of sodium and potassium in the body to help preserve total body water and regulate blood pressure.

**Minute ventilation ($\dot{V}_E$):** A measure of the amount of air that passes through the lungs in 1 minute; calculated as the tidal volume multiplied by the ventilatory rate.

**Mitochondria:** An specialized organelle that synthesizes ATP aerobically and, often called the "power plant" of the cells.

**Mitral valve:** Heart valve that regulates blood flow from the left atrium to the left ventricle.

**Mobility:** The degree to which an articulation is allowed to move before being restricted by surrounding tissues or structures.

**Moderate altitude:** 1,500 to 2,500 m (4,950-8,250 ft); compared with high altitude, which is defined as greater than 2,500 m (8,250 ft).

**Moderate-to-vigorous physical activity (MVPA):** Moderate physical activity refers to activities equivalent in intensity to brisk walking or bicycling. Vigorous physical activity produces large increases in breathing or heart rate, such as jogging, aerobic dance, or bicycling uphill. MVPA is a term used in physical education to describe the type of physical activity required to prepare children to lead physically active lives and improve health and academic outcomes.

**Monosaccharides:** The simplest and only absorbable form of sugar; it cannot be broken down any further.

**Monounsaturated fats (MUFA):** A type of unsaturated fat (liquid at room temperature) containing one carbon-carbon double-bond within its carbon backbone that limits the ability of the carbon atoms to bind with hydrogen ions (e.g., oleic acid in olive oil).

**Morbidity:** The rate of incidence of a disease.

**Mortality:** The condition of being mortal, or susceptible to death; the number of deaths in a given population.

**Mortality rate:** A measure of the number of deaths in a population in a given time period. Typically expressed as the sum of deaths per 1,000 individuals per year.

**Motor neurons:** Nerve cells that conduct impulses from the central nervous system to the periphery signaling muscles to contract, regulating muscular movement.

**Motor unit:** A motor nerve and all of the muscle fibers it stimulates.

**Motor unit end plate:** A depression on the sarcolemma where it has synaptic contact with a nerve fiber and has a high density of neurotransmitter receptors.

**Multijoint movements:** Movement or exercises that incorporate simultaneous movement at multiple joints throughout the whole body (kinetic-chain) as opposed to single, isolated joints.

**Multiplanar training:** Training that includes movements in all three planes to reflect activities of daily living (ADL) more accurately.

**Muscle spindle:** The sensory organ located within a muscle that is sensitive to the rate and magnitude of stretching and serves to protect the muscle against stretching by triggering a muscle contraction; can also augment contractile strength during plyometric training.

**Muscular endurance:** The ability of a muscle or muscle group to exert force against a resistance over a sustained period.

**Muscular power:** The product of muscular force (strength) and speed of movement.

**Muscular strength:** The ability of a muscle or group of muscles to exert maximal levels of force.

**Myelin:** The fatty insulation of nerve fibers that is important for the conduction of nerve impulses. These fibers become damaged in individuals with multiple sclerosis.

**Myocardial infarction:** An episode in which some of the heart's blood supply is severely cut off or restricted, causing the heart muscle to suffer and die from lack of oxygen. Commonly known as a heart attack.

**Myocardial perfusion studies:** Nuclear medicine procedures that illustrate the function of the heart muscle (myocardium).

**Myocardium:** The muscle tissue of the heart.

**Myofascial release:** A technique involving the use of various tools to reduce adhesions (knots) within fascial (soft) tissue, which, in turn, helps restore tissue extensibility (movement) and reduce muscle discomfort.

**Myofibrils:** The portion of the muscle containing the thick (myosin) and thin (actin) contractile filaments; a series of sarcomeres where the repeating pattern of the contractile proteins gives the striated appearance to skeletal muscle.

**Myofilaments:** The arrangement of contractile and regulatory proteins that make up the sarcomeres of the myofibrils. Usually referred to as the thick and thin myofilaments.

**Myoglobin:** A compound similar to hemoglobin, which aids in the storage and transport of oxygen within the muscle cells.

**Myosin:** Contractile protein that makes up the thick filament in the sarcomere of a myofibril.

**Nasal cavity:** The large, air-filled space above and behind the nose in the middle of the face.

**Nasal meatus:** The passages in the nasal cavity formed by the projections of the nasal conchae.

**Negative energy balance:** A state of consuming fewer calories than are expended; leads to weight loss.

**Negative feedback system:** A corrective system that underlies the maintenance of homeostasis, where a disruption in constancy is detected and responses are activated that reverse the disruption and restore the constancy of function in the body.

**Neuromuscular coordination:** The ability to activate large and small muscles with the correct amount of force in the most efficient sequence to accomplish a task.

**Neuromuscular junction:** The site at which a motor neuron transmits information to a muscle fiber.

**Neurotransmitter:** A chemical substance such as acetylcholine or dopamine that transmits nerve impulses across synapses.

**Nia:** An expressive fitness and awareness movement program and a holistic approach to health that combines movements from tai chi, yoga, martial arts, and modern ethnic dances.

**Nicotinamide adenine dinucleotide (NAD⁺):** A coenzyme that transfers hydrogen to the electron transport chain.

**Nicotinamide adenine dinucleotide hydride (NADH):** The reduced form of nicotinamide adenine dinucleotide (NAD). NAD is a coenzyme found in all living cells that is involved in redox reactions, carrying electrons from one reaction to another. This reaction forms NADH, which can then be used as a reducing agent to donate electrons.

**Nitroglycerin:** A chemical substance used medically as a vasodilator to treat heart conditions, such as angina and chronic heart failure.

**Nociceptors:** Sensory neurons that respond to potentially damaging stimuli by sending nerve signals to the spinal cord and brain; usually involved in the perception of pain.

**Nonalcoholic fatty liver disease (NAFLD):** A cause of a fatty liver, occurring when fat is deposited in the liver not because of excessive alcohol use, but because of other compounds like excessive fructose in the diet; related to insulin resistance and the metabolic syndrome.

**Noncalorimetric techniques:** The measurement energy usage via any method other than calorimetry.

**Nonessential amino acid:** An amino acid that can be made by the body.

**Nonessential nutrients:** Nutrients that the body can produce internally from food sources.

**Nonexercise activity thermogenesis (NEAT):** Energy expended for everything we do that does not include sleeping, eating, physical activity or exercise—ranges from simple standing to fidgeting and moving about; physiological processes that produce heat; a relative newly discovered component of energy expenditure.

**Non-HDL cholesterol (non-HDL):** Total cholesterol minus high-density lipoproteins (HDL); the sum of the low-density lipoprotein (LDL), very low-density lipoprotein (VLDL), and intermediate-density lipoprotein (IDL). Non-HDL cholesterol is strongly associated with the development of cardiovascular disease, and non-HDL levels appear to be equal to or better than LDL levels at identifying atherogenic particles.

**Non-insulin-dependent diabetes mellitus (NIDDM):** Most common form of diabetes affecting 90% to 95% of all diabetics; typically develops in adulthood and is characterized by a reduced sensitivity of the insulin target cells to available insulin; usually associated with obesity. Also referred to as type 2 diabetes mellitus.

**Nonshivering thermogenesis:** Generation or production of heat, especially by physiological processes.

**Nonsteroid hormones:** Hormones not derived from steroid (fat) compounds, but from protein sources.

**Nonsteroidal anti-inflammatory drug (NSAID):** A class of drugs that can reduce inflammation, swelling, stiffness, and joint pain; examples include aspirin and ibuprofen.

**Nontropic hormones:** Hormones that stimulate target cells directly to induce effects.

**Norepinephrine:** A hormone released from the adrenal medulla and a neurotransmitter released from the terminal ends of sympathetic nerves as part of the body's sympathetic response to exercise.

**NSAID:** *See* Nonsteroidal anti-inflammatory drug.

**Nutrients:** Refer to compounds that contribute to cell growth, cell repair, and cell maintenance; considered either essential (obtained from food) or nonessential (manufactured within the body).

**O$_2$ difference:** The difference in the oxygen content of the blood between the arterial blood and the venous blood; an indication of how much oxygen is removed from the blood in capillaries as the blood circulates in the body.

**Obesity:** An excessive accumulation of body fat. Usually defined as more than 20% above ideal weight or greater than 25% body fat for men and greater than 32% body fat for women; also can be defined as a body mass index of more than 30 kg/m$^2$ or a waist girth greater than 40 in. (102 cm) in men and greater than 35 in. (89 cm) in women.

**Obesogenic:** An environment that tends to generate or create a state of obesity.

**Objective:** Pertaining to a phenomenon or clinical finding that is observed; not subjective. An objective finding is often described in health care as a sign that can be seen, heard, felt, or measured.

**Off-season:** The period between the post-season and approximately 6 weeks (although this may vary) before the first contest or competition of the following year's season.

**Oldest-old adults:** Those who are 86 to 120 years old.

**Oligosaccharides:** A carbohydrate chain containing between 3 to 10 simple sugar units (monosaccharides).

**Omega-3 fats:** An essential fatty acid that promotes a healthy immune system and helps protect against heart disease and other diseases; found in egg yolk and cold-water fish like tuna, salmon, mackerel, cod, crab, shrimp, and oyster. Examples include alpha-linolenic acid (ALA), eicosapentaenoic acid (EPA) and docosahexaenoic acid (DHA).

**One-repetition maximum (1 RM):** The maximal amount of resistance that can be moved through the range of motion for one repetition before the muscle is temporarily fatigued.

**Onset of blood lactate accumulation (OBLA):** The point in time during high-intensity exercise at which the production of lactic acid exceeds the body's capacity to eliminate it; after this point, oxygen is insufficient at meeting the body's demands for energy.

**Open drills:** Drills that require athletes to accurately respond to a variety of environmental stimuli to select an appropriate movement pattern based on the context of the situation.

**Operant conditioning:** A learning approach that considers the manner in which behaviors are influenced by their consequences.

**Oral cavity:** The cavity of the mouth, bounded by the jaw bones and associated structures (muscles and mucosa).

**Orographic uplift:** Forced lifting of air along a topographic barrier, such as a mountain range.

**Orthopnea:** Form of dyspnea in which the person can breathe comfortably only when standing or sitting erect, and not when in supine or prone positions; associated with asthma, emphysema, and angina.

**Osmolality:** A measure of the number of dissolved particles per kilogram of fluid.

**Osteoarthritis (OA):** Degenerative joint disease; characterized by pain and stiffness in the joints; most common form of arthritis.

**Osteoblasts:** Bone-forming cells.

**Osteoclasts:** Cells that reabsorb or erode bone mineral.

**Osteopenia:** A loss of bone density that predisposes an individual to development of osteoporosis.

**Osteoporosis:** A disorder, primarily affecting postmenopausal women, in which bone density decreases and susceptibility to fractures increases; can also affect female athletes with amenorrhea.

**Overload:** Manipulation of training variables to impose continued increases in stress placed on a system or systems being trained.

**Overtraining:** Constant intense training that does not provide adequate time for recovery; symptoms include increased resting heart rate, impaired physical performance, reduced enthusiasm and desire for training, increased incidence of injuries and illness, altered appetite, disturbed sleep patterns, and irritability.

**Overweight:** An excessive amount of weight for a given height, using height-to-weight ratios.

**Oxidation:** Process of oxidizing, or the addition of oxygen to a compound with a resulting loss of electrons.

**Oxidation-reduction reactions:** Reactions that involve electron transfer.

**Oxygen consumption ($\dot{V}O_2$):** The process by which oxygen is used to produce energy for cellular work; also called oxygen uptake.

**Oxygen debt:** Although a term no longer used is in exercise science, it represented the amount of extra oxygen required by the body to replenish the anaerobic energy pathways following vigorous exercise.

**Oxygen deficit:** The energy supplied to muscles through anaerobic mechanisms at the start of exercise, before a steady state of oxygen uptake is reached.

**Oxygen saturation:** The fraction of the hemoglobin molecules in a blood sample that are saturated with oxygen at a given partial pressure of oxygen; normal saturation is 95% to 100%.

**Oxyhemoglobin:** Hemoglobin that contains bound oxygen, a compound formed from hemoglobin on exposure to alveolar gas in the lungs.

**Oxytocin:** Hormone released by the posterior pituitary lobe that causes increased contraction of the uterus during labor, stimulates the ejection of milk into the ducts of the breasts following childbirth, and stimulates affiliate behaviors like a mother bonding to her child.

**P.R.I.C.E.:** Protection, Restricted Activity, Ice, Compression, and Elevation—describes a safe, early intervention strategy for an acute injury.

**Pacinian corpuscles:** A specialized bulblike mechanoreceptor located in the subcutaneous tissue of the skin responsible for detecting pressure; occur abundantly in the skin of palms, soles, and joints.

**Palpitations:** Irregular, rapid beating or pulsations of the heart.

**Parameters:** Measurable aspects of fitness or performance.

**Parasympathetic:** The part of the autonomic nervous system originating in the brainstem and the lower part of the spinal cord that opposes the physiological effects of the sympathetic nervous system; functions to promote rest, repair and recovery by stimulating digestive secretions, slowing heart rate contractility, constricting the pupils, and dilating blood vessels.

**Parasympathetic tone:** The parasympathetic nervous system's rate of firing under normal conditions.

**Parathyroid glands:** Small bodies in the region of the thyroid gland that secrete parathyroid hormone and are concerned chiefly with the metabolism of calcium and phosphorus.

**Paresthesias:** Tingling, prickling, and numbness.

**Parietal:** Relating to or forming the wall of any cavity.

**Parietal pleura:** The serous membrane that lines the different parts of the wall of the pulmonary cavity.

**Partial pressure (P$_x$):** The pressure exerted by a specific gas within a defined volume or space (e.g., such as in the blood or lungs).

**Partial pressure of inhaled oxygen (Po$_2$):** The pressure exerted by oxygen.

**Particulate matter (PM):** A small, discrete mass of solid or liquid matter that remains individually dispersed in gas or liquid emissions.

**Passive overeating:** The excessive eating of foods that are high in fat because the human body is slow to recognize the caloric content of rich foods.

**Passive system:** Defines the structures within and around the joint that essentially remain consistent in their size, shape, and length, and include the bony structures, joint capsule, ligaments, and tendons.

**Patellofemoral pain syndrome (PFPS):** A degenerative condition of the posterior surface of the patella, which may result from acute injury to the patella or from chronic friction between the patella and the groove in the femur through which it passes during motion of the knee.

**Pathogenesis:** Disease development.

**Peak height velocity (PHV):** The maximum rate of growth in stature during a growth spurt.

**Peak oxygen uptake (peak $\dot{V}O_2$):** The highest value of oxygen consumption detected during a cardiorespiratory fitness test.

**Peptide:** A compound consisting of two or more amino acids linked in a chain.

**Percent one repetition maximum (%1 RM):** The greatest amount of weight that can be lifted with proper form for one repetition.

**Pericardial space:** A space between the parietal pericardium and visceral layer; contains a supply of serous fluid.

**Pericardium:** The membrane enclosing the heart.

**Perimysium:** A sheath of connective tissue that covers a bundle of muscle fibers.

**Periodization:** The systematic manipulation of the acute variables of training like volume and load over a period that may range from days to years.

**Peripheral arterial disease:** All diseases caused by the obstruction of large peripheral arteries, which can result from atherosclerosis, inflammatory processes leading to stenosis, an embolism, or thrombus formation.

**Peripheral arterial occlusive disease (PAOD):** Disease caused by the obstruction of large arteries in the arms and legs.

**Peripheral chemoreceptors:** Structures in major arteries that detect variation of the oxygen concentration in the arterial blood, while also monitoring arterial carbon dioxide and pH.

**Peripheral nervous system (PNS):** The parts of the nervous system that are outside the brain and spinal cord (central nervous system).

**Peripheral vascular disease (PVD):** A painful and often debilitating condition, characterized by muscular pain caused by ischemia to the working muscles. The ischemic pain is usually due to atherosclerotic blockages or arterial spasms, referred to as claudication. Also called *peripheral vascular occlusive disease (PVOD)*.

**Perturbation training:** The use of randomized and unpredictable, yet controlled, multidirectional forces to create subtle disturbances in an individual's balance.

**Pharynx:** The muscular, membranous tube extending from the base of the skull to the esophagus.

**Phosphagen system:** A system that transfers chemical energy from the breakdown of creatine phosphate to regenerate adenosine triphosphate (ATP).

**Phosphocreatine:** A molecule located within skeletal muscle that is used in the phosphagen system to regenerate adenosine triphosphate (ATP).

**Phosphofructokinase (PFK):** The most important regulatory enzyme involved in the glycolysis pathway; the activity level of PFK probably limits the rate of glycolysis during maximal exercise.

**Physical activity:** Any bodily movement produced by skeletal muscles that results in energy expenditure.

**Physical activity epidemiology:** The formal study of epidemiological investigation into the associations of physical activity with many health outcomes.

**Physical Activity Readiness Questionnaire (PAR-Q):** A brief, self-administered medical questionnaire recognized as a safe pre-exercise screening measure for low-to-moderate (but not vigorous) exercise training for individuals between the ages of 15 and 69 years of age.

**Physical fitness:** The physical components of well-being that enable a person to function at an optimal level.

**Phytochemicals:** Naturally occurring protective substances that may help protect against myriad diseases and conditions.

**Pilates:** A method of mind-body conditioning that combines stretching and strengthening exercises; developed by Joseph Pilates in the 1920s.

**Pituitary gland:** A pea-sized gland located at the base of the brain responsible for controlling many of the other endocrine glands; for this reason, it is often called the *master gland*.

**Planning fallacy:** States that people consistently underestimate the time, energy, and other resources required to complete a given task.

**Plantar fasciitis:** An inflammatory condition of the plantar aponeurosis or fascia of the foot.

**Plasma:** The liquid portion of the blood.

**Plastic stretch:** Stretching to the point where deformation is temporarily permanent; plastic deformation occurs after excessive elastic deformation and results in increases in extensibility of non-elastic tissue (i.e., improvements in flexibility).

**Plasticity:** Capable of undergoing continuous deformation without rupture or relaxation.

**Pleura:** Thin membranes that line the thorax and envelop the lungs in humans.

**Pleural cavity:** The cavity in the thorax that contains the lungs and heart.

**Polymorphisms:** Natural variations in a gene, deoxyribonucleic acid (DNA) sequence, or chromosome.

**Polysaccharides:** A chain of monosaccharide (sugar) units composed of greater than 10 units.

**Polyunsaturated fats (PUFA):** A type of unsaturated fat (liquid at room temperature) containing two or more carbon-carbon double-bonds within its carbon backbone that limits the ability of the carbon atoms to bind with hydrogen ions (e.g., corn, safflower, and soybean oils).

**Pons:** Part of the brainstem responsible for multiple functions such as transferring signals between the cerebrum and the cerebellum.

**Positive energy balance:** A state of consuming more calories than are expended; leads to weight gain.

**Positive shin angle (PSA):** The lower leg contacting the ground in a position either directly underneath or slightly behind an individual's center of mass while starting or accelerating.

**Post-exercise hypotension:** Acute post-exercise reduction in both systolic and diastolic blood pressure.

**Postpartum:** The period after childbirth.

**Postseason:** Commences after the completion of the in-season period and is generally devoted to recovery, allowing athletes much-needed time to recover from the stress of competition (offloading).

**Power:** The amount of work performed per unit of time or the rate at which work is performed. This is often thought of in terms of the Olympic athlete demonstrating maximal levels of power, but power applies to any level of work performed.

**Power stroke:** A single movement of the myosin head toward the center of the sarcomere following attachment to the binding site on the thin filament. This movement causes the thin filament to slide over the thick filament, and results in sarcomere shortening and force production. Repeated power strokes are necessary for full shortening of the muscle fiber.

**Preadipocytes:** Precursor cells for adipocytes (fat cells).

**Prediabetes:** The state in which some, but not all, of the diagnostic criteria for diabetes are met (e.g., blood glucose levels are higher than normal but are not high enough for a diagnosis of diabetes).

**Preeclampsia:** A serious maternal-fetal disease that is diagnosed after 20 weeks of gestation and is characterized by persistent hypertension (>140/90 mm Hg) and proteinuria (24-hour urinary protein level ≥ 0.3 g).

**Pre-exhaustive sets:** Designed to pre-fatigue assistant muscles (synergists) to place more emphasis on the prime mover (e.g., triceps extensions performed before a barbell bench press fatigue the triceps, shifting more emphasis on the larger pectoralis major muscles).

**Prehypertension:** A systolic pressure of 120 to 139 mm Hg and/or a diastolic pressure of 80 to 89 mm Hg. Having this condition puts an individual at greater risk for development of hypertension.

**Preload:** The end volumetric pressure that stretches the right or left ventricle of the heart to its greatest geometric dimensions under variable physiological demand.

**Prenatal:** Relating to pregnant women and their unborn babies; also called *antenatal*.

**Preoptic/anterior hypothalamus (POAH):** The part of the brain responsible for core body temperature regulation.

**Preseason:** The period immediately following the off-season training program; lasts approximately 2 to 4 months for most sports.

**Pressor area:** The primary regulator of the sympathetic nervous system located in the medulla.

**Pressor response:** A disproportionate increase in heart rate during resistance training resulting from sympathetic nervous system reflex activity.

**Primary aging:** The innate processes of maturation and subsequent decline that occur in the body's cells and physiological systems throughout the life span and make the organism more susceptible to disease, injury, and death. This process is considered to be "hardwired" into the genetic code and cannot be altered.

**Primary amenorrhea:** The absence of menarche in girls 16 years or older.

**Primary prevention:** Measures provided to individuals to prevent the onset of a targeted condition.

**Processes of change:** Interventions and strategies that lead to the progression from one stage to the next in the transtheoretical model of behavioral change.

**Products:** Molecules manufactured from the substrates that are involved in enzymatically catalyzed reactions.

**Progesterone:** Hormone produced by the ovaries, adrenal cortex, and placenta, the function of which is to prepare the uterus for implantation following ovulation and facilitate growth of the embryo.

**Progression:** The systematic application of overload to promote long-term benefits or prepare an athlete or an individual for a specific event.

**Prolactin:** Hormone secreted from the anterior pituitary lobe that stimulates milk production after childbirth.

**Proprioception:** The sense of knowing where one's body or body part is in space relative to the ground; closely linked to balance and the core.

**Proprioceptive neuromuscular facilitation (PNF):** A method of promoting the response of neuromuscular mechanisms through the stimulation of proprioceptors in an attempt to gain more stretch in a muscle; often known as a contract/relax method of stretching.

**Proprioceptively enriched environments:** Unstable, yet controllable situations where exercises or movements are performed in such a manner that they place demands on the body to use its balance and stabilization mechanisms.

**Proprioceptors:** Somatic sensory receptors located within muscles, tendons, ligaments, joint capsules, and skin that gather information about body position and the direction and velocity of movement.

**Prostaglandins:** A potent substance that acts like a hormone and is found in many bodily tissues; produced in response to trauma and may affect pain, inflammation, and blood pressure.

**Protein Digestibility Corrected Amino Acid Score (PDCAAS):** A widely used and accepted scale to measure protein quality; score is based on the bioavailability and essential amino acid content of protein compared with a reference protein.

**Proton:** In bioenergetics, refers to a hydrogen ion.

**Puberty:** The period during which adolescents reach sexual maturity and become capable of reproduction.

**Pulmonary arteries:** Arteries that transport deoxygenated blood from the body to the right atrium of the heart.

**Pulmonary circulation:** The flow of blood from the right ventricle through the pulmonary artery to the lungs, where carbon dioxide is exchanged for oxygen, and back through the pulmonary vein to the left atrium.

**Pulmonary valve:** Regulates flow from the right ventricle to the pulmonary circulation.

**Pulmonary veins:** Four veins, two from each lung that transport oxygenated blood from the lungs to the left atrium of the heart.

**Pulmonary ventilation ($\dot{V}_E$):** The total volume of gas inspired or expired per minute.

**Pulse pressure:** The difference between systolic and diastolic pressures.

**Pyruvate:** The primary product of the glycolytic energy system; pyruvate can be reduced to lactate in the sarcoplasm or oxidized to acetyl-coenzyme A in the mitochondria.

**$\dot{Q}$:** See cardiac output.

**Q-angle:** The angle formed by lines drawn from the anterior superior iliac spine (ASIS) to the central patella and from the central patella to the tibial tubercle.

**Qigong:** A system of self-healing exercise and meditation that are executed at very low metabolic levels, usually between two and four metabolic equivalents (METs).

**Quantitative computed tomography (QCT):** A computerized x-ray technique that uses electronic systems to measure volumetric bone mineral density, plus other measures such as the stress-strain index (SSI) and the geometry of the bone.

**Quantitative ultrasound (QUS):** A bone density test using sound waves.

**Questionnaires:** A list of questions submitted for replies that can be analyzed for usable information.

**Radiation:** Heat transferred from one body to another via the passage of electromagnetic heat waves, without any direct contact between the two surfaces, such as heat transferring from the sun to a roof.

**Random practice sessions:** Once the athlete refines his or her technique and skills, random practice sessions may be used to further challenge the athlete's cognitive abilities.

**Range of motion (ROM):** The number of degrees that an articulation will allow one of its segments to move.

**Rate coding:** The frequency of impulses sent to a muscle. Increased force can be generated through an increase in the rate at which the impulses are received at the neuromuscular junction.

**Rate-pressure product (RPP):** Expressed as a product of heart rate in beats per minute times systolic blood pressure. Bears a close relationship with myocardial work or oxygen demand (myocardial $\dot{V}O_2$).

**Ratings of perceived exertion (RPE):** A scale, originally developed by noted Swedish psychologist Gunnar Borg, that provides a standard means for evaluating a participant's perception of exercise effort. The original scale ranged from 6 to 20; a revised category ratio scale ranges from 0 to 10.

**Reaction time:** The amount of time elapsed between the stimulus for movement and the beginning of the movement.

**Reactivity:** The ability to rapidly respond to stimuli; generally includes the time needed to process sensory information, plus the time needed to generate and execute the appropriate motor response.

**Reciprocal inhibition:** The reflex inhibition of the motor neurons of antagonists when the agonists are contracted.

**Recommended Dietary Allowances (RDAs):** The levels of intake of essential nutrients that, on the basis of scientific knowledge, are judged by the Food and Nutrition Board to be adequate to meet the known needs of practically all healthy persons.

**Recruitment:** The process of activating motor units to increase force production in a muscle.

**Reduction:** The addition of an electron to a molecule or an atom.

**Reflex:** An involuntary action or response.

**Regurgitant:** A surging up of partially digested food.

**Relative risk:** Compares the degree of risk for development of a disease in one group compared with the same risk within another group, where the two groups generally differ by one or multiple variables. The relative risk is expressed as a ratio that equates incidence or prevalence between two groups.

**Relative strength:** A measurement of maximum muscular force exerted in relationship to body weight or muscle size.

**Releasing factors:** Substances produced by the hypothalamus that are capable of accelerating the secretion of a given hormone by the anterior pituitary lobe.

**Renin-angiotensin mechanism:** A system that regulates blood pressure controlled by the release of renin from the kidney when renal blood flow or blood pressure is low. Renin converts angiotensinogen to angiotensin, which ultimately releases aldosterone from the adrenal cortex. Angiotensin is also a powerful vasoconstrictor, which also aids in increasing blood pressure.

**Residual volume (RV):** The volume of air remaining in the lungs following a maximal expiration.

**Resistance training:** A specialized method of conditioning that involves the progressive use of a wide range of resistive loads and a variety of training modalities.

**Resisted running:** Running with added resistance using a variety of tools, including resistance bands, a resistance harness, a resistance parachute, sled, or other accessories.

**Resorption:** The removal stage of the bone remodeling cycle, increasing blood levels of calcium and phosphate.

**Respiratory bronchioles:** The smallest bronchioles that connect the terminal bronchioles to alveolar ducts; permit the exchange of gases.

**Respiratory compensation point:** The instant during an aerobic exercise where minute ventilation starts becoming excessive with respect to carbon dioxide output; forms the boundary between the heavy and severe exercise intensity domains.

**Respiratory control center:** Located in the medulla oblongata; receives controlling signals of neural, chemical, and hormonal nature, and controls the rate and depth of respiratory movements of the diaphragm and other respiratory muscles.

**Respiratory exchange ratio (RER):** A ratio of the amount of carbon dioxide produced relative to the amount of oxygen consumed.

**Respiratory membrane:** The membrane that separates air within the alveoli from the blood within pulmonary capillaries; prevents each alveolus from collapsing as air moves in and out during respiration.

**Respiratory quotient (RQ):** A ratio of the amount of carbon dioxide produced relative to the amount of oxygen consumed.

**Respiratory rate (RR):** The rate at which a person inhales and exhales.

**Respiratory system:** The specific organs and structures used for the process of respiration; includes the trachea, bronchi, bronchioles, lungs, and diaphragm.

**Respiratory zone:** The site for oxygen and carbon dioxide exchange in the lung tissue with the blood.

**Resting heart rate (RHR):** The number of heartbeats per minute when the body is at complete rest; usually counted first thing in the morning in a supine position.

**Resting membrane potential:** A stable voltage across the membrane of a cell that is not being stimulated.

**Resting metabolic rate (RMR):** The number of calories expended per unit time at rest; measured early in the morning after an overnight fast and at least 8 hours of sleep; can be estimated using various formulas.

**Reverse elasticity:** The ability of a stretched material to return to its original resting state.

**Reversibility:** The partial or complete loss of any training-induced adaptation that occurs as a result of a decrease in a training stimulus.

**Rheumatoid arthritis (RA):** A chronic and systemic inflammatory disease.

**Right and left main coronary arteries:** The vessels that deliver oxygen-rich blood to the myocardium.

**Right bundle branch:** The bundle of cardiac nerves that feeds the right ventricle.

**Sarcomere:** The basic functional unit of the myofibril containing the myofilaments that generate skeletal muscle movements.

**Sarcopenia:** The degenerative loss of skeletal muscle mass and strength associated with aging.

**Saturated fatty acid (SFA):** A fatty acid that contains no carbon-carbon double bonds within its carbon backbone, allowing each carbon atom to maximally bind with hydrogen atoms; typically solid at room temperature and very stable.

**Scope of practice:** The range and limit of responsibilities normally associated with a specific job or profession.

**Second messenger:** Molecules that relay signals from receptors on the cell surface to target molecules inside the cell.

**Second ventilatory threshold (VT2):** A metabolic marker that represents the point at which high-intensity exercise can no longer be sustained because of an accumulation of lactate in the blood.

**Secondary aging:** Those age-related deteriorations that result from lifestyle behaviors (e.g., physical activity, nutrition, tobacco use, and alcohol consumption), disease processes (e.g., diabetes, cancer, and cardiovascular disease), environment (e.g., exposure to toxins, air pollution, and ultraviolet radiation), injury, and illness. These factors are highly variable and can be significantly controlled by the individual to delay some age-related processes.

**Secondary amenorrhea:** Missed menstrual cycles for longer than 3 to 6 months for female individuals of any age who once had regular menstrual cycles.

**Secondary bronchi:** Respiratory airways that arise from the primary bronchi, with each one serving as the passage to a specific lobe of the lung.

**Secondary prevention:** The identification and treatment of asymptomatic persons who have already developed risk factors or preclinical disease but in whom the condition is not clinically apparent.

**Secondary sex characteristics:** Features that appear during puberty, especially those that distinguish the two sexes of a species.

**Sedentary:** The absence of physical activity.

**Self-contained underwater breathing apparatus (SCUBA):** A device worn and carried entirely by an underwater diver that provides the diver with breathing gas at the ambient pressure.

**Self-efficacy:** One's perception of his or her ability to change or to perform specific behaviors (e.g., exercise regularly).

**Semilunar valves:** The heart valves at the beginning of the aorta and of the pulmonary artery that prevent the blood from flowing back into the ventricle.

**Sense of effort:** The sense of exertion experienced during physical effort.

**Serial task:** A combination of discrete tasks.

**Serous pericardium:** The membranous sac filled with serous fluid that encloses the heart and the roots of the aorta and other large blood vessels.

**Shoulder impingement:** Occurs when the soft-tissue structures (e.g., bursa and rotator cuff tendons) get abnormally compressed.

**Shuttles:** Specialized transporters that move molecules across membranes from one environment to another.

**Simple carbohydrates:** Short saccharide (sugar) chains consisting of monosaccharides and disaccharides that are rapidly digested.

**Simple reaction:** Defined as the display of a single stimulus that has only one correct response, such as a coach yelling "go" to signal an athlete to run a 40-yard dash.

**Sinoatrial node (SA node):** A group of specialized myocardial cells, located in the wall of the right atrium, that controls the heart's rate of contraction; the "pacemaker" of the heart.

**Size principle:** The scientific theory that to move a load, motor units are recruited from smallest to largest.

**Skeletal muscle:** A type of voluntary striated muscle tissue attached to the skeleton that provides movement at the joints when it contracts.

**Skinfold caliper:** A device that measures the thickness of a fold of skin with its underlying layer of fat; used in estimating body composition.

**Slow reversal-hold-relax:** A method of proprioceptive neuromuscular facilitation (PNF) composed of four stages: dynamic contraction of the antagonists involved, isometric contraction of the antagonists, brief voluntary relaxation, and dynamic contraction of the agonists; used to enhance functional flexibility.

**Slow-twitch motor unit:** A motor unit composed of slow-twitch muscle fibers; designed for use of aerobic glycolysis and fatty acid oxidation, recruited for low-intensity, longer-duration activities such as walking and swimming.

**Slow-twitch muscle fibers:** A muscle fiber type designed for use of aerobic glycolysis and fatty acid oxidation, recruited for low-intensity, longer-duration activities such as walking and swimming. Also called *type I muscle fiber.*

**SMART goals:** Goals that are specific, measurable, achievable, relevant, and time bound.

**Smooth muscle:** A type of involuntary nonstriated muscle tissue responsible for the contractility of hollow organs, such as blood vessels, the gastrointestinal tract, the bladder, or the uterus.

**Soluble:** The ability of a substance to be dissolved.

**Specificity:** Principle that states that training adaptations or outcomes are determined by the nature of the imposed demands or method of training placed on a system or systems being trained.

**Speed:** The distance covered per unit of time; usually subdivided further into speed-agility-quickness (SAQ).

**Speed-endurance:** The ability to maintain top, or near-top, speed performance. This includes the ability to withstand fatigue and sustain high intensities without significant reductions in speed.

**Speed of contraction:** How quickly a motor unit fires and subsequently causes its associated muscle fibers to contract.

**Spirometry:** Pulmonary function testing that measures lung function by assessing the amount (volume) and/or speed (flow) of air that can be maximally inhaled and exhaled; used in the diagnosis and management of asthma and other pulmonary disorders.

**Sprains:** Injuries that occur to a joint and the surrounding ligaments.

**Stability:** The ability to control the position or movement of a joint or series of joints.

**Stable angina:** Generally occurs with exertion and is reproducible at a given rate pressure product (heart rate × systolic blood pressure).

**Stages of maturation:** Stages of psychosocial development throughout the life span.

**Standard activity factor score (SAF):** A multiple of the energy required to perform a certain level of physical activity.

**Static balance:** Requires an individual to control, or alter his or her center of mass over an unchanging, or fixed, base of support.

**Static flexibility:** The range of motion about a joint with no emphasis on speed.

**Static posture:** The structural arrangement of the individual parts of the skeleton; often represented by how a person stands.

**Static stretching:** Holding a nonmoving (static) position to immobilize a joint in a position that places the desired muscles and connective tissues passively at their greatest possible length.

**Stenotic:** A constriction or narrowing of a duct or passage.

**Steroid hormones:** Signaling compounds or chemical messengers derived from cholesterol and involved in regulating many physiological functions within the body; examples include the sex hormones—estrogen and testosterone; mineralocorticoids—aldosterone; and glucocorticoids—cortisol.

**Stimulant:** A substance that activates the central nervous system and may be found in various forms, with perhaps the most commonly abused stimulant being caffeine.

**Stimulus control:** Involves learning how to avoid triggers such as the sight of food and wanting to eat, or dealing with cravings for food.

**Strains:** Injuries that occur to a muscle or a muscle-tendon unit.

**Stress:** A nonspecific response to any stimulus that overcomes, or threatens to overcome, the body's ability to maintain equilibrium between all its internal biological mechanisms.

**Stress fracture:** A fracture, often in one or more of the metatarsal bones, that occurs from abnormal or repeated stress and are common in distance runners and track athletes.

**Stretch reflex:** An involuntary motor response that, when stimulated, causes a suddenly stretched muscle to respond with a corresponding contraction.

**Stretch-shortening cycle:** A natural type of muscle function where an eccentric action of a muscle is followed closely by the concentric action of a muscle.

**Striated:** The appearance of skeletal and cardiac muscle tissue under a microscope such that a series of alternating light and dark bands (or striations) can be seen within the muscle fiber.

**Stride frequency:** The number of strides per unit time.

**Stride length:** The distance covered in a single stride.

**Stroke:** A sudden and often severe ischemic attack due to blockage of an artery feeding into the brain.

**Stroke volume:** The amount of blood pumped from the left ventricle of the heart with each beat.

**Subcutaneous:** Located or placed just beneath the skin.

**Subfibrils:** Structures that makes up the fibril in connective tissue.

**Subjective:** Particular to a given person; personal experience.

**Subserous fascia:** A type of fascia lying between the internal layer of deep fascia and the serous membranes lining body cavities in much the same manner as the subcutaneous fascia lies between the skin and the deep fascia.

**Substrates:** The material or substance on which an enzyme acts.

**Successful aging:** The ability to maintain a low risk for disease and disease-related disability, high mental and physical function, and active engagement with life.

**Summation:** The repeated stimulation of a muscle fiber when the fiber is not allowed to completely relax. Summation of the responses to the stimuli leads to an increase in tension compared with a single twitch.

**Superficial fascia:** The thin layer of loose, fatty connective tissue underlying the skin and binding it to the parts beneath.

**Supersetting:** Involves completing two exercises that are performed in sequence before taking a rest interval that traditionally target opposing muscle groups (e.g., one set of seated back rows followed immediately by one set of barbell chest press). However, many variations of supersetting exists.

**Supine:** Lying on the back, facing upwards.

**Surfactant:** A substance secreted by the alveolar cells of the lung, which serves to maintain the stability of pulmonary tissue by reducing the surface tension of fluids that coat the lung.

**Sympathetic nervous system:** A branch of the autonomic nervous system responsible for mobilizing the body's energy and resources during times of stress and arousal (i.e., the fight-or-flight response). Opposes the physiological effects of the parasympathetic nervous system (e.g., reduces digestive secretions, speeds the heart, and contracts blood vessels).

**Synapse:** The region at the end of an axon where it communicates with another cell (neuron, muscle, gland).

**Synaptic cleft:** The space between the end of an axon and an adjacent cell, across which a neurotransmitter diffuses to communicate to the other cell.

**Synchronization:** The simultaneous firing of motoneurons, which leads to more efficient motor unit recruitment.

**Syncope:** A transient state of unconsciousness during which a person collapses to the floor as a result of lack of oxygen to the brain; commonly known as fainting.

**Synergistic dominance:** Refers to the event where synergistic or assistance muscles at the joint assume the role of becoming the prime mover to move that joint.

**Systemic circulation:** The general circulation, carrying oxygenated blood from the left ventricle to the body tissues, and returning venous blood to the right atrium from the body.

**Systole:** The contraction phase of the cardiac cycle.

**Systolic blood pressure (SBP):** The pressure exerted by the blood upon the vessel walls during ventricular contraction.

**Tachycardia:** Elevated heart rate over 100 beats per minute.

**Tai chi:** One form of the more ancient practice of qigong. Tai chi chuan is a complex martial arts choreography of 108 flowing graceful movements that can be practiced for health, meditation, and self-defense.

**Talk test:** A method for measuring exercise intensity using observation of respiratory effort and the challenge associated with talk continuously while exercising.

**Tapering:** The intentional reduction in peak training load or volume over a short period to prepare the body for competition.

**Target organ:** A tissue or organ that is affected by a specific hormone.

**Tendinopathy:** A degenerative disease process that occurs in a tendon.

**Tendonitis:** A traditional term for inflammation of the tendon that often involves an overuse condition that commonly affects the elbows, knees, and ankles.

**Tendons:** Bands of fibrous tissue forming the termination of a muscle and attaching the muscle to a bone.

**Tensegrity:** A concept of muscular-skeletal relationships that refers to the forces of tension (provided by muscles, tendons, ligaments, and fascia) pulling on structures (bones and joints) that help keep the body both stable and efficient in mass and movement.

**Tensile deformation:** When a force is applied to tissue, its length is increased.

**Terminal bronchioles:** The last portion of a bronchiole that does not contain alveoli; it subdivides into respiratory bronchioles.

**Terminal cisternae:** Enlarged areas of the sarcoplasmic reticulum surrounding the transverse tubules within a muscle cell that store and secrete calcium when an action potential courses down the transverse tubules, eliciting muscle contraction.

**Tertiary bronchi:** Airways of the respiratory system that branch out from the secondary bronchi, which descend from the mainstream bronchi; also called the *segmental bronchi.*

**Testosterone:** The steroid hormone produced in the testes in male individuals and, in small amounts, in the adrenal cortex in male and female individuals; involved in growth and development of reproductive tissues, sperm, and secondary male sex characteristics.

**Tetanus:** The highest tension developed by a muscle in response to a high frequency of stimulation.

**Thermic effect of food:** An increase in energy expenditure due to digestive processes of chewing, swallowing, digesting, absorbing, and storing food. Also called *thermic effect of feeding.*

**Thermodynamics:** The science of the relationship between heat and other forms of energy (such as mechanical, electrical,

or chemical energy), and, by extension, of the relationship between all forms of energy.

**Thermogenesis:** Calories released from metabolism; the process of generating heat.

**Thermoregulation:** Regulation of the body's relatively constant core temperature.

**Thermoregulatory system:** The internal system that regulates an organism's body temperature to keep it within certain boundaries, even when the surrounding temperature is very different.

**Thyroid gland:** A large, butterfly-shaped, ductless gland in the neck that secretes hormones regulating growth and development through controlling the rate of metabolism.

**Thyroid-stimulating hormone (TSH):** Hormone secreted from the anterior pituitary lobe that stimulates the function of the thyroid gland; also called *thyrotropin.*

**Thyroxine (T4):** The main hormone produced by the thyroid gland, acting to increase metabolic rate and thus regulating growth and development.

**Tidal volume ($V_T$):** The volume of air inspired per breath.

**Time under tension (TUT):** The amount of time spent completing a full repetition.

**Titin:** A connecting filament thought to be responsible for maintaining myosin's position between the Z lines (even during sarcomere stretching), as well as maintaining some resting tension within the muscle fiber.

**Total body density:** The mass of the human body divided by its volume, where the volume represents the space occupied by the body. Used in the estimation of fat mass and fat-free mass in body composition.

**Total body water (TBW):** The total volume of water in the human body. Used in the estimation of hydration states and body composition.

**Total daily energy expenditure (TDEE):** Amount of energy expended in a 24-hour period, which includes resting metabolic rate (RMR), thermic effect of food (TEF) and the thermic effect of physical activity (TEPA—exercise, physical activity, NEAT).

**Total lung capacity (TLC):** The total volume of air contained within the lungs at the end of a maximal inspiration.

**Total peripheral resistance (TPR):** The resistance to the passage of blood through the small blood vessels, especially arterioles.

**Trachea:** The cartilaginous and membranous tube extending from the larynx to the bronchi; windpipe.

**Transamination:** The reversible exchange of the amino group found on an amino acid between different amino acids.

**Transient ischemic attack (TIA):** An incident in which the blood flow to a part of the brain stops for a brief period.

**Transporter:** A protein complex that is involved in active transport.

**Transtheoretical model of behavioral change (TTM):** A behavioral change theory that provides a framework to describe how people acquire and maintain healthy behaviors, moving between different stages and built upon the premise of readiness to change: precontemplation, contemplation, preparation, action, and maintenance. Also called the *stages-of-change model.*

**Tricuspid valve:** Regulates flow from the right atrium to the right ventricle.

**Triglyceride (TG):** The principal storage form of fat consisting of three molecules of fatty acid bound to a glycerol molecule backbone.

**Triiodothyronine (T3):** Thyroid hormone similar to thyroxine that exerts the same biological effects as thyroxine (T4); although released in smaller doses than T4, it is considered a more potent hormone.

**Triple extension:** Extension of the ankle, knee, and hip in lower-extremity, closed-chain movements. Typically involved in acceleration movements.

**Triple flexion:** Flexion of the ankle, knee, and hip in lower-extremity, closed-chain movements. Typically involved in deceleration movements.

**Trochanteric bursitis:** The painful inflammation of the bursa surrounding the greater trochanter of the femur.

**Tropic hormones:** Hormones that are produced and secreted by one endocrine gland that target other endocrine glands.

**Tropomyosin:** A regulatory protein involved in muscle contraction; located in parallel to the actin filaments and covers the active sites needed for myosin head attachment.

**Troponin:** A globular protein complex involved in muscle contraction; located along the tropomyosin strands and binds to calcium to initiate muscle contractions.

**Tumor necrosis factor (TNF):** A protein involved in systemic inflammation that when activated induces inflammation.

**Tumors:** Uncontrolled cell growth; formation of tissue masses.

**Twitch:** The tension-generating response following the application of a single stimulus to a muscle.

**Type 1 diabetes:** Previously called *insulin-dependent diabetes mellitus (IDDM);* develops when pancreatic beta cells that are responsible for producing insulin are destroyed by the body's immune system.

**Type 2 diabetes:** Most common form of diabetes; typically develops in adulthood and is characterized by a reduced sensitivity of the insulin target cells to available insulin; usually associated with obesity; formerly known as *non-insulin-dependent diabetes mellitus (NIDDM)* and *adult-onset diabetes.*

**Universal athletic position (UAP):** A static, "ready" position when athletes stand in a quarter-squat with feet flat, hips flexed, shoulders positioned forward of the hips, torso inclined at an angle of about 45 degrees, hands in front with one or both placed on the ground supporting the body, and shoulders over the knees.

**Unsaturated fatty acid (UFA):** Fatty acids that contain one or more double bonds between the carbon atoms in the backbone; typically liquid at room temperature and fairly unstable, making them susceptible to oxidative damage and a shortened shelf life.

**Unstable angina:** Presents with periods of increasing frequency, low levels of intensity, and may even occur after meals and at rest.

**Upregulation:** A state in which target cells develop a greater number of receptors in response to decreasing hormone levels.

**Usual aging:** How the majority of individuals in a society "usually" or "typically" age. For example, the typical older adult is able to function independently, but has an increased risk for disease or disability. The disability risk is due, in large part, to the reduced functional reserve capacity of the individual and his or her downward aging trajectory. That is, the individual has a reduced capacity for performing more intense activities.

**Valgus collapse:** Characterized by an abnormal outward turning of a bone, especially of the hip, knee, or foot.

**Valsalva maneuver:** Breath-holding during exertion while bearing down on a closed glottis; increases thoracic stiffness for forcer production, but reduces venous return and subsequent blood circulation to the brain which may result in symptoms of light-headedness or dizziness.

**Vasoconstriction:** Narrowing of the opening of blood vessels (notably the smaller arterioles) caused by contraction of the smooth muscle lining the vessels.

**Vasodilation:** Increase in diameter of the blood vessels, especially dilation of arterioles, leading to increased blood flow to a part of the body.

**Vasopressin:** Hormone released by the posterior pituitary gland during exercise; reduces urinary excretion of water and prevents dehydration.

**Vectors:** Physical quantities that include both magnitude and direction.

$\dot{V}_E$: *See* Minute ventilation.

**Vegan:** A vegetarian who does not eat any animal products, including dairy products such as milk and cheese.

**Veins:** Blood vessels that carry deoxygenated blood toward the heart from vital organs and the extremities.

**Venoconstriction:** The narrowing of the opening of veins.

**Ventilatory equivalent for carbon dioxide:** The ratio of the volume of air ventilating the lungs to the volume of carbon dioxide produced.

**Ventilatory equivalent for oxygen:** The volume of gas breathed in liters per minute (ventilation) divided by the oxygen consumption in liters per minute over the same period: an index of the efficiency of oxygen uptake in the lungs.

**Ventral:** Relating to or situated on or close to the anterior aspect of the human body.

**Ventricular fibrillation:** Sudden cardiac death.

**Venules:** Smaller divisions of veins.

**Vertical banded gastroplasty:** A gastroplasty for the treatment of morbid obesity in which an upper gastric pouch is formed by a vertical staple line, with a cloth band applied to prevent dilation at the outlet into the main pouch.

**Very low-density lipoprotein (VLDL):** Synthesized in the liver, VLDL is the major carrier of triglyceride and cholesterol to the peripheral tissues. VLDL contains 10% to 15% of the body's total serum cholesterol.

**Vestibular system:** Part of the central nervous system that coordinates reflexes of the eyes, neck, and body to maintain equilibrium in accordance with posture and movement of the head.

**Vigorous:** A descriptive term used to characterize physical activity that feels challenging, causes deep and rapid breathing, and leaves the exerciser unable to say more than a few words without pausing for breath.

**Viscera:** The collective internal organs of the abdominal cavity.

**Visceral adiposity:** The fat located deep in the abdomen that surrounds the vital organs. Its accumulation is associated with insulin resistance, glucose intolerance, dyslipidemia, hypertension, and coronary artery disease.

**Visceral pleura:** The thin serous membrane around the lungs and inner walls of the chest.

**Viscoelasticity:** The property that allows tissues to exhibit both plastic and elastic behaviors.

**Vital capacity:** The volume of air that can be maximally inhaled after maximal expiration or maximally exhaled after maximal inspiration.

**Vitamin:** An organic micronutrient that is essential for normal physiological function.

$\dot{V}O_2$: *See* Oxygen consumption.

$\dot{V}O_2$**max:** *See* Maximal oxygen consumption.

$\dot{V}O_2$ **reserve ($\dot{V}O_2$R):** *See* Oxygen consumption reserve.

**Volume:** The amount of work performed in a training program; in resistance training, it is generally measured by multiplying the number of sets times the number of repetitions completed; in aerobic training it is generally measured by multiplying the frequency of training times the duration of training.

**Volume training:** Involves the use of submaximal or lighter loads until some defined endpoint is achieved (e.g., number of repetitions) or until momentary muscle fatigue is achieved.

**Waist-to-hip ratio:** A useful measure for determining health risk due to the site of fat storage. Calculated by dividing the waist measurement by the hip circumference.

**Wet suits:** Close-fitting garments made of permeable material worn in cold water to retain body heat.

**Wet-bulb globe thermometer (WBGT):** A composite temperature used to estimate the effect of temperature, humidity, and solar radiation on humans.

**Wet-bulb temperature:** Considers the amount of moisture in the air and reflects the cooling effect of evaporation.

**Whey:** The soluble milk protein remaining after milk has been curdled and strained; more rapidly digested and absorbed with a high ability to stimulate muscle protein synthesis.

**Wind chill index:** A chill factor created by the increase in the rate of heat loss via convection and conduction caused by the wind.

**Wingate anaerobic test:** An anaerobic fitness test, most often performed on a cycle ergometer, that is used to measure peak anaerobic power and anaerobic capacity.

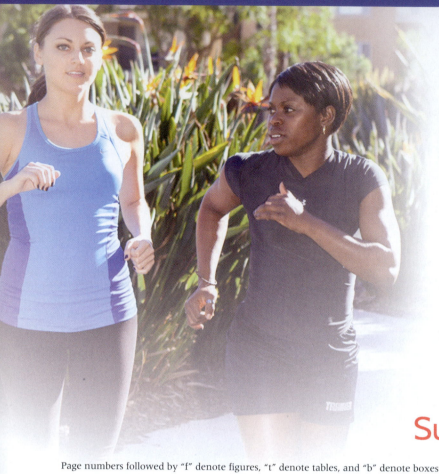

# Subject Index

Page numbers followed by "f" denote figures, "t" denote tables, and "b" denote boxes

## A

A bands, 234, 234f
A-March and skip drill, 510b
a-vO$_2$. *See* Arterial-venous oxygen difference (a-vO$_2$)
AACPR. *See* American Association for Cardiovascular and Pulmonary Rehabilitation (AACPR)
Abdominal circumference, 636f, 649
Abdominal obesity, 718
Abdominal skinfold measurements, 639f, 652
ABI. *See* Ankle–brachial index (ABI)
Absolute oxygen consumption, 107, 109f
A1c test. *See* Glycohemoglobin (HbA1c)
Academy of Nutrition and Dietetics, 546
Acai, 578t
Acceleration
    description of, 483, 485, 486f
    posture, arm, and leg action during, 508t
Accelerometers, 103–104
Acclimatization, to high-altitude environments, 808
Acetyl-CoA, 86
Acetyl-coenzyme A, 79, 81
Acetylcholine, 183–184, 198, 238, 249, 344
Acetylcholinesterase, 344
Achilles tendinopathy, 852f, 852f
Acid salts, 76
Acid–base balance, 155
Acidosis, 75–76
ACSM. *See* American College of Sports Medicine (ACSM)

ACTH. *See* Adrenocorticotropic hormone (ACTH)
Actin, 234, 452
Action potential, 238, 249
Action stage, of behavioral change, 661t, 663–664
Active aging, 714b, 715
Active flexibility training, 464
Active isolated stretching, 457, 459t, 460–461, 461f
Active overeating, 611, 611b–612b
Active resistance, 482b, 491
Active sites, 234
Active stretching, 260, 260f, 458, 458f
Active system, of stability, 354–355
Actively passive system, 355
Activities of daily living (ADLs), 535, 839
Acute mountain sickness (AMS), 813
Acute musculoskeletal injuries, 836, 837f
Acute myocardial infarction, 758
Acyl-CoA synthetase, 84
Adductor strain, 833
Adenosine diphosphate (ADP), 68–69, 73
Adenosine triphosphate (ATP)
    ATPase for breakdown of, 237
    carbohydrates as source of, 83f, 83–84
    chemical structure of, 68f
    components of, 68
    deficiency of, 79
    energy from, 67, 78, 692
    exercise-induced demand for, 66
    hydrolysis of, 68, 68f
    lipids as source of, 85–86

palmitate as source of, 86t
phosphagen system for generation of, 69–70
regeneration of, 69f
rephosphorylation of, 70f
synthesis of, 68
Adenosine triphosphate-phosphocreatine (ATP-PC) system, 692
Adipocytes
    hyperplasia of, 605
    in lean and obese individuals, 608f
Adipogenesis, 605, 608f
Adipose cells, 54
Adipose tissue
    aging effects on placement of, 631
    body density of, 654
    free fatty acids manufactured in, 84
Adiposity, 717t, 791
Adolescence, 689b
Adolescents. *See also* Boys; Children; Girls
    aerobic fitness in, 694–695
    exercise training in
        aerobic exercise, 700–701
        aerobic metabolism, 691–693
        anaerobic metabolism, 691–693
        cardiorespiratory responses to, 692t, 693–695
        dynamic warm-up, 703–704
        flexibility exercise, 702
        fluid intake during, 695
        fundamental movement skills, 696, 697f, 701, 704–706
        guidelines for, 697